Perioperative Critical Care

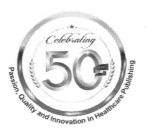

Perioperative Critical Care

Editors

Atul Prabhakar Kulkarni
MD (Anesthesiology) FISCCM PGDHHM FICCM
Professor and Head
Division of Critical Care
Department of Anesthesiology
Critical Care and Pain
Tata Memorial Hospital
Homi Bhabha National Institute
Mumbai, Maharashtra, India

Sohan Lal Solanki
MD (Anesthesiology) PDCC (Organ Transplant Anesthesiology) MAMS
Professor
Department of Anesthesiology
Critical Care and Pain
Tata Memorial Hospital
Homi Bhabha National Institute
Mumbai, Maharashtra, India

Jigeeshu Vasistha Divatia
MD (Anesthesiology) FICCM FCCM
Professor and Head
Department of Anesthesiology
Critical Care and Pain
Tata Memorial Hospital
Homi Bhabha National Institute
Mumbai, Maharashtra, India

JAYPEE BROTHERS MEDICAL PUBLISHERS
The Health Sciences Publisher
New Delhi | London

Jaypee Brothers Medical Publishers (P) Ltd

Headquarters
Jaypee Brothers Medical Publishers (P) Ltd
4838/24, Ansari Road, Daryaganj
New Delhi 110 002, India
Phone: +91-11-43574357
Fax: +91-11-43574314
E-mail: jaypee@jaypeebrothers.com

Overseas Office
JP Medical Ltd
83 Victoria Street, London
SW1H 0HW (UK)
Phone: +44 20 3170 8910
Fax: +44 (0)20 3008 6180
E-mail: info@jpmedpub.com

Website: www.jaypeebrothers.com
Website: www.jaypeedigital.com

© 2021, Jaypee Brothers Medical Publishers

Perioperative Critical Care

First Edition: **2021**

ISBN: 978-93-90020-50-8

Printed at: Replika Press Pvt. Ltd.

Contributors

Aakanksha Chawla Jain MD IDCCM
Attending Consultant
Department of Respiratory
Critical Care and Sleep Medicine
Indraprastha Apollo Hospitals
New Delhi, India

Abdullah Zoheb Azhar MD Anesthesia, Fellow Intensive Care
Medicine (QAH, Portsmouth, UK)
Resident Physician
Department of Internal Medicine
Metropolitan Hospital Center
New York Medical College
New York, USA

Abhilash Chandra MD (Medicine) DM (Nephrology)
Associate Professor
Department of Nephrology
Dr Ram Manohar Lohia Institute of Medical Sciences
Lucknow, Uttar Pradesh, India

Ajay Kumar MD (Anesthesia & Critical Care) DM (Cardiac Anesthesia)
Associate Professor
Department of Anesthesia
All India Institute of Medical Sciences
Rishikesh, Uttarakhand, India

Ajeeta Mohan Kulkarni BSC (PT) MSc (Psychology)
Scientific Assistant
Department of Physiotherapy
Tata Memorial Hospital
Mumbai, Maharashtra, India

Ajmer Singh MD
Director, Cardiac Anesthesia
Medanta Institute of Critical Care and Anesthesiology
Gurugram, Haryana, India

Amish Jasapara MD (Anesthesiology)
Department of Anesthesiology
Fortis Hospital
Mumbai, Maharashtra, India

Amit Rastogi MD PDCC EDAIC
Associate Professor
Department of Anesthesiology
Intensive Care and Pain Medicine
Sanjay Gandhi Postgraduate Institute of Medical Sciences
Lucknow, Uttar Pradesh, India

Amlendu Yadav MD FNB (Critical Care)
Associate Professor
Department of Anesthesiology and Critical Care
Atal Bihari Vajpayee Institute of Medical Sciences (ABVIMS)
and Dr Ram Manohar Lohia Hospital
New Delhi, India

Amol Kothekar MD (Anesthesiology)
Professor
Department of Anesthesiology
Critical Care and Pain
Tata Memorial Hospital
Mumbai, Maharashtra, India

Amrit Kaur BSN RN
Senior Nursing Officer
Department of Pediatric Surgery
Postgraduate Institute of Medical Education and Research
Chandigarh, India

Anila Malde MD DA (Anesthesiology)
Professor and Head
Department of Anesthesiology
Lokmanya Tilak Municipal Medical College and Lokmanya
Tilak Municipal General Hospital
Mumbai, Maharashtra, India

Anshuman Sarkar MD
Associate Consultant
Department of Anesthesia and Critical Care
Tata Medical Center
Kolkata, West Bengal, India

Anudeep Jafra MD
Assistant Professor
Department of Anesthesia and Intensive Care
Postgraduate Institute of Medical Education and Research
Chandigarh, India

Anuja Bidkar DNB DA (Fellow Onco-anesthesia & Pain)
Associate Professor
Department of Anesthesia
DY Patil Medical College
Hospital and Research Center
Mumbai, Maharashtra, India

Anuja Jain DA DNB DESA MNAMS
Junior Consultant
Department of Anesthesia
Critical Care and Pain
National Cancer Institute
Nagpur, Maharashtra, India

Anuradha Abhijit Daptardar BSc (PT)
Officer-in-Charge
Department of Physiotherapy
Tata Memorial Hospital
Mumbai, Maharashtra, India

Arindam Chatterjee MD
Senior Resident
Department of Anesthesiology
Sanjay Gandhi Postgraduate Institute of Medical Sciences
Lucknow, Uttar Pradesh, India

Ashit Hegde MD MRCP
Consultant
Department of Medicine and Critical Care
PD Hinduja Hospital
Mumbai, Maharashtra, India

Atul Prabhakar Kulkarni
MD (Anesthesiology) FISCCM PGDHHM FICCM
Professor and Head
Division of Critical Care
Department of Anesthesiology
Critical Care and Pain
Tata Memorial Hospital
Homi Bhabha National Institute
Mumbai, Maharashtra, India

Balakrishnan KR MS Mch
Director
Institute of Heart and Lung Transplant and Mechanical
Circulatory Support Services
MGM HealthCare
Chennai, Tamil Nadu, India

Balkrishna Nimavat MD DNB (Anes) IDCCM FNB EDIC EDAIC
(Critical Care)
Intensivist
Department of Internal Medicine and Intensive Care
Apollo Hospital
Navi Mumbai, Maharashtra, India

Bharathram Vasudevan MD
Resident Physician
Department of Anesthesiology
John H Stroger Hospital
Cook County Health
Chicago, Illinois, USA

Bindiya Salunke MD (Anesthesiology)
Assistant Professor
Department of Anesthesiology
Critical Care and Pain
Tata Memorial Hospital
Mumbai, Maharashtra, India

Chandan Biswas MD
Associate Consultant
Department of Critical Care Medicine
Advanced Medicare Research Institute
Kolkata, West Bengal, India

Debashree P Lahiri DNB (Anesthesia)
Assistant Professor
Department of Anesthesiology
Critical Care and Pain
Tata Memorial Hospital
Mumbai, Maharashtra, India

Deeksha Singh Tomar DA IDCCM IFCCM EDICM
Consultant, Critical Care
Narayana Superspecialty Hospital
Gurugram, Haryana, India

Deepak Govil MD EDIC FCCM
Director
Department of Critical Care Medicine
Medanta—The Medicity
Gurugram, Haryana, India

Devangi Parikh MD (Anesthesiology)
Associate Professor
Department of Anesthesiology
Lokmanya Tilak Municipal Medical College and Lokmanya
Tilak Municipal General Hospital
Mumbai, Maharashtra, India

Devendra Gupta MD PDCC (Neuro-anesthesia)
Professor
Department of Anesthesiology
Sanjay Gandhi Postgraduate Institute of Medical Sciences
Lucknow, Uttar Pradesh, India

Dilip R Karnad MD FACP FRCP
Senior Consultant
Department of Critical Care
Jupiter Hospital
Thane, Maharashtra, India

Divya Srivastava MD (Anesthesiology) PDCC (Organ Transplant
Anesthesia)
Assistant Professor
Department of Anesthesiology
Sanjay Gandhi Postgraduate Institute of Medical Sciences
Lucknow, Uttar Pradesh, India

Ganesh Kumar Munirathinam MD DM (Cardiac Anesthesia)
Assistant Professor
Department of Cardiac Anesthesia
Postgraduate Institute of Medical Education and Research
Chandigarh, India

Gauri Raman Gangakhedkar DA DNB (Anesthesiology)
Fellowship in Neuro-anesthesia
Assistant Professor
Department of Anesthesiology
Seth GS Medical College and KEM Hospital
Mumbai, Maharashtra, India

Gauri Saroj MD EDIC
Consultant
Department of Critical Care
Jupiter Hospital
Thane, Maharashtra, India

Harish MM MD DM (Critical Care Medicine, TMH) DNB IDCCM EDIC (Dublin)
MBA (Healthcare Management)
Consultant Incharge
Department of Critical Care Medicine
Narayana Hrudayalaya
Bengaluru, Karnataka, India

Jeson Rajan Doctor MD DNB MNAMS
Professor
Department of Anesthesiology
Critical Care and Pain
Tata Memorial Hospital
Mumbai, Maharashtra, India

Jigeeshu Vasistha Divatia MD (Anesthesiology) FICCM FCCM
Professor and Head
Department of Anesthesiology
Critical Care and Pain
Tata Memorial Hospital
Homi Bhabha National Institute
Mumbai, Maharashtra, India

Joseph Monteiro MD
Program Director Neuroanesthesia
Consultant Neuroanesthesiologist
Department of Anaesthesiology
PD Hinduja Hospital
Mumbai, Maharashtra, India

Jyotsna Goswami MD
Senior Consultant and Head
Department of Anesthesia and Critical Care
Tata Medical Center
Kolkata, West Bengal, India

Kapil Zirpe MD FICCM FCCM
Director
Neuro Trauma Unit
Ruby Hall Clinic
Pune, Maharashtra, India

Karishma Shah BPTh
Trainee Physiotherapist
Tata Memorial Hospital
Mumbai Maharashtra, India

Kelika Prakash MD DM (Liver Transplant Anesthesia)
Assistant Professor
Department of Anesthesia and Critical Care Medicine
Institute of Liver and Biliary Sciences
New Delhi, India

Khalid Ismail Khatib MD FICCM
Professor
Department of Medicine
Smt Kashibai Navale Medical College
Pune, Maharashtra, India

Kishore Mangal MD DNB IDCCM IFCCM EDIC
Senior Consultant
Department of Critical Care Medicine
Eternal Heart Care Center
Jaipur, Rajasthan, India

Kushal R Kalvit MD (General Medicine)
Senior Resident
Division of Critical Care
Department of Anesthesiology
Critical Care and Pain
Tata Memorial Hospital
Mumbai, Maharashtra, India

Lalita Gauri Mitra DA DNB MNAMS
Associate Professor
Department of Anesthesia and Critical Care Medicine
Institute of Liver and Biliary Sciences
New Delhi, India

Madhavi Shetmahajan MD (Anesthesiology) FRCA
Professor
Department of Anesthesiology
Critical Care and Pain
Tata Memorial Hospital
Mumbai, Maharashtra, India

Madhusudan Jaju DNB IDCCM EDIC
Director
Department of Critical Care Medicine
CARE Institute of Medical Sciences
Hyderabad, Telangana, India

Mahima Gupta MD
Senior Resident
Department of Onco-Anesthesiology and Palliative Medicine
All India Institute of Medical Sciences
New Delhi, India

Malini P Joshi MD (Anesthesiology)
Professor
Department of Anesthesiology
Critical Care and Pain
Tata Memorial Hospital
Mumbai, Maharashtra, India

Martin Jose Thomas MD DNB (Anesthesia)
Advanced Trainee
Department of Medicine
Dubbo Base Hospital
Dubbo, New South Wales, Australia

Mekhala Paul MD
Senior Resident
Department of Anesthesiology
Sanjay Gandhi Postgraduate Institute of Medical Sciences
Lucknow, Uttar Pradesh, India

Mozammil Shafi MD FNB EDIC
Consultant
Department of Critical Care Medicine
Medanta Institute of Critical Care and Anesthesiology
Medanta—The Medicity
Gurugram, Haryana, India

Nagarajan Ramakrishnan
AB (Int Med) AB (Crit Care) AB (Sleep Med) MMM FACP FCCP FCCM FICCM
FISDA
Director
Department of Critical Care Medicine
Apollo Hospitals
Chennai, Tamil Nadu, India

Nandhakishore Jampala DA IDCCM EDIC
Consultant Critical Care
Medicover Hospital
Hyderabad, Telangana, India

Natesh Prabu R
MD DNB (Anesthesiology) DM (Critical Care Medicine) EDIC
Assistant Professor
Department of Critical Care Medicine
St John's Medical College Hospital
Bengaluru, Karnataka, India

Nayana Amin MD (Anesthesiology)
Professor
Department of Anesthesiology
Critical Care and Pain
Tata Memorial Hospital
Mumbai, Maharashtra, India

Neerja Bhardwaj MD
Professor
Department of Anesthesia and Intensive Care
Postgraduate Institute of Medical Education and Research
Chandigarh, India

Neeti Vijay Dogra MD
Assistant Professor
Department of Anesthesia and Intensive Care
Postgraduate Institute of Medical Education and Research
Chandigarh, India

Neha Singh MD CCEPC
Associate Professor
Department of Anesthesiology
All India Institute of Medical Sciences
Bhubaneswar, Odisha, India

Nileena NKM MD FSM
Associate Consultant
Department of Sleep Medicine and Psychiatry
Sri Ramachandra Medical College and Hospital
Chennai, Tamil Nadu, India

Nishant Agrawal MD (Anesthesia)
Senior Resident
Critical Care Medicine
Bharati Vidyapeeth (Deemed to be University) Medical
College
Pune, Maharashtra, India

Nitasha Mishra MD DNB DM
Assistant Professor
Department of Anesthesiology and Critical Care
All India Institute of Medical Sciences
Bhubaneswar, Odisha, India

Parnandi Bhaskar Rao MD PDCC FIPM
Associate Professor
Department of Anesthesiology
All India Institute of Medical Sciences
Bhubaneswar, Odisha, India

Pon Thelac AS MD
Senior Resident
Department of Respiratory Medicine
Nithra Institute of Sleep Sciences
Chennai, Tamil Nadu, India

Poojitha Reddy Gunnam MD (Anesthesia & Critical care)
Senior Resident
Department of Anesthesia
All India Institute of Medical Sciences
Rishikesh, Uttarakhand, India

Pradnya Atul Kulkarni MBBS DPB
Blood Transfusion Officer
Department of Pathology (Blood Bank)
KJ Somaiya Hospital and Research Center
Mumbai, Maharashtra, India

Prashant Nasa MD FNB (Critical Care Medicine) EDICM CIC
Specialist and Head Critical Care Medicine
Chairman Prevention and Control of Infection
NMC Specialty Hospital
Al Nahda, Dubai, UAE

Praveen Kumar G MD EDIC FNB
Associate Consultant
Department of Critical Care Medicine
Medanta—The Medicity
Gurugram, Haryana, India

Priya Ranganathan MD (Anesthesiology)
Professor
Department of Anesthesiology
Critical Care and Pain
Tata Memorial Hospital
Mumbai, Maharashtra, India

Rahul Pandit FCICM FJFICM EDICM FCCP FICCM MD DA
Director
Intensive Care Unit
Fortis Hospital
Mumbai, Maharashtra, India

Rajeev Chauhan MD DM (Neuro-anesthesia)
Assistant Professor
Department of Anesthesia and Intensive Care
Postgraduate Institute of Medical Education and Research
Chandigarh, India

Rajesh Chawla MD FCCM FCCP
Senior Consultant
Department of Respiratory
Critical Care and Sleep Medicine
Indraprastha Apollo Hospitals
New Delhi, India

Rakesh Garg MD DNB FICA Fellowship in Palliative Medicine
Additional Professor
Department of Onco-anesthesiology and Palliative
Medicine
All India Institute of Medical Sciences
New Delhi, India

Ramya BM MD (Anesthesiology)
Associate Consultant
Department of Anaesthesia
Mazumdar Shaw Medical Centre
Narayana Hrudayalaya
Bommasandra
Bengaluru, Karnataka, India

Reshma P Ambulkar MD (Anesthesiology) FRCA
Professor
Department of Anesthesiology, Critical Care and Pain
Tata Memorial Hospital
Mumbai, Maharashtra, India

Riddhi Joshi MD (Anesthesia)
Registrar
Department of Anesthesia
Dubbo Base Hospital
Dubbo, New South Wales, Australia

Robert James Premkumar MD
Fellow in Critical Care
Department of Critical Care Medicine
Narayana Hrudayalaya
Bengaluru, Karnataka, India

Ruchi Jain
MD (Anesthesiology) Postdoctoral fellowship in Neuro-anesthesiology
Assistant Professor
Department of Anesthesiology
Lokmanya Tilak Municipal Medical College and Lokmanya
Tilak Municipal General Hospital
Mumbai, Maharashtra, India

Ruchira Wasudeo Khasne MBBS DA DNB IDCCM EDAIC & EDAIC
Consultant and Head
Department of Critical Care Medicine
Ashoka-Medicover Hospital
Nashik, Maharashtra, India

Rupesh Yadav MD
Associate Professor
Department of Anesthesiology and Critical Care
Atal Bihari Vajpayee Institute of Medical Sciences (ABVIMS)
and Dr Ram Manohar Lohia Hospital
New Delhi, India

Sachin Gupta MD IDCCM IFCCM EDICM FCCM FICCM
Head
Department of Critical Care Medicine
Narayana Superspecialty Hospital
Gurugram, Haryana, India

Sandeep Sahu MD DNB PDCC FICCM
Professor
Department of Anesthesiology
Sanjay Gandhi Postgraduate Institute of Medical Sciences
Lucknow, Uttar Pradesh, India

Sapna Annaji Nikhar MD
Associate Professor
Department of Anesthesia and Intensive Care
Nizam's Institute of Medical Sciences
Hyderabad, Telangana, India

Sapna Ravindranath MD
Clinical Assistant Professor
Clerkship Co-Director
Department of Anesthesia
University of Lowa Hospital and Clinics
Lowa City, California, USA

Shagun Bhatia Shah DA DNB
Consultant Anesthesiologist
Department of Anesthesia and Critical Care
Rajiv Gandhi Cancer Institute and Research Center
New Delhi, India

Shashi Srivastava MD
Professor
Department of Anesthesiology
Sanjay Gandhi Postgraduate Institute of Medical Sciences
Lucknow, Uttar Pradesh, India

Sheila Nainan Myatra MD (Anesthesiology)
Professor
Department of Anesthesiology
Critical Care and Pain
Tata Memorial Hospital
Mumbai, Maharashtra, India

Shilpushp Bhosale DNB (Anesthesiology) DM
Associate Professor
Department of Anesthesiology
Critical Care and Pain
Tata Memorial Hospital
Mumbai, Maharashtra, India

Shivacharan Patel MD
Senior Resident
Department of Anesthesiollogy, Critical Care and Pain
Tata Memorial Hospital
Mumbai, Maharashtra, India

Shivakumar Iyer MD DNB EDIC
Professor and Head
Critical Care Medicine
Bharati Vidyapeeth (Deemed to be University) Medical College
Pune, Maharashtra, India

Shwetal Goraksha MD PDF (Neuroanesthesia and Critical Care)
Consultant
Department of Anesthesiology
PD Hinduja Hospital
Mumbai, Maharashtra, India

Sohan Lal Solanki
MD (Anesthesiology) PDCC (Organ Transplant Anesthesiology) MAMS
Professor
Department of Anesthesiology
Critical Care and Pain
Tata Memorial Hospital
Homi Bhabha National Institute
Mumbai, Maharashtra, India

Sonali Saraf DA DNB FRCA
Consultant
Department of Anesthesia
Jupiter Hospital
Thane, Maharashtra, India

Sree Kumar EJ MD DNB
Assistant Professor
Department of Anesthesiology
Sri Ramachandra Institute of Higher Education and Research
Chennai, Tamil Nadu, India

Srinivas Monanga MD (Anesthesia) FNB (Critical Care)
Junior Consultant
Department of Critical Care Medicine
Care Hospital
Visakhapatnam, Andhra Pradesh, India

Srinivas Samavedam MD DNB FRCP FNB EDIC FICCCM DMLE MHA
Head
Department of Critical Care
Virinchi Hospitals
Hyderabad, Telangana, India

Sritam Swarup Jena MD DM
Associate Professor
Department of Anesthesiology and Critical Care
All India Institute of Medical Sciences
Bhubaneswar, Odisha, India

Subha Padakannaya MD (Anesthesia)
Clinical Assistant
Department of Critical Care
PD Hinduja Hospital and Medical Research Institute
Mumbai, Maharashtra, India

Subhal Bhalchandra Dixit MD IDCCM FICCM FICP FCCM
Consultant Critical Care and Director ICU
Department of Critical Care
Sanjeevan and MJM Hospitals
Pune, Maharashtra, India

Subhash Todi MD MRCP
Director
Department of Critical Care Medicine
Advanced Medicare Research Institute
Kolkata, West Bengal, India

Sudhindra Prakash Kanavehalli MD FNB
Post Doctoral Fellow in Critical Care
Department of Critical Care Medicine
Mazumdar Shaw Medical Center
Narayana Hrudayalaya Health City
Bengaluru, Karnataka, India

Sudipta Mukherjee MD (Anesthesia) IDCCM FNB (Critical Care) EDICM
Junior Consultant
Department of Anesthesia and Critical Care
Tata Medical Center
Kolkata, West Bengal, India

Suhail Sarwar Siddiqui MD Fellow Critical Care DM EDIC
Assistant Professor
Department of Critical Care Medicine
King George's Medical University
Lucknow, Uttar Pradesh, India

Sunder L Negi MD DM (Cardiac Anesthesia)
Assistant Professor
Department of Anesthesia and Intensive Care
Postgraduate Institute of Medical Education and Research
Chandigarh, India

Suresh Ramasubban AB (Internal Medicine, Pulmonary and Critical Care)
Senior Consultant
Department of Respiratory, Critical Care
and Sleep Medicine
Apollo Gleneagles Hospital
Kolkata, West Bengal, India

Suresh Rao KG MD
Co-Director
Institute of Heart and Lung Transplant and Mechanical
Circulatory Support Services
MGM Healthcare Pvt Ltd
Chennai, Tamil Nadu, India

Sureshkumaran K MD (Anesthesia) PDF (Cardiac Anesthesia) FICCC
Consultant
Department of Cardiac Anesthesia
Institute of Heart and Lung Transplant and Mechanical
Circulatory Support
MGM Healthcare Pvt Ltd
Chennai, Tamil Nadu, India

Sushan Gupta MD
Senior Resident
Department of Anesthesiology
Critical Care and Pain
Tata Memorial Hospital
Mumbai, Maharashtra, India

Sushil Ambesh MD FICA FICCM FAMS
Professor
Department of Anesthesiology
Intensive Care and Pain Medicine
Sanjay Gandhi Postgraduate Institute of Medical Sciences
Lucknow, Uttar Pradesh, India

Swapnil Parab MD (Anesthesiology)
Professor
Department of Anesthesiology
Critical Care and Pain
Tata Memorial Hospital
Mumbai, Maharashtra, India

Swetha RD MD Fellowship in Neonatal Intensive Care (PGDDN)
Junior Consultant
Department of Pediatrics and Neonatology
Rainbow Children's Hospital
Bengaluru, Karnataka, India

Uma Hariharan MBBS DNB PGDHM
Associate Professor
Department of Anesthesiology and Intensive Care
Atal Bihari Vajpayee Institute of Medical Sciences (ABVIMS)
and Dr Ram Manohar Lohia Hospital
New Delhi, India

Usha Yadav MS
Specialist
Department of Obstetrics and Gynecology
Deen Dayal Upadhyay Hospital
New Delhi, India

Vaibhav Bhargava MD FNB (Critical Care) EDIC
Senior Consultant
Department of Critical Care Medicine
Eternal Heart Care Center
Jaipur, Rajasthan, India

Vandana Agarwal MD (Anesthesiology) FRCA
Professor
Department of Anesthesiology, Critical Care and Pain
Tata Memorial Hospital
Mumbai, Maharashtra, India

Vijay Chakkaravarthy KR DNB (Internal Medicine) IDCCM
Associate Consultant
Department of Critical Care Medicine
Apollo Hospitals
Chennai, Tamil Nadu, India

Vijaya Patil MD (Anesthesiology) Dip (Hosp Adminis)
Professor
Department of Anesthesiology
Critical Care and Pain
Tata Memorial Hospital
Mumbai, Maharashtra, India

Vincent Singh Parmanandam BPT MSc (Psychology) MSc in
Cancer Care (UK) PhD Scholar University of Sydney, NSW
Technical Officer
Department of Physiotherapy
Tata Memorial Hospital
Mumbai, Maharashtra, India

Virendra K Arya MD FRCPC (Canada) FASE
Professor
Department of Anaesthesia and Intensive Care
PGIMER
Chandigarh, India

Yatin Mehta MD MNAMS FRCA FAMS FIACTA FICCM FTEE
Chairman
Institute of Critical Care and Anesthesia
Medanta—The Medicity
Gurugram, Haryana, India

Preface

We take great pleasure in presenting to you the first edition of *Perioperative Critical Care*. There is an exponential growth in the complexity of surgeries that are being undertaken, as compared as little as 10 years back. The price of the progress in anesthesia and surgical techniques that we pay has increased manifold now, and this means we are anesthetizing patients, which were considered to be unfit to undergo anesthesia and any kind of surgery back then. So, the indications of surgery have expanded and so has the complexity of the management of these elderly, frail patients undergoing surgeries, which are now accompanied by myriad changes in the physiology and subsequent complications. The only advantage that the anesthetists and/or the intensivist, as the case may be depending on the set-up you work in, is that unlike a critically ill patient coming to you from ward, the timing of insult is known. You also have a chance to offer best possible optimization to these patients in the preoperative period. This does not mean however, that the surgical patient is easier to manage. This is because the complications that will be seen will be unique to these patients. This means that there are unique challenges and you need a definite skill set to manage these patients. A book covering these aspects was not available, so we decided to write this book. This meant we needed authors with different backgrounds specializing in care of these patients from different skill sets. Though the problems are different, the critical care that is needed is similar to other patients in the critical care units, so we needed authorities in the field of critical care. We were lucky that in India we are blessed with people with experience in these areas. Not only that, they are willing to spend the time and effort to write for the readers. So, we must thank all these contributors, many of them not from anesthesiology background, that they have spared the time and energy for us. Without them, the book could not have been written.

Our colleagues in the department have worked hard year over year and contributed significantly to the book. They also endured our time away from clinical duties, so we could work on the book, ungrudgingly. Our sincere thanks to all of them. Ms Chetna Malhotra Vohra (Associate Director–Content Strategy), an old friend, who works with M/s Jaypee Brothers Medical Publishers Pvt. Ltd and Ms Rajul Jain, Development Editor for the book, for their patience, help, and understanding. Big thanks to our families have been very supportive, without any nagging, while we worked on the book.

We hope you enjoy refreshing your knowledge, may be learn a few new things and see an improvement in patient outcomes. Please do get back to us with your suggestions and criticisms it is always welcome!

Atul Prabhakar Kulkarni
Sohan Lal Solanki
Jigeeshu Vasistha Divatia

Contents

Section 3: Neurosciences

Section 4: Pediatrics

Section 5: Obstetrics and Gynecology

Section 6: Gastrointestinal

Section 7: Genitourinary

Section 8: Orthopedics

Section 9: Head and Neck

Section 10: Transplantation

Section 11: Miscellaneous

General

SECTION OUTLINE

Critical Care in Perioperative Period—Need, Indications, Infrastructure, and Staffing

Harish MM, Robert James Premkumar, Ramya BM, Atul Prabhakar Kulkarni

INTRODUCTION

There has been a significant increase in the number of surgeries performed all over the world, across varying economic background. In 2004, there were globally 234.2 million surgical procedures, which had risen to 312.9 million in 2012, a documented 33.6% increase. About 30% of these surgeries in the poor health expenditure countries were cesareans. Each year, this number continues to grow. It has been observed that the increase in number of surgeries corresponds to a parallel increase in life expectancy.[1] But as the number of surgeries go up, the postoperative complications are also anticipated to increase.[2,3] Postoperative complications are associated with increased cost, mortality, and morbidity.[4-6]

NEED FOR SURGICAL CRITICAL CARE UNIT

Mortality following uncomplicated surgery is low.[7] But there is an ongoing change in demography resulting in a high-risk population. The average age of the general population continues to go up.[8] This older population has more comorbidities especially coronary artery disease, compared to the general population.[9] They also require surgery four times more than the general population.[10] A higher postoperative mortality is attributed to them.[11]

Overall, the postoperative complication is determined by a combination of the type of surgery, tissue injury associated with the surgery, and patient characteristics such as age and comorbidities. Some of the commonly seen complications that can be mitigated by good postoperative care are severe pain pneumonia, respiratory failure, myocardial infarction, arrhythmias, acute kidney injury, stroke, pulmonary thromboembolism, and delirium.[5]

Therefore, there is a need for enhancement of critical care in perioperative period, which involves identification of the surgical population at risk of developing complications; systematic preoperative assessment; optimization of comorbidities; and postoperative care.

INDICATIONS FOR ADMISSION TO SURGICAL INTENSIVE CARE UNIT

In order to provide optimal care, the vulnerable population needs to be identified. But it is easier said than done. It was noted in a study in UK, of all the surgeries performed in the hospitals, only about 12.5% were high-risk. But they contributed to 80% of mortality. Interestingly, only about 15% of them were admitted in intensive care unit (ICU) postoperatively.[11] This suggests that there are some lacunae in identifying high-risk patients and therefore, this is an avenue where there is scope for improvement, which may translate into improved outcomes.

Preoperative Identification

There are various scoring systems, some subjective and others objective, which are used to predict risk, with varying levels of accuracy. It has to be kept in mind that no single scoring system alone is absolute in predicting risk.

American Society of Anesthesiologists Physical Status Classification System

It is one of the oldest and most commonly used preoperative scoring system, which takes in to account the patient's comorbidities and clinical condition. It is graded from 1 for a normal healthy patient to 6 for a brain dead patient for organ donation. It is a better predictor of perioperative risk when combined with other factors like the type of surgery, deconditioning, and frailty.[12] The advantage of this scoring system is that it is convenient and does not consider laboratory parameters. The disadvantage is the interobserver variability in attributing score.[13] In spite of this, it is considered as a good predictor of perioperative morbidity and mortality.[14] It is noted that ASA IV or V constitutes about 50% of surgical mortality.[15]

Charlson Comorbidity Index

It is a weighted index, which was developed to stratify risk based on the comorbidities of the patient. Scoring is given for both the number and severity of the comorbid illness. The severity of the comorbid illness was also taken into consideration following the observation that certain illness such as malignancy and acquired immunodeficiency syndrome (AIDS) had a higher mortality than others; therefore attributing equal weightage to all comorbidities was bound to be inaccurate. More weightage is given to metastatic solid tumor, AIDS and moderate-to-severe liver disease compared to congestive cardiac failure, cerebrovascular disease, and chronic pulmonary disease.

One-year mortality with scores 0, 1–2, 3–4, and 5 and above was 12%, 26%, 52%, and 85%, respectively. The disadvantage of this index is that it was devised with a relatively small cohort of 559 patients and number of patients with certain illness and severity were small. Therefore, it needs further validation in larger population.[16]

Revised Cardiac Risk Index

It is an index used for predicting risk of major cardiac complication in patients undergoing noncardiac surgery. It incorporates six parameters; namely (1) High-risk surgery, (2) Ischemic heart disease, (3) History of congestive heart failure, (4) History of cerebrovascular disease, (5) Diabetes on insulin, and (6) Serum creatinine > 2 mg/dL preoperatively. Each of the parameter is assigned 1 score. Increase in score correlates with increase in cardiac complications.[17]

Surgical Mortality Score

It is a simple yet accurate risk stratification model developed from already available data from the database of 11,089 patients from a single institution. It takes into consideration, surgical specialty, age, sex, if the surgery is elective or emergency, onset time of surgery, and median operating time. Increasing scores were associated with increasing mortality.[18]

Modified Duke Activity Status Index

Functional capacity of the patient at baseline is a reliable predictor of perioperative cardiac events. The functional capacity and thereby cardiovascular risk can be estimated using the modified duke activity status index, as suggested by guidelines from the American College of Cardiology Foundation (ACCF) and the American Heart Association (AHA) in noncardiac surgery. It consists of a questionnaire regarding the various physical activities the patient is capable of, from which energy requirements are estimated. Along with the functional status, clinical risk factors and the type of surgery (high, intermediate, and low risk) are taken into consideration to assess perioperative risk.[19]

Intraoperative Identification

Similar to the preoperative parameters, the intraoperative parameters play a huge role in the development of postoperative complications. Emergency procedures and longer duration of surgeries have shown correlation with poor outcomes.[11,20,21]

P-POSSUM

Portsmouth-Physiological and Operative Severity Score for the Enumeration of Mortality and Morbidity (P-POSSUM) is a scoring system, which can be used preoperatively and intraoperatively to predict mortality in general surgical patients. It is an improvement over the original POSSUM score with better accuracy. It involves both physiological and operative parameters.[22-24]

Other scoring systems to predict mortality include the Estimation of Physiologic Ability and Surgical Stress (E-PASS) and Surgical Apgar Score (SAS).[25-27]

It must be kept in mind that most of these scoring systems are accurate while comparing a group of population rather than individuals since they were originally developed for the purpose of benchmarking and audit.[28]

Failure to Rescue

Failure to rescue is the fraction of the mortality amongst the patients with postoperative complications out of the total population with postoperative complications. It has been noted in studies that higher failure to rescue rates were associated with higher 30-day mortality even though postoperative complication rates were comparable.[29,30] Therefore, there needs to be more emphasis on improving the rescue rates.

Admission Criteria

According to *Society of Critical Care Medicine (SCCM)* guidelines, patients are classified into five priority groups. Priority 1 and 2 groups are to be provided ICU admission. Priority 1 includes patients on ventilator and organ support, requiring rigorous monitoring and treatment modalities that can only be imparted in the ICU. Priority 2 includes patient population as in priority 1, but whose survival chances are bleak and are not for cardiopulmonary resuscitation (CPR) in the event of cardiac arrest. Priority 3 includes patient population with organ dysfunction and need treatment modalities that can be provided in the Intermediate Medical Unit (IMU). They may require ICU admission in case of deterioration or lack of IMU facility in the hospital. Priority 4 includes patient population as in priority 3, with bleak survival chances and is not for CPR. Priority 5 includes patients for palliative care.[31]

The Intensive Care Society, in its "levels of critical care in adult patients" has defined levels of care from 0 to 3. Level 2 and/or 3 require ICU care.

Level 2 includes patients who need:

- Preoperative cardiovascular, respiratory, and renal optimization requiring central venous line and arterial line.
- Extended postoperative care:
  - Major surgeries
  - Surgery in high-risk patients
  - When complications are anticipated who might require intervention/monitoring
- Stepping down from level 3 who may have to be escalated back.
- Basic respiratory support:
  - Noninvasive ventilation/continuous positive airway pressure (NIV/CPAP)
  - Intubated for airway protection but do not require ventilation
  - More than 50% oxygen requirement via facemask
  - Anticipated worsening who would require advanced respiratory support
  - Recently extubated (24 hours) after being ventilated for >24 hours via endotracheal tube
  - Very frequent suctioning/physiotherapy to clear secretions
- *Basic cardiovascular support:* Use of central venous catheter (CVC)/arterial line; single intravenous (IV) vasoactive drug; or single/multiple IV rhythm control drugs.
- *Advanced cardiovascular support:* Multiple IV vasoactive or rhythm control drugs; continuous cardiac output, intra-aortic balloon pump (IABP), and other assist devices; and temporary pacemaker insertion.
- *Renal support:* Acute renal replacement therapy (RRT) or RRT in a chronic kidney disease patient who is requiring other organ support.
- *Neurological support:* Central nervous system (CNS) depression that may compromise airway protection; invasive neurological monitoring; continuous medication to control seizures; and therapeutic hypothermia.
- *Dermatological support:* Burns/extensive skin rashes/exfoliation affecting >30% bovine serum albumin (BSA).

Level 3 includes patients who need (1) advanced respiratory support alone [invasive mechanical ventilation via endotracheal or tracheostomy tube; bilevel positive airway pressure (BiPAP) via endotracheal or tracheostomy tube; CPAP via endotracheal tube or extracorporeal membrane oxygenation (ECMO)] or (2) a minimum of two organ support.[32]

INFRASTRUCTURE OF SURGICAL INTENSIVE CARE UNIT

The ICU/postanesthesia care unit should be designed and customized at its inception based on combined inputs from the anesthesia/critical care team along with the other departments the unit will be catering to; the management/administrative staff; and the architect/engineers involved in the construction process. It should be either in close proximity or should have easy access to the operating theater, emergency room, and the radiology suite. Provisions must be in place to rapidly procure medicines, blood products, and perform laboratory investigations.

Be it single rooms or common rooms, there must be adequate individual patient care area, enough to perform procedures and to accommodate, if needed, various accessories such as ventilators, echo/ultrasonography (USG) machines, defibrillator, X-ray machine, etc. There must be provisions for power supply, oxygen, vacuum, and compressed air. A trolley, with the patient's documentation must be available. Privacy of the patients must be ensured and provisions for curtains/screens should be available. At the same time, nurses should be able to visualize the patients always, including from the nurse station. The doorway should be wide enough to accommodate various equipment. Isolation rooms, if required, with negative pressure, should be available for specific patient groups such as post-transplant, burns, etc. Dedicated storage area for emergency drugs and equipment must be available. Computers equipped with picture archiving and communication system (PACS) should be available for rapid access to investigations and imaging.[33]

In order to ensure uninterrupted functioning of the various equipment, a reliable electricity supply is of paramount importance. Ideally, there must be appropriate electricity backup as rescue during power cuts. Voltage stabilizers are to be used to prevent damage to expensive equipment during power surges. Backup protocols should be in place to safely handle electrical outages.

Based on the size and requirement of the particular institution, source of oxygen in the form of cylinders, concentrators or pipeline supply must be in place.

Monitoring equipment should have electrocardiogram, noninvasive blood pressure, and pulse oximetry as the bare minimum for all beds. Capnography must be included in case of ventilated patient. Adequate number of ventilators should be available based on the requirement of the institution. NIV devices should also be available in adequate number. Point-of-care devices such as USG/echo machines, arterial-blood gas (ABG) machines, glucometers, etc., should be available.

STAFFING

The efficient functioning of ICU involves a team approach, which includes medical staff, nursing staff, physiotherapists, respiratory therapists, clinical pharmacists, dieticians, and administrative personnel. According to studies, a closed system of ICU, where the patients are completely managed by these especially trained physicians reduces the mortality and morbidity.[34,35]

Medical Staff[33]

Director

The head of the ICU must be a specialist specifically trained or experienced in intensive care medicine and is completely responsible for the medical and administrative aspect of the ICU. He preferably has a full-time commitment to the ICU and does not hold any other major responsibilities in the hospital.

Medical Staff Members

It includes physicians who are trained or experienced in intensive care medicine and ICU trainees. ICU trainees have a background in medical specialties and work/train in the ICU under supervision. Adequate number of staff should be in the team taking into account: (1) Total beds in the ICU, (2) Number of shifts, (3) Occupancy rate, (4) Holidays and illness, and (5) Overall workload. Consultant patient ratio exceeding 1:14 has shown to be deleterious in terms of patient care, staff well-being, and education.[36] Prolonged working hours have also shown a negative effect of medical and patient well-being.[37-39] Proper physician cover should be ensured during nights, weekends, and holidays.

Nursing Staff[33]

Nursing Head

A full-time head nurse is responsible for the efficient functioning and quality of the nursing staff. The head nurse should have training/experience in intensive care. Head nurse is responsible for the continuing education of the nursing staff and also for implementing policies in conjunction with the medical head.

Nurses

They are trained in intensive care medicine and are supervised by the head nurse. It must be ensured that they have a minimum standard by conducting regular training and examination. Nurse to patient ratio should be 1:1, 1:2, and 1:3 for level of care 3, 2, and 1, respectively.

Allied Healthcare Personnel[40]

Physiotherapists

Physiotherapists play a major role in the weaning and rehabilitation of complicated cases. Physiotherapists must have enough experience and be adequate in number.

Dietician

Dietician must be an integral part of the critical care team. The ICU dietician will be involved in the assessment of optimal nutritional need of the patient and also the appropriate route.

Speech and Language Therapist

Once the decision to wean a patient on tracheostomy, from the ventilator is made, speech and language therapist have to assess communication and swallowing aspects of the patient.

Clinical Pharmacist

A competent clinical pharmacist must be a part of the critical care unit. Clinical pharmacist's services must be available at least 5 days in a week. They must be preferably part of the consultant-led rounds, which has shown improvement in rectification of errors.

Psychologist

Anxiety, delirium, and post-traumatic stress disorders are common in the ICU. Therefore, the role of a psychologist is very important in assessing and alleviating of these conditions.

Radiology Technician

Radiology technicians must be available every day, in order to meet the increasing need for imaging, especially X-ray, CT, MRI, and other interventional procedures.

Critical Care Technician

The critical care technicians take on a wide variety of roles based on the institutional needs. They are knowledgeable about the functioning, setting-up, monitoring, and calibration of diverse equipment available in the unit such as ventilators, RRT devices, IABP, pulmonary artery (PA)/ CVC catheters, ECMO, and cardiac output monitors. They deliver these critical care services, in conjunction with the medical, nursing, and other paramedical staff.

Administrative Personnel

Secretaries have the role of typing report, certificates, and summaries. Other responsibilities may include organizing of admissions, discharges, and ward shifts. They also aid with the academic programs. Ideally one secretary is needed for 12 ICU beds.[33]

Cleaning Personnel

Cleaning and disinfection of the ICU is of paramount importance. It requires a group of individuals organized under one of more supervisors and is well versed with the infection control protocols of the institution.[33]

Biomedical Engineering Personnel

The role of biomedical engineers came into prominence when Ralph Nader published a report in 1971 about the high incidence of electrocutions in hospitals every year due to electrical accidents, leading to mortality and morbidity. Some of their important responsibilities include maintenance of an inventory of all equipment in use, regularly assessing if they are in working condition, servicing faulty devices, upgradation of devices, outsourcing of repair-work if required, and also in the education of the hospital staff about newly procured equipment.[41]

▌CONCLUSION

It is indisputable that there is a steady rise in the number of high-risk surgeries performed in a high-risk population, and as a direct consequence of which, there is a rise in the number of perioperative complications. High quality perioperative critical care involves the prevention or appropriate management of these complications by identifying the high-risk population early; risk stratifying them using the scoring systems; optimizing their comorbidities and safely conducting the surgical procedure; anticipating complications and shifting to ICU promptly; and exercising the expertise of a multifaceted medical, nursing, and paramedical team in an infrastructure which accommodates the necessary tools.

▌REFERENCES

1. Weiser TG, Haynes AB, Molina G, Lipsitz SR, Esquivel MM, Uribe-Leitz T, et al. Estimate of the global volume of surgery in 2012: an assessment supporting improved health outcomes. Lancet. 2015;385:S11.
2. Alkire BC, Raykar NP, Shrime MG, Weiser TG, Bickler SW, Rose JA, et al. Global access to surgical care: a modelling study. Lancet Glob Health. 2015;3(6):e316-23.
3. Meara JG, Greenberg SLM. The Lancet Commission on Global Surgery Global surgery 2030: Evidence and solutions for achieving health, welfare and economic development. Surgery. 2015;157(5):834-5.
4. Scally CP, Thumma JR, Birkmeyer JD, Dimick JB. Impact of surgical quality improvement on payments in medicare patients. Ann Surg. 2015;262(2):249-52.
5. Pearse RM, Holt PJE, Grocott MPW. Managing perioperative risk in patients undergoing elective non-cardiac surgery. BMJ. 2011;343:d5759.
6. International Surgical Outcomes Study group. Global patient outcomes after elective surgery: prospective cohort study in 27 low-, middle- and high-income countries. Br J Anaesth. 2016;117(5):601-9.
7. Pearse RM, Moreno RP, Bauer P, Pelosi P, Metnitz P, Spies C, et al. Mortality after surgery in Europe: a 7 day cohort study. Lancet. 2012;380(9847):1059-65.
8. Naughton C, Feneck RO. The impact of age on 6-month survival in patients with cardiovascular risk factors undergoing elective non-cardiac surgery. Int J Clin Pract. 2007;61(5):768-76.
9. Carroll K, Majeed A, Firth C, Gray J. Prevalence and management of coronary heart disease in primary care: population-based cross-sectional study using a disease register. J Public Health Med. 2003;25(1):29-35.
10. Crowe S. Anaesthesia and the older surgical patient: something old, something new, something borrowed. Age Ageing. 2004;33(1):4-5.
11. Pearse RM, Harrison DA, James P, Watson D, Hinds C, Rhodes A, et al. Identification and characterisation of the high-risk surgical population in the United Kingdom. Crit Care Lond Engl. 2006;10(3):R81.
12. ASA. (2019). ASA Physical Status Classification System. [online] Available from https://www.asahq.org/standards-and-guidelines/asa-physical-status-classification-system. [Last accessed February, 2020].
13. Owens WD, Felts JA, Spitznagel EL. ASA Physical Status Classifications: A Study of Consistency of Ratings. Anesthesiology. 1978;49(4):239-43.
14. Wolters U, Wolf T, Stützer H, Schröder T. ASA classification and perioperative variables as predictors of postoperative outcome. Br J Anaesth. 1996;77(2):217-22.
15. Callum KG, Gray AJG, Hargraves CMK, Hoile RW, Ingram GS, Martin IC, et al. National Confidential Enquiry into Perioperative Deaths. London: the 2001 Report of the National Confidential Enquiry into Perioperative Deaths; 2001.
16. Charlson ME, Pompei P, Ales KL, MacKenzie CR. A new method of classifying prognostic comorbidity in longitudinal studies: Development and validation. J Chronic Dis. 1987;40(5):373-83.
17. Lee TH, Marcantonio ER, Mangione CM, Thomas EJ, Polanczyk CA, Cook EF, et al. Derivation and prospective validation of a simple index for prediction of cardiac risk of major noncardiac surgery. Circulation. 1999;100(10):1043-9.
18. Hadjianastassiou VG, Tekkis PP, Poloniecki JD, Gavalas MC, Goldhill DR. Surgical mortality score: risk management tool for

auditing surgical performance. World J Surg. 2004;28(2):193-200.

19. Fleisher LA, Beckman JA, Brown KA, Calkins H, Chaikof EL, Fleischmann KE, et al. 2009 ACCF/AHA Focused Update on Perioperative Beta Blockade Incorporated Into the ACC/AHA 2007 Guidelines on Perioperative Cardiovascular Evaluation and Care for Noncardiac Surgery: A Report of the American College of Cardiology Foundation/American Heart Association Task Force on Practice Guidelines. Circulation. 2009;120(21):e169-276.

20. Turrentine FE, Wang H, Simpson VB, Jones RS. Surgical risk factors, morbidity, and mortality in elderly patients. J Am Coll Surg. 2006;203(6):865-77.

21. Leung JM, Dzankic S. Relative importance of preoperative health status versus intraoperative factors in predicting postoperative adverse outcomes in geriatric surgical patients. J Am Geriatr Soc. 2001;49(8):1080-5.

22. Copeland GP, Jones D, Walters M. POSSUM: a scoring system for surgical audit. Br J Surg. 1991;78(3):355-60.

23. Campillo-Soto A, Flores-Pastor B, Soria-Aledo V, Candel-Arenas M, Andrés-García B, Martín-Lorenzo JG, et al. The POSSUM scoring system: an instrument for measuring quality in surgical patients. Cirugia Espanola. 2006;80(6):395-9.

24. Guha A, Ramesh V, Mercer S. The P-POSSUM scoring systems for predicting the mortality of neurosurgical patients undergoing craniotomy: Further validation of usefulness and application across healthcare systems. Indian J Anaesth. 2013;57(6):587.

25. Yamashita S, Haga Y, Nemoto E, Nagai S, Ohta M. E-PASS (The Estimation of Physiologic Ability and Surgical Stress) scoring system helps the prediction of postoperative morbidity and mortality in thoracic surgery. Eur Surg Res Eur Chir Forsch Rech Chir Eur. 2004;36(4):249-55.

26. Tominaga T, Takeshita H, Takagi K, Kunizaki M, To K, Abo T, et al. E-PASS score as a useful predictor of postoperative complications and mortality after colorectal surgery in elderly patients. Int J Colorectal Dis. 2016;31(2):217-25.

27. Gawande AA, Kwaan MR, Regenbogen SE, Lipsitz SA, Zinner MJ. An Apgar score for surgery. J Am Coll Surg. 2007;204(2):201-8.

28. Higgins TL. Quantifying risk and benchmarking performance in the adult intensive care unit. J Intensive Care Med. 2007;22(3):141-56.

29. Ghaferi AA, Birkmeyer JD, Dimick JB. Complications, failure to rescue, and mortality with major inpatient surgery in medicare patients. Ann Surg. 2009;250(6):1029-34.

30. Ghaferi AA, Birkmeyer JD, Dimick JB. Variation in hospital mortality associated with inpatient surgery. N Engl J Med. 2009;361(14):1368-75.

31. Nates JL, Nunnally M, Kleinpell R, Blosser S, Goldner J, Birriel B, et al. ICU admission, discharge, and triage guidelines: a framework to enhance clinical operations, development of institutional policies, and further research. Crit Care Med. 2016;44(8):1553-602.

32. Intensive Care Society. (2009). Levels of Critical Care for Adult Patients. [online]. Available from http://icmwk.com/wp-content/uploads/2014/02/Revised-Levels-of-Care-21-12-09.pdf. [Last accessed February, 2020].

33. Valentin A, Ferdinande P, ESICM Working Group on Quality Improvement. Recommendations on basic requirements for intensive care units: structural and organizational aspects. Intensive Care Med. 2011;37(10):1575-87.

34. Wilcox ME, Chong CAKY, Niven DJ, Rubenfeld GD, Rowan KM, Wunsch H, et al. Do intensivist staffing patterns influence hospital mortality following ICU admission? A systematic review and meta-analyses. Crit Care Med. 2013;41(10):2253-74.

35. van der Sluis FJ, Slagt C, Liebman B, Beute J, Mulder JWR, Engel AF. The impact of open versus closed format ICU admission practices on the outcome of high risk surgical patients: a cohort analysis. BMC Surg. 2011;11:18.

36. Ward NS, Afessa B, Kleinpell R, Tisherman S, Ries M, Howell M, et al. Intensivist/patient ratios in closed ICUs: a statement from the Society of Critical Care Medicine Taskforce on ICU Staffing. Crit Care Med. 2013;41(2):638-45.

37. Arnedt JT, Owens J, Crouch M, Stahl J, Carskadon MA. Neurobehavioral performance of residents after heavy night call vs after alcohol ingestion. JAMA. 2005;294(9):1025-33.

38. Landrigan CP, Rothschild JM, Cronin JW, Kaushal R, Burdick E, Katz JT, et al. Effect of reducing interns' work hours on serious medical errors in intensive care units. N Engl J Med. 2004;351(18):1838-48.

39. Barger LK, Cade BE, Ayas NT, Cronin JW, Rosner B, Speizer FE, et al. Extended work shifts and the risk of motor vehicle crashes among interns. N Engl J Med. 2005;352(2):125-34.

40. NHS. (2002). The Role of Healthcare Professionals within Critical Care Services [online]. Available from http://www.wales.nhs.uk/sites3/Documents/768/AHPs%20%26%20HCS%202002.pdf. [Last accessed February, 2020].

41. Wilder DK. Clinical engineering support for the critical care unit. Crit Care Clin. 1993;9(3):501-9.

Oxygen Therapy in the Perioperative Period

Bindiya Salunke, Madhusudan Jaju, Amol Kothekar

INTRODUCTION

Oxygen is essential element required for aerobic metabolism for the synthesis of adenosine triphosphate (ATP) within mitochondria and for survival. ATPs are the primary energy source for all active metabolic processes. Concentration of oxygen in the air at or near sea level (21% or partial pressure of 160 mm Hg) is more than sufficient for healthy individuals with intact respiratory drive. Oxygen supplementation is often required in perioperative period due to wide range of pathophysiological effects of anesthesia and surgery on respiratory function and lung physiology. Hence, understanding the respiratory physiology in relation to oxygen and pathophysiology of conditions needing oxygen supplementation is vital for management of perioperative patient. Oxygen is considered as a lifesaving drug in various emergencies; however, there is a growing evidence of toxicities associated with excess oxygen use. Hence, it is equally important to avoid its use in the unindicated cases.

PHYSIOLOGY

Atmospheric oxygen enters the body by the process known as respiration, the process of carrying oxygen to the tissues, which is known as transportation. Oxygen utilization is the process of oxidation of glucose into ATP, water and carbon dioxide. The processes of respiration and transportation are described in brief.

Respiration

It deals with the transport of atmospheric oxygen from the alveoli and subsequently into the blood. Alveolar gas equation explains the physiology of the former component of transport of atmospheric oxygen to the alveoli. Alveolar arterial gradient (A–a gradient) deals with the later component of transport of alveolar oxygen into the arterial blood.

Alveolar Gas Equation

The simplified alveolar gas equation is described here:[1]
$$PAO_2 = (P_{atm} - PH_2O) FiO_2 - PaCO_2/R$$
where,

PAO_2 = partial pressures of O_2 in the alveolar gas

P_{atm} = the atmospheric pressure (At sea level average value = 760 mm Hg)

PH_2O = partial pressure of water (Average value = 45 mm Hg)

FiO_2 = the fraction of inspired oxygen (Average value = 0.21)

$PACO_2$ = partial pressures of CO_2 in the alveolar gas (average value = 40–45 mm Hg)

R = the respiratory exchange ratio VCO_2/VO_2, in which VCO_2 is the rate of CO_2 elimination from the lungs and VO_2 is the rate of O_2 uptake from the alveolar gas (average value = 0.8–0.82)

Putting all these values in the equation, alveolar oxygen pressure is calculated below:
$$PAO_2 = (760 - 47) 0.21 - 40/0.8 = 149 - 40/0.8$$
$$= 149 - 50 = 99 \text{ mm Hg (approximately)}$$

Clinical utility of alveolar gas equation: Alveolar gas equation highlights three key determinants of alveolar oxygen pressure, viz., atmospheric pressure, fraction of inspired oxygen (FiO_2), and partial pressure of carbon dioxide in alveoli (blood).

Decrease in the partial pressures of O_2 in the alveolar gas (PAO_2) at high altitude is due to drop in atmospheric pressure. Decrease in PAO_2 can also occur when there is drop in FiO_2. The older anesthesia machines without 'link 25' safety mechanism had potential risk for delivering hypoxic mixture by possible decrease in FiO_2 when incorrect flow settings of oxygen and nitrous oxide were used.

Alveolar gas equation beautifully explains decrease in PAO_2 in conditions which increase partial pressure of carbon dioxide (PCO_2), e.g., respiratory depression. For each 8 mm Hg increase in PCO_2, there is 10 mm Hg drop in PAO_2. When PCO_2 increases from 40 to 80 mm Hg, PAO_2 drops by 50 to the value of 49 mm Hg.

PAO_2 (at PCO_2 of 40) = (760 − 47) 0.21 − 40/0.8 = 149 − 40/0.8

= 149 − 50 = 99 mm Hg

PAO_2 (at PCO_2 of 48) = (760 − 47) 0.21 − 48/0.8 = 149 − 48/0.8

= 149 − 60 = 89 mm Hg]

PAO_2 (at PCO_2 of 80) = (760 − 47) 0.21 − 80/0.8 = 149 − 80/0.8

= 149 − 100 = 49 mm Hg

This is one of the common causes of perioperative hypoxemia. The physiological treatment of it is normalization of PCO_2 rather than supplemental oxygen. Alveolar gas equation is essential for calculation of alveolar–arterial or A–a gradient which can be used for identification of cause of hypoxemia (see later).

Alveolar–arterial Gradient (A–a Gradient)

Oxygen diffuses from the alveoli, against a pressure gradient into the mixed venous blood of the alveolar capillaries. Hence, partial pressure of oxygen in arterial blood (PaO_2) will always be lesser than the alveolar partial pressure of oxygen (PAO_2).

Oxygen diffuses from alveoli to the capillary blood through a membrane known as alveolar capillary membrane. As oxygen diffuses across a pressure gradient, the alveolar PAO_2 (upstream) will always be higher than arterial (downstream) PaO_2 **(Fig. 1)**.

Alveolar–arterial gradient (A–a gradient) is the difference between the partial pressure of oxygen in alveoli (A) and the artery (a), and can be calculated by the following formula:

$$\text{A–a gradient} = PAO_2 − PaO_2$$

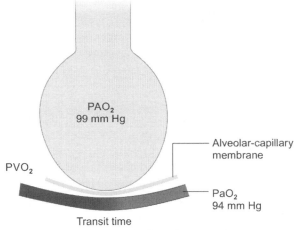

Fig. 1: Schematic diagram showing anatomy of alveolar unit. Oxygen gradient between alveolar and arterial blood is known as alveolar–arterial gradient (A–a gradient).

(PAO_2: partial pressures of oxygen in alveolar gas; PaO_2: partial pressure of oxygen in arterial blood; PVO_2: mixed venous partial pressures of oxygen)

Table 1: Alveolar–arterial gradient (A–a gradient) and efficacy of 100% oxygen to correct PaO_2 in various clinical conditions.[2]

Disease state	A–a gradient	Correctable with 100% oxygen	Causes
Low inspired pO_2	Normal	Yes	High altitude
Hypoventilation	Normal	Yes	CNS depression, neuromuscular disease, skeletal abnormalities of the chest wall, opiate and other CNS depressant use
Diffusion disorder	Elevated	Yes	Interstitial lung disease
V/Q mismatch	Elevated	Yes	• *Increased V/Q:* Chronic bronchitis, mucus plugging, pulmonary edema • *Decreased V/Q:* Pulmonary embolism, emphysema
Shunting	Elevated	No	• *Alveolar:* Pneumonia, severe pulmonary edema, atelectasis, ARDS • *Cardiac:* Eisenmenger syndrome, cyanotic heart disease • *Vascular:* Pulmonary AV shunt

(ARDS: acute respiratory distress syndrome; AV shunt: arteriolar venous shunt; CNS: central nervous system; V/Q: ratio between ventilation and perfusion of lungs; pO_2: partial pressure of oxygen; PaO_2: partial pressure of arterial oxygen)

A young nonsmoker adult has A–a gradient of 5–10 mm Hg when breathing room air. This gradient can go up to 30 at 100% FiO_2.

Clinical utility of alveolar–arterial gradient: Calculation of A–a gradient can help in diagnosis of underlying mechanism of decrease in PaO_2 (hypoxia). **Table 1** explains the A–a gradient in various disease states. It also differentiates clinical conditions based on the efficacy of 100% oxygen to correct PaO_2.

Oxygen Transportation

Oxygen Contents of Blood

The major component of oxygen binds with hemoglobin and minor component is dissolved in the plasma. Oxygen content of the blood can be measured by the formula given below:

Arterial oxygen content = bound oxygen + dissolved oxygen

CaO_2 = (SaO_2 × Hb × Oxygen combining capacity of hemoglobin) + (oxygen solubility × PaO_2)

= (SaO_2 × Hb × 1.31 × 0.01) + (0.0225 × PaO_2)

where,

- 1.31 = Hüfner's constant
- Hb = the amount of hemoglobin (g/dL)
- SaO_2 = the arterial hemoglobin saturation in percent
- 0.0225 = the solubility coefficient of oxygen at body temperature
- PaO_2 = the partial pressure of oxygen in arterial blood in kilopascals (kPa).

At Hb of 15 g/dL, saturation of 100% and PaO_2 of 99 mm Hg (13.19 kPa), oxygen content in the blood is 19.94 mL (almost 20 mL) for each 100 mL or 200 mL for each 1,000 mL or one liter, out of which 19.65 mL is carried by hemoglobin and 0.29 mL is dissolved.

Oxygen Delivery and Extraction

At cardiac output of 5 L/min, 1,000 mL of oxygen (SpO_2 100%) is delivered to the tissues out of which 250 mL is utilized and 750 mL (SvO_2 or mixed venous saturation of 75%) returns to the heart. Oxygen consumption is roughly 250 mL/min. Factors affecting oxygen consumption are listed in **Table 2**.

At higher altitude, inspired oxygen drops due to drop in atmospheric pressure leading to proportionate drop in PAO_2. Body compensates by CO_2 washout to reduce PCO_2 (see alveolar gas equation) and by increasing hemoglobin to increase oxygen content of the blood.

Physiologic Determinants of Oxygenation

Shunt fraction and Functional Residual Capacity play major role in the physiology of oxygenation.

Shunt Fraction

Pulmonary shunt is an area of the lung which gets perfusion in the absence of ventilation. The cardiac output reaching shunt area does not take part in oxygenation. Pulmonary shunt can be quantified in percentage, known as shunt fraction. The normal range of shunt fraction for an adult is around 4–10%. In pathological conditions, the shunt fraction is significantly greater and even breathing 100% oxygen does not fully oxygenate the blood. Classic example is acute respiratory distress syndrome (ARDS), application of positive end-expiratory pressure (PEEP) "recruits" the collapsed alveoli reducing shunt fraction and hence improving oxygenation.[3]

Table 2: Factors affecting oxygen consumption (VO_2).

Increased VO_2	Decreased VO_2
Exercise and physiotherapy	General anesthesia: Sedation, muscle relaxants, analgesics
Trauma (Surgery)	Antipyretics
Shivering and agitation	Mechanical ventilation
Inflammation, sepsis, pyrexia	Shock state

Functional Residual Capacity (FRC)

The amount of air left in the lung at the end of normal expiration is called functional residual capacity (FRC). Two most important functions of FRC are:

1. It helps in prevention of alveolar collapse and in healthy lungs; most of the alveoli are open at FRC. In diseased lungs (pulmonary edema, ARDS, etc.) there is collapse of significant number of alveoli at FRC causing hypoxemia due to shunt. Addition of PEEP (either invasive or noninvasive) increases FRC which helps in opening of these alveoli, reduces shunt and improves oxygenation. PEEP may also improve lung compliance and reducing work of breathing as it is easy to inflate already opened alveoli than to reopen closed alveoli.

2. It represents the oxygen store available for gas exchange during the apnea. Preoxygenation or denitrogenation of FRC replaces air or nitrogen for oxygen. Adequate preoxygenation helps in providing safe apnea time for airway procedures like intubation or bronchoscopy.

Time required for the desaturation after apnea depends on FRC and oxygen consumption and hence varies from individual to individual. Larger FRC and reduced oxygen consumption provide longer apnea time.

HYPOXIA VS. HYPOXEMIA

Hypoxemia is defined as a decrease in the partial pressure of oxygen in the blood. Hypoxia is defined by reduced level of tissue oxygenation.

Types of Hypoxia

Following types of hypoxia are described:

1. *Hypoxic hypoxia:*[4] This is further divided into:
   a. Diminished oxygen content
   b. Obstruction of the airway
   c. Abnormal lung conditions
   d. Pulmonary shunt or extrapulmonary right to left shunt
2. *Anemic hypoxia*: Due to reduced hemoglobin
3. *Stagnant hypoxia*: due to reduced cardiac output or reduced regional blood flow
4. *Histotoxic hypoxia*: (e.g., cyanide poisoning)
5. *Cytopathic hypoxia*: (e.g., secondary to sepsis and inflammation)[5]

Pathophysiology and Management of Hypoxia and Hypoxemia in Perioperative Period

Hypoxemia during perioperative period can occur anytime; however, it is more common during induction or emergence of anesthesia. Common causes of hypoxemia during perioperative period are:

- *Obstruction of the airway:* Both mechanical (laryngospasm, bronchospasm, complete ventilation failure) and functional obstruction (respiratory depression, residual paralysis) of the airway.
- *Shunt:* Atelectasis, one lung ventilation. Inhalation anesthetics can increase severity of hypoxemia due to shunt by inhibiting hypoxic pulmonary vasoconstriction.
- Anemic hypoxia due to sudden massive blood loss.

Management of Hypoxia in Perioperative Period

Prevention: Prevention of hypoxia is of prime importance. Perioperative physician should anticipate, prevent and treat all possible causes of hypoxia.

Preoperative measures: Preoperative aerobic exercise and inspiratory muscle training, especially for patients with high risk of postoperative pulmonary complications.[6] This has been proven to reduce postoperative atelectasis and pneumonia. This can be achieved by:

- Incentive spirometry 10 times per hour.
- Deep breathing exercises.

Intraoperative measures:

- *Preoxygenation:* It increases the duration of safe apnea till definitive airway is achieved. The primary goal of preoxygenation is to denitrogenate FRC of the lungs and to achieve end-tidal oxygen concentration (ETO_2) of greater than 90%.[7] Following techniques can be utilized during preoxygenation.
  - Oxygen delivery 100% FiO_2 via anesthesia circuit with well-fitted mask. This can be achieved by either 3 minutes tidal volume breathing or eight vital capacity breaths.[8]
    - High-flow nasal cannula (HFNC) is another option and it continues to provide apneic oxygenation during the process of intubation.
    - If patient cannot achieve saturation greater than 93–95% before intubation with high FiO_2 alone, noninvasive positive pressure ventilation should be applied. Continuous positive airway pressure (CPAP) or PEEP will help decrease the degree of shunts and will also prevent absorption atelectasis caused due to high FiO_2.[9]
  - Position of patient
    - Supine position increases the risk of atelectasis of the dependent lung. Patients who are at high risk of hypoxemia (critically ill patients, patients having morbid obesity or abdominal distension) should be preferably preoxygenated in a propped up position. If the patient is immobilized (e.g., spine injury)

then reverse Trendelenburg position is ideal. Head elevated position additionally provides benefit of better laryngeal view on direct laryngoscopy.[10]

- *Bag-mask ventilation:* Periods of apneas should be avoided during induction by ventilating the patient with bag-mask ventilation. This will benefit in several ways like:
  - Increases oxygenation through distension of alveoli and decreases shunting
  - Minimizes accumulation of carbon dioxide by actively washing it out which will otherwise cause acidosis and cerebral vasodilatation.

Modified rapid sequence intubation allowed gentle mask ventilation in patients who are considered as full stomach. Care must be taken to prevent risk of regurgitation and aspiration by limiting inspiratory pressure below 25 cm of H_2O.[11,12]

- *Apneic oxygenation:* It extends the duration of safe apnea.[13] It can be provided either by a nasal cannula set at 15 L/min. Benefit of short-term apneic oxygenation during intubation procedure outweighs the risk of delivery of such high flows of dry and cold oxygen via nasal cannula both in patients with high risk for hypoxemia and the patient having difficult intubation. Alternatively, a HFNC with 100% FiO_2 and flow rate up to 70 L/min can be safely used.

Apneic oxygenation will work best with patent upper airway. Ideal position during apneic ventilation should aim at maximizing upper airway patency, and this is achieved by head elevated position and chin lift-jaw thrust position.[14]

- *Prevention of atelectasis:* Atelectasis can be prevented by the use of PEEP unless contraindicated. Recruitment maneuvers can be used for reversal of atelectasis during anesthesia.[15] It is prudent to avoid higher FiO_2 to reduce and prevent recurrence of atelectasis.[16]

Postoperative measures to prevent hypoxia[17]

- Continuation of incentive spirometry as advised preoperatively
- Deep breathing and cough every 2 hourly
- Early mobilization of patients
- Head end of bed elevated >30 degrees
- Use of bronchodilators for patients with chronic obstructive pulmonary disease (COPD) and asthma[18]
- Good postoperative analgesia
- Utilization of regional blocks (epidural or facial plane blocks) for analgesia as much as possible
- Opioid-free analgesia postoperatively as much as possible.

Treatment of Established Hypoxia

Supplementation of oxygen is the first line of treatment of hypoxia. Supplemental oxygen can be delivered to patient at normal atmospheric pressure and is referred as normobaric oxygen therapy or at higher than atmospheric pressure is known as hyperbaric oxygen therapy. Hyperbaric oxygen therapy is beyond the purview of this chapter.

Depending on the dependency of patients upon the oxygen delivery device to correct any oxygen delivery deficiency, they can be classified as:[19]

- *Low dependency*: When supplemental oxygen alone is effective to correct hypoxia in spontaneously breathing patient, e.g., nasal prongs, standard facemask.
- *Medium dependency*: When spontaneously breathing patient requires additional respiratory support along with supplemental oxygen to correct hypoxia, e.g., CPAP mask, HFNC, etc.
- *High dependency*: When patient requires supplemental oxygen and full respiratory support to maintain oxygenation, e.g. Noninvasive positive-pressure ventilation (NIPPV), Intermittent positive pressure ventilation (IPPV).

Continuous positive airway pressure, NIPPV, and IPPV are beyond the purview of this chapter. Here we are discussing low-dependency devices and HFNC.

Low-dependency devices can be further classified as variable performance devices or fixed performance devices depending on if fixed amount of oxygen is delivered to patient during both the phases of respiration or its variable depending on patient's respiratory rate, tidal volume or flow rate.

Depending on reservoir capacity, low-dependency oxygen delivery devices can be classified as:

- No capacity oxygen delivery devices, e.g., nasal cannulae
- Low-capacity oxygen delivery devices (Capacity < 100 mL), e.g., pediatric facemask, tracheostomy mask
- Medium-capacity oxygen delivery devices (Capacity = 100–250 mL), e.g., standard facemask
- High-capacity oxygen delivery devices (Capacity = 250–1,500 mL), e.g., rebreathing mask, nonrebreathing mask (NRBM)
- Very high-capacity oxygen delivery devices (Capacity > 1,500 mL), e.g., incubator, head tent.

Commonly available devices: Commonly available oxygen devices in day-to-day use are explained in detail here:

- *Nasal cannulae (Fig. 2)*: These deliver unhumidified oxygen to the nasopharynx. Its advantages being less

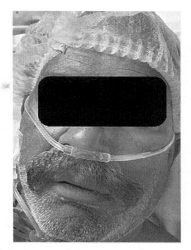

Fig. 2: Patient receiving oxygen via nasal prongs.

claustrophobic and allows easy accessibility to mouth for uninterrupted talking, and eating. But its major drawback being unpredictability of FiO_2 and oxygen delivery >2 L/min can be uncomfortable and can cause drying of nasal mucosa.

- *Facemask (Figs. 3A and B)*: Here oxygen flow of 2–5 L/min should be used and rebreathing is seen commonly if oxygen flow rate is kept <2 L/min or if patient has very high minute ventilation.
- *Nonrebreathing masks (Fig. 4)*: They have reservoir bag connected to the facemask via a flap valve which prevents rebreathing. Oxygen supply enters the reservoir bag first and then enters the facemask. Reservoir bag provides extra oxygen to match the patient's peak inspiratory flow rate (PIFR) which is higher than the oxygen supply flow rate. Presence of two one-way flap valve on the mask prevents entrainment of room air during inspiration and allows expiratory air to vent out to atmosphere. FiO_2 up to 75–90% can be achieved at oxygen flow rate of 12–15 L/min.[19] NRBM should be used with caution, they provide higher FIO_2 than the face mask and may mask severe respiratory failure. It should not be encouraged to use NRBM except for short-term use or use in patients with do-not-intubate (DNI) orders. If the patient's FiO_2 is in this range, need of ventilation should be assessed.
- *Partial rebreathing masks (Fig. 5)*: They are similar to the NRBM except for the absence of flap valve to the oxygen reservoir. These masks are supposed to allow rebreathing of the heated and humidified dead space gas while preventing rebreathing of alveolar gases. Dead space gas does not contain expired CO_2 and has oxygen concentration similar to fresh gas. Mapleson A breathing system (Magill circuit) also utilizes similar advantage of dead space rebreathing.

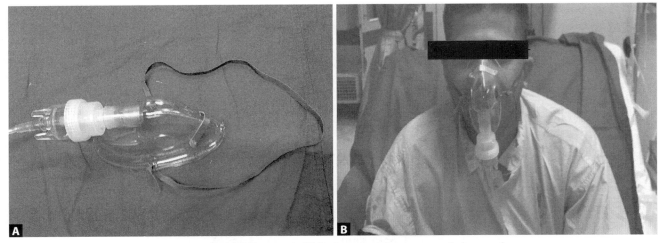

Figs. 3A and B: (A) Facemask; (B) Patient receiving oxygen via facemask.

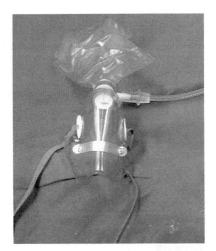

Fig. 4: Nonrebreathing mask.

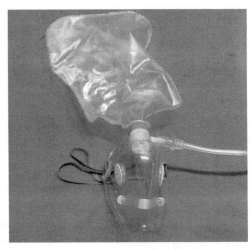

Fig. 5: Partial rebreathing mask.

- *Venturi mask (**Figs. 6A and B**):* This is an example of fixed performance device. It works on Bernoulli effect and Venturi principle. Here, mixing of room air and oxygen occurs due to delivery of oxygen at high velocity through a small orifice and shear forces. There is entrainment of room air but at fixed rate. Mask adapters are of different sizes and color-coded, which help us to adjust the FiO_2. To ensure target FiO_2 and adequate CO_2 clearance, oxygen flow rate should exceed patient's minute ventilation.[20] These masks can provide FiO_2 from 0.24 to 0.60% **(Table 3)**.

HIGH-FLOW NASAL CANNULA (FIG. 7)

Conventional oxygen delivery systems typically deliver variable and unreliable FiO_2 due to low flows (e.g., nasal cannula or facemask) leading to difficult in its monitoring and titration. High-flow systems like Venturi masks and NRBM can provide more or less fixed FiO_2, however, with delivery of cold and dry gases. Oxygen given by high-flow systems for prolonged periods is poorly tolerated by patients due to inadequate warming and humidification of inspired gas.

High-flow nasal cannula is an innovative oxygen delivery system which delivers high flows of heated and humidified gases which offer advantage of both fixed FiO_2 and better patient acceptance. HFNC provides heated and humidified oxygen at high flows to the patient. It can deliver FiO_2 of 0.21–1.00% at flow rates of up to 60 L/min. The flow rate and FiO_2 can be independently titrated based on the patient's flow and FiO_2 requirements.

High-flow nasal cannula may also be used in safe environment with less monitoring availability in stable cooperative patients who do not have severe hypoxemia.[21]

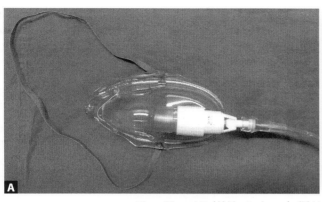
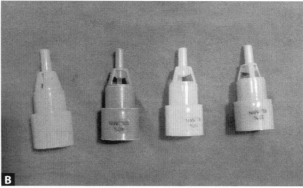

Figs. 6A and B: (A) Venturi mask; (B) Venturi connecters for different FiO_2.

Table 3: Venturi devices with color coding, oxygen flow rate, air entrainment and total flow to patient.[19]

Color of device	FiO₂ (Fraction of inspired oxygen)	Oxygen flow rate (L/min)	Air entrainment (L/min)	Total flow (L/min)
Blue	0.24	2	51	53
White	0.28	4	41	45
Orange	0.31	6	41	47
Yellow	0.35	8	37	45
Red	0.40	10	32	42
Green	0.60	15	15	30

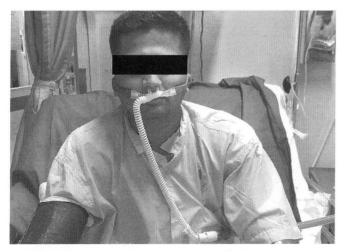

Fig. 7: Patient receiving oxygen via high-flow nasal cannula.

Physiology and Mechanics of High-flow Nasal Cannula

Washout of Nasopharyngeal Dead Space

High flows delivered by HFNC tend to washout dead space from the upper airway;[22] this improves the efficiency of ventilation as the proportion of alveolar to minute ventilation increases. HFNC in healthy volunteers lead to approximate 20% fall in minute ventilation due to a decrease in tidal volume without any change in respiratory rate during sleep.[23] This effect is probably due to lesser requirements of minute ventilation due to washout of nasopharyngeal dead space. In patients with PaO_2:FiO_2 ratio < 300 mm Hg; use of HFNC at 40 L/min lead to decrease in minute ventilation due to decreased respiratory rate and constant tidal volume without any change in arterial CO_2 levels.[24]

Positive End-expiratory Pressure

High-flow nasal cannula offers some resistance to expiratory flow leading to modest PEEP. The PEEP[25] effect is almost twice high when the mouth is closed compared to when mouth is open. At 50 L/min of inspiratory flow, PEEP of 3.31 ± 1.05 cm H_2O is generated with closed mouth and 1.73 ± 0.82 H_2O with open mouth.

Improvement of Mucociliary Clearance and Patient Comfort[26]

Warm and humidified gases prevent dryness of the upper airways, enhance the mucociliary clearance, and are generally well accepted by the patients.

Fixed Fraction of Inspired Oxygen

Higher flows close to the patients PIFR reduces room air dilution of oxygen providing fixed FiO_2. This may reduce the transient hypoxemic episodes.

Reducing Work of Breathing[22]

High-flow nasal cannula may help in reducing work of breathing by many mechanisms. It reduces inspiratory flow resistance. The PEEP effect may help in improving oxygenation and increasing compliance. Active heating and humidification reduces the metabolic demand of gas conditioning.

Indications of High-flow Nasal Cannula

Indications of HFNC are expanding; typical indications are listed below:[27]

- Postoperative respiratory failure
- Prevention or treatment of extubation failure
- Preoxygenation and apneic oxygen during intubation and airway procedures
- Comfort care in palliative patients

Postoperative Respiratory Failure

High-flow nasal cannula has been used both for prevention and treatment of postoperative extubation failure and respiratory failure. BiPOP[28] study has compared continuous HFNC (50 L/min with FiO_2 50%) versus BIPAP (pressure support 8 cm H_2O; PEEP 4 cm H_2O; FiO_2 50% at least 4 hours per day) in 830 postoperative cardiothoracic surgery patients who were either high risk for respiratory failure due to pre-existing risk factors or had failed spontaneous breathing trial or extubation. Both groups had similar treatment failure and mortality rates. BiPAP group had higher incidence of skin breakdown.

In a multicenter randomized controlled trial (OPERA study) comparing HFNC versus standard oxygen therapy via nasal prongs or facemask, in adults undergoing major abdominal surgery and having moderate-to-high risk of postoperative pulmonary complications, HFNC was not associated with improved pulmonary outcomes.[29]

Prevention or Treatment of Extubation Failure

High-flow nasal cannula is an attractive oxygenation strategy for reducing the risk of reintubation in the ICU. In patients with PaO_2/FiO_2 ratio less than or equal to 300,[30] HFNC compared with Venturi mask provides better oxygenation, better patient comfort, fewer episodes of desaturation and most importantly five times lower reintubation and ventilatory support. Benefits of HFNC for prevention of extubation failure are well demonstrated. In patients who are at low risk for reintubation, HFNC for 24 hours, compared to the conventional oxygen therapy[31] reduces postextubation respiratory failure and reintubation within 72 hours. In patients who are at high risk for reintubation, HFNC is as good as NIV for preventing both reintubation and postextubation respiratory failure. As HFNC is generally better tolerated than NIV, its role in prevention of postextubation failure looks promising. Patients having hypercapnia during the spontaneous[31] breathing trial were excluded in the study; hence, the result cannot be applied to these patients. HFNC has been studied for weaning and extubation in both, in patients with high risk and low risk for extubation. In high-risk and nonhypercapnic patients, HFNC is independently associated with lowering postextubation failure.[32]

Preoxygenation and Apneic Oxygen during Intubation and Airway Procedures

High-flow nasal cannula can be used for both preoxygenation and apneic oxygenation **(Fig. 8)** during intubation or other airway procedures. Advantage of HFNC over conventional preoxygenation is that there is no need to engage an operator to achieve a tight mask seal. Another important advantage is the same setup can be continued during intubation for apneic oxygen. Disadvantage is difficulty in monitoring endpoint of preoxygenation. Conventionally,[33] ETO_2 of 90% is considered as endpoint of maximal preoxygenation. With HFNC, capnography cannot be used due to dilution of excelled gases with the high flows. Transnasal humidified rapid insufflation ventilatory exchange (THRIVE)[34] technique has used HFNC for 3 minutes for preoxygenation. Initial flow rate was 30 L/min which was increased to 70 over the first minute. Apneic oxygen using THRIVE has shown to significantly increase safe apnea time for intubation.[35]

Comfort Care in Palliative Patients

High-flow nasal cannula can be used for comfort care of palliative patients having respiratory distress. Its detailed applications are beyond the purview of this chapter.

Success of HFNC does not necessarily mean end of NIV era. Combining use of high-flow nasal oxygen with noninvasive ventilation may improve gas exchange and reduce the work of breathing. HFNC-NIV combination in patients who are high risk for extubation failure is associated with decreased reintubation rates compared to HFNC alone.[36]

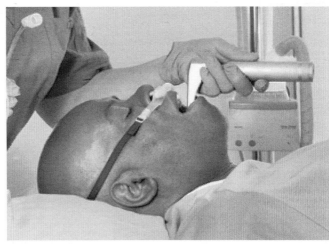

Fig. 8: High-flow nasal cannula (HFNC) during apneic ventilation.

Physiology of FiO$_2$ Delivery

For a device with a reservoir bag [NRBM, partial rebreathing mask (PRBM)], keeping the flow close to minute ventilation and ensuring proper functioning of the flap valves prevents drop in FiO$_2$ due to entrainment of air close to patient. For high-flow devices like Venturi, which do not have flap valve or a reservoir bag, ensuring the delivered flow close to the patient's PIFR prevents drop in FiO$_2$ due to entrainment of air close to patient. Venturi masks, especialy the one with high FiO$_2$ have total flow rates significantly lower than average PIFR of 60 L/min (*see* **Table 3**) and hence may deliver FiO$_2$ 5–10% lower than the actual setting.[19] For low-flow devices like face mask or nasal prongs, we can never achieve fixed FiO$_2$. HFNC ensures fixed FiO$_2$ by providing high flow rate close to patient's PIFR. They have additional benefit of washing out of nasopharyngeal dead space which increased alveolar ventilation without increasing total minute ventilation. **Table 4** shows the comparison of various oxygen devices described in the chapter.

SPECIAL SITUATIONS

- *Obesity:*[37] Obese patients are at more risk of hypoxia during induction, intubation and also after extubation due to following reasons:
  - Reduced FRC below closing capacity
  - Significant atelectasis and shunting in dependent lung regions

Table 4: Comparison of various oxygen devices.

Type	Flow rate (in L/min)	FiO$_2$ (in %)	Indication	Advantage	Disadvantage	Caution
Nasal cannula	1–2 L/min	Variable	Minimal oxygen supplementation	• Possible to give low flow rates like 1–2 L/min without rebreathing • Better patient acceptance as patient can talk, eat and drink • No claustrophobia	• No reservoir hence entrainment of room air • FiO$_2$ is unpredictable • Oxygen flow > 2 L/min causes drying of nasal mucosa	• Not for moderate and severe respiratory failure • Not for mouth breathers
Facemask	2–5 L/min	Variable	Moderate oxygen supplementation	Can be used for nebulized drug delivery	Rebreathing if oxygen flow rate is kept 2 L/min or if patient has very high minute ventilation	Lower flows can cause rebreathing
NRBM	12–15 L/min	75–90%	High oxygen supplementation	• Higher FiO$_2$ • Do not need electric supply • Good system for short term use, e.g., transport, remote location like MRI suite	• Cold dry gases • FiO$_2$ can vary	• Can mask severe respiratory failure • Patients who require such high FiO$_2$, generally need additional therapy like HFNC, NIV or IMV
PRBM	≥8 L/min	60–80%	Moderate-high oxygen supplementation	Partial humidification and heating duet to rebreathing of anatomical dead space	Rebreathing of alveolar gas if flow rate is not adequate	• Can mask severe respiratory failure. • See NRBM
Venturi mask	• Flow meter setting 2–15 L/min • Total flow delivered to the patient 30–53 L/min	24–60%		• Gives precise oxygen concentration • Can be used in COPD patients requiring oxygen supplementation as FiO$_2$ does not exceed	• Skin irritation • Uncomfortable for patient due to cold dry gases	Delivered FiO$_2$ is lower than the set FiO$_2$ (Especially for high FiO$_2$ setting) since total flow rates are significantly lower than average PIFR of 60 L/min
HFNC	Up to 70 L/min	21–100%	Moderate respiratory failure	• Fixed FiO$_2$ • Heated humidified • Patient comfort	• Requires electric power source and distilled water supply • Difficult to use during transport • Not MRI compatible	Cautious to use in patients with altered consciousness and excessive secretion (risk of aspiration), and hemodynamic instability

(COPD: chronic obstructive pulmonary disease; FiO$_2$: fraction of inspired oxygen; HFNC: high-flow nasal cannula; IMV: invasive mechanical ventilation; NIV: noninvasive ventilation; NRBM: nonrebreathing mask; PIFR: peak inspiratory flow rate; PRBM: partial rebreathing mask)

– Increased resting metabolic rate and increased oxygen consumption

Following precautions can help in avoiding hypoxia in these patients:

- Induction of anesthesia
  - Preoxygenation in head up or ramped position
  - Adequate preoxygenation ensuring $ETO_2 > 80–90\%$
  - Use of NIV during preoxygenation especially in critically ill patients
  - Avoiding apnea during induction
- Intubation
  - Apneic oxygenation during laryngoscopy
- Extubation
  - Head up position
  - Chest physiotherapy and intensive spirometry
  - Oxygen administration
  - Use of CPAP/NIV if patient was using one preoperatively or whose hypoxia postoperatively is not responding to chest physiotherapy

- Effect of regional blocks of respiratory function
  - *Interscalene block*: Phrenic nerve block is commonly associated with this block and is usually well tolerated unless patient has compromised respiratory system (COPD, morbid obesity). That is why, it is recommended to avoid this block in patients with contralateral respiratory pathology.
  - *Epidural analgesia*: It is boon for major thoracic and abdominal surgeries. It resulted in pain-free ventilation and increased abdominal ventilation and ability to cough in the postoperative period.[38] Even high thoracic epidural anesthesia (sensory blockade from C4 to T8) was not detected by patients as respiratory distress, even when it showed no change in FRC and reduced both forced expiratory volume in one second (FEV1) and vital capacity by 8–10%.[39]

- *Flail chest:* It generally occurs following trauma. It is characterized by either double fractures of three or more contiguous ribs or combined sternal and rib fractures resulting in an unstable segment of the chest wall, which moves paradoxically with respiration. It results in reduction in effective ventilation leading to hypoventilation.[40]

CURRENT EVIDENCE FOR USE OF SUPPLEMENTAL OXYGEN THERAPY IN PERIOPERATIVE AND CRITICALLY ILL PATIENTS

Oxygen is a drug and should be used only in indicated cases at a particular dose (flow rate of FiO_2) and duration. Evidence suggest indiscriminate use of oxygen leading to

hyperoxia causes increased production of reactive oxygen species (ROS), which promote a deleterious inflammatory response leading to secondary tissue damage and/or apoptosis. Oxygen has direct lung toxicity causing atelectasis and tracheobronchitis. The studies looking at effect of various oxygenation strategies in critically ill patients are listed in **Table 5**.

Guidelines for Use of Supplemental Oxygen Therapy

Following recommendations are suggested by British Thoracic Society Guideline for oxygen use in adult in 2017:

Recommendation of use of oxygen in perioperative care:[41]

- Target saturation recommended for most of the patients is 94–98%, except for those at risk of hypercapnic respiratory failure, where recommendation is 88–92%.
- Pulse oximetry monitoring is recommended in all postoperative patients.
- For patients using the *patient-controlled analgesia* (PCA), oxygen saturation should be monitored every two hourly with oximetry and if needed oxygen should be administered to keep patient within recommended saturation range.

Weaning and discontinuation of oxygen therapy[41]

- If patient is clinically stable and maintaining oxygen saturation above or near upper limit of recommended target saturation for around 4–8 hours, then oxygen concentration should be steadily lowered and eventually weaned off.
- Before cessation of oxygen therapy, patients should be stepped down to lowest oxygen concentration, i.e., 2 L/min via nasal cannula and 1 L/min for patients at risk of hypercapnic respiratory failure.
- Oxygen therapy should be stopped when the patient is clinically stable on low-concentration oxygen with the oxygen saturation within the recommended range on two consecutive observations.
- After stopping oxygen therapy, oxygen saturation on air should be monitored for 5 minutes and again at 1 hour, if it remains in the desired range.
- After 1 hour, if oxygen saturation remains within target range, then patient can be safely discontinued from oxygen therapy. However, if saturation drops below the patient's target range after stopping oxygen therapy, we should restart oxygen therapy to maintain the patient in the target range and the patient should be clinically re-evaluated to establish the cause for deterioration.

Table 5: Effect of various oxygen strategies on outcome in critically ill patients.

Name of trial or author / Year	Study type	Patient population	Intervention	Comparison	Endpoints	Outcome	Conclusion
AVOID[42] 2015	• RCT • 9 metropolitan hospitals • Melbourne	441 patients with ST-elevation myocardial infarction	• No oxygen therapy (No O_2, unless O_2 saturation falls below 94%)	• Routine oxygen therapy (Prehospital supplemental O_2 at 8 L/min and in hospital as per hospital protocol)	• *Primary endpoint:* myocardial infarct size as assessed by cardiac enzymes, troponin I, and creatine kinase	• Statistically significant reduction in creatine kinase • Non statistically significant decrease in infarct size	• No significant benefit of routine oxygen therapy for reducing myocardial infarct size, improving patient hemodynamic, or alleviating symptoms • Possible harm with routine oxygen therapy due to larger myocardial infarct size at 6 months and also higher frequency of myocardial infarction recurrence
DETO2X-AMI[43] Published in 2017	• RCT (multicenter) • 35 Swedish hospitals	6,629 patients with suspected myocardial infarction and O_2 saturation ≥90%	Ambient room air	Supplemental oxygen (6 L/min for 6–12 hours)	• Primary endpoint: All-cause mortality at 1 year • Secondary endpoint: All-cause mortality within 30 days after randomization, and rehospitalization with myocardial infarction or heart failure	No significant difference	No benefit of supplemental oxygen in suspected infarction patients with O_2 saturation ≥ 90%
SO2S trial[44] 2017	• RCT • 136 participating centers in the United Kingdom	8,003 nonhypoxic patients with acute stroke	• Continuous oxygen • Nocturnal oxygen	*Control group:* Oxygen only if clinically indicated	The primary outcome: Death or disability at 3 months using the modified Rankin Scale score	No statistically significant difference in primary outcome in primary and subgroup analysis	The prophylactic use of low-dose oxygen supplementation in nonhypoxic patients with acute stroke did not reduce death or disability at 3 months
Oxygen-ICU[45] 2016	RCT (single center) Modena University Hospital, Italy	• Adult patients admitted to ICU with an expected length of stay of 72 hours or longer	Conservative oxygen therapy (Target SpO2 = 94–98%, PaO2 = 70–100 mm Hg)	Conventional oxygen therapy (Target SpO2 = 97–100%, PaO2 up to 150 mmHg, FiO2 ≥0.4	• *Primary outcome:* ICU mortality. • *Secondary outcome:* occurrence of new organ failure and infection 48 hours or more after ICU admission	• Conservative oxygen therapy lead to statistically significant 43% relative risk (RR) reduction in mortality	Striking mortality and organ failure benefit in critically ill patients given a conservative oxygen regimen Contd...

Contd...

Name of trial or author Year	Study type	Patient population	Intervention	Comparison	Endpoints	Outcome	Conclusion
		• Originally planned sample size 660 patients (unplanned early termination of the trial due to difficulty in patient enrolment) • Final sample size 480 patients				• New organ failure and infection were also less common in conservative oxygen therapy group	
HYPRESS[46] 2017	• Two-by-two factorial, multicenter, randomized, clinical trial • 22 centers in France	• 442 patients • Septic shock (stopped prematurely for safety reasons)	FiO_2 of 1.0 for first 24 hours (hyperoxia)	FiO_2 set to target an arterial oxygen saturation of 88–95% (normoxia) during the first 24 hours	*The primary endpoint:* Mortality at day 28	The trial was stopped prematurely due to observation of significant increase in 28-day mortality and doubled incidence of ICU acquired weakness and atelectasis in hyperoxia group	In patients with septic shock, setting FiO_2 to 1.0 to induce arterial hyperoxia might increase the risk of mortality
ICU-ROX[47] 2019	• RCT • 21 ICUs in Australia and New Zealand	1,000 patients	• Conservative oxygen group SPO_2 90–96% • Decreasing FIO_2 if SPO_2 97% or above	• Usual oxygen therapy • Maintaining SPO_2 above 90% with no upper limit	*The primary outcome:* The number of ventilator-free days from randomization to day 28	No difference in primary endpoint	Conservative oxygen therapy did not reduce number of ventilator-free days
Jonge et al.[48] 2019	Meta-analysis of 17 RCT comparing the effect of high (80%) vs. standard (30–35%) FiO_2 on the incidence of SSI		Surgical patients receiving 80% FiO_2 intraoperatively	Surgical patients receiving 30–35% FiO_2 intraoperatively	Incidence of surgical site infection (SSI)	No overall reduction in SSI with high FiO_2. Significant reduction in SSI in intubated patients {RR: 0.80 [95% confidence interval (CI): 0.64–0.99]}	No definite benefits with SSI with high FiO_2 in adult surgical patients undergoing general anesthesia
IOTA[49] 2018	• Systemic review and meta-analysis • 25 RCTs comparing liberal and conservative oxygen therapy in acutely ill adults (aged ≥18 years)	16,037 patients	Liberal oxygen group (median FiO_2 of 0.52 for a median duration of 8 hours)	Conservative oxygen group (median FiO_2 0.21)	*Outcomes:* Mortality and morbidity (disability, risk of any hospital-acquired infection, and hospital length of stay)	• Increased mortality – In-hospital (RR 1.21, 95% CI 1.03–1.43), – At 30 days (RR 1.14, 95% CI 1.01–1.29), – At longest reported follow-up (RR 1.10, 95% CI 1.00–1.20) • Morbidity out-comes were similar between groups	In a heterogeneous group of ICU patients hyperoxia increased mortality without improving other patient-important outcomes

ACKNOWLEDGMENT

We would like to acknowledge Dr Vijay Kumar Kandala for his help in writing this chapter.

REFERENCES

1. Kavanagh BP, Hedenstierna G. Respiratory physiology and pathophysiology. In: Miller RD, Cohen NH, Eriksson LI, Fleisher LA, Young WL, Kronish JW (Eds). Miller's Anesthesia, 8th edition. Philadelphia: Saunders Elsevier; 2015. pp. 444-72.
2. Hantzidiamantis PJ. Physiology, Alveolar to Arterial Oxygen Gradient (Aa Gradient). Treasure Island (FL): StatPearls; 2020. Available from https://www.ncbi.nlm.nih.gov/books/NBK545153/. [Last accessed March, 2020].
3. Coruh B, Luks AM. Positive end-expiratory pressure. When more may not be better. Ann Am Thorac Soc. 2014:1327-31.
4. Cafaro RP. Hypoxia: Its causes and symptoms. J Am Dent Soc Anesthesiol. 1960;7:4-8.
5. Dunn JOC, Mythen MG, Grocott MP. Physiology of oxygen transport. BJA Educ. 2016;16:341-8.
6. Bhatia PK, Bhandari SC, Tulsiani KL, Kumar Y. End-tidal oxygraphy and safe duration of apnoea in young adults and elderly patients. Anaesthesia. 1997;52:175-8.
7. Baraka AS, Taha SK, Aouad MT, El-Khatib MF, Kawkabani NI. Preoxygenation: comparison of maximal breathing and tidal volume breathing techniques. Anesthesiology. 1999;91:612-6.
8. Baillard C, Fosse JP, Sebbane M, Chanques G, Vincent F, Courouble P, et al. Noninvasive ventilation improves preoxygenation before intubation of hypoxic patients. Am J Respir Crit Care Med. 2006;174:171-7.
9. Lee BJ, Kang JM, Kim DO. Laryngeal exposure during laryngoscopy is better in the 25 degrees back-up position than in the supine position. Br J Anaesth. 2007;99:581-6.
10. Weingart SD, Levitan RM. Preoxygenation and prevention of desaturation during emergency airway management. Ann Emerg Med. 2012;59:165-75.
11. Ruben H, Knudsen EJ, Carugati G. Gastric inflation in relation to airway pressure. Acta Anaesthesiol Scand. 1961;5:107-14.
12. Rothen HU, Neumann P, Berglund JE, Valtysson J, Magnusson A, Hedenstierna G. Dynamics of re-expansion of atelectasis during general anaesthesia, Br J Anaesth. 1999;82:551-6.
13. Lawes EG, Campbell I, Mercer D. Inflation pressure, gastric insufflation and rapid sequence induction. Br J Anaesth. 1987;59:315-8.
14. Dixon BJ, Dixon JB, Carden JR, Burn AJ, Schachter LM, Playfair JM, et al. Preoxygenation is more effective in the 25° head-up position than in the supine position in severely obese patients. Anesthesiology. 2005;102:1110-5.
15. Rothen HU, Sporre B, Engberg G, Wegenius G, Högman M, Hedenstierna G, et al. Influence of gas composition on recurrence of atelectasis after a reexpansion maneuver during general anesthesia. Anesthesiology. 1995;82:832-44.
16. Brueckmann B, Villa-Uribe JL, Bateman BT, Grosse-Sundrup M, Hess DR, Schlett CL, et al. Development and validation of a score for prediction of postoperative respiratory complications. Anesthesiology. 2013;188:1276-85.
17. Kelkar KV. Post-operative pulmonary complications after non-cardiothoracic surgery. Indian J Anaesth. 2015;59:599-605.
18. Karcz M, Papadakos PJ. Respiratory complications in the postanesthesia care unit: A review of pathophysiological mechanisms. Can J Respir Ther. 2013;49:21-9.
19. Wheeler DW. Equipment for the inhalation of oxygen and other gases. In: Davey AJ, Diba A (Eds). Ward's Anaesthetic Equipment, 5th edition. Philadelphia: Saunders Elsevier; 2005. pp. 215-30.
20. Campbell EJ. A method of controlled oxygen administration which reduces the risk of carbon-dioxide retention. Lancet. 1960;2:12-4.
21. Spoletini G, Alotaibi M, Blasi F, Hill NS. Heated humidified high-flow nasal oxygen in adults: mechanism of action and clinical implications. Chest. 2015;148:253-61.
22. Dysart K, Miller TL, Wolfson MR, Shaffer TH. Research in high flow therapy: mechanisms of action. Respir Med. 2009;103:1400-5.
23. Mündel T, Feng S, Tatkov S, Schneider H. Mechanisms of nasal high flow on ventilation during wakefulness and sleep. J Appl Physiol. 2013;114:1058-65.
24. Mauri T, Turrini C, Eronia N, Grasselli G, Volta CA, Bellani G, et al. Physiologic effects of high-flow nasal cannula in acute hypoxemic respiratory failure. Am J Respir Crit Care Med. 2017;195:1207-15.
25. Parke RL, Eccleston ML, McGuinness SP. The effects of flow on airway pressure during nasal high-flow oxygen therapy. Respir Care. 2011;56:1151.
26. Renda T, Corrado A, Iskandar G, Pelaia G, Abdalla K, Navalesi P. High-flow nasal oxygen therapy in intensive care and anaesthesia. Br J Anaesth. 2018;120:18-27.
27. Kashani NA, Kumar R. High-flow nasal oxygen therapy. BJA Educ. 2017;17:57-62.
28. Stéphan F, Barrucand B, Petit P, Rézaiguia-Delclaux S, Médard A, Delannoy B, et al. High-flow nasal oxygen vs noninvasive positive airway pressure in hypoxemic patients after cardiothoracic surgery: A randomized clinical trial. JAMA. 2015;313:2331-9.
29. Futier E, Paugam-Burtz C, Godet T, Khoy-Ear L, Rozencwajg S, Delay JM, et al. Effect of early postextubation high-flow nasal cannula vs conventional oxygen therapy on hypoxaemia in patients after major abdominal surgery: a French multicentre randomised controlled trial (OPERA). Intensive Care Med. 2016;42:1888-98.
30. Maggiore SM, Idone FA, Vaschetto R, Festa R, Cataldo A, Antonicelli F, et al. Nasal high-flow versus Venturi mask oxygen therapy after extubation. Effects on oxygenation, comfort, and clinical outcome. Am J Respir Crit Care Med. 2014;190:282-8.
31. Hernández G, Vaquero C, González P, Subira C, Frutos-Vivar F, Rialp G, et al. Effect of postextubation high-flow nasal cannula vs conventional oxygen therapy on reintubation in low-risk patients: a randomized clinical trial. JAMA. 2016;315:1354-61.
32. Fernandez R, Subira C, Frutos-Vivar F, Rialp G, Laborda C, Masclans JR, et al. High-flow nasal cannula to prevent postextubation respiratory failure in high-risk non-hypercapnic patients: a randomized multicenter trial. Ann Intensive Care. 2017;7:47.

33. Nimmagadda U, Salem MR, Crystal GJ. Preoxygenation: physiologic basis, benefits, and potential risks. Anesth Analg. 2017;124:507-17.

34. Mir F, Patel A, Iqbal R, Cecconi M, Nouraei SA. A randomised controlled trial comparing transnasal humidified rapid insufflation ventilatory exchange (THRIVE) pre-oxygenation with facemask pre-oxygenation in patients undergoing rapid sequence induction of anaesthesia. Anaesthesia. 2017;72: 439-43.

35. Patel A, Nouraei SA. Transnasal Humidified Rapid-Insufflation Ventilatory Exchange (THRIVE): a physiological method of increasing apnoea time in patients with difficult airways. Anaesthesia. 2015;7:323-9.

36. Thille AW, Muller G, Gacouin A, Coudroy R, Decavèle M, Sonneville R, et al. Effect of postextubation high-flow nasal oxygen with noninvasive ventilation vs high-flow nasal oxygen alone on reintubation among patients at high risk of extubation failure: a randomized clinical trial. JAMA. 2019;322:1465-75.

37. Sharmeen L, Bellamy MC. Anaesthesia and morbid obesity. Contin Educ Anaesth Crit Care Pain. 2008;8:151-6.

38. Anderson MB, Kwong KF, Furst AJ, Salerno TA. Thoracic epidural anesthesia for coronary bypass via left anterior thoracotomy in the conscious patient. Eur J Cardiothorac Surg. 2001;20:415-7.

39. Groeben H, Schwalen A, Irsfeld S, Tarnow J, Lipfert P, Hopf HB. High thoracic epidural anesthesia does not alter airway resistance and attenuates the response to an inhalational provocation test in patients with bronchial hyperreactivity. Anesthesiology. 1994;81:868-74.

40. McCool DF. Diseases of the Diaphragm, Chest Wall, Pleura, and Mediastinum. In: Goldman L, Schafer A (Eds). Goldman's Cecil Medicine, 24th edition. Philadelphia: Saunders Elsevier; 2012. pp. 603-13.

41. O'Driscoll BR, Howard LS, Earis J, Mak V. British Thoracic Society Guideline for oxygen use in adults in healthcare and emergency settings. BMJ Open Resp Res. 2017;4:1-20.

42. Stub D, Smith K, Bernard S, Nehme Z, Stephenson M, Bray JE, et al. Air versus oxygen in ST-segment-elevation myocardial infarction. Circulation. 2015;131:2143-50.

43. Hofmann R, James SK, Jernberg T, Lindahl B, Erlinge D, Witt N, et al. Oxygen therapy in suspected acute myocardial infarction. N Engl J Med. 2017;377:1240-9.

44. Roffe C, Nevatte T, Sim J, Bishop J, Ives N, Ferdinand P, et al. Effect of routine low-dose oxygen supplementation on death and disability in adults with acute stroke: the stroke oxygen study randomized clinical trial. JAMA. 2017;318:1125-35.

45. Girardis M, Busani S, Damiani E, Donati A, Rinaldi L, Marudi A, et al. Effect of conservative vs conventional oxygen therapy on mortality among patients in an intensive care unit. JAMA. 2016;316:1583-9.

46. Asfar P, Schortgen F, Boisramé-Helms J, Charpentier J, Guérot E, Megarbane B, et al. Hyperoxia and hypertonic saline in patients with septic shock (HYPERS2S): a two-by two factorial, multicentre randomised, clinical trial. Lancet Respir Med. 2017;5:180-90.

47. ICU-ROX Investigators and the Australian and New Zealand Intensive Care Society Clinical Trials Group, Mackle D, Bellomo R, Bailey M, Beasley R, Deane A, et al. Conservative oxygen therapy during mechanical ventilation in the ICU. N Engl J Med. 2020;382:989-98.

48. De Jonge S, Egger M, Latif A, Loke YK, Berenholtz S, Boermeester M, et al. Effectiveness of 80% vs 30-35% fraction of inspired oxygen in patients undergoing surgery: an updated systematic review and meta-analysis. Br J Anaesth. 2019;122(3):325-34.

49. Chu DK, Kim LH, Young PJ, Zamiri N, Almenawer SA, Jaeschke R, et al. Mortality and morbidity in acutely ill adults treated with liberal versus conservative oxygen therapy (IOTA): a systematic review and meta-analysis. Lancet. 2018;391:1693-705.

Airway Management in Critical Care Unit

Sheila Nainan Myatra

INTRODUCTION

Tracheal intubation (TI) is one of the most commonly performed procedures in the intensive care unit (ICU). Airway management in critically ill patients is more challenging and more likely to be associated with life-threatening complications as compared to that in the operating room.[1,2] This chapter will highlight the complexities of airway management in ICU, give a stepwise approach to airway management, along with a detailed description of the preparation, assessment, procedure, precautions, maintenance, and complications associated with TI. Emergency management of a patient with a tracheostomy and extubation of a difficult airway will also be covered.

CHALLENGES DURING TRACHEAL INTUBATION IN ICU

The ICU is regarded as "a hostile environment" for airway procedures. Unlike the operating room (OR), the ICU environment is not designed for anesthetizing patients. In addition, the different base specialties of the airway operators, varying level of training and experience in airway management along with the critically ill patient having a physiologically difficult airway, make airway management in ICU a high-risk procedure.[3] The challenges faced during TI in ICU are summarized in **Table 1**.

The Physiologically Difficult Airway

The anatomically difficult airway is one in which obtaining a glottic view or passing a tracheal tube is challenging. Critically ill patients have a physiologically difficult airway. The physiologically difficult airway is one in which physiologic derangements such as hypoxemia, hypotension, severe metabolic acidosis, right ventricular failure, etc. place the patient at higher risk of cardiovascular collapse during TI and conversion to positive pressure ventilation.[4]

Table 1: Challenges during tracheal intubation in ICU.	
Environmental factors	
Infrastructure	Poor access to patient's head end, lack of space around the patient, poor lighting, unavailability of trained help
Equipment	Airway devices such as flexible bronchoscope, supraglottic airways devices, video laryngoscope, capnography, etc. may not be readily available in the ICU
Monitoring	Patient monitors are usually placed at the head end of the bed and may not be visible to the airway operator
Timing	Urgent intubation may be required at any time in the day or night
Patient factors	
Airway assessment	May be difficult or impossible due to lack of time or patient being uncooperative
Challenging anatomy	Maxillofacial trauma, cervical spine injury, airway injuries, burns, retropharyngeal abscess, etc.
Risk of aspiration	Full stomach, gastroparesis associated with critical illness or patient not fasted and requiring emergency intubation
Preoxygenation	Insufficient time for preoxygenation when progressive illness requires rapid TI. Inefficient preoxygenation caused by ventilation perfusion mismatch due to the underlying illness. Lack of physiological reserves may lead to rapid oxygen desaturation allowing less safe apnea time for tracheal intubation
Physiologically difficult airway	Presence of hypotension, hypoxemia, metabolic acidosis, right ventricular failure, etc. may increase the risk of complications during TI
Waking up the patient	Unlike in the operating room, waking up the patient and postponing airway management is not possible as the critical illness mandates a definitive airway
Operator factors	
Training	Limited airway training and poor airway management skills
Experience	An inexperienced junior doctors may be performing intubation alone
Human factors	The patient, ICU or operator-related factors, alone or in combination may produce a stressful situation for the operator which may affect performance

In addition to this, if the patient also has an anatomically difficult airway, the risk of life-threatening complications further increases.

Critically ill patients have an increased risk of desaturation and hypotension during airway management. These physiologic derangements in the patient should be addressed during TI even if an anatomic difficulty is not anticipated. Measures that can reduce the risk of desaturation include proper positioning, preoxygenation with noninvasive ventilation (NIV) or high-flow nasal oxygen (HFNO), apneic oxygenation or mask ventilation between induction of anesthesia and laryngoscopy and measures that can increase first pass success in TI. Fluid loading, proper selection of drugs for induction of general anesthesia for TI and early use of vasopressor agent to treat hypotension may be useful.[5,6]

HISTORY, EXAMINATION, AND STABILIZATION

- Provide oxygen therapy while evaluating the patient. Initiate cardiorespiratory monitoring (ECG, noninvasive blood pressure, pulse oximetry, etc.) and secure an intravenous line if not already present.
- A quick history and assessment of the airway, breathing and circulation is required. History should include that related to the present illness, presence of comorbidities, fasting status, and contraindications to use succinylcholine/other drugs and previous history of a difficult intubation. Examination of the cardiorespiratory system and other systems should be performed.
- Critically ill patients, requiring airway support often present with hypotension and may be hypovolemic. The induction of general anesthesia for intubation and the increase in the intrathoracic pressure during positive pressure ventilation, may further worsen the hemodynamic status, especially in a hypovolemic patient, leading to precipitous fall in blood pressure, arrhythmias and sometimes cardiac arrest. Keeping this in mind, it is important to provide adequate volume support unless contraindicated and keep vasopressor agents ready for use prior to TI.

ASSESS THE NEED FOR TRACHEAL INTUBATION[7]

- Look for clinical signs of acute respiratory failure—anxiousness, sweating, restlessness, cyanosis, shortness of breath, rapid breathing and air hunger, use of accessory muscles of ventilation, paradoxical abdominal breathing, exhaustion, confused state or drowsiness. The respiratory system examination findings are important.
- Lung ultrasound facilitates fast and accurate bedside examinations of most of the acute respiratory disorders.

- The oxygen saturation by pulse-oximetry, an arterial blood gas analysis and a chest X-ray/CT scan if performed, can help assess the disease severity. However, this should not replace clinical evaluation or delay an airway intervention.
- *Common indications for TI are as follows:*
  - Facilitation of invasive mechanical ventilation (inadequate oxygenation/ventilation, shock, cardiac arrest, avoidance of hypercarbia, controlled hyperventilation, need for neuromuscular paralysis, postoperative elective ventilation)
  - Protection of the respiratory tract from aspiration of gastric contents
  - Relief of upper airway obstruction
  - Tracheobronchial toilet

AIRWAY ASSESSMENT

Airway assessment to identify difficult intubation has a low positive predictive value and specificity. Nevertheless, identification of a patient at risk for a difficult airway management helps in better planning and preparation. Several methods and tests are available; however, they are often impractical to use and also difficult to assess in the ICU unlike in the operating room, especially during emergency airway management.

- Generally accepted, independent predictors of difficult airway in controlled setting which can be quickly and easily assessed are as follows. However, this may not be feasible in all ICU patients:
  - Length of upper incisor—relatively long
  - Inter-incisor distance—less than two fingers (3 cm)
  - Overbite—maxillary incisors override mandibular incisors
  - Temporomandibular joint translation—cannot place mandibular incisors anterior to maxillary incisors
  - Mandibular space compliance—small, stiff, indurated, or occupied by mass
  - Thyromental distance—less than three fingers (6 cm)
  - Mallampati class—III and IV
  - Neck—short, thick
  - Limited neck mobility—cannot touch chin to chest or cannot extend neck
- *MACOCHA score:* This is a simple score developed for use in ICU patients which has been shown able to identify difficult airway in ICU patients.[8,9] The MACOCHA score has seven easily identifiable variables. It takes into account not only the anatomical difficulty, but also physiological derangements (such as hypoxia and coma) and the skill of the airway operator. This makes it very relevant for use in ICU **(Table 2)**
- Some medical conditions may make intubation difficult **(Table 3)**

- A history of difficult intubation is a reliable predictor of future difficult intubation.
- Call for help in advance if difficulty in mask ventilation or TI is anticipated.

PREPARATION FOR TRACHEAL INTUBATION IN ICU

Tracheal intubation should be attempted once all necessary preparation has been made. It is useful to use a checklist to ensure that patient setup, equipment check and team preparation is adequate. Use of preintubation checklists have been recommended for ICU patients.[10,11]

Janz et al. performed the first randomized trial comparing the use of a written checklist prior to TI in ICU compared to usual care.[11] There was no difference in lowest oxygen saturation and lowest systolic blood pressure from induction up to 2 minutes after TI between the groups. However, the checklist used did not include interventions aiming at physiological optimization (e.g., vasopressors, noninvasive ventilation, fluid loading, etc.), possibly explaining why the checklist did not influence the selected outcomes. Moreover, the center in which the study was conducted had significant experience in the use of checklist for other ICU procedures, thus a high penetrance of checklist items may have been already present in the control group. Nevertheless, a preintubation checklist may be more effective in less experienced hands. It is helpful to use a checklist before intubation which may be adapted to your needs and situation. The checklist should be used whenever possible.

A suggested checklist is detailed here:
- *Patient setup:*
  - Patient history taken, examination performed (including airway) and investigations reviewed
  - Adequate space between bed and wall for airway operator
  - Head board removed
  - Side rails down
  - Patient well-positioned (centered in bed, vertex at the head of bed)
  - Monitoring should include at least blood pressure, heart rate, continuous ECG, and pulse-oximetry
  - Gastric contents suctioned (if gastric tube in place)
  - Suction catheter and apparatus ready for use
  - Secure patent intravenous line
  - Fluid preloading in absence of cardiogenic pulmonary edema
- *Equipment check:* Ensure that there is personal protection equipment for the airway operators (gown, gloves, mask, and eye protection). The following equipment should be checked before initiating TI:
  - Oxygenation and ventilation:
    ♦ Bag with reservoir-valve-mask connected to oxygen (>10 L/minute)/ventilator circuit with face mask to provide NIV (Pressure support + PEEP)/high-flow nasal cannula oxygen device or simple nasal cannula (for apneic oxygenation)
    ♦ Face masks of appropriate size
    ♦ Oropharyngeal and nasopharyngeal airways of appropriate size
    ♦ Mechanical ventilator checked and ready
  - *Tracheal intubation:*
    ♦ Appropriate sizes and types of direct laryngoscope (DL) blades and handles/videolaryngoscope (VL)/flexible bronchoscope (if awake intubation is planned)
    ♦ Appropriate sizes of tracheal tubes. Tracheal tubes with subglottic suction should be preferably used for all adult patients in whom prolonged intubation is anticipated.
    ♦ Lignocaine jelly
    ♦ Magill forceps
    ♦ Tracheal tube stylet
    ♦ Tracheal tube introducer (Bougie)

Table 2: MACOCHA score.

Factor	Points
Factors related to patients	
Mallampati score III or IV	5
Obstructive sleep **A**pnea syndrome	2
Reduced mobility of **C**ervical spine	1
Limited mouth **O**pening <3 cm	1
Factors related to pathology	
Coma	1
Severe **H**ypoxemia	1
Factors related to operator	
Non-**A**nesthesiologist	1
Total	12
Score from 0 to 12: 0 = easy; 12 = very difficult	

Table 3: Medical conditions that may make intubation difficult.

Rheumatoid arthritis	Restricted movement of the small joints of the airway
Diabetes	Small joints of the airway are diseased in 30% of long standing diabetes cases leading to restricted neck extension, fixed arytenoids
Ankylosing spondylitis	Limited or no neck extension, inability to lie supine, kyphosis
Acromegaly	Thick tongue and intraoral tissue
Radiotherapy of head and neck tumors	Postradiation fibrosis can fix the structures in the neck

- ◆ Syringe for inflating tracheal tube cuff
- ◆ Tube fixator/tapes and ties
- ◆ Waveform capnography monitor
- – *Drugs:*
  - ◆ Appropriate anesthetic agents and neuromuscular blocking agent
  - ◆ Topical anesthetics
  - ◆ Vasopressor agents to treat hypotension
  - ◆ Drugs for resuscitation (e.g., atropine, adrenaline, etc.)
- – *Rescue devices:*
  - ◆ Supraglottic airway device (SGA)
  - ◆ Equipment to perform emergency cricothyroidotomy (commercial cricothyroidotomy set/scalpel, bougie and tracheal tube size 6/needle cricothyroidotomy device with jet ventilation)
- ● *Team preparation:*
  - – Airway plan verbalized
  - – Roles and responsibilities of team members assigned
  - – Rescue strategy discussed
  - – Questions and concerns raised have been addressed.

THE "INTUBATION BUNDLE"

Jaber and colleagues proposed an "intubation bundle".[12] In before and after study, they showed that adherence to this bundle resulted in significant reduction in life-threatening complications such as severe hypoxemia, severe hypotension, and cardiac arrest (21% vs. 34%). Though this bundle needs to be validated externally at other centers and with more patients. It provides objective criteria for the clinicians to prepare better for TI and preventing associated complications.

The ten components of intubation bundle are discussed here.

Pre-intubation

1. Presence of two operators
2. Loading patient with fluid—500 mL of isotonic saline or 250 mL starch (in absence of cardiogenic pulmonary edema) to prevent or minimize hypotension following intubation.
3. Preparation of long-term sedation
4. Preoxygenation for 3 minutes with NIPPV in case of acute respiratory failure—FiO_2 100%, PSV level between 5 and 15 cm H_2O to obtain an expiratory tidal volume 6–8 mL/kg with PEEP 5 cm

During Intubation

5. Rapid sequence intubation—ketamine 1.5–3 mg/kg or etomidate 0.2–0.3 mg/kg followed by succinylcholine 1–1.5 mg/kg
6. Sellick's maneuver

Post-intubation

- ● Immediate confirmation of the tube placement using capnography
- ● Norepinephrine, if diastolic pressure remains low
- ● Initiate long-term sedation
- ● Initial lung protective ventilation—tidal volume 6–8 mL/kg, PEEP 5 cm H_2O, plateau pressures <35 cm H_2O, FiO_2 1.

PERFORMING TRACHEAL INTUBATION IN THE CRITICALLY ILL

Patient Positioning for Tracheal Intubation

Optimal positioning help to keep the upper airway patent, improved access and increases the functional residual capacity, and may reduce the risk of aspiration.[13] The head elevated laryngoscopy position (HELP), a 25° head elevation improves glottic visualization during laryngoscopy compared with the supine position.[14] Ramping (aligning the external auditory meatus with sternal notch) has been shown to be useful in obese and non-obese patients[15] **(Figs. 1A and B).** The head should be extended on the neck such that the face is horizontal. Ramped position can be achieved by using folded towels under the head and shoulder until the alignment is achieved.

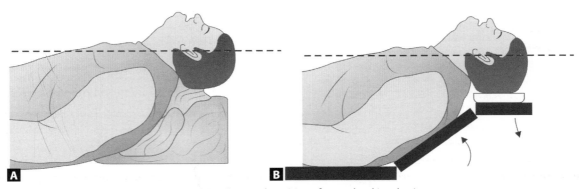

Figs. 1A and B: Ramped positions for tracheal intubation.

Preoxygenation and Apneic Oxygenation during Tracheal Intubation

Hypoxemia is the most common complications during TI of critically ill patients. Preoxygenation is of paramount importance to mitigate the risk of hypoxemia especially during a difficult intubation in the ICU population where the majority of patient population are limited with poor oxygen reserve.

There are three distinct phases of the TI where oxygenation and ventilation can be provided: (1) Preoxygenation, (2) induction to laryngoscopy, and (3) laryngoscopy to TI. Recent studies have evaluated the use of conventional oxygen therapy (COT), HFNO, and NIV in these phases of TI.[16]

Balliard et al. compared NIV for preoxygenation with COT using valve-bag facemask in ICU patients needing intubation and reported that NIV improved oxygenation at the end of preoxygenation and markedly decreased the proportion of patients with severe oxygen desaturation during intubation (from 46% to only 7%, $p < 0.01$) as compared with COT.[17] NIV may prevent the severe hypoxemia probably due to higher FiO_2 and to increased end-expiratory lung volume induced by PEEP.

The PROTRACH study[18] conducted in patients undergoing TI in the ICU without pre-existing hypoxemia (PaO_2/FiO_2 ratio ≥ 200 mm Hg) randomized 192 patients to HFNO (which was continued during laryngoscopy) or to COT by face mask (removed during laryngoscopy). The study failed to increase the lowest oxygen saturation during intubation (the primary outcome). However, several secondary outcomes including mild hypoxemia (oxygen saturation < 90%) favored the HFNO.

The FLORALI-2 study,[19] randomized 322 hypoxemic, critically adults undergoing TI to NIV (from induction to laryngoscopy) or HFNO (from induction to TI). The incidence of severe hypoxemia during TI was 23.2% in the NIV group and 27.5% in the HFNC group ($p = 0.39$). However, in the subgroup analyzes there was a potential benefit for NIV among patients with a P/F ratio < 200. Taken together with prior trials, the results of the FLORALI-2 trial suggest that NIV may be the best method of preoxygenation to reduce oxygen desaturation during TI of critically ill patients, particularly among patients at high risk.[16].

The OPTINIV study,[20] a proof of concept study by Jaber et al. showed that the using apneic oxygenation via high-flow nasal cannula oxygen combined with NIV for preoxygenation prevented desaturation during TI in hypoxemic patients compared to using NIV alone for preoxygenation and may provide the ideal combination of preoxygenation and apneic oxygenation. However, this needs to be tested in a larger study.

While the PROTRACH and FLORALI trials focused on preoxygenation, management of the period from induction to laryngoscopy has been similarly controversial. Following induction there is a period where the patient may be apneic. Bag-mask ventilation during this period may prevent hypoxemia but has been proposed to increase the risk of gastric insufflation and pulmonary aspiration. In the PREVENT study, Casey et al.[21] randomized 401 patients to receive bag-mask ventilation from induction to laryngoscopy or no ventilation, except as treatment of hypoxemia. Bag-mask ventilation reduced the incidence of severe hypoxemia (oxygen saturation < 80%) by more than half, without increasing the rate of pulmonary aspiration. The trial, however, was not powered to provide a definitive assessment of the relationship between bag-mask ventilation and pulmonary aspiration.

Choice of Drugs to Facilitate Tracheal Intubation

The choice of agents depends on the hemodynamic status of the patient and the anticipated nature of difficult airway. Administration of sedation and/or anesthetic agent causes decrease in sympathetic activity catecholamine release. This invariably leads to significant hypotension in hemodynamically unstable patients. Vasodilatation leads to precipitous fall in blood pressure especially in hypovolemic patients. Therefore, drugs are to be administered to the effect and not strictly as per body weight.

- Intravenous ketamine or etomidate, being cardiostable agents unless contraindicated, are the preferred induction agent.
- Propofol can cause profound hypotension and myocardial depression and should be used with extreme caution; better to avoid in hemodynamically unstable, hypovolemic patients and in patients with ischemic heart disease, cardiomyopathy, poor ventricular function.
- Intravenous midazolam in combination with opioid (fentanyl, morphine) is relatively cardiostable.
- Rapidly acting muscle relaxants such as succinylcholine and rocuronium (higher doses of 1.2 mg/kg) may be used for rapid sequence intubation. Fasciculations following administration of succinylcholine increases serum potassium levels by 0.5 mEq/L in normal individual. In patients with acidosis and hypokalemia, serum potassium levels may rise by 3 mEq/L. This rise may lead to sudden cardiac arrest and therefore is to be avoided in severe acidosis, acute or chronic neuromuscular disease, burn patients, and cervical trauma.

Doses, advantages, and disadvantages of various agents are detailed in **Table 4.**

Table 4: Drugs used to facilitate tracheal intubation.[7]

Name	Usual IV dose	Advantages	Disadvantages
Anesthetic, amnesic, and analgesic drugs			
Midazolam	0.02–0.2 mg/kg	Relatively cardiostable	Optimum intubation condition may not be obtained when used alone
		Better amnesia	
		Sedation	
Fentanyl	0.05–0.4 mg	Fast-acting	Optimum intubation condition may not be obtained when used alone
		Relatively cardiostable	
		Analgesia	
		Cough suppression	
		Useful in combination with midazolam	
Morphine	0.05–0.2 mg/kg	Analgesia	Optimum intubation condition may not be obtained when used alone
		Cough suppression	
		Useful in combination with midazolam	Hypotension
Ketamine	1–2 mg/kg	Cardiostable	Increased intracranial/intraocular pressure
		Bronchodilator	Does not suppress airway reflexes
		Potent analgesic	Hypertension and tachycardia
		Safe induction of anesthesia	
Propofol	1–2.5 mg /kg	Bronchodilatation useful in COPD/asthma	Can cause profound hypotension and bradycardia
		Suppression of airway reflexes	
		Reduces ICP	
Etomidate	0.2–0.6 mg/kg	Cardiostable	Adrenal suppression
Thiopentone sodium	5–7 mg/kg	Rapid induction	Hypotension
		Reduces ICP	Can precipitate laryngospasm and bronchospasm
Neuromuscular blocking agents			
Succinylcholine	0.5–2 mg/kg	Rapid action (1 min) and short duration (up to 10 min) hence ideal for RSI	Hyperkalemia and cardiac arrest
			Contraindicated in severe acidosis, acute or chronic neuromuscular disease, burn patients and cervical spine trauma (up to 6 months),lower motor neuron disease
			Malignant hyperthermia
Rocuronium bromide	0.4–2.0 mg/kg	Rapid action (60–90 sec) hence ideal for RSI	Long acting (30–90 min)
		No complications associated with Scoline	
Vecuronium bromide	0.05–0.1 mg/kg	Cardiostable	Long acting (30–60 min)
		Delayed action	
Atracurium besylate	0.4–0.5 mg/kg	Not metabolized by liver or kidney	Long acting (20–30 min)
		Delayed action	Histamine release
			Hypotension

Device Selection during Tracheal Intubation

Three recent systematic review comparing VL with traditional DL for TI in ICU did not improve time to intubation or first attempt success rate.[22-24] Some studies included in these meta-analyses showed higher incidence of life-threatening complications with VL use. Nevertheless, though recent evidence does not support the routine use of VL for all TI in ICU, VL improves the glottic visualization as compared to DL, making it an important tool for difficult airway management in ICU, especially in expert hands. Future trials will better define the role of VL in ICU, especially with respect to optimal patient position, use of airway adjuncts, ideal glottis view required for a successful VL intubation, etc.[25]

A recent large randomized study compared the use of a bougie with a tracheal tube and a stylet for TI in the emergency department in patients with at least one difficult airway characteristic.[26] There was higher first-attempt intubation success in patients in whom a bougie was used. This was a single center study with operators experienced with bougie use. Nevertheless, given the low cost and absence of harm, it seems reasonable to suggest that a bougie may be used to facilitate the initial TI in those experienced with its use.

Rapid Sequence Induction

Most critically ill patients are at a risk of aspiration. These patients may be not fasted or have a slower gastric emptying (gastroparesis of critical illness, other medical conditions such as diabetes, etc.). Thus, conventionally, a rapid sequence induction (RSI), i.e., administration of induction agents, followed immediately by a neuromuscular blocking drugs with rapid onset of action [to minimize the time between the patient being asleep and the endotracheal tube (ETT) in situ] and avoidance of ventilation between induction and intubation to limit gastric insufflations to avoid aspiration. Cricoid pressure (at 20–40 N or 2–4 kg) is applied before loss of consciousness to avoid aspiration. The goal is to intubate the trachea as quickly and safely as possible.

However, hypoxemia during this period is a concern these patients. Bag-mask ventilation during this period may prevent hypoxemia but has been proposed to increase the risk of gastric insufflation and pulmonary aspiration. In the PREVENT study,[21] a randomized control study, Casey et al. showed that the incidence of severe hypoxemia (oxygen saturation < 80%) decreased by more than half when gentle mask ventilation was used during the apneic period during TI, compared to when it was not, without increasing the rate of pulmonary aspiration. Though this study was not powered to provide a definitive assessment of the relationship between bag-mask ventilation and pulmonary aspiration, it gives us some confidence to use gentle mask ventilation, especially in high-risk patients and those which desaturate during apnea.

The cricoid pressure may obscure proper glottis visualization and should be released if this is the case. Otherwise, the cricoid pressure is released only after intubation, cuff inflation, and confirmation of tube placement.

Confirmation of Tracheal Tube Position

The gold standard to confirm tube placement in the trachea is by using end-tidal CO_2 using waveform capnography (wait to see 5-6 waveforms before confirmation). Disposable calorimetric CO_2 detector devices which work on the principle of litmus reaction may also be used instead, but are not as reliable.

Checking the proper position of the tube is usually done by visual inspection or palpation of symmetrical chest rise and auscultation of bilaterally equal air entry in the lungs. In addition to this, tube fixation at a depth of 20 and 22 cm at the level of the incisor for females and males, respectively; had 100% sensitivity for preventing endobronchial intubations. Bronchoscopic visualization is the gold standard to confirm position of the tip of the tracheal tube. However, this is not required routinely. Secure the tracheal tube adhesive tapes and a tube tie or a commercially available tube fixator.

Delayed Sequence Intubation

Delayed sequence intubation (DSI) may be a useful technique to preoxygenate agitated patients who cannot tolerate preoxygenation (via nasal cannula, nonrebreather mask, bag-valve-mask, or NIV) or in whom another procedure is required before intubation, but the patient will not tolerate it, such as nasogastric tube placement before intubation in the setting of a gastrointestinal bleeding or when rapid sequence intubation would be otherwise unsafe because of the risk of hypoxemia.

The ideal agent to be used is ketamine, (1 mg/kg) slowly over 15–30 seconds to prevent apnea. If intubation is required, administer the neuromuscular blockade, leaving the preoxygenation devices in place for 45–60 seconds while the paralytic takes effect. During intubation leave the nasal cannula in place to provide apneic oxygenation. Following TI, confirm tracheal tube placement and initiate mechanical ventilation if required with appropriate use of sedation.

Steps after Tracheal Intubation

- Initiate mechanical ventilation if required and use appropriate sedation.
- Make a note of the exact distance of the ETT at the angle of mouth or nose on the case notes and ICU chart. Tube position should be checked and noted daily during each nursing shift.
- Tracheal tube position has to be always confirmed by X-ray (tip 2.5–4 cm above carina).
- Do not start feeding until position of oro/nasogastric tube is confirmed on chest radiograph.
- Check the tracheal cuff pressure using the cuff pressure gauge and maintain it below 20 mm Hg at all times **(Fig. 2)**.
- Following an unanticipated difficult TI, postprocedure monitoring for complications is required. Watch for airway edema. Documentation of airway difficulty along with counseling of the patient/family is essential.

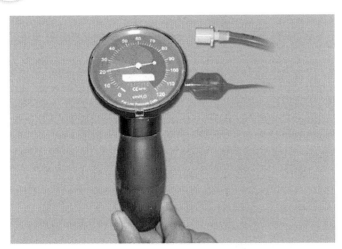

Fig. 2: Tracheal tube cuff pressure monitoring device.

COMPLICATIONS OF TRACHEAL INTUBATION IN ICU

Complications during TI in the critically ill patients in ICU are significantly higher than in the operating room. Approximately one in three patients experience moderate complications, and almost one in four experience severe complications.[27,28] Peri-intubation cardiac arrest occurs in 2–4% of cases, and is highly associated with peri-intubation oxygen desaturation and hypotension.[28]

Immediate Complications

- Esophageal intubation/endobronchial intubations/accidental ETT disconnections—atelectasis formation/collapse in the unventilated lung and hyperinflation and barotrauma with development of pneumothorax of the intubated lung (in endobronchial intubations) can cause profound hypoxemia manifesting as bradycardia and even progressing to cardiac arrest
- Hypertension, tachycardia, raised intracranial pressure, raised intraocular pressure and myocardial ischemia due to stimulation from laryngoscopy and intubation
- Hypotension due to loss of sympathetic tone from drugs for intubation or dynamic hyperinflation due to hyperventilation or relative dehydration
- Pulmonary aspiration of gastric contents
- Airway trauma and bleeding associated with laryngoscopy and TI—lip injury, dental or denture dislodgment, facial trauma and bleed, uvular hematoma, nasal bleed, and fracture of nasal turbinates (during nasal intubation)
- Negative pressure pulmonary edema after sudden relief of severe airway obstruction
- Cardiac arrest
- Toxic and adverse effects of drugs
- Death

Long-term Complications of Intubation

- Sore throat
- Hoarseness of voice
- Sinusitis
- Granuloma
- Vocal cord paralysis
- Arytenoid subluxation or fracture
- Tracheal stenosis
- Tracheomalacia
- Tracheoesophageal fistula (more associated with tracheostomy)

ROLE OF SUPRAGLOTTIC AIRWAY DEVICES IN ICU

Supraglottic airway devices (SADs) are devices that can be used to ventilate patients above the level of the vocal cords. These devices are used ventilate patients electively during short duration surgery in the operating room. However, they can also be in an emergency in cases of difficult mask ventilation or when there is a failed intubation (two failed attempts at TI in ICU). A second generation SAD such as LMA® Proseal, LMA® supreme or LMA® protector, i-gel®, Ambu® AuraGain or Baska mask® should be preferably used, as these devices have a higher sealing pressure and thus give better protection against aspiration compared to a first generation device, e.g., LMA classic.[29,30] Contraindication for use an SAD are of a mouth opening two fingers, intraoral tumors, trauma, or bleeding.

This device should therefore be an integral component of the difficult airway cart in ICU. Ventilation through SAD in ICU is temporary to ensure adequate oxygenation till a definitive airway such as tracheostomy (surgical or percutaneous) or TI through the SAD is performed. If an anesthetist who has the expertise to intubate through the SAD with a flexible bronchoscope is available, this may be considered and a tracheostomy may be avoided. However, blind intubation through the SAD should not be performed.

An SAD may also be inserted in a patient temporarily for ventilation to perform a percutaneous tracheostomy. This procedure requires the patient to be completely immobilized using general anesthesia with neuromuscular blockade.

EMERGENCY CRICOTHYROIDOTOMY

Emergency cricothyroidotomy is a rescue procedure to be performed when there is complete ventilation failure. Complete ventilation failure is as a situation where TI, ventilation using SAD and face mask have all failed after giving the best attempt, even if oxygenation may be maintained.[29]

Multiple attempts at TI may convert a *cannot-intubate* but *can-ventilate* situation into a *complete ventilation failure.* Thus it is prudent to expedite the decision to perform emergency cricothyroidotomy. Proper planning, preparation and skill training in cricothyroidotomy is essential. Emergency cricothyroidotomy can be performed by a surgical incision (surgical cricothyroidotomy) or puncture of the cricothyroid membrane using a needle cricothyroidotomy or using a wide-bore (usually internal diameter ≥4 mm) commercially available cricothyroidotomy kits.[29] Following needle cricothyroidotomy, jet ventilation is required, which is not available in ICU. Hence, surgical cricothyroidotomy (scalpel bougie technique) or a wide bore cannula cricothyroidotomy using various commercially available cricothyroidotomy kits is usually preferred.

GUIDELINES FOR TRACHEAL INTUBATION IN ICU

Recognizing the high risk of airway management in ICU, guidelines for TI in ICU have been recently formulated by various international societies.[31-33] These guidelines have subtle differences; however, the broad principles are the similar with a focus on strategies to enhance safety during TI.

The first guidelines on TI in ICU was published by the All India Difficult Airway Association (AIDAA) in 2016.[31] This guideline gives a stepwise approach to TI in ICU using evidence-based recommendations. This includes continuation of mask ventilation, insertion of a supraglottic airway, one last attempt at mask ventilation if this fails and finally performing an emergency cricothyroidotomy to maintain the oxygenation while a tracheostomy is performed to establish a definite airway management. Unlike in the operating room, waking up the patient and postponing the surgery is not an option. The AIDAA 2016 algorithm for management of TI in ICU is given in **Flowchart 1.**

EMERGENCY MANAGEMENT OF THE TRACHEOSTOMY PATIENT[34,35]

Some patients may come to the ICU with a tracheostomy tube in situ after surgery or a tracheostomy may be performed in these patients in the ICU. Great care must be taken of the tracheostomy tubes to prevent blockage and dislodgement. Patients with tracheostomies are vulnerable to airway problems. Deterioration can be rapid in critically ill patients, those who are receiving mechanical ventilation or having an abnormal upper airway and may lead to a life-threatening emergency.

Many tracheostomy problems are predictable and often involve warning signs. Common warning signs include the following:

- An agitated patient without any other obvious cause
- Inability to pass a suction catheter
- Obstructed or partially obstructed tracheostomy tube
- Increasing airway pressure during mechanical ventilation
- Absence or change of chest wall movement during mechanical ventilation
- Loss of tidal volume during mechanical ventilation
- Obvious air leak during mechanical ventilation
- Absence or change of capnography waveform if used
- Surgical emphysema
- Vocalization with tracheostomy tube in situ with cuff inflated
- Need for frequent reinflation, of the pilot balloon
- Bleeding from the tracheostomy tube

Bleeding from the tracheostomy is usually related to trauma related to tracheal suction. However, this may herald arterial bleeding. Hyperinflation of the tracheostomy tube cuff, resuscitation of the patients and urgent surgical intervention are warranted.

Management of a Blocked or Displaced Tracheostomy Tube

Maintaining oxygenation should be the high priority in these patients. If the patient is breathing, apply high flow oxygen to the face and the tracheostomy. If a metal tracheostomy is used, remove the blocked inner tube. With nonmetallic tracheostomy tubes check patency by passing a suction catheter. If suction catheter can be passed, the tracheostomy tube is patent or may be partially obstructed. If partially obstructed, repeat suction with saline followed by manual ventilation using a self-inflating resuscitator bag to restore patency. If you cannot pass the suction catheter through the tracheostomy tube, deflate the tracheostomy tube cuff.

Removal of a blocked or displaced tracheostomy tube should be performed as soon as identified. A patient with a recent tracheostomy performed for weaning from mechanical ventilation, should be managed using an oral intubation. Oral intubation will depend on the indication for which the tracheostomy was performed. In patients with an end tracheostomy, upper air obstruction or altered/difficult upper airway anatomy, oral intubation may be possible.

If oral intubation is not possible ventilation through a tracheostomy stoma can be performed using a pediatric face mask and manual ventilation with a self-inflating resuscitator bag to restore patency. A smaller size tracheotomy tube or a cut size 6 tracheal tube should be used. Consider using an airway exchange catheter or a flexible bronchoscope while inserting the tracheostomy tube. An otolaryngologist surgeon should preferably be involved for reintubation through recently formed stoma, as the stoma is not well formed and chances of inserting the tracheostomy tube into a false passage are high. Use of tracheal dilators and

Flowchart 1: The AIDAA 2016 guidelines for tracheal intubation in ICU.

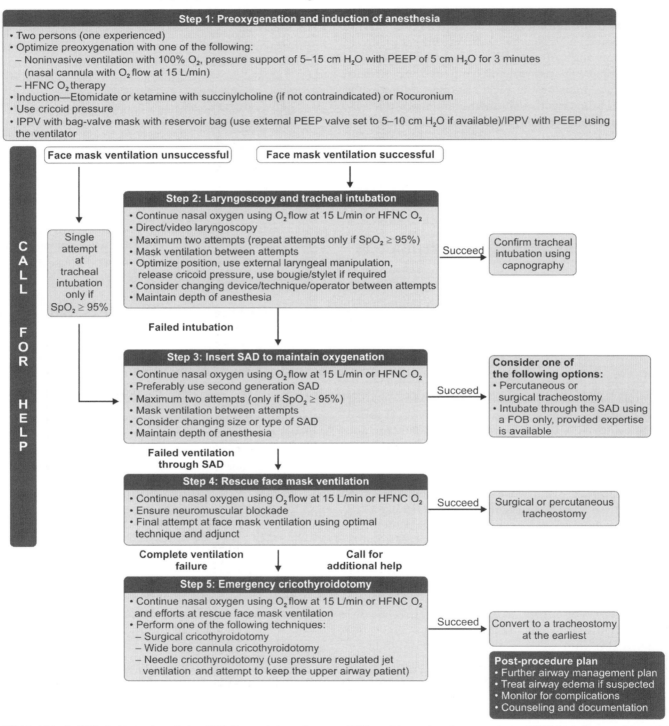

(AIDAA: All India Difficult Airway Association; FOB: fiberoptic bronchoscope; PEEP: positive end-expiratory pressure; HFNC: high-flow nasal cannula; SAD: supraglottic airway device; IPPV: intermittent positive pressure ventilation; SpO₂: oxygen saturation)

other instrument may be warranted in these patients. Use waveform capnography to confirm proper tracheal position and airway patency, once a tracheostomy tube has been reinserted.

EXTUBATION OF THE DIFFICULT AIRWAY

Surgical patients that are intubated in ICU in the postoperative period when they become critically ill, will require extubation

Flowchart 2: The AIDAA 2016 algorithm for the management of anticipated difficult extubation.

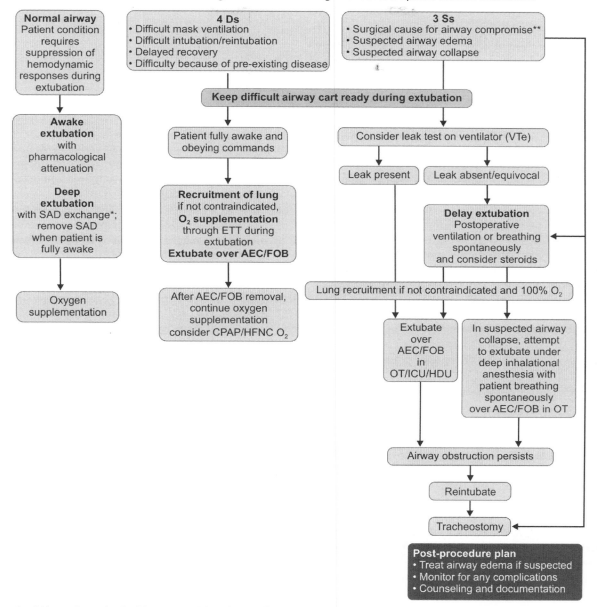

*Exchange should be performed only if the patient did not have difficult mask ventilation, difficult intubation and is not a case of full stomach (obese, pregnant, recent ingestion of food or raised intra-abdominal pressure).

**Suspected nerve damage/structural damage to airway.

(AIDAA: All India Difficult Airway Association; AEC: airway exchange catheter; CPAP: continuous positive airway pressure; ETT: endotracheal tube; HDU: high dependency unit; FOB: fiberoptic bronchoscope; HFNC: high-flow nasal cannula; SAD: supraglottic airway device; VTe: expired tidal volume)

at some stage. Following major surgery some patients may be electively ventilated due to major blood loss, hemodynamic instability, hypothermia or due to complications that may have occurred in the intraoperative period. Patients undergoing major intraoral surgery or other airway surgery may be shifted to the ICU with a tracheal tube in situ to maintain airway patency with a plan for a delayed extubation.

Extubation failure is defined as the inability of the patient to maintain a patent airway with effective spontaneous ventilation after purposeful removal of the previously placed tracheal tube within a specified time. Although the incidence of extubation failure or reintubation after surgery is relatively uncommon with an incidence of 0.1–0.45%, it leads to an overall increased mortality.

The 2016 AIDAA guidelines for the management of anticipated difficult extubation encompass various strategies for a safe extubation following surgery, which are easily executable and modifiable as per the local requirements. The AIDAA algorithm for the management of anticipated difficult extubation is given in **Flowchart 2**.

▌REFERENCES

1. Nolan JP, Kelly FE. Airway challenges in critical care. Anaesthesia. 2011;66(Suppl)2:81-92.

2. Cook TM, Woodall N, Harper J, Benger J. Fourth National Audit Project. Major complications of airway management in the UK: results of the Fourth National Audit Project of the Royal College of Anaesthetists and the Difficult Airway Society. Part 2: intensive care and emergency departments. Br J Anaesth. 2011;106(5):632-42.

3. Myatra SN, Ahmed SM, Kundra P, Garg R, Ramkumar V, Patwa A, et al. The All India Difficult Airway Association 2016 guidelines for tracheal intubation in the intensive care unit. Indian J Anaesth. 2016;60(12):922-30.

4. Mosier JM, Joshi R, Hypes C, Pacheco G, Valenzuela T, Sakles JC. Airway. West J Emerg Med. 2015;16(7):1109-17.

5. Russotto V, Myatra SN, Laffey JG. What's new in airway management of the critically ill. Intensive Care Med. 2019; 45(11):1615-8.

6. Scott JA, Heard SO, Zayaruzny M, Walz JM. Airway management in critical illness: an update. Chest. 2019;(19):34193-5.

7. Myatra SN, Lodh N, Divatia JV. Airway management. In: Chawla R, Todi S (Eds). ICU Protocols. Singapore: Springer; 2020.

8. De Jong A, Molinari N, Terzi N, Mongardon N, Arnal JM, Guitton C, et al. Early identification of patients at risk for difficult intubation in the intensive care unit. Development and validation of the MACOCHA score in a Multicenter Cohort Study. Am J Respir Crit Care Med. 2013;187(8):832-9.

9. Mayo PH, Hegde A, Eisen LA, Kory P, Doelken P. A program to improve the quality of emergency endotracheal intubation. J Intensive Care Med. 2011;26(1):50-6.

10. Choudhary A, Angurana SK. Pre-intubation checklist: need of the hour. Chest. 2018;153(4):1075-6.

11. Janz DR, Semler MW, Joffe AM, Casey JD, Lentz RJ, deBoisblanc BO, et al. A multicenter randomized trial of a checklist for endotracheal intubation of critically ill adults. Chest. 2018;153:816-24.

12. Jaber S, Jung B, Corne P, Sebbane M, Muller L, Chanques G, et al. An intervention to decrease complications related to endotracheal intubation in the intensive care unit: a prospective, multiple-center study. Intensive Care Med. 2010;36(2):248-55.

13. Myatra SN. Optimal position for laryngoscopy: time for individualization? J Anaesthesiol Clin Pharmacol. 2019;35(3): 289-91.

14. Lee BJ, Kang JM, Kim DO. Laryngeal exposure during laryngoscopy is better in the 25 degrees back-up position than in the supine position. Br J Anaesth. 2007;99:581-6.

15. Lebowitz PW, Shay H, Straker T, Rubin D, Bodner S. Shoulder and head elevation improves laryngoscopic view for tracheal intubation in non-obese as well as obese individuals. J Clin Anesth. 2012;24:104-8.

16. Casey JD, Semler MW. Ventilation before intubation: how to prevent hypoxaemia? Lancet Respir Med. 2019;7:284-5.

17. Baillard C, Fosse JP, Sebbane M, Chanques G, Vincent F, Courouble P, et al. Noninvasive ventilation improves preoxygenation before intubation of hypoxic patients. Am J Respir Crit Care Med. 2006;174(2):171-7.

18. Guitton C, Ehrmann S, Volteau C, Colin G, Maamar A, Jean-Michel V, et al. Nasal high-flow preoxygenation for endotracheal intubation in the critically ill patient: a randomized clinical trial. Intensive Care Med. 2019;45:447-58.

19. Frat JP, Ricard JD, Quenot JP, Pichon N, Demoule A, Forel JM, et al. Non-invasive ventilation versus high-flow nasal cannula oxygen therapy with apnoeic oxygenation for preoxygenation before intubation of patients with acute hypoxaemic respiratory failure: a randomised, multicentre, open-label trial. Lancet Respir Med. 2019;7:303-12.

20. Jaber S, Monnin M, Girard M, Conseil M, Cisse M, Carr J, et al. Apnoeic oxygenation via high-flow nasal cannula oxygen combined with non-invasive ventilation preoxygenation for intubation in hypoxaemic patients in the intensive care unit: the single-centre, blinded, randomised controlled OPTINIV trial. Intensive Care Med. 2016;42:1877-87.

21. Casey JD, Janz DR, Russell DW, Vondehaar DJ, Joffe AM, Dischert KM, et al. Bag-mask ventilation during tracheal intubation of critically ill adults. N Engl J Med. 2019;380:811-21.

22. Huang HB, Peng JM, Xu B, Liu GY, Du B. Video laryngoscopy for endotracheal intubation of critically ill adults: a systemic review and meta-analysis. Chest. 2017;152:510-7.

23. Jiang J, Ma D, Li B, Yue Y, Xue F. Video laryngoscopy does not improve the intubation outcomes in emergency and critical patients—a systematic review and meta-analysis of randomized controlled trials. Crit Care. 2017;21(1):288.

24. Cabrini L, Landoni G, Baiardo Redaelli M, Saleh O, Votta CD, et al. A tracheal intubation in critically ill patients: a comprehensive systematic review of randomized trials. Crit Care. 2018;22(1):6.

25. Jaber S, De Jong A, Pelosi P, Cabrini L, Reignier J, Lascarrou JB. Videolaryngoscopy in critically ill patients. Crit Care. 2019;23:221-7.

26. Driver BE, Prekker ME, Klein LR, Reardon RF, Miner JR, Fagerstrom ET, et al. Efect of use of a bougie vs endotracheal tube and stylet on frst-attempt intubation success among patients with difcult airways undergoing emergency intubation: a randomized clinical trial. JAMA. 2018;319:2179-89.

27. Griesdale DE, Bosma TL, Kurth T, Isac G, Chittock DR. Complications of endotracheal intubation in the critically ill. Intensive Care Med. 2008;34(10):1835-42.

28. De Jong A, Rolle A, Molinari N, Paugam-Burtz C, Constantin JM, Lefrant JY, et al. Cardiac arrest and mortality related to intubation procedure in critically ill adult patients: a multicenter cohort study. Crit Care Med. 2018;46(4):532-539.

29. Myatra SN, Shah A, Kundra P, Patwa A, Ramkumar V, Divatia JV, et al. All India Difficult Airway Association 2016 for the management of unanticipated difficult tracheal intubation in adults. Indian J Anaesth. 2016;12:885-98.

30. Frerk C, Mitchell VS, McNarry AF, Mendonca C, Bhagrath R, Patel A, et al. Difficult airway society 2015 guidelines for management of unanticipated difficult intubation in adults. Br J Anaesth. 2015;115:827-48.

31. Myatra SN, Ahmed SM, Kundra P, Garg R, Ramkumar V, Patwa A, et al. Republication: all India difficult airway association 2016 guidelines for tracheal intubation in the intensive care unit. Indian J Crit Care Med. 2017:21:146-53.

32. Higgs A, McGrath BA, Goddard C, Rangasami J, Suntharalingam G, Gale R, et al. Guidelines for the management of tracheal intubation in critically ill adults. Br J Anaesth. 2018;120:323-52.

33. Quintard H, I'Her E, Pottecher J, Adnet F, Constantin JM, De Jong A, et al. Intubation and extubation of the ICU patient. Anaesth Crit Care Pain Med. 2017;36:327-41.

34. McGrath BA, Bates L, Atkinson D, Moore JA. National Tracheostomy Safety Project. National Tracheostomy Safety Project. Multidisciplinary guidelines for the management of tracheostomy and laryngectomy airway emergencies. Anaesthesia. 2012;67:1025-41.

35. Bontempo LJ, Manning SL. Tracheostomy Emergencies. Emerg Med Clin North Am. 2019;37:109-19.

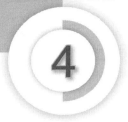

4

Pain, Agitation, and Delirium in Postoperative Period

Srinivas Samavedam, Nandhakishore Jampala

INTRODUCTION

In the postoperative setting, pain, agitation, delirium often occur as interrelated parts of a "syndrome" rather than as separate entities and it is difficult for the clinicians to recognize and treat each of these variants due to the similarities in presentation.[1] The challenge is greater in older patients due to underlying comorbidities, inability to report pain, and age-related physiologic changes that may affect the metabolism of certain medications. Data has shown that up to 60% of hospitalized patients receive inadequate analgesia and sedation during the postsurgical period as these symptoms are extremely subjective with variable tolerability.[2] In this chapter we will discuss each aspect of this syndrome, their clinical considerations related to the assessment, and treatment.

PAIN

Pain is defined as "an unpleasant sensory and emotional experience associated with potential tissue damage affecting the functioning and quality of life".[1] Inadequate pain control is associated with increased morbidity and increase length of hospital stay, on the other hand optimal perioperative pain relief provides early ambulation and enhanced recovery.[2]

Factors influencing Pain[1]

- *Procedure related*:
  - Type of procedure/surgery (e.g., chest tube removal/postcardiac surgery)
  - Preprocedural pain intensity
  - Injury type and location of surgery
- *Nonprocedure related*:
  - Psychologic (anxiety, depression, and cognitive function)
  - Demographic (young age, female sex, comorbidities, and past surgeries)

Assessment of Pain[1,3,4]

The reference standard measure of pain is the patient's self-report, if they can communicate reliably.

- *In patients who can self-report pain*:
  - 0–10 numerical rating scale in a visual format (NRS-V)
  - 0–10 numerical rating scale in oral format (NRS-O)
  - 0–10 visual analog scale (VAS)
  - Verbal rating scale/verbal descriptor scale (VRS/VDS)
  - Faces pain scale-revised (FPS-R)

Among the above pain assessment scales, NRS-V has shown to be more affective considering its ease of use and highest success rate in terms of response obtained.

- *In patients who cannot self-report pain/who cannot communicate*:
  - Behavioral pain scale (BPS) has international validation
  - Critical-care pain observation tool (CPOT)
- In the absence of patient's self-reporting of pain, behavioral observation is recommended (looking at various behavioral patterns like facial grimacing, moaning or groaning, agitation, irritability, and combativeness).
- International Association for the Study of Pain (IASP) and American Society of Pain management have developed clinical guidelines that address the use of behavioral measures to assess pain.
- Vital signs [like heart rate, blood pressure (BP), respiratory rate, and percutaneous arterial oxygen saturation (SpO_2)] should not be used alone to assess pain, rather should be used only as an indicator to make further assessment.

Management of Pain in Postoperative Patients

It is always preferable to use an "assessment-driven, protocol-based, and stepwise approach" for management of pain in postoperative patients. A multimodal strategy including nonpharmacological measures should be considered for effective pain control.[5]

Table 1: Options for perioperative analgesia

Medication	Considerations

Opioids[4,7,8]	• *Parenteral*:
	  – *Fentanyl*: 0.5 µg/kg IV bolus followed by 0.7–10 µg/kg/h as IV infusion. Most commonly used agents due to its fewer side effects
	  – *Sufentanil*: 0.5 µg/kg IV bolus followed by 0.5–1.5 µg/kg/h as continuous infusion
	    ♦ Has less context-sensitive half-life than fentanyl (but more than remifentanil)
	  – *Remifentanil*: 1.5 µg/kg IV loading dose followed by 0.5–15 µg/kg/h as continuous infusion
	    ♦ Ultrashort-acting with a very rapid onset of action
	    ♦ It has very less context-sensitive half-life (3–4 minutes)
	    ♦ Hydrolyzed by plasma esterases
	    ♦ No accumulation in hepatic/renal failure
	  – *Morphine*: 2–4 mg/IV/2nd hourly or 2–30 mg/h as continuous infusion
	    ♦ *Side effects*: Accumulation with hepatic and renal impairment; histamine release
	• *Oral*:
	  – *Hydromorphone*: 7.5 mg/BID
	    ♦ Therapeutic option in patients tolerant to morphine/fentanyl
	  – *Morphine*: 30 mg/OD

Nonopioids[6]	• *IV acetaminophen*: 650–1,000 mg IV every 6 hours (maximum dose < 4 gr/day)
	  – Short onset of action (<5 minutes) with IV formulation
	• *Oral/rectal acetaminophen*: 325–1,000 mg every 4–6 hours (maximum dose < 4 gr/day)
	  – Contraindicated in hepatic dysfunction
	  – Rectal suppositories are helpful in patients who have GI intolerance
	• *NSAIDs (nonselective COX inhibitors)*:
	  – *Ketorolac*: 30 mg IM/IV, then 15–30 mg every 6 hours (maximum dose—120 mg/day)
	  – *Ibuprofen*: 400–800 mg IV every 6 hours infused over 30 minutes (max dose—3.2 gr/day)
	    ♦ Oral formulation (400 mg/every 4 hours; maximum dose—2.4 gr/day)
	    ♦ Avoid in conditions like renal dysfunction, GI bleeding, platelet abnormality, asthma, post-CABG, concomitant treatment with ACE inhibitors
	• *NSAIDs (selective COX-2 inhibitors)*: Celecoxib and etoricoxib
	• *Ketamine*: NMDA receptor antagonist
	  – *Dose*: 0.1–0.5 mg/kg/IV loading dose, followed by 0.05–0.4 mg/kg/h
	  – Reduces the development of acute tolerance to opioids. May cause hallucinations and psychiatric disturbances
	• *Gabanoids, gabapentin, and pregabalin*: Inhibit the α-2-δ subunit of calcium-gated channels on presynaptic axons

Regional analgesia	Neuraxial opioid → intrathecal opioid, epidural opioid Epidural analgesia with local anesthetics
Peripheral nerve blocks	Field blocks (intercostal nerve block, vertebral plexus block, and incisional site infiltration)
Patient-controlled analgesia (PCA)[1,9]	Allows the patients to administer the analgesic (usually opioid) themselves, most commonly in the vein or epidural space Basic parameters are set by the physician in advance and cannot be changed by the patient, which include bolus dose administered when the patient pushes the button. There is a lockout interval—time during which the machine will not administer a further dose, despite any further demands made by the patient, and usually the maximum dose to be given per 4 or 6 hours

(ACE: angiotensin-converting enzyme; CABG: coronary artery bypass grafting; GI: gastrointestinal; IV: intravenous; IM: intramuscular; NMDA: N-methyl-D-aspartate; NSAIDs: nonsteroidal anti-inflammatory drugs)

Preoperative Optimization

Effective postoperative pain management begins even before surgery. Continuation of previous medications to avoid withdrawal, optimization of comorbid conditions is the mainstay of preoperative optimization.[2]

Pharmacological Options (Table 1)

- As per the American Society of Anesthesiologists (ASA) and American Pain Society (APS) task force recommendations, opioids remain the mainstay of therapy for pain management in most of the postoperative care settings.[5,6]

- Acetaminophen, nonsteroidal anti-inflammatory drugs (NSAIDs) (selective COX-2 inhibitors), and calcium channel α-2-δ antagonists (gabapentin and pregabalin) should be considered concurrently with opioids as an integral part of multimodal postoperative analgesia program.[6]
- Whenever possible (if patient's characteristics allow), regional blockade with local anesthetics should also be considered (e.g., epidural analgesia and field blocks).[6]
- The scientific rationale behind such multimodal approach is to block all the possible pain-related pathways and inhibit molecular mechanisms of acute pain. It also helps in reducing the usage of opioids and their unwanted side effects.

POSTOPERATIVE AGITATION

Postoperative agitation (POA) is a well-described phenomenon seen especially during the recovery phase (emergence) of anesthesia. It usually lasts for a short time, but can be harmful to the patient leading to potential injuries ranging from abnormal movements requiring physical restraints to life-threatening accidental pull-outs of invasive lines, catheters, and tubes. It can also lead to violence against staff and increased resource utilization.[10]

Precipitating Factors[10,11]

- Inadequate pain relief
- *Metabolic*: Hypoglycemia and hyponatremia
- Hypotension and hypoxia
- Alcohol and smoking withdrawal
- Too rapid emergence from anesthesia
- Lighter planes of anesthesia during extubation
- Premedication with atropine and phenergan
- Use of rapid emergence inhalational anesthetics (sevoflurane and desflurane)
- Presence of invasive lines (tracheal tube, nasogastric tube, and urinary catheter)
- Nasal packing
- Male gender and young age
- Preexisting mental health problems

Pathophysiology of Agitation

Two main events combined together trigger the onset of agitation. The first being incomplete recovery from anesthesia. The second being a constant source of discomfort/pain (irritation by catheter, tubing or alcohol withdrawal).[11]

Assessment of Agitation[8,10,11]

- The return of mental status to normal preprocedural levels (after postanesthesia recovery) is a standard criterion to be achieved before a patient is being moved from an surgical intensive care unit (SICU) to a lower level of care.
- A balance must be maintained in the recovery room between the levels of sedation given (to calm down an agitated patient) and to make sure there is no complication related to the sedation. To strike it correctly, we need to perfectly recognize agitation and the depth of sedation through certain assessment tools.
- Richmond Agitation-Sedation Scale (RASS) and Sedation-Agitation scale (SAS) are the most reliable easy tools available for the assessment of agitation and the need for depth of sedation in postoperative patients.
- Emergence agitation was defined as a RASS score of +3 or +4.

Management of Agitation[4,10]

Preoperative Optimization

- Using dexmedetomidine instead of benzodiazepines for preoperative sedation has shown to reduce the emergence symptoms.
- Substitution of atropine by glycopyrrolate [as it does not cross the blood-brain barrier (BBB)].

Prevention

- Providing adequate postoperative analgesia.
- Avoiding rapid emergence inhalational agents.
- Prompt early removal of invasive lines.
- Correction of metabolic parameters.

Pharmacological Measures

- *Nonbenzodiazepine sedatives*: Propofol or dexmedetomidine are preferred to produce sedation not at a very deep level, but just to calm the agitated patient.
- Postoperative patients with agitation stay longer in the recovery area and are more likely to have subsequent delirium and respiratory complications. Hence prior anticipation of high-risk patients could reduce the incidence of agitation and can prevent these untoward events.

POSTOPERATIVE DELIRIUM

- Delirium is defined as "an acute, but fluctuating disturbance in the sensorium characterized by a patient's inability to focus, maintain or shift attention which is often associated with cognitive dysfunction and change in perception" that is precipitated due to an underlying medical illness.[12]
- The incidence of delirium was found to be 15–25% following a major elective surgery and as high as 50% with cardiac surgery and fractures of hip. It is most commonly seen typically during the first 3 postoperative days.[12,13]
- It is usually manifested in the form of → new onset altered level of consciousness/inattention/disorientation or disorganized thinking/hallucination or delusion/psychomotor agitation/inappropriate speech, mood or behavior/sleep-wake cycle disturbance.

Pathophysiology of Delirium[12,14]

- Pathophysiology of delirium is multifactorial, where multiple brain systems are disrupted. There is biochemical as well as electrophysiologic derangement.
- Cholinergic pathways play a significant role. There is decrease in the acetylcholine function (increased anticholinergic activity correlates with severity of delirium).

- Changes in various neurotransmitters, hormones, and cytokines also contribute to delirium. There are abnormal levels of endorphins, serotonin, and neuropeptides seen in the circulating cerebrospinal fluid (CSF). Hence delirium represents a global brain dysfunction.[12]

Risk Factors for Delirium[14-16]

- Advanced age (due to preexisting dementia, decreased cognitive ability, decreased ability to metabolize drugs, polypharmacy, visual or hearing impairment, underlying brain disease, and psychiatric illness especially depression)
- History of alcohol intake and nicotine abuse
- Preoperative use of benzodiazepines and opioids
- Use of physical restraints
- Duration of mechanical ventilation
- Past history of cognitive dysfunction (dementia) and stroke
- ASA Grade III-IV patients
- Increased acute physiologic assessment and chronic health evaluation-II (APACHE-II) and sequential organ failure assessment (SOFA) scores at the time of SICU admission
- Anticholinergics, antipsychotics, and sedatives
- Intraoperative blood loss and blood transfusions
- Intraoperative adverse events (hypotension and hypoxia)
- Type of surgery—emergency > elective/trauma, cardiac
- Duration of surgery
- Sleep deprivation

Assessment of Delirium[14,15]

- All postoperative patients must be assessed daily for delirium using validated tools.

- Delirium can be classified into three subtypes; hypoactive (with low psychomotor behavioral activity), hyperactive (with high psychomotor activity), and mixed.
- In postoperative patients, "hypoactive form" is just as common as the hyperactive form and the prognosis seems to be worse with this type due to under recognition by the treating team, resulting in delayed treatment.
- The most commonly used validated tools are the confusion assessment method for the ICU (CAM-ICU) and intensive care delirium screening checklist (ICDSC).
- Diagnosis of delirium is purely clinical. Diagnostic tests are used not to establish the diagnosis of delirium, but to identify the potentially correctable factors contributing to it.

Management of Delirium[13-15]

Most important aspect in the management of delirium is early identification and treatment of the precipitating factor. Symptom control though important must never delay the correction of the precipitating cause.

Preoperative Optimization

- Identification of the potential modifiable risk factors in patients before surgery and treating them has shown to decrease the incidence of postoperative delirium (POD).
- There is no pharmacological agent which has shown to prevent POD and prophylactic administration of antipsychotics has no role in the prevention.

Supportive Measures (Multidisciplinary Aspects)

- Optimization of comorbidities
- Aggressively treat the pain
- Maintain adequate lighting and space

Table 2: Options for perioperative delirium	
Medication	*Consideration*
Dexmedetomidine	<ul><li>α2 agonist</li><li>Has all the combined effects like anxiolysis, analgesia, sedation, and sympatholysis</li><li>Ideal drug to treat symptoms and reduce the duration of delirium</li><li>*Dose*: 1 µg/kg loading dose over 10 minutes, followed by maintenance dose as continuous infusion 0.2–0.7 µg/kg/h</li><li>*Adverse effects*: Bradycardia, hypotension, and arrhythmias</li></ul>
Haloperidol	<ul><li>Typical antipsychotic</li><li>It should not be used as the first choice of agent due to its adverse effects</li><li>*Dose*: 0.5 mg TID/QID (totally <5 mg/day is safe). Should be tapered in 3–5 days</li><li>*Adverse effects*: Extrapyramidal symptoms and neuroleptic malignant syndrome</li></ul>
Benzodiazepines	<ul><li>Have rapid onset of action, but can worsen sedation and can cause paradoxical agitation</li><li>Lorazepam and midazolam are preferred (short-acting)</li><li>*Dose*: 0.5–2 mg TID</li><li>Drug of choice to treat delirium secondary to alcohol withdrawal</li></ul>
Atypical antipsychotics	<ul><li>Quetiapine, olanzapine, ziprasidone, aripiprazole, and risperidone</li><li>Shown to reduce the duration of delirium in postoperative patients</li><li>*Adverse effects*: QT prolongation and torsades de pointes</li></ul>

- Avoid unnecessary noise, especially during nights
- Avoid sleep interruption
- Early mobilization and ambulation
- Avoiding physical restraints and early removal of catheters
- Promote orientation by using clocks, calendars, and familiar objects
- Ensure use of hearing aids and glasses

Symptom Control through Pharmacological Agents[17] *(Table 2)*

Outcomes of Delirium[15,18]

Delirium is associated with increased morbidity and mortality. It is an independent predictor of negative outcomes including increased length of hospital stay, cost of care, and long-term cognitive dysfunction.

Though agitation and delirium manifest in a similar way in a postoperative patient (both having excitation and confusion), both are different in their course and progression. Agitation is short lived. The onset is rapid but does not last long and responds quickly on removal of the inciting stimulus. Whereas delirium is more fatal and lasts long and is difficult to treat.

▌REFERENCES

1. Málek J, Ševčík P, Bejšovec D, Gabrhelík T, Hnilicová M, Křikava I, et al. Postoperative Pain Management. Prague, Czechia: Mladá fronta; 2017.
2. Garimella V, Cellini C. Postoperative pain control. Clin Colon Rectal Surg. 2013;26(3):191-6.
3. Chou R, Gordon DB, de Leon-Casasola OA, Rosenberg JM, Bickler S, Brennan T, et al. Management of Postoperative Pain: A Clinical Practice Guideline From the American Pain Society, the American Society of Regional Anesthesia and Pain Medicine, and the American Society of Anesthesiologists' Committee on Regional Anesthesia, Executive Committee, and Administrative Council. J Pain. 2016;17(2):131-57.
4. Iakovou A, Wong Lama KM, Tsegaye A. Update on sedation in the critical care unit. Open Crit Care Med J. 2013;6(Suppl 1: M5):66-79.
5. American Society of Anesthesiologists Task Force on Acute Pain Management. Practice Guidelines for Acute Pain Management in the Perioperative Setting: An Updated Report by the American Society of Anesthesiologists Task Force on Acute Pain Management. Anesthesiology. 2012;116:248-73.
6. Wardhan R, Chelly J. Recent advances in acute pain management: Understanding the mechanisms of acute pain, the prescription of opioids and the role of multimodal pain therapy. F1000Res. 2017;6:2065.
7. Casserly E, Alexander JC. (2020). Perioperative Uses of Intravenous Opioids in Adults. [online] Available from https://www.uptodate.com/contents/perioperative-uses-of-intravenous-opioids-in-adults. [Last accessed March, 2020].
8. Barr J, Fraser GL, Puntillo K, Ely EW, Gélinas C, Dasta JF, et al. Clinical practice Guidelines for the management of Pain, Agitation, and Delirium in Adult patients in the Intensive Care Unit. Crit Care Med. 2013;41(1):263-306.
9. Edward R Mariano. (2020). Management of Acute Perioperative Pain. [online] Available from https://www.uptodate.com/contents/management-of-acute-perioperative-pain. [Last accessed February, 2020].
10. Fields A, Huang J, Schroeder D, Sprung J, Weingarten T. Agitation in adults in the post-anesthesia care unit after general anesthesia. Br J Anesth. 2018;121:1-7.
11. Hyun-Chang K, Eugene K, Young-Tae J, Jung-Won H, Young-Jin L, Jeong-Hwa S, et al. Postanesthetic emergence agitation in adult patients after general anesthesia for urological surgery. J Int Med Res. 2015;43:226-35.
12. Chaiwat O, Chanidnuan M, Pancharoen W, Vijitmala K, Danpornprasert P, Toadithep P, et al. Postoperative delirium in critically ill surgical patients: incidence, risk factors and predictive scores. BMC Anesthesiol. 2019;19:39.
13. Vlisides P, Avidan M. Recent Advances in Preventing and Managing Postoperative Delirium. F1000Res. 2019;8:F1000.
14. Pandharipande P, Cotton BA, Shintani A, Thompson J, Pun BT, Morris JA Jr, et al. Prevalence and risk factors for development of delirium in surgical and trauma intensive care patients. J Trauma. 2008;65:34-41.
15. Amador LF, Goodwin JS. Postoperative Delirium in the older patent. J Am Coll Surg. 2005;200:767-73.
16. Robinson TN, Raeburn CD, Tran ZV, Angles EM, Brenner LA, Moss M. Postoperative delirium in the elderly: risk factors and outcomes. Ann Surg. 2009;249:173-8.
17. Reade MC, Finfer S. Sedation and delirium in the intensive care unit. N Engl J Med. 2014;370:444-54.
18. Sprung J, Roberts RO, Weingarten TN, Cavalcante AN, Knopman DS, Petersen RC, et al. Postoperative delirium in elderly patients is associated with subsequent cognitive impairment. Br J Anaesth. 2017;119(2):316-23.

Goal Directed Fluid Therapy in Perioperative Critical Care

Kushal R Kalvit, Atul Prabhakar Kulkarni

INTRODUCTION

Fluid therapy in the perioperative period is a seemingly innocuous part of patient management. Fluids are like any other drugs and each type has its own dose, effects, adverse effects, indications, and contraindications. Apart from selecting appropriate fluid for each patient, and from the same patient at different stages of illness, achieving appropriate balance between intake and output is necessary to prevent adverse outcomes. The subject of fluid therapy is a matter of debate since decades, but still remains unresolved. The perioperative period is a period of differing requirements for the patient and involves many dynamic changes in fluid balance. It is affected by many factors such as preoperative fluid status, comorbidities, type and duration of surgery, blood loss, and hemodynamic deterioration during surgery, and postoperative complications. This can be further complicated by the type of amount of fluid chosen for therapy during this period.

The consequences of under-resuscitation and fluid overload are well known. Persistent fluid deficit eventually leads to reduced cardiac output (CO) and impaired organ perfusion and can cause organ dysfunction. Fluid overload, on the other hand, causes interstitial edema and organ dysfunction. The association between perioperative morbidity and fluid administered is a typical U-shaped curve with increased morbidity and mortality occurring with too little or too much fluid **(Fig. 1)**.[1] A meta-analysis (29 trials with 4,805 patients) showed that advanced hemodynamic monitoring with pre-emptive intervention (with fluid therapy alone or/and vasoactive medications) to achieve preset goals, significantly reduced mortality [OR 0.48 (95% CI: 0.33–0.78); $p = 0.0002$] and surgical complications [OR 0.43 (95% CI: 0.34–0.53); $p < 0.0001$], emphasizing the fact that such strategies can improve postoperative outcomes.[2] Miller and colleagues comment on this systematic review is quite thought provoking. They suggest that optimization may not be that different from restrictive fluid therapy. Other

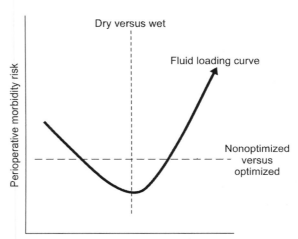

Fig. 1: Fluid loading and risk of perioperative mortality.

factors that are stressed upon are that with the availability of newer less invasive monitors of CO, and absence of tissue oxygenation monitor, oxygen delivery index (DO_2I) can still be used, if not to achieve the 650 mL/m/m^2 in all patients but in an individualized manner.[3] With some evidence coming to fore with the long-term benefits of perioperative optimization[4] (due to reduced immediate postoperative complications), it is essential for us to use advanced hemodynamic monitoring with pre-emptive intervention to improve postoperative outcomes.

GOAL-DIRECTED FLUID THERAPY

The term goal-directed fluid therapy (GDT) has been used since more than three decades and has been extensively studied. Unfortunately, it has not been standardized yet. The "goals" in GDT are still unclear. Blood pressure and urine output were used as markers of adequate perfusion in yesteryears. However, it has been shown time and again that these do not reliably predict volume status or organ perfusion. Jarisch, in 1928, quoted—"It is a source of regret that the measurement of flow (stroke volume) is so much more difficult than pressure. This has led to an undue interest in the blood pressure manometer. Most organs, however, require flow rather than pressure."[5] In reality, organs need both, but physiology maintains pressure first at the expense of flow.

PRACTICE OF GOAL-DIRECTED FLUID THERAPY

The story of GDT in the perioperative fluid therapy has been a story of changing goalposts. In the 1980s, fluid therapy was directed at increasing the oxygen delivery to the tissues by augmenting the CO using fluid infusion and vasoactive medications. This supranormal approach coexisted for some time with the liberal fluid infusion strategy used by the anesthesiologist who calculated intraoperative fluid requirement by using various factors such as fluids for preoperative fasting, maintenance fluids, third space losses, and replacement of the blood lost. Following this, came the period of restrictive fluid therapy when the disadvantages of excessive fluid infusion were realized. Recently, an individualized approach for fluid optimization has been adopted in most places. The following sections give a brief overview of each approach.

SUPRANORMAL OXYGEN DELIVERY

The first systematic approach at GDT was made by Shoemaker and colleagues in 1988.[6] They noted that survivors of supramajor surgeries achieved high cardiac index (CI) and delivery and consumption of oxygen. They hypothesized that since the supramajor surgeries evoked a strong systemic inflammatory response, which produces oxygen debt. Those who can overcome this debt survive, while those who could not perished. To test this, they inserted a pulmonary artery catheter (PAC) in patients undergoing high-risk surgery and used a combination of fluids, blood transfusion, vasopressors, and inotropes (principally dobutamine). The predefined goals in the intervention group were CI > 4.5 L/min/m^2, DO$_2$I > 600 mL/min/m^2, and oxygen consumption index (VO$_2$I) > 170 mL/min/m^2. The study showed that there was significant reduction in the morbidity (leading to decreased duration mechanical ventilation and ICU and hospital LOS) and mortality in PAC group as compared to the control group. The remaining patients either survived but had organ dysfunction or developed organ failure and died. The patient who developed organ dysfunction had deficient oxygen delivery and consumption and they termed this as "Oxygen Debt". They subsequently published a study demonstrating the effect of oxygen debt, where nonsurvivors had significantly higher oxygen debt as compared to those

who survived with and without development of organ failure.[7] Studies conducted by various groups later showed improved outcomes with this approach.[8-10] A meta-analysis published by Kern and Shoemaker later showed that supranormal oxygen delivery worked in high-risk patients undergoing supramajor surgeries (mortality rate >20%), provided optimization was achieved before development of organ failure.[11] Attempts to extrapolate this approach in critically ill patients did not result in better outcomes in the intervention group.[12] As remarked by Shoemaker in response to this study, dead cells cannot be resuscitated even with oxygen![13] Connors and colleagues in a prospective trial on the efficacy of PAC (with propensity score matched historical controls) showed that the use of PAC resulted in higher 30-day mortality (OR: 1.24; 95% CI: 1.03–1.49), higher mean cost and longer ICU LOS (14.8 vs. 13 days).[14] A multicenter Canadian study, which randomized 1,994 patients between 1990 and 1999, to either GDT with the use of PAC or a control group, found that there was no difference in inhospital mortality in the groups.[15] However, the goals of therapy (CI: 3.5–4.5 mL/m/m^2 and DO$_2$I - mL/m/m^2) were achieved in only in 18.6% and 21.0%, at study entry, while after surgery, they were achieved in 79% and 62.9% patients. The study was criticized for this low-goal achievement and for not having any goals in the control group. Also, the goals were not similar to those described by Shoemaker and colleagues. Following this study and as a result of the Connors study, the use of PAC and supranormal oxygen delivery declined. The use of PAC in the operating rooms (barring the cardiac surgery OTs) has declined following the advent of newer less invasive and noninvasive CO monitors. However, as Gelman puts it succinctly in his editorial—"Is goal-directed hemodynamic therapy dead?" the answer has to be negative.[16]

THE ERA OF RESTRICTIVE FLUID THERAPY

The tussle between liberal and restrictive fluid strategy has been going on for two decades and we still have not found the "sweet spot". Large amounts of fluid were infused in the past especially in abdominal surgeries for perceived "third space" losses. The presence of this "third space" is now being questioned.[17] We encourage the readers to read this excellent piece of work. The proponents of restrictive fluid therapy quote this "lack of presence of the third space" and the adverse effects of fluid overload on the postoperative outcomes.

Brandstrup et al. compared liberal versus restrictive strategy in patients undergoing colorectal surgery.[18] In this study, patients in the liberal group (LG) received 6 liters of fluid on the day of surgery with a postoperative weight gain of 4 kg, while the restrictive group received 4 liters fluid with a resultant weight gain of 1 kg. The "restrictive" regimen was aimed at maintaining the preoperative body weight. This regimen significantly reduced the rate of complications both by intention-to-treat (33% vs. 51%; $p < 0.013$) and per-protocol (30% vs. 56%; $p < 0.03$) analyses. Nisanevich et al. in 2005 examined the effects of liberal (bolus of 10 mL/kg followed by 12 mL/kg/h) versus restrictive (4 mL/kg/h) fluid therapy on postoperative mortality in patients undergoing abdominal surgeries.[19] They found that although the gastrointestinal (GI) complications and length of stay were less in the restrictive group, the mortality was not significantly different. Subsequently, there have been more studies with different primary endpoints (postoperative pulmonary complications[20] and postoperative recovery).[20] Showing better postoperative outcomes with restrictive fluid therapy.

All these studies favored the restrictive regimen. However, there was an increasing concern on the adverse effects of restrictive fluid therapy, especially acute kidney injury. This formed the basis of a recent multicenter RELIEF trial[21] ($n = 3,000$), which compared a restrictive and liberal fluid approach. The patients in the restrictive group (RG) received a fluid bolus of maximum 5 mL/kg during induction, followed by 5 mL/kg/hour till the end of surgery, followed by 0.8 mL/kg/hour for 24 hours. The patients in the LG received a fluid bolus of 10 mL/kg followed by 8 mL/kg/hour till the end of the surgery and 1.5 mL/kg/hour for 24 hours. The primary endpoint, the rate of disability-free survival at 1 year, was not different in the two groups, [81.9% RG vs. 82.3% LG (HR for death or disability, 1.05; 95% CI: 0.88–1.24; $p = 0.61$)]. However, there was a significantly higher risk of acute kidney injury in the RG (8.6% vs. 5.0%; $p < 0.001$). The important secondary outcomes were higher in the RG, but were not statistically significant [a composite of septic complications, surgical site infection, or death (21.8% vs. 19.8%; $p = 0.19$; RRT at 90 days (0.9% vs. 0.3%; $p = 0.048$)]. Bandstrup makes very keen and important comments in the editorial accompanying the trial.[22] Instead of being truly restrictive in trying to achieve zero fluid balance, we tend to forget the basic physiological principles that hypovolemia causing oliguria must be recognized and corrected with fluid. He emphasizes that in the current era where minimally invasive surgeries are common, a modestly liberal administration of fluids will not cause significant fluid retention. Importantly, the findings of the RELIEF trial do not support excessive intravenous fluid administration and that a modestly liberal fluid regimen is safer than a truly restrictive regimen.

INDIVIDUAL OPTIMIZATION

There are no established criteria for "euvolemic status" and every individual reacts differently at different times to a fluid challenge. This essentially means that one size does not fit all. Therefore, the concept of individual optimization of fluid therapy. It depends on monitoring of the stroke volume (SV) or stroke volume variation (SVV) of an individual and infusing fluids with the aim of optimizing (some would say maximizing) the SV for that individual at that point of time. This strategy, however, demands the use of advanced hemodynamic monitoring. It can be done using various less invasive or even noninvasive monitors, but the most studied monitor is the esophageal Doppler.

The OPTIMISE was the first multicenter trial ($n = 734$) of individualized GDT.[23] Authors used a CO-guided algorithm for fluid and dopexamine infusion during and 6 hours following surgery. The trial also included an updated systematic review and meta-analyses of similar trials published from 1966 to 2014. OPTIMISE showed that there was no significant difference in 30 days major complications or mortality after using the CO-guided algorithm [30-day mortality (intervention, 4.9% vs. control group 6.5%; RR: 0.82 (95% CI 0.67–1.01)]. However, inclusion of the results in the meta-analysis showed that individual optimization was associated with significantly reduced complications and mortality as well. This paved the way for further large studies focusing on hemodynamic monitor-guided therapy.

The multicenter FEDORA[24] trial group (2018) conducted a similar study in which they first optimized the fluid status to achieve maximum SV using esophageal Doppler-guided hemodynamic monitoring algorithm. The intraoperative goals were to maintain a maximal SV with mean arterial pressure > 70 mm Hg and CI > 2.5 L/min/m^2. This group was then compared to the control group to study the postoperative complications and mortality. Although there was no difference in the mortality in GDHT group, there were significantly fewer complications including acute kidney injury, pulmonary edema, and respiratory distress syndrome and wound infections in the same group. The ICU and hospital LOS and time to ambulation were also reduced significantly.

These trials show that esophageal Doppler-guided individual optimization is associated with fewer complications, even if there is no decrease in mortality. There is growing evidence that even a short duration of intraoperative hypotension is associated with renal and cardiac injury. For this, fluid therapy alone might not be enough, and some patients may need vasopressor therapy, in addition. This formed the basis of the INPRESS[25] (Intraoperative Norepinephrine to control Arterial Pressure) trial (2017), which compared the effect of individualized versus standard blood pressure target strategies using norepinephrine on postoperative organ dysfunction. They aimed at achieving individualized target of systolic blood pressure (SBP) within 10% of the reference value (i.e., patient's resting SBP) versus standard strategy of treating

SBP < 80 mm Hg or lower than 40% from the reference value. There were no significant differences in the adverse events or 30-day mortality but the postoperative organ dysfunction was significantly lower in the intervention group [46.3% vs. 63.4%; adjusted HR 0.66; 95% CI: 0.52–0.84; $p = 0.001$].

STRIKING THE RIGHT BALANCE

Despite having a plethora of controlled trials and observational studies, we are still facing with the two basic questions: How much fluid to give? When to give fluid bolus?

Based on the results of RELIEF trial, it is safe to say that a modestly liberal approach would be a better alternative. Intraoperatively, maintenance fluid therapy should aim to achieve a positive balance of 1–2 liters at the end of surgery. The total amount of fluid infused or the rate of infusion will obviously vary depending on various factors. Intraoperative fluid boluses usually consist of 250-mL fluid infused over a very short time and should always be given in the face of an objective evidence of hypovolemia. The timing of fluid bolus is also an important consideration given the results of INPRESS trial. It would be wise to use specific hemodynamic monitoring of SV and accordingly give the fluid bolus before significant hypotension develops.[26] This is mostly applicable in case of high-risk surgeries, while its utility in low-risk (less extensive) surgeries is questionable.

Individual optimization of fluid therapy is the counterpart of "personalized" medicine in the perioperative period. Future multicenter large randomized controlled trials (RCTs) on similar subject using different surgical populations would help to refine the current recommendations and improve surgical outcomes as well.

REFERENCES

1. Bellamy MC. Wet, dry or something else? Br J Anaesth. 2006;97:755-7.
2. Hamilton MA, Cecconi M, Rhodes A. A systematic review and meta-analysis on the use of preemptive hemodynamic intervention to improve postoperative outcomes in moderate and high-risk surgical patients. Anesth Analg. 2011;112: 1392-402.
3. Miller TE, Roche AM, Gan TJ. Poor adoption of hemodynamic optimization during major surgery: are we practicing substandard care? Anesth Analg. 2011;112:1274-6.
4. Sun Y, Chai F, Pan C, Romeiser JL, Gan TJ. Effect of perioperative goal-directed hemodynamic therapy on postoperative recovery following major abdominal surgery-a systematic review and meta-analysis of randomized controlled trials. Crit Care. 2017;21:141.
5. Prys-Roberts C. The measurement of cardiac output. Br J Anaesth. 1969;41:751-60.
6. Shoemaker WC, Appel PL, Kram HB, Waxman K, Lee TS. Prospective trial of supranormal values of survivors as therapeutic goals in high-risk surgical patients. Chest. 1988;94:1176-86
7. Shoemaker WC, Appel PL, Kram HB. Role of oxygen debt in the development of organ failure sepsis, and death in high-risk surgical patients. Chest. 1992;102:208-15.
8. Boyd O, Grounds RM, Bennett ED. A randomized clinical trial of the effect of deliberate perioperative increase of oxygen delivery on mortality in high-risk surgical patients. JAMA. 1993;270:2699-707.
9. Wilson J, Woods I, Fawcett J, Whall R, Dibb W, Morris C, et al. Reducing the risk of major elective surgery: randomised controlled trial of preoperative optimisation of oxygen delivery. BMJ. 1999;318:1099-103.
10. Pearse R, Dawson D, Fawcett J, Rhodes A, Grounds RM, Bennett ED. Early goal-directed therapy after major surgery reduces complications and duration of hospital stay. A randomised, controlled trial. Crit Care. 2005;9:R687-693.
11. Kern JW, Shoemaker WC. Meta-analysis of hemodynamic optimization in high-risk patients. Crit Care Med. 2002;30: 1686-92.
12. Gattinoni L, Brazzi L, Pelosi P, Latini R, Tognoni G, Pesenti A, et al. A trial of goal-oriented hemodynamic therapy in critically ill patients. SvO2 Collaborative Group. N Engl J Med. 1995;333:1025-32.
13. Shoemaker WC. Goal-oriented hemodynamic therapy. N Engl J Med. 1996;334:799-800.
14. Connors AF Jr, Speroff T, Dawson NV, Thomas C, Harrell FE Jr, Wagner D, et al. The effectiveness of right heart catheterization in the initial care of critically ill patients. SUPPORT Investigators. JAMA. 1996;276:889-97.
15. Sandham JD, Hull RD, Brant RF, Knox L, Pineo GF, Doig CJ, et al. Canadian Critical Care Clinical Trials Group. A randomized, controlled trial of the use of pulmonary-artery catheters in high-risk surgical patients. N Engl J Med. 2003;348:5-14.
16. Gelman S. Is goal-directed haemodynamic therapy dead? Eur J Anaesthesiol. 2020;37:159-61.
17. Jacob M, Chappell D, Rehm M. The "third space"–fact or fiction? Best Pract Res Clin Anaesthesiol. 2009;23:145-57.
18. Brandstrup B, Tonnesen H, Beier-Holgersen R, Hjortso E, Ording H, Lindorff-Larsen K, et al. Effects of intravenous fluid restriction on postoperative complications: comparison of two perioperative fluid regimens: a randomized assessor-blinded multicentre trial. Ann Surg. 2003;238:641-8.
19. Nisanevich V, Felsenstein I, Almogy G, Weissman C, Einav S, Matot I. Effect of Intraoperative Fluid Management on Outcome after Intraabdominal Surgery. Anesthesiology. 2005;103:25-32.
20. Holte K, Foss NB, Andersen J, Valentiner L, Lund C, Bie P, et al. Liberal or restrictive fluid administration in fast track colonic surgery: a randomized, double blind study. Br J Anaesth. 2007;99(4):500-8.
21. Myles PS, Bellomo R, Corcoran T, Forbes A, Peyton P, Story D, et al. Australian and New Zealand College of Anaesthetists Clinical Trials Network and the Australian and New Zealand Intensive Care Society Clinical Trials Group, Restrictive *versus* liberal fluid therapy for major abdominal surgery. N Engl J Med. 2018;378:2263-74.

22. Brandstrup B. Finding the right balance. N Engl J Med. 2018;378(24):2335-6.

23. Pearse RM, Harrison DA, MacDonald N, Gillies MA, Blunt M, Ackland G, et al. OPTIMISE study group, effect of a perioperative, cardiac output-guided hemodynamic therapy algorithm on outcomes following major gastrointestinal surgery: A randomized clinical trial and systematic review. JAMA. 2014;311:2181-90.

24. Calvo-Vecino JM, Ripollés-Melchor J, Mythen MG, Casans-Francés R, Balik A, Artacho JP, et al. FEDORA Trial Investigators Group, Effect of goal-directed haemodynamic therapy on postoperative complications in low-moderate risk surgical patients: A multicentre randomised controlled trial (FEDORA trial). Br J Anaesth. 2018;120:734-44.

25. Futier E, Lefrant JY, Guinot PG, Godet T, Lorne E, Cuvillon P, et al. INPRESS Study Group, Effect of individualized vs standard blood pressure management strategies on postoperative organ dysfunction among high-risk patients undergoing major surgery: a randomized clinical trial. JAMA. 2017;318:1346-57.

26. Miller TE, Myles PS. Perioperative Fluid Therapy for Major Surgery. Anesthesiology. 2019;130:825-32.

Shock in Postoperative Period

Ashit Hegde

DEFINITION AND RECOGNITION OF SHOCK

Shock is defined as a circulatory dysfunction resulting in an inability of the circulatory system to meet the requirements of the peripheral metabolizing tissue. Shock is usually recognized by the presence of hypotension along with evidence of tissue hypoperfusion. [Oliguria, altered sensorium, decreased capillary refill time (CRT), increased lactate levels]; however, an occult state of hypoperfusion may exist without hypotension.[1]

PATHOPHYSIOLOGY OF POSTOPERATIVE SHOCK

Postoperative shock may be caused by any of the four pathophysiologic mechanisms of shock (either alone or in combination).[2]

Hypovolemic Shock

Hemorrhage is the commonest cause of postoperative shock and should always be considered in the differential diagnosis no matter what the timing of shock.

Pure fluid deficit causing hypovolemic shock in the absence of hemorrhage is rare. Patients with a pheochromocytoma are often very fluid depleted and may develop hypovolemic shock if they have not received adequate fluids during surgery. In other situations, a diagnosis of hypovolemic shock purely due to fluid depletion should be made with caution.

Vasodilatory Shock

Septic shock is probably the second most common cause of shock after surgery. The patient might be one who has undergone surgery for source control of an infective focus (such patients might temporarily deteriorate after surgery) or the patient might develop septic shock as a result of a surgical complication or due to a nosocomial infection.

Vasoplegia[3] is a condition where there is as low systemic vascular resistance and severe hypotension despite a high cardiac output and aggressive therapy with fluids and vasopressors. It is most often encountered after cardiac surgery but may occur after any major prolonged surgery. The mechanism of loss of vasomotor tone is most probably a severe inflammatory response.

Anaphylactic shock is a rare cause of postoperative shock but needs to be considered in patients with vasodilatory shock in whom the cause is obscure.

Hypoadrenalism is another rare cause of postsurgery shock and must be considered in patients with known adrenal insufficiency or in patients who have been taking prolonged courses of corticosteroids or in patients who have undergone adrenal or pituitary surgery.

Cardiogenic Shock

Myocardial dysfunction may be the primary cause of or may contribute to shock in patients who have undergone cardiac surgery. High-risk patients might develop a fresh myocardial ischemic event postoperatively and may end up with cardiogenic shock.

Obstructive Shock

Pulmonary embolism may cause shock any time in the postoperative period. Patients undergoing cancer surgery, or knee or hip replacements, are at the highest risk but no patient is exempt from this lethal complication. *Cardiac tamponade* may contribute to shock in patients who have undergone cardiac surgery. A *tension pneumothorax* may rarely cause shock in patients who have undergone cardiac or lung surgery.

The abdominal compartment syndrome (ACS) may be an under-recognized cause of shock especially in patients who have undergone surgery for trauma, abdominal aneurysms or other major abdominal surgery. ACS is more common in patients who have received aggressive resuscitation with crystalloids.

EVALUATION OF A PATIENT WITH POSTOPERATIVE SHOCK[4]

The initial evaluation of the patient who presents with shock after surgery is not much different from the assessment of any other patient with shock. Of course, resuscitation of the patient must go hand-in-hand with evaluation. The nature of surgery, the timing of shock, the patient's comorbidities, the presence of any accompanying symptoms (e.g. chest pain, dyspnea, fever), a general examination of the patient, an examination of the surgical site and a few simple investigations should enable the clinician to quickly diagnose the cause of shock in most cases.

For example, bleeding is the first consideration in a patient who develops hypotension, cold extremities, pallor and a narrow pulse pressure immediately after cardiac surgery. Conversely, a patient who has hypotension, warm extremities and a bounding pulse post cardiac surgery most probably has vasoplegia. In a patient who develops shock 4 days after abdominal surgery with warm extremities and a bounding pulse, septic shock is the most likely cause. Pulmonary embolism is the most likely cause of shock in an obese patient who develops shock 6 days after a knee replacement. The presence of pulsus paradoxus leads to a suspicion of tamponade or ACS. Laboratory investigations, electrocardiography (ECG) and a chest X-ray may be helpful but an ultrasound examination (including echocardiography) is probably the single most important diagnostic tool.

UTILITY OF ULTRASONOGRAPHY FOR DIAGNOSIS OF SHOCK[5,6]

The ultrasound can reveal the volume depleted status of the patient and may reveal collections of blood at the surgical site confirming the diagnosis of hemorrhagic shock. The sonography may reveal collections of pus in abdomen in patients with suspected septic shock. The cardiac ultrasound revealing hypovolemia in bleeding patients will confirm a suspicion of tamponade, and will help to confirm or exclude the diagnosis of pulmonary embolism. The cardiac ultrasound will also help diagnose fresh myocardial dysfunction contributing to shock. A pneumothorax can be quickly excluded by lung ultrasound. The ultrasound also allows safe central venous access if necessary and helps to guide fluid resuscitation. More sophisticated hemodynamic tools are sometimes needed when combined causes of shock (for example, cardiogenic and septic) are suspected.

MANAGEMENT OF THE PATIENT WITH POSTOPERATIVE SHOCK

Hemorrhagic Shock[7]

A patient who has developed shock as a result of bleeding will almost certainly need definitive control of the source of bleeding. The patient will simultaneously need adequate resuscitation and correction of any coagulopathy. Under-resuscitation may contribute to organ dysfunction, especially in elderly patients with coexisting cardiac, neurologic or renal disease and with poor reserves, but may be tolerated well by younger healthier patients.

Over-resuscitation with crystalloids may also cause more harm than good. Aggressive crystalloid therapy may worsen coagulopathy by causing hypothermia, acidosis (with use of normal saline) and a dilutional coagulopathy. Intra-abdominal hypertension might also result from over-infusion of crystalloids. The targets of resuscitation, therefore, need to be tailored to each patient. Along with moderate doses of crystalloids, blood definitely needs to be transfused in patients with hemorrhagic shock. Blood transfusions are usually accompanied by platelet and plasma infusions to correct coagulopathy. Vasopressors may be administered to patients with hemorrhagic shock and very low blood pressures in order to maintain organ perfusion. Norepinephrine seems to be the vasopressor of choice for this purpose.

Coagulopathy is common after prolonged major surgery[8] and may be due to various causes—platelet dysfunction, effect of heparin, hypothermia and acidosis. Conventional tests of coagulation might be normal in the hypothermic patient and thromboelastography (TEG) provides a more accurate estimate of the need for specific blood products. All infused fluids must be warmed to prevent further hypothermia, and the bleeding hypothermic patient will need to be warmed because the coagulation cascade is not very effective in the presence of hypothermia. Acidosis needs to be corrected. Calcium might need to be supplemented in patients who have received a lot of blood products. Factor VII concentrates might be considered in those patients who continue to ooze from the surgical site in spite of correction of hypothermia, acidosis, and administration of blood products. Even if the patient has a coagulopathy, and if the bleeding is from only one source, it usually indicates that the patient needs definitive control of the bleeding source, the presence of a coagulopathy should therefore not lead to a delay in any procedure needed for definitive control of the bleeding (*coagulopathy needs to be corrected simultaneously, of course*).

Septic Shock

Septic shock might develop after surgery either as a result of a surgical complication leading to infection (especially abdominal or urologic surgery) or because of a nosocomially acquired pneumonia, urinary tract infection, or central line-related infection. The principles of management[9] are the same as those for any other patient with septic shock—appropriate cultures and imaging, adequate fluid resuscitation, vasopressors (norepinephrine is the vasopressor of choice), and early appropriate antibiotics. Source control is very important in the management of postoperative septic shock and all attempts must be made to detect and remove a potential focus of infection. In patients who have undergone abdominal surgery, a CT scan might be more sensitive than an ultrasound in detecting infected collections which might need drainage (radiologically or surgically).

Vasoplegic Shock[10]

It is fairly common after cardiac surgery but may occur after other major surgeries as well. Norepinephrine has traditionally been used as the initial vasopressor in this condition but many patients might need to be administered vasopressin infusions as well. Methylene blue has been recommended as salvage therapy for patients who are refractory to vasopressin. Recent anecdotal reports suggest that the addition of intravenous (IV) hydroxocobalamin to methylene blue might be even more effective.

Obstructive Shock

Massive pulmonary embolism can occur in any postsurgical patients, but the high-risk groups [hip and knee surgery, cancer surgery, obesity, previous history of deep vein thrombosis (DVT), etc.] are more vulnerable. The presence of new onset right ventricular (RV) dysfunction in a patient with shock is very suggestive of pulmonary embolism but ideally the diagnosis should be confirmed by a computed tomography pulmonary angiography (CTPA). Conversely, normal RV function in a patient with shock rules out pulmonary embolism as the cause of shock. Thrombolysis is generally contraindicated in postsurgical patients. Percutaneous catheter-guided clot extraction or surgical embolectomy are the options in the management of patients who have developed a massive pulmonary embolism after surgery.[11]

Cardiac tamponade: This is a serious complication of cardiac surgery and may need surgical intervention in up to 5% of cases. Cardiac tamponade usually presents within the first 24 hours after surgery; however, some patients may present late. Cardiac tamponade presents with rapid deterioration for which there is no other explanation. The chest tube drainage may suddenly cease. There may be a paradoxical pulse initially which is replaced by a narrow pulse pressure. Most cases occur in patients who have had substantial bleeding or were on anticoagulants. Echocardiography is the most useful method to diagnose cardiac tamponade. TEE may be required in the diagnosis of late tamponade. Immediate drainage of the pericardial fluid (sometimes in the ICU itself) is the only treatment.[12]

Abdominal compartment syndrome: Intra-abdominal pressures should be measured in patients who are at risk for ACS. Patients with ACS and shock will need urgent decompression.[13]

Cardiogenic Shock[14]

Patients undergoing coronary artery bypass grafting (CABG) may develop temporary worsening of cardiac function (probably due to myocardial stunning) leading to shock. High-risk patients undergoing major noncardiac surgery may develop a myocardial ischemic event after surgery and go on to develop cardiogenic shock. Norepinephrine is the vasopressor of choice in the patient with cardiogenic shock. More advanced hemodynamic monitoring might be needed in patients who do not respond because many of these patients have combined causes of shock. Patients who develop cardiogenic shock following noncardiac surgery may be taken up for early revascularization after weighing the pros and cons of revascularization in the early postoperative period. Patients who develop shock after CABG due to myocardial stunning and who do not respond to pharmacologic therapy are candidates for an intra-aortic balloon pump (IABP) or even extracorporeal membrane oxygenation (ECMO) because the stunning of the myocardium is likely to reverse soon.

SUMMARY

Some of the common causes of shock in the postoperative period (bleeding, vasoplegia, tamponade) are different from the usual causes of shock. The approach to the diagnosis and management, however, is not much different. Most cases of shock can be diagnosed and managed using a bit of clinical acumen, a few investigations (chiefly ultrasound) and lots of common sense.

REFERENCES

1. Vincent JL, De Backer D. Circulatory Shock. N Engl J Med. 2013;369:1726-34.

2. Weil MH, Shubin H. Proposed reclassification of shock states with special reference to distributive defects. Adv Exp Med Biol. 1971;23:13-23.

3. Lambden S, Creagh-Brown BC, Hunt J, Summers C, Forni LG. Definitions and pathophysiology of vasoplegic shock. Crit Care. 2018;22:174.

4. Kim AW, Maxhimer JB. Hypotension in the Postoperative Patient. In: Myers JA, Millikan KW, Saclarides TJ (Eds). Common Surgical Diseases. New York, NY: Springer; 2008.

5. Mok KL. Make it SIMPLE: enhanced shock management by focused cardiac ultrasound. J Intensive Care. 2016;4:51.

6. Perera P, Mailhot T, Riley D, Mandavia D. The RUSH exam: Rapid Ultrasound in SHock in the evaluation of the critically ill. Emerg Med Clin North Am. 2010;28:29-56.

7. Cannon JW. Hemorrhagic Shock. N Engl J Med. 2018;378:370-9.

8. Grottke O, Fries D, Nascimento B. Perioperatively acquired disorders of coagulation. Curr Opin Anaesthesiol. 2015;28:113-22.

9. Rhodes A, Evans LE, Alhazzani W, Levy MM, Antonelli M, Ferrer R, et al. **Surviving Sepsis Campaign: International** Guidelines for Management of Sepsis and Septic Shock: 2016. Intensive Care Med. 2017;43(3):304-77.

10. Busse LW, Barker N, Petersen C. Vasoplegic syndrome following cardiothoracic surgery—review of pathophysiology and update of treatment options. Crit Care. 2020;24(1):36.

11. Konstantinides SV, Meyer G, Becattini C, Bueno H, Geersing GJ, Harjola VP, et al. The Task Force for the diagnosis and management of acute pulmonary embolism of the European Society of Cardiology (ESC). Eur Heart J. 2020;41(4):543-603.

12. Carmona P1, Mateo E, Casanovas I, Peña JJ, Llagunes J, Aguar F, et al. Management of cardiac tamponade after cardiac surgery. J Cardiothorac Vasc Anesth. 2012;26(2):302-11.

13. Luckianow GM, Ellis M, Governale D, Kaplan LJ. Abdominal compartment syndrome: risk factors, diagnosis, and current therapy. Crit Care Res Pract. 2012;6:908169.

14. Lomivorotov VV, Efremov SM, Kirov MY, Fominskiy EV, Karaskov AM. Low cardiac-output syndrome after cardiac surgery. J Cardiothorac Vasc Anesth. 2017;31(1):291-308.

Fluid and Electrolyte Disturbances in the Perioperative Period

Kishore Mangal, Vaibhav Bhargava

INTRODUCTION

The stress of surgery and physiologic insult of the perioperative period may lead to a wide variety of fluid and electrolyte imbalances, which in turn can impact outcomes, especially in high-risk surgeries. As the aim of any fluid therapy is to restore or maintain fluid and electrolyte homeostasis in tissues and effective circulating blood volume, hence optimal fluid and electrolyte management is a cornerstone therapy of perioperative medicine.[1]

FLUID PHYSIOLOGY

Water is distributed into all compartments of body but the electrolyte content of these compartments is varied. So, the fluid infused in a patient is distributed according to the electrolyte component of the fluid.

Fluid Compartments

Total body water (TBW) content in an adult is around 60%, which may vary according to age, sex, and body composition. TBW is further divided into intra- and extracellular fluid (ECF) compartments. The intracellular component has around 55% of TBW and is largely regulated by movement of free water, whereas extracellular component has 45% and is regulated by movement of sodium. The extracellular volume can be subdivided into:

1. *Interstitial fluid (20%)*: Fluid occupying spaces in between cells and lymphatics.
2. *Intravascular fluid (7.5%)*: Plasma volume, including subglycocalyceal fluid.
3. *Transcellular fluid (2.5%)*: It is an important compartment with fluids of widely varying composition by being formed from the secretions of epithelial cells by epithelia-lined spaces and regulated by active cellular transport. It includes gastrointestinal (GI) tract fluid, bile, urine, cerebrospinal fluid, aqueous humor, joint fluid, and pleural, peritoneal, and pericardial fluid.

4. *Bone and connective tissue (15%)*: It contains 15% of total body fluid but they are slow to mobilize and largely nonfunctional ECF.[2]

Physiology of Fluid Movement

The movement of fluid and solutes in different compartments is governed by diffusion and osmosis. Diffusion is the process by which movement of solute occurs from high to low concentration. Osmosis is the movement of water through a semipermeable membrane (through which solute cannot move) to the side with higher solute concentration.

Osmotic pressure is the hydrostatic pressure required to resist the movement of solvent molecules. This pressure directly depends on the number rather than the type of osmotically active particles in a solution. The total osmotic pressure of plasma is approximately 5,545 mm Hg.

Oncotic pressure is the component of total osmotic pressure exerted by large-molecular-weight particles, predominantly proteins (albumin, globulins, and fibrinogen). Plasma oncotic pressure is 25–28 mm Hg. Albumin is responsible for 65–75% of plasma oncotic pressure.

Osmolality and osmolarity: Osmolality of the solution is the number of osmoles (each containing 6×10^{23} of any type of particle present) present in 1 kg of solvent, whereas osmolarity is number of osmoles in 1 L of solvent. Normal body osmolality is 285–290 mOsmol/kg and is the same in intracellular and extracellular compartments because of the free movement of water between compartments.

Tonicity: There are some osmoles which can move across cell membranes like urea and glucose and so are ineffective, whereas sodium and chloride do not cross and hence are effective osmotic force across these membranes. Tonicity is the effective osmolality of a solution with respect to a particular semipermeable membrane. It can be estimated by subtracting urea and glucose concentrations from measured osmolality. Tonicity is important in determining in vivo distribution of fluids across a cell membrane and is sensed by the hypothalamic osmoreceptors.[2]

STARLING'S PRINCIPLE AND ITS REVISION

Classic Starling's principle was expressed by the following equation:

$$J_v/A = L_p (P_c - P_i) - \sigma (\pi_c - \pi_i)$$

Where J_v/A is the filtration rate per area, L_p is the hydraulic conductance, P_c is the intravascular hydrostatic pressure, P_i is the interstitial hydrostatic pressure, σ is the osmotic reflection coefficient, π_c is the plasma oncotic pressure, and π_i is the interstitial oncotic pressure.

P_c is the force favoring filtration, whereas P_i and colloidal oncotic pressure gradient $(\pi_c - \pi_i)$ opposes filtration (P_{co}). The net fluid movement depends on a balance between these forces. Based on few assumptions, it was concluded that filtration of fluid predominates at the arteriolar end of capillaries, while absorption emerges at the venular end.[3]

However, this equation could not explain clinical and experimental observations. When better techniques became available, it was shown that P_c remains above P_{co} throughout the entirety of capillaries. So, no reabsorption takes place at venular end. Notable exception to this rule occurs in tissues like intestinal mucosa and kidneys.[2,3]

Another mismatched observation was the amount of fluid predicted to be filtered in lymphatics was found to be higher than actually filtered. This paradox was resolved with the introduction of the glycocalyx-cleft model. It appears now that colloid oncotic pressure is not transendothelial force per se, rather an intraendothelial force.[3,4]

Starling's principle was thus revised (**Fig. 1**) to the following:

$$J_v/A = L_p (P_c - P_i) - \sigma (\pi_c - \pi_{sg})$$

Where π_{sg} is the subglycocalyx oncotic pressure.

The endothelial glycocalyx layer (EGL) consists of various types of glycosaminoglycans covalently attached to plasma membrane-bound core proteoglycans. EGL repels other negatively charged molecules like red blood cell (RBC), white blood cell, and platelets and also acts as a sieve, restricting passage of molecules >70 kDa, mainly proteins. However, albumin is able to bind glycocalyx because it is amphoteric in nature and size is 67 kDa. Thus, a cell free and protein poor subglycocalyceal layer (SGL) is formed within the capillaries. SGL is part of intravascular volume, with content different from plasma, and may be as much as 1,700 mL. The SGL is in dynamic equilibrium with plasma and is essential for vascular homeostasis. It also helps in attenuation of leukocyte and platelet adhesion, binding of cytokines/chemokines, hormones, etc.[3-5]

Normally, π_{sg} is quite low, but this force is entirely within the capillary such that J_v across the endothelium is

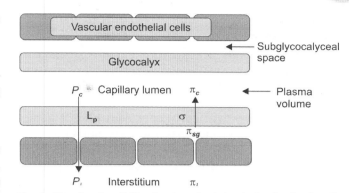

Fig. 1: The "revised" Starling's principle. L_p is the hydraulic conductance, P_c is the intravascular hydrostatic pressure, P_i is the interstitial hydrostatic pressure, σ is the osmotic reflection coefficient, π_c is the plasma oncotic pressure, π_i is the interstitial oncotic pressure and π_{sg} is the subglycocalyx oncotic pressure.

dependent on P_c and P_i, and colloid osmotic pressure (COP) across glycocalyx $(\pi_c - \pi_{sg})$ simply retards filtration.[5,6]

Clinical Relevance of Revised Starling's Equation

- Intravascular volume comprises circulating RBC volume, plasma volume and glycocalyx volume instead of only plasma and cellular elements.
- During steady state, ultrafiltrate is produced due to filtration across glycocalyx and no venous reabsorption occurs at the venous end.
- Lymph forms the major route for removal of the fluid from the interstitial space and return into circulation.
- Artificially raising COP by infusing colloids may reduce filtration but will not lead to reabsorption of fluid from the interstitium into the plasma. Thus, administering exogenous albumin or other colloids neither reduce peripheral or pulmonary edema, nor improve overall outcomes in sepsis.
- Acutely reduced capillary pressure (e.g., acute hemorrhage) can result in transient absorption of fluid to the plasma volume, up to approximately 500 mL of autotransfusion. This exception to no reabsorption rule, though remains for few minutes only.[3]
- *Intravascular effects of crystalloids and colloids*: If capillary pressures (P_c) remain low (e.g., hypovolemic shock) beyond autotransfusion, filtration (J_v) will approach zero, and ongoing reabsorption does not occur. Infusion of fluids in this context (with J_v close to zero) will remain intravascular until capillary pressure rises to normal or supranormal levels. Thus, colloids will expand plasma volume only and not SGL, but crystalloid will expand both plasma and SGL volume. This may help in explaining why during early resuscitation phase, intravascular volume effect of isotonic crystalloid is

similar to those from isotonic colloid in the ratio 1:1.5 rather than the predicted 1:3.

On the other hand, at supranormal capillary pressures, fluid infusion will further raise capillary pressures and thus filtration. Though colloids, by nature, maintain the oncotic pressure, crystalloids decrease oncotic pressure, hence filtration will increase to a greater extent with crystalloids and thus will result in lower half-life of crystalloids.[2,7]

PATHOPHYSIOLOGICAL CHANGES DURING PERIOPERATIVE PERIOD

Perioperatively, fluid homeostasis can be altered by several mechanisms. Different stages of perioperative period bring different challenges for the anesthesiologist. The central goal in the management of patient remains maintenance of fluid and electrolyte balance with avoiding both excess and deficiency of them.

Preoperative Period

Preoperative fasting strategies should not only aim to reduce the risk of aspiration, but also emphasize that the patient arriving in the operating room is not in a hypovolemic or dehydrated state. The effects of preoperative fasting on fluid balance have perhaps been overstated, with studies showing that despite overnight fasting, healthy volunteers remain normovolemic.[8] Still careful assessment of volume status must be made in patients with bowel obstruction, ongoing bleed, on chronic diuretic therapy, ongoing sepsis or who have received mechanical bowel preparation. More severe abnormalities can be seen in acutely ill patients. These patients might require appropriate intravenous (IV) fluid and electrolyte replacement preoperatively. On the other hand, patients of end-stage renal disease dependent on dialysis for fluid removal, the timing of dialysis relative to surgery is critical in preoperative stabilization.[9]

Intraoperative Period

This is a period where maximum manipulation in hemodynamics occurs and several factors can be responsible for instability.

Anesthesia-related Factors

1. Most drugs used for induction or maintenance of anesthesia may cause dose-dependent vasodilation and myocardial depression that may lead to hypotension. Thus, carefully avoiding unnecessary deep anesthesia may avoid the problem.
2. Sympathetic blockade during neuraxial anesthesia results in increased venous capacitance and dilation of arteriolar resistance vessels, leading to relative hypovolemia, with resultant hypotension.

Based on these two factors, prophylactic administration of fluids has long been advocated to counteract this hypotension. However, this practice cannot be recommended, due to role of EGL and studies also refute efficacy of this practice.[4,5]

3. *Avoiding hypervolemia*: Hypervolemia can result in the shedding of the EGL, which is induced by the release of atrial natriuretic peptide, due to atrial stretch. This can result in interstitial space edema.[10]

Surgery-related Factors

1. Major surgery involves tissue insult which induces an inflammatory response that results in vasodilatation and favors redistribution of fluid from the intravascular to the extracellular compartment.
2. *Leaking to interstitial space*: Inflammatory response during surgery, alters EGL, leading to pathological shifting of protein-rich fluid crossing vascular endothelial barrier.[6]

   Contemporary surgery, often with minimal access or laparoscopically assisted, probably triggers much less physiological stress response and thus lesser fluids shifting can be expected with newer techniques.
3. *Third space loss*: The third space is a term for spaces in which body fluids lose their function to affect fluid balance between intravascular and extravascular compartments, i.e., nonfunctional ECV. Older studies attempted to show significant third space fluid loss following trauma or surgery, but improved methodology proved that functional ECV levels do not decrease in or after surgery. Thus, concept of third space loss of fluid has been rebutted.[6,11-13]
4. *Hemorrhage*: There can be direct volume loss due to bleeding during surgery.
5. *Insensible losses*: Major laparotomies can lead to exposure of organs, especially intestines to operating room environment leading to perioperative deficits and insensible losses. This fluid loss is measured at 0.5–1.0 mL/kg/h during major abdominal surgery.[1,6,14]
6. *Urine output*: Perioperative oliguria is commonly interpreted as hypovolemia and prompts infusion of yet more sodium-containing fluids. However, in the absence of complications, it is usually a normal physiological stress response to surgery due to increased secretion of hormones like vasopressin, catecholamines and the renin-angiotensin-aldosterone system (RAAS). Thus, clinical evaluation, and in severe cases, invasive monitoring must be done to determine whether the oliguric patient has significant intravascular hypovolemia needing treatment and avoid unnecessarily side effects of fluids.[10,11]

Table 1: Composition of common crystalloids.

Fluid	Plasma	0.9% NaCl	5% dextrose	Lactated Ringer's	PlasmaLyte 148	Sterofundin ISO
Sodium (mmol/L)	135–145	154	0	130	140	145
Potassium (mmol/L)	3.5–5.0	0	0	4	5	4
Chloride (mmol/L)	98–106	154	0	109	98	127
Calcium (mmol/L)	2.2–2.6	0	0	1.5	0	2.5
Magnesium (mmol/L)	0.8–1.0	0	0	0	1.5	1
Bicarbonate (mmol/L)	24	0	0	0	0	0
Lactate (mmol/L)	1	0	0	28	0	0
Acetate (mmol/L)	0	0	0	0	27	24
Gluconate (mmol/L)	0	0	0	0	23	0
Malate (mmol/L)	0	0	0	0	0	5
Glucose	3.5–5.5	0	50 g	0	0	0
Osmolarity (mOsm/L)	291	308	278	273	294	309
Actual osmolality (mOsmol/kg H$_2$O) or tonicity	287	286	Very low	256	271	290
Strong ion difference (SID)	42	0	0	28	47	37
pH	7.35–7.45	6	4.5	6.5	4–6.5	5.1–5.9

Postoperative Period

An underappreciated facet of perioperative care is that much of the fluid that patients receive during a surgical admission is delivered postoperatively.[12]

Postoperative fluid therapy is primarily determined by events in pre- and intraoperative periods, along with systemic inflammation, immune response, catabolic state and need for increased substrate delivery to tissue for healing. Replacement of ongoing losses from hemorrhage, sepsis, GI tract and others must be done. Intraoperative antidiuretic hormone (ADH) release and RAAS activation lead to postoperative retention of water and salt.

Thus, careful re-evaluation by clinical examination, close monitoring and laboratory valuation must be done for their hemodynamic and fluid status. Early oral intake is recommended. Maintenance postoperative fluid should generally be salt poor and contain a modest volume of free water and should be able to replace electrolyte requirement.[2,9,13]

COMPOSITION OF FLUID THERAPY: CRYSTALLOIDS AND COLLOIDS

Crystalloids

Crystalloids are fluids that contain crystal-forming elements, i.e., electrolytes. Crystalloids can be classified by their composition and osmolality.

Normal saline (NS) or 0.9% saline: It is a widely used crystalloid over the globe. Although referred to as "normal", 0.9% saline is not physiologically "normal". Sodium and particularly chloride concentration are higher than plasma.

Strong ion difference (SID) of 0.9% saline is zero, whereas the SID of ECF is approximately 40 mEq/L. Thus, large volume of "NS" may lead to metabolic acidosis and hyperchloremia. It is often regarded as slightly hypertonic solution at 308 mOsmol/L, but in vivo, it is isotonic. Sodium and chloride are partially active with a coefficient 0.926, which means effective tonicity is 285 mOsmol/kg of water, equal to plasma.[15]

Balanced salt solutions: Buffered/balanced crystalloids have additional cations (potassium, calcium, magnesium) and anions, such as lactate, acetate, gluconate and/or malate, acting as physiological buffers to generate bicarbonate. The SID of these various fluids is also comparable to ECF.[15] **(Table 1)**.

Ringer's lactate is hypotonic solution with a calculated in vivo osmolality (tonicity) of approximately 254 mOsmol/kg of water. Their use can lead to significant free water load leading positive fluid balance and are contraindicated in patients at risk of cerebral edema.[15,16]

PlasmaLyte is the most balanced isotonic electrolyte solution and has an osmolality of 294 mOsmol and tonicity of around 271. It aims to mimic "normal physiology" as much as possible. It contains both acetate and gluconate as buffers.

Dextrose solutions: They have a very limited role perioperatively. Since it is a hypotonic solution with very large volume of distribution and negligible effect on plasma expansion, it is mainly used as maintenance solution rather than resuscitation fluid.[11]

Crystalloid selection should be based upon individual patient need with clinical consideration of osmolality, ionic composition, and pH. Balanced salt solutions are increasingly recommended as a pragmatic initial resuscitation fluid for the majority of acutely ill patients, 0.9% saline is recommended in patients with alkalosis and in patients with traumatic brain injury.[16]

Colloids

Colloids are human plasma derivatives (e.g., human albumin, fresh frozen plasma) or semisynthetic preparations [e.g., hydroxyethyl starch (HES), gelatins]. They are dissolved in either isotonic saline or with a balanced salt solution. They exert a COP across the microvascular tissue barrier and retain fluid in the intravascular bed. The only rational indication for a colloid is acute intravascular hypovolemia.[17]

Albumin: Isotonic human albumin (4–5%) in saline is considered to be the standard colloidal solution, as plasma albumin is majorly responsible for intravascular osmotic pressure. It is manufactured by the fractionation of blood and is heat treated to prevent transmission of pathogenic viruses. It is available in different concentrations like 5% and 25% solutions or in some parts of the world, as 4% and 20% solutions. Despite being more expensive than other solutions, and it has not been shown to be safer or more efficacious than synthetic colloids (e.g., HES) or balanced crystalloid solutions. In a trial, 4% albumin solution was harmful for patients with increased intracranial pressure.[16]

Hydroxyethyl starches: HES solutions are most commonly used semisynthetic colloids, identified by three numbers corresponding to concentration, molecular weight, and molar substitution. A high degree of molar substitution helps in prolonging intravascular time by protection from amylases in blood, but it also increases risk of HES-induced renal toxicity. Various trials on HES in critically ill patient population have showed higher risk of acute kidney injury. However, the results cannot be directly extrapolated to surgical population, as the duration and quantity of HES usage in perioperative period is limited. Thus, despite warning, starches continue to be used perioperatively, but its use must be avoided in patients with sepsis and renal dysfunction.[1,16]

Other semisynthetic colloids include succinylated gelatin, polygeline preparations, and dextran solutions. There is no evidence to support these colloids.[7,18]

PERIOPERATIVE ELECTROLYTE DISTURBANCES

In order to understand the regulating mechanism of electrolyte homeostasis, we have extracellular and intracellular compartments. Sodium (Na^+), chloride (Cl^-), calcium (Ca^{2+}), and bicarbonate (HCO_3^-) are mainly present in extracellular space, whereas potassium (K^+), phosphate (PO_4^{3-}), magnesium (Mg^{2+}), and proteins are in intracellular compartments. Understanding of basic physiology is essential for good perioperative electrolyte management.

Sodium

Sodium, known to be principal extracellular cation and solute, is essential for generating action potential in neurological and cardiac tissues.[19] Daily ingestion has wide range of 50–300 mEq/day. Normal plasma sodium concentration is 135–145 mEq/L. Sodium and its accompanying anions are responsible for maintaining 87% of plasma osmolality. Normal plasma osmolality is 285–295 mOsmol/kg. It is calculated by $2 \times (Na^+ + K^+) + (BUN/2.8) + (glucose/18)$.[20] Sodium balance is related to ECF volume and water balance. Disorders of sodium, hyponatremia and hypernatremia, result mainly because of excess or deficit of water, respectively. There is hypothalamo-renal feedback mechanism to maintain the serum sodium concentration in narrow range. With rise in serum sodium, osmoreceptors in hypothalamus respond by signaling the posterior pituitary gland to secrete the ADH also called vasopressin.[21] ADH acts on renal collecting duct, via V_2 receptors, to increase water permeability, which leads to antidiuresis hence called as ADH. This leads to increase in blood volume increases and brings back sodium to normal which further turn off osmoreceptors in hypothalamus.[22]

Hyponatremia

Defined as serum sodium concentration <135 mEq/L. It can lead to wide spectrum of clinical symptoms, from subtle to life-threatening. It is associated with increased mortality, morbidity, and increased hospital stay.

Classification of hyponatremia:[23]
1. *Based on biochemical severity*:
    a. *Mild*: Serum sodium between 130 and 135 mEq/L
    b. *Moderate*: Serum sodium between 125 and 129 mEq/L
    c. *Severe*: Serum sodium <125 mEq/L.
2. *Based on time of development*:
    a. *Acute*: Hyponatremia that exists for <48 hours.
    b. *Chronic*: Hyponatremia that exists for at least 48 hours.
3. *Based on symptoms*:
    a. *Moderately severe symptomatic hyponatremia*: It is associated with symptoms like nausea without vomiting, confusion and headache.
    b. *Severely symptomatic hyponatremia*: It is associated with symptoms like vomiting, cardiorespiratory distress, abnormal and deep somnolence, seizures, coma [Glasgow Coma Scale (GCS) ≤8].

Flowchart 1: Evaluation of hyponatremia.

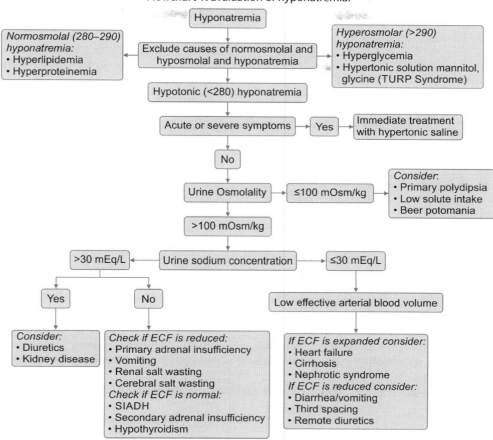

(ECF: extracellular fluid; SIADH: syndrome of inappropriate antidiuretic hormone)

Evaluation of hyponatremia: The evaluation of hyponatremia has been shown in **Flowchart 1**.

Etiologies of special importance:

1. *Transurethral resection of the prostate (TURP) syndrome*: During TURP procedure, the prostatic tissue is resected in small strips using diathermy loops. The bladder is continuously irrigated with irrigating fluid to allow direct vision and to wash away blood and debris. Glycine 1.5% (osmolality 220 mOsmol/kg) is most commonly used as irrigation fluid, and is hyposmolal to plasma, leading to hyponatremia and affect central nervous system (CNS). Acute hyponatremia is initially produced by dilutional effect of large volume of absorbed irrigation fluid but later caused by natriuresis. Since, hyposmolality is more important than hyponatremia in CNS disturbance, patients who are hyponatremic but normosmolal are likely to be asymptomatic, hence no intervention is required to correct Na⁺. Rapid correction of hyponatremia may lead to cerebropontine-myelinolysis. Approximately 10–15% of TURP procedures may be complicated by this syndrome within 15 minutes to 24 hours of onset of resection. Risk factors include prolong resection, high intravesical pressure, hypotonic irrigants, and open prostatic sinuses.

Measures to prevent TURP syndrome:
- The use of isotonic conducting irrigants like saline with bipolar diathermy.[24]
- Close monitoring of duration of surgery and amount of fluid absorbed. Terminate surgery if > 2,000 mL has been absorbed.[2,25,26]
- Limiting intravesical pressure to <15–25 mm Hg.
- Monitoring the patient's neurologic status by using regional anesthetic techniques.

2. *Syndrome of inappropriate antidiuretic hormone (SIADH)*: Underlying cause of SIADH is nonosmotic vasopressin secretion from posterior pituitary or ectopic source. These patients are euvolemic, so true or perceived volume deficit is not the cause of high ADH secretion.

Common causes:
- CNS related
- Infections

- Bleed
- Mass
- Hydrocephalus
- Carcinomas
- Lung (small cell, mesothelioma)
- Gastrointestinal (stomach, duodenum, pancreas)
- Genitourinary (prostate, endometrial)
- Pulmonary
- Infection
- Cystic fibrosis
- Asthma
- Drugs [valproate, selective serotonin reuptake inhibitors (SSRIs)]

Diagnostic criteria:

- Urine osmolality greater than plasma osmolality
- Serum osmolality <275 mOsmol/kg
- Euvolemia in clinical examination
- In the setting of normal sodium dietary intake, urine sodium >20 mEq/L
- Normal renal, thyroid, cardiac, and adrenal function
- No recent use of diuretics.

3. *Postoperative hyponatremia*: Postoperatively, at least 4% patients experience sodium below 130 mEq/L. Although neurological manifestations usually do not accompany mild postoperative hyponatremia, signs of hypervolemia are occasionally present. Postoperative hyponatremia is usually attributable to IV administration of hypotonic fluids, secretion of ADH hormone, drugs and altered renal function. If ADH is persistently increased, hyponatremia can develop even with administration of isotonic fluids. Women appear to be more vulnerable than men. Premenopausal women are more vulnerable than postmenopausal women for brain damage secondary to postoperative hyponatremia.[27]

4. *Cerebral salt-wasting syndrome*: Central nervous system (CNS) trauma (especially subarachnoid hemorrhage) and neurosurgery may lead to enhanced release of brain natriuretic peptide or loss of renal sympathetic tone. Increased sodium loss encourages volume depletion which leads to nonosmotic release of ADH. Hypovolemia or volume depletion is the main feature differentiating cerebral salt wasting (CSW) from SIADH. Hyponatremia does not get corrected with fluid resuscitation perhaps because of concomitant ADH release from the damaged brain.

Treatment of hyponatremia:

1. *Symptomatic hyponatremia*: In patients with moderate symptoms like confusion, lethargy and nausea, 3% saline can be used at an initial rate of 1 mL/kg/h with the goal of increasing Na+ by 1 mEq/L/h for initial 3–4 hours, after which electrolytes should be rechecked.

The Adrogue–Madias equation can be used to estimate expected change in sodium after 1 L of infusion. The equation is:

$$\text{Change in serum Na}^+ = [(\text{Infusate Na}^+ + \text{infusate K}^+) - \text{Serum Na}^+]/(\text{Total body water (kg)} + 1)$$

This anticipated change can be spread over number of hours to prevent rapid correction. This equation does not take into account ongoing urinary losses and is notoriously inaccurate. The infusion rate should be modified to ensure that Na+ is increased by no >10 mEq/L in the first 24 hours of treatment. Electrolytes and osmolality should be rechecked initially may be every 1–2 hours, later on every 6 hourly.

For severe hyponatremia with symptoms like coma and seizures and sodium <120 mEq/L, bolus of 100 mL of 3% saline should be given with the aim of increasing sodium by 2–3 mEq/L. If unsuccessful, it may be repeated once or twice at 10 minutes interval. Otherwise treatment remains same as for moderately symptomatic hyponatremia.

2. *Chronic, asymptomatic hyponatremia*: No acute intervention for asymptomatic hyponatremia is required. Always treat the underlying cause. Fluid restriction, loop diuretics, and ADH antagonists (lithium, demeclocycline) can be tried.

3. *Hypovolemic hyponatremia*: Symptoms are unusual. ECF volume should be restored with isotonic saline, which will also reduce ongoing ADH release.

4. *Hypervolemic hyponatremia*: Focus on restricted water intake and optimization of underlying disease along with use of diuretics should be followed. Vaptan, a combined V_1a/V_2 receptor antagonist, has been approved for the treatment of euvolemic and hypervolemic hyponatremia.[28]

Hypernatremia

Hypernatremia is defined as serum sodium concentration >145 mEq/L. It is almost always result of relative water deficit. This is defined by water intake being less than water losses or deficiency of ADH or excessive salt intake. Major symptoms are thirst, confusion, neuromuscular excitability, seizures, and coma. In case of severe hypernatremia (Na+ >160 mEq/L), risk of mortality increases depending on the severity of the underlying disease process.[29,30]

Diabetes insipidus: It is caused by lack of ADH action with consequent failure to concentrate urine and excretion of large quantities of inappropriately dilute urine. There are two types of diabetes insipidus: (1) central and (2) nephrogenic.

- *Central diabetes insipidus*: It is characterized by decreased release of ADH, resulting in polyuria. Deficiency of ADH is caused by diseases which affect one or more below mentioned sites that are involved in ADH secretion.

– Hypothalamic osmoreceptors
– Supraoptic or paraventricular nuclei
– Superior portion of the supraoptic hypophyseal.

It is usually seen after subarachnoid hemorrhage, pituitary surgery, traumatic brain injury, and brainstem death.

- *Nephrogenic diabetes insipidus*: It is defined as decrease in urinary concentrating ability that results from resistance at the site of action of ADH. It may be collecting tubules, or interference with the countercurrent mechanism due to medullary injury. Nephrogenic diabetes insipidus may be found in renal disease or due to drugs like lithium, foscarnet, amphotericin B, demeclocycline.

Clinical features of hypernatremia: With acute hypernatremia, the rapid decrease in brain volume can cause rupture of the cerebral veins, leading to focal intracerebral and subarachnoid hemorrhages and possibly irreversible neurologic damage. Acute hypernatremia may also result in demyelinating brain lesions similar to those associated with overly rapid correction of chronic hyponatremia.[31-33] Important clinical features are lethargy, weakness, and irritability, and which may progress to twitching, seizures, and coma.

Diagnosis: Diagnosis of hypernatremia depends upon Na^+ concentration, intravascular volume status, and urinary osmolality. Diagnostic criteria for diabetes insipidus has an inappropriately dilute urine (urine osmolality < 800 mOsmol/kg) in combination with hypernatremia and high serum osmolality (>305 mOsmol/kg).

Evaluation of hypernatremia: The evaluation of hypernatremia has been shown in **Flowchart 2**.

Treatment: Treatment is decided as per intravascular volume status, but correction of the Na^+ concentration should not be >10 mEq/L/day. The Adrogue–Madias equation is also used for correcting hypernatremia.

1. *Hypovolemic hypernatremia*: Correction of the intravascular volume deficit with isotonic saline and correction of the underlying cause is main treatment. Then correction of the water deficit is to be done with 0.45% saline, 5% dextrose or enteral water to cover the deficit and ongoing losses.

2. *Euvolemic hypernatremia*: Use of 0.45% saline, 5% dextrose, or enteral water to replace the deficit and ongoing losses. In central diabetes insipidus, in which urine output is >250 mL/h and risk exists for hypovolemia, titrated IV doses of 0.4–1 µg desmopressin acetate or 5–40 µg desmopressin nasal puff twice daily should be given to reduce the urine output.

3. *Hypervolemic hypernatremia*: As patient is hypervolemic, stop giving exogenous Na^+, administer furosemide with 5% dextrose or free water enterally. Dialysis may be required in the presence of renal failure.

Potassium Disorders

Potassium (K^+) is the most abundant cation in the body. Of the total body potassium content [about 3,500 mmol (mEq)], 90% is sequestered within cells.[34] This compartmental distribution depends on active transport through the cell membrane by a sodium-potassium pump. Normal serum potassium level roughly lies between 3.6 and 5.0 mEq/L. Even loss of just 1% of total body potassium content seriously disturbs the potassium balance in body and results in profound physiologic changes.[35]

Hypokalemia and hyperkalemia are electrolyte disturbances which are caused by altered potassium intake or excretion, or transcellular shifts. Both types of

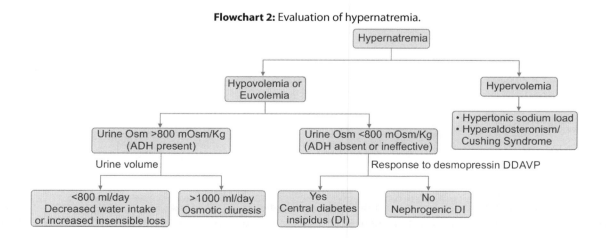

Flowchart 2: Evaluation of hypernatremia.

potassium disorders can lead to life-threatening cardiac conduction disturbances and neuromuscular dysfunction. Hence, they should be treated on priority basis through a combination of history, physical examination, laboratory, and electrocardiography (ECG) findings.[36] Although not uncommon, sampling artifacts in laboratory tests of K[+] also occur. Anticoagulated samples typically give results 0.4–0.5 mEq/L less than those from clotted samples because of erythrocyte K[+] release during clotting. Hemolysis also artificially increases K[+] levels and may be introduced by poor sampling technique or delayed processing of samples.

Hypokalemia

Patients with hypokalemia are often asymptomatic, particularly when it is mild hypokalemia (serum K[+] 3.0–3.5 mEq/L). With more severe hypokalemia, nonspecific symptoms, such as generalized weakness, lassitude, and constipation, are more common. When serum potassium decreases to <2.5 mEq/L, muscle necrosis (rhabdomyolysis) can occur, and at serum concentrations of <2.0 mEq/L, an ascending paralysis can develop, with eventual impairment of respiratory function. ECG does not correlate well with serum potassium levels but patient may have ST segment depression, T wave depression, U wave elevation and arrhythmias like atrial fibrillation and ventricular extrasystoles.

Hypokalemia can be the result of:
- Shifting of potassium into the cells
- Renal wasting
- Extrarenal losses.

Calculating the transtubular potassium gradient (TTKG) may help distinguish renal from extrarenal losses of potassium. It can be calculated by the formula

$$TTKG = (Urine\ K^+ \times Plasma\ osmolality)/(Plasma\ K^+ \times Urine\ osmolality)$$

Normal value range falls between 8 and 9. Levels < 3 reflect renal conservation and some extrarenal cause whereas levels > 3 suggest inappropriate renal wasting.

Evaluation of hypokalemia: The evaluation of hypokalemia has been shown in **Flowchart 3**.

1. *Transcellular shift*:
   - *Insulin*: It stimulates Na[+]/K[+]-ATPase thus driving to more potassium into the cell.
   - *Beta-2 agonist*: It acts via cyclic adenosine monophosphate (cAMP), stimulates Na[+]/K[+]-ATPase results in intracellular shifting.
   - *Alkalemia*: As extracellular pH goes up, cells will pump out H[+] ions to try to drive it back down. In order to neutralize the H[+] loss, potassium will move into the cell.
   - *Hypokalemic periodic paralysis*: After exercise or stress (things that cause insulin or catecholamine release), potassium suddenly moves into the cells, lowers plasma K[+] to 1.5–2.5 mEq/L.
2. *Renal wasting*:
   - Diuretics (loop and thiazides)—stimulate aldosterone via volume depletion, increasing distal Na[+] delivery and causing more potassium excretion. Blood pressure is normal or low.

Flowchart 3: Evaluation of hypokalemia.

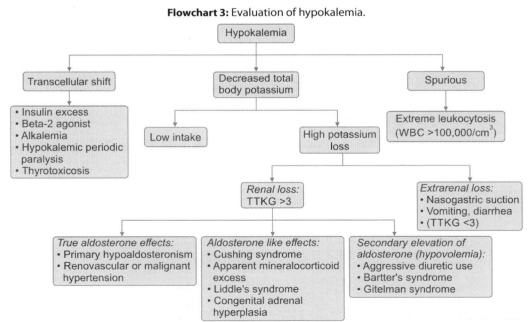

(WBC: white blood cell; TTKG: transtubular potassium gradient)

- Salt-wasting nephropathies—behave as diuretics, associated with hypotension, e.g., Bartter's syndrome, Gitelman's syndrome.
- Mineralocorticoid excess is associated with hypertension:
  - Primary hyperaldosteronism (adrenal tumor, bilateral hyperplasia)
  - Renovascular disease (renal artery stenosis)
  - Congenital adrenal hyperplasia
  - Liddle's syndrome
- *Renal tubular acidosis (RTA)*:
  - Distal hypokalemic RTA (type I)—defect in K^+/H^+ exchanger in the collecting duct; cannot reabsorb K^+—e.g., Sjögren's syndrome or rheumatoid arthritis
  - Proximal RTA (type II)—defect in bicarbonate reabsorption in the proximal tubule
- Hypokalemia occurs in 40–60% of cases of hypomagnesemia, so always correct Mg deficit to restore K^+.

3. *Gastrointestinal losses*:
- Vomiting and nasogastric tube output
  - Causes metabolic alkalosis due to loss of hydrochloric acid (HCl)
  - Potassium loss from emesis is 5–10 mEq/L
  - Aldosterone is activated due to volume loss; aldosterone increases sodium reabsorption and potassium secretion in the principal cells of the collecting duct.
  - Due to higher levels of bicarbonate, bicarbonate exceeds its reabsorption threshold in the proximal tubule; bicarbonate has a negative charge and pairs with Na^+, carrying more sodium to the distal nephron. High Na^+ concentration to the distal nephron increases Na^+ reabsorption distally but also increases potassium secretion.
- Diarrhea and laxatives
  - Causes normal anion gap metabolic acidosis due to loss of bicarbonate from the GI tract.

Treatment: Potassium replacement is the mainstay of treatment. Patients with hypokalemia may also have hypomagnesemia, which should be corrected simultaneously.

Mild-to-moderate hypokalemia:
- Serum potassium 3–3.4 mEq/L.
- *Treatment depends upon the cause of hypokalemia and acid-base status*:
  - *Patient with GI loss*:
    - *Treatment with potassium chloride*: In presence of metabolic alkalosis (vomiting) or with normal bicarbonate

- *Treatment with potassium citrate*: In presence of metabolic acidosis (diarrhea or RTA).
  - *Patient with renal loss*:
    - *Potassium sparing diuretic*: Spironolactone or eplerenone.

Severe hypokalemia:
- Serum potassium <2.5–3.0 mEq/L or symptomatic with arrhythmias, marked muscle weakness.
- Intravenous potassium chloride in nondextrose solutions with careful potassium monitoring. Rates as high as 40 mEq/h have been used for life-threatening hypokalemia. Rates above 20 mEq/h are highly irritating to peripheral veins and should be infused into a large central vein.

Hyperkalemia (Serum K^+ >5.5 mEq/L)

Three main mechanisms of hyperkalemia are (1) pseudohyperkalemia, (2) transcellular shift, and (3) reduced urinary excretion.

1. *Pseudohyperkalemia*:
   - Movement of K^+ out of the cells during or after drawing blood specimen
   - Occurs due to hemolysis (from technique during blood draw), thrombocytosis, or leukocytosis (acute leukemia)
2. *Transcellular shift*:
   - *Metabolic acidosis*: H^+ ions enter the cell to raise the extracellular pH; K^+ leaves the cell in order to maintain electroneutrality.
   - *Hyperglycemia and hyperosmolality*: As the serum osmolality increases, water moves from the intracellular fluid (ICF) to the ECF. This causes the intracellular potassium concentration to go up; some potassium will move down its concentration gradient to the ECF.
   - *Nonselective beta-blockers*: They interfere with K^+ uptake into the cell by beta-adrenergic receptors (prevent stimulation of the Na^+-K^+-ATPase).
   - *Tissue breakdown*: Rhabdomyolysis, postchemotherapy, and burns cause release of intracellular potassium into the ECF.
   - *Digitalis toxicity*: It inhibits the Na^+-K^+-ATPase pump.
   - *Hyperkalemic familial periodic paralysis*: Reasons are cold, fasting, rest after exercise, potassium ingestion (mutation in skeletal muscle Na^+ channel).
3. *Decreased urinary excretion*:
   - *Renal failure*: Serum potassium levels are maintained as long as both distal flow rate and aldosterone secretion are maintained. When distal flow rate decreases and potassium load is too high, hyperkalemia ensues.
   - Volume depletion with decreased distal delivery of sodium occurs during hypovolemia, effective arterial volume depletion with extracellular volume excess (liver cirrhosis with ascites, heart failure).

- *Functional hypoaldosteronism*: Either low aldosterone or aldosterone-resistant state
  - *Mineralocorticoid deficiency*: It occurs due to primary adrenal insufficiency (high renin, low aldosterone), or hyporeninemic hypoaldosteronism type IV RTA (low plasma renin, aldosterone levels; diabetic nephropathy).
  - *Tubulointerstitial diseases*: Sickle cell disease and urinary tract obstruction impair the Na^+ reabsorption in the principal cell, reducing K^+ and H^+ secretion (normal renin, high aldosterone).
- *Drugs*: Angiotensin-converting enzyme (ACE) inhibitors, angiotensin receptor blockers (ARBs), and aldosterone antagonists block conversion to aldosterone or binding to the aldosterone receptor. Nonsteroidal anti-inflammatory drugs (NSAIDs) decrease renin release. Amiloride, triamterene, trimethoprim, and pentamidine bind to the epithelial sodium channel (ENaC) channel in principal cells.

Clinical manifestations of hyperkalemia
- Muscle weakness or paralysis, ascending weakness (flaccid paralysis)
- *ECG abnormalities and cardiac arrhythmias:* Bundle branch block, advanced atrioventricular (AV) block, sinus bradycardia, sinus arrest, slow idioventricular rhythm, ventricular tachycardia and fibrillation, asystole
  - *Early changes*: tall peaked T waves, shortened QT interval
  - *Late ECG changes*: prolongation of PR and QRS interval, P wave may be lost with widened QRS, sine wave and finally flat line with asystole.

Diagnosis of hyperkalemia:
- Clinical history and physical examination
- Measure of plasma potassium in suspected pseudohyperkalemia
- Plasma renin activity and aldosterone concentration
- *Role of TTKG in identifying hypoaldosteronism as a cause for hyperkalemia*: Value <5, suggestive of hypoaldosteronism.

Evaluation of hyperkalemia: The evaluation of hyperkalemia has been shown in **Flowchart 4**.

Treatment of hyperkalemia: The treatment of hyperkalemia has been shown in **Table 2**.

Calcium

Calcium ions are most widely used intracellular messengers. Approximately 98% of calcium is stored in bone.

Normally, the level of calcium in the cell is very low (around 100 nM) with two main depots in the cell:
1. The ECF, where the concentration is ~ 2 mM or 20,000 times higher than in the cytosol
2. Endoplasmic reticulum ("sarcoplasmic" reticulum in skeletal muscle).
- *Calcium homeostasis*: Serum calcium homeostasis is maintained by largely by vitamin D and parathyroid hormone (PTH) in the range of 4.5 and 5 mEq/L or 2.2–2.5 mmol/L (8.5–10.5 mg/dL). Around 50% of circulating Ca^{2+} is in the biologically active ionized form (normal range 2–2.5 mEq/L or 1–1.5 mmol/L), 40% bound to

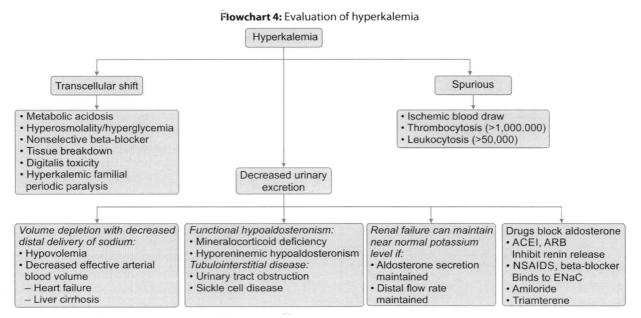

Flowchart 4: Evaluation of hyperkalemia

(ACEI: angiotensin-converting enzyme inhibitor; ARB: angiotensin receptor blocker; ENaC: epithelial sodium channel; NSAIDs: nonsteroidal anti-inflammatory drugs)

Table 2: Treatment of hyperkalemia.

Drug/therapy	Mechanism of action	Dose	Onset/duration	Amount of K^+ decline
Calcium gluconate or calcium chloride	Antagonize cardiac toxicity	1 g of 10% infused over 2–3 minutes	Immediate/30–60 min	None
Insulin	Intracellular potassium shift	10-unit regular insulin in D50	15 min/6–8 hours	Around 1 mEq/L
Albuterol	Intracellular potassium shift	10–20 mg by nebulization over 15 min	10–30 min/3–6 hours	Around 1–1.5 mEq/L
Sodium bicarbonate	Increase renal excretion	2–4 mEq/min in drip until bicarbonate normalizes	At 4 hours/>6 hours	0.5–0.75 mEq/L
Loop/thiazide diuretics	Increase renal excretion	Dose depends on glomerular filtration rate (GFR)	30–60 min/4–6 hours	Depends on diuretic response
Sodium polystyrene sulfonate	Gastrointestinal resin exchange	25–50 g mixed in 100 mL 20% sorbitol PO or 50 g in 200 mL 30% sorbitol per rectum	1–2 hours/4–6 hours	0.5–1 mEq/L
Hemodialysis	Extracorporeal removal	Based on starting potassium	Immediate/lasting until dialysis completion	Variable, based on dialysis dose and dialysate potassium

proteins, predominantly albumin and globulins, and 10% complexed to anions such as HCO_3^-, citrate, sulfate, PO_4^{3-}, and lactate.

Hypoalbuminemia decreases the total serum Ca^{2+} but has less effect on the ionized form. In order to calculate the corrected total Ca^{2+} concentration, 0.8 mg/dL is added per 1 g/dL decrease in albumin concentration below 4 g/dL.

- *Parathormone and calcium*: Hypercalcemia is sensed by the extracellular domain of a G-coupled receptor expressed on parathyroid cells (the Ca^{2+}/Mg^{2+}-sensing receptor), inhibiting PTH release.[37]

  Parathyroid hormone responds to hypocalcemia by:
  - Stimulating osteoclast bone resorption, releasing Ca^{2+} into the ECF
  - Stimulating distal tubule calcium reabsorption
  - Stimulating the renal conversion of 25-(OH)-vitamin D to 1,25-$(OH)_2$-vitamin D.
- *Vitamin D and Calcium*: Synthesis of active vitamin D involves cholecalciferol formation in the skin during exposure to ultraviolet light, which then undergoes hepatic hydroxylation to 25-hydroxycholecalciferol, then renal hydroxylation under the influence of PTH to 1,25-dihydroxycholecalciferol (calcitriol). As with PTH, calcitriol stimulates osteoclastic bone resorption and additionally stimulates absorption of Ca^{2+} from the GI tract.

Hypocalcemia

It is defined as corrected calcium <8.4 mg/dL or ionized calcium <2.1 mEq/L.

Causes of hypocalcemia: The causes of hypocalcemia are related to:

- *Reduced regulatory hormones*: Hypoparathyroidism, pseudohypoparathyroidism
- Vitamin D deficiency
- *Chelation*: Massive transfusion, pancreatitis, cell lysis
- Pseudohypocalcemia (reduced albumin bound calcium)
- *Increased bone deposition*: Prostate and breast cancer.

Clinical features: The clinical features of hypocalcemia are mainly related to cardiac and neuromuscular systems.

- *Cardiac*: Impaired inotropy, prolonged QT, ventricular fibrillation and heart block
- *Neuromuscular*: Circumoral or distal paresthesias, tetany, muscle cramps, laryngospasm, Chvostek's sign (facial twitching induced by tapping on the facial nerve), Trousseau's sign (forearm muscular spasm induced by inflating a pressure cuff), seizures.

Calcium ion plays very important role in coagulation. Coagulopathy attributable to hypocalcemia occurs only at ionized Ca^{2+} concentrations <1.2 mEq/L. In this situation, supplemental Ca^{2+} should be given to support cardiac inotropy and neuromuscular function, targeted for ionized Ca^{2+} >1.8 mEq/L.[38]

After parathyroidectomy, Ca^{2+} levels should be checked more frequently until they are stabilized. Vitamin D and Ca^{2+} supplementation may be required in both the short and long term.

Evaluation of hypocalcemia: The evaluation of hypocalcemia has been shown in **Flowchart 5**.

Treatment of hypocalcemia: In critically ill patients, total Ca^{2+} levels may be reduced because of hypoalbuminemia. Ca^{2+} supplementation should be required only if the ionized levels are low.

Flowchart 5: Evaluation of hypocalcemia.

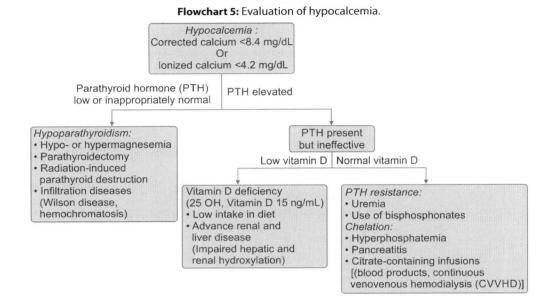

If ECG changes or neuromuscular symptoms are present:

- Injection calcium gluconate (10%) or injection calcium chloride (10%) can be given over 10 minutes. Calcium gluconate is preferred for peripheral administration due to less tissue injury on inadvertent extravasation.
- *Continuous calcium infusion*: 6 g diluted in 500 mL of 5% dextrose or saline infuse at 1 mg elemental calcium/kg/h.
- Follow ionized calcium or corrected calcium until calcium normalizes.
- 1–2 g of elemental calcium PO TID, separate from meals.
- Bolus 2 g magnesium sulfate IV over 15 minutes if hypomagnesemia present or empirically if renal function is normal.
- Add calcitriol in vitamin D deficient states.

Hypercalcemia

It is defined as corrected calcium >10.3 mg/dL or ionized calcium >2.6 mEq/L.

Causes of hypercalcemia

- *Bone resorption:*
  - *Primary hyperparathyroidism*: It is caused by tumor within the parathyroid gland. Parathyroid adenoma is most common reason.
  - *Secondary hyperparathyroidism*: Excessive secretion of parathormone in response to hypocalcemia with hyperplasia of these glands, e.g., severe kidney disease.
  - *Tertiary hyperparathyroidism*: State of excessive secretion of parathormone after a long period of secondary hyperparathyroidism which causes hypercalcemia. It occurs most commonly after renal transplant.
- *Malignancy*: Cause hypercalcemia through production of PTH like substance [PTH-related protein (PTHrP)]

or lytic destruction of bone with release of calcium into circulation.

- *Thyrotoxicosis*: Thyroid mediated increase in bone resorption
- Vitamin D intoxication
- Granulomatous disease (sarcoidosis)
- *Other less common causes:*
  - Immobilization
  - Paget's disease
  - Hypervitaminosis A
  - Acromegaly
  - Milk-alkali syndrome
  - Thiazide diuretics
  - Adrenal insufficiency.

Clinical manifestations:

- *Mild hypercalcemia (calcium <12 mg/dL)*: It may be asymptomatic, or may have nonspecific symptoms, such as constipation, fatigue, and depression.
- *Moderate hypercalcemia (calcium 12–14 mg/dL)*: It may be well tolerated chronically, while an acute rise to these concentrations may cause marked symptoms, including polyuria, polydipsia, dehydration, anorexia, nausea, muscle weakness, and changes in sensorium. ECG changes reveal short QT interval or variable degree AV block.
- *Severe hypercalcemia (calcium >14 mg/dL)*: Progression of above-mentioned symptom.

Evaluation of hypercalcemia: The evaluation of hypercalcemia has been shown in **Flowchart 6**.

Treatment of hypercalcemia: The treatment of hypercalcemia has been shown in **Table 3**.

Flowchart 6: Evaluation of hypercalcemia.

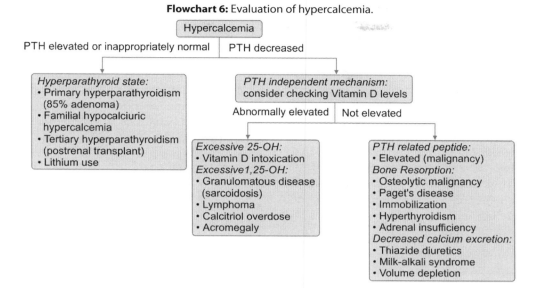

Table 3: Treatment of hypercalcemia.

Treatment	Mechanism of action	Dose	Onset/duration
Isotonic saline	Promotes calcium excretion	Bolus until euvolemia, then adjust to achieve U/O 100–150 mL/h	2–4 hours
Calcitonin	Increases renal calcium excretion and decreases bone resorption	4–8 IU/kg IM or SC q6-12 hours	4–6 hours/tachyphylaxis at 2–3 days
Bisphosphonates	Inhibit calcium release from bones	• Zoledronate 4 mg IV over at least 15 minutes • Pamidronate 60–90 mg IV over 2–4 hours	Onset after 2 days, peak effects at 4–6 days/lasts 2–4 weeks
Prednisolone (in granulomatous disease, e.g., sarcoidosis)	Decreases calcitriol production by the activated mononuclear cells in the lung and lymph nodes	20–40 mg/day	Onset in 5–10 days
Denosumab (zoledronate failure or contraindicated)	Prevent development of osteoclast	60–120 mg SC	Onset in 3 days, half-life of 25 days
Hemodialysis	Extracorporeal removal of calcium	Variable, based on starting calcium	Immediate onset, last till dialysis completion

General guidelines:
1. Always correct volume depletion first, with isotonic NS.
2. If ECG changes are present, begin with most rapid-acting therapies in combination (NS and calcitonin).
3. If rapid improvement is not seen, consider adding long-acting treatment (bisphosphonates) early.

Magnesium

Around 50% of magnesium is in bone and, 20% is in muscle, and the rest in heart, liver and other tissues. Only 1% is within the ECF, and normal plasma levels may be maintained in the face of total body Mg^{2+} depletion. Within the plasma, total Mg^{2+} concentration is 1.5–2.1 mEq/L, of which approximately 25% is mainly albumin bound, 65% is in the biologically active ionized form and the remainder is complexed to phosphates, citrates, and other anions.[39]

Magnesium is responsible for three main cellular functions:[2]
1. *Ion transport*: Mg^{2+} supports the activity of ion-pumping ATPases through which it helps in maintaining normal transmembrane electrochemical gradients which is responsible for effectively stabilizing cell membranes and organelles. Mg^{2+} has physiologic competitive antagonism with Ca^{2+} which is mediated through inhibition of L-type Ca^{2+} channels and extracellular local modification of membrane potential, preventing the intracytoplasmic influx of Ca^{2+} from both the ECF and within intracellular sarcoplasmic reticulum stores. Mg^{2+} also antagonizes N-methyl-D-aspartate

(NMDA) receptors within the CNS which reduces Ca^{2+} entry by specific ion channels. This results in inhibition of excitable tissue cellular actions, including neurotransmitter release, muscular contraction, cardiac pacemaker and action potential activity, and pain signal transmission.

2. *Nucleotide and protein production*: Mg^{2+} acts as a cofactor in every step of DNA transcription and replication and also in translation of messenger RNA.
3. *Energy metabolism*: Mg^{2+} is required for ATP phosphorylation reactions.

Unlike calcium and phosphorus, no hormonal feedback mechanism controls Mg^{2+} balance. The main determinant which influences the Mg^{2+} balance is Mg^{2+} itself. Hypomagnesemia stimulates renal tubular resorption of Mg^{2+} and hypermagnesemia inhibits this process.

Hypomagnesemia

Hypomagnesemia most commonly occurs in intensive care unit (ICU) settings. Symptoms of hypomagnesemia usually do not occur until Mg^{2+} is <1 mEq/L. Common manifestations are confusion, ataxia, lethargy, nystagmus, fasciculations, tremors, tetany, and seizures. Atrial and ventricular arrhythmias may be found, especially in patients on digoxin. ECG may show prolonged PR and QT intervals with wide QRS waves. Torsades de pointes is classically associated with hypomagnesemia. Hypomagnesemia is often associated with hypocalcemia (both lower down parathormone secretion) and hypokalemia (due to urinary potassium wasting). Urinary losses in renal wasting have a fractional excretion of Mg^{2+} > 2%. This is calculated by:

$$\text{Urine } Mg^{2+} \times \text{Serum creatinine}/0.7 \times \text{Serum } Mg^{2+} \times \text{Urine creatinine}$$

There are three main mechanisms of hypomagnesemia:
1. Renal wasting
2. Extrarenal loss
3. Chelation.

Evaluation of hypomagnesemia: The evaluation of hypomagnesemia has been shown in **Flowchart 7**.

Treatment of hypomagnesemia: The route of Mg^{2+} replacement depends upon clinical manifestations of Mg^{2+} deficiency and not on actual Mg^{2+} levels. Oral supplementation should be preferred in asymptomatic or without ECG changes as IV supplementation stimulates renal Ca^{2+}/Mg^{2+} sensing receptor, reducing Mg^{2+} reabsorption and leading to renal excretion of much of the acute dose. Replacement dosage should be reduced in renal insufficiency.

- *Patients who are asymptomatic and without ECG changes*:
  - *Mild hypomagnesemia*: 240 mg elemental Mg^{2+} per oral per day in divided doses
  - *Severe hypomagnesemia*: up to 720 mg elemental Mg^{2+} per oral per day in divided doses
  - *If per oral is not possible or in case of diarrhea*: 2–6 mg IV $MgSO_4$ infused at 1 g/h or less.
- *Patients with ECG changes or symptomatic*:
  - 1–2 g $MgSO_4$ IV over 15 minutes, followed by infusion of 6 g in 1 L of NS over 24 hours
  - Continuous infusion may be required for 3–7 days to replenish total body stores. Measure frequently and target <2.5 mEq/L.
- For chronic hypomagnesemia from renal wasting, consider high-dose amiloride.

Hypermagnesemia

The Mg^{2+} has limited GI absorption and increased renal excretion, so rise in Mg^{2+} is commonly iatrogenic. Symptoms are typically seen if serum Mg^{2+} levels >4 mEq/L (1 mEq/L = 2.36 mg/dL) and system involvement is level-dependent.

- *Serum levels 5–7 mg/dL*: Therapeutic required for treatment of preeclampsia

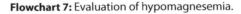

Flowchart 7: Evaluation of hypomagnesemia.

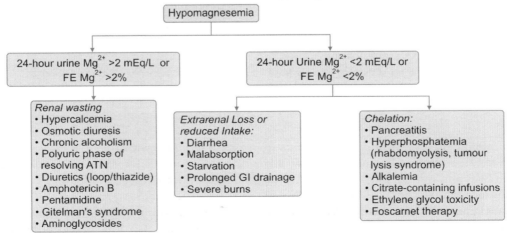

- *Serum levels 5–10 mg/dL*: Cardiac conduction impaired (wide QRS, long PR)
- *Serum levels 20–34 mg/dL*: Neuromuscular involvement (reduced deep tendon reflexes, muscle weakness)
- *Serum levels 20–48 mg/dL*: Hypotension (diffuse vasodilatation)
- *Serum levels 48–72 mg/dL*: Coma, respiratory paralysis.

The Mg^{2+} should be cautiously administered in patients with:
- Neuromuscular transmission diseases (myasthenia gravis, Lambert–Eaton myasthenic syndrome)—high Mg^{2+} increases weakness
- Coadministration of paralyzing agents (both depolarizing and nondepolarizing agents) during anesthesia—Mg^{2+} potentiates their effect
- Renal disease.

Causes of hypermagnesemia:
- *Exogenous sources*:
  - Magnesium-containing laxatives in renal failure
  - Antacids in renal failure
  - Over aggressive IV Mg^{2+} in case of treatment of eclampsia and preeclampsia.
- *Endogenous sources*:
  - Tumor lysis syndrome
  - Diabetic ketoacidosis
  - Theophylline intoxication
  - Adrenal insufficiency.

Treatment of hypermagnesemia:
- Forced saline resuscitation
- *If ECG changes are present*: IV calcium gluconate 1–2 g over 10 minutes to antagonize effect of high Mg^{2+} and avoid diuretic-induced hypocalcemia
- Definitive treatment with hemodialysis—especially in case of kidney disease.

▌ REFERENCES

1. Navarro LH, Bloomstone JA, Auler JO Jr, Cannesson M, Rocca GD, Gan TJ, et al. Perioperative fluid therapy: a statement from the International Fluid Optimization Group. Perioper Med (Lond). 2015;4:3.
2. Miller RD, Cohen NH, Eriksson LI, Fleisher LA, Wiener-Kronish JP, Young WL. Miller's Anesthesia, 8th edition. Philadelphia: Elsevier Saunders; 2015.
3. Woodcock TE, Woodcock TM. Revised Starling equation and the glycocalyx model of transvascular fluid exchange: an improved paradigm for prescribing intravenous fluid therapy. Br J Anaesth. 2012;108:384-94.
4. Kundra P, Goswami S. Endothelial glycocalyx: role in body fluid homeostasis and fluid management. Indian J Anaesth. 2019;63:6-14.
5. Song JW, Goligorsky MS. Perioperative implication of the endothelial glycocalyx. Korean J Anesthesiol. 2018;71:92-102.
6. Chappell D, Jacob M, Hofmann-Kiefer K, Conzen P, Rehm M. A rational approach to perioperative fluid management. Anesthesiology. 2008;109:723-40.
7. Lira A, Pinsky MR. Choices in fluid type and volume during resuscitation: impact on patient outcomes. Ann Intensive Care. 2014;4:38.
8. Danielsson EJ, Lejbman I, Åkeson J. Fluid deficits during prolonged overnight fasting in young healthy adults. Acta Anaesthesiol Scand. 2019;63:195-9.
9. Miller TE, Myles PS. Perioperative fluid therapy for major surgery. Anesthesiology. 2019;130:825-32.
10. Chappell D, Bruegger D, Potzel J, Jacob M, Brettner F, Vogeser M, et al. Hypervolemia increases release of atrial natriuretic peptide and shedding of the endothelial glycocalyx. Crit Care. 2014;18:538.
11. MacDonald N, Pearse RM. Are we close to the ideal intravenous fluid? Br J Anaesth. 2017;119(Suppl 1):i63-71.
12. Minto G, Mythen MG. Perioperative fluid management: science, art or random chaos? Br J Anaesth. 2015;114:717-21.
13. Kayilioglu SI, Dinc T, Sozen I, Bostanoglu A, Cete M, Coskun F. Postoperative fluid management. World J Crit Care Med. 2015;4:192-201.
14. Voldby AW, Brandstrup B. Fluid therapy in the perioperative setting: a clinical review. J Intensive Care. 2016;4:27.
15. Reddy S, Weinberg L, Young P. Crystalloid fluid therapy. Crit Care. 2016;20:59.
16. Myburgh JA, Mythen MG. Resuscitation fluids. N Engl J Med. 2013;369:1243-51.
17. Chappell D, Jacob M. Hydroxyethyl starch—the importance of being earnest. Scand J Trauma Resusc Emerg Med. 2013;21:61.
18. Raghunathan K, Murray PT, Beattie WS, Lobo DN, Myburgh J, Sladen R, et al. Choice of fluid in acute illness: what should be given? An international consensus. Br J Anaesth. 2014;113:772-83.
19. Kraut JA, Madias NE. Serum anion gap: its uses and limitations in clinical medicine. Clin J Am Soc Nephrol. 2007;2:162-74.
20. Gravenstein D. Transurethral resection of the prostate (TURP) syndrome: a review of the pathophysiology and management. Anesth Analg. 1997;84:438-46.
21. Antunes-Rodrigues J, de Castro M, Elias LL, Valença MM, McCann SM. Neuroendocrine control of body fluid metabolism. Physiol Rev. 2004;84:169-208.
22. Baylis PH, Thompson CJ. Osmoregulation of vasopressin secretion and thirst in health and disease. Clin Endocrinol (Oxf). 1988;29:549-76.
23. Spasovski G, Vanholder R, Allolio B, Annane D, Ball S, Bichet D, et al. Clinical practice guideline on diagnosis and treatment of hyponatraemia. Intensive Care Med. 2014;40:320-31.
24. Mamoulakis C, Skolarikos A, Schulze M, Scoffone CM, Rassweiler JJ, Alivizatos G, et al. Results from an international multicentre double-blind randomized controlled trial on the perioperative efficacy and safety of bipolar vs monopolar transurethral resection of the prostate. BJU Int. 2012;109:240-8.

25. Olsson J, Hahn RG. Ethanol monitoring of irrigating fluid absorption in transcervical resection of the endometrium. Acta Anaesthesiol Scand. 1995;39:252-8.

26. American College of Obstetricians and Gynecologists. ACOG technology assessment in obstetrics and gynecology, number 4, August 2005: hysteroscopy. Obstet Gynecol. 2005;106: 439-42.

27. Lien YH, Shapiro JI. Hyponatremia: clinical diagnosis and management. Am J Med. 2007;120:653-8.

28. Aditya S, Rattan A. Vaptans: a new option in the management of hyponatremia. Int J Appl Basic Med Res. 2012;2:77-83.

29. Kumar S, Berl T. Sodium. Lancet. 1998;352(9123):220-8.

30. Tisdall M, Crocker M, Watkiss J, Smith M. Disturbances of sodium in critically ill adult neurologic patients: a clinical review. J Neurosurg Anesthesiol. 2006;18:57-63.

31. Chang L, Harrington DW, Milkotic A, Swerdloff RS, Wang C. Unusual occurrence of extrapontine myelinolysis associated with acute severe hypernatraemia caused by central diabetes insipidus. Clin Endocrinol (Oxf). 2005;63:233-5.

32. van der Helm-van Mil AH, van Vugt JP, Lammers GJ, Harinck HI. Hypernatremia from a hunger strike as a cause of osmotic myelinolysis. Neurology. 2005;64:574-5.

33. Ismail FY, Szóllics A, Szólics M, Nagelkerke N, Ljubisavljevic M. Clinical semiology and neuroradiologic correlates of acute hypernatremic osmotic challenge in adults: a literature review. AJNR Am J Neuroradiol. 2013;34:2225-32.

34. Mandal AK. Hypokalemia and hyperkalemia. Med Clin North Am. 1997;81:611-39.

35. Cohn JN, Kowey PR, Whelton PK, Prisant LM. New guidelines for potassium replacement in clinical practice: a contemporary review by the National Council on Potassium in Clinical Practice. Arch Intern Med. 2000;160:2429-36.

36. Viera AJ, Wouk N. Potassium disorders: hypokalemia and hyperkalemia. Am Fam Physician. 2015;92:487-95.

37. Brown EM, Pollak M, Seidman CE, Seidman JG, Chou YH, Riccardi D, et al. Calcium-ion-sensing cell-surface receptors. N Engl J Med. 1995;333:234-40.

38. Lier H, Krep H, Schroeder S, Stuber F. Preconditions of hemostasis in trauma: a review. The influence of acidosis, hypocalcemia, anemia, and hypothermia on functional hemostasis in trauma. J Trauma. 2008;65:951-60.

39. Dubé L, Granry JC. The therapeutic use of magnesium in anesthesiology, intensive care and emergency medicine: a review. Can J Anaesth. 2003;50:732-46.

Acid-base Disturbances in the Perioperative Period

Atul Prabhakar Kulkarni, Jigeeshu Vasistha Divatia

INTRODUCTION

Acid-base disturbances are quite common in the perioperative period and all four types of primary acid-base disturbances can occur. Of these, metabolic acidosis is the most common.[1] An older study described a very high incidence (51%) of postoperative metabolic alkalosis and also suggested its role in mortality.[2] In a prospective, multicenter observational study involving 618 high-risk surgical patients, in three hospitals in Brazil, 59.1% of patients admitted to the intensive care unit (ICU) had metabolic acidosis on admission.[1] Of these, 23.9% had hyperchloremic acidosis, 21.3% had lactic acidosis, and 13.9% had increased anion gap (AG) acidosis. Of the patients who continued to have metabolic acidosis at 12 hours after admission, a large number developed complications (69% in hyperlactatemia and increased AG group, 66% in those with hyperchloremia vs. 59% in those without acidosis). The hazard ratio (HR) for 30 days mortality was HR = 1.74, 95% [confidence interval (CI) = 1.02–2.96] for those with lactic acidosis. The chance of developing renal failure by 7th day was also higher in patients with persistent acidosis. Persistent hyperlactatemia has been commonly quoted to lead to poor outcomes; some studies also found that hyperchloremic acidosis can be equally bad.[3-7]

An interesting study of 98 patients found that metabolic alkalosis defined as pH > 7.45 and standard base excess (SBE) > +3 was more common than metabolic acidosis (49% vs. 23%, $p < 0.0001$) and was correlated with hypochloremia.[8] While metabolic acidosis occurred intraoperatively and in the ICU, the incidence of alkalosis decreased from preoperative to postoperative periods (13% vs. 3%, $p = 0.003$).

BASICS OF ACID-BASE BALANCE

Definitions

An acid is a substance that can donate hydrogen ions (H^+). A base is a substance that can accept H^+ ions. Strong acids are completely ionized while weak acids are incompletely ionized. In the body (H^+—normal 40 nEq/L), concentration of hydrogen is strictly regulated within a narrow range, as at higher range, H^+ may interact with enzymes, and impair their actions. The normal HCO_3^- concentration is 24 mEq/L. Three processes ensure this strict control: (1) use of extracellular and intracellular buffers, (2) alveolar ventilation that controls the arterial carbon dioxide (CO_2) and (3) H^+ excretion by the kidneys to control carbonic acid concentration (HCO_3^-). It is evident that CO_2 control is faster than the renal excretion of H^+. **Flowchart 1** shows how the respiratory system helps in the regulation of the acid-base homeostasis of the body.

Flowchart 1: Respiratory regulation of acid-base homeostasis.

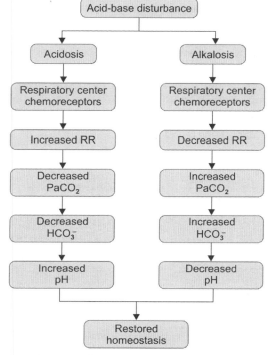

(PaCO$_2$: partial pressure of arterial carbon dioxide; RR: respiratory rate)

The average individual generates approximately 15,000 mmol of CO_2 and 50–100 mEq of H^+ from the catabolism of carbohydrates, fats, and proteins. An appropriate response to this acid load is essential as the range of extracellular H^+ concentration compatible with life (150–15 nmol/L and respective pH of 6.8–7.8) is fairly narrow. Disorders of the acid-base system and the appropriate management are best understood by examining the equation for the bicarbonate-CO_2 buffer system:

$$H_2O + CO_2 \leftrightarrow H_2CO_3 \leftrightarrow H^+ + HCO_3^-$$

Indeed, critically ill patients often suffer from compound acid-base and electrolyte disorders. Successful evaluation and management of such patients requires recognition of common patterns (e.g., hypokalemia and metabolic alkalosis) and an ability to recognize one disorder from another.

Buffers

These are molecules that donate or accept protons (H^+) to prevent changes in pH as acids or bases are added to the solution. A buffer consists of a weak acid and its conjugate base or a weak base and its conjugate acid. The common buffering systems in the body are cell and plasma proteins, hemoglobin, phosphates, bicarbonate ions, and carbonic acid. Of these, bicarbonate buffer is the most important buffering system.

Renal Regulation of Acid-base Homeostasis (Fig. 1)

Essentially while the respiratory system maintains acid-base homeostasis by controlling the CO_2 levels, the kidneys regulate the levels of bicarbonates (HCO_3^-) in the body. A large amount of acids comprising of volatile (e.g., carbonic) and nonvolatile acids are added to the body fluids as a result of metabolism of proteins [i.e., sulfur-containing amino acids—sulfuric acid (H_2SO_4)] and dietary phosphate [phosphoric acid (H_2PO_4)].

The kidneys conserve the bicarbonate in four steps. The first step is reabsorption of the Na^+ ions from filtrate while H^+ is excreted in the renal tubule. Second step is the production of bicarbonate ions, which go to the peritubular capillaries. In the third step, CO_2 forms carbonic acid, which dissociates to form HCO_3^- and H^+. Step 4. This H^+ is either excreted in the urine, or takes part in formation of H_2O while the HCO_3^- returns to the body.[9,10]

Anion Gap

The AG is the difference between the concentration of the major measured cation Na^+ and the major measured anions Cl^- and HCO_3^-.[11]

Table 1 below shows the primary acid-base disturbances and their secondary response.

APPROACHES TO EVALUATION OF ACID-BASE DISTURBANCES

Three approaches can be used for interpretation of acid-base disorders:
1. Approach centered on serum bicarbonate (HCO_3^-) concentration and the AG
2. Approach centered on "base excess (BE)/deficit"
3. Stewart's physicochemical approach.

In this chapter, we will be discussing acid-base disorders using the first two approaches.

The classical steps used to interpret arterial blood gas (ABG) are as follows.

Steps in the Interpretation of Arterial Blood Gas for Acid-base Disturbances

- *Step 1*: Assess the internal consistency of the values using the Henderson–Hasselbalch equation:

$$(H^+) = \frac{24\,(PaCO_2)}{HCO_3^-}$$

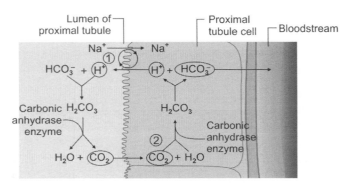

Fig. 1: Renal regulation of acid-base homeostasis.

Table 1: Primary acid-base disturbances and their secondary response.				
Acid-base disorders	**pH**	**Primary change**	**Secondary change**	**Mechanism of secondary change**
Metabolic acidosis	<7.40	↓HCO_3^-	↓pCO_2	Hyperventilation
Metabolic alkalosis	>7.40	↑HCO_3^-	↑pCO_2	Hypoventilation
Respiratory acidosis	<7.40	↑pCO_2	↑HCO_3^-	↑HCO_3^- reabsorption
Respiratory alkalosis	>7.40	↓pCO_2	↓HCO_3^-	↓HCO_3^- reabsorption

(pCO_2: partial pressure of carbon dioxide)

If the pH and the H^+ are inconsistent, the ABG is probably not valid.

- *Step 2*: Is there alkalemia or acidemia present?
  - pH < 7.35 (acidemia)
  - pH > 7.45 (alkalemia).
- *Step 3:* Is the disturbance respiratory or metabolic? What is the relationship between the direction of change in the pH and the direction of change in the partial pressure of arterial carbon dioxide ($PaCO_2$)? In primary respiratory disorders, the pH and $PaCO_2$ change in opposite directions; in metabolic disorders, the pH and $PaCO_2$ change in the same direction.
- *Step 4*: Is there any appropriate compensation for the primary disturbance? Usually, compensation does not return the pH to normal (7.35–7.45) (**Table 2**).

  If the observed compensation is not the expected compensation, it is likely that more than one acid-base disorder is present.
- *Step 5*: Calculate the AG (if a metabolic acidosis exists):

  $$AG = Na^+ - (Cl^- + HCO_3^-) - 12 \pm 2$$

  A normal AG is approximately 12 mEq/L.

  In patients with hypoalbuminemia, the normal AG is lower than 12 mEq/L; the "normal" AG in patients with hypoalbuminemia is about 2.5 mEq/L lower for each 1 g/dL decrease in the plasma albumin concentration (for example, for a patient with a plasma albumin of 2.0 g/dL, the AG would be approximately 7 mEq/L).

  If the AG is elevated, consider calculating the osmolal gap in compatible clinical situations.
  - Elevation in AG is not explained by an obvious case [diabetic ketoacidosis (DKA), lactic acidosis, and renal failure]
  - Toxic ingestion is suspected.

    OSM gap = Measured OSM – [2Na⁺ – glucose/18 – blood urea nitrogen (BUN)/2.8]
  - The OSM gap should be <10.

- *Step 6*: If an increased AG is present, assess the relationship between the increase in the AG and the decrease in HCO_3^-.

  Assess the ratio of the change in the ΔAG to the change in ΔHCO_3^-.

  $$\Delta HCO_3^- : \Delta AG / \Delta HCO_3^-$$

  This ratio should be between 1.0 and 2.0 if an uncomplicated AG metabolic acidosis is present.

  If this ratio falls outside of this range, then another metabolic disorder is present.

  If $\Delta AG / \Delta HCO_3^- < 1.0$, then a concurrent non-AG metabolic acidosis is likely to be present.

  If $\Delta AG / \Delta HCO_3^- > 2.0$, then a concurrent metabolic alkalosis is likely to be present.
- *Step 7*: Urine AG:

  $$(Urine\ Na^+ + K^+) - (Urine\ Cl^-) = Urine\ AG$$

  Diagnose metabolic acidosis due to renal excretory failure.

  NH_4^+ is most important unmeasured ion in urine.

  Urine NH_4^+ excretion is accompanied by Cl^-

  Negative urine AG = Increased NH_4^+ excretion.

  In a metabolic acidosis without a serum AG:

  Negative urine AG suggests diarrhea

  Positive urine AG suggests renal tubular acidosis.

CAUSES OF PERIOPERATIVE ACID-BASE DISORDERS

Acid-base disturbances may be seen in the preoperative, intraoperative, and postoperative periods due to various causes and some of these may be asymptomatic with no effects. Hyperlactatemia is a common cause of acidosis in the perioperative period and in the critically ill patients. The various causes of lactic acidosis are given in **Box 1**.[12]

Preoperative Period

Preoperatively fasting and saline infusion can lead to asymptomatic hyperchloremic metabolic acidosis. Patients undergoing emergency surgeries will often have tissue hypoperfusion due to septic shock and may have acidosis due to lactic acidosis and renal dysfunction. Preexisting comorbidities can also cause metabolic derangements. Patients with gastric outlet obstruction due to cancer may have metabolic alkalosis due to vomiting and loss of acid and potassium while those with acute intestinal obstruction with dehydration can have lactic acidosis and electrolyte derangements renal dysfunction (due to prerenal causes). Patients with severe chronic obstructive pulmonary disease (COPD) may have chronic CO_2 retention and respiratory acidosis. Hypovolemia due to bleeding in a trauma victim can also have similar problems.

Table 2: Various disorders with their expected compensation.

Disorders	Expected compensation	Correction factor
Metabolic acidosis	Partial pressure of arterial carbon dioxide ($PaCO_2$) = (1.5 × HCO_3^-) + 8	±2
Acute respiratory acidosis	Increase in HCO_3^- = $\Delta PaCO_2$/10	±3
Chronic respiratory acidosis (3–5 days)	Increase in HCO_3^- = 3.5($\Delta PaCO_2$/10)	–
Metabolic alkalosis	Increase in $PaCO_2$ = 40 + 0.6(ΔHCO_3^-)	–
Acute respiratory alkalosis	Decrease in HCO_3^- = 2($\Delta PaCO_2$/10)	–
Chronic respiratory alkalosis	Decrease in HCO_3^- = 5($\Delta PaCO_2$/10) to 7($\Delta PaCO_2$/10)	–

Box 1: Causes of hyperlactatemia.[12]

Type A:
- Severe anemia
- Septic, hemorrhagic, and cardiogenic shock
- CO poisoning
- Organ ischemia
- Convulsions
- Intense physical exercise

Type B:
- *Subtype B1—underlying primary diseases*:
  - Cancer and hemopathy
  - Decompensated diabetes
  - HIV infection
  - Liver failure
  - Sepsis
  - Severe malaria attack.
- *Subtype B2—medication and toxins*:
  - Alcohol
  - Beta-adrenergic agents
  - Cyanide and cyanogenic compounds
  - Diethyl ether
  - 5-fluorouracil (5-FU)
  - Halothane
  - Iron
  - Isoniazid
  - Linezolid
  - Metformin
  - Nalidixic acid
  - Niacin (vitamin B_3 or nicotinic acid)
  - Nucleoside reverse transcriptase inhibitors
  - Paracetamol
  - Propofol
  - *Psychostimulants*: Cocaine, amphetamines, and cathinones
  - Salicylates
  - Strychnine
  - *Sugars*: Fructose, sorbitol, and xylitol
  - Sulfasalazine
  - Total parenteral nutrition
  - Valproic acid
  - *Vitamin deficiency*: Thiamine (vitamin B_1) and biotin (vitamin B_8).
- *Subtype B₃—inborn errors of metabolism*:
  - Fructose-1,6-diphosphatase deficiency
  - Glucose-6-phosphatase deficiency (von Gierke disease)
  - Kearns–Sayre syndrome
  - MELAS syndrome
  - MERRF syndrome
  - Methylmalonic acidemia (methylmalonyl-CoA mutase deficiency)
  - Pearson syndrome
  - Pyruvate carboxylase deficiency
  - Pyruvate dehydrogenase deficiency

(CO: carbon monoxide; HIV: human immunodeficiency virus; MELAS: mitochondrial myopathy, encephalopathy, lactic acidosis, and stroke; MERRF: myoclonic epilepsy with ragged red fibers)

Preoperative Drug Therapy

Drugs, which may cause metabolic acidosis and alkalosis in the preoperative period, are as follows.[13,14]

Drugs likely to cause metabolic acidosis:
- *Oral hypoglycemic agents*: Metformin, sodium-glucose cotransporter-2 (SGLT2) inhibitors (gliflozins): dapagliflozin, canagliflozin, and empagliflozin

- Angiotensin-converting enzyme (ACE) inhibitors, angiotensin receptor blockers
- *Antimicrobial agents*: Linezolid, netilmicin, flucloxacillin, zidovudine, pentamidine, trimethoprim, zalcitabine, tenofovir, abacavir, didanosine, etc.
- *Cancer chemotherapeutic agents*: Cisplatin, ifosfamide, etc.
- *Analgesics and antipyretics*: Salicylate, acetaminophen
- *Sedatives and hypnotics*: Intravenous diazepam and lorazepam, propofol
- *Immunosuppressants*: Cyclosporine, tacrolimus
- *Others*: Cholestyramine, amiloride, trimeterene, ketoconazole, and heparin.

Drugs likely to cause metabolic alkalosis:
- *Thiazide and loop diuretics*: Indapamide, hydrochlorothiazide, chlorthalidone, furosemide, bumetanide, and torsemide
- *Antimicrobial agents*: Carbenicillin, other penicillins, and gentamicin
- *Steroids*: Fludrocortisone
- Laxatives.

Intraoperative and Postoperative Periods

The common acid-base disorder seen in intraoperative and postoperative periods is metabolic acidosis. Hyperlactatemia, increased AG, and hyperchloremia are the common etiological factors. Park and colleagues reported that the metabolic acidosis in the postoperative period, in patients undergoing major abdominal surgery, was largely due to either hyperchloremia due to intraoperative use of normal saline (NS) and lactic acidosis due to lactate production. The patients who received NS had a significantly lower SBE, strong ion difference, and higher corrected chloride.[15]

In another large study by Silva and colleagues, nearly 60% patients had acidosis at the time of admission to the ICU.[1] As compared to the patients who did not have metabolic acidosis, patients who had persistent acidosis at 12 hours had increased incidence of renal dysfunction starting at day 1, lasting up to day 8 in ICU. Patients with lactic acidosis had significantly higher mortality as compared to those with no acidosis (30% vs. 10%, $p < 0.001$). These patients had higher risk of dying (HR 1.739, 95% CI: 1.021–2.975), but not those with increased AG (HR 1.684, 95% CI: 0.851–3.321) and hyperchloremic acidosis (HR 1.471, 95% CI: 0.747–2.901). The authors concluded that patients who develop lactic acidosis have poorer outcomes as compared to those with other types of acidosis.

A more recent study, the Bradford Anaesthetic Department Acidosis Study, looked at the prevalence of metabolic acidosis and evolution of acidosis over time in patients undergoing major elective surgical procedures.[16] They also aimed at defining causes and outcomes of patients with metabolic acidosis. The incidence of metabolic acidosis (defined as an SBE < 2 mEq/L), at the time of ICU admission following surgery, was 78%, out of which many patients (41) had significant metabolic acidosis (SBE < 2 mEq/L). Interestingly metabolic acidosis was seen in many patients before surgical incision (38%). In 34% of patients, the metabolic acidosis persisted till after 24 hours of ICU admission. The authors discuss the reasons behind development of metabolic acid-base disturbances after induction. Administration of any type of fluid seemed to have a protective effect before induction of anesthesia and the SBE increased (by approximately +1 mEq/L) before induction. Metabolic acidosis began developing within the first hour of surgery before the incision was taken; this was most likely due to use of desflurane for maintenance of anesthesia. Acidosis continued to occur during the intraoperative period, but did not seem to be associated with hyperchloremia or any unmeasured ions, but seemed mainly to correlate with the use of gelofusine and blood. The acidosis continued to be present in 38% of patients at 24 hours. There were only three deaths in the study group. The authors state that though there seemed to be a trend toward increased hospital stay, this was not statistically significant.

There are multiple studies, which have demonstrated that infusion of NS as intraoperative maintenance fluid leads to development of metabolic acidosis in the postoperative period.[17,18] As compared to a balanced salt solution, the NS group showed a significant lower BE (–3.20 vs. –1.35, $p = 0.049$), more hyperchloremia (115.12 mmol/L vs. 111.74 mmol/L, $p < 0.001$), and hypokalemia (3.36 mmol/L vs. 3.70 mmol/L, $p < 0.001$) in patients who had undergone surgeries for traumatic brain injury in postoperative period at the end of 24 hours.[17]

In patients undergoing gynecological surgeries, infusion of large volumes of NS (30 mL/kg) intraoperatively led to development of metabolic acidosis, which was not seen in patients receiving Ringer's lactate (RL) solution.[19]

Contrary to the other studies mentioned above, a prospective observational study in 97 pediatric patients who had undergone cardiopulmonary bypass surgery for various reasons found that most children had mild metabolic acidosis (median standard bicarbonate 20.1 mmol/L, BE 5.1 mEq/L) characterized by hyperchloremia (median corrected Cl^- 113 mmol/L) and hypoalbuminemia (median albumin 30 g/L).[20] The major determinants of net BE were chloride and albumin components (chloride effect –4.8 mEq/L, albumin effect +3.4 mEq/L). Metabolic acidosis occurred in 72 children (74%), but was not associated with increased morbidity. Hyperchloremia was a causative factor in 53

children (74%) with metabolic acidosis. Hyperchloremic children required less adrenaline infusion support while those who had hypoalbuminemia needed longer duration of inotropic therapy and ICU stay.

The exact effect of hyperchloremic acidosis in this group of patients on postoperative period is not known. In a study involving 206 patients, 42 (20.4%) patients developed postoperative acute kidney injury (AKI) (AKI group) and 164 (79.6%) did not (non-AKI group). As compared to those whose renal function remained normal, the patients who developed AKI had lower BE-Cl^- difference and strong ion difference (SID) (<31 mmol/L, $p < 0.05$). In multivariate logistic regression analysis, postoperative BE-Cl^- difference of >7 mEq/L, i.e., SID < 31 mEq/L was an independent risk factor for AKI (odds ratio: 2.8, 95% CI: 1.2–6.4, $p = 0.01$). The patients who developed AKI had longer ICU and hospital length of stay (LOS) ($p < 0.05$). It is thus possible that hyperchloremic acidosis may have harmful effects on postoperative outcomes.[18] Further studies will probably bring more clarity to this matter, however it seems prudent from the current evidence to suggest that the use of intravenous balanced salt solutions such as RL or other newer fluids is safe, provided cost is not an issue.

The French Intensive Care Society [Société de Réanimation de Langue Française (SRLF)] and the French Emergency Medicine Society [Société Française de Médecine d'Urgence (SFMU)] have developed formalized recommendations from experts using the GRADE methodology for the diagnosis, assessment, and management of patients with metabolic acidosis in Intensive Care and Emergency Medicine.[12] These, however, are equally applicable to patients undergoing major surgeries. The algorithm for diagnosis of patient with metabolic acidosis can be seen in **Flowchart 2**. The important applicable recommendations are given below.

▍DIAGNOSIS

- The experts suggest that ABG measurements can be performed in patients with a decreased plasma bicarbonate level so as to eliminate respiratory alkalosis, confirm the diagnosis of metabolic acidosis, and test for mixed acidosis.
- The AG corrected for albumin should probably be used rather than the uncorrected AG to differentiate acidosis related to acid load from acidosis related to base deficit.
- The experts suggest using an algorithm to improve the etiological diagnosis of metabolic acidosis.
- The experts suggest that a normal value of venous lactate discounts hyperlactatemia.
- Arterial lactate should probably be measured to confirm hyperlactatemia in case of increased venous lactate.

Flowchart 2: Algorithm for diagnosis and management of metabolic acidosis.[12]

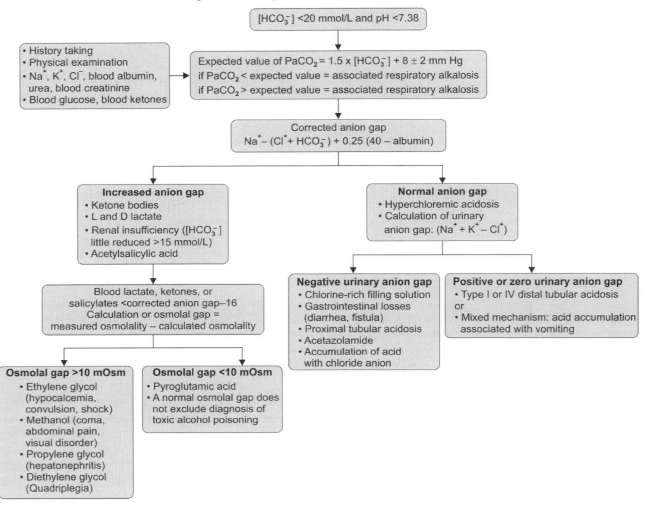

(PaCO₂: partial pressure of arterial carbon dioxide)

- Capillary blood lactate should not be measured to diagnose hyperlactatemia.
- Capillary blood ketones rather than urine ketones should be measured when diagnosing ketoacidosis.

PATIENT ASSESSMENT AND REFERRAL

- The pH value should probably not be used alone to identify critically ill patients.
- Hyperlactatemia, whatever its value, should be considered as a marker of severity in initial treatment. Diagnostic and therapeutic management should be rapid and multidisciplinary if needed.
- Increase in blood lactate should probably be controlled in the first hours of management so as to assess the response to treatment.
- The experts suggest close monitoring of patients with DKA, ideally in an ICU.

MANAGEMENT

The first four recommendations are about management of diabetic acidosis, which we have not included here, since they are relevant to topic at hand. We have also omitted some other recommendations as not being pertinent to the perioperative period.

1. The experts suggest administering sodium bicarbonate to compensate for gastrointestinal or renal base loss in case of poor clinical tolerance.

2. Sodium bicarbonate should probably be administered to intensive care patients with severe metabolic acidemia (pH 7.20, PaCO₂ < 45 mm Hg) and moderate-to-severe acute renal insufficiency, so as to improve prognosis.

3. Sodium bicarbonate should not be administered routinely in the therapeutic management of circulatory arrest, apart from preexisting hyperkalemia or poisoning by membrane stabilizers.

4. The experts suggest compensating for acidemia by increasing respiratory frequency without inducing intrinsic positive end-expiratory pressure with a maximum of 35 cycles/min and/or a tidal volume up to 8 mL/kg of body mass and by monitoring plateau pressure. The aim of ventilation is not to normalize pH. A target pH $\geq$ 7.15 seems reasonable. Medical treatment of metabolic acidosis and of its cause should be envisaged concomitantly, as ventilatory compensation can only be symptomatic and temporary.

SUMMARY

Acid-base disturbances are common in the perioperative period. The clinician should be able to diagnose these disorders and a systematic stepwise approach is useful for this purpose. Metabolic acidosis, caused by either hyperchloremia or lactate production, is the predominant disorder seen in the perioperative period. Hyperchloremic acidosis is mainly iatrogenic and can be easily prevented by avoiding excessive administration of NS. Lactic acidosis needs to be promptly diagnosed and the causative problem tackled as soon as possible so as to improve outcomes of the patients.

REFERENCES

1. Silva JM, Ribas Rosa de Oliveira AM, Mendes Nogueira FA, Vianna PM, Amendola CP, Carvalho Carmona MJ, et al. Metabolic Acidosis Assessment in High-Risk Surgeries: Prognostic Importance. Anesth Analg. 2016;123:1163-71.

2. Okusawa S, Aikawa N, Abe O. Postoperative metabolic alkalosis following general surgery: its incidence and possible etiology. Jpn J Surg. 1989;19:312-8.

3. Matteucci M, Ferrarese S, Cantore C, Cappabianca G, Massimi G, Mantovani V, et al. Hyperlactatemia during cardiopulmonary bypass: risk factors and impact on surgical results with a focus on the long-term outcome. Perfusion; 2020. [Epub ahead of print].

4. Duval B, Besnard T, Mion S, Leuillet S, Jecker O, Labrousse L, et al. Intraoperative changes in blood lactate levels are associated with worse short-term outcomes after cardiac surgery with cardiopulmonary bypass. Perfusion. 2019;34:640-50.

5. Hajjar LA, Almeida JP, Fukushima JT, Rhodes A, Vincent JL, Osawa EA, et al. High lactate levels are predictors of major complications after cardiac surgery. J Thorac Cardiovasc Surg. 2013;146:455-60.

6. Oh TK, Do SH, Jeon YT, Kim J, Na HS, Hwang JW. Association of Preoperative Serum Chloride Levels With Mortality and Morbidity After Noncardiac Surgery: A Retrospective Cohort Study. Anesth Analg. 2019;129:1494-501.

7. McCluskey SA, Karkouti K, Wijeysundera D, Minkovich L, Tait G, Beattie WS. Hyperchloremia after noncardiac surgery is independently associated with increased morbidity and mortality: a propensity-matched cohort study. Anesth Analg. 2013;117:412-21.

8. Boaz M, Iskhakov A, Tsivian A, Shimonov M, Berkenstadt H, Izakson A, et al. Perioperative metabolic alkalemia is more frequent than metabolic acidemia in major elective abdominal surgery. J Clin Monit Comput. 2011;25:223-30.

9. Hamm LL, Nakhoul N, Hering-Smith KS. Acid-Base Homeostasis. Clin J Am Soc Nephrol. 2015;10:2232-42.

10. Anatomy and Physiology. (2019). Fluid, Electrolyte, and Acid-base Balance. [online] Available from https://opentextbc.ca/anatomyandphysiology/chapter/26-4-acid-base-balance/. [Last accessed March, 2020].

11. Kraut JA, Madias NE. Serum anion gap: its uses and limitations in clinical medicine. Clin J Am Soc Nephrol. 2007;2:162-74.

12. Jung B, Martinez M, Claessens Y, Darmon M, Klouche K, Lautrette A, et al. Diagnosis and management of metabolic acidosis: guidelines from a French expert panel. Ann Intensive Care. 2019;9:92.

13. Pham AQ, Xu LH, Moe OW. Drug-Induced Metabolic Acidosis. F1000Res. 2015;4:F1000.

14. Kitterer D, Schwab M, Alscher MD, Braun N, Latus J. Drug-induced acid-base disorders. Pediatr Nephrol. 2015;30:1407-23.

15. Park CM, Chun HK, Jeon K, Suh GY, Choi DW, Kim S. Factors related to post-operative metabolic acidosis following major abdominal surgery. ANZ J Surg. 2014;84:574-80.

16. Lawton TO, Quinn A, Fletcher SJ. Perioperative metabolic acidosis: The Bradford Anaesthetic Department Acidosis Study. J Intensive Care Soc. 2019;20:11-7.

17. Hassan MH, Hassan WMNW, Zaini RHM, Shukeri WFWM, Abidin HZ, Eu CS. Balanced Fluid Versus Saline-Based Fluid in Post-operative Severe Traumatic Brain Injury Patients: Acid-Base and Electrolytes Assessment. Malays J Med Sci. 2017;24:83-93.

18. Toyonaga Y, Kikura M. Hyperchloremic acidosis is associated with acute kidney injury after abdominal surgery. Nephrology (Carlton). 2017;22:720-7.

19. Scheingraber S, Rehm M, Sehmisch C, Finsterer U. Rapid saline infusion produces hyperchloremic acidosis in patients undergoing gynecologic surgery. Anesthesiology. 1999;90:1265-70.

20. Hatherill M, Salie S, Waggie Z, Lawrenson J, Hewitson J, Reynolds L, et al. Hyperchloraemic metabolic acidosis following open cardiac surgery. Arch Dis Child. 2005;90:1288-92.

CHAPTER

9

Acute Respiratory Failure in Postoperative Patient

Rajesh Chawla, Prashant Nasa, Aakanksha Chawla Jain

INTRODUCTION

Postoperative pulmonary complications (PPCs) are common and can increase overall surgical and anesthesia risk. Postoperative respiratory failure (PRF) is the most common PPC with significantly morbidity, mortality, unplanned admissions to the intensive care unit (ICU), increased hospital length of stay (LOS), and overall costs. The majority of these PPCs occur within 24 hours after surgery and many of them are preventable. The risk stratification and identification of vulnerable patients, perioperative optimization, and adequate postoperative management can prevent or improve outcome of PRF. In this chapter, we will discuss the incidence, risk factors, and predictors of patients with high risk of PRF and preoperative optimization of such patients.

DEFINITION OF POSTOPERATIVE RESPIRATORY FAILURE

There are myriads of definition available in the literature for PRF **(Box 1)**.[1-16] The heterogeneous definitions impact the identification of true incidence of the problem, and appropriate tools for prediction and management of PRF.

Box 1: Different definitions of postoperative respiratory failure used in literature.

- Postoperative PaO_2 < 8 kPa (60 mm Hg) on room air, a PaO_2:FIO_2 ratio < 40 kPa (300 mm Hg), or arterial oxyhemoglobin saturation measured with pulse oximetry < 90% and requiring oxygen therapy[1]
- Reintubation after surgery or ventilator dependence for > 1 postoperative day[2,3]
- Need for postoperative mechanical ventilation > 48 hours[4-7]
- Unplanned reintubation within 30 days of surgery because of respiratory distress, hypoxia, hypercarbia, or respiratory acidosis[4,5,7-9]
- Reintubation within 3 days and requiring mechanical ventilation[10]
- Postoperative acute lung injury or ARDS[11-13]
- Requiring mechanical ventilation within 7 days of surgery[14,15]
- Requiring NIV after surgery[16]

The variations in the definitions are mainly on different time frame used from surgical–anesthetic effect to respiratory failure (RF) and physiological tools used to define RF. The diagnosis of PRF has implications on not only patient outcomes but also on medicolegal, regulatory liabilities, and quality of patient care. The RF started preoperatively and continued postoperatively which is attributed primarily to a preexisting medical condition such as heart failure or severe chronic obstructive pulmonary disease is not included in this definition. The patients requiring postoperative ventilation for nonpulmonary illness, such as sepsis, heart failure, head injury, are also excluded from this definition despite the time frame of ventilation.

We have used the definition recommended by European Society of Anaesthesiology (ESA) and European Society of Intensive Care Medicine (ESICM) joint task force on RF which define PRF as postoperative PaO_2 < 60 mm Hg (8 kPa) on room air, a PaO_2 to FiO_2 ratio < 300 mm Hg (40 kPa), or arterial oxyhemoglobin saturation measured with pulse oximetry < 90% and requiring oxygen therapy.[1]

PERIOPERATIVE CONSIDERATIONS OF RESPIRATORY PHYSIOLOGY

The intraoperative and postoperative period causes significant alterations on respiratory physiology. The effect of anesthesia and surgery on pulmonary functions is dependent on many factors like type of anesthesia (general versus regional), anesthetic agents and drugs, mode of ventilation (spontaneous or mechanical) including loss of consciousness, posture of patient, type of surgery, and postoperative pain management. The understanding of these changes helps anesthesiologist in risk assessment, preoperative patient optimization, and plan for appropriate postoperative pain management. The effect of anesthesia on pulmonary system can be seen as direct effect of anesthesia intraoperatively and postoperative alterations.

Effect of Anesthesia on Respiratory System

Anesthetics affect all aspects of respiratory system—control of breathing, airway and respiratory muscles, and mechanics including lung volumes. Anesthesia decreases central respiratory drive and blunt compensatory respiratory response to hypoxia and hypercarbia by effect of anesthetic agents on carotid and aortic body chemoreceptors.[17] There is a dose dependent decrease in minute ventilation by decreasing both tidal volume and respiratory rate.

Anesthesia reduces upper airways muscle tone and reflexes, can precipitate anatomic airway obstruction, or laryngospasm and bronchospasm in patients with hyperreactive airways.[18] The loss of muscle tone and inadequate minute ventilation decrease lung volumes especially functional residual capacity (FRC) and forced expiratory volume in 1 second (FEV1) resulting in ventilation and perfusion mismatch.[19] The reduction of FRC causes small airways collapse and atelectasis as FRC approaches closing capacity. Pulmonary blood flow during anesthesia remains unaltered and is dependent mainly on patient position which is not matched with altered ventilation causing further mismatch. Hypoxic pulmonary vasoconstriction (HPV) a natural homeostatic response to divert the pulmonary blood flow from poorly ventilated areas to better-ventilated areas is also blunted by inhalational anesthetic agents.[20] The supine position during anesthesia altered the shape and motion of rib cage along with diaphragmatic paralysis and caused further decrease in FRC and ventilation-perfusion mismatch.

POSTOPERATIVE RESPIRATORY PHYSIOLOGY ALTERATIONS

These changes observed during anesthesia continue to persist even postoperatively to varying degrees. The compensatory ventilatory response to hypoxia and hypercarbia continued to remain blunted especially when opioids are used for pain management postoperatively. Studies have shown postoperative atelectasis on CT scan up to 24 hours postoperatively and resultant effect on FRC and other pulmonary function tests (PFTs).[21] The position of surgery such as thoracic and upper abdominal surgery also causes reduction in vital capacity by 50% and in FRC by 30%.[21] The postoperative reduction of FRC is caused by diaphragmatic dysfunction, postoperative pain, and splinting in these cases. FRC is most affected with its nadir reached at 1–2 days postoperatively, and it remains diminished for up to 5–7 days.[21] The residual effects of anesthesia and postoperative opioids may inhibit cough, mucociliary clearance, and increase the risk of postoperative pneumonia.[22]

The normalization of respiratory physiology may take up to 6 weeks in few patients.[22]

INCIDENCE AND OUTCOMES

The pulmonary complications are common after surgery and PRF is the most common PPC.[21,23] The incidence of PRF varies from 0.3 to 17% depending upon the definition used to measure RF.[21,22,24,25] PPCs contribute to significant postoperative morbidity and mortality. There is around 10-fold increased risk of dying in first month after surgery in patients with PPC as compared to those without PPC (14–30% vs. 0.2–3%).[22,23,26] The PPCs also increases risk of reintubation, ICU admission, and hospital LOS.[27-29] The increase in hospital LOS significantly increases the healthcare costs. This highlights the importance of PRF for anesthetists and surgeons to evaluate risk and adopt preventive strategies for reduction of morbidity, mortality, and healthcare costs.

RISK FACTORS AND PREOPERATIVE PREDICTION OF POSTOPERATIVE RESPIRATORY FAILURE

The preoperative risk stratification using risk factors scoring is an important pre-emptive measure which can identify patients at high risk of complications. The risk factors can be modifiable or nonmodifiable which helps in perioperative optimization and also in prognostication during informed consent.[21,30] There is another classification based on factors specific to patient or procedure **(Table 1).** The high-risk procedures for PRF are aortic aneurysm, neurosurgery and thoracic, abdominal, upper abdominal, head and neck, and vascular surgery.[31]

These risk factors are used in various prediction models in heterogeneous patient populations for specific risk assessment. Irrespective of origin, these models have some common variables based on either patients at risk such as American Society of Anesthesiologists (ASA) classification (3 or greater), obesity, obstructive sleep apnea (OSA), chronic obstructive pulmonary disease (COPD), congestive heart failure (CHF), anemia, malnutrition or surgical risk factors such as site of surgery, surgical duration, and emergency surgery.[21,23,30,32-38]

Some of the popular and extensively validated models are discussed in **Table 2.**

The SPORC is validated to predict for reintubation but sensitivity for identifying patients with PRF who require less invasive intervention is not calculated.[22] The STOP-BANG questionnaire is another validated tool to identify patients with high risk of OSA and have higher PPCs and higher LOS in hospital.[35-37] Seven factors ARISCAT score has been extensively validated in a multicenter (63 European hospitals) in PERISCOPE Prospective evaluation of a Risk score for postoperative pulmonary complications in Europe (PERISCOPE) study.[38] Recently another score using

Table 1: Risk factors for postoperative respiratory failure.

Procedure specific	Patient specific
Modifiable	
Perioperative ventilation strategy	Smoking
Residual neuromuscular block: Use of long-acting NMBDs and TOF ratio < 0.7 in PACU	Obstructive airway disease (COPD and asthma)
Type of anesthesia (GA versus regional)	Comorbidities (CCF, CLD, CKD, DM)
Use of Sugammadex for reversal	Anemia
Avoiding intubation	OSA (BMI > 27 kg/m²)
Neostigmine	Preoperative sepsis
Open versus laparoscopic surgery	Alcohol
Duration of surgery	
Perioperative blood transfusion	
Nonmodifiable	
Type of surgery	Age and Sex
Emergency (vs. elective)	ASA class > 2
Reoperative	Functional dependence (frailty)
	Comorbidities (cerebrovascular accident, malignancy)
	Weight loss > 10% (within 6 months)
	Acute respiratory infection (within 1 month)
	Impaired sensorium
	Long-term steroid use

(COPD: chronic obstructive pulmonary disease; CCF: congestive heart failure; CLD: chronic liver disease; CKD: chronic kidney disease; DM: diabetes mellitus; OSA: obstructive sleep apnea; BMI: body mass index; PACU: postanesthesia care unit)

13 independent risk factors, Las Vegas score is validated in more than 6,000 patients with moderate discrimination ability.[39]

The models have been validated in heterogeneous cohorts and are helpful in assessing patients with comorbidities. However, each of the tools though useful in subset of populations has its own limitations and no single tool can predict risk in every patient. There are other significant factors which also need to be considered like impact of intraoperative and postoperative events, anesthetic medications, and monitoring strategies which are not included in these preoperative risk prediction models.

Laboratory Investigations in Preoperative Risk Assessment

The preoperative evaluation of the patients for anesthesia includes laboratory and various other investigations. The following tests are commonly used to assess patients for the risk of PRF.

Table 2: Preoperative risk prediction models.

Score for the prediction of Postoperative Respiratory Complications (SPORC)	Components	Interpretation
	ASA score ≥ 3: 3 points	0 points: RI 0.1%
	Emergency procedure: 3 points	3 points: RI 0.5%
	High-risk service: 2 points	5 points: RI 1.5%
	Congestive heart failure: 2 points	7 points: RI 4.2%
	COPD: 1 points	9 points: RI 11.2%
Assess respiratory risk in surgical patients in Catalonia (ARISCAT)	Age ≤50 years: 0 points 51–80 years: 3 points >80 years: 16 points	<26 points: Low risk 26–44 points: Moderate risk ≥45 points: High risk
	Preoperative oxygen saturation ≥96%: 0 points 91–95%: 8 points ≤90%: 24 points	
	Other clinical risk factors: Respiratory infection (in prior month): 17 points Preoperative Hb ≤ 10 g/dL: 11 points	
	Surgical incision Upper abdominal: 15 points Intrathoracic: 24 points	
	Duration of surgery <2 hours: 0 points 2–3 hours: 16 points >3 hours: 23 points	
	Emergency procedure No: 0 points Yes: 8 points	
STOP-BANG Questionnaire	Snoring: Do you snore loudly? Tired: Do you often feel tired, fatigued, or sleepy during the daytime Observed: Has anyone observed you stop breathing during sleep? Pressure: Has anyone observed you stop breathing during sleep? BMI: >35 kg/m² Age: >50 years Neck: >40 cm Gender: Male	Answer to any question: 1 point Score < 3 points: Low risk of OSA >3 points: High risk of OSA

(Hb: hemoglobin; OSA: obstructive sleep apnea; COPD: chronic obstructive pulmonary disease; ASA: American Society of Anesthesiologist)

Pulmonary Function Tests

The PFT is commonly used to assess the respiratory reserve and to predict PPCs. Abnormal PFT may be associated with increased duration of postoperative mechanical ventilation. The FEV1:FVC < 0.7 and FEV1 < 80% of predicted is correlated with increased risk of PRF. Routine PFT is of marginal benefit in predicting PRF other than patients undergoing lung resection.[40,41]

Arterial Blood Gases

Preoperative arterial blood gas (ABG) is usually done to predict postoperative risk of RF. However in a systematic review, ABG was found to be inadequate to predict this complication.[16] The National Institute for Health and Care Excellence (NICE) guidance on spirometry and ABGs is to be done in ASA score III or IV patients with confirmed or suspected respiratory disease.[42]

Chest X-ray

The preoperative chest X-ray (CXR) is very common test advised during anesthesia assessment of operative patients. The advantage of CXR over clinical assessment is however doubtful and adds very little value in preoperative assessment.[30] In a systematic review on preoperative screening CXR, the rate of PPC was not higher in patients with no preoperative CXR.[43]

The NICE guidance on preoperative CXRs is that it should not be performed routinely before elective surgery without risk factors.[42]

Preoperative Oxygen Saturation

There is recent interest in simple beside tests such as oxygen saturation (SpO_2) to predict PPCs. Age adjusted low preoperative SpO_2 assessed in supine position and on breathing room air is independently associated with increased risk of PPCs.[23,38]

The patients with preoperative SpO_2 91–95% were two times more likely and those with $SpO_2 \leq 90\%$ were 10 times more likely to get PPCs as compared to patients with SpO_2 > 95%.[34]

There are other few laboratory tests which have been found to be associated with increased risk of PPCs, high urea > 7.5 mmol/L, increased creatinine, abnormal liver function tests, preoperative anemia (hemoglobin < 10 g/dL), low serum albumin, and predicted maximal oxygen uptake.[44]

Preoperative Risk Reduction

The preoperative strategy to reduce risk of PRF can either be optimization and control of modifiable risk factors or preoperative lung preparation for anesthesia and surgery.

Optimization of Modifiable Risk Factors

The prevention of PRF starts with preoperative optimization of modifiable risk factors. The optimization requires time besides other resources. Postponing a surgery for optimization should be done on patient–patient basis with risk of delaying surgery versus developing a PPC and needs input from all stakeholders.

Smoking: Current/active smoking is an independent risk factor for PPCs. The smokers are more likely to have PPCs as compared to ex-smokers and which in-turn have higher risk as compared to the ones who never smoked.[45,46] The incidence of complications is also increased with number of pack-years of smoking.[47]

Smoking cessation can reduce postoperative morbidity but the timing of cessation is a matter of debate. There was speculated risk of bronchospasm and increased secretions when cessation is done close (less than 8 weeks) to the surgery. In two systematic reviews on timing of smoking cessation, there is definitely benefit of smoking cessation for at least 4 weeks before surgery but less than that the evidence is not robust for any benefit or increased risk.[48,49] The patients should be encouraged to quit smoking anytime before surgery.

Comorbidities: Comorbidities like COPD, OSA, CHF, or chronic liver disease (CLD), diabetes mellitus (DM) are independently associated with increased risk of PPCs.[23,50] Preoperative optimization of some of these chronic illnesses is beneficial whenever feasible. COPD and asthma should be optimally controlled with bronchodilators, inhaled or oral steroids, and treatment of any active respiratory infection.[51] The CHF can also be pharmacologically optimized involving a cardiologist and maximizing functional capacity.[52]

Alcohol: Daily alcohol consumption especially within 2 weeks before surgery increases the risk of PPCs and PRF.[22]

Type of surgery and anesthesia: Minimally invasive surgery like laparoscopic abdominal surgery is associated with fewer PPCs as compared to open laparotomy.[22] General anesthesia and its effect on respiratory function as discussed increase the incidence of PPCs and regional anesthesia is a better choice wherever feasible.[53] The duration of surgery is also important and risk of PPCs increases significantly with duration more than 2 hours.[34]

Preoperative Preparation for Surgery

The preoperative preparation of surgery is increasing the functional capacity and endurance of lung to reduce the risk of PPCs. These measures work along with patient education and compliance and optimization of modifiable risk factors wherever feasible.

Preoperative physiotherapy: Physiotherapy such as preoperative aerobic exercises and inspiratory muscle training (IMT) are simple, uncomplicated, and cost-effective strategy that reduce PPCs especially in patients with cardiac and abdominal surgeries but not joint replacement surgeries.[54]

A recent meta-analysis confirmed that IMT may halve the PPCs in patients undergoing cardiac and abdominal surgery.[55]

Correction of anemia: Patients with preoperative anemia defined as hemoglobin less than 10 g/dL have threefold increased risk of PPC undergoing any type of surgery.[34] Parenteral iron if patient is intolerant to oral therapy or surgery is due for less than 4 weeks. The blood transfusions should be reserved for emergencies or for symptomatic decompensated anemia.[56]

CONCLUSION

Postoperative respiratory failure is a common but serious complication of anesthesia and surgery with significant morbidity and mortality. The preoperative identification of patients at risk helps in risk assessment, preparation, and prognostication. The prediction of PRF using range of risk factors: preoperative comorbidity, type and duration of surgery, perioperative respiratory status, smoking status, and multiple hits to the lung during surgery have been found to be consistent in many studies. The prediction models can be used for preoperative risk assessment but no single tool has been validated enough to identify all patients at risk. The preoperative optimization of both modifiable risk factors and patient preparation using IMT or aerobic exercise are effective method of risk reduction of PRF.

REFERENCES

1. Jammer I, Wickboldt N, Sander M, Smith A, Schultz MJ, Pelosi P, et al. Standards for definitions and use of outcome measures for clinical effectiveness research in perioperative medicine: European Perioperative Clinical Outcome (EPCO) definitions: a statement from the ESA-ESICM joint taskforce on perioperative outcome measures. Eur J Anaesthesiol. 2015;32:88-105.
2. Lawrence VA, Hilsenbeck SG, Mulrow CD, Dhanda R, Sapp J, Page CP. Incidence and hospital stay for cardiac and pulmonary complications after abdominal surgery. J Gen Intern Med. 1995;10:671-8.
3. Lawrence VA, Dhanda R, Hilsenbeck SG, Page CP. Risk of pulmonary complications after elective abdominal surgery. Chest. 1996;110:744-50.
4. Arozullah AM, Daley J, Henderson WG, Khuri SF. Multifactorial risk index for predicting postoperative respiratory failure in men after major non cardiac surgery. The National Veterans Administration Surgical Quality Improvement Program. Ann Surg. 2000;232:242-53.
5. Gupta H, Gupta P, Fang X, Miller WJ, Cemaj S, Forse RA, et al. Development and validation of a risk calculator predicting postoperative respiratory failure. Chest. 2011;140:1207-15.
6. Yang CK, Teng A, Lee DY, Rose K. Pulmonary complications after major abdominal surgery: National surgical quality improvement program analysis. J Surg Res. 2015;198:441-9.
7. Gupta H, Gupta PK, Schuller D, Fang X, Miller WJ, Modrykamien A, et al. Development and validation of a risk calculator for predicting postoperative pneumonia. Mayo Clin Proc. 2013;88:1241-9.
8. Hua M, Brady J, Guohua L. A scoring system to predict unplanned intubation in patients having undergone major surgical procedures. Anesth Analg. 2012;115:88-94.
9. Ramachandran SK, Nafiu OO, Ghaferi A, Tremper KK, Shanks A, Kheterpal S. Independent predictors and outcomes of unanticipated early postoperative tracheal intubation after nonemergent, noncardiac surgery. Anesthesiology. 2011;115:44-53.
10. Brueckmann B, Villa-Uribe JL, Bateman BT, Grosse-Sundrup M, Hess DR, Schlett CL, et al. Development and validation of a score for prediction of postoperative respiratory complications. Anesthesiology. 2013;118:1276-85.
11. Kor DJ, Warner DO, Alsara A, Fernández-Pérez ER, Malinchoc M, Kashyap R, et al. Derivation and diagnostic accuracy of the surgical lung injury prediction model. Anesthesiology. 2011;115:117-28.
12. Li C, Yang WH, Zhou J, Wu Y, Li YS, Wen SH, et al. Risk factors for predicting post-operative complications after open infrarenal abdominal aortic aneurysm repair: Results from a single vascular center in China. J Clin Anesth. 2013;25:371-8.
13. Blum JM, Stentz MJ, Dechert R, Jewell E, Engoren M, Rosenberg AL, et al. Preoperative and intraoperative predictors of postoperative acute respiratory distress syndrome in a general surgical population. Anesthesiology. 2013;118:19-29.
14. McAlister FA, Bertsch K, Man J, Bradley J, Jacka M. Incidence of and risk factors for pulmonary complications after non-thoracic surgery. Am J Respir Crit Care Med. 2005;171:514-7.
15. Grosse-Sundrup M, Henneman JP, Sandberg WS, Bateman BT, Uribe JV, Nguyen NT, et al. Intermediate acting non-depolarizing neuromuscular blocking agents and risk of postoperative respiratory complications: prospective propensity score matched cohort study. BMJ. 2012;345:e6329.
16. Fisher BW, Majumdar SR, McAlister FA. Predicting pulmonary complications after nonthoracic surgery: a systematic review of blinded studies. Am J Med. 2002;112:219-25.
17. Pandit JJ. Effect of low dose inhaled anaesthetic agents on the ventilatory response to carbon dioxide in humans: a quantitative review. Anaesthesia. 2005;60:461-9.
18. Parameswara G. Anesthetic concerns in patients with hyper-reactive airways. Karnataka Anaesth J. 2015;1:8-16.
19. Saraswat V. Effects of anaesthesia techniques and drugs on pulmonary function. Indian J Anaesth. 2015;59(9):557-64.
20. Lumb AB, Slinger P. Hypoxic pulmonary vasoconstriction: Physiology and anesthetic implications. Anesthesiology. 2015;122:932-46.

21. Miskovic A, Lumb AB. Postoperative pulmonary complications. Br J Anaesth. 2017;118(3): 317-34.

22. Rao VK, Khanna AK. Postoperative respiratory impairment is a real risk for our patients: The intensivist's perspective. Anesthesiol Res Pract. 2018;2018:3215923.

23. Canet J, Sabaté S, Mazo V, Gallart L, de Abreu MG, Belda J, et al. Development and validation of a score to predict postoperative respiratory failure in a multicentre European cohort. A prospective, observational study. Eur J Anaesthesiol. 2015;32:458-70.

24. Respiratory Compromise is Common, Costly and Deadly, White Paper Covidien, Boulder, CO, USA, 2014. [online] Available from http://www.medtronic. com/content/dam/covidien/library/us/en/legacyimport/patient monitoringrecovery/patient-monitoring/17/respiratory-compromise- common-costly-deadly-white-paper.pdf [Last accessed March, 2020].

25. Shander A, Fleisher LA, Barie PS, Bigatello LM, Sladen RN, Watson CB. Clinical and economic burden of postoperative pulmonary complications: patient safety summit on definition, risk-reducing interventions, and preventive strategies. Crit Care Med. 2011;39(9):2163-72.

26. Kim M, Brady JE, Li G. Interaction effects of acute kidney injury, acute respiratory failure, and sepsis on 30-day postoperative mortality in patients undergoing high-risk intraabdominal general surgical procedures. Anesth Analg. 2015;121:1536-46.

27. Khan NA, Quan H, Bugar JM, Lemaire JB, Brant R, Ghali WA. Association of postoperative complications with hospital costs and length of stay in a tertiary care center. J Gen Intern Med. 2006;21:177-80.

28. Smith PR, Baig MA, Brito V, Bader F, Bergman MI, Alfonso A. Postoperative pulmonary complications after laparotomy. Respiration. 2010;80:269-74.

29. Nafiu OO, Ramachandran SK, Ackwerh R, Tremper KK, Campbell DA Jr, Stanley JC. Factors associated with and consequences of unplanned post-operative intubation in elderly vascular and general surgery patients. Eur J Anaesthesiol. 2011;28:220-4.

30. Smetana GW, Lawrence VA, Cornell JE. Preoperative pulmonary risk stratification for non-cardiothoracic surgery: Systematic review for the American College of Physicians. Ann Intern Med. 2006;144:581-95.

31. Mazo V, Sabaté S, Canet J. How to optimize and use predictive models for postoperative pulmonary complications. Minerva Anestesiol. 2016;82(3):332-42.

32. Ramachandran SK, Pandit J, Devine S, Thompson A, Shanks A. Postoperative respiratory complications in patients at risk for obstructive sleep apnea: a single-institution cohort study. Anesth Analg. 2017;125(1):272-9.

33. Kodra N, Shpata V, Ohri I. Risk factors for postoperative pulmonary complications after abdominal surgery. Open Access Maced J Med Sci. 2016;4(2):259-63.

34. Canet J, Gallart L, Gomar C, Paluzie G, Vallès J, Castillo J, et al. Prediction of postoperative pulmonary complications in a population-based surgical cohort. Anesthesiology. 2010;113(6): 1338-50.

35. Chung F, Abdullah HR, Liao P. STOP-BANG questionnaire: a practical approach to screen for obstructive sleep apnea. Chest. 2016;149(3):631-8.

36. Nagappa M, Patra J, Wong J, Subramani Y, Singh M, Ho G, et al. Association of STOP-BANG questionnaire as a screening tool for sleep apnea and postoperative complications: a systematic review and Bayesian meta-analysis of prospective and retrospective cohort studies. Anesth Analg. 2017;125(4):1301-8.

37. Khanna AK, Sessler DI, Sun Z, Naylor AJ, You J, Hesler BD, et al. Using the STOP-BANG questionnaire to predict hypoxaemia in patients recovering from noncardiac surgery: a prospective cohort analysis. Br J Anaesth. 2016;116(5):632-40.

38. Mazo V, Sabaté S, Canet J, Gallart L, de Abreu MG, Belda J, et al. Prospective external validation of a predictive score for postoperative pulmonary complications. Anesthesiology. 2014;121(2):219-31.

39. Neto AS, da Costa LGV, Hemmes SNT, Canet J, Hedenstierna G, Jaber S, et al. The LAS VEGAS risk score for prediction of postoperative pulmonary complications: an observational study. Eur J Anaesthesiol. 2018;35(9):691-701.

40. Bart S, Weinel L, Chan J, Nguyen P, Johnston S, Finnis M, et al. Pulmonary function testing does not predict post-operative ventilation requirements after elective cardiac surgery accurately to guide individual patient resource allocation. Aust Crit Care. 2019;32:S8.

41. Ivanov A, Yossef J, Tailon J, Worku BM, Gulkarov I, Tortolani AJ, et al. Do pulmonary function tests improve risk stratification before cardiothoracic surgery? J Thorac Cardiovasc Surg. 2016;151(4):1183-9.e3.

42. Routine preoperative tests for elective surgery. 2016. NICE guidelines [NG45]. [online] Available from https://www.nice. org.uk/guidance/ng45. [Last accessed March, 2020].

43. Joo HS, Wong J, Naik VN, Savoldelli GL. The value of screening preoperative chest x-rays: a systematic review. Can J Anaesth. 2005;52(6):568-74.

44. Scholes RL, Browning L, Sztendur EM, Denehy L. Duration of anaesthesia, type of surgery, respiratory co-morbidity, predicted VO$_2$max and smoking predict postoperative pulmonary complications after upper abdominal surgery: an observational study. Aust J Physiother. 2009;55:191-8.

45. Schmid M, Sood A, Campbell L, Kapoor V, Dalela D, Klett DE, et al. Impact of smoking on perioperative outcomes after major surgery. Am J Surg. 2015;210:221-9.

46. Hawn MT, Houston TK, Campagna EJ, Graham LA, Singh J, Bishop M, et al. The attributable risk of smoking on surgical complications. Ann Surg. 2011;254:914-20.

47. Musallam KM, Rosendaal FR, Zaatari G, Soweid A, Hoballah JJ, Sfeir PM, et al. Smoking and the risk of mortality and vascular and respiratory events in patients undergoing major surgery. JAMA Surg. 2013;148:755-62.

48. Myers K, Hajek P, Hinds C, McRobbie H. Stopping smoking shortly before surgery and postoperative complications: a systematic review and meta-analysis. Arch Intern Med. 2011;171(11):983-9.

49. Wong J, Lam DP, Abrishami A, Chan MT, Chung F. Short-term preoperative smoking cessation and postoperative complications: A systematic review and meta-analysis. Can J Anaesth. 2012;59(3):268-79.

50. Arozullah AM, Conde MV, Lawrence VA. Preoperative evaluation for postoperative pulmonary complications. Med Clin North Am. 2003;87(1):153-73.

51. Lumb A, Biercamp C. Chronic obstructive pulmonary disease and anaesthesia. Contin Educ Anaesth Crit Care Pain. 2013;14:1-5.

52. Ponikowski P, Voors AA, Anker SD, Bueno H, Cleland JGF, Coats AJS, et al. ESC Guidelines for the diagnosis and treatment of acute and chronic heart failure. Eur Heart J. 2016;37:2129-2200.

53. Guay J, Choi P, Suresh S, Albert N, Kopp S, Pace NL. Neuraxial blockade for the prevention of postoperative mortality and major morbidity: an overview of Cochrane systematic reviews. Cochrane Database Syst Rev. 2014;1:CD010108.

54. Valkenet K, van de Port IG, Dronkers JJ, de Vries WR, Lindeman E, Backx FJ. The effects of preoperative exercise therapy on postoperative outcome: a systematic review. Clin Rehabil. 2011;25(2):99-111.

55. Mans CM, Reeve JC, Elkins MR. Postoperative outcomes following preoperative inspiratory muscle training in patients undergoing cardiothoracic or upper abdominal surgery: a systematic review and meta-analysis. Clin Rehabil. 2015;29(5):426-38.

56. Kotzé A, Harris A, Baker C, Iqbal T, Lavies N, Richards T, et al. British Committee for Standards in Haematology Guidelines on the Identification and Management of Pre-Operative Anaemia. Br J Haematol. 2015;171(3):322-31.

Venous and Pulmonary Thromboembolism

Ruchira Wasudeo Khasne, Atul Prabhakar Kulkarni

INTRODUCTION

Venous thromboembolism (VTE) encompasses superficial, deep vein thrombosis (DVT) and pulmonary embolism (PE) manifest as a spectrum and can lead to high morbidity and mortality. Acute PE is a consequence of DVT in which a portion of thrombus breaks, travels to the lung and may be fatal. Spectrum of disease can vary from a silent extremity or pelvic vein thrombus to massive PE. Clinically PE presents in variable fashion with nonspecific symptomatology. Perioperatively, the symptoms are often lost in the plethora of changes due to surgery which makes the recognition and diagnosis even more challenging. Therefore, a high index of suspicion for occurrence of perioperative PE is necessary so that appropriate treatment can be instituted to prevent morbidity and improve survival.

Intraoperatively, PE will often present with hemodynamic instability and if it progresses quickly, can lead to circulatory collapse and death. Presence of right ventricle (RV) dysfunction and shock are suggestive of adverse outcome.[1] Surgery itself is a procoagulant state and therefore the patients are at a high-risk of developing DVT. This is particularly common with surgeries for major trauma, lower-limb fractures and joint replacements, spinal cord injury and prostate and other pelvic surgeries. As there are limited therapeutic options, since most of these can cause bleeding, we have to weigh the risks and benefits of these therapies. In this chapter, we will discuss the risk factors for PE, methods for perioperative DVT prophylaxis, diagnostic challenges, and management of PE using various reperfusion strategies.

INCIDENCE

Venous thromboembolism with DVT and PE are globally the third most frequent cardiovascular events which may be lethal in acute phase and may lead to chronic disease and disability. In epidemiological studies, annual incidence of DVT is 53–162/100,000 population and for PE from 39–115/100,000 population.[1] As per the International Cooperative Pulmonary Embolism Registry (ICOPER) study reported that the 90-day mortality of PE is as high as 45.1%.[2] The incidence of PE seems to be increasing, probably because of increasing awareness and recognition, advances in imaging modalities and improved diagnostic accuracy.

Surgical patients have additional risk of development of PE as they have specific risk factors which lead to a fivefold increase in incidence of PE. It is highest in orthopedic surgeries such as total hip arthroplasty (0.7–30%), hip fracture repair (4.3–24%) and total knee arthroplasty (1.8–7%) followed by multisystem trauma (2.3–6.2%) and acute spinal cord injury (4.6–9%).[3] In contrast, laparoscopic surgeries have minimum incidence of PE (0.06–0.9%) because of early mobilization, less surgical trauma and less pronounced prothrombotic state compared to open surgical procedures.[3] VTE is estimated to be four to seven times greater in patients with cancer. Cancer is the most common prevailing factor in patients who develop PE (27%), and the mortality is higher as well in these patients [30.3% vs. those without cancer (3.7% per patient-year)].[4] PE can also arise from DVT in nonlower extremity veins including renal and upper extremity veins, embolization rarely occurs from these veins.

STRATIFICATION OF PULMONARY EMBOLISM BASED ON SEVERITY

The American Heart Association (AHA) has classified PE into three classes: (1) massive PE, (2) submassive PE, and (3) low-risk PE.[5] Presence or absence of hemodynamic instability is an important factor for patient outcomes and deciding management strategy.

- *Massive PE*: Acute PE with sustained hypotension [systolic blood pressure (SBP) <90 mm Hg for at least 15 minutes or requiring inotropic support, not due to a cause other than PE, such as arrhythmia, hypovolemia, sepsis, or left

Table 1: Simplified version of Pulmonary Embolism Severity Index (PESI) score.

Variable	Score
Age	1
Cancer	1
Chronic cardiopulmonary disease	1
Pulse rate >110/min	1
Systolic BP <100 mm Hg	1
Oxygen saturation <90%	1

Table 2: Risk factors for deep vein thrombosis (DVT).

History	Blood diseases	Systemic diseases
Venous thromboembolism (VTE) history/malignancy (active or occult)	Thrombophilia	Acute heart failure, respiratory failure
Advanced age, tobacco, smoking	Protein C/protein S deficiency	Acute myocardial infarction/stroke/spinal cord disease
Prolonged immobility	Antithrombin deficiency/factor V Leiden	Obesity, pregnancy
Medications Estrogen therapy, oral contraceptives, chemotherapy, radiotherapy, antipsychotics	Hyperhomocystein-emia	• Multisystem trauma, surgery (cancer-related surgery, hip and knee surgery, prostatic) • General anesthesia
Varicose veins, prior thromboembolism	Hyperfibrinogenemia	Inflammatory bowel disease, autoimmune diseases
• Thrombocytosis • Myeloproliferative disorders	Prothrombin gene deficiency	Chronic kidney disease

ventricular (LV) dysfunction], pulselessness, or persistent profound bradycardia [heart rate (HR) <40 bpm with signs or symptoms of shock].

- *Submassive PE*: Acute PE without systemic hypotension (SBP ≥90 mm Hg) but with either RV dysfunction or myocardial necrosis.[6] RV dysfunction means the presence of at least one of the following:
  - RV dilation (apical 4-chamber ratio of RV to LV diameter >0.9) or RV systolic dysfunction on echocardiography
  - RV dilation on computed tomography (CT) (4-chamber RV diameter divided by LV diameter >0.9) or elevation of brain-type natriuretic peptide (BNP) (>90 pg/mL)/elevation of N-terminal proBNP (>500 pg/mL)
  - Electrocardiographic changes (new complete or incomplete right bundle branch block, ST elevation or depression, or anteroseptal T-wave inversion)
  - Myocardial necrosis is defined as either of elevation of troponin I (>0.4 ng/mL) or elevation of troponin T (>0.1 ng/mL).
- *Definition for low-risk PE*: Acute PE and the absence of the clinical markers of adverse prognosis that define massive or submassive PE.

Pulmonary Embolism Severity Index Score

The Pulmonary Embolism Severity Index (PESI) score is used to the risk of mortality after PE (11 variables). A simplified version of PESI score for rapid bedside assessment includes six variables, and presence of any one variable is associated with increased risk of mortality **(Table 1)**.

RISK FACTORS

Surgical patients can have one or more risk factors and are categorized into having low, intermediate and high-risk of PE. It is primarily due to release of thromboplastin during surgery leading to generalized hypercoagulable state. It is important for the anesthesiologist to identify the patient related and surgical risk factors and take

necessary preventive measures. These should be initiated preoperatively and continued postoperatively. Even the choice of anesthesia technique (i.e., regional anesthesia vs. general anesthesia) has profound impact on the risk of PE.

Table 2 enumerates the risk factors for development of DVT. Lower limb fractures, hospitalization for congestive heart failure (CHF) or atrial fibrillation/flutter (within previous 3 months), hip or knee replacement, major trauma, myocardial infarction (MI) (within previous 3 months), previous VTE, spinal cord injury are strong risk factors.[1] Hypercoagulable state associated chemotherapeutic agents, oral contraceptives, hormone replacement therapy, antipsychotics, obesity and smoking are the additional risk factors for PE.

Pulmonary Embolism Risk Prediction Tools

Caprini score: It is the most widely used prediction tool for perioperative PE risk.[6] Based on this score, one can categorize patient into high-risk group which warrants PE prophylaxis preoperatively itself **(Table 3)**.

The interpretation of the score is as follows:
- *Score 0*: Lowest risk of VTE
- *Score 1–2*: Low risk of VTE
- *Score 3–4*: Moderate risk of VTE
- *Score 5–6*: High risk of VTE
- *Score 7–8*: High risk of VTE
- *Score ≥ 9*: Highest risk of VTE.

Table 3: Caprini score.

Condition	Caprini score
Age >75 years	3
Postpartum	1
Major trauma	5
Hospitalization on a medical service	0
Cancer	3
Surgery	3
Pregnancy	1
Prolonged bed rest	1
Oral contraception	1
Factor V Leiden (heterozygous)	3
Hormone replacement therapy	1
Prothrombin 20210G (heterozygous)	3
Obesity [body mass index (BMI) >30]	1
Family history	3
Travel >4 hours	0
Elevated homocysteine level	3

Table 4: Revised Geneva score.[7]

Criteria	Point
Age >65 years	1
Previous deep vein thrombosis or pulmonary embolism	3
Surgery or fracture within 1 month	2
Active malignant condition	2
Unilateral lower limb pain	3
Hemoptysis	2
Heart rate	2
Pain on lower limb deep palpation and unilateral edema	4
Low probability: 0–3 points	
Intermediate probability: 4–10 points	
High probability: ≥11 points	

Table 5: Modified Wells criteria for pulmonary embolism (PE).[8]

Clinical criteria	Points
Tachycardia (>100 bpm)	1
Hemoptysis	1
History of deep vein thrombosis/PE	1
DVT symptoms/signs	1
Immobilization/surgery with 4 weeks	1
Cancer treated with 6 months/metastatic	1
Alternative diagnosis less likely than PE	1
Cutoff for PE unlikely ≤1	

Assessment of Clinical Probability of Pulmonary Embolism

Clinical probability of PE is based on clinical judgment or as per revised Geneva score and Wells criteria (**Tables 4 and 5**). Simultaneous application of PE rule out criteria (PERC) is validated to identify low-risk group. This criteria is not a screening tool but it helps to reduce unnecessary D-dimer testing.

PATHOPHYSIOLOGY

Perioperative PE can be and may go undiagnosed or it may be symptomatic and lead to life-threatening hemodynamic instability. Whenever the natural anticoagulation system is overwhelmed by procoagulant factors, intravascular thrombosis causing DVT occurs. The "Virchow's triad" is as follows:[9]
- Acute inflammatory reactions (acute infections, cancers, smoking)
- Hypercoagulability (activation of clotting cascade by surgery, oral contraceptives, cancer, antiphospholipid antibody syndrome)
- Stasis (surgery, pregnancy, heart failure) which worsens the venous stasis and promotes formation of thrombus.

The formed thrombus in the deep veins of leg dislodges and travels up to the pulmonary vasculature through the inferior vena cava and to the pulmonary vasculature through the right side of heart causes dead space ventilation (by cutting off flow in pulmonary artery and/or its branches. Cascades of events are as per **Flowchart 1**.

Clinical Presentation

The clinical signs and symptoms of acute PE are nonspecific. It may be asymptomatic and discovered incidentally or it can present with life-threatening hemodynamic instability, worsening hypoxemia, leading to cardiac arrest. Awake perioperative patient can present with dyspnea, anxiety, tachycardia, tachypnea, chest pain, presyncope or syncope, or hemoptysis, but if patient is under general anesthesia, PE may present with sudden hypotension, tachycardia, hypoxemia with sudden drop in end-tidal CO_2 ($EtCO_2$). Intraoperatively, these findings can be subtle and masked, and the first sign of PE may be sudden cardiopulmonary collapse. Key to diagnosis is high index of suspicion, and one should identify the event promptly and rule out the potential causes of hypoxemia and hypotension, including medication effect, surgical bleeding, infection, tension pneumothorax, cardiac tamponade, MI, CHF, or electrolyte imbalance, etc. One can assess the clinical probability of the disease by Geneva score or Simplified Wells score (**Tables 4 and 5**). On physical examination, with small emboli there will be no signs but with large-sized thrombus,

Flowchart 1: Pathophysiology of pulmonary embolism (PE).

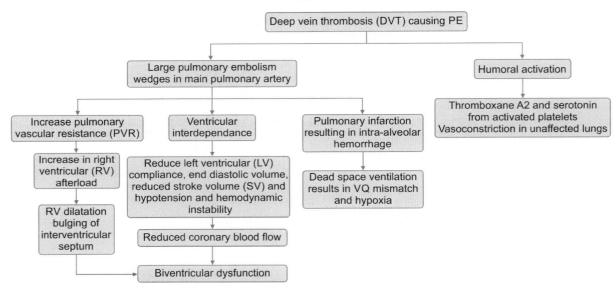

signs of RV pressure overload, raised jugular venous pressure (JVP), tender hepatomegaly, parasternal heave, loud P2, tricuspid regurgitation (TR) may be present. The guidelines have defined high-risk PE by hemodynamic instability and encompasses the three forms of presentation.[1]

1. Cardiac arrest requiring cardiopulmonary resuscitation (CPR)
2. Obstructive shock when SBP < 90 mm Hg or vasopressors required to achieve a blood pressure (BP) ≥90 mm Hg despite adequate filling status and end-organ hypoperfusion (altered mental status; cold, clammy skin; oliguria/anuria; increased serum lactate)
3. Persistent hypotension when SBP <90 mm Hg or SBP drop ≥40 mm Hg, lasting longer than 15 minutes and not caused by new-onset arrhythmia, hypovolemia, or sepsis.

DIAGNOSIS

Diagnosis of PE remains a challenge due to poor sensitivity and specificity of symptomatology and if it occurs intraoperatively. It is very challenging for the anesthesiologist as the symptoms are subtle and masked under anesthesia and mechanical ventilation. For any hypotension and tachycardia, best approach is to have high index of suspicion about the possibility of PE with clinical prediction scores and categorize the patient into low, intermediate and high risk. Implement necessary diagnostic modalities suitable for the situation to facilitate the definitive diagnosis. Myriads of diagnostic tests are available and each has its own limitations **(Table 6)**. Immediate simple diagnostic tests such as electrocardiogram (ECG), chest X-ray (CXR), transthoracic echocardiography (TTE)/ transesophageal echocardiography (TEE) and D-dimer assay can be done. Though these tests are nonspecific and highly insensitive, one can have a presumptive diagnosis and correlate clinically. D-dimer test has got a high negative predictive value to rule out PE with low clinical probability, but in perioperative period it has limited role.

Transthoracic echocardiography and/or TEE are the point-of-care investigations when shifting patient for CT pulmonary angiography (CTPA) is not safe or feasible. Any patients presenting with hemodynamic instability, TTE should be done as a fast, immediate step to differentiate between suspected high-risk PE and other acute life-threatening situations. According to the consensus statement of the American Society of Echocardiography and the Society of Cardiovascular Anesthesiologists, TEE is indicated when "unexplained life-threatening circulatory instability persists despite corrective therapy".[10] Besides that TEE is useful to rule out other conditions which can lead to hemodynamic collapse such as aortic dissection, valvular insufficiency, pericardial diseases, MI, etc. **(Table 6)**. Usefulness of intraoperative TEE is more as a monitoring tool to evaluate PE-induced hemodynamic compromise rather than as a primary diagnostic technique. The role of TEE to evaluate its role in diagnosis of acute PE via direct visualization has been found to be very limited. TTE could find direct evidence of PE in only 46% of the patients. The sensitivity for direct visualization of thromboemboli at any specific location was only 26%.[11]

Supportive investigation such as D-dimer assay has a very low positive predictive value and it is not useful as multiple conditions such as perioperative patients, infection, cancer, trauma, surgery, other inflammatory states also have elevated D-dimer levels.[12] But its negative

Table 6: Diagnostic modalities.

Diagnostic test	Parameters	Advantages	Limitations
Electrocardiogram (ECG)	Sinus tachycardia, arrhythmias (atrial) Nonspecific ST-T changes, right bundle branch block (RBBB), right axis deviation, RV strain, S1Q3T3, P-pulmonale	Available easily Low cost MI can be ruled out (as a differential diagnosis)	Nonspecific Low sensitivity Always need to correlate clinically
Arterial blood gas	Hypoxemia, hypocapnia	Can detect hypoxia, associated ongoing metabolic acidosis, rising lactates	<40% patients have normal arterial oxygen saturation (SaO_2) and 20% have a normal alveolar-arterial oxygen gradient
Highly sensitive plasma D-dimer tests	Fibrin degradation product by using enzyme-linked immunosorbent assays (ELISA) Recommended in outpatient or emergency department with low or intermediate clinical probability or those with PE is unlikely Clinicians should not obtain a D-dimer measurement in patients with a high pretest probability of PE	Have high negative predictive value. Negative D-dimer rules out PE The European Society of Cardiology (ESC) new recommendation to use age-adjusted cutoffs (age > 50 years × 10 is taken as upper limit cutoff) to improve the performance of D-dimer testing in the elderly[1]	Sensitivity of point-of-care D-dimer assays is low: 88% (95% CI 83–92%) whereas conventional laboratory-based D-dimer testing has sensitivity of at least 95%. Do not measure D-dimers in patients with high clinical probability, as a normal result does not safely exclude PE
Troponin I and T	Elevated in RV strain	Can help in predicting worst prognosis	Not helpful for diagnosis
B-type natriuretic peptide (BNP) and N-terminal (NT)-proBNP	Increased myocardial stretch, which leads to the release of BNP	Reflect the severity of RV dysfunction and hemodynamic compromise in acute PE	Sensitivity 60% Specificity 62%
Chest radiograph	Helps to rule out other causes of hypoxia and hypotension Focal oligemia (Westermark's sign) Dilated descending pulmonary artery (PA) (Palla's sign) Enlarged PA (Fleischner's sign) Dilated right descending PA with sudden cutoff (Chang sign) Peripheral wedge of airspace opacity and implies lung infarction (Hampton's hump)	It is mainly used bedside to rule out other causes of respiratory distress	Nonspecific Very low sensitivity and specificity Not very helpful to establish diagnosis of PE
Compression ultrasonography (CUS)	Suspected PE, simple four-point examination (bilateral groin and popliteal fossa) Look for incomplete compressibility of the vein	Useful point-of-care procedure in the diagnostic strategy of patients with contraindications CTPA It is recommended to perform CUS, in patient with clinical suspicion of PE Accept the diagnosis of VTE if CUS shows a proximal DVT in a patient with clinical suspicion of PE	Further testing is needed if CUS shows distal DVT The high diagnostic specificity (96%) along with a low sensitivity (41%) of CUS
Transthoracic echocardiography (TTE)	Echocardiography is useful bedside tool in differential diagnosis of acute dyspnea, evaluation of shock, justify emergency reperfusion treatment for PE if immediate CT angiography is not feasible in a patient with high clinical probability and no other obvious causes for RV pressure overload	Point-of-care, noninvasive Readily available No radiation exposure Reproducible enlarged right ventricle Dilated RV with basal RV/LV ratio, flattened interventricular septum, distended inferior vena cava with diminished inspiratory collapsibility, right heart mobile thrombus, decreased tricuspid annular plane systolic excursion (TAPSE) (<16 mm), decreased peak systolic (S') velocity of tricuspid annulus (<9.5 cm/s), patterns describing RV ejection which is highly specific, including "McConnell's sign" (e.g., RV free wall hypokinesis with preserved contraction of the apex) and the "60-60 sign" (e.g., a tricuspid regurgitation gradient < 60 mm Hg with pulmonary flow acceleration < 60 ms)	Subjective Interobserver variability Negative results cannot exclude PE Association of RV dysfunction or overload can be associated with concomitant cardiac or respiratory diseases Limited view in poor acoustic window

Contd...

Contd...

Investigation	Features	Advantages	Limitations/Notes
Ventilation-perfusion (V/Q) scan	Categorized into low, intermediate and high probability of PE	Lower radiation than CTPA, effective dose ~2 mSv compared to CTPA Reject the diagnosis of PE (without further testing) if the perfusion lung scan is normal Should be considered to accept the diagnosis of PE if result is with high probability for PE	The sensitivity 50–98% Specificity 20–60% Not useful perioperatively Interobserver variability Results reported as likelihood ratios Inconclusive in 50% of cases Cannot provide alternative diagnosis if PE excluded
CT pulmonary angiography (CTPA)	Visualize filling defect in pulmonary artery recommended to confirm the diagnosis of PE Gold standard Reject the diagnosis of PE (without further testing) if CTPA is normal in a patient with low or intermediate clinical probability, or if the patient is PE unlikely	Rapid accurate Other pathologies can pick up Readily available Excellent accuracy Strong validation in prospective management outcome studies Low rate of inconclusive results (3–5%) Short acquisition time Less invasive compared to pulmonary angiography if it shows segmental or more proximal filling defect with intermediate or high clinical probability	Not available bedside Invasive contrast exposure Contraindicated in severe renal failure Radiation effective dose 3–10 mSv Risks in pregnant and breastfeeding women Limited use in iodine allergy, hyperthyroidism The Prospective Investigation of Pulmonary Embolism Diagnosis II (PIOPED II)[13] study observed a sensitivity of 83% and specificity of 96% for (mainly four-detector) CTPA in PE diagnosis Sensitivity and specificity for PE of 95% to 100% in patients with low or intermediate pretest probability and a sensitivity of 85–95% in patients with high pretest probability
Magnetic resonance angiography	Thrombus in pulmonary artery	No risk of radiation	Not readily available Low sensitivity Not validated Should not be used to rule out PE
Pulmonary angiography	Can visualize thrombus directly As filling defect or as amputation of pulmonary arterial branch Reserved in patients where the diagnosis is still uncertain after CT angiography or V/Q scan Invasive	Historical gold standard Can perform catheter-directed therapies Excellent for those who cannot hold breath	Shifting if unstable is not possible Invasive contrast exposure, radiation exposure Highest radiation, effective dose 10–20 mSv Not readily available 85% sensitivity and 94% specificity in diagnosis of PE

predictive value is very high which helps in ruling out PE specially in nonsurgical settings. In perioperative settings where CTPA is not feasible, one can use compression ultrasound (CUS) of the leg veins. Demonstration of lack of vein compressibility in painful calf is the diagnostic of DVT which can be a surrogate for PE.[1] However, absence of DVT on CUS does rule out PE as there is no evidence of DVT in up to 50% of cases. Thus, negative CUS needs close monitoring and repeat evaluation.

Based on above-mentioned bedside tests and hemodynamic status, the presumptive diagnosis of PE should be made with simultaneous application of clinical probability scores such as Wells score or Geneva score as follows:

- *In hemodynamic stable patient with low intermediate probability and negative D-dimer*: PE is ruled out.
- *In hemodynamic stable patient with high clinical probability and elevated D-dimer*: Go for CTPA if possible to confirm diagnosis.
- *In hemodynamic unstable patient with suspected PE*: CTPA.
- *If CTPA unavailable or patient cannot be moved for CTPA*: TTE/TEE and CUS both lower limbs and look for RV dysfunction and DVT. If positive, treat it and do CTPA once stable and if negative search for alternative diagnosis.

MANAGEMENT DILEMMA IN THERAPEUTIC OPTIONS OF PE MANAGEMENT

Therapeutic options are limited in perioperative patients as there is always an increased risk of associated bleeding. Treatment needs a multidisciplinary approach and should be individualized. Thrombolysis is the choice of therapeutic strategy in hemodynamically unstable high-risk PE and has better outcome but this option is associated with more complications particularly in perioperative group. Other reperfusion techniques such as catheter-based thrombolysis or surgical embolectomy are preferred options. If PE presents with near arrest situation, immediate CPR support should be initiated as per the current guidelines of advanced cardiac life support. It should be continued for 60–90 minutes before termination of resuscitation attempts with simultaneous consideration of thrombolysis has shown better outcome.[14] CPR is not a contraindication for thrombolysis if the cause of cardiac arrest is suspected PE but avoid thrombolysis if PE is unlikely a cause of cardiac arrest. Whenever any patient has high clinical probability of PE, till confirmation of definitive diagnosis, one can initiate anticoagulation treatment.

Immediate management comprises the following:
1. Maintenance of oxygenation and ventilation
2. Hemodynamic stabilization

3. Reperfusion treatment:
   a. Anticoagulation
   b. Thrombolysis
   c. Catheter-based thrombolysis
   d. Surgical embolectomy

Maintenance of Oxygenation and Ventilation

Pulmonary embolism leading to hypoxia is due to ventilation-perfusion mismatch which indicates the severity of PE and should be managed by giving 100% oxygen. If the patient is not already intubated, secure the airway and initiate lung-protective ventilation (keep plateau pressure < 30 cm H_2O). One has to be very vigilant at initiation of intermittent positive pressure ventilation (IPPV) as it may precipitate RV failure. If hypoxia occurs intraoperatively under general anesthesia, first step is to put off inhalational anesthetic agents and start 100% oxygen. Positive end-expiratory pressure (PEEP) should be cautiously applied as it can worsen hemodynamics and cause circulatory collapse. Obtain arterial blood gas and modify oxygen therapy.

Hemodynamic Stabilization

Hemodynamic management of PE is complex and not clearly understood. Hemodynamic instability is a major risk factor for mortality. Cautious volume loading may be appropriate in case of low central venous pressure (CVP), low arterial pressure combined with low RV end-diastolic volume (RVEDV) to improve cardiac index. However, volume loading should not over distend RV, and/or worsen ventricular dysfunction (which occurs due to ventricular interdependence) and compromise cardiac output. With increased filling pressures, enthusiastic volume expansion should be avoided and vasopressors should be initiated.[15] Norepinephrine and/or dobutamine should be considered in patients with high-risk PE.[1] Norepinephrine (0.2–1.0/kg/min) is the vasopressor of choice which improves RV inotropy and systemic BP, promotes ventricular systolic interaction and coronary perfusion, without causing a change in pulmonary vascular resistance (PVR). But excessive doses may cause vasoconstriction and worsen tissue perfusion. Inodilators like dobutamine (2–20 mg/kg/min) may be considered for those with low cardiac index, and normal BP. It increases RV inotropy, lowers filling pressures. But it may aggravate arterial hypotension due to associated vasodilatation if used alone; it may trigger or aggravate arrhythmias. Levosimendan may restore RV-pulmonary arterial coupling in acute PE along with pulmonary vasodilation with improved RV contractility but there is no evidence to support this practice. Vasodilators reduce pulmonary artery pressure (PAP) and PVR but may worsen hypotension and systemic hypoperfusion as systemic side effects as they are not selective to pulmonary circulation. Theoretically, inhaled nitric oxide may improve hemodynamic status, reduce PVR and RV afterload but there is no evidence with regard to its safety.[16]

Initial Anticoagulation

According to Joint Working Group (JCS),[17] AHA,[5] the American College of Chest Physicians (ACCP),[18] the European Society of Cardiology (ESC) guidelines[1] recommended parenteral anticoagulation as a first-linetherapy for an acute high or intermediate clinical probability of PE without delay while awaiting the results of diagnostic tests **(Table 7)**. Any delay in anticoagulation can lead to an increase in morbidity and mortality. Anticoagulation serves to prevent further clot propagation and effective thrombolysis with clot dissolution. This is usually done with parenteral anticoagulants such as subcutaneous, weight-adjusted low-molecular-weight heparin (LMWH) or fondaparinux or intravenous (IV) unfractionated heparin (UFH). Advantage of UFH is rapid reversal if needed particularly in perioperative patients although frequent activated partial thromboplastin time (APTT) monitoring is required which is cumbersome

and costly. LMWH is associated with early attainment of therapeutic anticoagulation and is preferred in patients who are at low risk of hemodynamic instability and do not have renal dysfunction. Regarding oral anticoagulation, recently EINSTEIN study 2012[19] showed that fixed-dose regimen of rivaroxaban was noninferior and had superior safety, with less incidence of major bleeding to standard therapy for the initial and long-term treatment of PE.

Following are the ESC guidelines 2019 recommendations for anticoagulation:[1]

- Initiation of anticoagulation is recommended without delay in patients with high or intermediate clinical probability of PE, while diagnostic workup is in progress.
- If anticoagulation is initiated parenterally, LMWH or fondaparinux is recommended (over UFH) for most patients (Recommendation IA)
- When oral anticoagulation is started in a patient with PE who is eligible for a non-vitamin K oral anticoagulants (NOACs), e.g., apixaban, dabigatran, edoxaban, or rivaroxaban. A NOAC is recommended in preference to a vitamin K antagonist (VKA) (Recommendation IA).
- When patients are treated with a VKA, overlapping with parenteral anticoagulation is recommended until an INR of 2.5 (range 2.0–3.0) is reached (Recommendation IA).

Table 7: Available anticoagulant agents for thromboprophylaxis and treatment.

Agent	Route of administration	Thromboprophylaxis dose	Treatment of PE dose	Mechanism of action	Therapeutic monitoring
Unfractionated heparin (UFH)	Subcutaneous	5,000 IU every 8–12 hours	80 units/kg bolus followed by 18 units/kg/h infusion	Inhibits factor Xa and thrombin	APTT and platelets
Enoxaparin	Subcutaneous	40 mg once daily	1 mg/kg every 12 hours	Predominantly inhibits factor Xa	No
Dalteparin	Subcutaneous	5,000 IU once daily	200 IU/kg/day once daily	Factor Xa inhibitor	No
Fondaparinux	Subcutaneous	2.5 mg once daily	If heparin-induced thrombocytopenia (HIT): <50 kg: 5 mg once daily 50–100 kg: 7.5 mg once daily > 100 kg: 10 mg once daily	Selective Xa inhibitor	No
Warfarin	Oral	2.5 mg once daily		Vitamin K antagonist	Required monitoring by international normalized ratio (INR). Target INR ranges 1.5–2.5
Dabigatran etexilate	Oral	150 mg twice daily	150 mg twice a day. It must be preceded by LMWH for at least 5 days	Thrombin inhibitor	No
Rivaroxaban	Oral	20 mg once a day	15 mg twice a day for 21 days	Factor Xa inhibitor	No
Apixaban	Oral	2.5 mg twice a day	10 mg twice day	Factor Xa inhibitor	No

- NOACs are not recommended in patients with severe renal impairment, during pregnancy and lactation, and in patients with antiphospholipid antibody syndrome.
- Regarding the duration of anticoagulation as per ACCP, in patients with a proximal DVT of the leg or PE provoked by surgery, treatment with anticoagulation for either 3 months over (1) treatment of a shorter period (Grade 1B), or (2) treatment of a longer time-limited period for 6, 12, or 24 months (Grade 1B), or (3) extended therapy (no scheduled stop date) (Grade 1B).[20]

Reperfusion Treatment

Reperfusion treatment comprises the following:
- Systemic thrombolysis
- Catheter-based thrombolysis
- Surgical embolectomy

These therapeutic options of reperfusion have limitation during perioperative period but whenever feasible should be opted by weighing the risk of bleeding and therapeutic benefit. Risk of bleeding is highest within first week of surgery which progressively reduces in subsequent days.

Surgical embolectomy and/or catheter-directed treatment are other alternatives, rescue thrombolytic therapy for patients who deteriorate hemodynamically.[1]

Systemic Thrombolysis

The US Food and Drug Administration (FDA) for acute PE recommends use of recombinant tissue-type plasminogen activator (tPA, alteplase), streptokinase (SK) and recombinant human urokinase (UK) for thrombolysis **(Table 8)**.

As per the AHA guidelines, thrombolysis is reasonable for patients with massive acute PE and acceptable risk of bleeding complications (IIa B recommendation). The ACCP 2016 suggests thrombolytic therapy for PE with hypotension (Grade 2B), and systemic therapy over catheter-directed thrombolysis as reperfusion therapies (Grade 2C).[20] A recent Cochrane review analyzed 17 randomized controlled trials (RCTs) in patients (2,197) with massive and submassive PE who were treated with either heparin alone, systemic thrombolytic therapy, or placebo. In setting of massive PE, systemic thrombolysis has been found to be associated with reduced mortality despite increase in hemorrhage rates compared to heparin alone.[21] Thrombolytic therapy is associated with improved hemodynamics and improved echo findings. But one must rule out absolute contraindications for thrombolytics before initiation **(Table 8)** and certain surgeries such as intracranial, spine, eye, and trauma surgery, and active surgical bleeding complicate a patient's candidacy for systemic thrombolysis. The patient needs to be critically considered when systemic thrombolysis is indicated perioperatively. In case of submassive PE, thrombolysis may be considered based on clinical judgment and associated evidence like new hemodynamic instability, worsening respiratory insufficiency, severe RV dysfunction, or major myocardial necrosis and low risk of bleeding complications. But guidelines do not support thrombolysis for normotensive patients who have a submassive PE, because of the risk of bleeding superseding the potential

Table 8: The US Food and Drug Administration (FDA) and the European Society of Cardiology (ESC) guidelines approved thrombolytic agents.

Thrombolytic agent	Recommended dosage	Accelerated regimen	Contraindications to fibrinolysis
Streptokinase First generation Not clot specific	250,000 IU as a loading dose over 30 min, followed by 100,000 IU/h over 12–24 hours	1.5 million units over 2 hours	*Absolute* History of hemorrhagic stroke or stroke of unknown origin Ischemic stroke in previous 6 months
Urokinase First generation Not clot specific	4,400 IU/kg over 10 minutes, then 4,400 IU/kg/h over 12–24 hours	3 million IU over 2 hours	Central nervous system neoplasm Major trauma, surgery, or head injury in previous 3 weeks Bleeding diathesis and active bleeding
Recombinant tissue-type plasminogen activator (rtPA) Second generation Clot specific	10 mg bolus, then 90 mg over 2 hours	0.6 mg/kg over 15 minutes Maximum dose 50 mg	*Relative* Transient ischemic attack in previous 6 months Oral anticoagulation Pregnancy or first postpartum week Noncompressible puncture sites Traumatic resuscitation Refractory hypertension (systolic BP > 180 mm Hg) Advanced liver disease Infective endocarditis Active peptic ulcer

benefit of the medications. Rescue thrombolytic therapy is recommended for patients who deteriorate hemodynamically on anticoagulation treatment.[1]

The major concern of thrombolytics in perioperative period is risk of bleeding and intracerebral hemorrhage. Unsuccessful thrombolysis can be seen by persistent clinical instability and unchanged RV dysfunction on echocardiography after 36 hours. Low-dose thrombolysis trial [Moderate Pulmonary Embolism Treated with Thrombolysis (MOPETT)][22] was conducted with intention that it could result in faster resolution of pulmonary hypertension with no significant increase in bleeding rates but was criticized by small sample size and the use of echocardiography to assess pulmonary hypertension. Other methods of reperfusion therapy are percutaneous catheter-directed treatment and surgical embolectomy when thrombolytic therapy is contraindicated and hemodynamic status does not improve with medical treatment. Approach to the patient of PE for reperfusion therapy is seen in **Flowchart 2**.

Catheter-based Thrombectomy

The decision to proceed with catheter-based thrombectomy requires interdisciplinary teamwork and local expertise. It should be considered for patients with high-risk massive or submassive PE associated with high risk of bleeding, failed thrombolysis or when it is contraindicated, life-threatening shock before systemic thrombolysis can take effect, provided appropriate expertise and resources are available.[1,20,23] The goal of catheter-based therapy is to rapidly reduce PAP, RV strain, PVR to improve systemic perfusion and facilitate RV recovery. Hybrid therapy which includes both catheter-based clot fragmentation and local thrombolysis is an emerging strategy.[5] These procedures are not recommended for patients with low-risk PE or submassive acute PE with minor RV dysfunction, minor myocardial necrosis, and no ongoing clinical worsening.[5]

Flowchart 2: Approach to the patient of pulmonary embolism (PE) for reperfusion therapy.

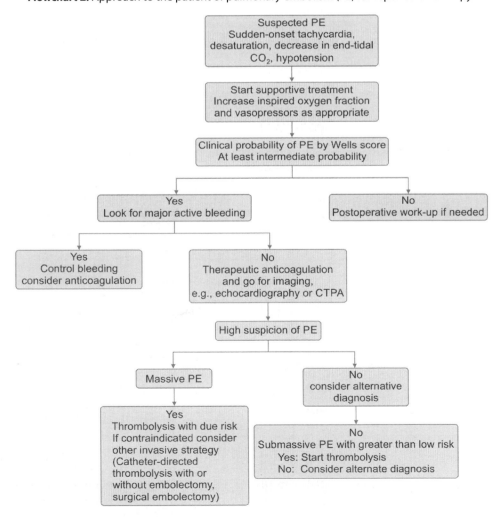

Percutaneous catheter-directed thrombolysis treatment comprises direct administration of thrombolytics into a clot. It requires low-dose thrombolytics and is effective in distal clots.

Ultrasound-assisted thrombolysis (USAT) where catheter-directed high-frequency ultrasound is used to break the clot with simultaneous administration of local thrombolytics. It requires less thrombolytics compared to catheter-directed therapies. ULTIMA[24] was an industry-sponsored randomized control trial of UFH plus catheter-directed thrombolysis with USAT and tPA dose of 10–20 mg over 15 hours in submassive PE. USAT regimen is found to be superior to anticoagulation with heparin alone in reversing RV dilatation at 24 hours, without an increase in bleeding complications.

Other trials like SEATTLE and PERFECT trials had come up with same conclusion for those with massive and submassive PE where systemic thrombolysis is contraindicated. However, robust evidence is lacking till date and there is risk of potential complications such as pulmonary hemorrhage and right atrial or ventricular perforation leading to cardiac tamponade and death. Other catheter-guided techniques such as rheolytic thrombectomy (with high saline Jetto macerate the thrombus), suction thrombectomy (direct aspiration of thrombus) and rotational thrombectomy (rotating screw-guided aspiration of thrombus) are available for effective thrombus removal but these are not free of complications and need expertise. These techniques are less invasive compared to surgical embolectomy but there is no evidence to support one technique over other.

Surgical Embolectomy

It is recommended for patients with high-risk PE with RV failure, in whom thrombolysis is contraindicated or has failed provided appropriate expertise and resources are available.[1,25] Surgical embolectomy is preferred in patients with PE refractory to thrombolysis and is carried out with patient on cardiopulmonary bypass. The pulmonary arteries are incised and clot is removed with suction. Major complications of surgical embolectomy are inability to wean from cardiopulmonary bypass because of primary RV dysfunction, persistent severe pulmonary hypertension, or severe hypoxia and need of extracorporeal membrane oxygenation (ECMO) as a bridge to recovery. ECMO may be considered, in combination with surgical embolectomy or catheter-directed treatment, in patients with PE and refractory circulatory collapse or cardiac arrest.[1] Prompt emboli removal facilitates RV load with improvement is cardiopulmonary function in early post operative period. It reduces hypoxia-induced pulmonary vasoconstriction, improves systemic BP, coronary perfusion and optimizes afterload thus improving biventricular function. It is safe and effective therapy in unstable patients with acute massive PE and offers acceptable outcomes.[26] Further RCTs are awaited. ECMO is associated with complications, if used over longer periods (>5–10 days), such as bleeding and infections and there is no clinical benefit unless combined with surgical embolectomy.

PREVENTION OF PULMONARY EMBOLISM

Thromboprophylaxis is not only extremely efficacious at preventing DVT but also highly effective in reducing burden of the disease. For low-risk surgeries, the ACCP recommends against specific thromboprophylaxis unless associated with major risk factors and encourages early frequent ambulation. For moderate-risk group, thromboprophylaxis with LMWH, UFH, or fondaparinux is recommended and for high-risk surgeries pharmacological method plus optimal use of a mechanical method are recommended. Those with a high risk of bleeding, optimal use of mechanical thromboprophylaxis with properly fitted graduated compression stocking (GCS) or intermittent pneumatic compression (IPC) and when the high bleeding risk decreases, pharmacologic thromboprophylaxis should be substituted for or added to the mechanical thromboprophylaxis. The ENDORSE study, a multinational cross-sectional study, found that only 58.5% of at-risk surgical patients (n = 11,613) and 39.5% at-risk medical patients (n = 6,119) received thromboprophylaxis. The ACCP guidelines recommend that every institution should develop their own individual PE prevention policy and frequent training program should be arranged for clinicians awareness and strict adherence to guideline is warranted.[27] The ACCP strongly recommends that every patient undergoing major surgery should receive thromboprophylaxis as therapeutic options are very limited and are not without complications.

- *Basic measures*: It includes early postoperative ambulation, active or passive limb physiotherapy and avoidance of preoperative dehydration, reduction in hypercoagulability by stopping hormone replacement therapy or oral contraceptives (if already ongoing).
- *Mechanical thromboprophylaxis*: These devices are used alone or along with pharmacological thromboprophylaxis. They act by augmenting venous blood flow and preventing venous stasis in the legs. It includes GCS, IPC, and foot pumps. It reduces the risk of proximal vein thrombosis by about one-half and the risk of PE by two-fifths.[28] A meta-analysis including 2,270 postoperative patients among which 427 were general surgery patients found that IPC reduced DVT risk by 60% as compared with no prophylaxis.[29] For DVT, the ACCP suggests not using compression stockings routinely to prevent post-thrombotic syndrome (Grade 2B).[20]

- *Pharmacological thromboprophylaxis*: Routine treatments with UFH, LMWH or fondaparinux have been studied extensively and are recommended for thromboprophylaxis **(Table 8)**. Perioperatively, one needs to identify surgical and patient-related risk factors before initiating thromboprophylaxis as there is obvious risk of bleeding. However, pharmacologic prophylaxis with anticoagulants may pose specific challenges in clinical practice related to surgical hemorrhage as well as regional anesthetic techniques. There has been always a concern related to neuraxial bleeding (spinal and epidural hematoma) and perioperative pharmacological prophylaxis although the incidence of bleeding is very low. The American Society of Regional Anesthesia and Pain Medicine (ASRAPM) guidelines have given specific recommendations regarding the use of antithrombotic and thrombolytics.[30] Optimum duration of thromboprophylaxis is still unclear. The ACCP guideline has following recommendations for the prophylaxis with moderate to high risk of PE.[20]

  – *In noncancer PE*: As long-term anticoagulant therapy, we suggest dabigatran (Grade 2B), rivaroxaban (Grade 2B), apixaban (Grade 2B), or edoxaban (Grade 2B) over VKA therapy, and suggest VKA therapy over LMWH (Grade 2C).

  – For VTE and cancer, we suggest LMWH over VKA (Grade 2B), dabigatran (Grade 2C), rivaroxaban (Grade 2C), apixaban (Grade 2C), or edoxaban (Grade 2C).

  – We have not changed recommendations for who should stop anticoagulation at 3 months or receive extended therapy.

  – In recurrent PE, LMWH is recommended over UFH.

Role of Antiplatelet Agents in Prevention of DVT or Pulmonary Embolism

The ACCP has suggested to use aspirin in patients with an unprovoked proximal DVT or PE who are stopping anticoagulant therapy and do not have any contraindication to aspirin (Grade 2B).[20] The ACCP guideline clearly mentions that aspirin is not a reasonable alternative to anticoagulant therapy for extended therapy but those who have stopped anticoagulants, aspirin can be used by weighing the risk of bleeding. Its use should be re-evaluated frequently.

Role of Inferior Vena Cava Filters in Prevention of Perioperative Pulmonary Embolism

Inferior vena cava filters (IVCFs) should be considered in patients with acute PE or proximal DVT with absolute contraindications to anticoagulation and in cases of recurrence of PE despite of therapeutic anticoagulation.[31] However, evidence does not support routine use of IVCF in prevention of PE in the perioperative setting and for PE treated with anticoagulants[1] (Grade 1B).[20]

Inferior vena cava filter is percutaneously inserted which is a mesh-like structure designed to trap thrombus in inferior vena cava and prevents its upward migration toward pulmonary vasculature. Potential complications such as penetration of the caval wall or embolization to the right heart cavities, generation of thrombus (if made up of metal) are noted. PREPIC-2 trial[32] (Prevention du Risque d'Embolie Pulmonaire par Interruption Cave-2) compared patients of proximal DVT with filter or without filter in addition to standard anticoagulant treatment. Out of 396 patients, symptomatic PE occurred in 9 patients in the filter group (6.2%) compared to 24 patients in without filter group (P = 0.008) showing reduced risk of PE. But 57 patients (35.7%) developed DVT in the filter group compared to 41 (27.5%) in the no-filter group (P = 0.042). In addition, there was no survival benefit [201 patients (50.3%) had died (103 in the filter and 98 in no-filter group)]. Subsequently, one systematic review and meta-analysis which included 11 studies (2,055 patients IVCF vs. 2,149 with no filter). IVCF placement was associated with a 50% reduction in the incidence of PE but around ~70% increase in the risk of DVT over time. Neither all-cause mortality nor PE-related mortality differed among the groups.[33] In nutshell, the beneficial effect of IVCF for preventing recurrent PE, in patients with DVT at high risk for PE, was offset by an increased incidence of recurrent DVT with no effect on overall mortality.[5] In case of submassive PE and proximal DVT, routine placement of IVCF is not supported by current evidence. Retrievable filters which can be removed within the recommended time can be considered.[34]

CONCLUSION

Perioperative PE is a preventable but devastating complication causing morbidity and mortality. One must always have a high index of suspicion in any perioperative patient with sudden onset of hemodynamic instability. Diagnosis can be challenging to anesthesiologist if it occurs intraoperatively, as symptoms are masked by anesthesia. High-risk group and high-risk surgery should be identified preoperatively and preventive measures should be instituted preoperatively. The anesthesia techniques can also be modified. As there are limited therapeutic options available, and those too with their own complications, best approach to PE is implement preventive strategies. Prompt diagnosis and early anticoagulation treatment can improve the survival of the patient. If PE is massive, it may warrant additional therapy, including consideration for systemic thrombolysis by weighing the risk-benefit ratio with interdisciplinary approach.

REFERENCES

1. Konstantinides SV, Meyer G, Becattini C, Bueno H, Geersing GJ, Harjola VP, et al. 2019 ESC Guidelines for the diagnosis and management of acute pulmonary embolism developed in collaboration with the European Respiratory Society (ERS). The Task Force for the diagnosis and management of acute pulmonary embolism of the European Society of Cardiology (ESC). Eur Heart J. 2019;1-61.

2. Goldhaber SZ, Visani L, De Rosa M. Acute pulmonary embolism: clinical outcomes in the International Cooperative Pulmonary Embolism Registry (ICOPER). Lancet. 1999;353(9162):1386-9.

3. Matthew C. Desciak DE. Perioperative pulmonary embolism: diagnosis and anesthetic management. J Clin Anesth. 2011;23:153-65.

4. Nakamura M, Yamada N. Current management of venous thromboembolism in Japan: current epidemiology and advances in anticoagulant therapy. J Cardiol. 2015;66:451-9.

5. Jaff MR, Mcmurtry MS, Archer SL, Cushman M, Goldenberg N, Goldhaber SZ, et al. Management of massive and submassive pulmonary embolism, iliofemoral deep vein thrombosis, and chronic thromboembolic pulmonary hypertension: a scientific statement from the American Heart Association methods. Circulation. 2011;123:1788-830.

6. Caprini JA. Thrombosis risk assessment as a guide to quality patient care. Dis Mon. 2005;51(2-3):70-8.

7. Le Gal G, Righini M, Roy PM, Sanchez O, Aujesky D, Bounameaux H, et al. Prediction of pulmonary embolism in the emergency department: the revised Geneva score. Ann Intern Med. 2006;144(3):165-71.

8. Wells PS, Anderson DR, Rodger M, Stiell I, Dreyer JF, Bernes D, et al. Excluding pulmonary embolism at the bedside without diagnostic imaging: management of patients with suspected pulmonary embolism presenting to the emergency department by using a simple clinical model and D-dimer. Ann Intern Med. 2001;135:98-107.

9. Virchow R. "Thrombose und Embolie. Gefässentzündung und septische Infektion". Gesammelte Abhandlungen zur Wissenschaftlichen Medicin (in German). Frankfurt, Germany: Meidinger Sohn; 1856. pp. 219-732.

10. Reeves ST, Finley AC, Skubas NJ, Swaminathan M, Whitley WS, Glas KE, et al. Basic perioperative transesophageal echocardiography examination: a consensus statement of the American Society of Echocardiography and the Society of Cardiovascular Anesthesiologists. Anesth Analg. 2013;117:543-58.

11. Rosenberger P, Shernan SK, Eltzschig HK, Body SC. Utility of intraoperative transesophageal echocardiography for diagnosis of pulmonary embolism. Anesth Analg. 2004;99:12-6.

12. Dindo D, Breitenstein S, Hahnloser D, Seifert B, Yakarisik S, Asmis LM, et al. Kinetics of D-dimer after general surgery. Blood Coagul Fibrinolysis. 2009;20:347-52.

13. Stein PD, Fowler SE, Goodman LR, Gottschalk A, Hales CA, Hull RD, et al. Multidetector computed tomography for acute pulmonary embolism. N Engl J Med. 2006;354:2317-27.

14. Truhlar A, Deakin CD, Soar J, Khalifa GE, Alfonzo A, Bierens JJ, et al. European Resuscitation Council guidelines for resuscitation 2015: Section 4. Cardiac arrest in special circumstances. Resuscitation. 2015;95:148-201.

15. Ventetuolo CE, Klinger JR. Management of acute right ventricular failure in the intensive care unit. Ann Am Thorac Soc. 2014;11:811-22.

16. Summerfield DT, Desai H, Levitov A, Rrt DA, Marik PE. Case reports inhaled nitric oxide as salvage therapy in massive pulmonary embolism: a case series. Respir Care. 2012;57:444-8.

17. JCS Joint Working Group. Guidelines for the diagnosis, treatment and prevention of pulmonary thromboembolism and deep vein thrombosis (JCS 2009). Circ J. 2011;75:1258-81.

18. Guyatt GH, Akl EA, Crowther M, Gutterman DD, Schünemann HJ, Lewis SZ. Introduction to the 9th edition: antithrombotic therapy and prevention of thrombosis, 9th Ed: American College of Chest Physicians—evidence-based clinical practice guidelines. Chest. 2012;141:7S-47S.

19. EINSTEIN–PE investigators, Büller HR, Prins MH, Lensin AW, Decousus H, Jacobson BF, et al. Oral rivaroxaban for the treatment of symptomatic pulmonary embolism. N Engl J Med. 2012;366:1287-97.

20. Kearon C, Akl EA, Ornelas J, Blaivas A, Jimenez D, Bounameaux H, et al. Antithrombotic therapy for VTE disease: CHEST Guideline and Expert Panel Report. Chest. 2016;149:315-52.

21. Hao Q, Dong Bi R, Yue J, Wu T, Liu GJ. Thrombolytic therapy for pulmonary embolism. Cochrane Database Syst Rev. 2015;(9):CD004437.

22. Shari M, Bay C, Skrocki L, Rahimi F. Moderate pulmonary embolism treated with thrombolysis (from the "MOPETT" trial). Am J Cardiol. 2013;111:273-7.

23. Devcic Z, Kuo WT. Percutaneous Pulmonary embolism thrombectomy and thrombolysis: technical tips and tricks. Semin Intervent Radiol. 2018;35:129-35.

24. Kucher N, Boekstegers P, Müller OJ, Kupatt C, Beyer-Westendorf J, Heitzer T, et al. Randomized, controlled trial of ultrasound-assisted pulmonary embolism. Circulation. 2014;129:479-86.

25. Iaccarino A, Frati G, Schirone L, Saade W, Iovine E, Abramo D, et al. Surgical embolectomy for acute massive pulmonary embolism: state of the art. J Thorac Dis. 2018;10:5154-61.

26. O'Malley TJ, Choi JH, Maynes EJ, Wood CT, D'Antonio ND, Mellado M, et al. Outcomes of extracorporeal life support for the treatment of acute massive pulmonary embolism: a systematic review. Resuscitation. 2020;146:132-7.

27. Cohen AT, Tapson VF, Bergmann J, Goldhaber SZ, Kakkar AK, Deslandes B, et al. Venous thromboembolism risk and prophylaxis in the acute hospital care setting (ENDORSE study): a multinational cross-sectional study. Lancet. 2008;371:387-94.

28. Zurawska U, Parasuraman S, Goldhaber SZ. Prevention of pulmonary embolism in general surgery patients. Circulation. 2007;115:e302-7.

29. Urbankova J, Quiroz R, Kucher N, Goldhaber SZ. Intermittent pneumatic compression and deep vein thrombosis prevention.

A meta-analysis in postoperative patients. Thromb Haemost. 2005;94:1181-5.

30. Horlocker TT, Vandermeulen E, Kopp SL, Gogarten W, Leffert LR, Benzon HT. Regional anesthesia in the patient receiving antithrombotic or thrombolytic therapy: American Society of Regional Anesthesia and Pain Medicine Evidence-Based Guidelines (Fourth Edition). 2018;43:263-309.

31. Comes RF, Mismetti P, Afshari A, ESA VTE Guidelines Task Force. European guidelines on perioperative venous thromboembolism prophylaxis: inferior vena cava filters. Eur J Anaesthesiol. 2018;35:108-11.

32. PREPIC Study Group. Eight-year follow-up of patients with permanent vena cava filters in the prevention of pulmonary embolism: The PREPIC randomized study. Circulation. 2005;112:416-22.

33. Bikdeli B, Chatterjee S, Desai NR, Kirtane AJ, Desai MM, Bracken MB, et al. Inferior vena cava filters to prevent pulmonary embolism: systematic review and meta-analysis. J Am Coll Cardiol. 2017;70:1587-97.

34. Condliffe R, Elliot CA, Hughes RJ, Hurdman J, Maclean RM, Sabroe I, et al. Management dilemmas in acute pulmonary embolism. Thorax. 2014;69:174-80.

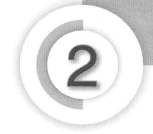
Cardiothoracic and Vascular

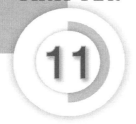

Perioperative Management of Coronary Artery Bypass Grafting

Yatin Mehta, Ajmer Singh

INTRODUCTION

Coronary artery bypass graft (CABG) surgery is the most commonly performed adult cardiac surgical procedure. There are two ways of performing CABG surgery: (1) conventional on-pump CABG (CCAB) which uses cardiopulmonary bypass (CPB); and (2) off-pump CABG (OPCAB) that does not require the use of CPB. The first few CABG procedures in early 1960s were performed on the beating heart without CPB. This technique, however, was soon abandoned due to developments in the extracorporeal circulation and improvement in myocardial protection that made the CCAB safer, standardized, and reproducible. The CABG *per se* is a potent triggering factor for cardiovascular events because it elicits major endocrine stress and systemic inflammatory responses, which involve the release of inflammatory cytokines and sepsis like symptoms in the postoperative recovery phase. The inflammatory response during CABG may be related, in part, to the use of CPB.[1] OPCAB was popularized to offset the potential deleterious effects of CPB, and was aimed to provide improved outcome with reduced inflammatory response, lesser renal dysfunction, reduced incidence of stroke, less coagulopathy, less blood transfusion requirement, and reduced lengths of intensive care unit (ICU) and hospital stay.

With the advances in anesthetic and surgical techniques, there has been a parallel advancement in the postoperative care of CABG patients. OPCAB comprises 15–20% of all CABG procedures in the United States and about 16% in the United Kingdom.[2,3] On the other hand, OPCAB forms approximately 60% of all CABG procedures performed in India.[4] A minority of surgeons and centers in Japan too continue to perform OPCABs in most of their patients. OPCAB procedures include: (1) off-pump multivessel CABG, (2) minimally invasive direct coronary artery bypass (MIDCAB) surgery in which left anterior descending

(LAD) artery is bypassed using a small anterolateral thoracotomy, (3) total endoscopic coronary artery bypass (TECAB) surgery, (4) robotic-assisted CABG in which robotic technique is used not only for internal mammary artery (IMA) harvesting and but also for the anastomosis, (5) hybrid cardiac revascularization, which combines left IMA (LIMA) to LAD artery anastomosis with percutaneous coronary intervention to other territories. The concept of hybrid cardiac revascularization has come from the fact that LIMA to LAD graft is superior to stenting of the LAD, while stenting is noninferior to venous bypass grafts for non-LAD territories.

Patients undergoing CABG develop alteration in cardiovascular function which can manifest in the form of low cardiac output (CO), myocardial ischemia, arrhythmias, bleeding, or cardiac tamponade.[5] The goals in the immediate postoperative period include: monitoring and assurance of hemodynamic and respiratory stability, preservation of other organ functions, restoration of normal body temperature, monitoring of fluid, electrolytes and blood loss from the chest tubes. Most of these patients are admitted in a cardiac surgical ICU, which is managed by an anesthesiologist, a surgeon and an intensivist all working as a team. Essentially all cardiac surgical units have a structured, written handover protocol enumerating intraoperative details, and briefing from surgical and anesthesia teams to the ICU team.[5]

Coyle has described several salient points that should be remembered in patients undergoing cardiac surgical procedures.[6] Although, these points are described for procedures involving CPB, they are equally relevant for off-pump procedures, which are: (1) Postoperative course is determined by intraoperative events, (2) Managing cardiovascular function is key to recovery of other organ systems, (3) Respiratory care is directed at restoring lung volume and minimizing lung water, (4) Preservation of renal function is essential in minimizing postoperative morbidity, (5) Management of postoperative pain is aimed to avoid chronic pain, infection, immunosuppression, etc., and (6) Coordination of care is required to facilitate immediate and timely intervention.

INTRAOPERATIVE EVENTS AND THEIR INFLUENCE ON POSTOPERATIVE OUTCOME

Intraoperative events that can influence the postoperative course of a patient include invasiveness of the procedure, anesthetic management including choice of neuromuscular blocking (NMB) agents and monitoring of neurotransmission, hypothermia, use of blood products, hemodilution, and pain management. MIDCAB, a less invasive technique, when compared with ONCAB, has shown benefits in terms of shorter ICU and hospital stay, as well as less transfusion requirement.[7] Port-access surgery or TECAB consists of small anterior thoracotomy incision and insertion of several small ports to view the heart and operate using endoscopic instruments. This technique involves a prolonged learning curve, extensive training of surgeons and staff, and extended operating times. Robotic-assisted CABG has the potential for quicker recovery and return to functional activity within a week after cardiac surgery. Potential benefits of robotic surgery include better tissue stabilization, lack of surgical tremors, lower risk of infection, faster recovery, and shorter hospital stay. Anaortic off-pump technique consists of complete avoidance of aortic manipulation. This technique may prevent dislodgement and embolization of atheromatous plaques into the aorta and reduce the risk of perioperative stroke.[8] A recent meta-analysis comparing CCAB, OPCAB with a partial-occlusion clamp, OPCAB with a Heartstring "clampless device," and anaortic OPCAB, has shown superior short-term outcomes in the anaortic technique.[9] Anaortic OPCAB resulted in statistically significant reductions in postoperative stroke, atrial fibrillation, renal failure, bleeding complications and early mortality.[9] Another issue that affects postoperative outcome and mortality, is emergent conversion of OPCAB to CCAB due to hemodynamic instability. An urgent or emergent conversion from OPCAB to CCAB is associated with greater risk of postoperative cardiac arrest, multisystem organ failure, and mortality than the patients undergoing elective CCAB.[10] When compared with successful OPCAB (not converted) and OPCAB converted to an CCAB, the latter resulted in significantly higher in-hospital mortality (10.3% vs. 0.7%, p < 0.001) in the recently published ART (Arterial Revascularization Trial) study.[11]

Some of the newer surgical procedures require one-lung ventilation for prolonged periods of time to optimize surgical exposure. This can result in hypoxia, hypercarbia, atelectasis, ventilation-perfusion mismatch, and higher risk of postoperative pulmonary complications.[12] Application of continuous positive airway pressure (CPAP) to the collapsed lung, and intermittent two-lung ventilation can help improve oxygenation and reduce shunt fraction. Adequate intraoperative analgesia by use of short-acting opioids and regional techniques (discussed later in detail) not only provides intraoperative hemodynamic stability, but also reduces surgical stress and postoperative pain. Fast-track cardiac anesthesia protocol consisting of use of short-acting anxiolytics/hypnotics/narcotics/NMB agents, and maintenance of normothermia help in early tracheal extubation, shorter durations of ICU and hospital stay, and better utilization of resources without affecting the quality of care. A recent, retrospective study (n = 609) has shown that remifentanil is more effective in reducing the time to tracheal extubation (80 min vs. 122 min, p = <0.001) and length of ICU stay when compared with sufentanil.[13] Residual paralysis after cardiac surgery is an important reason for delayed tracheal extubation, and no extubation should occur without verification of normal neuromuscular transmission. The risk of residual paralysis is higher when longer acting NMB agent, such as pancuronium is used, or a continuous infusion of NMB drug is used.

MANAGEMENT OF CARDIOVASCULAR FUNCTION

The common cardiovascular complications seen after CABG include hypotension, low CO, cardiac arrhythmias, myocardial ischemia (ST-T changes), cardiac tamponade, and excessive bleeding.

- *Hypotension:* Hypotension can result from hypovolemia, arrhythmias, vasodilatation, low CO, or impaired myocardial contractility. Treatment of hypotension is based on its etiology, which can be diagnosed with clinical evaluation and hemodynamic data derived from pulmonary artery catheter (PAC) and/or transesophageal echocardiography (TEE).

- *Low cardiac output:* Low CO (defined as cardiac index < 2.2 L/min/m^2), may occur in the immediate postoperative period or later on during periods of stress. Independent risk-factors for low CO include advanced age, impaired left ventricular (LV) function, OPCAB converted CCAB, emergency surgery, and incomplete revascularization.[14] Low CO is associated with high incidence of LV dysfunction, respiratory failure, renal dysfunction, neurological dysfunction, disseminated intravascular coagulation, gastrointestinal ischemia, and death. Low CO is managed by optimization of heart rate, preload, afterload, and contractility. Lactated Ringer's solution or balanced salt solutions are considered as first-line volume expanders. Synthetic colloids are not preferred over crystalloids as they can worsen coagulopathy and renal failure. Patients with LV hypertrophy, such as those with systemic hypertension require higher filling pressure for optimization of CO. Central venous pressure (CVP), PA diastolic pressure (PADP), and pulmonary capillary wedge pressure (PCWP) are commonly used parameters as surrogates for preload. While static intravascular pressures poorly predict fluid responsiveness, dynamic parameters such as pulse pressure variation (PPV) and stroke volume variation (SVV) require controlled mechanical ventilation, absence of spontaneous respiration, and sinus rhythm to predict fluid responsiveness.[15] The dynamic parameters are considered inaccurate in open chest conditions. Dynamic inferior vena cava (IVC) derived parameters such as IVC-collapsibility index, IVC-distensibility index, and IVC/aorta index do not predict fluid responsiveness in the first 6 hours after cardiac surgery.[16] Afterload reduction is essential to control blood pressure in patients with hypertension and in those at risk of postoperative bleeding. Short-acting vasodilators such as nitroglycerine and sodium nitroprusside are preferred for afterload reduction to avoid risk of sudden hemodynamic collapse.

Use of PAC is controversial even in high-risk patients such as those with severe LV dysfunction, right ventricular (RV) failure, pulmonary hypertension, and renal failure.[17,18] Alternative techniques of CO measurement, such as pulse contour analysis, transesophageal Doppler, and transpulmonary thermodilution, have shown conflicting results in cardiac surgical patients.[19] Patients who do not respond to optimization of preload and afterload, may need inotropic support to augment CO. Commonly used inotropes for low CO state include dopamine, dobutamine, and adrenaline. Dobutamine, an inodilator, often needs to be used in combination with vasopressor such as noradrenaline to maintain mean arterial pressure. A combination of dobutamine and noradrenaline is probably safer than adrenaline. Phosphodiesterase-III inhibitors (milrinone, amrinone, enoximone) or levosimendan (calcium sensitizer) may be required in situations of low CO with vasoconstriction, and with RV dysfunction.

Phosphodiesterase-V inhibitors (sildenafil, tadalafil, vardenafil) and inhaled pulmonary vasodilators [inhaled nitric oxide (iNO), iloprost, epoprostenol] may be useful in the settings of RV failure and pulmonary hypertension. Pulmonary hypertension and RV failure may reduce LV filling, LV systolic and diastolic pressures and CO, and lead to systemic hypotension. Decreased arterial blood pressure may compromise LV and RV coronary perfusion at a time when RV end-diastolic pressure and RV myocardial oxygen consumption are increased due to increased RV

wall tension, thereby leading to RV ischemia. RV ischemia exacerbates RV failure, causing a further reduction in CO and blood pressure. Concomitant LV dysfunction further impairs RV performance due to the loss of the interventricular septal contributions to RV function which are largely determined by LV function. One of the key interventions to break this vicious cycle is to reduce the RV afterload, for example by decreasing pulmonary vascular resistance (PVR), thereby enabling the RV to pump more blood forward. Although systemic vasodilators may reduce PVR, concomitant reduction of systemic blood pressure not only decreases the RV coronary perfusion pressure but also decreases LV contraction, which adversely affects RV function. Inhalation of NO produces selective pulmonary vasodilation without reducing the systemic arterial pressure in patients with pulmonary hypertension. A meta-analysis of 10 randomized controlled trials has shown a physiological benefit of inhaled pulmonary vasodilators (i.e., significantly increased RVEF) compared to intravenously administered vasodilators, but it fell short of determining whether or not inhaled vasodilators improve clinical outcome (i.e., length of ICU stay and mortality).[20] Vasopressors (noradrenaline, vasopressin, methylene blue) are useful agents for vasoplegic syndrome, or in the face of inodilator-induced vasodilation. Mechanical circulatory support using intra-aortic balloon counter pulsation (IABC), venoarterial extracorporeal membrane oxygenation (VA-ECMO), or ventricular assist device (VAD) is needed when low CO fails to respond to conventional therapy. Options for VAD in refractory shock include pneumatic pumps (Abiomed BVS, Danvers, MA), axial pumps (Impella, Abiomed), and centrifugal pumps (TandemHeart, Centrimag, Thoratec).[21]

- *Cardiac arrhythmias:* Postoperative arrhythmias are associated with hemodynamic instability, prolonged ICU and hospital stay, and risk of venous thromboembolism (VTE). Arrhythmias are potentiated by diuresis-induced hypokalemia and hypomagnesemia. Arrhythmias peak between the second and fifth postoperative days. Bradyarrhythmias occur commonly after inferior wall myocardial infarction. They can also be drug-induced or reflexly-mediated from hemorrhagic shock. Pacing may be required for hemodynamically significant bradyarrhythmias. Supraventricular tachyarrhythmias occur in 20–50% of patients after cardiac surgery.[22] AF is the most commonly seen supraventricular arrhythmia; and it can be prevented and treated with beta-blockers and amiodarone. Shehata et al., in their study have shown no significant difference between CCABG and OPCAB regarding incidence of postoperative tachyarrhythmias.[23] They also found higher incidence of supraventricular tachycardia among OPCAB patients and higher incidence of AF among CCAB group of patients. Ventricular arrhythmias (ectopics, tachycardia, fibrillation) can be prevented by lignocaine and magnesium; however, the benefit has not been seen in randomized clinical trials. Ventricular arrhythmias, though occur less commonly than supraventricular arrhythmias, are more ominous and may indicate myocardial ischemia. Patients with severe LV dysfunction and repeated ventricular arrhythmia may benefit from implantation of cardioverter/defibrillator (ICD).

- *Myocardial ischemia:* Nonspecific ST-T changes are not seen infrequently after OPCAB, and may reflect pericardial inflammation. ST-T changes seen in two or more contiguous leads indicate an acute graft failure, and may need further evaluation by TEE, cardiac enzyme studies, and/or coronary angiogram. New q-waves on a 12-lead ECG denote myocardial injury, and predict mortality.[24] In the absence of contraindications, all patients following CABG should be readministered aspirin, clopidogrel (for aspirin-sensitive patients), statin, and beta-blockers. Benefits of aspirin, at recommended daily doses of 100–325 mg, include better long-term graft patency, reduced incidence of myocardial infarction, stroke, bowel infarction, renal failure, and overall mortality.[25] Aspirin should be administered to all patients preoperatively, readministered within 6 hours postoperatively and continued indefinitely. Statins have the potential to decrease the incidence of AF, graft occlusion, renal dysfunction, adverse coronary events, and mortality.[26] Statins should be started postoperatively as soon as patient can take oral medications, and continued indefinitely. Beta-blockers prevent AF, and cause reduction in myocardial ischemia and all-cause mortality. It is reasonable to start low-dose beta-blocker (such as metoprolol 25 mg twice daily) and increase the dose as tolerated by the patient. Postoperative hypercoagulability and nonuse of CPB puts OPCAB patients at higher risk of VTE. Prophylaxis against VTE is suggested using a combination of mechanical and pharmacological methods. For patients at low risk of VTE, mechanical prophylaxis is suggested; and it can be achieved by either pneumatic compression devices or elastic compression stockings. High-risk patients should receive pharmacological prophylaxis (unfractionated heparin or low molecular weight heparin) in addition to mechanical compression.[26]

- *Cardiac tamponade:* Cardiac tamponade is suspected by worsening of hemodynamic status (i.e., tachycardia, hypotension, low CO), equalization of filling pressures (CVP, PCWP and PADP all being equal), and loss of the y-descent on the CVP or PCWP tracing. It should also be suspected when low CO is accompanied by sudden cessation of chest tube drainage. Transthoracic

echocardiography (TTE) has a poor sensitivity for the diagnosis of cardiac tamponade. Furthermore, a normal TTE does not exclude tamponade. TEE is a more sensitive tool than TTE for cardiac tamponade; and re-exploration is warranted if suspicion of tamponade is high. At the authors' institution, in a prospective study, TEE led to quick (9.6 min ± 2.8 min) diagnosis of cause of hemodynamic instability in 126 hypotensive patients after OPCAB.[27] Furthermore, TEE was helpful in preventing unnecessary surgical intervention. In another study, TEE not only prevented unnecessary surgical re-exploration in 19 out of 30 (63.3%) patients, but it also helped in locating the specific site of bleeding in six out of 11 (54.5%) patients who were re-explored.[28]

- *Cardiac arrest:* Cardiac arrest can occur as a complication of acute, massive blood loss, cardiac tamponade, malignant ventricular arrhythmia, or loss of pacing in a pacing-dependent patient. The treatment of cardiac arrest in ICU generally begins with up to three attempts of defibrillation in the event of ventricular fibrillation/tachycardia, epicardial pacing for severe bradycardia or asystole, reopening of chest cavity and internal cardiac massage. Return to the operating room is contemplated if the clinical situation does not improve despite these maneuvers. Chest compressions can cause cardiac lacerations and disruption of suture lines. Moreover, chest compressions should not be performed in patients on ECMO or VAD support. Cardiopulmonary resuscitation can cause dislodgement of cannulae and malfunctioning of the device in these patients. For the ICU resuscitation of postoperative cardiac arrest, the reader is suggested to review the guidelines published in "Cardiac Advanced Life Support-Surgical Guideline" or "Cardiac Surgical Unit-Advanced Life Support".[29,30]

POSTOPERATIVE BLEEDING

Excessive bleeding is defined as chest tube drainage ranging from more than 200 mL/hour to 1,500 mL in 8 hours.[31] An alternative definition is more than 400 mL in the first hour, 300 mL/hour for first 2 hours, or 200 mL/hour for 3 consecutive hours. Threshold for bleeding should be lower for OPCAB procedures compared to CCAB, because of absence of CPB-induced coagulopathy in the former. Risk factors for excessive bleeding include age more than 65 years, preoperative anemia, preoperative dual antiplatelet therapy, emergency surgery, use of IMA during CABG, lower body mass, decreased cardiac function, and poor attention to hemostasis. Postoperative bleeding can be termed either "Medical" or "Surgical". 'Medical bleeding' occurs secondary to disorders in coagulation system, platelet function, fibrinogen, or residual heparin effect. Treatment of "medical bleeding" depends on the cause;

and consists of the following: (1) Desmopressin 0.2–0.4 µg/kg intravenously for Hemophilia A, vonWillebrand's disease, or platelet dysfunction, (2) Platelet transfusion, to keep functional platelet count above 100,000 per µL, (3) Fresh frozen plasma (FFP), to keep prothrombin time normal, (4) Cryoprecipitate for hypofibrinogenemia, and (5) Antifibrinolytics for fibrinolysis. Based on the literature from trauma, it is reasonable to use packed red cells, FFP, and platelets in a ratio of 2:2:1 in an actively bleeding patient.[32] Alternatively, thromboelastography (TEG) or other point of care (POC) viscoelastic testing may be used to obtain information regarding activity of clotting factors, platelets, fibrinogen, and plasminogen. "Surgical bleeding" occurs secondary to leaks at the anastomotic sites or from small mediastinal vessels, in the absence of hemostatic disorders. For patients undergoing minimally invasive procedures, the threshold for bleeding should be lower due to inadequate hemostasis complicated by smaller incisions.

RESPIRATORY SYSTEM AND PREVENTION OF PULMONARY COMPLICATIONS

Changes in respiratory system that occur with median sternotomy include a decrease in functional residual capacity and approximately 50% decrease in vital capacity, both of which reach nadir on second or third postoperative day. Atelectasis (subsegmental, segmental, or lobar) and pleural effusion are seen in more than 90% of postoperative cases. Harvesting of IMA is associated with more pulmonary impairment than the saphenous vein harvesting.[33] Causes of respiratory failure after CABG include pneumonia, pulmonary edema, phrenic nerve injury, and acute respiratory distress syndrome (ARDS). The primary goals of respiratory care include provision of adequate oxygenation and ventilation; while the secondary goals are avoidance of barotrauma, volutrauma, infection, and pain. Extubation within 4–6 hours can be achieved in most patients after CABG, unless there is LV dysfunction, neurological injury, fluid overload, sepsis, renal failure, or exploration for bleeding/tamponade. Mechanical ventilation for more than 16 hours after cardiac surgery is associated with poorer postoperative prognosis.[34] Standardized institutional protocol regarding sedation and analgesia has shown shorter ventilation times. Moreover, an ICU managed by an intensivist has shown a reduced postoperative intubation time (61% extubated within 6 hours vs. 12%, p = 0.004), reduced blood product consumption, shorter ICU stay (by 0.28 days), shorter hospital stay (by 0.54 days), and decreased total costs (2285 USD/patient).[35]

A combination of preoperative physiotherapy interventions consisting of inspiratory muscle training, muscle strengthening with aerobic exercises at low intensity, deep breathing exercises, assisted coughing, and holistic therapy aimed at stress reduction, have all shown reduced incidence of postoperative pulmonary complications following CABG.[36] The beneficial effects are seen as decrease in the incidence of postoperative pneumonia, atelectasis, respiratory failure, reduction in ventilation time, anxiety, depression, and length of hospitalization. An observational study with 263 participants undergoing OPCAB, has shown a 52% relative risk reduction of atelectasis (17% vs. 36%, p = 0.001) in those who received prophylactic physiotherapy and education in respiratory exercises.[36]

GASTROINTESTINAL SYSTEM COMPLICATIONS

Dysfunction of gastrointestinal (GI) system, although seen less commonly following CABG, is associated with about 50% in-hospital mortality.[37] GI system dysfunction can be seen in the form of paralytic ileus, bowel perforation, upper GI bleeding, cholecystitis, pancreatitis, or hyperbilirubinemia. Mesenteric malperfusion during cardiac procedures generally results from hypovolemia, low-flow state, or overuse of vasoconstrictors. Acute mesenteric ischemia is suspected by abdominal pain, unexplained metabolic acidosis, elevation of lactate and D-dimer levels, decreased oxygenation, hypotension, and oliguria with or without peritoneal signs. The high risk of infection among patients with acute mesenteric ischemia outweighs the risks of antibiotic resistance, and therefore broad-spectrum antibiotics should be administered early in the course of treatment. Intestinal ischemia leads to early loss of the mucosal barrier, which facilitates bacterial translocation and the risk of septic complications. The multidetector computed tomography angiography is the diagnostic study of choice for acute mesenteric ischemia. Centers equipped with hybrid operating room can offer endovascular therapy (embolectomy/angioplasty/stent placement) and simultaneous laparoscopy or laparotomy if needed for such patients. The mortality rates after acute mesenteric ischemia are reported as 95% in medically treated patients, and about 57% in surgically treated patients.[37]

INFECTION AND SEPSIS

Sternal wound infection, mediastinitis, pneumonia, urinary tract infection, central line associated bloodstream infection (CLABSI), and sepsis can occur after CABG surgery. Mediastinitis, though occurs in only 1–2% of cases following cardiac surgery, is associated with 50% mortality. Risk factors for surgical site infection (SSI) include diabetes mellitus, obesity, blood transfusion, use of bilateral IMA, use of IABC, re-exploration, and prolonged ventilatory support.[5] Hyperglycemia is complicated in the postoperative period by surgical stress and catecholamine support used for hemodynamic optimization. With improved hyperglycemia management by devising a sliding scale for glycemic control, the immediate outcome in patients with diabetes is similar to those without diabetes.[38] After van den Berghe's article, tight blood sugar control (blood sugar less than 110 mg/dL) became the norm, till NICE-SUGAR study moderated it to 110–180 mg/dL.[39,40] The Society of Thoracic Surgeons (STS) practice guidelines recommend the blood sugar level to be kept below 180 mg/dL in the intraoperative and immediate postoperative period (class I, level of evidence C).[41] Sepsis is the most common cause of death, with the mortality rates as high as 20–60% in ICU patients. Gram-negative bacteria are responsible for 50–80%, while gram-positive organisms result in 6–24% of septic shock. The source of bacteremia leading to sepsis must be identified by culture and sensitivity tests, and the specific organism should be treated by appropriate antibiotic therapy.

RENAL DYSFUNCTION

The risk-factors associated with renal dysfunction include preexisting renal disease, perioperative hypotension, advanced age, diabetes mellitus, use of blood and blood-products, pharmacological or mechanical circulatory support, and use of nephrotoxic agents. The common nephrotoxic agents used in cardiac patients include contrast dye during angiography leading to contrast-induced nephropathy (CIN), nonsteroidal anti-inflammatory agents (NSAIDs), and angiotensin converting enzyme (ACE) inhibitors. The incidence of acute kidney injury (AKI) ranges from 0.7 to 4.3% in cardiac surgical patients.[42] Among the various biomarkers available for predicting AKI postoperatively, urine neutrophil gelatinase-associated lipocalin (NGAL) has shown promise as a sensitive marker of impending AKI in OPCAB patients.[43] AKI requiring renal replacement therapy (RRT) increases the length of ICU and hospital stay, and the risk of mortality by 27-times compared with patients without AKI.[44] Preventive measures to avoid AKI include avoidance of dehydration, maintenance of adequate perfusion pressure, and avoidance of nephrotoxic agents. If any signs of dehydration are present, positive input-output balance (about 500 mL) is achieved using potassium-free fluid after surgery. Drug dosages should be strictly adjusted based on estimated glomerular filtration rate (eGFR), especially when using antibiotics.

NEUROLOGICAL DYSFUNCTION

Neurological complications after CABG surgery range from mild cognitive dysfunction to cerebrovascular accident (CVA). Delirium after cardiac surgery is a major problem and occurs in up to 50% of patients over 60 years of age following surgery. Delirium is associated with cognitive decline, poor 1-year functional recovery, five-fold increased risk of nosocomial infection, and ten-fold increased risk of mortality.[45] Use of dexmedetomidine, an α-2 receptor agonist, has been shown to be associated with reduced incidence of delirium after cardiac surgery in a meta-analysis of 11 randomized, controlled trials.[46]

The incidence of stroke after CABG (off-pump or on-pump) is approximately 2–4%. Although OPCAB may have theoretical advantage of avoiding embolic atheromatous burden due to avoidance of aortic cannulation and CPB, there are case reports describing dislodgement of mobile atheroma even during OPCAB.[47] Epiaortic scanning should be performed in such cases to further delineate the site of severe atherosclerosis so that surgical modifications can be made. Anaortic technique is the most definitive way to reduce the risk of stroke in patients with atheromatous or porcelain aorta.[48] Recently, a successful outcome after simultaneous transcatheter aortic valve implantation (TAVI) and OPCAB surgery for Takayasu arteritis with porcelain aorta has been reported.[49] Stroke is usually embolic in nature and treatment is supportive. Amputation/occlusion of left atrial appendage (LAA), along with OPCAB surgery has been shown to reduce the incidence of emboli-associated neurological complications.[50] Currently, percutaneous devices for closure of LAA are available, and are considered noninferior to systemic anticoagulation with warfarin for stroke prophylaxis in patients with AF.[51]

POSTOPERATIVE ANALGESIA

Ineffective postoperative pain management may result in chronic pain, immunosuppression, infection, respiratory dysfunction (atelectasis, pneumonia, hypoxemia), activation of sympathetic nervous system, deep vein thrombosis (DVT), and poor wound healing. Chronic pain is a serious issue and is seen in about 20–80% patients after thoracic surgery.[52] Higher pain intensity is observed in female patients, younger and obese individuals; and in patients undergoing surgery with the use of CPB compared to off-pump surgery. Most patients undergoing cardiac procedures require multimodal analgesic techniques consisting of simultaneous use of systemic analgesics with different mechanisms of action, along with regional analgesic technique. Frequently used regional analgesic techniques include thoracic epidural analgesia (TEA), continuous unilateral thoracic paravertebral block, intrapleural block, and intercostal nerve block. A meta-analysis of 15 studies enrolling 1,178 patients undergoing CABG, randomized to receive either general anesthesia

(GA) or GA combined with TEA, demonstrated that the latter group had reduced incidence of dysrhythmias, pain, pulmonary complications, and ventilation times without any effect on the incidence of perioperative myocardial infarction or mortality.[53] Another study has found TEA to be beneficial technique in patients with chronic obstructive pulmonary disease (COPD) and obesity (body mass index of more than 30 kg/m^2) undergoing OPCAB surgery with better analgesia and pulmonary function test postoperatively.[54] Nonanalgesic benefits of TEA include decreases in stress and inflammatory markers in the form of interleukin-6, tumor necrosis factor-α, leukocyte count, procalcitonin, cortisol and catecholamine surge.[55]

HYPOTHERMIA

Patients undergoing CABG are prone to hypothermia due to low ambient operating room temperature, use of cold intravenous fluids/blood/blood products, cold saline lavage, and heat loss from open body cavities during surgery. Adverse effects of hypothermia include: (1) sympathetic hyperactivity with risk of arrhythmias and lowering of ventricular fibrillation threshold; (2) increases in systemic vascular resistance, afterload, and myocardial workload; (3) splanchnic vasoconstriction leading to mesenteric and renal ischemia, (4) shivering with increased oxygen consumption; and (5) coagulopathy with impaired platelet function. Hypothermia induced coagulopathy, is the reason why rewarming is an important part of the treatment of a bleeding patient. Rewarming in the postoperative period is generally achieved by "forced air warming".

WEANING AND DE-ESCALATION

Weaning from the ventilatory support following most uncomplicated CABG procedures can be achieved within 4–6 hours. If the swallowing function is normal, intake of clear liquids can be allowed shortly after tracheal extubation. Weaning of inotropic support, removal of PAC, removal of chest drains and Foley catheter can be accomplished on postoperative day one in most of the patients. Central venous catheter should be removed at the earliest to reduce the risk of infection. Most patients can be ambulated and discharged from the ICU within 24–48 hours after surgery. Cardiac rehabilitation and physiotherapy form integral parts of postoperative care.

CONCLUSION

Postoperative management of CABG procedures requires a comprehensive understanding of the multisystem pathophysiology, as the sequele of the procedures can affect virtually every organ system. Good outcomes can be achieved by protocol-driven approach and high-quality care. With ever increasing number of high-risk cases, a cardiac intensivist must keep abreast of the latest advances in technology, newer procedures, and their specific management concerns. The use of minimally invasive and hybrid approaches is promising, particularly in high-risk patients.

REFERENCES

1. Strüber M, Cremer JT, Gohrbandt B, Hagl C, Jankowski M, Völker B, et al. Human cytokine responses to coronary artery bypass grafting with and without cardiopulmonary bypass. Ann Thorac Surg. 1999;68:1330-5.
2. Bakaeen FG, Shroyer AL, Gammie JS, Sabik JF, Cornwell LD, Coselli JS, et al. Trends in use of off-pump coronary artery bypass grafting: Results from the Society of Thoracic Surgeons Adult Cardiac Surgery Database. J Thorac Cardiovasc Surg. 2014;148:856-64.
3. Taggart DP. Off-pump coronary artery bypass grafting (OPCABG)—a "personal" European perspective. J Thorac Dis. 2016;8:S829-S831.
4. Kaul U, Bhatia V. Perspective on coronary interventions and cardiac surgeries in India. Indian J Med Res. 2010;132:543-8.
5. Stephens RS, Whitman GJ. Postoperative critical care of the adult cardiac surgical patient. Part I: Routine postoperative care. Crit Care Med. 2015;43:1477-97.
6. Coyle JP. Sedation, pain relief, and neuromuscular blockade in the postoperative cardiac surgical patient. Semin Thorac Cardiovasc Surg. 1991;3:81-7.
7. Zenati M, Domit TM, Saul M, Gorcsan J 3rd, Katz WE, Hudson M, et al. Resource utilization for minimally invasive direct and standard coronary artery bypass grafting. Ann Thorac Surg. 1997;63:S84-7.
8. Seco M, Edelman JJ, Van Boxtel B, Forrest P, Byrom MJ, Wilson MK, et al. Neurologic injury and protection in adult cardiac and aortic surgery. J Cardiothorac Vasc Anesth. 2015;29:185-95.
9. Zhao DF, Edelman JJ, Seco M, Bannon PG, Wilson MK, Byrom MJ, et al. Coronary artery bypass grafting with and without manipulation of the ascending aorta: a network meta-analysis. J Am Coll Cardiol. 2017;69:924-36.
10. Edgerton JR, Dewey TM, Magee MJ, Herbert MA, Prince SL, Jones KK, et al. Conversion in off-pump coronary artery bypass grafting: an analysis of predictors and outcomes. Ann Thorac Surg. 2003;76:1138-43.
11. Benedetto U, Altman DG, Gerry S, Gray A, Lees B, Flather M, et al. Arterial Revascularization Trial investigators. Off-pump versus on-pump coronary artery bypass grafting: Insights from the Arterial Revascularization Trial. J Thorac Cardiovasc Surg 2018;155:1545-53.
12. Ganapathy S. Anaesthesia for minimally invasive cardiac surgery. Best Practice & Research: Clinical Anaesthesiology. 2002;16:63-80.
13. Zakhary WZA, Turton EW, Flo Forner A, von Aspern K, Borger MA, Ender JK. A comparison of sufentanil vs remifentanil in fast-track cardiac surgery patients. Anaesthesia. 2019;74:602-8.

14. Lomovorotov VV, Efremov SM, Kirov MY, Fominskiy EV, Karaskov AM. Low cardiac output syndrome after cardiac surgery: Review article. J Cardiothorac Vasc Anesth. 2017;31:291-308.

15. Marik PE, Cavallazzi R, Vasu T, Hirani A. Dynamic changes in arterial waveform derived variables and fluid responsiveness in mechanically ventilated patients: a systematic review of the literature. Crit Care Med. 2009;37:2642-7.

16. Sobczyk D, Nycz K, Andruszkiewicz P. Bedside ultrasonographic measurement of the inferior vena cava fails to predict fluid responsiveness in the first 6 hours after cardiac surgery: a prospective case series observational study. J Cardiothorac Vasc Anesth. 2015;29:663-9.

17. Ranucci M. Which cardiac surgical patients can benefit from placement of a pulmonary artery catheter? Crit Care. 2006;10:S6.

18. Bein B, Worthmann F, Tonner PH, Paris A, Steinfath M, Hedderich J, et al. Comparison of esophageal Doppler, pulse contour analysis, and real-time pulmonary artery thermodilution for the continuous measurement of cardiac output. J Cardiothorac Vasc Anesth. 2004;18:185-9.

19. Sharma J, Bhise M, Singh A, Mehta Y, Trehan N. Hemodynamic measurements after cardiac surgery: Transesophageal Doppler versus pulmonary artery catheter. J Cardiothorac Vasc Anesth. 2005;19:746-50.

20. Ichinose F, Zapol WM. Inhaled pulmonary vasodilators in cardiac surgery patients-Correct answer is NO. Anesth Analg. 2017;125:375-7.

21. Stephens RS, Whitman GJ. Postoperative critical care of the adult cardiac surgical patient. Part II: Procedure-specific considerations, management of complications, and quality improvement. Crit Care Med. 2015;43:1945-2014.

22. Kirklin JW, Barratt-Boyes BG. Cardiac Surgery, 2nd edition. New York: Churchill Livingstone; 1993. pp. 195-247.

23. Shehata M, AbdElhalim B, Hanna H, Nabih M. Postoperative tachyarrhythmias: on-pump versus off-pump coronary artery bypass grafting. ISRN Vascular Medicine. 2014;2014:1-7.

24. Yokoyama Y, Chaitman BR, Hardison RM, Guo P, Krone R, Stocke K, et al. Association between new electrocardiographic abnormalities after coronary revascularization and five-year cardiac mortality in BARI randomized and registry patients. Am J Cardiol. 2000;86:819-24.

25. Mangano DT. Multicenter Study of Perioperative Ischemia Research Group: Aspirin and mortality from coronary bypass surgery. N Eng J Med. 2002;347:1309-17.

26. Cartier R, Robitaille D. Thrombotic complications in beating heart operations. J Thorac Cardiovasc Surg. 2001;121:920-2.

27. Wasir H, Mehta Y, Mishra Y, Shrivastava S, Mittal S, Trehan N. Transesophageal echocardiography in hypotensive post-coronary bypass patients. Asian Cardiovasc Thorac Ann. 2003;11:139-42.

28. Wasir H, Mittal S, Mishra Y, Mehta Y, Trehan N. Site-specific detection of bleeder using transesophageal echocardiography. Asian Cardiovasc Thorac Ann. 2005,13:366-8.

29. Dunning J, Fabbri A, Kolh PH, Levine A, Lockowandt U, Mackay J, et al. EACTS Clinical Guidelines Committee: Guideline for resuscitation in cardiac arrest after cardiac surgery. Eur J Cardiothorac Surg. 2009;36:3-28.

30. Herrmann C. Cardiac advanced life support-surgical guideline: Overview and implementation. AACN Adv Crit Care. 2014;25:123-9.

31. Ranucci M, Baryshnikova E, Castelvecchio S, Pelissero G. Major bleeding, transfusions, and anemia: the deadly triad of cardiac surgery. For the surgical and clinical outcome research (SCORE) group. Ann Thorac Surg. 2013;96:478-85.

32. Zink KA, Sambasivan CN, Holcomb JB, Chisholm G, Schreiber MA. A high ratio of plasma and platelets to packed red blood cells in the first 6 hours of massive transfusion improves outcomes in a large multicenter study. Am J Surg. 2009;197:565-70.

33. Berrizbetia LD, Tessler S, Jacobowitz IJ, Kaplan P, Budzilowicz L, Cunningham JN. Effect of sternotomy and coronary bypass surgery on postoperative pulmonary mechanics. Comparison of internal mammary and saphenous vein bypass grafts. Chest. 1989;96:873-6.

34. Cannon MA, Beattie C, Speroff T, France D, Mistak B, Drinkwater D. The economic benefit of organizational restructuring of the cardiothoracic intensive care unit. J Cardiothorac Vasc Anesth. 2003;17:565-70.

35. Kumar K, Zarychanski R, Bell DD, Manji R, Zivot J, Menkis AH, et al. Impact of 24-hour in-house intensivists on a dedicated cardiac surgery intensive care unit. Cardiovascular Health Research in Manitoba Investigator Group. Ann Thorac Surg. 2009;88:1153-61.

36. Diez MP, Lourido BP. Prevention of postoperative pulmonary complications through preoperative physiotherapy interventions in patients undergoing coronary artery bypass graft: literature review. J Phys Ther Sci. 2018;30:1034-8.

37. Schoots IG, Koffeman GI, Legemate DA, Levi M, van Gulik TM. Systematic review of survival after acute mesenteric ischaemia according to disease aetiology. Br J Surg. 2004;91:17-27.

38. Beena B, Mithal A, Carvalho P, Mehta Y, Trehan N. Medanta insulin protocols in patients undergoing cardiac surgery. Indian J Endocr Metab. 2014;18:455-67.

39. van den Berghe G, Wouters P, Weekers F, Verwaest C, Bruyninckx F, Schetz M, et al. Intensive insulin therapy in critically ill patients. N Eng J Med. 2001;345:1359-67.

40. Finfer S, Chittock DR, Su SY, Blair D, Foster D, Dhingra V, et al. Intensive versus conventional glucose control in critically ill patients. NICE-SUGAR Study Investigators. N Eng J Med. 2006;360:1283-97.

41. Lazar HL, McDonnell M, Chipkin SR, Furnary AP, Engelman RM, Sadhu AR, et al. The Society of Thoracic Surgeons practice guideline series: Blood glucose management during adult cardiac surgery. Society of Thoracic Surgeons Blood Glucose Guideline Task Force. Ann Thorac Surg. 2009;87:663-9.

42. Bhat JG, Gluck MC, Lowenstein J, Baldwin DS. Renal failure after open heart surgery. Ann Intern Med. 1976;84:677-82.

43. Jain V, Mehta Y, Gupta A, Sharma R, Raizada A, Trehan N. The role of neutrophil gelatinase-associated lipocalin in predicting acute kidney injury in patients undergoing off-

pump coronary artery bypass graft: a pilot study. Ann Card Anaesth. 2016;19:225-30.

44. Kuitunen A, Vento A, Suojaranta-Ylinen R, Pettila V. Acute renal failure after cardiac surgery: evaluation of the RIFLE classification. Ann Thorac Surg. 2006;81:542-6.

45. O'Neal JB, Shaw AD. Predicting, preventing, and identifying delirium after cardiac surgery. Perioper Med. 2016;5:1-8.

46. Lin YY, He B, Chen J, Wang ZN. Can dexmedetomidine be a safe and efficacious sedative agent in post-cardiac surgery patients? A meta-analysis. Crit Care. 2012;16:R169.

47. Mehta Y, Khanna S, Juneja R, Trehan N. Cardiac surgery in patients with mobile aortic atheromas. J Cardiothorac Vasc Anesth. 2001;15:778-84.

48. Kowalewski M, Suwalski P, Pawliszak W, Benetti F, Raffa GM, Malvindi PG, et al. Risk of stroke with "no-touch" - As compared to conventional off-pump coronary artery bypass grafting. An updated meta-analysis of observational studies. Int J Cardiol. 2016;222:769-71.

49. Yamashita K, Kobayashi J, Fujita T, Hata H, Shimahara Y, Kumeet Y, et al. Simultaneous transcatheter aortic valve implantation and off-pump coronary artery bypass grafting for Takayasu arteritis. J Cardiol Cases. 2017;15:158-60.

50. Kuroda K, Kato TS, Kuwaki K, Kajimoto K, Lee SL, Yamamoto T, et al. Early postoperative outcome of off-pump coronary artery bypass grafting: a report from the highest-volume center in Japan. Ann Thorac Cardiovasc Surg. 2016;22:98-107.

51. Reddy VY, Doshi SK, Sievert H, Buchbinder M, Neuzil P, Huber K, et al. Percutaneous left atrial appendage closure for stroke prophylaxis in patients with atrial fibrillation: 2.3-Year Follow-up of the PROTECT AF (Watchman Left Atrial Appendage System for Embolic Protection in Patients with Atrial Fibrillation) Trial. Circulation. 2013;127:720-9.

52. Kampe S, Geismann B, Weinreich G, Stamatis G, Ebmeyer U, Gerbershagen HJ. The influence of type of anesthesia, perioperative pain, and preoperative health status on chronic pain six months after thoracotomy: a prospective cohort study. Pain Med. 2017;18:2208-13.

53. Liu SS, Block BM, Wu CL. Effects of perioperative central neuraxial analgesia on outcome after coronary artery bypass surgery: A meta-analysis. Anesthesiology. 2004;101:153-61.

54. Sharma M, Mehta Y, Sawhney R, Vats M, Trehan N. Thoracic epidural analgesia in obese patients with body mass index of more than 30 kg/m² for off pump coronary artery bypass surgery. Ann Card Anaesth. 2010;13:28-33.

55. Zawar BP, Mehta Y, Juneja R, Arora D, Raizada A, Trehan N. Nonanalgesic benefits of combined thoracic epidural analgesia with general anesthesia in high risk elderly off pump coronary artery bypass patients. Ann Card Anaesth. 2015;18:385-91.

Perioperative Management of Pediatric Cardiac Surgeries

Virendra K Arya, Ganesh Kumar Munirathinam

INTRODUCTION

With the estimated incidence of 8–10 per 1,000 live birth, congenital heart disease (CHD) forms the most common birth defects constituting almost one-third of all major birth anomalies.[1] It can be defined as an anatomic malformation of the heart or great vessels which occurs during intrauterine development, irrespective of the age at presentation.[2] Surgical correction forms the mainstay of treatment in such children. With the first successful CHD surgery by Robert E Gross, performing patent ductus arteriosus (PDA) ligation in 1938, the field has seen tremendous development such that almost all the CHDs are either totally corrected or palliated to a better physiological condition nowadays.[3] The surgery for the CHD forms the major bulk of cardiac surgeries performed in pediatric population with the rare exceptions where surgeries are performed for traumatic causes. The complete understanding of each patient—cardiac anatomy, physiology and surgical corrections performed—is essential for the better management and improved outcome in the perioperative settings. This chapter reviews the types of CHDs with its altered physiology, its surgical correction and postoperative management of such patients along with the expected complications and its management.

CLASSIFICATION OF CONGENITAL HEART DISEASES

The broad spectrum of lesions and the underlying physiology in these patients make the classification of CHDs difficult. Even though the international nomenclature and database project precisely defines the lesions according to anatomy/morphology, for a better and easy understanding, CHDs can be classified functionally into acyanotic, cyanotic, and obstructive lesions. Cyanotic lesions can be further subclassified into cyanotic with increased pulmonary blood flow, with decreased pulmonary blood flow, and with single ventricular physiology.[4] This functional classification helps in deciding the therapeutic implications as to go with complete repair/biventricular repair or single ventricular repair or palliation and does not give much details on the anatomical details of the lesion. The different CHDs along with its incidence are given in **Table 1**.

The International Congenital Heart Surgery Nomenclature and Database project allows for a hierarchical system, with up to five levels of anatomical detail and additional modifiers.[5] Authors suggest the readers to go through the database for complete details on anatomical classification of CHDs.

PATHOPHYSIOLOGY OF CONGENITAL HEART DISEASES

Acyanotic Congenital Heart Diseases

The lesions with left-to-right shunts such as atrial septal defects (ASD), ventricular septal defects (VSD), PDA, aortopulmonary windows (APW) and left-sided obstructive lesions such as coarctation of aorta (COA) constitutes this group. These lesions with left-to-right shunts create conditions for increase of pulmonary blood flow as compared to systemic blood flow. The ASD imposes flow (volume)-related hemodynamic load while the defects in the ventricular septum and great vessels (PDA, AP window) enforce both the flow (volume) and pressure-related load on the pulmonary vasculature. In case of ASD, the magnitude of shunt is determined by:

- The size of the defect
- The comparative compliances of the ventricles
- The comparative resistances within the pulmonary and systemic vascular beds.[6]

These shunts increase as the age advances but it takes several years for the development of pulmonary vascular disease since it is not exposed to any pressure stress. In case of VSD, the amount of shunting is determined by:

- The size of the defect relative to left ventricular outflow tract (LVOT) diameter

Table 1: Functional classification of congenital heart lesions and incidence.

Acyanotic congenital heart diseases	
• Left-to-right shunts	
– Ventricular septal defects	20%
– Atrial septal defects	10%
– Patent ductus arteriosus	10%
– Atrioventricular septal defects	2–5%
– Aortopulmonary windows	<2%
• Left-sided obstructed lesions	
– Coarctation of aorta	10%
– Congenital aortic stenosis	10%
– Interrupted aortic arc	1%
– Congenital mitral stenosis	<1%
Cyanotic congenital heart diseases	
• Lesions associated with decreased pulmonary blood flow (Right-to-left shunt)	
– Tetralogy of Fallot	10%
– Pulmonary stenosis	10%
– Pulmonary atresia	5%
♦ With intact ventricular septum	
♦ With ventricular septal defect	
– Tricuspid atresia	3%
– Ebstein's anomaly	0.5%
• Lesions associated with increased pulmonary blood flow (Complete mixing lesions)	
– Transposition of great arteries	5–8%
♦ With intact ventricular septum	
♦ With ventricular septal defect	
– Double outlet right ventricle (DORV)	
– Truncus arteriosus	3%
– Total anomalous pulmonary venous connection	2%
Single ventricle physiology	
• Hypoplastic left heart syndrome	2%
• Double inlet ventricle	

- The comparative resistances across the outflow tracts [VSD vs. LVOT and aortic valve (AV)].

If the VSD is of nonrestrictive type meaning VSD area is bigger than LVOT area, the left-to-right shunt is determined by relative resistances across the pulmonary and systemic vascular beds and this shunt increases as the pulmonary vascular resistance (PVR) decreases after birth. The children with significant VSD usually start showing the symptoms of heart failure by about 4–8 weeks of life when the volume-overloaded left ventricle fails to overcome the added hemodynamic burden imposed by physiologic anemia.[7]

Likewise, in PDA the size of the ductus arteriosus and the comparative difference between the systemic vascular resistance and PVR govern the degree of left-to-right shunting. Similar to unrestrictive VSD, the pulmonary blood flow (PBF) increases considerably with postnatal decline in PVR and leads to left ventricular dilation and failure in large PDA. However, in children with complete obstruction of either systemic or pulmonary ventricular outflow such as interrupted aortic arch and pulmonary atresia respectively,

PDA plays an obligatory role for survival. Pathophysiology of APW is analogous to other lesions that have a large left-to-right shunt where the PBF increases as PVR declines and cardiac failure develops early.

Cyanotic Congenital Heart Diseases

In these conditions, there occurs cyanosis due to the shunting of deoxygenated blood from the right-sided chambers to the left-sided cardiac chambers. In lesions with decreased PBF, there exists some form of obstruction in the right-sided chambers such as tricuspid atresia (TA), Ebstein anomaly, right ventricular outflow tract (RVOT) obstruction or pulmonary valve (PV) stenosis and atresia. In such lesions, presence of shunt is obligatory for survival which usually presents in the form of ASD or VSD. The degree of right-to-left shunting depends on the severity of right-sided obstruction and size of the shunt. Due to prolonged cyanosis, such children are exposed to the consequences of cyanosis like clubbing, erythrocytosis, polycythemia, cerebrovascular accidents, cerebral abscess, hypercyanotic spells, hyperuricemia and coagulations abnormalities.[8] In addition these children exhibit right ventricular hypertrophy in case of obstruction at the level of RVOT and PV thereby leading to right ventricle (RV) diastolic dysfunction and increase of chance ischemia due to reduction in the effective perfusion pressure of RV.

In conditions such as transposition of great arteries (TGA) and double outlet right ventricle (DORV) with sub-pulmonary VSD, the child presents with cyanosis in spite of increased PBF due to the presence of parallel circulation where the systemic venous return is pumped to the aorta and pulmonary venous return is pumped to the pulmonary arteries (PAs). In such conditions, the presence of mixing of both the parallel circulations is mandatory for the survival of the child which can occur in the form of ASD, VSD, and PDA alone or combination of any of the three. This presence of mixing leads to appearance of cyanosis in such children and due to increased PBF, they may develop irreversible changes in the pulmonary vasculature.

▌MANAGEMENT

Management of Acyanotic Congenital Heart Diseases

Almost all the acyanotic CHDs are correctable either by surgery or by interventional procedures in catheterization laboratory before the development of irreversible changes in the pulmonary vascular bed (**Flowchart 1**). Surgical closure of the defect by patch is needed for patients with ostium primum and sinus venosus ASDs, as well as for patients with secundum ASDs whose anatomy is unfavorable for

Flowchart 1: Management of acyanotic CHD.

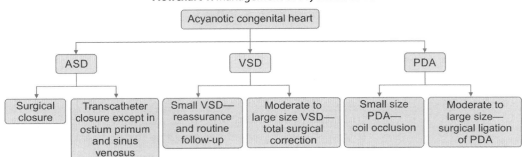

(ASD: atrial septal defects; CHD: congenital heart disease; PDA: patent ductus arteriosus; VSD: ventricular septal defects)

device closure.[9] The device closure has become the optimal treatment for secundum ASDs in most centers of the developed world.[10] Unsuitability criteria for device closure of secundum ASDs are:

- Defect dimensions >36 mm
- Inadequate atrial septal rims to allow stable device deployment
- Atrial septal defects with proximity of the defect to the AV valves or the coronary sinus, or the vena cava.

These are usually referred for surgical repair.

Among VSDs, particularly perimembranous type, conventionally surgical closure has been recognized as a low-risk highly successful procedure despite the fact that it is associated with some morbidity, pain, and a sternotomy scar. Patients with muscular VSDs constitute a high-risk surgical repair group in whom surgery is related with substantial morbidity and mortality, in addition to a high incidence of residual defects.[11] For these reasons percutaneous device closure of muscular VSDs appears as an appealing alternative to surgery offering high complete closure rates and avoiding morbidity associated with the surgery.

Surgical ligation or division of the PDA remains the treatment of choice for the rare very large ductus. Rarely, a large, window-type PDA may have insufficient length to permit ligation, and the appropriate surgical procedure is patch closure on cardiopulmonary bypass (CPB).[12] Small ductus <4 mm in diameter are closed by Gianturco stainless coils and larger ones by Amplatzer PDA device. An optimal candidate for the coil occlusion has the ductus 2.5 mm or less in size but the use of multiple coils can close a ductus up to 5 mm. Amplatzer device may be used for PDAs varying in size from 4 to 10 mm (with 100% closure rate).

Management of Cyanotic Congenital Heart Diseases

All the cyanotic CHDs can undergo any of the following three pathways. It can be totally corrected into a complete double ventricular repair where there will be a systemic and pulmonary ventricle to pump the blood into the systemic and pulmonary circulation without any communication between the two thereby forming a series circulation. The second pathway is the palliative procedures such as Blalock–Taussig (BT) shunts in case of tetralogy of Fallot (TOF) for improving the growth of PAs and the blood saturation, PA banding in case of multiple VSDs to prevent the development of irreversible changes in the pulmonary circulation. All these palliative procedures will be followed by a complete double ventricular repair once the patient becomes suitable for the surgery. Third pathway is the Fontan pathway which is usually followed in children with CHDs where the complete double ventricular repair is not possible due to hypoplastic ventricles such as TA. The first step in this pathway will be either BT shunt or bidirectional (BD) Glenn procedure based on the size of the PAs and the PA pressure (**Flowchart 2**).

The arterial switch operation (ASO), introduced in the early 1980s, for TGA with intact ventricular septum (IVS) in newborns was based on the assumption that the neonatal left ventricle would be suitable for systemic work after having withstood systemic pressure throughout fetal life.[13] The neonatal ASO has since been developed as the desired technique of repair for TGA with IVS and is presently feasible with an average surgical mortality rate of 2–5%.[14]

The ideal timing for an ASO in babies with TGA with IVS has been proven from the first few days to 3 weeks of life.[15] The optimal surgical management of neonates and infants with TOF remains controversial. Evidence suggests that early repair of CHD minimizes the secondary damage to the heart and other organ systems.[16] Palliative procedures are suggested to increase PBF in infants with severe cyanosis or uncontrollable hypoxic spells on whom the corrective surgery cannot be performed safely, and in children with hypoplastic PA on whom the corrective surgery is technically difficult. CPB is used to carry out total repair of the defect that includes patch closure of the VSD, widening of the RVOT by resection of the infundibular muscle tissue, and

Flowchart 2: Three-pathway approach for cyanotic CHD management.

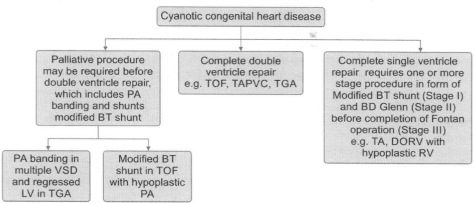

(BD: bidirectional; BT: Blalock–Taussig; CHD: congenital heart disease; DORV: double outlet right ventricle; LV: left ventricular; PA: pulmonary arteries; RV: right ventricle; TA: tricuspid atresia; TAPVC: total anomalous pulmonary venous connection; TGA: transposition of great arteries; TOF: tetralogy of Fallot; VSD: ventricular septal defects)

usually placement of a fabric patch to widen the RVOT. Some centers advocate placement of a monocusp valve at the time of initial repair, whereas some other centers recommend PV replacement at a later time if indicated.[17]

There is no palliative procedure for total anomalous pulmonary venous connection (TAPVC) and only corrective surgery is indicated for all these patients. Neonates with pulmonary venous obstruction are operated soon after the diagnosis, with a surgical mortality rate of about 20%, and infants without pulmonary venous obstruction are operated on by 4–12 months of age, with a mortality rate of 5–10%.

The definitive surgery for TA is a Fontan-type operation [superior vena cava (SVC) and inferior vena cava (IVC) joined to PAs] which could be fenestrated (flap valve provision from IVC baffle to RA to allow right-to-left shunt in event of pulmonary hypertensive crisis) or nonfenestrated. One or more palliative procedures such as Glenn (SVC connection to right PA) are required before Fontan operation to reduce the risk of the procedure. Risk factors for the failure of Fontan operation are:

- High PVR (>2 WU/m^2) or high mean PA pressure (>18 mm Hg)
- Distorted or stenotic PAs secondary to previous shunt operations
- Poor left ventricular (LV) systolic and diastolic functions (LV end-diastolic pressure >12 mm Hg or an ejection fraction <60%)
- Atrioventricular valve regurgitation.

The presence of two or more of these risk factors constitutes a high-risk situation for Fontan failure.

Postoperative Care in ICU

Fluid and Electrolyte Management

Hypotonic fluids have been commonly used in perioperative pediatric patients. However, it results in increasing incidence of hyponatremia after cardiac surgery. Neonates and young infants require 2.5–10% dextrose containing fluids with maintenance electrolytes. For the first 24 hours 50% maintenance fluid is to be given. Hypotension secondary to hypovolemia is managed with 5–10 mL/kg bolus infusions of 5% albumin, ringer lactate or fresh frozen plasma (FFP).[18] Fragile and anemic pediatric patients should receive packed red blood cells (pRBC), and those with persistent bleeding will require FFP or Octaplex (prothrombin complex concentrate that contains human coagulation factor II, VII, IX, X, protein C and protein S) 1–2 mL/kg for international normalized ratio (INR) values >1.4, cryoprecipitate or fibrinogen concentrate (Haemocomplettan®) 15–20 mg/kg for fibrinogen levels less than 2.5 g/L and platelets for functional platelet counts <50,000. Thromboelastometry or thromboelastography (TEG) testing should be used to guide blood component therapy in bleeding coagulopathic postcardiac surgery in pediatric patients. Octaplex and fibrinogen concentrate have the advantage of delivering low volume highly concentrated coagulation factors that are crucial in bleeding neonates to prevent fluid overload. Special consideration should be given in maintaining ionic calcium level ≥1.2 mEq/L, pH 7.30–7.45, and temperature ≥36°C in bleeding coagulopathic patient. On postoperative day 2, fluids may be increased to 75% of requirements and then to 100% from day 3 onward in pediatric patients.

Tetralogy of Fallot

Post TOF repair common major issues faced in the ICU could be low cardiac output (CO) state, desaturation episodes or persistent low arterial oxygen saturation, conduction abnormalities, and coagulopathy. Possible causes of a low CO state may be a result of right ventricular diastolic failure,[19] residual significant RVOT obstruction or distal PA stenosis, systolic failure of relatively hypoplastic LV exposed to volume overload from persistent major aortopulmonary collateral arteries (MAPCA). Resection of RVOT tract leads to significant pulmonary regurgitation that is usually very well tolerated by hypertrophied RV. RV dysfunction during immediate postoperative period is often caused by exposure of the hypertrophied RV to poor myocardial protection on CPB and reperfusion injury. Inotropic agents are of little benefit in the setting of RV diastolic failure. During diastole, the high pressure in RV alters the normal transeptal pressure gradient, leading the interventricular septum to bulge into the left ventricle.[20] Significant residual RVOT gradient or PA stenosis cannot be managed medically and need immediate surgical intervention to relieve obstruction or to create patent foramen ovale (PFO) if obstruction is not correctable. In this setting if surgical correction is not done, RV systolic dysfunction develops rapidly as there is no venting of blood from RV post repair due to VSD closure. This leads to high CVP and consequently systemic congestion and low perfusion pressure leading to multiple organ failure. The common causes of post-TOF repair hypoxia associated with unstable hemodynamics and high CVP are VSD patch dehiscence, major MAPCA, LV dysfunction, and endobronchial intubation. In case of persistent low arterial saturation after TOF repair with stable hemodynamics and normal CVP, most likely possibility is that persistent left-sided SVC with missed unroofing of coronary sinus must be considered. This can be easily diagnosed in ICU using bedside transthoracic echo by injecting air-agitated saline into left-sided intravenous access and appearance of air bubbles in left atrium in apical four-chamber view. Invariably some degree of right bundle branch block is present after TOF surgery and cardiac resynchronization therapy has been indicated to recover hemodynamics in some patients who are difficult to separate from bypass.[21]

Total Anomalous Pulmonary Venous Connections

The pulmonary vasculature often has a thickened medial layer after birth which persists longer in patients with increased pulmonary flow such as in TAPVC; thus, PVR does not decline normally after repair and the RV has to work against an augmented afterload. After correction of this condition, another reason for pulmonary hypertensive crisis is that left atrium and the left ventricle are unable to support the circulation probably because they are underfilled and underutilized prior to correction and remain small in size. Moreover, residual gradient across the connection of common chamber with left atrium can also lead to back congestion in pulmonary circulation. LV function is also impeded by inter ventricular septal shift toward LV in pulmonary hypertensive crisis. Thus, the postoperative period is complicated by existence of a low output state, persistence of pulmonary hypertension (PHT) (reactive or secondary to back pressure) and a highly reactive pulmonary vasculature.[22] This abnormal pulmonary vasculature responds very briskly to the changes in blood gases and lung mechanics. It has been shown that a 50% rise in PAP happens when the $PaCO_2$ is increased from less than 30 to 40–45 mm Hg during the postoperative period in these children with reactive pulmonary vasculatures.[23] Thus, mechanical ventilation to a $PaCO_2$ to 30–35 mm Hg is required in the postoperative period. However, in recent years inhaled nitric oxide (NO) has surfaced as a relatively specific pulmonary vasodilator which quickly disseminates through the alveolar capillary membrane and activates soluble guanylate cyclase leading to smooth muscle relaxation. Due to its direct actions on vascular smooth muscle, it remains effective in reducing PVR despite the post-CPB endothelial injury faced commonly in children. Its usefulness in controlling PHT has been frequently proven and it has been confirmed as the treatment of choice in this setting.[24] In cases of TAPVC where there is residual gradient at anastomosis of common chamber with left atrial (LA) or severely hypoplastic LA, vertical vein may not be ligated to allow left-to-right shunting of blood to prevent pulmonary congestion and hypertension.

Transposition of Great Arteries

Surgical and medical bleeding is a usual postoperative problem in patients after ASO. Blood loss in the ICU implies the requirement for suitable drainage from the mediastinum to prevent cardiac tamponade while rectifying a tenacious coagulopathy. Low cardiac output syndrome (LCOS) can occur in neonates after ASO with cardiac index dropping to less than 2 L/min/m² during the first operative night, while PVR and systemic vascular resistance increase.[25] The various causes for LCOS include:
- Arrhythmias
- Left ventricular dysfunction
- Myocardial ischemia/reperfusion injury
- Pulmonary hypertension
- Residual cardiac anomaly.

Issue of coronary artery buttons implantation and especially right coronary artery implantation getting kinked should always be kept in mind if arrhythmias and cardiac dysfunction had also occurred during separation from bypass. Transesophageal echocardiography (TEE) or epicardiac echo can help to diagnose this problem. The use of high-dose milrinone (0.75 µg/kg/min) after pediatric congenital heart surgery is described to reduce the risk of LCOS especially in uncomplicated surgical repair.[26] Maintaining a normal sinus rhythm is essential as losing atrial-ventricular sequential pacing results in a 15–20% reduction in CO. Neonates with edematous heart and thorax may require keeping their chest open for 24–48 hours till fluid overload is corrected by diuresis. During this phase, patients need to be kept completely paralyzed and spontaneous efforts completely abolished as these efforts can lead to increasing lung collapse and atelectasis in the setting of open chest leading to hypoxemia and worsening of PHT and hemodynamic collapse.

Parental or eternal nutrition is vital to meet high-energy demand of neonate, to maintain normal intestinal microflora and prevent gut-originated sepsis, to promote wound healing and to help weaning from the ventilator effectively. Maternal breast expressed milk feeding through nasogastric tube should be promoted within 4 hours postsurgery in all neonatal cardiac surgical patients until contraindication for eternal feeding exists such as suspicion of bowel ischemia. Keeping open chest is no contraindication to eternal feeding in neonates and infants. Mother's breast milk contains immunoglobulin G (IgG) antibodies also that provide immunological protection to neonate. Malnutrition is usual in neonates and infants post ASO, particularly in those who have severe underlying diseases and poor nutritional status preoperatively.

Bidirectional Glenn

Hypoxemia is major challenge after the bidirectional Glenn surgery. Various predisposing factors include:
- Pulmonary venous admixture
- Systemic venous collaterals
- Pulmonary arteriovenous malformations.[27]

One approach to recover pulmonary circulation output (Qp) and oxygenation is permissive hypercapnia that uncouples cerebral blood flow from cerebral metabolism allowing for an increase in SVC flow and thus Qp.[28] Hoskote et al. validated that gradual increases in $PaCO_2$ led to increases in Qp and oxygenation without increasing PVR.[29] These alterations were coupled with a decrease in systemic vascular resistance and increase in systemic CO (Qs) and a striking increase in systemic oxygen delivery (DO_2). In the absence of systemic hypotension, manipulation of systemic blood pressure will not affect cerebral blood flow and oxygenation because cerebral pressure autoregulation is intact.[30] Negative pressure ventilation and early extubation should be a priority in BD Glenn patient in early postoperative period to promote PBF.

Fontan Procedure

A low CO state is the major challenge after the Fontan procedure that is secondary to inadequate ventricular filling volume. LV or common ventricular diastolic dysfunction may be present to unpredictable levels. In contrast to the BD Glenn shunt, in Fontan all systemic venous return must overcome the PVR without any prepulmonary ventricular support that further compromises systemic ventricular filling.[31] Inotropic support provides minimal help as a result

of inadequate venous return and ventricular filling. In Fontan also alike BD Glenn, negative pressure ventilation promotes ventricular filling and systemic CO by augmenting venous return and the ventricular diastolic transmural pressure. This is in part the justification for an early extubation after Fontan surgery.[32] Increasing mean systemic filling pressure either by volume administration or by capacitance vascular system squeeze rises the upstream driving pressure for venous return and improves hemodynamics, whereas venodilators by increasing venous capacitance and reducing mean systemic filling pressure compromise venous return and systemic hemodynamics. Even modest increases in pulmonary vascular resistance may not be tolerated and normalizing the functional residual capacity, pH, and alveolar PO_2 may improve Qp.[33] Some of the patients may respond to inhaled NO.[34] In rapidly deteriorating hemodynamics refractory to vasopressors and inotropes; abdominal pressure may temporarily increase venous return and improve hemodynamics and make vasoactive medications to cross lung and reach on systemic side of their site of action. This abdominal compression maneuver may be crucial to prevent cardiac arrest or hemodynamic collapse in post-Fontan surgery. Fenestrated Fontan will be less prone for hemodynamic collapse but more prone for hypoxemia in the event of rising pulmonary vascular resistance whereas nonfenestrated Fontan will be more prone for hemodynamic collapse in similar situation.

Hypoxemia is another common problem complicating the postoperative course of Fontan surgery and may be due to systemic venous collaterals.[35] Transudative and chylous pleural and pericardial effusions are also common after the Fontan procedure and may result from traumatic injury to a lymphatic tributary or elevated systemic or pulmonary venous pressure impeding lymphatic drainage.[36]

Common Postoperative Complications of Congenital Heart Surgery and Their Management

Low Cardiac Output Syndrome

One of the main postoperative problems after CPB is LCOS and usually appears within the first 6–12 hours postsurgery. Reported incidence is around 25% among patients undergoing CPB for congenital heart surgery. LCOS has been defined by a collective signs and symptoms of low CO state that includes tachycardia, markers of poor peripheral perfusion, and oliguria. LCOS requiring increasing inotropic support may finally result in cardiac arrest.[26] The factors accountable for LCOS are:
- Hemodynamically significant residual lesions postsurgery

- Myocardial dysfunction resulting from poor myocardial preservation as a result of prolonged periods of cardioplegia delivery intervals
- Myocardial ischemia
- Reperfusion injury
- Cardiac arrhythmias.

Other contributing factors include inflammatory response to CPB, with a resulting increase in systemic vascular resistance, PVR, capillary leak, and pulmonary dysfunction.[37]

The risk of LCOS is highest among neonates undergoing intricate surgeries. Additional risk factors are prolonged CPB time, prolonged cross-clamp time, preoperative circulatory collapse, and preoperative ventricular dysfunction.[38] Refractory cases of LCOS not responding to medical therapy may require extracorporeal membrane oxygenation (ECMO) support.

In ICU setup, transthoracic echo is very useful tool to diagnose residual lesions such as VSD or AV valve regurgitation or residual stenosis. Laboratory evaluation such as worsening acidosis, rising lactate levels, falling mixed venous saturation, and widening arterial-to-end tidal CO_2 gap helps to make the diagnosis of LCOS and to distinguish the clinical repercussions of the LCOS, such as worsening acidosis and resultant end-organ dysfunction. Lactic acidosis could be secondary to gut ischemia or use of high doses of epinephrine infusions. A normal arterial-to-end tidal CO_2 gradient ($PaCO_2 - EtCO_2$) <5 mm Hg in the setting of lactic acidosis most likely rules out LCOS as cause of lactic acidosis. A rising lactate level with rising or normal mixed venous saturation in the setting of LCOS suggests refractory LCOS and poor prognosis. This is an indicator of inability of tissues to utilize oxygen and oxidative metabolic decoupling. Diagnosis of residual surgical lesions is often accurately made in the ICU by echocardiogram, but their absolute contribution to a patient's clinical deterioration may be difficult to ascertain. Therefore, the intensivist may need to err on the side of being more aggressive, which may include cardiac catheterization with angiography for further evaluation and establishing the diagnosis.

After workup, LCOS must be stratified into two main groups—those requiring surgical intervention and those responsive to medical therapy. For example, neonates undergoing TOF repair usually do not tolerate a significant residual VSD or RVOT obstruction, and infants who have undergone AV canal defect repair mostly do not tolerate a persistent PDA. These clinical scenarios present significant hemodynamic problems with refractory LCOS and often require urgent reoperation.

Low cardiac output syndrome management and therapy should be customized and a patient's response to interventions closely monitored. Medical therapy is directed toward the apparent cause; however, all patients must be adequately fluid resuscitated to maintain preload and systemic blood pressure followed by suitable use of inotropic agents to support myocardial contractility and afterload decreasing agents to reduce ventricular workload, improve CO, and recover perfusion.[39] The prophylactic intravenous use of milrinone after cardiac operation in pediatrics (PRIMACORP) study has recommended the use of milrinone prophylactically to prevent postoperative LCOS.[26] Institutional differences exist in use of agents to prevent or treat LCOS, including low-dose epinephrine alone or in combination with milrinone. Drugs such as milrinone, dopamine, and epinephrine also have been shown to have significant arrhythmogenicity in the postoperative period.[40] In the absence of a surgical cause, medical therapy resistant LCOS requires mechanical support such as ECMO that has been used with good results in postoperative cardiac patients, including those placed on ECMO for an inability to wean from CPB.[41] The timing of ECMO poses a major decision challenge due to associated morbidity. This requires an early engagement of the multidisciplinary team, involving critical care, surgery, anesthesiology, and cardiology.

Pulmonary Arterial Hypertension

Pulmonary arterial hypertension (PAH) resulting from elevated PVR is a common postoperative complication after congenital heart surgery. This can acutely raise RV afterload with subsequent RV dysfunction and is a common reason for cardiac arrest in the postoperative period. One of the important factors among numerous causes contributing for elevated PVR is prolonged CPB leading to a systemic inflammatory response syndrome, involving mediators, such as interleukin 6, interleukin 10, tumor necrosis factor α, P-selectin, E-selectin, leptin, soluble intercellular adhesion molecule and vascular cell adhesion molecule, fractalkine, etc.[42] Other patient factors that are responsible for PAH include comorbid conditions, some genetic syndromes like Down syndrome and following cardiac pathophysiologies:

- An increased pressure load to the pulmonary arterial system, such as truncus arteriosus, VSD, AV canal defect, aortopulmonary window and PDA
- Impaired egress of blood from the pulmonary arterial tree (obstructed TAPVCs), mitral valve stenosis, hypoplastic LA, or restrictive atrial communication in cases of hypoplastic left heart syndrome (HLHS)
- Pulmonary vessels compressing major trachea-bronchial tree leading to hypoplasia of lung tissue or atelectasis in postoperative period
- Heart transplant patients with preexisting PHT (e.g., restrictive cardiomyopathy)
- Comorbid conditions, such as congenital diaphragmatic hernia, may also pose an independent risk to the development of PAH.

The major postoperative repercussion of PAH is pulmonary vascular reactivity. In this situation, a potentially fatal episodic pulmonary hypertensive crisis can be initiated by a vasospastic stimulus that can end in acute RV failure, tricuspid regurgitation, decreased CO, and myocardial ischemia.[43] The primary approach to postoperative PAH is prevention by minimizing noxious stimuli such as endotracheal suctioning should be accomplished judiciously in a mechanically ventilated patient. This might mean limiting suctioning to the tip of the endotracheal tube and dispensing additional sedation/analgesia/ neuromuscular blockade in labile patients. Hypercarbia should be avoided, and supplemental oxygen should be used cautiously for its pulmonary vasodilatory benefit.

Despite debatable prophylactic use of inhaled NO to prevent PAH,[44] it is an effective agent in the treatment of PAH in the postoperative period by its vascular tone reducing effect on pulmonary circulation. Preemptive use of NO should be considered in those critically ill patients who are less likely to tolerate an acute decompensation. Other agents used to treat postoperative PAH include inhaled illoprost[44] and intravenous sildenafil.[45]

Postoperative Arrhythmias

The reported incidence of cardiac arrhythmias varies between 15% and 50% after congenital heart surgery. While most arrhythmias are clinically inconsequential, junctional ectopic tachycardia (JET), reentrant supraventricular tachycardia, ectopic atrial tachycardia (EAT), and ventricular tachycardia can cause substantial hemodynamic instability when they occur. These can result in continued mechanical ventilation, increased inotrope use, lengthy ICU stay, increased danger of cardiac arrest, and reduced survival.[46] Risk factors for the genesis of tachyarrhythmia include younger age, prolonged CPB and cross-clamp times, and use of deep hypothermic circulatory arrest.[47] Ventricular tachycardia presenting as a wide complex tachycardia, although uncommon in the postoperative period, must be quickly differentiated from an aberrantly conducted supraventricular tachycardia as former can lead to rapid hemodynamic collapse.

Optimal management of postoperative arrhythmia requires precise diagnosis. Narrow complex tachycardia could be automatic or reentrant rhythm. Reentrant arrhythmias have abrupt onset and respond to pharmacologic agents such as adenosine or electrical cardioversion. They also respond to overdrive pacing and have the characteristic of sudden termination. The automatic arrhythmias (JET and EAT) display warmup and cooldown phenomena (i.e., slow increase and slow decline in heart rate); they are catecholamine responsive and do not respond to overdrive pacing or cardioversion. A 12-lead or 15-lead ECG with rhythm strip may be necessary to make the diagnosis, and in some cases an atrial electrocardiogram is necessary to identify the location of P waves.

The cornerstone for aggressive prevention of JET and other postoperative tachyarrhythmia is insistent repletion of electrolytes and treatment of significant acid-base disturbances. There is some recommendation for prophylactic use of amiodarone for prevention of postoperative JET.[48] The automatic arrhythmias require minimizing a patient's catecholamine state such as prevention of fever, establishing applicable sedation when indicated, and adequate neuromuscular blockade that may be able to lessen the risk of arrhythmia. Once arrhythmia occurs, the treatment algorithm is predominantly decided by the hemodynamic state of the patient whether stable or unstable.

Ventricular tachycardia is managed as per the guidelines of Pediatric Advanced Life Support algorithm. Supraventricular tachycardia with aberrant conduction may appear similar to ventricular tachycardia on ECG. The recommended treatment of stable reentrant tachycardia is vagal maneuvers, adenosine, or β-blockers. Unstable patients should be treated with adenosine (if it can be administered promptly) or synchronized cardioversion. For EAT, β-blockers (e.g., esmolol) are effective initial therapy.[49] For JET, the conventional therapeutic modalities include cooling to approximately 36°C, decreasing catecholamine infusions as tolerated, adequate sedation, and appropriate neuromuscular blockade. Cooling must be carefully accomplished because shivering can cause a catecholamine surge and counteract the therapy. Amiodarone is a suggested first-line pharmacologic therapy for JET.[50] It can be effective, but its dose-related adverse effects (i.e., α-blockade related hypotension) should be considered.[51]

Common bradyarrhythmias seen in the postoperative period are sinus bradycardia, as seen in sick sinus syndrome, and varying degrees of AV node block. These respond well to pacing using temporary pacing wires placed at the time of surgery. In isolated sick sinus syndrome, atrial pacing alone is adequate. AV node block often requires AV sequential pacing.

▌REFERENCES

1. Marian AJ. Congenital heart disease: the remarkable journey from the "Post-Mortem Room" to adult clinics. Circ Res. 2017;120(6):895-7.

2. Rao PS. Diagnosis and management of cyanotic congenital heart disease: Part I. Indian J Pediatr. 2009;76(1):57-70.

3. Chalphin AV, Yeo CJ, Cowan SW, Milan S. Robert Edward Gross (1905-1988): ligation of a patent ductus arteriosus and the birth of a speciality. Am Surg. 2014;80(11):1087-8.

4. Dodge-Khatami A. The classification and nomenclature of congenital heart disease. In: Wheeler DS, Wong HR, Shanley TP (Eds). Pediatric Critical Care Medicine. London: Springer-Verlag; 2014. pp. 335-41.

5. Mavroudis C, Jacobs JP. Congenital heart surgery nomenclature and database project: overview and minimum dataset. Ann Thorac Surg. 2000;69(4 Suppl):S2-17.

6. Rudolph A. Congenital Diseases of the Heart: Clinical Physiological Considerations, 3rd edition. Chichester, UK: Wiley-Blackwell; 2009. pp. 1-544.

7. Lister G, Hellenbrand WE, Kleinman CS, Talner NS. Physiologic effects of increasing hemoglobin concentration in left-to-right shunting in infants with ventricular septal defects. N Engl J Med. 1982;306(9):502-6.

8. Rao PS. Pathophysiologic consequences of cyanotic congenital heart disease. Indian J Pediatr. 1983;50(406):479-87.

9. Vida VL, Barnoya J, O'Connell M, Leon-Wyss J, Larrazabal LA, Castañeda AR. Surgical versus percutaneous occlusion of ostium secundum atrial septal defects: results and cost-effective considerations in a low-income country. J Am Coll Cardiol. 2006;47(2):326-31.

10. Mullen MJ, Dias BF, Walker F, Siu SC, Benson LN, McLaughlin PR. Intracardiac echocardiography guided device closure of atrial septal defects. J Am Coll Cardiol. 2003;41(2):285-92.

11. Seddio F, Reddy VM, McElhinney DB, Tworetzky W, Silverman NH, Hanley FL. Multiple ventricular septal defects: how and when should they be repaired? J Thorac Cardiovasc Surg. 1999;117(1):134-40.

12. Grünenfelder J, Bartram U, Van Praagh R, Bove KE, Bailey WW, Meyer RA, et al. The large window ductus: a surgical trap. Ann Thorac Surg. 1998;65(6):1790-1.

13. Quaegebeur JM, Rohmer J, Ottenkamp J, Buis T, Kirklin JW, Blackstone EH, et al. The arterial switch operation. An eight-year experience. J Thorac Cardiovasc Surg. 1986;92(3 Pt 1):361-84.

14. Sarris GE, Chatzis AC, Giannopoulos NM, Kirvassilis G, Berggren H, Hazekamp M, et al. The arterial switch operation in Europe for transposition of the great arteries: a multi-institutional study from the European Congenital Heart Surgeons Association. J Thorac Cardiovasc Surg. 2006;132(3):633-9.

15. Duncan BW, Poirier NC, Mee RB, Drummond-Webb JJ, Qureshi A, Mesia CI, et al. Selective timing for the arterial switch operation. Ann Thorac Surg. 2004;77(5):1691-7.

16. Castaneda AR, Mayer JE Jr, Jonas RA, Lock JE, Wessel DL, Hickey PR. The neonate with critical congenital heart disease: repair—a surgical challenge. J Thorac Cardiovasc Surg. 1989;98(5 Pt 2):869-75.

17. Touati GD, Vouhé PR, Amodeo A, Pouard P, Mauriat P, Leca F, et al. Primary repair of tetralogy of Fallot in infancy. J Thorac Cardiovasc Surg. 1990;99(3):396-403.

18. Arya VK. Basics of fluid and blood transfusion therapy in paediatric surgical patients. Indian J Anaesth. 2012;56(5): 454-62.

19. Cullen S, Shore D, Redington A. Characterization of right ventricular diastolic performance after complete repair of tetralogy of fallot. Restrictive physiology predicts slow postoperative recovery. Circulation. 1995;91(6):1782-9.

20. Mikesell CE, Bronicki RA, Domico M. Right ventricular synchronization therapy following repair of tetralogy of Fallot. Pediatr Crit Care Med. 2010;11(Suppl):S102.

21. Janousek J, Vojtovic P, Hucín B, Tláskal T, Gebauer RA, Gebauer R, et al. Resynchronization pacing is a useful adjunct to the management of acute heart failure after surgery for congenital heart defects. Am J Cardiol. 2001;88(2):145-52.

22. Raisher BD, Grant JW, Martin TC, Strauss AW, Spray TL. Complete repair of total anomalous pulmonary venous connection in infancy. J Thorac Cardiovasc Surg. 1992;104(2):443-8.

23. Morray JP, Lynn AM, Mansfield PB. Effect of pH and PCO2 on pulmonary and systemic hemodynamics after surgery in children with congenital heart disease and pulmonary hypertension. J Pediatr. 1988;113(3):474-9.

24. Russell IA, Zwass MS, Fineman JR, Balea M, Rouine-Rapp K, Brook M, et al. The effect of inhaled nitric oxide on postoperative pulmonary hypertension in infants and children undergoing surgical repair of congenital heart disease. Anesth Analg. 1998;87(1):46-51.

25. Hoffman TM, Wernovsky G, Atz AM, Kulik TJ, Nelson DP, Chang AC, et al. Efficacy and safety of milrinone in preventing low cardiac output syndrome in infants and children after corrective surgery for congenital heart disease. Circulation. 2003;107(7):996-1002.

26. Hoffman TM, Wernovsky G, Atz AM, Bailey JM, Akbary A, Kocsis JF, et al. Prophylactic intravenous use of milrinone after cardiac operation in pediatrics (PRIMACORP) study. Prophylactic intravenous use of milrinone after cardiac operation in pediatrics. Am Heart J. 2002;143(1):15-21.

27. Chang RK, Alejos JC, Atkinson D, Jensen R, Drant S, Galindo A, et al. Bubble contrast echocardiography in detecting pulmonary arteriovenous shunting in children with univentricular heart after cavopulmonary anastomosis. J Am Coll Cardiol. 1999;33(7):2052-8.

28. Bradley SM, Simsic JM, Mulvihill DM. Hypoventilation improves oxygenation after bidirectional superior cavopulmonary connection. J Thorac Cardiovasc Surg. 2003;126(4):1033-9.

29. Hoskote A, Li J, Hickey C, Erickson S, Van Arsdell G, Stephens D, et al. The effects of carbon dioxide on oxygenation and systemic, cerebral, and pulmonary vascular hemodynamics after the bidirectional superior cavopulmonary anastomosis. J Am Coll Cardiol. 2004;44(7):1501-9.

30. Simsic JM, Bradley SM, Mulvihill DM. Sodium nitroprusside infusion after bidirectional superior cavopulmonary connection: preserved cerebral blood flow velocity and systemic oxygenation. J Thorac Cardiovasc Surg. 2003;126(1):186-90.

31. Myers CD, Ballman K, Riegle LE, Mattix KD, Litwak K, Rodefeld MD. Mechanisms of systemic adaptation to univentricular Fontan conversion. J Thorac Cardiovasc Surg. 2010;140(4):850-6,e1-6.

32. Cooper DS, Costello JM, Bronicki RA, Stock AC, Jacobs JP, Ravishankar C, et al. Current challenges in cardiac intensive care: optimal strategies for mechanical ventilation and timing of extubation. Cardiol Young. 2008;18(Suppl 3):72-83.

33. Williams DB, Kiernan PD, Metke MP, Marsh HM, Danielson GK. Hemodynamic response to positive end-expiratory pressure following right atrium-pulmonary artery bypass (Fontan procedure). J Thorac Cardiovasc Surg. 1984;87(6):856-61.

34. Goldman AP, Delius RE, Deanfield JE, Miller OI, de Level MR, Sigston PE, et al. Pharmacological control of pulmonary blood flow with inhaled nitric oxide after the fenestrated Fontan operation. Circulation. 1996;94(9 Suppl):II44-8.

35. Buheitel G, Hofbeck M, Tenbrink U, Leipold G, vd Emde J, Singer H. Possible sources of right-to-left shunting in patients following a total cavopulmonary connection. Cardiol Young. 1998;8(3):358-63.

36. Mellins RB, Levine OR, Fishman AP. Effect of systemic and pulmonary venous hypertension on pleural and pericardial fluid accumulation. J Appl Physiol. 1970;29(5):564-9.

37. Nagashima M, Imai Y, Seo K, Terada M, Aoki M, Shinóka T, et al. Effect of hemofiltrated whole blood pump priming on hemodynamics and respiratory function after the arterial switch operation in neonates. Ann Thorac Surg. 2000;70(6):1901-6.

38. Brown KL, Ridout DA, Hoskote A, Verhulst L, Ricci M, Bull C. Delayed diagnosis of congenital heart disease worsens preoperative condition and outcome of surgery in neonates. Heart. 2006;92(9):1298-302.

39. Butts RJ, Scheurer MA, Atz AM, Zyblewski SC, Hulsey TC, Bradley SM, et al. Comparison of maximum vasoactive inotropic score and low cardiac output syndrome as markers of early postoperative outcomes after neonatal cardiac surgery. Pediatr Cardiol. 2012;33(4):633-8.

40. Smith AH, Owen J, Borgman KY, Fish FA, Kannankeril PJ. Relation of milrinone after surgery for congenital heart disease to significant postoperative tachyarrhythmias. Am J Cardiol. 2011;108(11):1620-4.

41. Beiras-Fernandez A, Deutsch MA, Kainzinger S, Kaczmarek I, Sodian R, Ueberfuhr P, et al. Extracorporeal membrane oxygenation in 108 patients with low cardiac output—a single-center experience. Int J Artif Organs. 2011;34(4):365-73.

42. Avni T, Paret G, Thaler A, Mishali D, Yishay S, Tal G, et al. Delta chemokine (fractalkine)—a novel mediator of pulmonary arterial hypertension in children undergoing cardiac surgery. Cytokine. 2010;52(3):143-5.

43. Adatia I, Beghetti M. Immediate postoperative care. Cardiol Young. 2009;19(Suppl 1):23-7.

44. Ofori-Amanfo G, Hsu D, Lamour JM, Mital S, O'Byrne ML, Smerling AJ, et al. Heart transplantation in children with markedly elevated pulmonary vascular resistance: impact of right ventricular failure on outcome. J Heart Lung Transplant. 2011;30(6):659-66.

45. Fraisse A, Butrous G, Taylor MB, Oakes M, Dilleen M, Wessel DL. Intravenous sildenafil for postoperative pulmonary hypertension in children with congenital heart disease. Intensive Care Med. 2011;37(3):502-9.

46. Shamszad P, Cabrera AG, Kim JJ, Moffett BS, Graves DE, Heinle JS, et al. Perioperative atrial tachycardia is associated with increased mortality in infants undergoing cardiac surgery. J Thorac Cardiovasc Surg. 2012;144(2):396-401.

47. Delaney JW, Moltedo JM, Dziura JD, Kopf GS, Snyder CS. Early postoperative arrhythmias after pediatric cardiac surgery. J Thorac Cardiovasc Surg. 2006;131(6):1296-300.

48. Imamura M, Dossey AM, Garcia X, Shinkawa T, Jaquiss RD. Prophylactic amiodarone reduces junctional ectopic tachycardia after tetralogy of Fallot repair. J Thorac Cardiovasc Surg. 2012;143(1):152-6.

49. Garnock-Jones KP. Esmolol: A review of its use in the short-term treatment of tachyarrhythmias and the short-term control of tachycardia and hypertension. Drugs. 2012;72(1):109-32.

50. Kovacikova L, Hakacova N, Dobos D, Skrak P, Zahorec M. Amiodarone as a first-line therapy for postoperative junctional ectopic tachycardia. Ann Thorac Surg. 2009;88(2):616-22.

51. Saul JP, Scott WA, Brown S, Marantz P, Acevedo V, Etheridge SP, et al. Intravenous amiodarone for incessant tachyarrhythmias in children: a randomized, double-blind, antiarrhythmic drug trial. Circulation. 2005;112(22):3470-7.

13

Perioperative Management of Valvular Heart Surgeries

Neeti Vijay Dogra, Ganesh Kumar Munirathinam

EPIDEMIOLOGY

Valvular heart disease (VHD) remains a major cause of morbidity and mortality globally with an estimated prevalence of 2.5% in a population-based study on 11,911 subjects on echocardiographic examination.[1] This prevalence increases to 13% at 75 years of age[1] due to primarily degenerative VHDs in industrialized countries.

In developing nations, rheumatic valvular diseases account for the major burden with recent reports of approximately 15 million cases detected on clinical screening,[2] and the number is likely to increase with echocardiographic screening.

PHYSIOLOGY

The pressure–volume (PV) loops are used to characterize the ventricular function (**Fig. 1**). As shown in **Figure 1**, labels correspond to (a) ventricular filling, (b) isovolumetric contraction, (c) ventricular systole, and (d) isovolumetric relaxation; (1) mitral valve closing, (2) aortic valve opening, (3) aortic valve closing, and (4) mitral valve opening. S is the width of the PV loop representing stroke volume. Line 4 to 1 represents the ventricular end-diastolic PV relationship (EDPVR) and is inversely related to ventricular compliance or diastolic function of the heart. This slope may increase with decrease in ventricular compliance as may occur in ventricular hypertrophy [hypertension and aortic stenosis (AS)]. Line 3 represents ventricular end-systolic PV relationship (ESPVR) and is a measure of ventricular contractility or systolic function of the heart. Volume is related to ventricular compliance. ESPVR gives a load-insensitive index of contractility. PV loops specific to individual lesions are discussed subsequently. Chronic volume load leads to ventricular dilatation disproportionate to hypertrophy, i.e., eccentric hypertrophy, while chronic pressure overload results in concentric hypertrophy where the chamber size may be normal or reduced as compared to increase in ventricular mass.

PREOPERATIVE OPTIMIZATION

Patient evaluation must be done to identify the etiology, severity, symptomatic status, risk prognostication, and risk-to-benefit ratio of the proposed intervention with regard to valvular disease. The evaluation must also aim to find the optimal treatment modality (valve replacement, valve repair, or less invasive catheter intervention) with an eye on local resources for planned intervention.

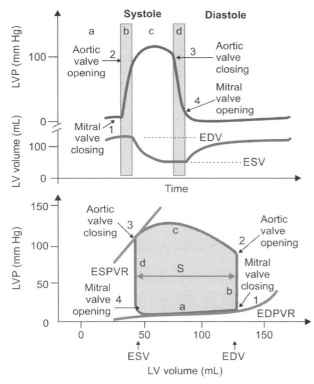

Fig. 1: Pressure–volume loops explained as per the cardiac cycle.

(EDPVR: end-diastolic press–volume relationship; ESPVR: end-systolic PV relationship; EDV: end-diastolic volume; ESV: end-systolic volume; LV: left ventricular; LVP: left ventricular pressure)

Clinical evaluation must obtain history to assess the symptoms, chronicity, and associated comorbidity. Of note is the assessment of lifestyle to detect any changes in the daily activity which may be progressive causing functional limitation. Patients who have been treated for heart failure and are currently asymptomatic should still be classified as symptomatic. In patients receiving chronic anticoagulant therapy as for atrial fibrillation (AF), evidence of bleeding and embolic complications as syncope should be carefully included in the history. Clinical examination must look for murmurs, prosthetic valve clicks, and signs of heart failure. It must also look for renal and hepatic dysfunction, chronic obstructive pulmonary disease, and peripheral vascular disease which are commonly associated comorbidities. Electrocardiogram (ECG) and chest X-ray (CXR) compliment the clinical examination.

Echocardiography

Echocardiography is the investigation of choice to confirm the diagnosis of VHD and to assess its severity, etiology, mechanism, and prognosis. The assessment of regurgitant lesions should include vena contractas and effective regurgitant orifice area (EROA) which are less flow dependent than color Doppler jet size. The assessment of stenotic lesions should combine the estimation of valve area with mean pressure gradients. Left ventricular (LV) and right ventricular (RV) dimensions, ejection fraction (EF), and pulmonary artery pressures provide important prognostic information. Transesophageal echocardiography (TEE) is useful to monitor the results of surgical intervention and percutaneous procedures as well as when transthoracic examination is limited by poor window or when infective endocarditis (IE) or prosthetic valve dysfunction is suspected. Stress echocardiography is indicated to identify an increase in mitral regurgitation (MR), pulmonary artery pressures, or aortic gradient for the evaluation of dyspnoea.[3] Dobutamine stress echocardiography is used for the assessment of low-flow low-gradient AS.

Computed tomography (CT) coronary angiography is used to exclude coronary artery disease (CAD) in low-risk patients and preprocedural assessment of annular size for transcatheter aortic valve implantation (TAVI).[4,5]

Coronary angiography is indicated in the detection of suspected CAD when valvular surgery is planned.

Risk Stratification

Operative mortality can be estimated by various scores such as Euro-SCORE II and the Society of Thoracic Surgeons (STS) score which have been used for risk stratification in valvular heart surgery.[6,7] Of the two scores, STS[8,9] is more specific to predict outcomes after valvular heart surgery. Mitral valve replacement (MVR) with coronary artery bypass

grafting (CABG) carries the highest operative mortality of 9.9% after surgery for VHDs followed by mitral valve repair with CABG (5.1%) and MVR without CABG (4.9%).[10] Aortic valve replacement (AVR) with CABG has an operative mortality of 3.9%.[10]

Endocarditis and Rheumatic Fever Prophylaxis

Patients with a prior history of IE and those with a prosthetic valve have a higher risk of IE, and they must be given antibiotic prophylaxis.[11] Intramuscular benzathine penicillin is given for at least 10 years after the last episode of acute rheumatic fever or till 40 years of age, whichever is longer for the prevention of relapse.[12]

Management of Atrial Fibrillation and Anticoagulation

Warfarin is a routinely used anticoagulant in patients with native valve disease and AF to maintain a target international normalized ratio (INR) of 2–3.[13] Nonvitamin K oral anticoagulants (NOAC) such as rivaroxaban and apixaban are approved for nonvalvular AF,[14] and they may be used in AF associated with bioprosthesis after the third postoperative month.[15] NOAC are contraindicated in patients with mechanical prosthesis.[16] Cardioversion is not advised in patients with uncorrected VHD unless there is a hemodynamic compromise.

INDIVIDUAL MANAGEMENT OF SPECIFIC VALVULAR LESIONS

Aortic Stenosis

Pathophysiology

The normal aortic valve area is 3–4 cm^2.[17] Valve area <1 cm^2 or <0.6 cm^2/m^2 is considered severe AS. AS may be rheumatic with symptom appearing between second and fourth decades, bicuspid with symptom onset between fourth and sixth decades, and degenerative with symptom appearing after the sixth decade. Dyspnea on exertion, angina on exertion, and syncope are common symptoms. The PV loop in AS shows an increased peak systolic pressure generated as the ventricle is contracting against an increased resistance. ES volume and ED volume increase as the venous return left after each cardiac cycle is added to the next one leading to rightward and upward shift of the PV loop. The width of the PV loop (stroke volume) decreases progressively as the severity of AS increases due to increased afterload. The slope of EDPVR is increased, and the ventricle displays poor compliance where increase in ED volume is limited by ventricular hypertrophy (**Fig. 2**).

Echocardiography is the key diagnostic tool to assess the severity of AS, valve calcification, and associated aortic pathology (**Figs. 3A to C**). Dobutamine echocardiography helps to differentiate true AS where low-dose dobutamine results in increase in pressure gradients without any change in valve area from pseudo-severe AS where the valve area increases significantly without any change in gradient across the valve.[18] See the hemodynamic grid (**Table 1**) for the perioperative management.

Management

All symptomatic AS patients should undergo surgery; asymptomatic patients with EF < 50% or abnormal exercise test should undergo intervention. Surgical AVR (SAVR) is the preferred modality of intervention, with transcatheter AVR (TAVR) being reserved for elderly patients with high surgical risk. The cardiac grid for the maintenance of hemodynamics in AS is shown in **Table 1**. Preload augmentation is necessary for the maintenance of cardiac output. Excessive tachycardia can impede coronary perfusion while bradycardia may limit cardiac output. The goal of anesthetic induction includes maintenance of

cardiac output by maintaining systemic vascular resistance (SVR) which preserves coronary blood flow. Phenylephrine is commonly used for the same. In critical AS, it is always prudent to connect the defibrillator pads to the patient. The cardiac surgeon and the perfusionist should be ready for emergency bypass should any hemodynamic instability occur. Myocardial preservation with anterograde as well as retrograde cardioplegia helps in preserving myocardial integrity.

Aortic Regurgitation

Pathophysiology

Aortic regurgitation (AR) may be acute if it is due to trauma, IE, or aortic dissection or it may be chronic (rheumatic and degenerative). Acute severe AR is a surgical emergency and may rapidly lead to pulmonary edema. Chronic AR can cause both volume and pressure overload leading to eccentric as well as concentric hypertrophy. The increased diastolic volume due to AR augments the preload preserving contractility till late in the disease. The disease tends to progress rapidly once the LVES diameter exceeds 50 mm and the ED diameter exceeds 70 mm, and LV failure may ensue if compensatory mechanisms are over rided[19] (**Figs. 4A to E**). The PV loop shows no true isovolumetric relaxation phase as blood begins to enter the ventricle during active relaxation. ED volume increases due to continuous blood ingress from the aorta leading to increased preload and activation of the Frank–Starling mechanism, leading to increased stroke volume and peak systolic ventricular pressures (**Fig. 5**). Echocardiography is the cornerstone to establish the diagnosis, mechanism, severity of AR as well as the morphology of the ascending aorta and LVEF.[20] Vena contracta > 0.6 cm and regurgitation fraction > 50% are indicators of severe AR.[20] TEE is superior to transthoracic echocardiography, especially if IE or aortic dissection is suspected[19] (**Figs. 6A to C**).

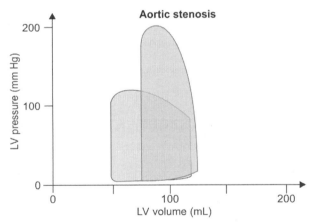

Fig. 2: Left ventricular (LV) pressure–volume loop in aortic stenosis.

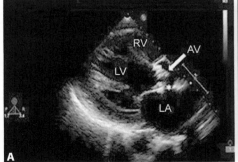
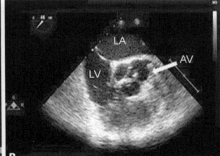
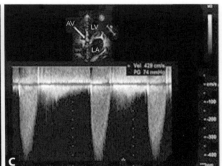

Figs. 3A to C: Transthoracic parasternal long-axis view showing heavily calcified aortic valve (AV) with echo dropouts due to calcium marked by * (A), aortic valve short axis view showing calcified AV in short axis with restricted opening (B), and aortic valve gradient measured using continuous wave Doppler in an apical four-chamber view (C).

Table 1: Hemodynamic goals for perioperative management of valvular heart diseases.

Valvular lesion	Preload	Systemic vascular resistance	Pulmonary vascular resistance	Heart rate	Contractility
AS	↑	↑	↔	↓	↔
AR	↑	↓	↔	↑	↔
MS	↑	↔	↓	↓	↔
MR	↑,↓	↑	↓	↔	↔
TR	↑	↔	↓	↔	↔

(AS, aortic stenosis; AR, aortic regurgitation; MS, mitral stenosis; MR, mitral regurgitation; TR, tricuspid regurgitation)

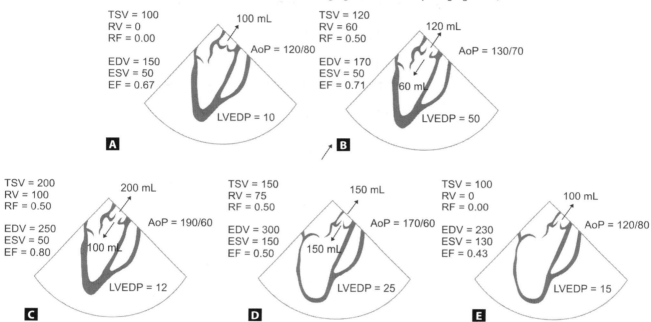

Figs. 4A to E: Hemodynamic changes in chronic Aortic regurgitation (AR). (A) Normal; (B)Severe Acute AR; (C) Chronic compensated AR; (D) Chronic decompensated AR; (E) Following AVR.

TSV: total stroke volume ; RV: residual volume ; RF: regurgitant fraction ; EDV: end diastolic volume ; ESV: end systolic volume ; EF: ejection fraction.

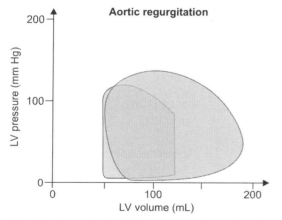

Fig. 5: Left ventricular (LV) pressure–volume loop in aortic regurgitation.

Management

Acute AR is a medical emergency with rapid development of pulmonary edema. Treatment consists of rapid decongestion with loop diuretics such as furosemide.

Selective arterial dilators such as nitroprusside may be used under hemodynamic monitoring for afterload reduction and decrease in regurgitant flow, thus improving cardiac output and decreasing LV filling pressures.[21] Acute severe AR is a surgical emergency requiring prompt valve replacement. Chronic AR with decreased EF requires vasodilator therapy: Angiotensin-converting enzyme (ACE) inhibitors, angiotensin receptor blockers (ARB), and dihydropyridine calcium channel blockers are preferred over beta blockers.[20] AVR is indicated in patients with symptomatic severe AR, patients with asymptomatic severe AR with LV dysfunction, and patients with severe AR undergoing cardiac surgery for other indications.[20]

Mitral Stenosis

Pathophysiology

The normal mitral valve area (MVA) is 4–6 cm². The most common etiology of mitral stenosis (MS) is rheumatic followed by degenerative with predominantly annular

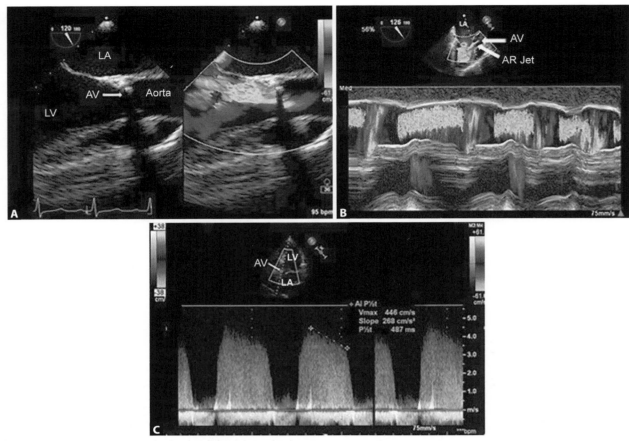

Figs. 6A to C: Transesophageal aortic valve (AV) long-axis view showing aortic regurgitation (AR) jet in color Doppler (A), with the color M-mode showing AR jet present throughout the diastole (B), and with the continuous wave Doppler across AV measuring its pressure half time not pulmonary hypertension of 487 ms equivalent to moderate AR (C).

calcification.[20] Rheumatic MS is characterized by commissural fusion and progressive narrowing of the valve orifice, leading to a characteristic funnel-shaped valve. Left atrial pressure increases progressively with increasing MS, leading to the development of pulmonary artery hypertension (PAH). An increase in left atrial size occurs gradually and leads to the development of AF which increases the risk of systemic embolization. Development of rapid ventricular rates with AF also leads to a decrease in cardiac output due to loss of the atrial component of cardiac filling.[20] Maintenance of sinus rhythm in MS is therefore necessary. MS can also worsen with anemia, pregnancy, and thyrotoxicosis, the conditions that increase the cardiac output and transvalvular pressure gradient.[19] PV loops show impaired LV filling with a decrease in ED volume/preload, resulting in decreased stroke volume and cardiac output. ED volume often decreases due to decreased afterload (**Fig. 7**). Echocardiographic features of severe MS (**Figs. 8A to C**) include MVA <1 cm^2 and diastolic pressure half time >220 ms. It also estimates PAH and left atrial size along with interrogation of other valves. Echocardiographic

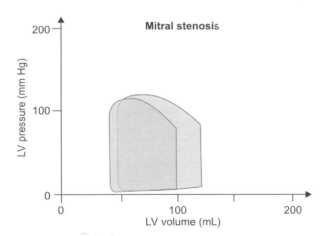

Fig. 7: Left ventricular (LV) pressure–volume loop in mitral stenosis.

assessment of mitral valve anatomy by Wilkins score helps in deciding whether to choose percutaneous intervention or not.[22] TEE is superior for diagnosing left atrial thrombus if transthoracic examination is inadequate.

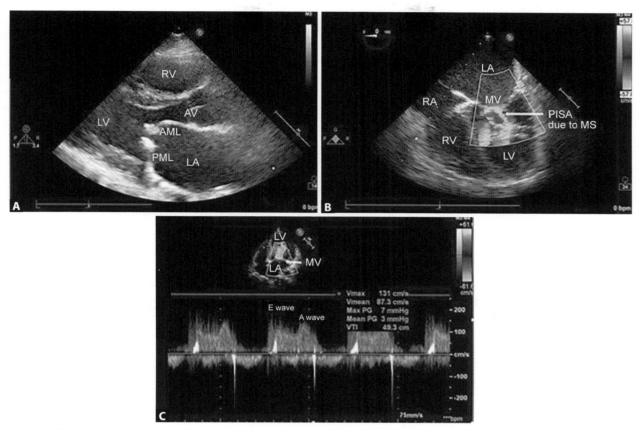

Figs. 8A to C: Transthoracic parasternal long-axis view showing heavily calcified, thickened mitral valve leaflets (AML and PML) (A), midesophageal four-chamber view showing turbulence across the mitral valve (MV) leading to the formation of PISA (B), and gradient across the stenosed MV measured using Doppler, which shows the fusion of E and A waves (C).

(AML: anterior mitral leaflet; PISA: proximal isovelocity surface area; PML: posterior mitral leaflet)

Intervention

Anticoagulation with warfarin is indicated in MS with AF, MS with a prior embolic event, and MS with left atrial thrombus.[23] Heart rate control is indicated in MS patients with AF with a fast ventricular rate[24] or in MS patients who are symptomatic on exercise.[25] Rate control is achieved with digoxin and beta blockers; cardioversion is indicated in acute AF with uncontrolled rates if medical therapy fails. MS with congestive heart failure/pulmonary edema is treated with oxygen and diuresis and may require mechanical ventilation. Percutaneous transmitral balloon commissurotomy (PTMC) is indicated in severe symptomatic MS with favorable valve morphology and the absence of moderate-to-severe MR or left atrial thrombus.[20] PTMC is indicated in pregnant patients with severe MS. MVR is indicated in severe symptomatic MS with unfavorable valve anatomy, failed PTMC, and patients undergoing cardiac surgery for other reasons.[20] In senile calcific MS, annular debridement, supra-annular valve replacement, and anchoring of the valve with felt around the mitral orifice may be needed.[20]

Mitral Regurgitation

Pathophysiology

Acute MR may be secondary to IE causing leaflet perforation, chest trauma leading to chordal rupture, and papillary muscle dysfunction/rupture secondary to myocardial ischemia/infarction.[20] Chronic MR may be primary due to the involvement of mitral valve apparatus (rheumatic MR and myxomatous degeneration) or may be secondary (ischemic MR and functional MR). While in primary MR mitral apparatus is involved, in secondary MR the dilated left ventricle causes papillary muscle displacement, leaflet tethering, and annular dilatation.[20] LV progressively dilates in chronic MR. Since the afterload is reduced, the EF increases above normal. Regressing of increased EF to normal values in fact heralds impairment of myocardial function. An EF < 40% implies poor prognosis after valve intervention. Chronic MR leads to PAH, left atrium enlargement, and AF (**Figs. 9A to D**). PV loops show elevated LV diastolic volume and compliance in chronic MR. There is no true isovolumetric contraction and relaxation phase. The stroke volume is increased, but the forward flow into the

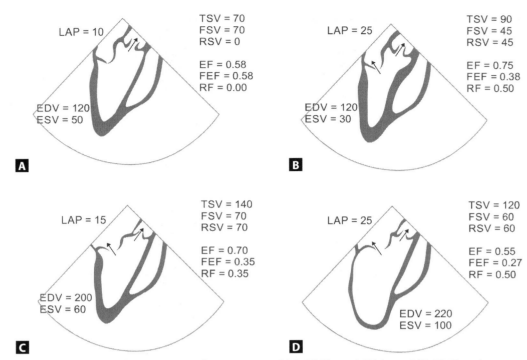

Figs. 9A to D: Hemodynamic changes in mitral regurgitation (MR). (A) Normal; (B) Acute MR; (C) Chronic compensated MR; (D) Chronic decompensated MR.

aorta is decreased as a part of the stroke volume is ejected back into the left atrium (**Fig. 10**). Echocardiography can be used to diagnose the etiology, severity of MR as well as LV/RV functions, PAH, and left atrial size. Vena contracta >0.7 mm, central regurgitant jet occupying >40% of left atrium area, and eccentric pansystolic murmur signify severe MR (**Figs. 11A to C**).

Intervention

Patients presenting with acute MR with congestive cardiac failure/pulmonary edema typically respond to antifailure measures as described above. Digoxin is helpful with LV dysfunction and AF with rapid rates. Intra-aortic balloon counter-pulsation (IABP) and other LV assist devices reduce the afterload and decrease MR. Acute severe MR is a surgical emergency, and early intervention is needed if the MR is traumatic; there is a flail leaflet secondary to myxomatous disease or papillary muscle rupture secondary to ischemia.[19] ACE inhibitors may be used for patients with chronic primary MR and cardiac failure. Beta blockers and spironolactone may be added for further control. Mitral valve repair is generally preferred over replacement if the pathology is limited and correctable with a durable repair.[20] MVR is done in symptomatic or asymptomatic patients with chronic primary severe MR. General anesthesia can severely alter the loading conditions and the severity of MR; therefore, the decision to intervene must be taken prior to anesthesia induction.[26] Chronic severe secondary MR is secondary to

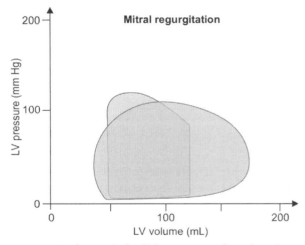

Fig. 10: Left ventricular (LV) pressure–volume loop in mitral regurgitation.

LV pathology and carries a poorer prognosis.[27] Diuretics, beta blockers, ACE inhibitors, aldosterone antagonists, and ARBs are used for the treatment of heart failure.[28-30] Cardiac resynchronization therapy may be indicated if left bundle branch block or other cardiac conduction abnormalities are the cause of MR.[31] Surgical intervention is recommended in patients with severe secondary MR with LVEF > 30% undergoing CABG[26] where valve repair is in preference to valve replacement.

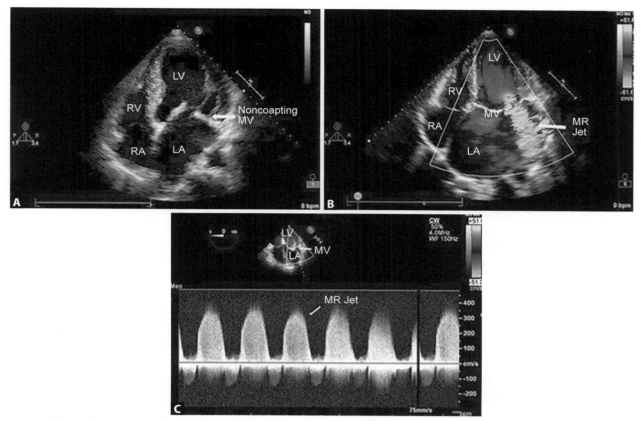

Figs. 11A to C: Transthoracic apical four-chamber view showing noncoapting mitral valve (MV) leaflets (A), with the mitral regurgitation (MR) jet demonstrated using color Doppler across MV (B), and transesophageal view with continuous wave Doppler placed across MV showing high-density MR Doppler jet indicating severe MR (C).

Tricuspid Stenosis

Pathophysiology and Intervention

Tricuspid stenosis (TS) is almost always rheumatic in origin, but may be congenital, drug induced, or functional secondary to right atrial mass. On echocardiography, a mean gradient > 5 mm Hg at the normal heart rate is indicative of severe stenosis.[17] Diuretics have a limited role in medical management. Surgical intervention for organic TS with replacement with a biological prosthesis is preferred because of better durability and high incidence of thrombosis with the mechanical valve in tricuspid position.[32]

Tricuspid Regurgitation

Pathophysiology

Tricuspid regurgitation (TR) may be due to the primary involvement of the tricuspid valve due to rheumatic disease, congenital (Ebstein anomaly), or IE in intravenous drug abusers or may be secondary to chronic volume/pressure overload of the right ventricle due to primary pulmonary hypertension or left-sided valvular disease.[33] Acute severe

TR could be because of trauma and RV procedures (biopsy and pacemaker lead extraction) and may lead to acute RV failure.[19] Chronic TR (usually secondary to left-sided lesions) leads to elevation of RV ED pressures and increase in RV size. Annular dilatation may occur in long-standing cases where TR begets TR. Coagulopathy and derangements of hepatic function are common in such patients. Echocardiography (**Figs. 12A and B**) has a central role in the evaluation of etiology, annular dilatation, RV dimensions, EF, and PAH.[33] Tricuspid annular dilation > 40 mm warrants surgical repair.

Intervention

Medical management with loop diuretics with the addition of spironolactone can be done. Digoxin is specifically helpful in improving RV contractility and controlling ventricular rate.[19] Inotropic support with dobutamine or milrinone decreases pulmonary artery pressures and increases forward flow. Surgical intervention is needed for severe primary or secondary TR when left-sided valve surgery is indicated and in patients with isolated severe primary TR without severe RV dysfunction.[26] In secondary TR, annular repair (preferably ring annuloplasty) improves

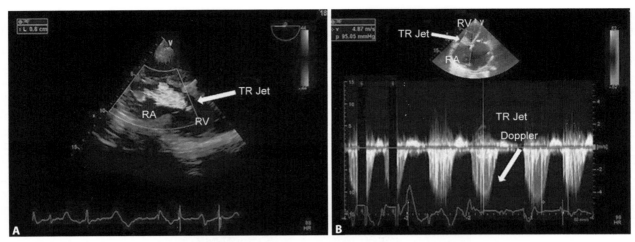

Figs. 12A and B: Midesophageal four-chamber view showing tricuspid regurgitation (TR) jet in color Doppler across tricuspid valve (A) and transthoracic apical four-chamber view showing measurement of gradient across tricuspid valve from TR jet using continuous wave Doppler across it (B).

the functional status of the patient and can even lead to RV remodeling and better long-term outcomes without any increase in surgical mortality.[34]

POSTOPERATIVE CRITICAL CARE MANAGEMENT IN THE INTENSIVE CARE UNIT

Postoperative Management of Individual Valvular Lesions

Aortic Stenosis

Patients with AS typically have concentric hypertrophy and diastolic heart failure which persists in the immediate postoperative period and takes 6–12 months to regress.[35] These patients benefit by higher preload which helps the hypertrophied LV filling. Adequate preload can be assessed by systolic pressure variation of the arterial pressure and by passive leg raising which increases the systemic venous return. Any increase in arterial pressure by these maneuvers signifies that cardiac output will increase by judicious volume loading. Along with higher preload, sinus rhythm with the avoidance of tachycardia is desired. Tachycardia decreases the available diastolic time and hence coronary perfusion of the hypertrophied myocardium which occurs primarily during diastole.[35] Rate control thus avoids subendocardial ischemia and hemodynamic compromise in the hypertrophied ventricle.[36] Among the beta blockers, esmolol is a prudent choice in the perioperative period because of its rapid onset and short duration should any worsening of hemodynamics ensue. Phenylephrine is the drug of choice if the patient is hypotensive with tachycardia.[35] It is to be noted that due to chronic elevation of LV ED pressures, the pulmonary

artery wedge pressures are also elevated in these patients and thus do not signify fluid overload. They may still be higher in patients with PAH and RV ischemia, especially in those with multivalvular lesions. These patients may benefit with milrinone or dobutamine with the maintenance of SVR. Clinical parameters such as lactate, urine output, and mixed venous oxygen saturation are helpful in assessing the response to inotropes.[35] Perivalvular leak may be recognized on echocardiography in the immediate post-bypass period, especially if replacement was done for calcific AS. Systolic anterior motion (SAM) of the mitral valve may be precipitated in AS with nonjudicious use of the diuretics and inotropes causing increased contractility and tachycardia. Treatment consists of rate control and volume to stent open the LV outflow tract.[35] AF is a common postoperative feature usually reversed with amiodarone. Cardioversion is indicated in recent AF or AF with hemodynamic instability.[37] Postoperative conduction disturbances may occur due to ischemia, edema, or surgical trauma to atrioventricular (AV) node or left bundle branch which is located in close proximity to noncoronary cusp. The surgeon may place AV sequential temporary pacing wires to preserve the atrial kick to hypertrophied LV. A permanent pacemaker may be required in 1% patients, the incidence increasing to 8% with advanced age and pre-existing conduction blocks.[38,39] Clinical stroke occurs in 17% and transient ischemic attacks occur in 2% of patients post AVR.[35] Silent infarcts were detected in MRI in 54% of patients who were stroke free.[40]

Aortic Regurgitation

Conduction abnormalities are the same as in AS. Inotropic support is often required by the dilated heart to maintain rate and contractility. If aortic root replacement was done, coagulopathy and neurological assessment are additional points to ponder, especially when circulatory arrest was employed.[41]

Mitral Stenosis

With long-standing MS, pulmonary hypertension, AF with its thromboembolic complication, and decreased cardiac output due to poor ventricular function are common complications.

Pulmonary hypertension: Left atrial pressure rises to pump against increasing obstruction leading to pulmonary venous hypertension (PVH) which is transmitted backward in long-standing MS to cause PAH.[35] A transpulmonary pressure gradient can distinguish between PAH and PVH (normal value < 12 mm Hg).[35] It is elevated in PAH and normal in PVH; this distinction is important as pulmonary vasodilators if used in PVH can worsen it by increasing pulmonary blood flow. Long-standing PAH may lead to RV dysfunction. Pain, hypothermia, hypoxia, and hypercarbia should be avoided as these can increase PAH. Medical therapy consists of dobutamine, milrinone, sildenafil, and bosentan. Prostacyclin analogs such as Iloprost and Epoprostenol are limited by systemic vasodilatation.[42] Inhaled nitric oxide may be added in refractory cases and has the advantage of selective pulmonary vasodilatation without systemic hypotension.[43]

Atrial fibrillation: Increase in left atrial pressure and size secondary to MS may lead to AF in up to 60% of cases in patients >50 years of age.[44] Since chronic AF will not revert with cardioversion, the aim is to control rate with beta blockers, verapamil, amiodarone, or digoxin.[45]

Mitral Regurgitation

In primary chronic MR, after the intervention (either mitral valve repair or replacement), the left ventricle has to eject against a competent valve, therefore increasing the afterload on an already dilated ventricle. The goals of postoperative management are therefore afterload reduction achieved by inodilators (milrinone and dobutamine) in the perioperative period. Additional inotropic support may be required if there is LV systolic dysfunction. In cases of severe LV dysfunction, IABP may be required to decrease the afterload till the ventricular function recovers.[35] Treatment of PAH is the same as in MS. SAM of the mitral valve may occur in 4–5% of cases with mitral valve prosthetic ring repair, especially in myxomatous mitral leaflets and hyperdynamic LV.[35] Management is the same as discussed in AS. AF is managed as above.

General Postoperative Management

Prosthetic Valve Considerations

Choice of prosthesis: A bioprosthetic valve is indicated in patients >70 years of age, when mechanical prosthesis is contraindicated and when there is thrombosis of the mechanical prosthesis despite adequate anticoagulation. A mechanical prosthetic valve (**Figs. 13A and B**) is indicated in younger patients with no contraindications to anticoagulation and accelerated structural deterioration of the bioprosthetic valve.

Anticoagulation: For mechanical prosthesis, life-long anticoagulation with vitamin K antagonists (VKA) is recommended. Bridging with unfractionated heparin or low-molecular-weight heparin is indicated till the effect of VKA starts in the postoperative period or as bridging therapy whenever VKA are discontinued for surgery or other indications. It is prudent to maintain an INR of 2.5 for mechanical prosthesis at aortic position. An INR of 3 is desired for mechanical prosthesis at aortic position with high risk of thromboembolism (AF, LV dysfunction, and previous

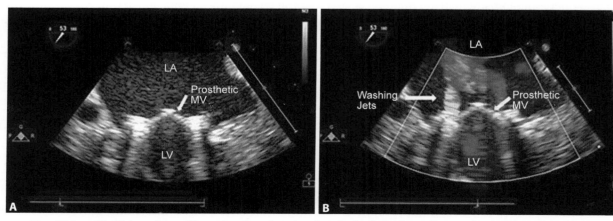

Figs. 13A and B: Midesophageal four-chamber view showing the leaflets of metallic prosthetic mitral valve (MV) (A), with color Doppler across the MV showing normal washing jets (B).

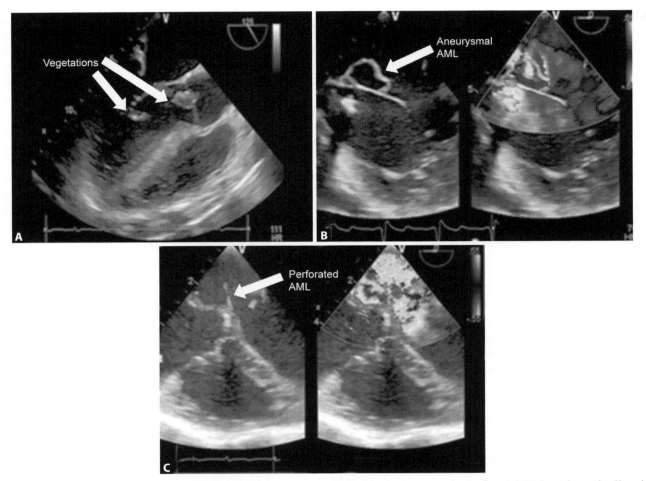

Figs. 14A to C: TEE Midesophageal long axis showing vegetations on Mitral valve and Aortic valve leaflets (A), Midesophageal 4 Chamber View showing aneurysmal anterior Mitral valve leaflet (AML) (B), Midesophageal 4 Chamber View showing perforation in AML (C).

thromboembolic episodes) or at mitral position.[46] Aspirin 75–100 mg is recommended in addition to VKA in patients with mechanical thrombosis. Acute mechanical prosthetic valve thrombosis is treated with low-dose fibrinolytic therapy or emergency surgery with a deteriorating hemodynamic profile. Severe peri-/paraprosthetic regurgitation causing heart failure or intractable hemolysis requires surgical intervention.[46]

Infective Endocarditis

Early surgical intervention is indicated in patients with IE who are experiencing symptoms of heart failure due to valve dysfunction, IE complicated by periannular abscess, heart block, IE with highly virulent organisms, persistent bacteremia despite antibiotic therapy, and prosthetic valve dehiscence.[46] Echocardiography is the investigation of choice to detect the complications of IE (**Figs. 14A to C**).

Pregnancy

Management during pregnancy may be decided by a multidisciplinary team consisting of the cardiologist,

obstetrician, and anesthesiologist as per the guidelines.[47] Transthoracic echocardiography with clinical evaluation should always be performed to assess the severity of the lesion. Elective cesarean section is recommended for severe MS, severe AS, in Marfan syndrome with ascending aortic dilatation > 45 mm, and severe PAH. PTMC should be considered in severe symptomatic MS and in those with pulmonary artery pressures > 50 mm Hg after the 20th week of gestation.[47] Chronic MR and AR are well tolerated and usually do not require any intervention if LVEF is maintained. Surgery with cardiopulmonary bypass if indicated in cases of severe maternal distress/hemodynamic instability carries a 15–30% fetal mortality.[48]

REFERENCES

1. Nkomo VT, Gardin JM, Skelton TN, Gottdiener JS, Scott CG, Enriquez-Sarano M. Burden of valvular heart diseases: a population-based study. Lancet. 2006;368:1005-11.
2. Carapetis JR, Steer AC, Mulholland EK, Weber M. The global burden of group A streptococcal diseases. Lancet Infect Dis. 2005;5:685-94.

3. Picano E, Pibarot P, Lancellotti P, Monin JL, Bonow RO. The emerging role of exercise testing and stress echocardiography in valvular heart disease. J Am Coll Cardiol. 2009;54:2251-60.

4. Neglia D, Rovai D, Caselli C, Pietila M, Teresinska A, Aguade-Bruix S, et al. Detection of significant coronary artery disease by noninvasive anatomical and functional imaging. Circ Cardiovasc Imaging. 2015;8:e002179.

5. Messika-Z D, Serfaty JM, Brochet E, Ducrocq G, Lepage L, Detaint D, et al. Multimodal assessment of the aortic annulus diameter: implications for transcatheter aortic valve implantation. J Am Coll Cardiol. 2010;55:186-94.

6. Ambler G, Omar RZ, Royston P, Kinsman R, Keogh BE, Taylor KM. Generic, simple risk stratification model for heart valve surgery. Circulation. 2005;112:224-31.

7. Van Gameren M, Kappetein AP, Steyerberg EW, Venema AC, Berenschot EA, Hannan EL, et al. Do we need separate risk stratification models for hospital mortality after heart valve surgery? Ann Thorac Surg. 2008;85:921-30.

8. O'Brien SM, Shahian DM, Filardo G, Ferraris VA, Haan CK, Rich JB, et al. The Society of Thoracic Surgeons 2008 cardiac surgery risk models: part 2 – isolated valve surgery. Ann Thorac Surg. 2009;88:S23-42.

9. Shahian DM, O'Brien SM, Filardo G, Ferraris VA, Haan CK, Rich JB, et al. The Society of Thoracic Surgeons 2008 cardiac surgery risk models: part 3 – valve plus coronary artery bypass grafting surgery. Ann Thorac Surg. 2009;88:S43-62.

10. Thourani VH, Suri RM, Gunter RL, Sheng S, O'Brien SM, Ailawadi G, et al. Contemporary real-world outcomes of surgical aortic valve replacement in 141,905 low-risk, intermediate-risk, and high-risk patients. Ann Thorac Surg. 2015;99:55-61.

11. Lalani T, Chu VH, Park LP, Cecchi E, Corey GR, Durante-Mangoni E, et al. In-hospital and 1-year mortality in patients undergoing early surgery for prosthetic valve endocarditis. JAMA Intern Med. 2013;173:1495-504.

12. Remenyi B, Carapetis J, Wyber R, Taubert K, Mayosi BM. Position statement of the World Heart Federation on the prevention and control of rheumatic heart disease. Nat Rev Cardiol. 2013;10:284-92.

13. Kirchhof P, Benussi S, Kotecha D, Ahlsson A, Atar D, Casadei B, et al. 2016 ESC Guidelines for the management of atrial fibrillation developed in collaboration with EACTS: The Task Force for the management of atrial fibrillation of the European Society of Cardiology (ESC). Developed with the special contribution of the European Heart Rhythm Association (EHRA) of the ESC Endorsed by the European Stroke Organisation (ESO). Eur Heart J. 2016:37:2893-962.

14. De Caterina R, Camm AJ. What is 'valvular' atrial fibrillation? A reappraisal. Eur Heart J. 2014;35:3328-35.

15. Heidbuchel H, Verhamme P, Alings M, Antz M, Diener HC, Hacke W, et al. Updated European Heart Rhythm Association Practical Guide on the use of non-vitamin K antagonist anticoagulants in patients with non-valvular atrial fibrillation. Europace. 2015;17:1467-507.

16. Eikelboom JW, Connolly SJ, Brueckmann M, Granger CB, Kappetein AP, Mack MJ, et al. Dabigatran versus warfarin in patients with mechanical heart valves. N Engl J Med. 2013;369:1206-14.

17. Baumgartner H, Hung J, Bermejo J, Edwardsen T, Goldstein S, Lancellotti P, et al. Focus update on the echocardiographic assessment of aortic valve stenosis: EAE/ASE recommendations for clinical practice. Eur J Echocardiogr. 2017;18:254-75.

18. Monin JL, Quéré JP, Monchi M, Petit H, Baleynaud S, Chauvel C, et al. Low-gradient aortic stenosis, operative risk stratification and predictors for long-term outcome: a multicenter study using dobutamine stress hemodynamics. Circulation. 2003;108:319-24.

19. Hall JB, Schmidt GA, Kress JP. Hall, Schmidt and Press's Principles of Critical Care, 4th edition. New York: McGraw Hill Education; 2015.

20. Nishimura RA, Otto CM, Bonow RO, Carabello BA, Erwin JP, Guyton RA, et al. ACC/AHA Task Force Members. 2014 AHA/ACC guideline for the management of patients with valvular heart disease: a report of the American College of Cardiology/American Heart Association Task Force on Practice Guidelines. Circulation. 2014;129:e521-643.

21. Miller RR, Vismara LA, DeMaria AN, Salel AF, Mason DT. Afterload reduction therapy with nitroprusside in severe aortic regurgitation: improved cardiac performance and reduced regurgitant volume. Am J Cardiol. 1976;38:564.

22. Wilkins GT, Weyman AE, Abascal VM, Block PC, Palacios IF. Percutaneous balloon dilatation of the mitral valve: an analysis of echocardiographic variables related to outcome and the mechanism of dilatation. Br Heart J. 1988;60:299-308.

23. Perez-Gomez F, Alegria E, Berjon J. Comparative effects of antiplatelet, anticoagulant, or combined therapy in patients with valvular and nonvalvular atrial fibrillation: a randomized multicentre study. J Am Coll Cardiol. 2004;44:1557-66.

24. Wood P. An appreciation of mitral stenosis. I. Clinical features. Br Med J. 1954;1:1051-63.

25. Stoll BC, Ashcom TL, Johns JP. Effects of atenolol on rest and exercise hemodynamics in patients with mitral stenosis. Am J Cardiol. 1995;75:482-4.

26. Baumgartner H, Falk V, Bax JJ, De Bonis M, Hamm C, Holm PJ, et al. 2017 ESC/EACTS Guidelines for the management of valvular heart disease. The Task Force for the Management of Valvular Heart Disease of the European Society of Cardiology (ESC) and the European Association for Cardio-Thoracic Surgery (EACTS). Eur Heart J. 2017; 38:2739-91.

27. Kang DH, Kim MJ, Kang SJ. Mitral valve repair versus revascularization alone in the treatment of ischemic mitral regurgitation. Circulation. 2006;114:I499-503.

28. Yusuf S, Pitt B, Davis CE, Hood WB Jr, Cohn JN. Effect of enalapril on mortality and the development of heart failure in asymptomatic patients with reduced left ventricular ejection fractions. The SOLVD Investigators. N Engl J Med. 1992;327:685-91.

29. Granger CB, McMurray JJ, Yusuf S. Effects of candesartan in patients with chronic heart failure and reduced left-ventricular systolic function intolerant to angiotensin-converting-enzyme inhibitors: the CHARM-Alternative trial. Lancet. 2003;362:772-6.

30. Eriksson SV, Eneroth P, Kjekshus J. Neuroendocrine activation in relation to left ventricular function in chronic severe congestive heart failure: a subgroup analysis from the Cooperative North Scandinavian Enalapril Survival Study (CONSENSUS). Clin Cardiol. 1994;17:603-6.

31. van Bommel RJ, Marsan NA, Delgado V. Cardiac resynchronization therapy as a therapeutic option in patients with moderate-severe functional mitral regurgitation and high operative risk. Circulation. 2011;124:912-9.

32. Filsoufi F, Anyanwu AC, Salzberg SP, Frankel T, Cohn LH, Adams DH. Long term outcomes of tricuspid valve replacement in the current era. Ann Thorac Surg. 2005;80:845-50.

33. Lancellotti P, Tribouilloy C, Hagendorff A, Popescu BA, Edvardsen T, Pierard LA, et al. Scientific Document Committee of the European Association of Cardiovascular Imaging. Recommendations for the echocardiographic assessment of native valvular regurgitation: an executive summary from the European Association of Cardiovascular Imaging. Eur Heart J Cardiovasc Imaging. 2013;14:611-44.

34. Van de Veire NR, Braun J, Delgado V, Versteegh MI, Dion RA, Klautz RJ, et al. Tricuspid annuloplasty prevents right ventricular dilatation and progression of tricuspid regurgitation in patients with tricuspid annular dilatation undergoing mitral valve repair. J Thorac Cardiovasc Surg. 2011;141:1431–9.

35. Miller S, Flynn BC. Valvular heart diseases and postoperative considerations. Seminars in Cardiothoracic and Vascular Anesthesia 2015;19:130-42.

36. DiNardo JA. Anesthesia for valve replacement in patients with acquired valvular heart disease. In: DiNardo JA (Ed). Anesthesia for Cardiac Surgery, 2nd edition. Stamford, CT: Appleton & Lange; 1998. pp. 109-40.

37. January CT, Wann LS, Alpert JS, Calkins H, CiCleveland JC Jr. 2014 AHA/ACC/HRS guideline for the management of patients with atrial fibrillation: a report of the American College of Cardiology/American Heart Association Task Force on Practice Guidelines and the Heart Rhythm Society. J Am Coll Cardiol. 2014;64(21):e1-76.

38. Merin O, Ilan M, Oren A. Permanent pacemaker implantation following cardiac surgery: indications and long-term follow-up. PACE. 2009;32:7-12.

39. Dawkins S, Hobson AR, Kalra PR, Tang AT, Monro JL, Dawkins KD. Permanent pacemaker implantation after isolated aortic valve replacement: incidence, indications, and predictors. Ann Thorac Surg. 2008;85:108-12.

40. Messe SR, Acker MA, Kasner SE. Stroke after aortic valve surgery: results from a prospective cohort. Circulation. 2014;12:2253-61.

41. Griepp EB, Griepp RB. Cerebral consequences of hypothermic circulatory arrest in adults. J Card Surg. 1992;7:134-55.

42. Akagi S, Ogawa A, Miyaji K, Kusano K, Ito H, Matsubara H. Catecholamine support at the initiation of epoprostenol therapy in pulmonary arterial hypertension. Ann Am Thorac Soc. 2014;11:719-27.

43. Mahoney PD, Loh E, Blitz LR, Herrmann HC. Hemodynamic effects of inhaled nitric oxide in women with mitral stenosis and pulmonary hypertension. Am J Cardiol. 2001;87:188-92.

44. Hernandez R, Banuelos C, Alfonso F. Long-term clinical and echocardiographic follow-up after percutaneous mitral valvuloplasty with the Inoue balloon. Circulation. 1999;99:1580-6.

45. Fuster V, Ryden LE, Cannom DS. 2011 ACCF/AHA/HRS focused updates incorporated into the ACC/AHA/ESC 2006 guidelines for the management of patients with atrial fibrillation: a report of the American College of Cardiology Foundation/American Heart Association Task Force on practice guidelines. Circulation. 2011;123:e269-e367.

46. Nishimura RA, Otto CM, Bonow RO, Carabello BA, Erwin JP, Fleisher LA, et al. 2017 AHA/ACC focused update of the 2014 AHA/ACC guideline for the management of patients with valvular heart disease: a report of the American College of Cardiology/American Heart Association Task Force on Clinical Practice Guidelines. Circulation. 2017;135:e1159-e95.

47. Regitz-Zagrosek V, Blomstrom Lundqvist C, Borghi C, Cifkova R, Ferreira R, Foidart JM, et al. European Society of Gynecology (ESG), Association for European Paediatric Cardiology (AEPC), German Society for Gender Medicine (DGesGM). ESC Committee for Practice Guidelines. ESC Guidelines on the management of cardiovascular diseases during pregnancy: the Task Force on the Management of Cardiovascular Diseases during Pregnancy of the European Society of Cardiology (ESC). Eur Heart J. 2011;32:3147-97.

48. Elassy SM, Elmidany AA, Elbawab HY. Urgent cardiac surgery during pregnancy: a continuous challenge. Ann Thorac Surg. 2014;97:1624-9.

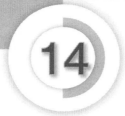

CHAPTER

14

Perioperative Management of Blunt Trauma Chest Injuries

Sandeep Sahu, Mekhala Paul, Arindam Chatterjee

INTRODUCTION

Chest trauma has significant mortality and morbidity. Most of the deaths due to chest trauma can be prevented with early diagnosis and aggressive treatment. Most of the cases can be treated by prioritizing and timely managing by Airway with cervical spine control, Breathing and ventilation management, managing Circulatory shock and simultaneous hemorrhage control (by stopping the bleeding), accessing neuro-Disability, Exposure to find possible missed injuries and environmental control to prevent hypothermia and its consequences (ABCDE approach) of trauma resuscitation as per the advanced trauma life support (ATLS) approach by airway management and intercostal drainage (ICD), or chest tube placement. Very few cases (<10% of blunt and only 15–30% of penetrating chest trauma) require operations.[1]

Lethal triad (hypoxia, hypercarbia, and acidosis) prevention and accordingly aggressive management are the cornerstones in chest trauma patients. Tissue hypoxia occurs because of inadequate supply of oxygen [because of blood loss, pulmonary ventilation/perfusion mismatch (lung contusion, hematoma, or alveolar collapse) and because of changes in the intrathoracic pressure (pneumothorax)]. This tissue hypoxia and hypoperfusion leads to metabolic acidosis. Hypercarbia can be because of inadequate ventilation, due to intrathoracic pressure changes and low level of consciousness.[2]

As per the ATLS, the initial assessment and treatment in chest trauma consist of a primary survey that includes the resuscitation of vital functions in the form of airway with cervical spine restriction, breathing and ventilation, circulation and hemorrhage control, neurological disability management followed by a detailed secondary survey and up to definitive care. Immediate threatening injuries are to be treated urgently and as early as possible. The secondary survey is affected by the mechanism of injury and a high

degree of suspicion for specific possible injuries.[1,2] Blunt chest trauma leading to different complications in the perioperative period is presented in **Table 1**.[3]

MANAGEMENT OF LIFE-THREATENING SCENARIOS IN THE PERIOPERATIVE PERIOD

Airway

If there is any preoperative evidence or suspicion of a partial laryngeal injury which may be associated with severe blunt chest trauma, assessment for requirement of any repair and/or reduction of upper airway edema before extubation or any airway manipulation must be done very cautiously. Triads of clinical signs are usually present in laryngeal trauma with partial or complete airway obstruction—hoarseness, subcutaneous emphysema, and palpable fracture. In postoperative-intubated patients, increasing subcutaneous emphysema always indicates the presence of larangeal and tracheo bronchial tree injury. If extubation or tracheostomy is planned, a leak test should be done to rule out upper airway edema.[4,5]

If any instability of the sternoclavicular joint with posterior dislocation of the clavicular head causes upper airway obstruction, immediate closed reduction should be done.

Breathing

Life-threating conditions and their management are given in the following text.

Tension Pneumothorax

As postoperatively patients usually remain intubated with positive-pressure ventilation (PPV), minimal pneumothorax or visceral pleural injury without ICD or dislodged ICD

Table 1: Chest trauma leading to different complications in the perioperative period.

Organ- or injury-specific complications	Types of complications
Wound complications	Wound infection
	Wound dehiscence (mainly for sternal wounds)
Cardiac complications	Myocardial infarction
	Arrhythmia
	Pericarditis
	Pericardial effusion/tamponade
	Ventricular aneurysm
	Septal defect
Pulmonary and bronchial complications	Atelectasis
	Pneumonia
	Lung abscess
	Empyema
	Pneumatocele
	Clotted hemothorax
	Bronchial repair disruption
	Bronchopleural fistula
	Fibrothorax
Vascular complications	Graft infection
	Graft thrombosis
	Pseudoaneurysm
	Deep venous thrombosis
	Pulmonary embolism
Neurologic complications	Stroke
	Paraplegia (after ruptured thoracic aorta repair)
	Causalgia (after brachial plexus injury)
Esophageal complication	Mediastinitis
	Esophageal fistula
	Esophageal stricture
	Leakage of repair

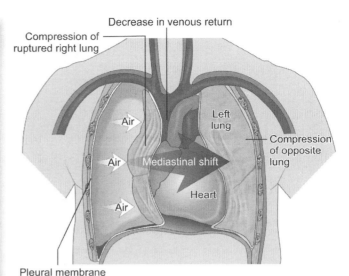

In a tension pneumothorax, air from a ruptured lung enters the pleural cavity without a means of escape. As air pressure builds up, the affected lung is compressed and all of the mediastinal tissues are displaced to the opposite side of the chest

Fig. 1: Pathophysiologic changes in right-sided tension pneumothorax leading to mediastinal shift causing compression of both the ventricles leading to sudden cardiac arrest.

[*Source*: Adapted from www.alamy.com, Nucleus Medical Media Inc/Alamy Stock Photo (Image ID: ADTTP2)]

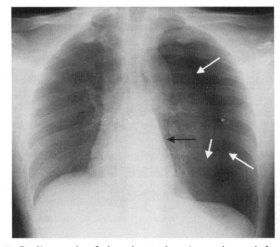

Fig. 2: Radiograph of the chest showing a large left-sided pneumothorax (white arrows) which is under tension as manifest as displacement of the heart to the right (black arrow) and depression of the left hemidiaphragm.
(*Source*: adapted from http://www.learningradiology.com/

may result in tension pneumothorax (**Figs. 1 and 2**). A misguided attempt at subclavian or internal jugular vein catheterization can also result in tension pneumothorax. So, continuous vital monitoring is very important.[6]

The clinical signs are as follows:
- Tachycardia, tachypnoea
- Hypotension
- Hypoxia (desaturation)
- Unilateral absence of breath sound
- Increased central venous pressure (CVP)
- *Ultrasound*: Lung-absent lung sliding, absence of B-line, barcode sign on M-mode, lung point
- Cardiac arrest

Management: Tension pneumothorax can be managed by immediate insertion of a wide-bore needle (ideally an 8-cm needle reaches the pleural space in >90% time) in the second intercostal space in the mid-clavicular line of the affected hemithorax. It converts the injury to simple pneumothorax. This must be followed by insertion of ICD into the fifth intercostal space just anterior to the mid-axillary line (usually at the nipple level) as soon as possible (**Fig. 3**). It is the definitive treatment. Otherwise, prolonged needle decompression may increase the risk of subsequent pleural injury by needle stick resulting in further pneumothorax.[7]

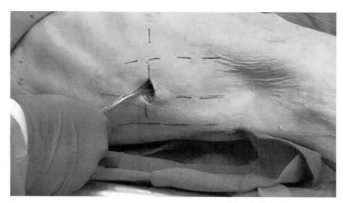

Fig. 3: Intercostal drainage placement to relive tension pneumothorax in the fifth intercostal space just medial to the midclavicular line.

Bronchopleural Fistula

Bronchopleural fistula (BPF) occurs in case of chest trauma with tracheobronchial tree disruption, after ipsilateral thoracotomy, right-sided pneumonectomy or lower lobectomy, and spontaneous pneumothorax. It increases mortality, morbidity and intensive care unit (ICU) stay significantly. The most common risk factors are as follows:

- Age > 60 years
- Diabetes mellitus
- Heavy smoker and chronic obstructive pulmonary disease (COPD)
- Low nutrition/poor wound healing
- Steroid use
- Prolonged postoperative mechanical ventilation
- Ventilator-induced barotrauma
- Associated infection with organisms such as *Streptococcus, Staphylococcus, Pseudomonas, Klebsiella,* and *Aspergillus*
- Acute respiratory distress syndrome (ARDS)

   Presentation may be *acute* life-threatening or subacute/chronic.

Acute BPF usually presents with the following symptoms:

- Sudden-onset dyspnea with chest pain
- Coughing up blood (just after trauma) or purulent fluid (in post-operative patients with prolonged stay in ICU with empyema) sputum
- Hemodynamic instability (hypotension, tachycardia)
- Subcutaneous emphysema
- Tracheal/mediastinal shift to the opposite side
- Persistent large/new air leak through ICD. It may be the only sign. If the patient is on ventilator, the desired tidal volume will never be achieved and continuous alarm of leak will be there. Large air leak also results in autotriggering which causes severe hyperventilation without adequate removal of carbon dioxide and needs

unnecessary use of a large dose of sedatives and muscle relaxants.
- Reduction/disappearance of pleural collection in chest X-ray (CXR).

Management: Diagnosis should be confirmed on the basis of clinical findings, radiographic findings, and bronchographic findings. Computerized tomography (CT) scan may reveal pneumothorax, pneumomediastinum, and underlying pathology with a fistulous tract. A discussion regarding bronchographic findings is beyond the scope of this chapter.

Treatment

- *General:* Life-threatening tension pneumothorax, pulmonary and endobronchial flooding with blood or pus should be addressed first.

   If it occurs after trauma with blood flooding with significant hypoxia, then the patient should undergo surgical repair. Video-assisted thoracoscopy and surgical repair are preferred if there is no massive bleeding as it has significantly lesser morbidity, mortality, and ventilator and ICU stay in comparison to thoracotomy.[8,9]

   If it occurs in association with infection (empyema or bronchial stump infection) in the post-operative period, some general measures must be taken:[10]

   – The patient should be placed with the affected side in dependent position and drainage of air and fluid from the pleural space by chest tube thoracostomy. This postural drainage should be continued till chest tube drainage is <30 mL/day.

   – In patients who are on mechanical ventilation, a chest tube is helpful for adding positive end-expiratory pressure (PEEP) during expiration, thus increasing air leak and occlusion during the inspiratory phase and decreasing BPF flow during inspiration. Sclerosing agents may also be applied through the chest tube.

   – Broad-spectrum antibiotics and appropriate nutritional supplement are recommended.

- *Ventilator management*

   – *Target:* Mean airway pressure should be maintained at or below the critical opening pressure of the fistula to promote healing providing adequate alveolar ventilation and thus adequate gas exchange. This target can be achieved by:

      ◆ Minimum and peak airway pressures are to be kept as minimum as possible (including minimal PEEP).

      ◆ Low tidal volume, decreasing respiratory rate, and shortening inspiratory time at the cost of permissive hypercapnia.

      ◆ Other techniques of ventilator strategies may be achieved—independent lung ventilation with a double-lumen tube, selective intubation of the unaffected lung, single-lumen tube with bronchial blocker, and high-frequency jet ventilation with hypercapnia.

- *Definitive therapy:* Small fistula < 5 mm in diameter—bronchoscopic intervention (application of occlusive agents) is preferable if size more than 8 mm than closure with airway stent, coil or amplatzer devices is more effective.

To limit the airflow across the fistula, the following procedures can be done:

- – Direct closure
- – Decortication
- – Thoracoplasty
- – Omental/muscle transposition
- – Complete pneumonectomy

Pulmonary Contusion

This injury is very common in blunt chest trauma (25–35%). It especially occurs when the moving chest hits a fixed solid object. There is accumulation of blood and excessive inflammation-induced fluid in interstitium and alveoli of the affected segment of lung. This causes ventilation-perfusion mismatch, increased intrapulmonary shunt, and loss of compliance Thus, the extent of severity of symptoms and signs, mortality, and morbidity are proportional to the degree/area of pulmonary contusion.[11]

The resulting clinical features are as follows:

- Hypoxia
- Hypercarbia
- Labored breathing with dyspnea (tachypnea)
- Tachycardia
- Cyanosis and eventually cardiorespiratory arrest
- Rales, wheeze, and decreased breath sound in severe contusion
- Blood-streak sputum or blood-tinged secretion from the endotracheal tube (ETT)

Respiratory distress usually peaks around 72 hours after trauma. Pulmonary contusion is an independent risk factor for the development of ARDS, pneumonia, and long term respiratory dysfunction. BPF is associated with 18–67% mortality.

Diagnosis

Clinical and radiological: CXR has low sensitivity to diagnose the size and extent of pulmonary contusion. Moreover, the actual picture and extent of contusion are apparent in the CXR 24–48 hours after the beginning of symptoms. Unlike the CXR, the CT scan not only determines the size and three-dimensional extent of pulmonary contusion but also differentiates contusion from areas of atelectasis or

aspiration with high sensitivity. The CT scan can identify minimal contusion even when the patient is clinically asymptomatic.

Bedside lung ultrasonography: The sensitivity of bedside ultrasonography for contusion is 94.6%.[12,13]

- Segment of multiple B lines
- Irregular hypoechoic area with indistinct margin without change/movement during respiration
- Subpleural, irregular bordered area without air inlets

Management: The Eastern Association for the Surgery of Trauma (EAST) practice management guideline reviewed 129 articles on pulmonary contusion with flail chest and published six level-2 and eight level-3 recommendations.[14]

i. Avoid fluid overload.

ii. Obligatory mechanical ventilation in absence of respiratory failure should be avoided.

iii. Lung-protective ventilation strategy (according to the ARDS net protocol) should be followed, i.e., low tidal volume and high PEEP. FiO_2 just to maintain oxygen saturation at 88–94%. This lung protective-ventilation is at the cost of permissive hypercapnia.

iv. Optimal analgesia and aggressive chest physiotherapy to prevent further respiratory failure. Epidural analgesia is the preferred mode until and unless it is contraindicated.

v. Steroid should not be used in pulmonary contusion therapy.

vi. Diuretics may be used in case of hydrostatic fluid overload in lung only when the patient is hemodynamically stable or with concurrent congestive cardiac failure.

vii. Independent lung ventilation may be considered in severe unilateral pulmonary contusion when the shunt cannot be corrected owing to maldistribution of ventilation.

viii. High-frequency oscillatory ventilation (HFOV) may be considered if conventional ventilatory modes are not effective.

Flail Chest

In this case, at least three consecutive ribs are fractured in two or more places compromising thoracic cage integrity. Morbidity and mortality increase with increased age, bilateral flail chest, and in cases of associated pulmonary contusion.

Management

- According to studies, surgical rib fixation definitely decreases ventilator days and length of stay in an ICU and in comparison to nonoperative management.

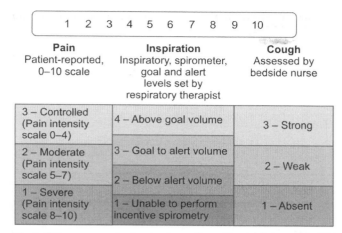

Fig. 4: PIC score monitoring tool monitored bedside hourly in ICU
(PIC: pain, inspiratory capacity, and cough)

(*Source*: Adapted from Harborview Medical Center PIC scoreboard)

- Proper multimodal analgesia including intravenous narcotics, nonsteroidal anti-inflammatory drugs (NSAIDs), and patient-controlled analgesia (intravenous or epidural, intercostal, or paravertebral blocks). According to studies, epidural analgesia reduces ventilator days, pain, and mortality more than other modes of analgesia.[15]
- *Pain, inspiratory capacity, and cough (PIC) score tool monitoring:* PIC are the three components of this tool which are monitored by nurse's bedside hourly in ICU patients and 4 hourly in lesser critical patients (**Fig. 4**).[16]

In case of inspiratory capacity, "GOAL" is at least 80% of the expected inspiratory capacity and "ALERT" level is 15 mL/kg. It should be assessed by a respiratory therapist every hourly in ICU patients. The PIC score was originally developed by the WellSpan York Hospital, York, Pennsylvania, USA. It should be notified and managed accordingly if a patient receives a score of 1 in any category or an overall score of ≤4 despite interventions.

Hemothorax

Surgical exploration should be performed in the following situations:

- Evacuation of >1,500 mL of blood immediately after tube thoracostomy (it is massive hemothorax)
- Continuous bleeding from chest cavity 150–200 mL/h for 4 hours
- Requirement of repeated blood transfusion/hemodynamic instability and decreasing hemoglobin even after blood transfusion

First, coagulopathy should be ruled out. Thromboelastography (TEG) is the most important point-of-care test which precisely identifies the type of coagulopathy based upon which we can transfuse blood and specific blood component. If the patient is on any anticoagulation therapy or has chronic liver disease, coagulopathy should be corrected first according to the protocol.[17]

Even after successful tube thoracostomy, the patient should be frequently examined and monitored for further sequelae in postoperative ICU:

- Retained clot (undrained collection of 500 mL or more as estimated by the CT scan thorax or one third or more of the chest on CXR)
  - *Clinical features:* Persistent hypoxia, tachypnoea, tachycardia, persistent requirement of high ventilator support, failure of weaning, and decreased breath sound on the affected side. It should be evacuated as early as possible as blood/clot acts as a very good medium for bacteria proliferation and consequent empyema and sepsis. Besides empyema, it can lead to fibrothorax.
- Video-assisted thoracoscopic surgery (VATS) is well accepted and there is less invasive intervention which can:
  - Identify and control the source of bleeding
  - Directly remove clot
  - Help to place the chest tube precisely

  It is mainly successful when done within 7 days of initial drainage of hemothorax.[18]
- *Thoracotomy:* When there is massive hemothorax with persistent heavy bleeding and/or VATS has failed or is not possible, thoracotomy should be done for bleeding vessels' identification and control and clot removal. In case of refractory empyema with sepsis not responding to antibiotic and thoracostomy drainage, thoracotomy should be done for empyema drainage or decortication.[19]

MASSIVE BLOOD TRANSFUSION MANAGEMENT IN PERIOPERATIVE PATIENTS[20]

Definition of massive blood transfusion (MBT)

- Replacement of one blood volume within 24 hours

or

- More than four units of packed red blood cell (PRBC) transfusion in 1 hour when the ongoing need of transfusion is predicted

or

- ≥50% of total blood volume (TBV) within 3 hours

When loss of TBV exceeds 30%, then there is a risk of critical hypoperfusion.

The results of over-resuscitation are as follows:

- Dilutional anemia
- Dilutional coagulopathy
  - Platelet count becomes 50,000 when TBV loss ≥ 200%
  - Critical hypofibrinogenemia (1 g/L when TBV loss > 150%)

– Critical deficiency of factors 2, 5, and 7 when TBV loss is 200%
- *Inadequate resuscitation*: It results in shock, multiorgan dysfunction syndrome (MODS), and disseminated intravascular coagulation (DIC).

Avoid the lethal triad of MBT, i.e., acidosis + hypothermia + coagulopathy.

Overzealous resuscitation can lead to:
- Dislodgement of hemostatic clots resulting in more bleeding
- Circulatory overload resulting in heart failure, pulmonary edema, and interstitial edema. Severe interstitial edema can cause abdominal compartment syndrome.

MANAGEMENT OF MASSIVE BLOOD LOSS

- Try to resuscitate optimally. Avoid overzealous resuscitation. In case of ongoing massive blood loss, immediately activate blood bank personnel for immediate arrangements of all blood and blood components.
- PRBC:fresh frozen plasma (FFP):platelet should be transfused in a 1:1:1 ratio to prevent dilutional coagulopathy.
- In case of life-threatening bleeding, recombinant factor 7a should be given bolus 200 µg/kg followed by 100 µg/kg at 1 and 3 hours.
- Tranexamic acid use [CRASH-2 (Clinical Randomisation of an Antifibrinolytic in Significant Haemorrhage 2) trial adult trauma patients with, or at risk of, significant bleeding within 8 hours of injury are given a loading dose of 1 g over 10 minutes followed by infusion of 1 g over 8 hours] as antifibrinolytics.[21]
- In case of unanticipated and ongoing massive blood loss or in case of rare blood group, the cell salvage technique must be considered, definitely with asepsis.

CARDIAC COMPLICATIONS OF BLUNT CHEST TRAUMA AND POSTOPERATIVELY[22]

Arrhythmia

The most common tachyarrhythmias are atrial fibrillation (AF) and supraventricular tachycardia (10–20% after lobectomy and 40% after pneumonectomy and also after cardiopulmonary bypass with cardiovascular repair). The risk factors are explained in **Table 2**.

Treatment

Hemodynamically unstable: Do the cardioversion [low-dose direct current (DC) shock under sedation with synchronization of R wave on electrocardiogram (ECG)].

Hemodynamically stable: Diltiazem or selective β-1 blocker is the best option. Usually, it is resolved automatically

Table 2: Risk factors for cardiac arrythmias.

Patient related	Surgery related	Treatment related
Pre-existing cardiovascular disease	Extensive procedure	Previous thoracic irradiation
Older age	Major bleeding	
Limited pulmonary reserve	Intrapericardial pneumonectomy	
	Extrapleural pneumonectomy	
	Anesthetic agents	

within 24 hours. If even after that there is recurrence or persistence of tachyarrhythmias, amiodarone has to be added. But it should be kept in mind that there is a 11% chance of ARDS in the amiodarone group in comparison to 1.8% in the nonamiodarone group as amiodarone has got pulmonary toxicity. It is exacerbated in the presence of traumatic lung injury including contusion, laceration, pneumonitis, or ventilator-associated pneumonia.

If ≥2 risk factors are present with postoperative AF for >48 hours among patient >75 years of age/hypertension/impaired left ventricular (LV) function/prior stroke/transient ischemic attack (TIA), anticoagulation therapy should be considered provided hemostasis is achieved and there is no active bleeding.

Cardiac Tamponade

Trauma and postcardiac surgery or thoracotomy procedure(s) where the pericardium has been injured is one of the most common causes of pericardial tamponade.

Clinical Features

Beck's triad comprises hypotension, heart sounds, and increased CVP. The diagnosis of this complication again requires a high index of suspicion. Echocardiography is the diagnostic study of choice to visualize impaired filling of the tight ventricle (**Figs. 5 and 6**).

Management

Pericardiocentesis is a life-saving emergency procedure. It may be a blind technique, under imaging guidance (ultrasonography or fluoroscopy guidance).

Blind technique

Patient position: Semirecumbent at a 30–45° angle.
Support: At least one wide-bore intravenous access for fast fluid therapy, oxygen therapy, and all vital monitors, with a nasogastric tube insertion to decompress stomach (if time is available).

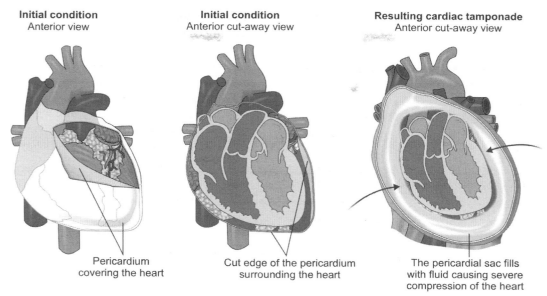

Fig. 5: Stages of pericardial tamponade.
(*Source*: Adapted from http://www.nucleuscatalog.com)

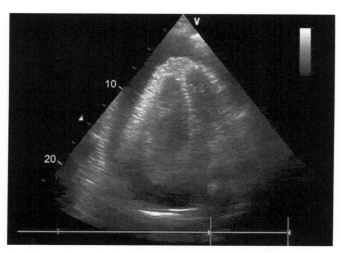

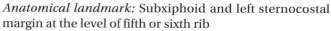

Fig. 6: Ultrasonography of the subxiphoid window of pericardium showing pericardial tamponade in the form of black shadow surrounding the heart chambers.

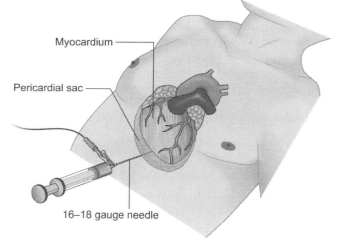

Fig. 7: Pericardiocentesis in the subxiphoid window. It can be done blind by the landmark technique or USG guided with ECG monitoring to drain blood from pericardium using a long needle with catheter and triway in pericardial tamponade.

Anatomical landmark: Subxiphoid and left sternocostal margin at the level of fifth or sixth rib

Technique: Take a spinal needle attached with a 20-mL syringe filled with 5-mL normal saline (NS) to check the patency of the needle. The direction of insertion is 45° angle to the abdominal wall and 45° off the midline sagittal plane. After advancement of 5 cm, it should be advanced slowly by maintaining continuous negative pressure until free fluid/blood comes (**Fig. 7**). If there is any ECG change suggestive of myocardial injury, like new ST changes, the needle should be slowly withdrawn until the ECG pattern returns to normal.[22]

Right-to-left Shunt

After pulmonary resection, a right-to-left shunt develops through patent foramen ovale (PFO) (PFO is persistently present in 20% of the general population) mainly after right lung resection, most probably because of pulmonary arterial hypertension.[23]

Clinical Features

- Refractory hypoxia in the postoperative period
- May present with platypnea and orthodeoxia (hypoxia in upright position) because of mediastinal shift

which modifies relationship between right atrium and left atrium and distorts foramen ovale. It resolves in recumbent position.

- Decrease in right ventricular (RV) compliance and hydrostatic pressures in left lateral decubitus and upright position increases the shunt.
- Associated COPD/PPV/RV infarction/pulmonary emboli/increased intrathoracic pressure increases the shunt.

Diagnosis can be done by nuclear lung perfusion scan, echocardiography, magnetic resonance imaging (MRI), and cardiac catheterization.

Cardiac Herniation

Cardiac herniation is a grave but rare complication. It manifests in the early postoperative period.

Clinical Features

- Cardiovascular collapse with elevated jugular venous pressure
- Ventricular fibrillation
- Mostly occurs after intrapericardial pneumonectomy or lobectomy with partial pericardiectomy
- Sudden postoperative superior vena cava syndrome with heart sound heard on the right side should alert the postoperative ICU intensivist for cardiac herniation.

Treatment

Urgent thoracotomy with defect repair.

Heart Failure and Pulmonary Edema

- RV dysfunction is very common, mainly in the early postoperative period, because of increased pulmonary arterial hypertension and increased RV afterload.
- LV dysfunction is because of RV dysfunction or myocardial infarction (MI).
- *Postpneumonectomy pulmonary edema*: Severe respiratory failure within 48 hours of surgery along with typical CXR findings suggestive of pulmonary edema. The incidence is approximately 2.5–4%.

Risk Factors

Age of patient, extent of resection, preoperative lung function, and other comorbidities.

Treatment

- Total positive fluid balance should not exceed 20 mL/kg [restriction of in vitro fertilization (IVF) with or without diuretics maintaining stable hemodynamic]
- Urinary output > 0.5 mL/kg is unnecessary

- Hyperinflation of the residual lung should be avoided
- Keeping the residual lung in a prolonged dependent position should be avoided.
- Factors contributing to increased pulmonary venous pressure should be avoided.
- Invasive monitoring is necessary to monitor tissue perfusion monitor [serial monitoring of lactate, CVP, mixed venous oxygen saturation (SvO_2) or central venous oxygen saturation ($ScvO_2$), and arterial oxygen pressure (PaO_2)].

Chylothorax

Chylothorax occurs due to thoracic duct injury following blunt chest trauma, after pleuropulmonary procedures and intrapericardial and mediastinal procedures, even after subclavian vein catheterization. There is huge loss of fluid, calories, and proteins resulting in dehydration, nutritional deficiency, and immunodeficiency. Chylothorax can cause respiratory compromise. It usually occurs 2 days to 4 weeks postoperatively.[24]

Conservative Treatment

Administration of low-fat medium-chain triglycerides by mouth. It is directly absorbed into the portal system bypassing the intestinal lymph system. Thus, chyle flow to the thoracic duct is decreased. If even after that chyle flow is not decreased in chest drain, the patient should be put on nil per mouth and total parenteral nutrition (TPN) should be started.

Somatostatin and octreotide decrease intestinal chyle production; hence, they can be considered. Chemical pleurodesis with talc can be done.

Surgery recommended when in spite of conservative therapy

- Drain is >1.5 L/day in an adult or >100 mL/kg/day in a child
- Persistent chyle flow for >2 weeks

Thoracoscopic thoracic duct ligation is done.

Prolonged Air Leak

This is different from BPF or bronchial repair disruption. In this after lung resection, there is heavy air leak from alveoli. This often requires re-exploration. When air leak persists for >5 days, it is called prolonged air leak. It increases atelectasis, pneumonia, empyema, and overall prolonged ventilation days and ICU stay. Usually, most cases stop within 2–3 weeks.[24]

Treatment

Autologous blood patch, instillation of sclerosing agents through tube thoracostomy, and VATS with parenchymal stapling or chemical pleurodesis are options of therapy.

HEART AND THORACIC VESSELS PSEUDOANEURYSM OR RUPTURE

Rapid deceleration of body during blunt chest trauma forces heart against the chest wall and creates excessive shear force on cardiac structures. It results in increased intraventricular pressure causing acute rupture of the free ventricular wall, septum, or valve cusps.[25] Heart and thoracic vessels injury should be suspected when:

- Motor vehicle collision from front with imprint on the front of chest/death of another vehicle's occupants/ airbag deployment
- Scapular/sternal/thoracic spine/multiple rib, especially including first and second rib fracture
- Absent/decreased upper extremity pulse and differential upper extremity blood pressure
- Any thrills/bruit—these are alerting signs
- Brachial plexopathy which is highly associated with subclavian artery injury
- Hemispheric neurologic findings

Ventricular Pseudoaneurysm

Cardiac rupture is contained by adherent pericardium or scar tissue. Even in severe blunt trauma, signs may be occult initially. So, in the postoperative ICU, high suspicion is required. Hence, the symptoms and signs should be known vividly.[25]

Clinical Features

- Gradually worsening chest pain, shortness of breath, and palpitation
- Unexplained sinus tachycardia, tachypnoea
- Diffuse systolic thrust over precordium with new murmur
- *CXR:* Cardiomegaly [though it is difficult to comment on the anteroposterior (AP) view], any radio-opacity beyond the border of cardiac silhouette
- *Echocardiography with Doppler study:* Sharp discontinuity in endocardial image at the site of communication of pseudoaneurysm with LV cavity and narrow orifice in comparison to diameter of pseudoaneurysm (maximum internal diameter of orifice/maximum internal diameter of cavity should not exceed 0.5). High-velocity, turbulent, bidirectional flow between LV and pseudoaneurysm in Doppler
- Multislice cardiac CT scan is diagnostic.

Treatment

Median sternotomy with cardiopulmonary bypass followed by defect repair. If the defect is small, closure of neck is sufficient. If the defect is large or near the base of heart, a patch should be applied to avoid traction on myocardium or distortion of circumflex artery and coronary sinus.

Postoperative Care

Serial echocardiography for assessment of serial cardiac function, graft function, and any structural distortion or delayed rupture.

Major Arteries Pseudoaneurysm and Rupture

The period of time between the accident and the initial diagnosis of pseudoaneurysm varies. It may be 7 days or years. Fifty percent of minimal injury lesions (intimal flap of <1 cm with or without minimal periaortic hematoma) can develop into pseudo-aneurysms within 8 weeks.

Clinical Features

Thoracic aorta: Precordial discomfort, angina, dyspnea, tachycardia, tachypnoea.

Compression signs: Dysphagia (esophageal compression), hoarseness (recurrent laryngeal nerve compression)

CXR: Ill-defined dense area in upper mediastinum with widening.

Multislice CT scan/MRI is diagnostic. It precisely detects the size and location.

Treatment

Surgical resection and patch repair or endovascular aortic stenting are done.

Aorta Pseudoaneurysm Rupture[25]

Clinical Features

- Chest or interscapular pain
- Dyspnea, tachypnoea, tachycardia, hypotension, dysphagia
- Left supraclavicular hematoma
- Upper extremity relative hypertension (pseudocoarctation)
- New cardiac or interscapular murmur

Radiological Findings

- *CXR:* Hemothorax, pneumothorax, mediastinum widening (>8 cm), important bony fractures (mentioned earlier), loss of aortopulmonary window, tracheal deviation to right, depression of the left mainstem bronchus
- *Biplanar angiography:* Though it is a diagnostic modality for blunt great vessel or aortic injury, it is invasive and time-consuming. In a number of scenarios, patients have associated acute kidney injury too.
- *Multislice CT scan:* It has got high sensitivity and specificity.

Treatment

Initially, in hemodynamically stable patients, we should keep mean arterial pressure (MAP) low (target 60–70 mm Hg). We should try to start a beta-blocker to decrease aortic shear force. The target heart rate is <100/min. Operative repair after sternotomy or thoracotomy with graft implant or endoluminal stent graft is done.

Outcome Assessment

Regular assessment of limb function is done as decreased blood flow to spinal cord can cause paraplegia. The required treatment and prognostication of the patient's relatives are very important. Restricted fluid therapy should be considered in cardiac injury.

Innominate Artery Pseudoaneurysm[25]

Tracheal Compression

Dyspnea, stridor, hoarseness of voice. Fiberoptic bronchoscopy confirms tracheal compression/stenosis and its location, length, and minimum tracheal diameter.

Diagnosis: Multislice CT scan is diagnostic.

Innominate artery rupture within trachea with innominate artery tracheal fistula causes hemoptysis.

Mediastinitis

Causes of blunt chest trauma

- Blunt chest trauma causing tracheobronchial disruption or esophageal perforation
- After sternotomy, sternal deep wound infection and dehiscence.

Risk factors

- Emergency life-saving surgery
- Postoperative shock, especially in case of multiple blood transfusion
- Prolonged bypass or operation room time
- Re-exploration
- Poor glycemic control
- Preoperative corticosteroid
- Obesity (>20% of ideal body weight)

Clinical features

- High fever with tachycardia and tachypnoea. In an advanced stage, signs of sepsis and septic shock are seen.
- Sternal pain—gradually increasing since surgery
- Increased drainage from the wound site
- Audible click due to sternal nonunion
- Hamman sign—crunchy sound heard with a stethoscope over the precordium during systole

- *CXR*: Pneumomediastinum, air-fluid level within the mediastinum. Mediastinum widening is not a reliable sign in the postoperative period.
- *CT scan*: Along with CXR features, sternal separation with substernal fluid collection is confirmatory. Later, after 2 weeks' postoperative period, it has sensitivity and specificity of 100%.

Treatment: Two-third cases are seen within 14 days of surgery. Most causative organisms are *Staphylococcus aureus* and *S. epidermidis* (70–80%) followed by 40% mixed (gram-positive and gram-negative) infection.[26]

Broad spectrum antibiotics with or without exploration of wound is recommended. It has got very high mortality.

Bronchial Repair Disruption

The cause is postoperative anastomotic dehiscence.[27]

Clinical features

- Massive air leak with increasing subcutaneous emphysema.
- If the patient is on ventilator, then he/she is unable to achieve desired tidal volume causing tachypnoea, hypoxia, and hypercapnia.
- Development of pneumothorax and pneumomediastinum.

Postoperative care for patients who underwent airway repair surgery[28]

- Healing is actually hindered by ETT cuff resting on injury with positive airway pressure. So, ideally the lesion should be bypassed using selective bilateral mainstem bronchus intubation with a small ETT passed through a large tracheotomy.
- Airway pressure should be maintained as low as possible.
- If the situation is associated with ARDS, then high-frequency jet ventilation with deflated cuff and low endobronchial pressure may be an alternative.

GENERAL PERIOPERATIVE CARE IN ALL TRAUMA PATIENTS IS TO BE CONTINUED IN ICU

Thromboprophylaxis

Trauma patients who received "no prophylaxis" and "only mechanical prophylaxis" have incidence of venous thromboembolism (VTE), of 12 and 7%, respectively. It is a leading cause of mortality in trauma patients.[29]

Risk Factors

- Age > 40 years
- High injury severity score

- Ventilator days > 3
- Major operative procedure (>2 hours)
- ≥4 transfusions in the first 24 hours
- Femoral vein line insertion
- The Glasgow Coma Scale (GCS) < 8 for >4 hours
- Associated spinal cord injury, lower extremity, and/or pelvic fracture
- Prolonged immobilization and hospital stay
- Delay of thromboprophylaxis > 48 hours

Recommendations in Treatment[29]

- For patients with low risk of bleeding: Combined pharmacologic and mechanical [intermittent pneumatic compression (IPC) device] prophylaxis rather than mechanical or pharmacologic prophylaxis alone.
- In patients with high risk of bleeding where pharmacological prophylaxis cannot be given, mechanical prophylaxis in the form of IPC must be applied provided there is no contraindication (external fixation, extremity ischemia). Pharmacological prophylaxis should be started as soon as the bleeding risk is resolved.
- Low molecular weight heparin (LMWH) is preferred to unfractionated heparin (UFH) because of its more effectiveness to prevent deep venous thrombosis (DVT) and lesser side effects. UFH is preferred in patients with severe renal dysfunction (creatinine clearance < 30 mL/min).
- Overall, pharmacologic prophylaxis should be started within 72 hours of trauma rather than later if there is no absolute contraindication.
- Prophylactic routine inferior vena cava (IVC) filter placement is not recommended. It is reasonable to put it in very high-risk patients with ongoing contraindication to anticoagulation.

Stress Ulcer Prophylaxis

Severely injured patients and intubated and coagulopathic patients, especially with a history of previous ulcer disease, are at a very high risk of stress ulceration. Without medication, the stress ulcer may present with mild to profuse bleeding, even gastric or duodenal perforation. Nowadays, proton-pump inhibitors are discouraged in those patients who tolerate targeted enteral feed because of strong association with *Clostridium difficile*-induced colitis. H2-receptor blockers are a better alternative for prophylaxis without an increasing chance of infective colitis.[30]

Prevention of Hypothermia

During initial evaluation, resuscitation in an operating room, mainly in a prolonged surgery with or without cardiopulmonary bypass, multiple blood transfusions, and trauma patients usually develop hypothermia. Hypothermia prevents clot formation and causes platelet dysfunction resulting in more generalized bleeding and worse outcome. Continuous temperature monitoring is essential.[30]

- Administration of warm fluid is necessary.
- Passive rewarming should be done with blankets and forced-air devices.
- In case of severe hypothermia with coagulopathy, central rewarming should be done.

Nutrition

Efforts should be made to start enteral nutrition as early as possible (within 48 hours). Enteral nutrition is always better than parenteral nutrition in view of lesser infection. 2 g of nitrogen per liter loss of abdominal fluid should be counted extra while calculating daily requirement in case of open abdomen.[31]

Indications of Parenteral Nutrition

- Persistent progressive ileus
- Bowel obstruction
- Massive bowel resection refractory to enteral therapy
- Gut hypoperfusion (shock with high vasopressor therapy) with a high risk of mesenteric ischemia and bowel necrosis
- High output enteral fistula
- Failure of enteral nutrition to meet caloric requirement

The details of nutrition therapy in critically ill trauma patients are out of the scope of this chapter for which the "ESPEN guideline on clinical nutrition in intensive care unit" has to be read.[32]

Prevention of Infection and Appropriate Antimicrobial Therapy[33]

- Maintaining all ICU bundle care to prevent hospital-acquired infection
- Maintaining an appropriate protocol for management of central line related blood stream infection (CRBSI), ventilator-associated pneumonia (VAP), and wound infection and catheter-associated urinary tract infection (CAUTI).
- Antibiotic stewardship
- To gain knowledge and its application on renal and liver dose adjustment of antimicrobials.

▌ SUMMARY

Blunt chest trauma management consists of urgent airway management, ICD placement with mechanical ventilation, support of respiratory and cardiac function, replacement of massive blood loss, and timely surgical intervention. In

postoperative ICU care by a multidisciplinary team with taken care of pulmonary complications and continuous hemodynamic monitoring, sepsis bundle care, pain and active physiotherapy. Recent advances in clinical practices based on the concept of damage control and balanced hemostatic resuscitation have made drastic changes in the outcome of hemorrhaging trauma patients. Recent evidence on use of extracorporeal membrane oxygenation for refractory hypoxemia and resuscitative endovascular balloon occlusion of the aorta (REBOA) for severe hemorrhage is coming in a big way with new promises to save life after complicated trauma.

REFERENCES

1. Committee on Trauma of the American College of Surgeons. Advanced Trauma Life Support: ATLS, 10th edition. Chicago: American College of Surgeons; 2018.
2. Duan Y, Smith CE, Como JJ. Cardiothoracic trauma. In: Wilson WC, Grande CM, Hoyt DB (Eds). Trauma. Volume 1. Emergency Resuscitation, Perioperative Anesthesia and Surgical Management. New York: Informa Healthcare; 2007. pp. 469-99.
3. Lang-Lazdunski L, Pons F, Jancovici R. Update on the emergency management of chest trauma. Curr Opin Crit Care. 1999;5: 488-99.
4. Wilson WC. Trauma airway management: as a difficult airway algorithm modified for trauma – and five common trauma intubation scenarios [online]. ASA Newsletter. 2005;69(11).
5. Kummer C, Netto FS, Rizoli S, Yee D. A review of traumatic airway injuries: potential implications for airway assessment and management. Injury. 2007;38:27-33.
6. Meredith JW, Hoth JJ. Thoracic trauma: when and how to intervene. Surg Clin North Am. 2007;87:95-118.
7. Mansky R, Scher C. Thoracic trauma in military settings: a review of current practices and recommendations. Curr Opin Anesthesiol. 2019;32(2):227-33.
8. Casos SR, Richardson JD. Role of thoracoscopy in acute management of chest injury. Curr Opin Crit Care. 2006;12:584-9.
9. Carrillo EH, Richardson JD. Thoracoscopy for the acutely injured patient. Am J Surg. 2005;190:234-8.
10. Salik I, Abramowicz AE. (2019). Bronchopleural fistula. Treasure Island, FL: StatPearls [Internet]. Available from https://www.ncbi.nlm.nih.gov/books/NBK534765/. [Last accessed March, 2020].
11. Rendeki S, Molnár TF. Pulmonary contusion. J Thorac Dis. 2019;11(Suppl 2):S141-151.
12. Soldati G, Testa A, Silva FR, Carbone L, Portale G, Silveri NG. Chest ultrasonography in lung contusion. Chest. 2006;130(2):533-8.
13. Nirula R, Allen B, Layman R, Falimirski ME, Somberg LB. Rib fracture stabilization in patients sustaining blunt chest injury. Am Surg. 2006;72(4):307-9.
14. Eastern Association for the Surgery of Trauma. EAST guidelines. [online] Available from www.east.org education practice-management-guidelines. [Last accessed March, 2020].
15. Unsworth A, Curtis K, Asha SE. Treatments for blunt chest trauma and their impact on patient outcomes and health service delivery. Scand J Trauma Resusc Emerg Med. 2015;23:17.
16. Witt CE, Bulger EM. Comprehensive approach to the management of the patient with multiple rib fractures: a review and introduction of a bundled rib fracture management protocol. Trauma Surg Acute Care Open. 2017;2(1):e000064.
17. Sengupta S. Post-operative pulmonary complications after thoracotomy. Indian J Anaesth. 2015;59(9):618-26.
18. Yeung WW. Post-operative care to promote recovery for thoracic surgical patients: a nursing perspective. J Thorac Dis. 2016; 8(Suppl 1):S71-7.
19. Shen KR, Wain JC, Wright CD, Grillo HC, Mathisen DJ. Postpneumonectomy syndrome: surgical management and long-term results. J Thorac Cardiovasc Surg. 2008;135:1210-6.
20. Patil V, Shetmahajan M. Massive transfusion and massive transfusion protocol. Indian J Anaesth. 2014;58(5):590-5.
21. The CRASH-2 Collaborators. The importance of early treatment with tranexamic acid in bleeding trauma patients: an exploratory analysis of the CRASH-2 randomised controlled trial. Lancet. 2011;377(9771):1096-101.
22. Moloney J, Fowler S, Chang W. Anesthetic management of thoracic trauma. Curr Opin Anaesthesiol. 2008;21(1):41-6.
23. Wanek S, Mayberry JC. Blunt thoracic trauma: flail chest, pulmonary contusion, and blast injury. Crit Care Clin. 2004;20:71.
24. Abu-Omar Y, Kocher GJ, Bosco P, Barbero C, Waller D, Gudbjartsson T, et al. European Association for Cardio-Thoracic Surgery expert consensus statement on the prevention and management of mediastinitis. Eur J Cardiothorac Surg. 2017;51(1):10-29.
25. Seitelman E, Arellano JJ, Takabe K, Barrett L, Faust G, George Angus LD. Chylothorax after blunt trauma. J Thorac Dis. 2012;4(3):327-30.
26. Gutierrez Romero DF, Barrufet M, Lopez-Rueda A, Burrel M. Ruptured intercostal artery pseudoaneurysm in a patient with blunt thoracic trauma: diagnosis and management. BMJ Case Rep. 2014;bcr2013202019.
27. Park IH, Lim HK, Song SW, Lee KH. Perforation of esophagus and subsequent mediastinitis following mussel shell ingestion. J Thorac Dis. 2016;8(8):E693-7.
28. Baumgartner F, Sheppard B, Virgilio C, Esrig B, Harrier D, Nelson RJ, et al. Tracheal and main bronchial disruptions after blunt chest trauma: presentation and management. Ann Thoracic Surg. 1990;50(4):569-74.
29. Chung SB, Lee SH, Kim ES, Eoh W. Incidence of deep vein thrombosis after spinal cord injury: a prospective study in 37 consecutive patients with traumatic or nontraumatic spinal cord injury treated by mechanical prophylaxis. J Trauma. 2011;71:867.
30. Sarani B. Overview of inpatient management of the adult trauma patient. 2018. available online on www.uptodate.com assessed on 20 Jan 2020.
31. ESPEN Guideline. ESPEN guideline on clinical nutrition in the intensive care unit. Clin Nutr. 2019;38:48-79.
32. Casaer MP, Hermans G, Wilmer A, Van den Berghe G. Impact of early parenteral nutrition completing enteral nutrition in adult critically ill patients (EPaNIC trial): a study protocol and statistical analysis plan for a randomized controlled trial. Trials. 2011;12:21.
33. Cook A, Norwood S, Berne J. Ventilator-associated pneumonia is more common and of less consequence in trauma patients compared with other critically ill patients. J Trauma. 2010;69:1083.

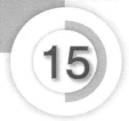
Perioperative Management of Mediastinal Mass Excision

Madhavi Shetmahajan

INTRODUCTION

Mediastinal mass surgeries, though relatively less common compared to other thoracic surgeries such as lung resections and esophagectomies, are important to an intensivist as they have unique perioperative implications. However, due to the heterogenous nature of the surgeries related to differences in size, location, histopathology, and involvement of surrounding structures, there is paucity of literature on incidence of adverse events and complications, as well as management protocols.

Mediastinum is the space between the pleural cavities extending from the root of the neck or the thoracic inlet superiorly to the diaphragm inferiorly. Though most of the masses arise from the mediastinal structures, some e.g. thyroid masses may extend from adjoining areas.

The location of the mediastinal mass is important for determining its etiology as well as for the pressure effects. The mediastinum can be divided into superior and inferior mediastinum or more commonly into anterior, middle, and posterior mediastinum.[1]

- *The superior and inferior mediastinum:* They are separated by an imaginary line joining the angle of Louis to the fourth thoracic vertebrae. The superior mediastinum packs major blood vessels and the trachea in a narrow area; therefore, masses in this area lead to early symptoms and worse complications compared to inferior mediastinum.
- *Anterior, middle, and posterior mediastinum:* The anterior or prevascular mediastinum extends from the undersurface of the sternum to the anterior pericardium. The middle or the visceral mediastinum extends from the anterior pericardium to the anterior surface of the thoracic vertebral bodies. The posterior or paravertebral mediastinum consists of the paravertebral sulci up to the lateral border of the transverse processes of the thoracic vertebrae.

Anterior mediastinum:

Contents: Thymus, lymph nodes

Tumors:
- *Thymic lesions*:
  - Thymoma may be associated with myasthenia gravis, neuroendocrine tumors may cause paraneoplastic syndromes
  - Thymic carcinoma.
- Retrosternal goiter
- Lymphoma
- Metastatic lymph nodes
- Germ cell tumors.

Middle mediastinum:

Contents: Major vessels—superior vena cava (SVC), aorta, pulmonary arteries, thoracic duct, trachea and proximal bronchi, esophagus, lymph nodes

Tumors: Most commonly lymphadenopathy

Posterior or paravertebral mediastinum:

Contents: Thoracic spine and paravertebral soft tissues

Tumors: Arising from the neural structures, e.g., schwannoma, neurofibroma.

As the anterior and middle mediastinum have vital vascular and airway structures closely packed in a relatively narrow space, mass lesions here tend to lead to significant cardiorespiratory problems. Anterior mediastinal masses constitute almost half of all mediastinal masses and are more likely to lead to severe life-threatening complications in the perioperative period. Posterior mediastinal masses are less common and usually have a more benign perioperative course.

Treatment of a mediastinal mass depends on the histopathology, size, and location of the tumor. Management strategies include chemotherapy, radiation, surgical excision or a combination of two or more modalities. Empirical use of steroids has been found to be effective in rapid reduction of tumor size and can be used in life-threatening airway obstruction by large tumors.[2]

Steroid administration may however confound the diagnosis and attempts should be made to obtain a biopsy before steroid administration.

Excision of mediastinal mass can be done by various approaches depending on the site of the tumor, its size, and involvement of adjoining structures. The most common approach is a median sternotomy incision.[3.]

Other approaches include a posterolateral thoracotomy or a clamshell incision. Video-assisted thoracic surgery and robot-assisted thoracic surgery are suitable for select cases viz. small tumors with well-defined margins. Minimally invasive approach has the advantage of less tissue trauma, less pain, and shorter hospital stay.[3.]

Use of extracorporeal circulation is described in complicated cases where the freedom to retract the heart, lung, and mediastinal mass without hemodynamic consequences helps in surgical exposure. Femorofemoral bypass is preferred as cannulation of vessels in the thoracic cavity may be difficult due to the mass. However, anticoagulation needed for the extracorporeal circulation may cause severe bleeding and hence the decision to use ECC needs careful consideration.[4]

Mediastinal masses present to the intensive care unit preoperatively mainly for airway obstruction and postoperatively for advanced monitoring.

Mediastinal masses have effects related to:
- *Mass effect on*:
  – Tracheobronchial tree
  – Cardiac and vascular structures, e.g., SVC syndrome
  – Lung parenchyma.
- *Production of hormones/antibodies, etc.*:
  – Thymoma—may be associated with myasthenia gravis
  – Retrosternal thyroid—hypothyroidism or hyperthyroidism
  – Neuroendocrine tumors—paraneoplastic syndromes, e.g., Cushing's syndrome, hypercalcemia

The details of management of specific diseases and syndromes are not discussed in this review.

▌AIRWAY OBSTRUCTION

Mediastinal masses most commonly present to the intensive care in the preoperative period for airway obstruction. Though most often the obstruction is due to extrinsic compression, occasionally there may be an infiltration into the trachea. Uncommonly, in addition to intrathoracic obstruction, there may be enlarged lymph node in the neck which can distort the laryngeal anatomy and increase the complexity of airway management.

Symptomatic patients with an obstructed airway with a luminal compromise of more than 50% and tumors involving the carina are at high risk of airway collapse and life-threatening hypoxemia during attempts to gain airway control.[3,5]

Signs and Symptoms

Dyspnea and stridor are initially present on exertion, which may progress to dyspnea at rest. Positional dyspnea is a characteristic finding. In patients with large anterior mediastinal masses, supine position is poorly tolerated. A detailed history to ascertain the best tolerated position is important for airway management in the perioperative period.[3]

Signs of SVC syndrome: Facial edema and dilated veins are suggestive of SVC obstruction. Severe airway edema may distort airway structures making their identification difficult. Also, a small size endotracheal tube will be required in these cases.

Investigations

- *CT scan:*
  – *Site of obstruction:* Distance from vocal cord and distance from the carina. In tumors close to carina, endobronchial intubation into the more patent bronchus may be the only option for airway control.
  – Length of obstruction
  – Narrowest diameter may help in choosing the size of endotracheal tube
  – *Lung fields:* To look for lung collapse or lung infiltration.
- *Arterial blood gas:* Hypercarbia and hypoxemia are indicators of a critically obstructed airway.

Management

Early involvement of an experienced anesthesiologist is essential when managing an obstructed airway. In symptomatic patients, airway management is best done in the operating room with meticulous preparation and planning.

Important points in management for a critically obstructed airway are as follows:
- The biggest risk is airway collapse due to the pressure of the tumor in supine position or loss of negative intrathoracic pressure.
- Awake fiberoptic intubation should be considered in case of a distorted upper airway anatomy.
- High flow oxygen administration should be used during airway manipulation to reduce the risk of life-threatening hypoxemia.

- Sedation should be given carefully and only after full preparation for airway control as loss of muscle tone can precipitate airway collapse.
- Spontaneous respiration helps to maintain patency of a dynamic intrathoracic obstruction and should be preserved during induction of anesthesia.
- A stiff endotracheal tube, preferably a reinforced tube, should be used and the tip is positioned beyond the obstruction using a fiberscope.
- A rigid bronchoscope with an experienced operator should be available to stent a collapsed airway. Also, resources to rapidly change the position of patient should be available.
- Very complicated cases should have femoral vessels cannulated and femorofemoral bypass circuit primed and ready to prevent hypoxic complications in case of a collapsed airway.
- Tracheostomy is of limited value as the obstruction due to a mediastinal mass is intrathoracic.

Finally, it is important to remember that not all symptomatic patients with obstructed airways will need an endotracheal tube which is placed across the obstruction. Some of the less obstructed airways can be managed by keeping the tube above the level of obstruction and instituting intermittent positive pressure ventilation (IPPV). Relieving the patient of the increased work of breathing helps to relieve the distress even if the obstruction is not bypassed.

One has to be watchful for development of auto positive end-expiratory pressure (PEEP) and dynamic hyperinflation as expiration is slow due to the constricted airway and adequate expiratory time has to be ensured.

Cardiovascular Effects

- *Involvement of SVC:* Obstruction of the SVC leads to SVC syndrome characterized by development of edema in the areas of SVC distribution viz. head, neck, and upper limbs, and development of collateral vessels in the upper part of the body which are visible as dilated veins. The internal and external jugular veins are distended. These patients are at a very high risk of major intraoperative bleeding. The airway management is also further complicated by edema of laryngeal structures which in its severest form distorts anatomy. These patients require a smaller size tube and airway needs gentle handling to prevent injury and bleeding.
- Compression of major vessels and cardiac structures can result in hypotension. Pericardial effusion may be present which may require drainage.
- A 2D echo and occasionally a cardiac MRI may help to diagnose involvement of cardiac structures.

Salient features of intraoperative management of mediastinal masses are:

- Lung isolation is often required. Double lumen tubes are preferred when lung resection is planned and the airway anatomy is normal. Bronchial blockers have an advantage in patients with airway involvement.
- VATS and RATS surgery may require use of capnothorax for improved surgical exposure. Extra care to avoid severe hypercapnia is needed when capnothorax is used during one lung ventilation.
- Large bore IV access is obtained in the legs or femoral veins as disruption in venous system in SVC distribution is possible.
- Intra-arterial blood pressure monitoring is required with advanced hemodynamic monitoring in complicated cases.

Other intraoperative complications in mediastinal mass:
Bleeding: Seen with large vascular tumors and tumors infiltrating vascular structures.

Postoperative Management

Postoperative concerns in patients operated for mediastinal mass excision:

- *Airway: Immediate postoperative management*—most patients would be extubated in the operating room as removal of tumor relieves the compression and improves the airway in most cases.

Reasons for patients requiring postoperative intubation are:

- *Airway related:* Airway edema, tracheomalacia, recurrent laryngeal nerve (RLN) injury causing vocal cord palsy
- *Need for ventilator support*
  - *Respiratory causes:* Preoperatively reduced lung function, extensive lung handling, transfusion related acute lung injury, transfusion associated circulatory overload, patients with myasthenia gravis
  - *Hemodynamic instability:* Major blood loss, preoperatively compromised cardiac function.

Patients with nonairway related indications can be extubated on improvement in their primary problem as per standard protocols.

Patients with airway related concerns should have an extubation plan based on anticipated problems as they may develop airway obstruction after extubation.

Postoperative Airway Complications

Airway edema: May be present preoperatively or may develop intraoperatively due to extensive airway handling. Head up position and steroids are useful in reducing edema. Presence of leak around the endotracheal tube on deflation of the cuff can be used as an indicator of absence of significant airway edema prior to extubation.

Tracheomalacia: Most commonly seen in long-standing tumors where pressure on the tracheal cartilages causes ischemia and softening. Diagnosis is by fiberscopy where dynamic collapse of the trachea is visible. In many patients, the tracheal wall will stabilize over days during which time endotracheal intubation is needed. Severe cases where there is no improvement may require procedures such as prosthetic stenting or tracheoplasty.

Vocal cord palsy could be due to inclusion of the RLN in the excision or inadvertent injury to the nerve or its blood supply during dissection. Some injuries may recover over time, commonly within 6 months but occasionally may recover over a longer period. Though many centers use steroids to treat RLN injury, evidence for its efficacy when given postoperatively is lacking.[6]

Unilateral injury: Unilateral vocal cord palsy causes hoarseness and a weak cough. Patients usually do not have significant airway obstruction. Risk of aspiration should be assessed before starting oral feeds. Compensatory hyperadduction by the opposite cord may allow adequate vocal and sphincter function over a period of time.

Bilateral injury: Bilateral partial injury of the RLN predominantly affects the abductors causing unopposed adduction of cords leading to complete glottic closure. Patient may need emergency tracheostomy. In bilateral complete denervation, the vocal cords assume paramedian (cadaveric) position. Patients have stridor and carry a very high risk of aspiration. These patients need endotracheal intubation and feeding with a nasogastric tube. The vocal cords are assessed after 24–48 hours. In absence of recovery, tracheostomy is performed after consultation with an ENT specialist.

Postoperative Respiratory Complications

When the lungs and the chest wall are involved in the mediastinal mass, they may have to be resected. This could involve a wedge resection, a segmentectomy, a lobectomy or rarely a pneumonectomy. Knowledge of the preoperative lung functions and the calculated predicted postoperative lung function is vital in guiding ventilatory strategy. Patients with borderline lung functions may benefit from noninvasive ventilatory support in the immediate postoperative period. Intensive physiotherapy and early recognition and treatment of lung infections reduce respiratory morbidity.

Patients with germ cell tumors may have received bleomycin as part of their chemotherapy regimen. Bleomycin toxicity comprises of pneumonitis and pulmonary fibrosis.

Though the evidence is not conclusive, high inspired concentration of oxygen and excessive fluid administration have been implicated in worsening of lung function in patients who have received bleomycin.[7,8]

Chest wall resections are repaired using a prosthetic mesh, cement or local tissue flaps depending on the site and extent of resection, and the risk of developing a flail chest. Those displaying flail segment after surgery are treated by strapping of the chest wall and positive pressure ventilation. Noninvasive ventilation is most appropriate in absence of other complications.

Close monitoring of the chest drains is required in the postoperative period both to watch for persistent air leak and to detect bleeding. Inadequate drainage of air from the pleural cavity can cause pneumothorax and partial collapse of the underlying lung. This can result in atelectasis, inadequate clearance of secretions, and pneumonia. In mechanically ventilated patients, parenchymal air leak can lead to tension pneumothorax if the chest drain is unable to vent adequately. Severe hypotension associated with high airway pressures should alert the clinician to the possibility of this life-threatening complication.

Phrenic nerve injury: During excision of large mediastinal masses, the phrenic nerve may be sacrificed or injured. This can present as failure to wean. An elevated dome of diaphragm and absence of diaphragmatic movement on ultrasound or fluoroscopy is diagnostic.[9]

Postoperative Cardiac Complication

- Arrhythmias
- Pericardial tamponade due to pericardial hematoma

Postoperative bleeding and anticoagulation-related complications: Postoperative bleeding is more likely in patients with large infiltrating vascular tumors where the intraoperative blood loss has been high. Extensive adhesions leave exposed raw surfaces which continue to bleed and ooze in the postoperative period. Such patients should be transferred to the high dependency unit after surgery to closely monitor the hemodynamics and drain output.

Hemoglobin levels and coagulation parameters should be monitored in at risk cases. Intrathoracic bleeds occasionally go undetected due to a blocked chest drain. Unexplained hypotension in the postoperative period with drop in hemoglobin should make one suspect a concealed bleed. A chest X-ray, an ultrasound or occasionally a CT scan of thorax may be ordered to confirm the diagnosis. Excision of a mediastinal mass involving large vessels such as the SVC, brachiocephalic, and subclavian vessels, necessitates vascular repair using native or prosthetic grafts. Prosthetic grafts in the low flow venous system often need therapeutic anticoagulation in the postoperative period to prevent graft thrombosis. Unfractionated heparin is the preferred anticoagulant in the immediate postoperative period particularly when the bleeding risk is high as it has a shorter half-life and its action can be easily terminated by administration of protamine in case of a catastrophic bleed. However, it needs monitoring of activated partial thromboplastin time (aPTT) levels to ensure optimum anticoagulation. All patients should receive deep venous thrombosis (DVT) prophylaxis in absence of specific contraindications.

Postoperative neurological complications: Injuries to spinal nerves or paraspinal plexii and rarely the spinal cord may complicate posterior mediastinal mass surgeries. Postoperative neurological monitoring is required in these cases.

Patients with myasthenia gravis are continued on their preoperative medications in the immediate postoperative period. Some will show improvement and need reduction in the drugs. However, the benefit is not uniform and treatment has to be individualized based on the response.

Postoperative pain management: Thoracic incisions especially lateral thoracotomies and clamshell incisions cause significant pain; inadequate pain control hampers effective chest physiotherapy and increases risk of postoperative pulmonary complications. Multimodal analgesia with thoracic epidural local anesthetics with systemic non-steroidal anti-inflammatory drugs is the most commonly used method for analgesia. Paravertebral blocks and patient controlled analgesia using intravenous opioids are other options. Removal of epidural catheter in an anticoagulated patient should be discussed with the acute pain service team as there is increased risk of epidural hematoma formation. Postoperative pain in minimally invasive thoracic surgery is generally amenable to simple systemic analgesics.

CONCLUSION

Management of mediastinal mass revolves around airway management in the preoperative period. The postoperative management focuses on cardiorespiratory stability and good pain control.

REFERENCES

1. Carter B, Benveniste M, Madan R, Godoy MC, de Groot PM, Truong MT, et al. ITMIG classification of mediastinal compartments and multidisciplinary approach to mediastinal masses. RadioGraphics. 2017;37:413-36.

2. Freedman J, Rheingold S. Lanzkowsky's Manual of Pediatric Hematology and Oncology, 6th edition; 2016. pp. 605-19.

3. Cosgun T, Kaba E, Toker A. Robotic approach for mediastinal diseases: state-of-the-art and current perspectives, Shanghai Chest. 2018;2:90.

4. Li W, van Boven W, Annema J, Eberl S, Klomp HM, de Mol Bas AJM. Management of large mediastinal masses: Surgical and anesthesiological considerations. J Thorac Dis. 2016;8:E175-E184.

5. Galvez C, Galiana M , Corcoles JM, Lirio F, Sesma J, Bolufer S. Current anesthesiological approach to mediastinal surgery. J Vis Surg. 2018;4:146.

6. Yan Jiang, Bo Gao, Xiaohua Zhang. Prevention and treatment of recurrent laryngeal nerve injury in thyroid surgery. Int J Clin Exp Med. 2014;7:101-7.

7. Allan N, Siller C, Breen A. Anaesthetic implications of chemotherapy, Continuing Education in Anaesthesia Critical Care & Pain. 2012;12:52-6.

8. Donat SM1, Levy DA: Bleomycin associated pulmonary toxicity: is perioperative oxygen restriction necessary?, J Urol. 1998;160:1347-52.

9. Kokatnur L, Rudrappa M. Diaphragmatic palsy. Diseases 2018;6:16.

Perioperative Management of Major Lung Resections

Swapnil Parab, Priya Ranganathan

INTRODUCTION

Surgical resection is the primary mode of treatment for stages 1 and 2 of nonsmall cell lung cancer. It includes removal of the lung parenchyma affected by the tumor and systematic evaluation of ipsilateral hilar and mediastinal lymph nodes. Although lung resection includes procedures such as wedge resection, metastasectomy, segmentectomy, lobectomy, and pneumonectomy, the latter two are often considered as "major pulmonary resection." Approaches for lung resection include open thoracotomy (anterolateral or posterolateral), median sternotomy, and minimally invasive techniques (video-assisted thoracoscopic and robotic surgeries). Perioperative management of a patient undergoing major pulmonary resection involves careful preoperative evaluation, adequate optimization, meticulous intraoperative management, and vigilant postoperative care.

PREOPERATIVE EVALUATION

The purpose of preoperative assessment for major pulmonary resection is to evaluate and identify the risk for postoperative complications and to implement measures for risk reduction in high-risk patients. Prethoracotomy assessment essentially involves all the factors that are part of complete preanesthesia checkup, which are past history, medications, history of allergies, and assessment of airway. However, there are a few additional tests which are focused on evaluation of the cardiorespiratory system. It is recommended that a multidisciplinary team, which includes a thoracic surgeon, anesthesiologist, and pulmonologist, should evaluate the patients scheduled for major pulmonary resection. The discussion regarding the preoperative evaluation for major lung resection in this chapter is based on the clinical practice guidelines by the American College of Chest Physicians (ACCP) (2013), British Thoracic Society (2010), and European Respiratory Society/European Society of Thoracic Surgery (ERS_ESTS) (2009).[1-3]

The specific tests include the following:
- Assessment of respiratory function
  - Assessment of mechanical function
  - Assessment of parenchymal function
  - Assessment of regional lung function
- Assessment of cardiorespiratory interaction
- Assessment of specific medical comorbidities

Assessment of Respiratory Function

The primary focus of the thoracic anesthesiologist during preoperative evaluation is to assess the risk of postoperative pulmonary complications. While it is possible to evaluate the respiratory function from the detailed history and the functional ability, quantitative measurement of respiratory functions helps in objective risk assessment and further monitoring for the improvement in the performance. The respiratory function test includes a variety of tests that assess mechanical function, parenchymal function, and regional lung function.

Assessment of Lung's Mechanical and Parenchymal Functions

The mechanical functions of the respiratory system are objectively assessed by spirometry, which is acceptable and reproducible for most of the patients. In addition, parenchymal function is tested by measuring the diffusing capacity for carbon monoxide (DLCO) and/or arterial blood gases (ABG). All patients undergoing pulmonary resection surgery should have baseline spirometry to measure forced expiratory volume in the 1st second (FEV1) and forced vital capacity (FVC). According to ACCP guidelines, patients with FEV1 > 80% of predicted (or >2 L), without evidence of dyspnea or interstitial lung disease, can undergo lung resection without any further testing.[1] Maximal voluntary ventilation (MVV) and residual volume/total lung capacity (RV/TLC) ratio have also shown correlation with post-thoracotomy outcomes. These values are always expressed as a percent of predicted volumes corrected for age, sex, and height of the patient.

- *FEV1 and DLCO:* FEV1 is the key test in the preoperative evaluation of surgical candidates with lung cancer. Various studies have shown that FEV1 is an independent predictor of respiratory complications [odds ratio (OR): 1.1 for every 10% decrease in FEV1] and cardiovascular complications (OR: 1.13 for every 10% decrease in FEV1).[4,5] Licker et al., after receiver-operating characteristic analysis, confirmed that the best cutoff value of preoperative FEV1 for predicting respiratory complications was 60%.[6] However, in patients with moderate-to-severe chronic obstructive pulmonary disease (COPD), FEV1 has a limited role in predicting postoperative complications.[7] In fact, due to "lobar volume reduction effect," the resection of affected parenchyma improves respiratory mechanics. DLCO has also been shown to be an independent predictor of cardiopulmonary complications, mortality, and long-term survival following lung resection.[8,9] Hence, guidelines recommend systematic measurement of DLCO, regardless of FEV1 value, prior to lung resection surgery.

- *Predicted postoperative (PPO) function:* Functionally, the lung is divided into 42 different segments or 19 anatomical segments. Accordingly, the calculation of ppoFEV1 and ppoDLCO is demonstrated in **Figure 1**. Nakahara et al. found that patients with ppoFEV1 > 40% had no or minor postoperative pulmonary complications following thoracic surgeries. In the same study, major complications after thoracic surgeries were observed in patients who had ppoFEV1 < 30%.[10] Historically, patients are considered fit for pulmonary resections if ppoFEV1 and ppoDLCO are >40% of predicted normal. Patients with ppoFEV1 < 40% are considered to have increased risk, and ppoFEV1 < 30% is considered as threshold for high risk. However, it must be noted that significant improvement in the areas of postoperative analgesia and minimally invasive surgeries have decreased the risk of postoperative pulmonary complications in high-risk group (ppoFEV1 < 30%) as well.[11] For patients whose ppoFEV1 and/or ppoDLCO is/are <40%, it is recommended to assess regional lung function and exercise capacity as additional preoperative risk-stratification methods. Also, alternate and/or limited therapies can be considered if surgical risk outweighs benefits.

Assessment of Regional Lung Function

Perfusion of the diseased lung varies from that of the normal lung. Hypoxic pulmonary vasoconstriction (HPV) drives the pulmonary blood flow away from the lung that receives less ventilation. Tumors, which obstruct

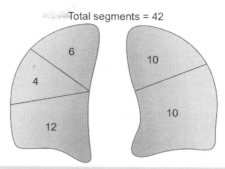

Ex 1. For left lower lobectomy, ppoFEV1 = preoperative postbronchodilator FEV1 x (1-10/42)
Ex 2. For right lower lobectomy, ppoDLCO = preoperative DLCO x (1-12/42)

Fig. 1: Anatomical segments of lung and estimation of postoperative function.
(DLCO: diffusing capacity for carbon monoxide)

the airways, create regional hypoxic segments within the lung, which then receive less pulmonary blood flow. Such nonfunctional areas within the lung may not correlate with anatomical segments. Hence, calculation of postoperative function based on anatomical segments may reveal lesser values than true postoperative function. Also, prediction of postoperative pulmonary function can be further improved by assessment of contribution of the diseased lung or lobe of the lung using imaging modalities. Regional lung function can be performed by three techniques:
1. Radionuclide ventilation/perfusion scanning (V/Q scan)
2. Quantitative computed tomography (CT) scanning
3. Three-dimensional dynamic perfusion magnetic resonance imaging (MRI)

Values of ppoFEV1 and ppoDLCO derived by the V/Q scan have higher correlation with actual postoperative values after pulmonary resection.[12] Quantitative CT scan works by quantification of each CT slice for areas of normal parenchyma, atelectasis, and emphysema. Hence, the total area of normal parenchyma or diseased lung can be estimated to predict postoperative function. Being a newer technique requiring expertise, the use of this technique is not common. Dynamic MRI works on the principle of estimation of regional pulmonary blood volume. This is the newest of the three techniques and is not used widely.

Split function tests are conducted to simulate postoperative respiratory situation by using a double-lumen tube or a bronchial blocker and/or by balloon occlusion of the branch of pulmonary artery to the diseased lung. Being not sufficiently valid with actual postoperative function, these tests are not used currently.[13]

Assessment of Cardiorespiratory Interaction

This is the most important part of preoperative assessment for thoracic surgery. Formal laboratory cardiopulmonary exercise testing (CPET) is the gold standard for the assessment of cardiopulmonary interaction. Maximal oxygen consumption (VO_2max) is the most useful predictor for post-thoracotomy risk. Postoperative morbidity and mortality are very high if preoperative VO_2max is <15 mL/kg/min, whereas patients with VO_2max >20 mL/kg/min are less likely to suffer postoperative complication following thoracic surgery.[14] VO_2max <10 mL/kg/min or <35% of predicted normal is considered a contraindication for any anatomical lung resection. Another parameter that has high correlation with the postoperative outcome is anaerobic threshold (AT).[15] It is the exercise level at which the anaerobic metabolism begins and takes over the aerobic metabolism. A value of AT < 11 mL/kg/min has been suggested as a marker of increased postoperative risk.[16] Apart from these, many other parameters have been studied for the prediction of postoperative risk. These include efficiency slope, oxygen pulse, and minute ventilation to CO_2 production ratio slope. Also, CPET is particularly useful to differentiate between respiratory and cardiac etiologies for poor effort tolerance. Those with primarily cardiac causes of poor effort tolerance show excessive increase in heart rate with exercise, whereas those with respiratory causes show excessive increase in minute ventilation with incremental exercise.

The facility for performing CPET may not be routinely available at all centers, especially in the developing countries. In such conditions, surrogate methods are used to assess cardiopulmonary interaction. These include stair climbing test, shuttle walk test (SWT), and 6-minute walk test (6MWT).

Stair climbing is a useful surrogate for CPET. It is an economic and widely applicable option, is simple to perform, and involves a larger muscle mass, resulting in greater values of VO_2max.[17] It is performed at a patient's own pace, without stopping, and is recorded as the number of flights is achieved. Although there is no exact definition of what each "flight of stairs" means, one flight involving 20 steps and each step measuring 6 inches is a widely accepted norm. The ability to climb 5 flights of stairs is considered to represent VO_2max of 20 mL/kg/min whereas the ability to climb <2 flights corresponds to VO_2max of <12 mL/kg/min and is associated with high postoperative risk.

In SWT, patients walk between the two markers which are set 10 m apart. The walking speed is gradually increased every minute by giving an audio signal to the patient. The test ends when the patient is unable to maintain the required speed. The inability to complete 25 shuttles on two occasions is shown to correspond with a VO_2max < 10 mL/kg/min.[18] All patients who walked > 400 m at the SWT have been shown to have VO_2max > 15 mL/kg/min.

For the 6-minute walk, patients are instructed to walk as far as possible in the time allotted. Patients can walk at their own speed and are allowed to rest if required during the test. The total distance covered at the end of 6 minutes is measured along with an increase in the heart rate and desaturation during the test. In a study of lobectomy patients, patients with a 6MWT distance of >500 m were found to have a significantly less rate of postoperative complications as compared to those who could walk <500 m (37% vs. 61%).[19] Patients who show desaturation by >4% during 6MWT are considered to have increased risk of morbidity and mortality.

Assessment of Cardiovascular Risk

Patients with lung cancer are predisposed to cardiovascular diseases because of the risk factors such as cigarette smoking, atherosclerosis, and old age. The prevalence of the underlying coronary artery disease is about 11–17% in patients with lung cancer.[20] The risk of major adverse cardiac events (myocardial ischemia, pulmonary edema, ventricular fibrillation or primary cardiac arrest, complete heart block, and cardiac-related death) is about 2–3% after lung resection.[21]

Similar to the "Revised Cardiac Risk Index" developed for all major noncardiac surgeries, a "Thoracic Revised Cardiac Risk Index" (ThRCRI) was developed by Ferguson et al. (**Table 1**). However, the predictive ability of this index in prospective studies is not high.[22] Noninvasive testing and treatment as per American Heart Association/American College of Cardiology guidelines should be carried out in these patients. Patients undergoing major lung resection are at risk of developing right ventricular dysfunction postoperatively. Biventricular function and pulmonary artery pressure should be assessed by transthoracic echocardiography preoperatively. Thus, in nutshell, prethoracotomy assessment can be summarized as "three-legged stool," as shown in **Flowchart 1**.[23]

Table 1: Anatomical changes following pneumonectomy.	
Within 24 hours	PPS fills with air, hemidiaphragm is elevated, and trachea remains central with no or minimal mediastinal shift toward PPS
1–5 days	Fluid accumulation occurs in PPS at the rate of 1–2 intercostal spaces per day
2 weeks	80–90% of PPS is filled with fluid
4 months	Complete radiological opacification of hemithorax

(PPS: postpneumonectomy space)

Flowchart 1: "Three-legged stool" for pre-thoracotomy assessment. Note that the bold font indicates the most valid test in each area. The threshold values are written in brackets.

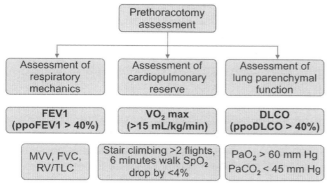

(DLCO: diffusing capacity for carbon monoxide; FVC: forced vital capacity; MVV: maximal voluntary ventilation; RV/TLC: residual volume/total lung capacity)

PREOPERATIVE OPTIMIZATION

Preoperative optimization of the patients scheduled for major pulmonary resection plays an important role in perioperative outcome. The following elements should be given attention for the optimal preoperative preparation of the patient:

- *Correction of malnutrition:* The incidence of preoperative severe malnutrition in patients with operable lung cancer [defined as at least three of the following conditions: weight loss >10–15% within the last 6 months, body mass index (BMI) < 18.5 kg/m², Subjective Global Assessment Grade C, and serum albumin level < 30 g/L with no coexisting hepatic or renal dysfunction] has been reported to be up to 28%.[24] Malnutrition is associated with impaired wound healing, immune dysfunction, and muscle wasting leading to respiratory fatigue in the postoperative period. Patients with severe malnutrition should be referred to a nutritionist at the earliest. High-protein diet (1.5–2 g/kg/day) along with adequate replacement of calories and supplementation of micronutrients should be the mainstay for the correction of malnutrition in the preoperative period.

- *Correction of anemia:* Anemia is a common incidental finding in patients with lung cancer and is known to increase perioperative morbidity and mortality. Enhanced Recovery After Surgery (ERAS) guidelines for thoracic surgery recommend that iron supplementation (oral and/or intravenous) should be the first-line therapy for treating anemia. Blood transfusion or erythropoietin treatment should be reserved for the patients with severe anemia (hemoglobin < 8 g/dL).

- *Cessation of smoking and alcohol:* Smoking is associated with an increased risk of postoperative morbidity (especially pulmonary complications) and mortality. It ideally should be stopped at least 4 weeks before surgery. Behavioral support, nicotine replacement, and

use of varenicline have been shown to be associated with smoking cessation, but their efficacy and effects on postoperative morbidity and mortality have not been studied.[25] Similarly, complete abstinence should be followed for alcohol for 4 weeks prior to thoracic surgery.

- *Preoperative information, education, and counseling:* Many studies have shown that preoperative counseling provides beneficial effects. In particular, formal education about physiotherapy, enteral nutrition, and postoperative pain management options helps to seek better compliance and cooperation from the patient.

- *Treatment of COPD:* COPD is the frequent finding in patients suffering with lung cancer. Four major complications of COPD, namely atelectasis, pulmonary edema, infection, and bronchospasm, should be screened for during initial preoperative evaluation. All COPD patients should receive maximum bronchodilator therapy as per their symptoms. Steroids may be considered in patients poorly controlled on beta-agonists and anticholinergic inhalers. In addition, adequate hydration and mucolytic drugs help in loosening the secretion and active expectoration.

- *Pulmonary physiotherapy and prehabilitation:* Patients with COPD are shown to have less postoperative pulmonary complications if an intensive physiotherapy program is initiated preoperatively.[26] The physiotherapy program may include cough and deep breathing exercises, incentive spirometry, and forceful exhalation methods. Pulmonary functions, performance in 6MWT, and muscle strength improve after a minimum of 4 weeks of a comprehensive physiotherapy program. All patients should be referred to a physiotherapist as soon as they are planned for thoracic surgery.

- *Special precautions in lung cancer patients:* All lung cancer patients should be assessed for 4 "M"s—mass effect, medications, metastasis, and metabolic effects. Use of preoperative chemotherapy drugs such as bleomycin should be sought. Pulmonary toxicity of bleomycin should be ruled out on CT scan and by measuring DLCO. Use of nephrotoxic drugs such as cisplatin and its effect on renal function should be noted in preoperative evaluation. Metabolic effects of the tumor (e.g., Cushing's syndrome, Lambert–Eaton syndrome, and hypercalcemia) should be noted. The mass effects of the tumors (e.g., recurrent laryngeal nerve palsy, phrenic nerve palsy, superior vena cava obstruction, and brachial plexopathy) should be documented during preoperative evaluation.

INTRAOPERATIVE MANAGEMENT

Plan of Anesthesia

Major pulmonary resections are usually carried out under general anesthesia supplemented by appropriate regional anesthesia. Various options of regional anesthesia include thoracic epidural analgesia, paravertebral block, erector spinae block, intercostal block, and serratus anterior plane block. The choice of regional anesthesia technique depends on the availability of devices, clinical expertise, and surgical approach. Studies have proven comparable efficacy and better safety profile for paravertebral and erector spinae block as compared to thoracic epidural analgesia for minimally invasive thoracic surgeries.[27,28]

Position of the Patient

Posterolateral thoracotomies for major lung resections are performed with the patient in lateral decubitus position. Median sternotomy and clamshell thoracotomy are performed in supine position with neck extension. The pressure points in the dependent portion of the body (ankle, knee, anterior superior iliac spine, chest wall, and elbow) should be carefully padded in lateral decubitus position.

Monitoring

In addition to standard monitoring (electrocardiogram, noninvasive blood pressure, pulse oximeter, capnometry, and temperature monitor) for general anesthesia, few additional methods of monitoring may be instituted. The central venous line (subclavian or internal jugular vein) is preferred on the side of the diseased lung, as potential complications of pneumothorax and hemothorax can worsen the function of the normal lung. It is useful for the administration of vasopressors, for monitoring central venous pressure (CVP), and for the estimation of mixed central venous oxygenation. Although not used in all lung surgeries, the central venous line is particularly useful when lung resections are associated with major blood loss. An arterial line is recommended for beat-to-beat blood pressure monitoring and to measure blood gases during and after the surgery. The dynamic indices of fluid monitoring (stroke volume variation and/or pulse pressure variation) give false results due to open thorax and use of low tidal volumes during most part of the surgery.[29] Cardiac output monitoring devices can be used for goal-directed fluid management during the intraoperative period. Cardiac output is calculated by different techniques such as measurement of flow velocity in descending aorta, pulse contour analysis, and thermodilution technique. The value of stroke volume may be targeted along with monitoring of downstream indices of perfusion like serum lactates. Indices such as extravascular lung water index (EVLWI) and pulmonary vascular permeability index (PVPI) are also useful for monitoring fluids in the postoperative period. These devices should be used in lung resection surgeries, complicated by major blood loss or significant cardiovascular comorbidity.

Airway Control

Major lung resection surgeries require lung isolation to prevent intraoperative contamination (by blood or secretions) and to facilitate the surgical exposure. All minimally invasive surgeries require lung isolation. Imaging modalities and bronchoscopy during preoperative workup reveal relevant information about the disease and airway anatomy.

Lung isolation can be provided by a suitable size of the double-lumen tube (DLT) or bronchial blocker. Endobronchial intubation is rarely required in adult patients. However, it is an important option in pediatric population < 2 years of age. The bronchial blocker is not preferred in case of involvement of bronchus by the disease. In such a case, DLT should also be placed in the opposite bronchus. Insertion of the lung isolation device and its confirmation must be done using pediatric fiberoptic bronchoscope before and after giving final position suitable for the surgery.

Plans of extubation depend largely on preoperative cardiorespiratory function, intraoperative course, surgical resection, hemodynamic stability, and adequacy of pain control. DLT should be replaced by a single-lumen tube at the end of the surgery, if postoperative ventilation is planned.

Intraoperative Ventilation

Acute lung injury (ALI) is an important cause of postoperative pulmonary complications. During thoracic surgery, both the lungs (ventilated and non-ventilated) are prone to ALI. The mechanisms of ALI in ventilated lung include volutrauma (by increased tidal volume), barotrauma (raised airway pressure for long time), biotrauma (due to inflammatory mediators such as interleukins), oxidative injury (due to high concentration of oxygen in inspired gases), and shearing stress on alveolar walls (by repetitive opening and collapse of the alveoli). Not only alveoli but also the capillaries are subjected to shearing stress, which may contribute to postoperative pulmonary edema. A non-ventilated lung, on the other hand, is subjected to surgical trauma, biotrauma, re-expansion injury, and re-perfusion injury. The ventilation strategy should be modified to minimize these mechanisms of ALI.

Two time points are important when one-lung ventilation is considered: at end inspiration, alveoli should not be overdistended (therefore use of low tidal volume) and at end expiration, alveoli should not be collapsed [use of optimal positive end expiratory pressure (PEEP)]. Accordingly, the below-given principles of ventilation are followed during thoracic surgery:

- One-lung ventilation is considered as "non-physiological." Hence, its use should be for the smallest duration possible.

- Postanesthesia induction and at the beginning of one-lung ventilation, recruitment maneuver should be applied to the ventilated lung (approximately 20 cm of water for 20 seconds)
- FiO_2 should be minimized as per the oxygenation status.
- Low tidal volume ventilation (4–5 mL/kg ideal body weight) should be followed.
- PEEP should be applied in incremental fashion (low PEEP to high PEEP), checking driving pressure (plateau pressure, PEEP) at all the levels of PEEP. The level at which the driving pressure is minimum should be selected as optimum PEEP.
- Mild hypercapnia (partial pressure of carbon dioxide in arterial blood—$PaCO_2$ between 55 and 60 mm Hg) should be accepted.

The incidence of hypoxia during one-lung ventilation (<5%) has decreased in the last two decades. This is due to better lung isolation devices, increased availability of pediatric bronchoscopes, and improved understanding of lung physiology. In case of hypoxemia, the following interventions are done to improve the oxygenation status:

- Increase the FiO_2.
- Confirm the position of lung isolation device by pediatric bronchoscope.
- Correct the hemodynamic instability, if present.
- Apply recruitment maneuver to the ventilated lung, keeping the watch on blood pressure.
- Increase the PEEP to the dependent lung.
- Apply continuous positive airway pressure (CPAP) of 1–2 cm of water to the operative lung.
- Consider surgical occlusion of the pulmonary artery to the diseased lung.
- Consider switching to two-lung ventilation.

Hypoxic pulmonary vasoconstriction is an important protective physiological reflex during one-lung ventilation. Modern inhalational anesthetic agents inhibit HPV minimally at minimum alveolar concentration (MAC) < 1.0. Intravenous anesthetic agents are not preferred as they inhibit HPV more.

Intraoperative Fluid Management

Excessive administration of intravenous fluids in thoracic surgical patients (>3 L in the first 24 hours) is an independent risk related to ALI.[30] Hence, patients undergoing major pulmonary resection should have restricted intraoperative fluid administration while preserving renal function. In some cases, inotropes/vasopressor may be required to maintain hemodynamic stability while restricting fluids. The below-given principles are followed, regarding intraoperative fluid administration:[31]

- The total positive fluid balance in the first 24 hours' perioperative period should not exceed 20 mL/kg.

- No fluid should be administered to replace third space fluid losses during pulmonary resection.
- Urine output > 0.5 mL/kg/h should not be targeted.
- Invasive monitoring should be used to guide fluids when lung resection is complicated by major blood loss or cardiovascular comorbidity.
- Inotropes should be carefully titrated along with fluids to achieve optimum tissue perfusion.

Extubation Plan

Preoperative evaluation plays an important role in decision-making about extubation of the patient. If a patient has ppoFEV1 > 40% of predicted normal, then the patient can be extubated in the operating room, provided the patient is awake, warm, and comfortable (AWaC). If PPO function is between 30 and 40% of normal, then extubation in the operating room should be decided by exercise tolerance, parenchymal function (ABG), and associated comorbidities. Patients with poor cardiopulmonary reserve should be considered for planned staged weaning in the intensive care unit, as increased postoperative demand of oxygen may not be met with spontaneous breathing. Patients with PPO function < 30% of the normal should be considered for staged weaning, under good analgesia provided by thoracic epidural.[23] Patients with minimally invasive surgery can be considered for early extubation. Patients with loss of diaphragmatic function (injury to phrenic nerve) or chest wall resection can be considered for postoperative positive pressure ventilation using noninvasive ventilation (NIV) methods or CPAP provided by high-flow nasal oxygen.

POSTOPERATIVE MANAGEMENT

Although major lung resection means resection of any large anatomical and/or physiological segment of lung, the discussion henceforth is as per the consideration of pneumonectomy.

Postoperative Analgesia

Adequate analgesia is of paramount importance in postoperative management of patients with lung resection. Lack of analgesia results in inadequate breathing efforts, poor clearance of tracheobronchial secretions, and delayed ambulation, leading to postoperative pulmonary complications such as atelectasis, pneumonia, and respiratory failure. Thoracic epidural analgesia to cover mid-thoracic dermatomes (T4–T8) works the best for posterolateral thoracotomies. Hypotension following the administration of epidural local anesthetic is the major drawback of epidural analgesia. Hence, it is important to choose low concentration of local anesthetic (e.g., 0.1–0.125% of levobupivacaine) and graded volume of the drug (4–5 mL). Continuous infusion of local anesthetic is required for 48–72 hours following surgery. Administration of enteral analgesics such as paracetamol and nonsteroidal anti-inflammatory drugs (NSAIDs) helps in providing multimodal analgesia. Patient-controlled boluses of strong opioids such as morphine and fentanyl are required when epidural analgesia is failed or inadequate. Other alternatives for epidural analgesia include paravertebral block, intercostal nerve block, and erector spinae block. Paravertebral block carries the advantages of unilateral analgesia and low incidence of hypotension. Higher volumes (up to 0.3 mL/kg) and concentration (0.125–0.25%) of local anesthetics are required for paravertebral block. A combination of intercostal block/paravertebral block/erector spinae block with oral analgesics works well for providing analgesia in minimally invasive surgeries.[32]

Postoperative Rehabilitation

Apart from analgesia, other important aspects of postoperative care include breathing exercises, early ambulation, enteral nutrition, and early removal of drain tubes. Physiotherapy plays an essential role in improving postoperative outcomes. Deep breathing exercises, chest wall percussion, wound support, management of position to facilitate gravity-assisted pulmonary toilet, and improvement of ventilation are the essential components of postoperative physiotherapy. Adequate calorie intake and protein supplementation are important to halt the catabolic state following major surgery. Thromboprophylaxis (mechanical and/or pharmacological) and early ambulation of the patient help in reducing the incidence of postoperative thromboembolic episodes. Postpneumonectomy changes are as follows:

- Postpneumonectomy anatomical changes
- Postpneumonectomy changes in pulmonary functions (**Table 1**):
  - Pulmonary function is decreased following pneumonectomy, although many of the changes are less than what is anticipated for the amount of lung tissue lost. Loss in the lung volumes following pneumonectomy is <50% because of overexpansion of the remaining lung. However, despite this overexpansion, the remaining lung does not show evidence of emphysema.
  - FEV1 and FVC decrease by not >50%.
  - DLCO also decreases by <50% and when corrected for lung volume, the value remains normal.
  - Lung compliance decreases and airway resistance increases.
  - Arterial oxygen saturation, PO_2, and PCO_2 at rest do not change if the other lung has no disease.

Risk Factors for Increased Morbidity and Mortality Following Pneumonectomy

Multiple retrospective and prospective studies on postoperative morbidity and mortality following pneumonectomy reveal 30 days' mortality rates of 2–11% across the world.[33,34] Certain risk factors have been identified to increase the mortality following pneumonectomy surgery. These are as follows:

- *Side of the pneumonectomy:* Higher mortality rates have been observed for right pneumonectomy than left (10–12% vs. 1–1.5%).[34] Higher complication rates [postpneumonectomy pulmonary edema, bronchopleural fistula (BFP), etc.] are observed after right pneumonectomy.
- *Nature of surgical resection:* Pleuropneumonectomy or pneumonectomy with chest wall resection is associated with a threefold increase in mortality rates as compared to simple pneumonectomy.[35] Similarly, pneumonectomy performed for trauma or massive hemoptysis as an emergency procedure carries higher mortality rates than an elective pneumonectomy.
- *Comorbidities:* Few comorbid conditions have been identified as risk factors for increased mortality following pneumonectomy surgeries; these include ischemic heart disease, underlying lung pathologies, new onset or worsening heart failure, atrial fibrillation, hypertension, history of stroke, active smoking, poor nutritional status, and weight loss (>10% prior to surgery).[35]

Postoperative Complications Following Major Lung Resection

- Pleural space complications
- Pulmonary complications
- Cardiovascular complications

Pleural Space Complications

Postpneumonectomy space (PPS) or contralateral pleural space can suffer from complications of infection, fistula formation, and accumulation of abnormal contents such as blood and chyle.

Postpneumonectomy empyema: Up to 5% of pneumonectomies develop empyema in the PPS. Early empyema occurs within 10–14 days after surgery and is associated with BFP. Empyema may present late as well (3 months to years after surgery) in the postoperative course and is associated with infection by the hematogenous route. Commonly isolated organisms are *Staphylococcus aureus* and *Pseudomonas aeruginosa*. It must be remembered that polymicrobial infections are not uncommon. Fever with expectorant cough is the common presenting symptom. Empyema may spread to chest wall and drain through the skin, known as "empyema necessitans." Late empyema may additionally present with weight loss and anorexia, in addition to persistent low-grade fever.

Immunosuppression, deranged sugar control, perioperative steroids, and prolonged preoperative hospital stay are likely risk factors for developing postoperative infective complications.

Chest radiographs are useful in diagnosing early empyema. Shifting of mediastinum away from PPS, development of new air fluid level, or sudden change in the air fluid level are common radiographic presentations. Bronchogram by using radiocontrast dye can detect BFP. Sampling of pleural fluid helps in the diagnosis of infection and in starting appropriate antibiotics.

Drainage of PPS, systemic antibiotics as per the culture sensitivity reports, and correction of the BFP are the mainstay of the treatment. Large BFPs are corrected by reopening of thoracotomy wound, surgical debridement, thorough irrigation of PPS, and repair of bronchial stump by omental patch.

Bronchopleural fistula: BFP is a potentially disastrous complication that carries high mortality. Early BPF occurring within a week after the surgery is not associated with empyema. However, those occurring after 2 weeks' postsurgery are associated with empyema. Fever, productive cough, hemoptysis, subcutaneous emphysema, and persistent air leak from the intercostal drain (ICD) are the common presenting signs and symptoms. Development of a new air fluid level in PPS and the presence of multiple air fluid levels are the common radiographic signs. Right-sided surgeries, large diameter (>25 mm) bronchial stump, preoperative chemoradiation, poor wound healing tendency, and prolonged postoperative mechanical ventilation are the risk factors for the development of BPF.[36,37]

Treatment of BPF includes drainage of PPS, systemic antibiotics, and repair of fistula following infection control. Fistulas in the early postoperative period can also be closed surgically. BPF associated with respiratory failure requires mechanical ventilation with lung isolation, in addition to drainage and antibiotics.

Chylothorax and hemothorax: These are relatively rare complications of major lung resection. Both present with rapid filling of PPS, along with signs of hypovolemia [hypotension, tachycardia, and raised jugular venous pressure (JVP)]. Hemothorax requires surgical re-exploration and management of bleeding source. Chylothorax can be managed conservatively with fat-free diet and adequate high-protein nutrition. Those with persistent chyle leak can be managed with lymphangiogram-guided localization of leak and surgical repair of the leak site.

Other rare pleural space complications include contralateral pneumothorax (occurs due to intraoperative damage to the contralateral mediastinal pleura or due to rupture of preexisting blebs or bullae) and esophagopleural fistula (occurs after right pneumonectomy, often due to recurrence of tumor). Contralateral pneumothorax can be diagnosed by chest radiography and requires intercostal drainage. An esophagopleural fistula presents late with empyema. Treatment includes drainage of empyema, surgical repair of fistula, and systemic antibiotics.

Pulmonary Complications

Pulmonary edema: With the reported incidence of 2–5%, postpneumonectomy pulmonary edema presents within 72 hours following surgery.[38] It occurs more commonly after right pneumonectomy than left pneumonectomy. Presentation is respiratory distress and hypoxemia in the postoperative period. Various etiologies have been proposed, which include acute respiratory distress syndrome, postoperative ventricular dysfunction, ischemia-reperfusion injury in the ventilated lung, and intraoperative ventilation-induced lung injury. Occurrence of pulmonary edema results in increased mortality (>50%).[38] Treatment includes positive pressure protective lung ventilation, systemic antibiotics, and hemodynamic supports.

Postpneumonectomy syndrome: It is a delayed complication that presents after 6 months following pneumonectomy. Right pneumonectomy has a higher incidence of postpneumonectomy syndrome than left pneumonectomy. It occurs due to extrinsic compression of the distal trachea and bronchus against the pulmonary artery, aorta or vertebral body due to shifting of mediastinum and hyperinflation of the remaining lung. Airway compression can be severe enough to produce symptoms of breathlessness and inspiratory stridor. Two other rare variants of the same syndrome involve compression of esophagus and compression of pulmonary vein. Treatment includes surgical repositioning of mediastinum by means of nonabsorbable expanders (e.g., saline expanders) placed in the empty PPS.

Acute respiratory failure: Acute respiratory failure (ARF) following thoracotomy is a major cause of morbidity and mortality. ARF is defined as the need for mechanical ventilation for >48 hours. The incidence is higher after right pneumonectomy (6.9–9.3%) than left pneumonectomy.[38] A higher incidence is also observed after extrapleural pneumonectomies than intrapleural pneumonectomies. Respiratory failure may be purely hypoxemic (type 1) or purely hypercapnic (type 2). However, the most common presentation is of the mixed type. Preoperative COPD is the most important patient-related factor for the development of ARF following lung resection.[39] Etiologies for ARF include pneumonia, pneumothorax, retained secretions, atelectasis, empyema, BFP, pulmonary embolism, pulmonary edema, and neurological injuries such as phrenic or recurrent laryngeal nerve injury. Early identification, mechanical protective lung ventilation, efficient toileting of pulmonary secretions (either by repeated bronchoscopy or by tracheostomy), antibiotics, and treatment of COPD form the mainstay of the treatment.

Cardiovascular Complications

Arrhythmias: Cardiac arrhythmias often present within 72 hours of the surgery; the incidence after pneumonectomy is approximately 20%. The commonest arrhythmia is atrial fibrillation. The reported risk factors for the development of a postoperative arrhythmia include older age (>65 years), right pneumonectomy, male gender, thoracotomy by clamshell incision, intrapericardial ligation of vessels, extrapleural pneumonectomy, preexisting coronary artery disease, and hypertension.[40,41]

Arrhythmias are commonly associated with hypotension and result in increased morbidity and longer hospital stay. Mechanical causes (e.g., ICD tube close to the pericardium and intrathoracic collections) should be looked for and should be treated immediately. Electrolyte abnormalities should be corrected. Arrhythmias with hemodynamic instability should be treated with urgent electrical synchronized cardioversion. For persisting arrhythmia, antiarrhythmic agents such as amiodarone should be used. For patients with stable hemodynamics, ventricular rate control should be achieved using beta-blockers or calcium channel blockers.

Pulmonary embolism: The reported incidence of thromboembolic disease following pneumonectomy is 9%.[42] In addition to pre-existing deep venous thrombosis in lower extremities, the thrombus can originate in the pulmonary artery stump. Intraoperative surgical repair of the pulmonary artery, right-sided pneumonectomy, and prothrombotic states (e.g., factor V mutation, protein C or protein S deficiency) can increase the risk of postoperative thromboembolism. In addition, tumor emboli can occur in patients with tumor invading the left atrium or the main pulmonary artery. CT with pulmonary angiography is the gold standard investigation. Bedside echocardiography can identify dilation of right-sided cardiac chambers and acute pulmonary hypertension. Management of pulmonary thromboembolism with obstructive shock requires mechanical thrombectomy with the help of interventional radiology. Successful treatment of pulmonary embolism after lung resection with recombinant tissue plasminogen activator (tPA) has been reported.[43] For stable patients, therapeutic anticoagulation and close monitoring are required.

Cardiac herniation: Cardiac herniation involves herniation of the heart through the defect in the pericardium into the empty pleural space, resulting in torsion and twisting of the heart. It is a rare complication that occurs within 3 days of surgery. It presents as sudden onset of hypotension, breathlessness, cyanosis, chest pain, and superior vena cava syndrome, often preceded by a precipitating event such as coughing or vomiting. Surgeries involving intrapericardial ligation of vessels and removal of pericardium are most commonly associated with this complication. Treatment involves emergent surgery to reposition the heart and close the pericardial defect.

REFERENCES

1. Brunelli A, Kim AW, Berger KI, Addrizzo-Harris DJ. Physiologic evaluation of the patient with lung cancer being considered for resectional surgery: diagnosis and management of lung cancer, 3rd ed: American College of Chest Physicians evidence-based clinical practice guidelines. Chest. 2013;143(suppl): e166S-90S.

2. Brunelli A, Charloux A, Bolliger CT, Rocco G, Sculier JP, Varela G, et al. ERS/ESTS clinical guidelines on fitness for radical therapy in lung cancer patients (surgery and chemo-radiotherapy). Eur Respir J. 2009; 34:17-41.

3. Lim E, Baldwin D, Beckles M, Duffy J, Entwisle J, Faivre-Finn C, et al. Guidelines on the radical management of patients with lung cancer. Thorax. 2010; 65(suppl 3):iii1-27.

4. Berry MF, Villamizar-Ortiz NR, Tong BC, Burfeind WR, Harpole DH, D'Amico TA, et al. Pulmonary function tests do not predict pulmonary complications after thoracoscopic lobectomy. Ann Thorac Surg. 2010;89(4):1044-51.

5. Ferguson MK, Siddique J, Karrison T. Modeling major lung resection outcomes using classification trees and multiple imputation techniques. Eur J Cardiothorac Surg. 2008;34(5):1085-9.

6. Licker MJ, Widikker I, Robert J, Frey JG, Spiliopoulos A, Ellenberger C, et al. Operative mortality and respiratory complications after lung resection for cancer: impact of chronic obstructive pulmonary disease and time trends. Ann Thorac Surg. 2006;81(5):1830-7.

7. Brunelli A, Al Refai M, Monteverde M, Sabbatini A, Xiumé F, Fianchini A. Predictors of early morbidity after major lung resection in patients with and without airflow limitation. Ann Thorac Surg. 2002;74(4):999–1003.

8. Liptay MJ, Basu S, Hoaglin MC, Freedman N, Faber LP, Warren WH, et al. Diffusion lung capacity for carbon monoxide (DLCO) is an independent prognostic factor for long-term survival after curative lung resection for cancer. J Surg Oncol. 2009;100(8):703-7.

9. Ferguson M, Dignam JJ, Siddique J, Vidneswaran WT, Celauro AD. Diffusing capacity predicts long-term survival after lung resection for cancer. Eur J Cardiothorac Surg. 2012;41(5):e81-6.

10. Nakahara K, Ohno K, Hashimoto J, Miyoshi S, Maeda H, Matsumura A, et al. Prediction of post-operative respiratory failure in patients undergoing lung resection for lung cancer. Ann Thorac Surg. 1988;46(5):549-52.

11. Lau KKW, Martin-Ucar AE, Nakas A, Waller DA. Lung cancer surgery in the breathless patient—the benefits of avoiding the gold standard. Eur J Cardiothorac Surg. 2010;38(1):6-13.

12. Slinger P, Darling G. Preanesthetic Assessment for thoracic surgery. In: Slinger P (Ed). Principles and Practice of Anesthesia for Thoracic Surgery, 2nd edition. Basel: Springer Nature Switzerland AG; 2019. p. 21.

13. Koegellenberg CFN, Bollinger CT. Assessing regional lung function. Thorac Surg Clin. 2008;18:19-29.

14. Walsh GL, Morice RC, Putnam JB, Nesbitt JC, McMurtrey MJ, Ryan MB, et al. Resection of lung cancer is justified in high risk patients selected by oxygen consumption. Ann Thorac Surg. 1994;58:704-10.

15. Nagamatsu Y, Shima I, Hayashi A, Yamana H, Shirouzu K, Ishitake T. Preoperative spirometry versus expired gas analysis during exercise testing as predictors of cardiopulmonary complications after lung resections. Surg Today. 2004;34:107-10.

16. Forshaw MJ, Strauss DC, Davies AR, Wilson D, Lams B, Pearce A, et al. Is cardiopulmonary exercise testing useful before esophagectomy? Ann Thorac Surg. 2008;85:294-9.

17. Holden DA, Rice TW, Stelmach K, Meeker DP. Exercise testing, 6-min walk, and stair climb in the evaluation of patients at high risk for pulmonary resection. Chest. 1992;102(6):1774-9.

18. Singh SJ, Morgan MDL, Scott S, Walters D, Hardman AE. Development of a shuttle walking test of disability in patients with chronic airways obstruction. Thorax. 1992;47(12):1019-24.

19. Marjanski T, Wnuk D, Bosakowski D. Patients who do not reach a distance of 500 meters during the 6-minute walk test have an increased risk of post-operative complications and prolonged hospital stay after lobectomy. Eur J Cardiothoracic Surg. 2015;47:e213-9.

20. Brunelli A, Varela G, Salati M, Jimenez MF, Pompili C, Novoa N, et al. Recalibration of the revised cardiac risk index in lung resection candidates. Ann Thorac Surg. 2010;90(1):199-203.

21. Brunelli A, Cassivi SD, Fibla J, Halgren LA, Wigle DA, Allen MS, et al. External validation of the recalibrated thoracic revised cardiac risk index for predicting the risk of major cardiac complications after lung resection. Ann Thorac Surg. 2011;92(2):445-8.

22. Ferfuson MK, Saha-Chaudhari P, Mitchell JD, Varela G, Brunelli A. Prediction of major cardiovascular events after lung resection using a modified scoring system. Ann Thorac Surg. 2014;97:1135-41.

23. Slinger PD, Johnston MR. Preoperative assessment: an anesthesiologist's perspective. Thorac Surg Clin. 2005;15:11.

24. Weimann A, Braga M, Harsanyi L, Laviano A, Ljungqvist O, Soeters P, et al. ESPEN Guidelines on Enteral Nutrition: Surgery including organ transplantation. Clin Nutr. 2006;25:224-44.

25. Wong J, Abrishami A, Yang Y, Zaki A, Friedman Z, Selby P, et al. A perioperative smoking cessation intervention with varenicline: a double-blind, randomized, placebo-controlled trial. Anesthesiology.2012;117:755–64.

26. Warner DO. Preventing post-operative pulmonary complications. Anesthesiology. 2009;92:1467-72.

27. Taketa Y, Irisawa Y, Fujitani T. Comparison of ultrasound-guided erector spinae plane block and thoracic paravertebral block for postoperative analgesia after video-assisted thoracic surgery: a randomized controlled non-inferiority clinical trial. Reg Anesth Pain Med. 2019;pii:rapm-2019-100827. doi: 10.1136/rapm-2019-100827. [Epub ahead of print]

28. Haager B, Schmid D, Eschbach J, Passlick B, Loop T. Regional versus systemic analgesia in video-assisted thoracoscopic lobectomy: a retrospective analysis. BMC Anesthesiol. 2019;19(1):183.

29. Jeong DM, Ahn HJ, Park HW, Yang M, Kim JA, Park J. Stroke volume variation and pulse pressure variation are not useful for predicting fluid responsiveness in thoracic surgery. Anesth Analg. 2017;125(4):1158-65.

30. Alam N, Park BJ, Wilton A, Seshan VE, Bains MS, Downey RJ, et al. Incidence and risk factors for lung injury after lung cancer resection. Ann Thorac Surg. 2007;84:1085-91.

31. Slinger P, Campos H. Anesthesia for thoracic surgery. In: Miller R (Ed). Miller's Anesthesia. 7th edition. Philadelphia, PA: Churchill Livingstone Elsevier.

32. Alzahrani T. Pain relief following thoracic surgical procedures: a literature review of uncommon techniques. Saudi J Anaesth. 2017;11(3):327-31.

33. Harpole DH, DeCamp MM, Daley J, Hur K, Oprian CA, Henderson WG, et al. Prognostic models of thirty-day mortality and morbidity after major pulmonary resection. J Thorac Cardiovasc Surg. 1999;117:969.

34. Watanabe S, Asamura H, Suzuki K, Tsuchiya R. Recent results of postoperative mortality for surgical resections in lung cancer. Ann Thorac Surg. 2004;78:999.

35. Wahi R, McMurtrey MJ, DeCaro LF, Mountain CF, Ali MK, Smith TL, et al. Determinants of perioperative morbidity and mortality after pneumonectomy. Ann Thorac Surg. 1989;48:33.

36. Ferguson MK, Reeder LB, Mick R. Optimizing selection of patients for major lung resection. J Thorac Cardiovasc Surg. 1995;109:275.

37. Darling GE, Abdurahman A, Yi QL, Johnston M, Waddell TK, Pierre A, et al. Risk of a right pneumonectomy: role of bronchopleural fistula. Ann Thorac Surg. 2005;79:433.

38. Jordan S, Mitchell JA, Quinlan GJ, Goldstraw P, Evans TW. The pathogenesis of lung injury following pulmonary resection. Eur Respir J. 2000;15:790.

39. Wendy S, Finley A, Ramsay J. Postoperative respiratory failure and treatment. In: Slinger P (Ed). Principles and Practice of Anesthesia for Thoracic Surgery, 2nd edition. Basel: Springer Nature Switzerland AG; 2019. p. 895.

40. Roselli EE, Murthy SC, Rice TW, Houghtaling PL, Pierce CD, Karchmer DP, et al. Atrial fibrillation complicating lung cancer resection. J Thorac Cardiovasc Surg. 2005;130:438.

41. Foroulis CN, Kotoulas C, Lachanas H, Lazopoulos G, Konstantinou M, Lioulias AG. Factors associated with cardiac rhythm disturbances in the early post-pneumonectomy period: a study on 259 pneumonectomies. Eur J Cardiothorac Surg. 2003;23:384.

42. Mason DP, Quader MA, Blackstone EH, Rajeswaran J, DeCamp MM, Murthy SC, et al. Thromboembolism after pneumonectomy for malignancy: an independent marker of poor outcome. J Thorac Cardiovasc Surg. 2006;131:711.

43. Kameyama K, Huang CL, Liu D, Okamoto T, Hayashi E, Yamamoto Y, et al. Pulmonary embolism after lung resection: diagnosis and treatment. Ann Thorac Surg. 2003;76:599.

Perioperative Management of Tracheal Tumor Surgeries

Sushan Gupta, Jigeeshu Vasistha Divatia

INTRODUCTION

Tracheal resection is uniquely challenging to the anesthesiologist in the perioperative period due to a compromised airway preoperatively, an intraoperatively shared airway with the surgeon and the risk of postoperative airway compromise.

Traditionally, the airway during tracheal surgeries is managed with cross-field ventilation, with a distal trachea ventilated using an endotracheal tube (ETT) inserted through the surgical field **(Figs. 1 to 3).** Even though it ensures adequate oxygenation, it limits surgical exposure that may even require intermittent retraction

during anastomosis. The emphasis lately has been on nonintubation ventilation techniques for tracheal resection surgeries. Case reports have highlighted the safety of this technique, associated better surgical field exposure and postoperative outcomes for patients. Also, it avoids the risk of bleeding and tumor shredding due to ETT insertion in the case of intratracheal tumors.

More so, tracheal resection surgeries require a comprehensive understanding of the disease pathology and associated airway compromise to formulate a comprehensive perioperative airway plan. In addition, an in-depth understanding of the surgical steps with back-up

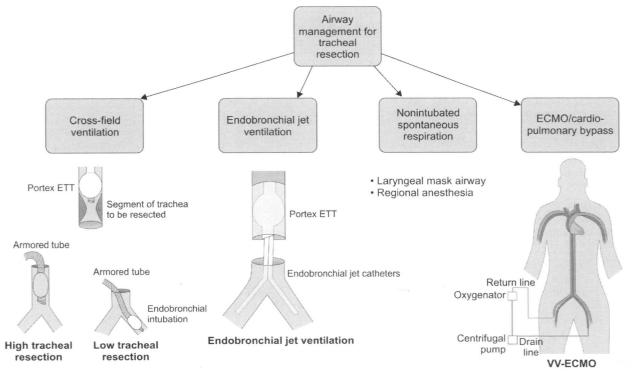

Fig. 1: Airway management in tracheal resection surgeries.
(ETT: endotracheal tube; VV-ECMO: Veno-venous extracorporeal membrane oxygenation)

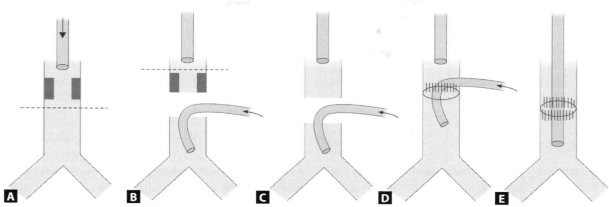

Figs. 2A to E: Schematic illustration to represent a cross-field airway management for high tracheal reconstructive surgery. (A) The lesion and the initial orotracheal intubation above the lesion. (B) After incision of the tracheal below the lesion, a sterile armored tube is placed in the distal airway through the surgical field. (C) Ventilation now proceeds through this distal tube. (D) After resection of the stenotic segment of trachea, construction of the anastomosis begins. When the posterior ends are being anastomosed, ventilation continues through the distal tube. (E) For the anterior anastomosis, the distal tube is removed, and the proximal endotracheal tube is pushed in. There is an initial leak which reduces as the anterior anastomosis is completed. On completion of the anastomosis, the oral endotracheal tube (ETT) is in situ with the cuff beyond the anastomosis with the tip of the tube in the distal airway. The surgery is completed by ventilation through this oral ETT.

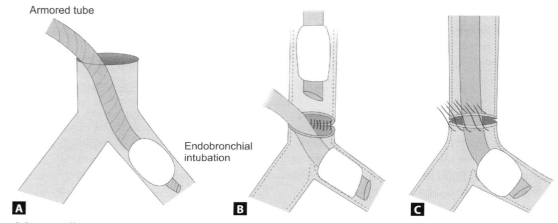

Figs. 3A to C: Schematic illustration to represent a cross-field airway management for low tracheal reconstructive surgery. (A) After tracheal incision, in preparation for resection of the stenotic segment, a sterile circuit is placed in the distal left endobronchial bronchus through the surgical field. (B) After resection of the stenotic segment of trachea, proximal and distal tracheas are approximated. (C) The return to oral intubation after anastomosis with the tip of the tube in the left mainstem bronchus.

plans to ensure oxygenation at each step is necessary to prevent hypoxemia-associated morbidity.

In this chapter, we will discuss the relevant airway anatomy and physiology associated with tracheal resection surgeries, and the perioperative management for these surgeries.

ANATOMY OF AIRWAY

The trachea is a D-shaped structure with cartilaginous rings that are incomplete anterolaterally and extends from the larynx to the carina before bifurcating into left and right bronchus. The trachea is approximately 2 cm in diameter in adult males, and 1.5 cm in females. It extends from below the cricoid at the level of C6 and extends to

the intervertebral disc between T4 and T5 in the thorax with approximately one-third lying in the extrathoracic region and two-thirds intrathoracic. The region around the vocal cords is narrowest with the region 2 cm below the cord constituting the subglottic region. The trachea is a mobile structure, deep inspiration and neck movement can bring about a change in its position. Neck flexion allows the trachea to become more mediastinal which is utilized during the surgery to improve exposure. Also, deep inspiration causes the carina to move down around the level of T6, clinically called tracheal tugging, that makes gaining control of tracheal stoma extremely difficult in patients presenting with respiratory distress.

The trachea is supplied by inferior thyroid, subclavian, innominate, internal thoracic, first intercostal, and bronchial arteries. Despite, its rich blood supply, circumferential pressures on tracheal mucosa by the tracheal tube cuff, may compromise the vascularity. The trachea is innervated by the vagus nerve through the superior and recurrent laryngeal nerves. The recurrent laryngeal nerve lies close to the trachea in the adjacent groove making it susceptible during surgical manipulation.

PHYSIOLOGY

Airflow is defined by the *Poiseuille equation,*

$$Flow = Q = \Delta P \pi r^4 / 8 \eta l$$

A decrease in the radius of the tracheal lumen can severely compromise the airflow between the atmosphere and the alveoli. To maintain this flow, the pressure gradient needs to increase between the alveoli and the atmosphere that leads to an increase in the work of breathing. Besides, any further compromise in the lumen by secretions, blood, and swelling can disproportionately decrease air entry. Al-Bazzaz et al. described that airway symptoms on exertion first appear when the airway diameter reduces to around 50%, and at rest when it decreases to 5–6 mm.[1] Apart from the degree of compromise, the severity of symptoms also depends on the rate of progression and site of obstruction.

On pulmonary function testing, a flow-volume loop with a fixed obstruction presents with limitation of airflow in both inspiration and expiration. Intrathoracic lesions are better tolerated by spontaneously breathing individuals, as thoracic pressures are lower than intratracheal pressures during inspiration that allows a continuous airflow. Flow volume loops in intrathoracic lesions show flattening of the curve in the expiration and vice-versa in case of extrathoracic lesions **(Fig. 4).**

ETIOLOGY

Most common indication of tracheal surgery is circumferential contracture secondary to inflammation,

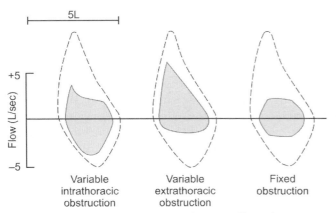

Fig. 4: Flow-volume loop showing effect of dynamic airway compression.

postprolonged intubation or excess cuff pressure. Other causes of tracheal stenosis include tracheal tumors, infection-inflammation, trauma, tracheal and tracheoesophageal fistulas.

Postintubation Tracheal Stenosis

Tracheal stenosis secondary to intubation or tracheostomy happens secondary to compromise in the blood supply of the surrounding mucosa. This can happen even after brief periods of intubation and tend to worsen over months with the formation of granuloma and fibrosis. Patients present with initial complaints of dyspnea of exertion, difficulty in clearing secretions progressing for weeks to months. These patients may develop recurrent pneumonia and present with acute decompensation.

Tracheal Tumors

These are rare forms of cancer that can be benign as well as malignant. The most common variety is squamous cell cancer and tends to have a poor prognosis. Other forms of the tracheal tumor are adenoid carcinoma, hemangioma, hamartomas, carcinoid, etc.

Congenital

Various congenital deformities present as a tracheal obstruction in childhood and are common causes of tracheal surgery in the pediatric population. These include vascular rings, tracheogenic cyst, congenital tracheal stenosis or malacia.

Infection

Infectious causes of tracheal obstruction include viral trachea-bronchitis, bacterial infection, papilloma, and rhinoscleroma.

Noninfectious

Traumatic tracheal obstructions are secondary to burns, laceration, airway hematoma, etc. Other causes include retrosternal goiter, mediastinal adenopathy, fibrosis, aortic aneurysms, etc.

SURGICAL REVIEW

A low collar incision is generally used for cervical tracheal surgeries, the incision may extend to involve the upper sternal border for distal lesions. Right thoracotomy may also be performed as an alternate technique for middle and lower tracheal lesion via a posterolateral incision, especially if right tracheal sleeve pneumonectomy is to be performed. Sternotomy followed by sternal retraction may be required for adequate exposure. Full sternotomy is rarely required. The surgery can be broadly categorized into three phases: (1) dissection to expose a diseased segment of the trachea, (2) resection of a part of the trachea, and finally (3) the anastomosis. After adequate exposure, the incision is made over the diseased section of the trachea and the resection is continued till the healthy portion of the trachea is reached. Most literature suggests that almost half of the trachea can be resected and reconstructed, however greater length above 4 cm requires release maneuvers such as suprahyoid, hilar and suprathyroid laryngeal release. In the case of the traditional cross-ventilation technique, a second ETT is placed in the distal trachea and sutured to ensure it stays in position **(Figs. 2 to 3)**. The distal divided trachea should be continuously suctioned to prevent seepage of blood or secretions. Finally, anastomotic sutures are placed between proximal and distal ends. The neck is flexed to allow approximation of the two ends. At the end of the surgery, the oral ETT is passed distal to the anastomotic site, more commonly under fiberoptic guidance. In some cases, a catheter is passed retrogradely into the proximal section of the trachea and is retrieved by the anesthesiologist. The distal end of ETT is tied across the catheter and ETT is advanced. The endotracheal tube is advanced distal to the suture line. Caution is ensured that the ETT does not entangle with the sutures, else reopening of anastomosis will be required.

An air leak test is then performed to ensure the patency of the suture line by deflating the cuff and ventilating using 20–40 cm H_2O pressures. There will be a gush of air through the mouth around the tube. Alternately, the trachea can be submerged in the saline, and the same process is repeated after covering the mouth and nose and ensure no bubbling is observed. A submental to presternal skin suture may be placed to maintain neck flexion and avoid tension on the suture line.

Preanesthesia Evaluation

All patients should undergo a routine preanesthetic examination, which includes a thorough history, general examination and clinical evaluation of the cardiovascular and pulmonary systems. Investigations required include hemogram, ECG, chest X-ray and estimation of serum electrolytes, creatinine and liver transaminases and bilirubin. Pulmonary function tests and arterial blood gas analysis can also be performed.

Clinical examination of airflow obstruction is the most important aspect of preoperative assessment of these sets of patients. We must assess the degree of breathing difficulty in terms of its onset and progression. Breathing difficulty persisting at rest is indicative of the narrowing of the tracheal lumen to less than 8 mm. Also, important is to evaluate the part of the breathing cycle, the difficulty increases. Distress at the time of inspiration is suggestive of the extrathoracic lesion and vice-versa. In patients with significant airway obstruction, induction of anesthesia may have to be performed in the sitting or semireclining position.

Surgical notes should also be tallied during preanesthesia evaluation. A lot of these patients may have had the airway assessed using fiberoptic bronchoscopy or rigid bronchoscopy. This gives an idea of the extent of airway compromise. However, it should be kept in mind, that these lesions may progress rapidly, and those findings may not be indicative of the true airway compromise.

Imaging

Also, the severity of airway obstruction, the site, and extent of the lesion should be determined by CT scan or magnetic resonance imaging of the neck and/or thorax.

Radiological evaluation using a CT scan with 3-D reconstruction or lately with virtual endoscopy identifies the level and extent of airway compromise. This is useful as an initial study to assess tracheal stenosis and also for follow-up after the surgery **(Fig. 5).** Indirect laryngoscopy and/or direct laryngoscopy were performed to assess the condition of the vocal cords and larynx.

At the start of surgery, bronchoscopic evaluation helps to assess the nature and extent of the problem, the

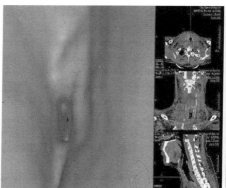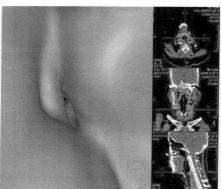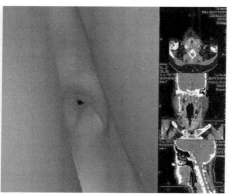

Fig. 5: CT scan and virtual endoscopy images of tracheal resection.

inflammation, tracheal mucosa, and the airway above and below the level of tracheal stricture.

A dynamic flow-volume loop may give an idea regarding the physiology of the limitation of airflow **(Fig. 4)**. However, this generally does not influence the clinical management plan in the presence of a CT scan and astute clinical examination.

Relative Contraindications

Patients with severe pulmonary disorders needing ventilatory support should not undergo this surgery. Apart from the risk of intraoperative hypoxemia, these patients might require ventilatory support postoperatively. This can compromise the surgical anastamosis. Such patients should undergo surgery after correction of the underlying medical disorder and weaning from the ventilator.

Patients with risk of wound dehiscence such as patients on steroids, recent radiation therapy should be given an adequate period of abstinence before taking the patient for surgery.

In patients with significant comorbidities, laryngotracheal resection with tracheostomy might be a better alternative.

Operation Room

A comprehensive airway plan with the necessary equipment and alternate back-ups should be available in the theater. The anesthesiologist and surgeon should be prepared and make a plan for cross-ventilation intraoperatively. All small size endotracheal tubes along with reinforced tubes for cross-ventilation across the surgical field should be present. Flexible and rigid bronchoscopes should also be available in case of an emergency. In case of severe and critical airway compromise, or distal airway involving carina, cardiopulmonary (CP) bypass or extracorporeal membrane oxygenation (ECMO) machines should be kept standby in the theater.

Monitoring

Apart from routine monitoring of ECG, pulse oximetry, capnography, temperature, and noninvasive blood pressure, an arterial line should be placed especially in the right hand, specifically to identify compression of the innominate artery, if the lesion is more distal in the trachea. In addition, an arterial line will help to measure $PaCO_2$ concentration levels to check for the adequacy of ventilation intraoperatively especially in cases where high-frequency jet ventilation (HFJV) is used as a method of ventilation. Adequate venous access should be present in these surgeries since arms will be tucked in intraoperatively. Depth of anesthesia monitoring is measured using bispectral index in case intravenous anesthesia is planned for all or part of the surgery. A peripheral nerve stimulator should also be present to ensure the adequate reversal of peripheral neuromuscular blockade at the end of the surgery.

Position

The patient is generally operated in a supine position with the neck slightly extended using bolsters kept under the shoulder. The hands of the patient are tucked in by the side. It is necessary to ensure the head is adequately supported.

Induction of Anesthesia

Most commonly these patients are induced using intravenous anesthetics. Superficial cervical plexus block, a cervical epidural can be used for adequate analgesia[2] along with local infiltration at the site of surgery and around the trachea during the surgery. Propofol, dexmedetomidine and opioid infusion can be titrated to maintain adequate depth of sedation.

Intravenous or Inhalation Induction of Anesthesia?

Inhalational anesthesia can also be used for induction of anesthesia. The theoretical advantage is the maintenance of spontaneous ventilation, and recovery of the patient from the effect of the inhalational agent should the patient become apneic secondary to the use of high dose inhalational agent, as the uptake of the agent from an anesthesia machine would cease during apnea. Also, intrathoracic lesions should be better tolerated in a spontaneously breathing patient. However, in the case of a critically obstructed airway, hypoventilation will lead to prolonged induction with inhaled agents. The work of breathing significantly increases necessitating the use of continuous positive airway pressure (CPAP) and positive end-expiratory pressure (PEEP) and sometimes even positive pressure ventilation to splint the airway open; as the partial airway obstruction progresses to complete airway obstruction, the egress of inhalational agents might not take place and the theoretical advantage is lost. Lack of muscle relaxation in this technique precludes the best attempt at both bag-mask ventilation as well as intubation. Inhalational induction is also associated with a higher incidence of coughing, breath-holding, airway obstruction, laryngospasm, failed intubation necessitating surgical airway procedure, and cardiac arrest in case of acute airway obstruction.[3]

Awake Intubation or Direct Laryngoscopy after Induction of Anesthesia?

Direct laryngoscopy (DL)[3] under anesthesia may be preferred over awake fiberoptic bronchoscopy (FOB)-guided intubation for several reasons. The FOB itself can cause a complete obstruction as the FOB is passed through a narrow lumen. It is difficult to overcome an obstruction using the malleable FOB, whereas DL will allow passage of a stiff stylet across the obstruction over which ETT can be railroaded. In addition, once an ETT is loaded, the size of ETT cannot be changed without removing the FOB. However, the advantage of FOB is it allows for visual assessment of the tracheal lesion. Depending on the extent of disease, close discussion with the surgeon, the airway plan should be made preoperatively.

Tracheal Tube Placement Proximal to the Lesion or Distal to it?

Initial placement of the ETT above lesion is associated with less risk of bleeding or tumor dislodgement, and allows and enables a larger ETT to be passed. Placing the ETT distal to the lesion definitively secures the airway, but may be associated with bleeding or dislodgement of the tumor. A small sized ETT may be required and the ETT lumen may be obstructed by a blood clot or tumor.

It may be a reasonable plan to place the ETT proximal to the tumor, examine the airway by an FOB through the ETT and attempt to pass the ETT distally if it is judged that it can be done atraumatically and without much maneuvering.

Role of Rigid Bronchoscopy

A rigid bronchoscopy may be performed just after induction of anesthesia and also at the end of the surgery to permit surgeons to evaluate the patency of anastomosis and perform airway toileting. This is extremely vital to understand the level, extent of disease, inflammation of tracheal mucosa and the presence of tracheomalacia. Also, the patient can be intubated with the largest possible ETT bypassing the constriction at the end of the bronchoscopy procedure. In case of severe stenosis, a pediatric rigid bronchoscope can be used to dilate the airway under direct vision. Excess endotracheal dilatation, however, can cause injury and should generally be avoided. A critical stricture of less than 6 mm diameter requires dilatation to allow for intubation with the small 5.5 endotracheal tubes.[4]

Airway Plan

This is the most critical aspect of anesthesia management in patients undergoing tracheal resection. A recent meta-analysis and systematic review by Schieren et al. described various techniques of airway management in tracheal resection surgeries and highlighted complications associated with them.[5] The most common airway management technique described was preoperative oral intubation followed by cross-field intubation of the distal trachea. Other methods included regional anesthesia

technique, use of supraglottic airway device, high-frequency jet ventilation, and ECMO support **(Fig. 1)**.

The first step in planning the airway is to decide whether to perform a tubeless surgery or to perform endotracheal intubation. While cross-field intubation is most commonly practiced, tubeless surgery provides an excellent surgical field and also, spontaneous breathing allows the reconstruction to be more physiological. Vocal cord movements can also be checked during the surgery. It also avoids the risk of restenosis although it is more difficult to perform for an anesthesiologist. It should generally be avoided in patients that may not tolerate apnea periods such as patients with pulmonary disease, cardiovascular diseases or obesity.

Cross-field Intubation

This is traditionally the most common technique for ventilation in patients undergoing tracheal resection surgeries. In this technique, the patient is intubated using a single lumen tube at the time of induction of anesthesia. During the phase of resection and reconstruction, the distal trachea is intubated by the surgeon using a flexometallic ETT, placed in the surgical field and ventilation is continued **(Figs. 2 to 3)**. Alternately, Schieren et al. have used laryngeal mask airway (LMA) for positive pressure ventilation of patients instead of ETT at the time of induction for cervical tracheal resection. Also, they used jet ventilation instead of ETT for cross-field ventilation to prevent hypoxemia.[5] LMA is particularly useful in the case of subglottic lesions where the placement of cuff proximal to stenosis or tumor might not be possible **(Figs. 6A to C)**.[6] It also avoids trauma,

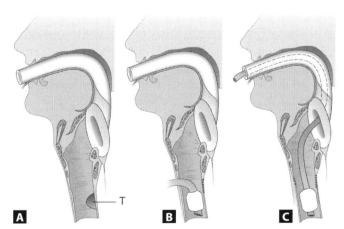

Figs. 6A to C: Airway management for subglottic tracheal reconstructive surgery using laryngeal mask airway. (A) Initial ventilation is through the laryngeal mask airway. (B) After tracheal incision, in preparation for resection of the stenotic segment, a sterile circuit is placed in the distal airway through the surgical field. (C) After resection of the stenotic segment of trachea, proximal and distal trachea are approximated and an endotracheal tube is passed through the LMA and pushed across the suture line.

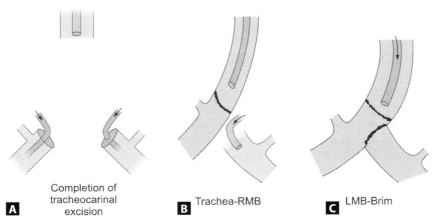

Completion of tracheocarinal excision

A

Trachea-RMB

B

LMB-Brim

C

Figs. 7A to C: Schematic illustration to represent a cross-field airway management for carinal reconstructive surgery. (A) After tracheal incision, in preparation for resection of the stenotic segment, a sterile circuit is placed in both mainstem bronchi through the surgical field. (B) After resection of the segment of the carina, the trachea and right bronchus are approximated and sutured. (C) Approximation of left main bronchus with the trachea, and ventilation is continued using single lumen tube.

bleeding and tumor fragmentation secondary to ETT placement.

Carinal Lesions

These are the most complex airway case scenarios that require extensive communication between surgeons and anesthesiologist. To begin with, the anesthesiologist can use a single lumen tube (SLT) to ventilate the patient. As SLT is kept above the lesion, high airway pressures might be required to ventilate the patient. In case SLT is passed across the stenotic part, one-lung ventilation should be accepted. In case, one is not able to ventilate the patient, rigid bronchoscopy should be performed and ETT passed across the lesion. Alternates like jet ventilation catheter or CP bypass should also be kept standby. Once the ventilation is achieved, resection is started and left mainstem bronchus is initially excised and cross-field ventilation is instituted through the left bronchus. Further resection part of the surgery is then completed. Once resection is complete, and anastomosis is started, the oral ETT can be pushed across into the left bronchus under vision, or a second ETT can be placed into the right bronchus and cross-field ventilation can be continued **(Figs. 7A to C).**

Jet Ventilation

Jet ventilation can be used as an alternate method for ventilation. A catheter is passed across the surgical field into the distal trachea to allow for oxygenation **(Figs. 8A to C).** This allows for better surgical exposure than ETT. The drawback is that there is no monitoring possible with the use of this technique, and constant arterial blood gas (ABG) is required to ensure $PaCO_2$ clearance. Also, there might be significant splashing of blood every time a jet is passed.

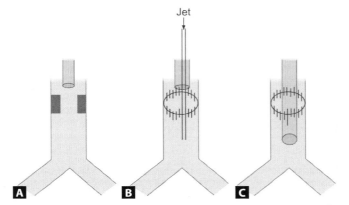

Jet

A   **B**   **C**

Figs. 8A to C: Schematic illustration to represent a jet ventilation for airway management of tracheal reconstructive surgery. (A) Patient is ventilated using single lumen tube proximal to the stenotic part of the trachea. (B) After tracheal incision, in preparation for resection of the stenotic segment, jet catheter is passed into the distal trachea. (C) After resection of the stenotic segment of trachea, proximal and distal tracheas are approximated and oral intubation is reinstated with the tip of the tube in the distal airway.

HFJV has been used in pediatric patients undergoing tracheal resection surgeries as well.[7]

Nonintubated Spontaneous Respiration

The safety of nonintubated anesthesia techniques has been documented in various studies with better postoperative outcomes and a lesser rate of airway complications associated with this technique. However, the management of spontaneously breathing patients might be difficult for the anesthesiologist. The most common complication is hypoxemia while the airway is exposed, and the management of hypercapnia. Also, it is difficult to perform air-leak test after reconstruction, there is a risk of airway obstruction due to blood and secretions into the distal airway.

Minimal invasive tracheal resection under general anesthesia has been commonly performed under cross-field ventilation. However, this requires placement of an extra port and placement of an ETT by the surgeon. This limits surgical exposure. Huang et al. highlighted the feasibility of nonintubated spontaneous respiratory anesthesia for tracheal surgeries in a case report of a 38 year, male with no cardiopulmonary risk factors, who underwent video-assisted thoracoscopic surgery (VATS) tracheal glomus tumor resection, under spontaneous ventilation using LMA and total intravenous anesthesia (TIVA) intraoperatively to maintain the depth of anesthesia. They performed a vagal nerve block using thoracoscopy before the operation.[8] Liu et al. reported a case of tracheal tumor resection, where 2 cm length of the trachea was resected with the patient spontaneously breathing throughout the surgery and oxygenated using a laryngeal mask.[2] Jiang et al. also presented a case series of 18 patients who underwent VATS tracheal and carinal surgeries under LMA and spontaneously breathing. They compared the respiratory and surgical parameters of these patients with a control group selected retrospectively who were intubated for similar procedures. They reported a shorter mean operative time with spontaneous ventilation. Also, there was similar partial pressure of oxygen between the two groups. However, the $PaCO_2$ was higher in the spontaneous ventilation (SV) group. The postoperative recovery was also faster in patients in SV-VATS group.[9] Similar case reports of tracheal surgery under nonintubated spontaneous ventilation have also been presented by other authors.[10-12]

Regional Anesthesia

Cervical Epidural

Macchiarini et al. reported a case series of 21 tracheal resections for benign stenosis performed under cervical epidural in awake spontaneously breathing patients.[13] Patients with subglottic lesions can be managed using cervical epidural placed at the C7-T1 level. The patient who does not require sternotomy is likely to benefit from this technique. Intraoperative sedation is maintained using intravenous anesthetics. Any desaturation intraoperatively can be managed using a catheter or ETT passed into the distal dissected trachea.[13,14]

Cervical epidural carries significant risk of a spinal block, epidural hematoma, bilateral nerve phrenic paralysis, and systemic hypotension. The distinct advantage of a spontaneously breathing patient is that it allows for testing of recurrent laryngeal nerve integrity during the surgery itself. However, there is a pertinent risk of aspiration as the airway is unsecured, and hence a careful resection of the trachea should be performed.

Bilateral Cervical Plexus Block

An ultrasound-guided bilateral superficial cervical plexus block can be performed to allow for intraoperative surgical anesthesia.[2,15] Intraoperative sedation is maintained using an intravenous anesthetic. Patients may require intermittent boluses of opioids. In the case of hypoxemia, a laryngeal mask airway or a cross-field intubation can be used.

Thoracic Epidural

Li et al. described the use of thoracic epidural in 25 patients undergoing VATS resection of tracheal stenosis. Thoracic epidural in this case series was supplemented with a preoperative intercostal nerve block and intraoperative sedation was maintained using propofol and sufentanyl infusion under LMA in spontaneously breathing patients.[10] Peng et al. also reported a case report where they carried out nonintubated thoracoscopic surgery for carinal resection using thoracic epidural at T6-T7 with laryngeal mask airway to maintain intraoperative airway under TIVA, with an intercostal nerve block and vagus nerve block.[16]

Local Anesthesia and Conscious Sedation

This was first reported by Loizzi et al. They described a case of an extrathoracic tracheal hamartoma occluding 80% of the lumen which was resected under ketamine and midazolam titrated boluses ensuring spontaneous breathing and local infiltration at various levels of surgical resection including transtracheal injection of local anesthetic.[17]

ECMO and CP Bypass

Cardiopulmonary bypass provides the best conditions for major tracheal resection surgery, as it avoids the presence of tubes in the airway. However, the risk of intrapulmonary hemorrhage following anticoagulation was a deterrent for elective CP bypass for major tracheal and carinal resections.

CP bypass and ECMO have been most commonly reported for carinal resections or as an emergency procedure when routine methods of airway management fail. The most common form of ECMO used has been venoarterial, although venovenous ECMO should be equally beneficial. The femoral cannulation has been the preferred site, and it can be done under local anesthesia or after induction of general anesthesia. ECMO most commonly used for the complete procedure, however, one could also use it till a specific airway or a cross-field intubation is secured.[5]

Tracheal resections have also been performed under CP bypass. Kar et al. reported a case of critical tracheal stenosis with a lesion at the level of the carina, blocking both the bronchus and trachea as well. Due to the uniquely difficult position of the lesion, they decided to go for femorofemoral bypass in awake patients. However, inadequate flows, followed by inability to ventilate the patient using ETT after induction of anesthesia, they instituted atriofemoral bypass in emergency and performed the surgery uneventfully further.[18]

As compared to CP bypass, ECMO generally requires less anticoagulation and known to generate a lesser systemic inflammatory response. It is also cheaper as compared to CP bypass.[19] However, the meta-analysis did not find any difference in complication rate in patients undergoing tracheal resection between these two techniques.

ECMO may have several advantages including lesser requirements for anticoagulation and risk for systemic inflammatory responses.

Emergence

It is an extremely critical part of the procedure. At the end of the surgery, the ETT is passed distal to the suture line. It is recommended to guide the ETT distal to the suture line under FOB guidance and ensure the cuff does not press against the suture line. In some cases, if required, an uncuffed ETT can also be passed, if the airway is a concern postoperatively like in rare cases of excess laryngeal edema during laryngotracheal surgery or in case of bilateral recurrent laryngeal nerve (RLN) palsy where a tracheostomy can also be performed, however, it is generally discouraged.[4] All patients should be reminded after emergence to ensure neck flexion and avoid any exaggerated movements to prevent suture give-away. There are certain other considerations for anesthesiologists. First and foremost, is to assess vocal function due to proximity of RLN to the trachea, there is a risk of vocal cord palsy postsurgery. Immediately after extubation, one could assess phonation in the patient to rule out RLN injury. Also important is airway toileting to suction and aspirate all the blood through the ETT, or in case of spontaneously breathing patient, by the surgeon before closure.

In the case of airway blockade postextubation, airway toileting is essential. It can be done using FOB guidance. At the same time, one could also assess the patency of sutures and tracheal lumen as well. Extubation can be delayed in case of evidence of laryngeal swelling. Nebulized epinephrine might be useful to relieve distress in such patients. Also, some patients will have neck sutures and head in a flexed position, smooth extubation is necessary for the integrity of the tracheal anastomosis in such patients.

At the time of extubation, all equipment for reintubation such as ETT, FOB both flexible and rigid, and laryngeal mask airway should be present. LMA might be used to provide for ventilation, while also as a conduit to perform FOB-guided intubation. If patient respiratory discomfort is severe, emergent intubation or even a tracheostomy might have to be performed. Having said that, intubating such patients might damage the suture line.

POSTOPERATIVE CARE

The patient is shifted to the postoperative room where these patients should be constantly evaluated for the pattern of breathing, secretions, and airway edema. The presence of airway edema, neck-flexion and pain may prevent the patient from adequately clear secretions. In addition, there might also be retained blood in the distal airway in the postoperative period. These patients should always be provided humidified oxygen that helps in clearing out secretions. Tracheal suction and gentle chest physiotherapy also prevents the accumulation of excess secretions and associated respiratory complications. Vigorous chest physiotherapy is discouraged to prevent large swings in intratracheal pressure that could disrupt the repair. In the case of visible airway obstruction, FOB can be performed to remove any left-over blood or secretions. Nausea/vomiting should be avoided using round the clock antiemetics. If extubation is to be performed, it is preferable to be done in a controlled setting like operation theater, in the presence of a rigid bronchoscope, flexible bronchoscope (including a pediatric FOB) and thoracic surgeon.

Patients can be sent to stepdown care after postoperative day (POD) 1 if recovery is uncomplicated. The patient can also resume feeding from POD 1. Speech physiotherapists should help in improving speech and swallowing functions of the patient. After about a week, a repeat bronchoscopy is performed to ensure patency of the airway.

COMPLICATIONS

Immediate complications are mainly airway blockade due to a variety of causes such as blood, secretions, vocal cord palsy. Delayed complications might happen if there is an anastomotic leak or hemoptysis.

Acute Respiratory Obstruction

In case of acute respiratory obstruction after extubation, differential diagnoses include vocal cord palsy, vocal cord edema or obstruction in the trachea secondary to the blood clot, mucosal flap, etc. The best technique in such a situation would be to lightly sedate the patient and immediately perform FOB with already loaded smallest size ETT. Spontaneous breathing should be preserved at all times. Bronchoscopy will help assess the vocal cords and also tracheal anastomosis and if required suction out clots or secretions. One could railroad the ETT, ensuring the cuff is away from the anastomosis. In the case of a neck-flexed position, one could perform pharyngoscopy and allow easier passage of FOB through the cords. In case of an inability to intubate, such patients should be tracheostomized.

Laryngeal Edema

This is commonly seen in cases of laryngotracheal resection.[8] Presenting symptoms in patients are hoarseness and sometimes stridor. The diagnosis can be confirmed by bronchoscopy. Primary management includes head elevation, voice rest, diuretics, helium-oxygen mixture, and nebulized epinephrine. Some centers routinely use pulsed high doses of steroids (20–40 mg/day) for a short time (5–7 days). Severe cases with the impending loss of the airway warrant intubation using a small-sized uncuffed ETT.

Recurrent Laryngeal Nerve Palsy

The function of the glottis should be documented preoperatively. Unilateral RLN injury may present with weak cough and hoarseness. Bronchoscopy can help determine the mobility of the vocal cords. Conservative management is followed for the first 6 months and the patient can be referred to a speech-language therapist to improve swallowing and phonation. Rare cases may involve B/L RLN palsy which requires an emergency tracheostomy.

Recurrent Aspiration

The risk of aspiration in these patients could be multifactorial. RLN injury may cause vocal cord palsy increasing the risk of aspiration. In addition, if the excess length of the trachea is resected, it may not sufficiently be able to elevate during deglutition. Laryngeal release procedures especially suprahyoid type, further predispose to aspiration.

Acute Respiratory Failure

This may occur due to pulmonary aspiration, decreased sputum clearance, atelectasis, and infection. Gentle chest physiotherapy and fiberoptic bronchoscopy may be required to clear secretions. Therapeutic antibiotics may be required.

Anastomotic Dehiscence

This is the most devastating complication and may present as stridor, cough, increased secretions, hemoptysis, persistent air leak, subcutaneous emphysema, mediastinal emphysema, pneumothorax, and mediastinitis. An attempt should be made to secure the airway by placing a tracheal tube distal to the anastomotic site under fiberoptic bronchoscopic guidance. Sometimes, however, the distal trachea may retract into the thoracic cavity and intubation under FOB guidance may not possible. Kim et al. reported a case of a post-tracheostomy patient who had trachea reconstruction surgery and had an anastomotic leak with distal trachea retracting into the mediastinum. They carrying out surgery under TIVA with the patient spontaneously breathing and used an oxygen blow-by system held by the assistant surgeon near the surgical site to provide oxygen through an endotracheal tube.[20]

Mode of Ventilation

The essence of ventilation in these patients is to avoid high airway pressures and prevent trauma to airway anastomosis. In the case of significant air leak, the rate of ventilation can be increased and allow for permissive hypercapnia. In the case of tracheostomy, anesthetist could use HFJV in the case when air leaks are high. One could also pass a catheter into the tracheostomy tube with the tip of the catheter beyond the anastomosis.

Tracheoinnominate Fistula

These patients manifest with massive hemoptysis and sudden respiratory and hemodynamic compromise which can be fatal. Tracheoinnominate fistula usually presents initially with small volume hemoptysis which can be evaluated with CT angiography and bronchoscopic evaluation. It occurs due to anterior sutural separation caused secondary to infection and inflammation that erodes into the innominate artery. However, significant hemoptysis should prompt emergency evaluation and immediate intervention.[10] Placement of a cuffed ETT can potentially seal the bleeding site while the patient is waiting for surgery.

Quadriparesis

This complication is related to a nonphysiological position of the neck secondary to the placement of guardian chin suture intraoperatively. This may develop due to neck flexion which could alter intraspinal blood supply and lead to quadriparesis. Kumar et al. reported a case of a young individual who developed quadriparesis post-tracheal resection surgery secondary to prolonged neck flexion. However, in their case report, the patient regained complete motor power 48 hours after the release of sutures.[21]

EMERGENT MANAGEMENT

Patients should be evaluated in the operation room under controlled settings. Elevation of bed, humidified oxygen, steroids, heliox or even nebulized epinephrine can be used to reduce the respiratory distress. A bronchoscope both rigid and flexible should be kept standby along with balloon dilator should the need arise.

BACKUP PLAN

It is equally important in the case of managing such patients. A rigid bronchoscope should be kept ready in case critical airway compromise. Jet ventilation can also be performed which might include transtracheal or supraglottic jet ventilation. CP bypass should be kept as the last resort in case of failure to maintain oxygenation by all other methods.

REFERENCES

1. Al-Bazzaz F, Grillo H, Kazemi H. Response to exercise in upper airway obstruction. Am Rev Respir Dis. 1975;111(5):631-40.

2. Liu J, Li S, Shen J, Dong Q, Liang L, Pan H, et al. Non-intubated resection and reconstruction of trachea for the treatment of a mass in the upper trachea. J Thorac Dis. 2016;8(3):594.

3. Walsh T, Wyncoll D, Stanworth S, Bateman A, McArdle F, Walsh T, et al. Fourth National Audit Project. Major complications of airway management in the UK: results of the Fourth National Audit Project of the Royal College of Anaesthetists and the Difficult Airway Society. J Intens Care Soc. 2015;16(4 Suppl):16-21.

4. Mathisen D. Distal tracheal resection and reconstruction: state of the art and lessons learned. Thorac Surg Clin. 2018;28(2):199-210.

5. Schieren M, Boehmer A, Dusse F, Koryllos A, Wappler F, Defosse J. New approaches to airway management in tracheal resections—a systematic review and meta-analysis. J Cardiothorac Vasc Anesth. 2017;31(4):1351-8.

6. Divatia J, Sareen R, Upadhye S, Sharma K, Shelgaonkar J. Anaesthetic management of tracheal surgery using the laryngeal mask airway. Anaesth Intens Care. 1994;22(1):69-73.

7. Alagöz A, Ulus F, Sazak H, ÇAmdal A, ŞAvkilioğlu E. High-frequency jet ventilation during resection of tracheal stenosis in a 14-year-old case. Pediatr Anesth. 2008;18(8):795-6.

8. Huang J, Qiu Y, Chen L, Liu H, Dong Q, Liang L, et al. Nonintubated spontaneous respiration anesthesia for tracheal glomus tumor. Ann Thorac Surg. 2017;104(2):e161-e3.

9. Jiang L, Liu J, Gonzalez-Rivas D, Shargall Y, Kolb M, Shao W, et al. Thoracoscopic surgery for tracheal and carinal resection and reconstruction under spontaneous ventilation. J Thorac Cardiovasc Surg. 2018;155(6):2746-54.

10. Li S, Liu J, He J, Dong Q, Liang L, Cui F, et al. Video-assisted transthoracic surgery resection of a tracheal mass and reconstruction of trachea under non-intubated anesthesia with spontaneous breathing. J Thorac Dis. 2016;8(3):575.

11. Guo M, Peng G, Wei B, He J. Uniportal video-assisted thoracoscopic surgery in tracheal tumour under spontaneous ventilation anaesthesia. Eur J Cardio-Thoracic Surg. 2017;52(2):392-4.

12. Caronia FP, Loizzi D, Nicolosi T, Castorina S, Fiorelli A. Tubeless tracheal resection and reconstruction for management of benign stenosis. Head Neck. 2017;39(12):E114-E7.

13. Macchiarini P, Rovira I, Ferrarello S. Awake upper airway surgery. Ann Thorac Surg. 2010;89(2):387-91.

14. Vachhani S, Tsai JY, Moon T. Tracheal resection with regional anesthesia. J Clin Anesth. 2014;26(8):697-8.

15. Cho AR, Kim HK, Lee EA, Lee DH. Airway management in a patient with severe tracheal stenosis: bilateral superficial cervical plexus block with dexmedetomidine sedation. J Anesth. 2015;29(2):292-4.

16. Peng G, Cui F, Ang KL, Zhang X, Yin W, Shao W, et al. Non-intubated combined with video-assisted thoracoscopic in carinal reconstruction. J Thorac Dis. 2016;8(3):586.

17. Loizzi D, Sollitto F, De Palma A, Pagliarulo V, Di Giglio I, Loizzi M. Tracheal resection with patient under local anesthesia and conscious sedation. Ann Thorac Surg. 2013;95(3):e63-e5.

18. Kar P, Malempati AR, Durga P, Gopinath R. Institution of cardiopulmonary bypass in an awake patient for resection of tracheal tumor causing near total luminal obstruction. J Anaesthesiol Clin Pharmacol. 2018;34(3):409.

19. Biscotti M, Yang J, Sonett J, Bacchetta M. Comparison of extracorporeal membrane oxygenation versus cardiopulmonary bypass for lung transplantation. J Thorac Cardiovasc Surg. 2014;148(5):2410-6.

20. Kim S, Khromava M, Zerillo J, Silvay G, Levine AI. Anesthetic management of a patient with tracheal dehiscence post–tracheal resection surgery. Seminars in cardiothoracic and vascular anesthesia. Los Angeles, CA: SAGE Publications; 2017.

21. Kumar A, Marwaha A, Pappu A, Sharma S, Sood J. Regressive quadriparesis following tracheal resection anastomosis: a rare debilitating but avoidable complication. J Clin Anesth. 2018;44:42-3.

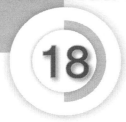

Perioperative Management of Major Vascular Surgeries

Sapna Annaji Nikhar

INTRODUCTION

Perioperative management of patients undergoing major vascular surgeries is always challenging. It is not only due to elderly patients but they are associated with multiple comorbidities, surgery itself induces hemodynamic and metabolic disturbances which results in increased perioperative morbidity and mortality. As such major vascular surgery patients have increased cardiac morbidity. So, the goal of this chapter is to review issues related to major vascular surgeries and take all necessary precautions in perioperative period to decrease overall morbidity and mortality.

ATHEROSCLEROSIS

Atherosclerosis is a disease of vascular intima, in which all the vascular system from aorta to coronary arteries can be involved and is characterized by intimal plaques.[1] The term *atherosclerosis* consists of two parts: (1) atherosis (accumulation of fat accompanied by several macrophages); and (2) sclerosis [fibrosis layer comprising of smooth muscle cells (SMCs), leukocyte, and connective tissue].[2] Connective tissue production by fibroblasts and deposition of calcium in the lesion cause sclerosis or hardening of the arteries. Finally, the uneven surface of the arteries results in clot formation and thrombosis, which leads to the sudden obstruction of blood flow.[3] Risk factors and changes during atherosclerosis have been shown in **Figures 1 and 2**, respectively. The exact risk factors and causes of atherosclerosis are unknown, however, certain conditions may favor the process of atherosclerosis.

Different mechanisms of development of atherosclerosis are the following:
- *Hypercholestrolemia*: It increases superoxide free radicals production and decreases endothelial-derived vasodilators, further causing nitric oxide (NO) deactivation.[2]
- *Apolipoproteins and lipoproteins*: Elevated plasma cholesterol levels are associated with elevated levels of chylomicrons, very low density lipoprotein (VLDL), and low density lipoprotein (LDL). Apolipoprotein B is the main transporter of cholesterol and responsible in forming LDL. It has been shown that increased apolipoprotein B levels indicate the future risk of heart disease more accurately than LDL.[4] Recently, there has been a challenge about the concept that increased high density lipoprotein (HDL) cholesterol concentrations will result in improved cardiovascular risk.[5] However, Onat et al.[6] indicated that high HDL cholesterol concentrations do not usually protect against future risk of coronary heart disease or diabetes. Research is going on to show the impact of apolipoprotein A (APOA-1) dysfunction and risk of atheroscelorosis.[7]
- *Hypertension*: Hypertension damages endothelium by increasing the permeability of arterial walls for lipoproteins. Elevated angiotensin II concentration stimulates smooth muscle cell growth, increases inflammation, and finally accelerates LDL oxidation in such patients.[8]

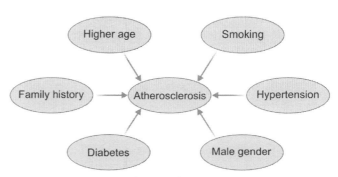

Fig. 1: Risk factors of atherosclerosis.

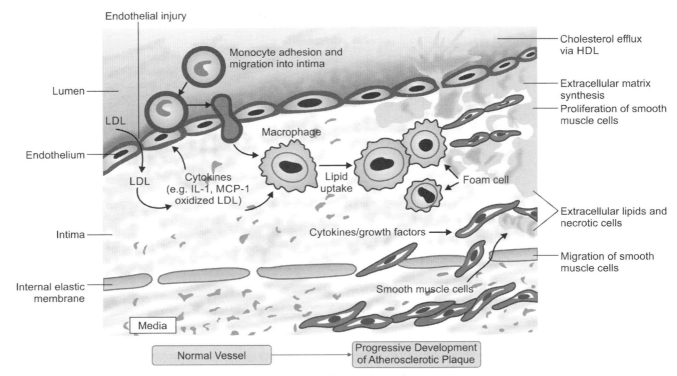

Fig. 2: Changes during atherosclerosis.

- *Decreased NO production or function*: NO has vascular tone adjustment capability, antiplatelet, and antiproliferating effect. It blocks cytokine-stimulated expression of endothelial adhesion molecules and decreases inflammatory activity.
- *Inflammation*: Different inflammatory markers are increased in coronary artery disease.[2] Numerous markers such as cytokines [tumor necrosis factor (TNF-α), interleukins (IL-6 and 18)], C-reactive protein (CRP), and adhesion molecules (intercellular adhesion molecule-1) are increased in plasma, following chronic inflammation. Matrix metalloproteinase (MMP-9 or gelatinase B) is identified in various pathological processes such as tumor metastasis, general inflammation, respiratory diseases, vascular aneurysms, myocardial injury, or remodeling. There is a strong association in IL-18 and baseline MMP-9 levels and future risk of cardiovascular death.[9,10]
- *Immune- and infection-mediated atherosclerosis*: There is a relationship between the pathophysiology of ischemic heart disease and infection as well as the severity of atherosclerosis.[11]
- *Hemostatic factors*: Currently, fibrinogen and factor VII (homeostatic factors) are known as confounding risk factors in cardiovascular diseases.
- *Homocysteine*: Homocysteine increases TNF expression, which enhances oxidative stress and induces a

proinflammatory vascular state that might contribute to the development of coronary atherosclerosis.[12]

Most risk factors including high cholesterol and LDL, low level of HDL in the blood, hypertension, smoking, diabetes mellitus, obesity, inactive lifestyle, and age can be controlled and atherosclerosis can be delayed or prevented.[13] Different antioxidants, such as vitamin E, selenium, and beta-carotene, have shown their beneficial effect as antioxidants and therefore, they can prevent atherosclerosis and vascular endothelium damage.[14]

Preoperative Evaluation

Patients with vascular disease have high incidence of cardiac disease and other coexisting diseases such as diabetes, hypertension, renal impairment, and chronic obstructive disease. All these conditions need to be assessed and optimized prior to surgery to reduce perioperative morbidity and mortality. With evidence from multiple studies, the overall prevalence of perioperative myocardial infarction (MI) and death is 4.9% and 2.4%, respectively. The assessment includes the following:

- *Define urgency and risk*: Emergent and high-risk procedures have higher risk of developing major adverse cardiac events (MACE). The reported rate of cardiac death or nonfatal MI is >5% in high-risk procedures, and emergency surgery is associated with particularly high

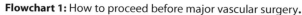

Box 1: Revised cardiac index.[17]

- Creatinine ≥2 mg/dL
- Insulin-dependent diabetes mellitus
- Intrathoracic, intra-abdominal, or suprainguinal vascular surgery
- History of cerebrovascular accident or transient ischemic attack (TIA)
- History of ischemic heart disease (Revised Cardiac Risk Index)
- History of heart failure

Flowchart 1: How to proceed before major vascular surgery.

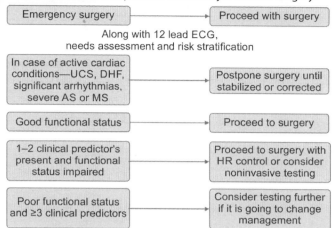

(UCS: unstable coronary syndromes; DHF: decompensated heart failure, significant arrhythmias are Mobitz type II or third-degree block, supraventricular tachycardia, atrial fibrillation with rapid ventricular rate, symptomatic ventricular arrhythmias or bradycardia, new ventricular tachycardia, AS: aortic stenosis; MS: mitral stenosis)

risk, as cardiac complications are 2–5 times more likely than with elective procedures.[15]

- *American Society of Anesthesiologists Physical Status Classification (ASA-PS)*: This gives some idea of general condition of a patient and whether coexisting diseases are controlled or not. "E" was added to indicate emergency surgery, adding risk to surgery.[16] Uncontrolled hypertension and diabetes have significant contribution toward increasing perioperative morbidity.

- *List of clinical predictors*: The different risk factors for ischemic heart disease may not be the same predictors for postoperative cardiac events. Revised Cardiac Risk Index (RCRI) gives risk factors associated with increased incidence of perioperative cardiac events.[17] The risk factors are given in **Box 1** and further plan till surgery is given in **Flowchart 1**.

- *Preoperative functional status*: Functional status can be expressed in metabolic equivalents. The ability to achieve four METs of activity without symptoms is thought to be a good prognostic indicator.[16] In the presence of significant risk factors and unknown functional status of a patient, consider pharmacologic stress testing (Class IIa). In case of abnormal test, coronary revascularization according to local clinical practice guidelines (Class I) is to be ensured. Once revascularization is done, there is a need to know the details of the procedure and drugs the patient is taking.

- *Assess pulmonary risk*: Many patients undergoing abdominal aortic surgery are current or former tobacco users with chronic obstructive pulmonary disease (COPD). Evaluation and optimization of COPD patients and abstinence from smoking will have beneficial effect.[18] Preoperative bronchodilator therapy and role of short course of glucocorticoids in case of severe obstructive pulmonary disease has been established.[19] Treatment with appropriate antibiotics in case of evident pulmonary infection helps to prevent postoperative complications. Use of incentive spirometer and continuous positive airway pressure are beneficial modalities to reduce postoperative pulmonary complications.[20,21]

- *Assess renal risk*: Elevated preoperative serum creatinine is the strongest predictor of postoperative renal dysfunction after open aortic surgery, and is also a predictor of cardiovascular complications and mortality. Prolonged aortic cross-clamping, embolism of atherosclerotic debris into the renal arteries, and/or hemodynamic instability may exacerbate or cause new renal dysfunction.[22,23] Perioperative uses of beta-blockers and statins have decreased risk of death in vascular surgery patients even with renal impairment.[24]

- Preoperative laboratory tests [complete blood count, tests of hemostasis, electrolytes, glucose, blood urea nitrogen (BUN), creatinine] provide baseline values for comparison with intraoperative point-of-care and postoperative tests. Echocardiography is strongly recommended (Class IA) before planned operative repair in patients with dyspnea of unknown origin or worsening dyspnea. Arterial blood gas sampling is indicated in COPD patients. Preoperative pulmonary function studies, including room air arterial blood gas determinations, in patients with a history of symptomatic COPD, long-standing tobacco use, or inability to climb one flight of stairs. Class II, C typing and cross matching for 2–4 units of red blood cells (RBCs) is performed; these should be available in the operating room prior to surgical incision. An increased incidence of myocardial ischemia and increased cardiac morbidity has been reported if hemoglobin concentration is <9 g/dL in the early postoperative period. Hence preoperative anemia management (hemoglobin above 9 g/dL) is very important in vascular surgery patients.

Preoperative Optimization

Perioperative cardiovascular, thrombotic, and infectious complications are minimized by continuing chronic

Table 1: Guidelines for different medications.[15]

Drugs/Medications	Regimen and remarks	Recommendations
Perioperative beta- blockade	1. Continue beta-blockers in patients who are on beta-blockers chronically	Class I
	2. In major vascular surgery with ≥3 Revised Cardiac Risk Index (RCRI) factors, it may be reasonable to begin beta-blockers before surgery.	Class IIb
Perioperative statins	1. Continue statins in patients currently taking statins	Class I
	2. Perioperative initiation of statin use is reasonable in patients undergoing vascular surgery.	Class IIb
Alpha-2 agonists	Alpha-2 agonists are not recommended for prevention of cardiac events.	Class III
Angiotensin converting enzyme (ACE) inhibitors	1. Continuation of ACE inhibitors or angiotensin receptor blockers (ARBs) is reasonable perioperatively.	Class IIa
	2. If ACE inhibitors or ARBs are held before surgery, it is reasonable to restart as soon as clinically feasible postoperatively	
Antiplatelet agents	1. Continue dual antiplatelet therapy (DAPT) in patients undergoing urgent noncardiac surgery during the first 4–6 weeks after BMS or DES implantation, unless the risk of bleeding outweighs the benefit of stent thrombosis prevention.	Class I, C
	2. In patients with stents undergoing surgery that requires discontinuation of P2Y12 (P2Y12 platelet receptor–inhibitor) inhibitors, continue aspirin and restart the P2Y12 platelet receptor–inhibitor as soon as possible after surgery.	Class I, B
Perioperative nitroglycerin	Prophylactic intravenous nitroglycerin is not effective in reducing myocardial ischemia in patients undergoing noncardiac surgery	Class III
Warfarin (vitamin K antagonist)	• Current guidelines recommend warfarin to be stopped 5 days before all elective operations. • In patients who are at high risk of thromboembolic events, bridging with low molecular weight heparin (LMWH) or unfractionated heparin is recommended.	

Quality of evidence ratings. Class I. Evidence provided by one or more well-designed randomized, controlled clinical trials—procedure should be performed. Class II. Evidence provided by one or more well-designed clinical studies, such as case control and cohort studies. Class III. Evidence provided by expert opinion, nonrandomized historical controls, or case reports of one or more—the procedure should not be performed. Class IIa indicates that the weight of evidence/opinion is in favor of usefulness or efficacy. It is reasonable to perform the procedure. Class IIb indicates that the usefulness or efficacy is less well established by evidence/opinion—the procedure may be considered. Grading of recommendations/Quality of evidence. A: based on hierarchy I evidence. B: based on hierarchy II evidence or extrapolated from hierarchy I evidence. C: based on hierarchy II evidence or extrapolated from hierarchy I or II evidence. D: directly based on hierarchy IV evidence or extrapolated from hierarchy I, II, or III evidence. (BMS: bare metal stent; DES: drug-eluting stents)

medications and managing administration of prophylactic medications. It depends on whether it is emergency or elective surgery. Patients who require emergency or urgent surgery are at increased risk of a perioperative cardiovascular event at any level of baseline risk. Time constraint is a big problem but all vascular patients undergoing elective or emergency surgery should have a full risk assessment performed prior to surgery in the appropriate time frame. Good diabetic control, smoking cessation, and management of any chronic lung disease, management of myocardial ischemia and function, and other cardiac risk factors help reduce perioperative risk. The two specific approaches— perioperative goal-directed therapy (GDT) and perioperative β-blockade are considered useful in major vascular surgery patients.[25] The perioperative goal-directed hemodynamic therapy involves the use of intravenous fluid and inotropic therapies aiming to achieve an oxygen delivery index of 600 mL/min/m² wherever possible, without causing tachycardia or myocardial ischemia. Central venous oxygen saturation has been shown to be a valid hemodynamic goal in high-risk surgery.[26] These modalities are thought to achieve both improved global oxygen delivery and maintain tissue perfusion.

- *Different medications and role before major vascular surgery[15]*: These should be used according to the American Heart Association Guidelines (**Table 1**).
- *Myocardial function and revascularization*: Perioperative assessment of myocardial function and detection of myocardial ischemia by electrocardiography (ECG), (Class I), echocardiography or transesophageal echocardiography (TEE), or use of PA (pulmonary artery) (Class IIb) catheter, although no controlled clinical trials have demonstrated reduction in morbidity by detecting myocardial ischemia but can definitely be used to optimize oxygen supply and demand. Even prophylactic percutaneous coronary intervention (PCI) and coronary artery bypass grafting in vascular surgery patients is controversial/no benefit and has less effect on long-

term outcome. Recent guidelines recommend the PCI in unstable active cardiac conditions or those develop inducible ischemia prior to their anaerobic threshold on a cardiopulmonary exercise test.[27] Few suggest coronary revascularization before aneurysm repair in patients with stable angina and two-vessel disease including the proximal left descending artery, and either inducible ischemia on noninvasive stress testing or reduced left ventricular (LV) systolic function (ejection fraction <50%).[28] If cardiologic revascularization is performed, we need to balance the risk of bleeding with thrombosis.

- *Timing of elective noncardiac surgery in patients with previous percutaneous coronary intervention*[15]: Elective noncardiac surgery should be delayed 14 days after balloon angioplasty and 30 days after bare metal stent (BMS) implantation. Elective open aneurysm surgery should optimally be delayed 365 days after drug-eluting stent (DES) implantation. We suggest deferring open aneurysm repair for at least 6 months after drug-eluting coronary stent placement or, alternatively, performing endovascular aneurysm repair (EVAR) with continuation of dual antiplatelet therapy.[28]

- *Role of transesophageal echocardiography*: The emergency use of perioperative TEE is reasonable in patients with hemodynamic instability undergoing noncardiac surgery to determine the cause of hemodynamic instability when it persists despite attempted corrective therapy.[15] It helps in detection of new onset regional wall motion abnormalities and deterioration of ventricular function after application of clamp. The TEE indicators such as poor global LV systolic or diastolic function predict postoperative congestive heart failure (CHF) and/or prolonged intubation after abdominal aortic surgery.[29,30]

- *Antimicrobial prophylaxis for vascular surgery in adults*: Parenteral prophylactic antimicrobials can be given as a single intravenous dose at least within 60 minutes before the procedure and repetition of dose is needed for every 4 hours if surgery is of long duration (>3 hours) and major blood loss is anticipated. Antibiotics are given prior to incision to have adequate tissue levels at the time of incision and to minimize the possibility of an infusion reaction close to the time of induction of anesthesia.[31]

Perioperative Strict Hemodynamic Monitoring

All patients of aneurysm need intensive care and use of continuous arterial blood pressure monitoring is a must over minimum standard monitoring due to massive fluid shifts, blood loss, and physiologic effects of clamping and unclamping. Intraoperative use of central venous pressure (CVP) and PA occlusion pressure may not give an accurate value.[32] Additional stroke volume or cardiac output (CO) monitoring may be useful if already cardiac function is

impaired but may respond slowly to hemodynamic changes with aortic cross-clamp application and release. The role of the TEE is expanded over the last decade.[29] A central venous catheter (CVC) is often inserted to provide port for fluid and blood administration and for vasoactive drug infusions.[28] Regular monitoring of arterial blood gases for pH, hemoglobin, electrolytes, and glucose along with tests of hemostasis are employed when there is an evidence of coagulopathy or significant bleeding. Activated clotting time (ACT) or thromboelastography (TEG) are the tests which are usually recommended. Patients with expected massive bleeding are at benefit from accurate assessment of functional state of coagulation system which is done by the TEG. This helps to provide optimal care and cost-effective replacement of blood components which are actually needed.[33]

Aortic Aneurysm Surgery

Management of Ruptured Abdominal Aortic Aneurysm

Ruptured abdominal aneurysm is both surgical and anesthetic emergency. There is very less or no time period to evaluate extensively and optimize the modifiable risk factors. Ultrasonography is helpful to diagnose the presence of an abdominal aortic aneurysm (AAA), but it cannot diagnose rupture.[28] Computed tomography (CT) is the most helpful special investigation to diagnose rAAA, but it should never delay patient transfer to a specialist vascular center. Few cases that come with cardiovascular collapse may need immediate shifting to operating theater. It is advised to do CT angiography if time permits and assess suitability of the endovascular approach.[34] Along with wide bore access strict hemodynamic monitoring is needed while mobilization. Traditionally, guidelines on the preoperative emergency management of patients with rAAA have always recommended the use of permissive (controlled) hypotension (systolic artery pressure >80 mm Hg) with restrictive fluid management is preferred in order to limit further blood loss and avoid dilution coagulopathy.[35,36] This is specifically found useful in patients with hypothermia and acidosis with pH ≤7.2. In ruptured abdominal aneurysm the main target is to have early hemorrhage control, adequate resuscitation, avoid hypothermia, dilutional coagulopathy, and acidosis and early hemostatic resuscitation.

During induction of anesthesia, the main aim is to maintain hemodynamic stability and avoid hypotension; a rapid sequence induction is the preferred mode of induction. Maintenance of normothermia is important as there is a high risk of perioperative cardiac complications.

In emergency cases, we do not get time to optimize the patients and most patients are on dual antiplatelet agents, vitamin K antagonist, or newer oral anticoagulants.

1. *Patient on antiplatelet agents*: In case of significant intraoperative bleeding, platelet concentrates with or without desmopressin can be administered. The transfusion of platelets is done to keep the counts above 50×10^3 cells/L in mild to moderate bleeding and above one lakh in severe or ongoing bleeding.[37]

2. *Vitamin K antagonist (warfarin)*: Recommendations emphasize to stop warfarin at least 5 days prior to elective surgical procedures and give bridging therapy with heparin but in case of emergency surgery and with severe bleeding, it is recommended to give 4-factor prothrombin complex concentrate to have complete reversal of anticoagulant effect and simultaneously vitamin K 10 mg intravenously for at least 3 days is to be given.[35]

3. *Newer oral anticoagulants*: These have better safety profile and do not warrant regular monitoring of coagulation but the main drawback is that they lack a specific antidote. Recommendations are to use prothrombin complex concentrate perioperatively in case of severe bleeding.

Intraoperative Measures to Control Bleeding

- *Rapid control of bleeding is a prerequisite of bleeding aneurysm*: EVAR, if technically feasible, is now preferred to open surgery. In the IMPROVE trial[38] EVAR under local anesthesia was associated with the lowest mortality and gives time for resuscitation even if there is a need for definitive repair.

- *Controlled hypotension with restrictive fluid strategy*: During initial resuscitation, guidelines recommend to have controlled hypotension and avoid loading patients with fluids. The recommended fluid of choice is balanced salt solution (IA recommendation) and colloid use has been restricted because of their adverse effects on hemostasis. Later management of fluid can be individualized targeting different parameters. We are not supposed to load the patient unnecessarily to get adequate urine output. Goal-directed fluid therapy has been advised for intraoperative fluid management.

- *Role of antifibrinolytics*: Antifibrinolytics prevent the process of fibrinolysis by preventing activation to fibrin and ultimately helping in wound healing. Drugs available in this regard are aprotinin, tranexamic acid, and epsilon aminocaproic acid. Aprotinin is a nonspecific serine protease inhibitor and multiple studies have shown that its use is associated with higher risk of renal, cardio, and cerebrovascular events. It is recommended to use prophylactic antifibrinolytics, tranexamic acid 20–25 mg/kg perioperatively with anticipated severe bleeding. Higher doses of tranexamic acid can cause seizures.[37]

- *Role of point to care testing*: Routine coagulation profiles are not useful and are mostly not accurate predictors in active bleeding and it takes on an average 30–60 min to be available which is too slow to support clinical decision making during vascular surgery in acute and profuse bleeding. Point of care testing is gaining popularity since few years and the tests included are TEG 5000 (Haemonetics Corporation, Braintree, MA) and rotational tromboelastometry (ROTEM) (TEM International GmbH, Munich, Germany). These are well-established viscoelastic methods for hemostatic testing in whole blood. They are very helpful to evaluate platelet function, fibrinogen, fibrinolysis, and are very cost-effective.[33,39]

- *Transfusion trigger and use of other blood components*: A restrictive transfusion trigger for red cells (≤7 g/dL) remains the mainstay of treatment except for the high-risk patients such as cardiac patients where the trigger should be individualized. (It is preferred to give transfusion ≤10 g/dL.) The PROPPR trial compared the effectiveness and safety in patients with severe trauma and major bleeding of using fresh-frozen plasma (FFP), platelets and RBC in a 1:1:1 ratio compared with a 1:1:2 ratio.[40] The use of fibrinogen concentrate is recommended in major bleeding where low circulating concentrations of fibrinogen have been demonstrated or are suspected. The use of rFVIIa should, therefore, be considered only for bleeding that cannot be stopped by conventional, surgical, or interventional radiological means and when comprehensive coagulation therapy has failed. In a Cochrane review, we recommend using cell salvage or an ultrafiltration device if large blood loss is anticipated (Class I, Quality of evidence B). Even autologous blood donation is advised for elective surgeries.[41]

Elective Aortic Aneurysm Surgeries

The core aim of anesthesia for elective open AAA repair is that the patient is managed to the end of surgery so as to be hemodynamically stable, comfortable, and normothermic. The use of goal-directed fluid therapy and prophylactic antifibrinolytics helps in avoiding dilutional coagulopathy and bleeding. Acid–base status and gas exchange values should be kept within norms. All this needs to target to have no immediate need for multiorgan support after operation. The hemodynamic instability is expected during aortic aneurysm surgery during:

- Aortic cross-clamping
- Aortic unclamping
- Blood loss with hypovolemia
- Vasodilation due to anesthetic agents, particularly the combined effects of epidural and general anesthetic agents
- Sympathetic stimulation with tracheal intubation during induction and extubation during emergence.

The thoracic aortic aneurysms are associated with increased morbidity and mortality. Hence, preferred is the endovascular approach. Spinal cord protection and monitoring becomes important in thoracic aortic aneurysm repair. The preferred anesthesia for aortic aneurysm repair is general anesthesia (GA) as a sole technique or with regional anesthesia. Few cases with severe respiratory compromise may need to get operated only under regional/epidural anesthesia.[42]

Role of Epidural Analgesia

Addition of intraoperative epidural anesthesia/analgesia during GA attenuates responses to painful stimuli to reduce intraoperative anesthetic and opioid requirement and provides optimal pain control that may facilitate early extubation in the operating room.[43] Continued use of epidural analgesia (the dose to be titrated to avoid hemodynamic instability) in the postoperative period reduces risk of MI, respiratory failure, and arterial graft occlusion, and facilitates early recovery of bowel function.[44] Different strategies can be used to avoid sudden rise in blood pressure during intubation and surgical incision and after clamp application. Vasodilators can help to lower the LV end diastolic volume, decreasing ventricular wall tension, decreasing the force of contraction, and improving endocardial perfusion. Intraoperative strict hemodynamic monitoring is needed and measures to be taken to maintain the blood pressures within range. Oxygen delivery markers such as mixed venous oxygen saturation (SvO_2) and serum lactate levels should also be monitored along with respiratory and metabolic status.

After aortic cross-clamp release, hypotension is expected due to peripheral vascular resistance decrease by 70–80%, causing a decrease in arterial pressure. Other mechanisms can be ischemia–reperfusion injury, and the washout of anaerobic metabolites causing metabolic (lactic) acidosis. This can cause direct myocardial suppression and profound peripheral vasodilatation. Coronary blood flow and LV end-diastolic volume also decrease (almost 50% from preclamp levels) after clamp release. Strategies to manage hypotension after aortic cross-clamp release include gradual release of the clamp, volume loading, vasoconstrictors, or positive inotropic drugs (e.g. ephedrine, metaraminol, phenylephrine, epinephrine, and norepinephrine). It is important to be aware that vasoactive drugs should only be used after adequate volume repletion.[27] Management of aortic cross-clamp application and release requires excellent communication with the surgeon in order to anticipate and manage the physiological effects. Blood products (FFP, platelets, and cryoprecipitate) are usually given according to the clinical need. Further, TEG testing can be used to monitor and help to manage coagulopathy.

Usually, heparin 75–150 unit/kg is given intravenously before aortic cross-clamp application. ACT can be used to guide heparin therapy (2–3 times more than baseline). Cell salvage equipment should be used when available. Facilities for the rapid infusion of warm fluids and blood should be available for immediate use. All efforts should be made to maintain normothermia. The limitations of CVP as a measure of intravascular volume are increasingly recognized; still it is a common practice to titrate fluids to maintain a CVP of 12–15 cm H_2O before cross-clamp release. Other monitors or measures of CO or fluid responsiveness such as pulse pressure variation or stroke volume variation may also be used, although few specific data are available in aortic surgery.

Spinal Cord Protection

In thoracic aneurysm surgery, modalities need to consider preserving spinal cord perfusion. Several techniques have been suggested to minimize anterior spinal cord ischemia: hypothermia, good perioperative oxygenation, cerebrospinal fluid drainage, arterial shunting, and pharmacological agents including papaverine and scavengers. Several monitoring techniques can detect patients at risk, including somatosensory-evoked potentials and motor-evoked potentials.

Perioperative Renal Protection

The main cause of renal complications after aortic aneurysm repair is the decrease in renal blood flow, increase in renal vascular resistance (by 30%) associated with aortic clamping, use of nephrotoxic drugs, and myoglobin release from ischemic tissues may contribute to acute tubular necrosis by decreasing local NO release, prostaglandin imbalance, and increased activity of renin–angiotensin system. Patients with intra-abdominal pressure (IAP) >25 mm Hg are at risk for compartment syndrome development as this may cause acute kidney injury. In this group of patients, it is important to maintain higher values of blood pressure and better oxygen delivery.[45] Even hypotension is associated with graft thrombosis and multiorgan failure, therefore, maintenance of adequate oxygen supply is crucial for kidneys, central nervous system (CNS), and spinal cord.[46]

Postoperative dialysis rates are similar in patients who have undergone either suprarenal or infrarenal aortic cross-clamping.[27] Often the renal injury can be managed with fluid management, inotropes, and occasionally temporary hemodiafiltration. Though, intraoperative urine output does not correlate with the degree of decrease in glomerular filtration rate (GFR) or the incidence of postoperative kidney failure, monitoring of urine output is must along with appropriate investigations to establish the cause (such as an ultrasound with Doppler to assess renal blood flow) should be done. Several drugs (dopamine, N-acetyl cysteine, mannitol, and furosemide) have been used in an attempt to protect against acute kidney injury, although none has been shown consistently to be beneficial, and all diuretics should be used only after adequate fluid replacement and volume loading.[27]

Ventilatory Strategies

Patients with aortic surgery are always benefited by protective lung ventilation strategy as most patients have associated chronic obstructive airway disease.

Protective ventilation includes the following[47,48]:

- Low tidal volumes of 6–8 mL/kg predicted body weight
- Respiratory rate at 8–10 breaths/min, with adequate expiratory time or more time for expiration to reduce breath stacking as most of the patients have COPD.[48]
- Maintenance of airway pressures—plateau pressures at <15–20 cm H_2O and peak airway pressures <35 cm H_2O
- Fraction of inspired O_2 (FiO_2) adjusted to maintain O_2 saturation >92%
- Cautious use of positive end-expiratory pressure (PEEP) at 5–8 cm H_2O to keep the small airways open without causing hemodynamic compromise.

Sometimes, recruitment of collapsed alveoli is needed. If there is a need for lung recruitment, after separating from the ventilator, it is preferable to use high flow oxygen therapy or intermittent nasal continuous positive airway pressure.[49]

Early Extubation and Enhanced Recovery

Most patients undergoing elective open abdominal aortic surgery will undergo tracheal extubation when surgery is complete.[50] In some patients, extubation may not be feasible due to failure to meet standard extubation criteria; hemodynamic instability; patients with multiple comorbidities, emergency procedure, massive blood loss, hypothermia (temperature <35.5°C); coagulopathy; or uncorrected hypoxemia, hypercarbia, or acidosis. These patients are transported to the intensive care unit (ICU) for a period of postoperative controlled ventilation. Enhanced recovery after vascular surgery is multimodal, evidence-based approach program and includes simultaneous optimization of preoperative status of patients, adequate selection of surgical procedure, and postoperative management.[46] The aim of this program is to reduce complications, the length of hospital stays, and to improve the patient outcome. The strategy is outlined in **Table 2**.

Postoperative Period

Patients are at high risk of cardiac, respiratory, and renal complications as well as intra-abdominal hypertension and

Table 2: Enhanced Recovery after Surgery (ERAS) recommendations for vascular surgery.[46]

System and therapy	Recommendations
Respiratory system	a. Preoperative antibiotics use b. Early extubation c. Protective modes of ventilation d. High flow oxygen therapy or intermittent nasal continuous positive airway pressure after extubation or noninvasive ventilation in postoperative period e. Breathing exercises
Cardiovascular system	a. Monitoring for signs of myocardial ischemia b. Goal-directed fluid therapy c. Maintaining the MAP above 80–90 mm Hg
Renal system	a. Monitoring of the amount of urine and creatinine clearance b. Maintaining the normovolemia and electrolyte balance c. Use diuretics with caution d. Avoid fluid overload and dopamine e. Adequate oxygen therapy
Abdominal and nutritional	a. Without preoperative mechanical bowel preparation b. Maintenance the glucose level <215 mg/dL c. Oral nutrition within the first 24–48 h after operation d. Use prokinetics (metoclopramide and erythromycin) e. Avoidance of nasogastric drainage or early removal f. Monitoring of intra-abdominal pressure (IAP)
Pain	a. Epidural analgesia 48 hours before and 48 hours after intervention b. Avoid systemic opioid use
Others	Consider thromboprophylaxis and early mobilization

ileus. Usually almost all patients are shifted to a critical care unit. We have to target to maintain hemodynamic goals to have good perfusion and oxygenation. Arterial blood gases and electrolyte levels should be measured frequently. Along with that renal function, coagulation, and hemoglobin should be closely monitored. Antifibrinolytics use can be extended in perioperative period for a short period. Maintenance of temperature plays an important role even in postoperative period for early recovery and avoiding coagulopathy. The lower limbs are closely monitored for signs of ischemia.

Postoperative Analgesia

Postoperative analgesia should be multimodal with combination of intravenous paracetamol, nonsteroidal anti-inflammatory drugs (NSAIDs), and local anesthetic agent along with opioid by epidural route. Paravertebral block may be preferred in some cases where epidural has not been placed or epidural is contraindicated. Patient controlled epidural analgesia is highly recommended. Opioid based patient controlled intravenous analgesia with opioids can also be given.

Deep Vein Thrombosis Prophylaxis

Prophylaxis against deep vein thrombosis (DVT) (hydration, compression stockings, and heparin therapy) should be started preoperatively and continued until the patient is fully mobile and no longer considered at risk of DVT.[18,46]

Nutrition

Earlier return of bowel function is associated with less pulmonary complications and also decreases malnutrition-related complications. Better glycemic control and early use of insulin to target blood sugars below 215 mg/dL is recommended to avoid delayed wound healing and graft-related infection.[46]

Postoperative Complications

1. *Hemodynamic instability*[49]: Development of hypertension is common after vascular surgery and if not controlled can lead to stroke or aortic dissection. Even hypotension is common and may be due to bleeding or vasoplegic state leading to multiorgan failure and graft thrombosis. So it is very crucial to maintain blood pressure to keep mean 80–100 mm Hg. Surgical cause should always be excluded before resuscitative measures. Vigilant monitoring of arterial blood pressure along with oxygen delivery markers such as SvO_2 and serum lactate levels should also be done. Transesophageal ultrasound should be available, especially during the periods of hemodynamic instability.[49] Maintenance of blood pressure is not always easy in practice and often requires the use of vasoconstrictors—noradrenaline and vasopressin, vasodilators—nitroglycerine and labetalol, and even inotropes such as dobutamine. Maintenance of adequate tissue perfusion along with adequate urine output and oxygen extraction index is targeted and adequate fluid replacement needs to be done. It has been showed that diuretics can improve venous drainage from the microcirculation, increase the oxygen extraction at cellular level, and improve mitochondrial function.[49,51] Risk of arrhythmias leading to hemodynamic instability is also there and common in patients with structural heart disease or may be due to electrolyte instability. Diagnosis of different rhythm disturbances and management to maintain tissue perfusion is must, only bradyarrhythmias should not be treated if they are not associated with hemodynamic instability.[52]

2. *Bleeding and coagulopathy*: The consequence of aortic surgery is coagulopathy leading to bleeding. So point of care testing and supplementation of deficient coagulation factor are ideal management practices. Blood transfusion is avoided if hemoglobin is above 9 g/dL. Antifibrinolytics can be continued in the postoperative period for a short period. Use of FFP as a plasma expander should be avoided.[45]

3. *Respiratory failure*: Respiratory complications are common in patients with pre-existing respiratory diseases, thoracoabdominal aortic surgery, at extremes of age, with multiple comorbidities, extensive surgery, prolonged use of muscle relaxants, and sedatives, postoperative hypothermia, and fluid overload. This can further lead to respiratory failure and prolonged ventilator support. Continuation of lung-protective strategies in postoperative period for those who are getting ventilated and prevention is possible by giving antibiotics and encouraging breathing exercises.[45]

4. *Myocardial ischemia*: Ischemic events are seen in up to 48% of vascular surgery patients postoperatively.[53] Postoperative ECG changes, increase of creatine phophokinase, increase of troponin-I, and troponin-T should all be followed closely. Ischemic events are manifested by an increased need for inotropic use, reduced CO, cardiac arrhythmias. Urgent angiography can be indicated after echocardiographic visualization of regional wall motion abnormality.[28,46] Once the diagnosis is confirmed rapid resuscitation should be done with supplemental oxygen, timely use of β-blockers, after load reduction agents, antiplatelets, anticoagulants, and PCI. Postoperatively fibrinolysis is a relative contraindication, but this decision must be individualized depending on the situation.[46]

5. *Renal injury*: This can be the result of bleeding, malposition of the stent, or importantly contrast-induced nephropathy. The best solution is to maintain adequate intravascular volume throughout perioperative period. Maintenance of adequate myocardial performance, volume status, and watch on urine output and urea/creatinine is must. Patients requiring chronic renal replacement therapy have bad prognosis.

6. *Others*: Neurological complications such as spinal cord ischemia and cognitive dysfunction and infection of the graft are also possible. Postoperative hyperglycemia occurs in 21–34% of the patients within 72 hours of surgery. Previous studies have shown that for every 40 mg/dL increase in PO glucose level leads to a 30% increase in risk of infection, graft failure, and longer ICU stay.[54] Hence, glucose monitoring and maintenance is needed. Intra-abdominal complications are rare but have high mortality (55–60%) and may exceed 90%

with colonic infarction.[46] Hence, critical observation of abdominal girth is needed along with vitals monitoring. The risk of DVT is also common among these patients and ranges from 0 to 20.5%. The predisposing factors such as elderly age and morbid obesity prolongs surgery and positive family history adds to the risk and ruptured aneurysm.[45] There are no adequate guidelines but most vascular surgeons recommend to start thromboprophylaxis.[55] The use of fractionated heparin reduces the rate of DVT with minor bleeding complications by more than 50%.[45]

Endovascular Aneurysm Repair and Hybrid Operations[28]

The endovascular approach can be done without extensive dissections and incision. Hence it is expected to have less fluid shifts, less bleeding, absence of aortic cross clamp, and less hemodynamic disturbances. Stent grafts have helped to extend the use of EVARs to a wide variety of cases. Aortic arch and descending aorta are being repaired using a hybrid several staged operations which combines open and endovascular approaches. Similar to open repair, cerebral, cardiac, renal, spinal, intestinal, or limb(s) injuries can occur with EVAR. Few late complications are device migration, endoleaks with/without aneurysm rupture and endograft infection.

CONCLUSION

Major vascular surgery continues to challenge the anesthesiologist as surgery itself is associated with multiple complications, superadded by elderly patients, comorbid conditions. Along with proper preoperative evaluation and optimization, critically managing these patients in intensive care preoperatively and postoperatively will definitely reduce mortality, morbidity, and help us to have better overall outcome.

REFERENCES

1. Hennekens CH, Gaziano JM. Antioxidants and heart disease: epidemiology and clinical evidence. Clin Cardiol. 1993;16(4 Suppl 1):I10-3.
2. Ross R. Atherosclerosis—an inflammatory disease. New England J Med. 1999;340:115-26.
3. Tavafi M. Complexity of diabetic nephropathy pathogenesis and design of investigations. J Renal Inj Prev. 2013;2:61-5.
4. McLean JW, Tomlinson JE, Kuang WJ, Eaton DL, Chen EY, Fless GM, et al. cDNA sequence of human apolipoprotein(a) is homologous to plasminogen. Nature. 1987;330:132-7.
5. Voight BF, Peloso GM, Orho-Melander M, Frikke-Schmidt R, Barbalic M, Jensen MK, et al. Plasma HDL cholesterol and risk of myocardial infarction: a Mendelian randomisation study. Lancet. 2012;380:572-80.
6. Onat A, Can G, Ayhan E, Kaya Z, Hergenç G. Impaired protection against diabetes and coronary heart disease by high-density lipoproteins in Turks. Metabolism. 2009;58:1393-9.
7. Onat A, Can G, Yüksel H. Dysfunction of high-density lipoprotein and its apolipoproteins: new mechanisms underlying cardiometabolic risk in the population at large. Turk Kardiyol Dern Ars. 2012;40:368-85.
8. Asgary S, Sahebkar A, Afshani MR, Keshvari M, Haghjooyjavanmard S, Rafieian-Kopaei M. Clinical evaluation of blood pressure lowering, endothelial function improving, hypolipidemic and anti-inflammatory effects of pomegranate juice in hypertensive subjects. Phytother Res. 2014;28:193-9.
9. Pasceri V, Willerson JT, Yeh ET. Direct proinflammatory effect of C-reactive protein on human endothelial cells. Circulation. 2000;102:2165-8.
10. Devaraj S, Xu DY, Jialal I. C-reactive protein increases plasminogen activator inhibitor-1 expression and activity in human aortic endothelial cells: implications for the metabolic syndrome and atherothrombosis. Circulation. 2003;107:398-404.
11. Gharavi EE, Chaimovich H, Cucurull E, Celli CM, Tang H, Wilson WA, et al. Induction of antiphospholipid antibodies by immunization with synthetic viral and bacterial peptides. Lupus. 1999;8:449-55.
12. Ames BN, Shigenaga MK, Hagen TM. Oxidants, antioxidants, and the degenerative diseases of aging. Proc Natl Acad Sci USA. 1993;90:7915-22.
13. Weber C, Noels H. Atherosclerosis: current pathogenesis and therapeutic options. Nat Med. 2011;17:1410-22.
14. Nasri H. Renoprotective effects of garlic. J Renal Inj Prev. 2012;2:27-8.
15. Fleisher LA, Fleischmann KE, Auerbach AD, Barnason SA, Beckman JA, Bozkurt B, et al. 2014 ACC/AHA guideline on perioperative cardiovascular evaluation and management of patients undergoing noncardiac surgery: executive summary: a report of the American College of Cardiology/American Heart Association Task Force on Practice Guidelines. Circulation. 2014;130(24):2215-45.
16. Practice advisory for preoperative evaluation: a report by American Society of Anaesthesiologists Task Force on Preanaesthetic evaluation. Anaesthesiology. 2002; 96:485-96.
17. Lee TH, Marcantonio ER, Mangione CM, Thomas EJ, Polanczyk CA, Cook EF, et al. Derivation and prospective validation of a simple index for prediction of cardiac risk of major noncardiac surgery. Circulation. 1999;100(10):1043-9.
18. Qaseem A, Snow V, Fitterman N, Hornbake ER, Lawrence VA, Smetana GW, et al. Risk assessment for and strategies to reduce perioperative complications for patients undergoing noncardiothoracic surgery: a guideline from the American College of Physicians. Ann Intern Med. 2006;144:575-80.
19. Hirshman CA. Perioperative management of the asthmatic patient. Can J Anaesth. 1991;38:R26-R38.
20. Bapoje SR, Whitaker JF, Schulz T, Chu ES, Albert RK. Preoperative evaluation of the patient with pulmonary disease. Chest. 2007;132(5):1637-45.

21. Crompton CN, Dillavou ED, Sheehan MK, Rhee RY, Makaroun MS. Is abdominal aortic aneurysm repair appropriate in oxygen-dependent chronic obstructive pulmonary disease patients? J Vasc Surg. 2005;42(4):650-3.

22. Zacharias M, Mugawar M, Herbison GP, Walker RJ, Hovhannisyan K, Sivalingam P, et al. Interventions for protecting renal function in the perioperative period. Cochrane Database Syst Rev. 2013;(9):CD003590. doi: 10.1002/14651858.CD003590.pub4

23. Ellenberger C, Schweizer A, Diaper J, Kalangos A, Murith N, Katchatourian G, et al. Incidence, risk factors and prognosis of changes in serum creatinine early after aortic abdominal surgery. Intensive Care Med. 2006;32(11):1808-16.

24. Welten GM, Chonchol M, Hoeks SE, Schouten O, Dunkelgrün M, van Gestel YR, et al. Statin therapy is associated with improved outcomes in vascular surgery patients with renal impairment. Am Heart J. 2007;154(5):954-61.

25. Pearse RM, Rhodes A, Grounds RM. Clinical review: how to optimize management of high-risk surgical patients? Crit Care. 2004;8(6):503-7.

26. Pearse RM, Dawson D, Rhodes A, Grounds RM, Bennett ED. Low central venous saturation predicts postoperative mortality. Intensive Care Med. 2003;29:S15.

27. Fleisher LA, Beckman JA, Brown KA, Calkins H, Chalkof E, Fleischmann KE, et al. ACC/AHA 2007 guidelines on perioperative cardiovascular evaluation and care for noncardiac surgery: a report of the American College of Cardiology/American Heart Association Task Force on Practice Guidelines (Writing Committee to Revise the 2002 Guidelines on Perioperative Cardiovascular Evaluation for Noncardiac Surgery): developed in collaboration with the American Society of Echocardiography, American Society of Nuclear Cardiology, Heart Rhythm Society, Society of Cardiovascular Anesthesiologists, Society for Cardiovascular Angiography and Interventions, Society for Vascular Medicine and Biology, and Society for Vascular Surgery. Circulation. 2007;116(17):e418-99.

28. Chaikof, EL, Dalman RL, Eskandari, MK, Jackson BM, Lee WA, Mansour MA, et al. The Society for Vascular Surgery practice guidelines on the care of patients with an abdominal aortic aneurysm. J Vasc Surg. 2018;67(1):2-77.

29. Matyal R, Hess PE, Subramaniam B, Mitchell J, Panzica PJ, Pomposelli F, et al. Perioperative diastolic dysfunction during vascular surgery and its association with postoperative outcome. J Vasc Surg. 2009; 50(1):70-6.

30. Mahmood F, Matyal R, Maslow A, Subramaniam B, Mitchell J, Panzica P, et al. Myocardial performance index is a predictor of outcome after abdominal aortic aneurysm repair. J Cardiothorac Vasc Anesth. 2008;22(5):706-12.

31. Bratzler DW, Dellinger EP, Olsen KM, Peri TM, Auwaerter PG, Bolon MK, et al. Clinical guidelines for antimicrobial prophylaxis in surgery. Surg Infect (Larchmt). 2013;14(1):73-156.

32. Gelman S. Venous function and central venous pressure: a physiologic story. Anasthesiology. 2008;108:735-48.

33. Verma A. Thromboelastography as a novel viscoelastic method for hemostasis monitoring: its methodology, applications, and constraints. Glob J Transfus Med AATM. 2017;2:8-18.

34. Hope K, Nickols G, Mouton R. Modern anesthetic management of ruptured abdominal aortic aneurysms. J Cardiothorac Vasc Anesth. 2016;30(6):1676-84.

35. Chee YE, Liu SE, Irwin MG. Management of bleeding in vascular surgery. Br J Anaesth. 2016;117(S2):ii85-ii94.

36. Rossaint R, Bouillon B, Cerny V, Coats TJ, Duranteau J, Fernández-Mondéjar E, et al. The European guideline on management of major bleeding and coagulopathy following trauma: fourth edition. Crit Care. 2016;20:100. doi: 10.1186/s13054-016-1265-x

37. Spahn DR, Bouillon B, Cerny V, Coats TJ, Duranteau J, Fernández-Mondéjar E, et al. Management of bleeding and coagulopathy following major trauma: an updated European guideline. Crit Care 2013;17(2):R76.

38. IMPROVE trial investigators. Endovascular or Open Repair Strategy for Ruptured Abdominal Aortic Aneurysm: thirty-day outcomes from IMPROVE randomized trial. Br Med J. 2014;348:f7661.

39. Inaba K, Rizoli S, Veigas PV, Callum J, Davenport R, Hess J, et al. 2014 Consensus conference on viscoelastic test-based transfusion guidelines for early trauma resuscitation: report of the panel. J Trauma Acute Care Surg. 2015;78(6):1220-9.

40. Holcomb JB, Tilley BC, Baraniuk S, Fox EE, Wade CE, Podbielski JM, et al. Transfusion of plasma, platelets, and red blood cells in a 1:1:1 vs a 1:1:2 ratio and mortality in patients with severe trauma: the PROPPR randomized clinical trial. JAMA. 2015;313(5):471-82.

41. Klein AA, Bailey CR, Charlton AJ, Evans E, Guckian-Fisher M, McCrossan R, et al. Association of Anaesthetists guidelines: cell salvage for peri-operative blood conservation 2018. Anaesthesia. 2018;73(9):1141-50.

42. Savas JF, Litwack R, Davis K, Miller TA. Regional anesthesia as an alternative to general anesthesia for abdominal surgery in patients with severe pulmonary impairment. Am J Surg. 2004;188:603.

43. Kaufman E, Epstein JB, Gorsky M, Jackson DL, Kadari A. Preemptive analgesia and local anesthesia as a supplement to general anesthesia: a review. Anesth Prog. 2005;52(1):29-38.

44. Davies MJ, Silbert BS, Mooney PJ, Dysart RH, Meads AC. Combined epidural and general anaesthesia versus general anaesthesia for abdominal aortic surgery: a prospective randomised trial. Anaesth Intensive Care. 1993;21(6):790-4.

45. Choudhury M. Postoperative management of vascular surgery patients: a brief review. Clin Surg. 2017;2:1584.

46. Stojanovic MD, Markovic DZ, Vukovic AZ, Dinic VD, Nikolic AN, Maricic TG, et al. Enhanced recovery after vascular surgery. Front Med (Lausanne). 2018;5:2.

47. Yang D, Grant MC, Stone A, Wu CL, Wick EC. A meta-analysis of intraoperative ventilation strategies to prevent pulmonary complications: is low tidal volume alone sufficient to protect healthy lungs? Ann Surg. 2016;263(5):881-7.

48. Ahmed SM, Athar M. Mechanical ventilation in patients with chronic obstructive pulmonary disease and bronchial asthma. Indian J Anaesth. 2015;59(9):589-98.

49. Shraag S. Postoperative management. Best Pract Res Clin Anaesthesiol. 2016;30:381-93.

50. Cohen J, Loewinger J, Hutin K, Sulkes J, Zelikovski A, Singer P. The safety of immediate extubation after abdominal aortic surgery: a prospective, randomized trial. Anesth Analg. 2001;93(6):1546-9.

51. Dünser MW, Takala J, Braunauer A, Bakker J. Re-thinking resuscitation: leaving blood pressure cosmetics behind and moving forward to permissive hypotension and tissue perfusion-based approach. Crit Care. 2013;17(5):326.

52. Heintz KM, Hollenberg SM. Perioperative cardiac issues: postoperative arrhythmias. Surg Clin North Am. 2005;85(6):1103-14.

53. Bryce GJ, Payne CJ, Gibson SC, Kingsmore DB, Byrne DS. The prognostic value of raised preoperative cardiac troponin I in major vascular surgery. Br J Cardiol. 2009;16:147-50.

54. Serio S, Clements JM, Grauf D, Merchant AM. Outcomes of diabetic and nondiabetic patients undergoing general and vascular surgery. ISRN Surg. 2013;2013:963930.

55. Scarborough JE, Cox MW, Mureebe L, Pappas TN, Shortell CK. A novel scoring system for predicting postoperative venous thromboembolic complications in patients after open aortic surgery. J Am Coll Surg. 2012;214:620-8.

19

Perioperative Management of Esophageal Surgeries

Priya Ranganathan, Swapnil Parab

UNDERSTANDING THE SURGERY[1]

Esophagectomy is the preferred modality of treatment for cancers of the middle and lower third esophagus. It is important to understand the various approaches to the surgery, since they will influence the anesthetic management.

Esophagectomy involves mobilization of the esophagus, total esophagectomy with lymph node dissection, and formation of a neoesophagus (usually a gastric conduit), which is then anastomosed to the remnant esophagus. The original Ivor Lewis technique involves two incisions—a right thoracotomy and an upper abdominal incision, with anastomosis in the mediastinum. The McKeown three-hole modification of this involves an additional left cervical incision with anastomosis in the neck. The thoracic and abdominal approaches to the surgery may be performed through minimal access (thoracoscopy/laparoscopy or robotic). Sometimes, due to patient factors or surgical reasons, the entire mobilization may be done via the abdominal route (transhiatal esophagectomy), thus avoiding a thoracotomy.

Since the gastric conduit continues to derive its blood supply from the celiac axis, the anastomosis at the extreme end of the gastric conduit is vulnerable to hypoperfusion. Therefore, anastomotic leaks and gastric conduit ischemia are potential complications after this surgery.

In revision esophagectomies, a pedicled segment of the colon is used in place of the gastric conduit to replace the esophagus.

The extent of lymphadenectomy during an esophagectomy is variable. Two-field (infracarinal and abdominal) and three-field (addition of supracarinal lymph nodes) lymphadenectomies have been described. Three-field lymphadenectomy may increase the risk of recurrent laryngeal nerve palsy and pulmonary complications. The other reasons for postoperative pulmonary complications following esophageal surgery are as follows:

- Ligation of the azygous vein in the thorax (may be done for access to the esophagus in some patients)
- Ligation of bronchial artery
- Lymphadenectomy.

All of these may lead to congestion of bronchial mucosa, sometimes denudation and decreased mucociliary clearance of secretions.

MORBIDITY AND MORTALITY AFTER SURGERY

Despite advances in surgery and anesthesia techniques and postoperative care, esophagectomy carries significant morbidity and mortality. It has been estimated that postoperative morbidity can occur in up to 60% of patients; of these, pulmonary complications are the most common (as high as 25%) and account for 50% of deaths after esophagectomy.[2-4]

PREOPERATIVE CONCERNS AND EVALUATION

- *Effects of neoadjuvant therapy*: Many patients presenting for esophagectomy would have received neoadjuvant chemotherapy or chemoradiation to downstage the tumor. The patients should be evaluated for the toxicities of the chemotherapeutic agents. Depending on the agent used, these toxicities could include renal and cardiac dysfunction, neuropathies, and hematological toxicity. In addition, it has been shown that neoadjuvant therapy decreases cardiopulmonary fitness in patients with esophagogastric cancers.[5-8]
- *Nutrition*: Patients with esophageal tumors have varying degrees of dysphagia, which may or may not respond to neoadjuvant therapy. This may cause malnutrition,

weight loss, and sarcopenia. Patients who have symptoms of obstruction may have episodes of vomiting, resulting in fluid and electrolyte imbalance. Depending on the degree of obstruction and response to neoadjuvant therapy, patients may need either oral high-protein supplements or enteral tube feeds preoperatively. It has been suggested that patients who are unable to take 75% of their target calories need nutritional supplements and those with intake <50% of their target calories need enteral feeds.[9] There is no evidence to support the routine use of immunonutrition in these patients.[10-11]

- *Pulmonary evaluation*: With a transthoracic (either open thoracotomy or minimally invasive) approach, there is handling of the lung. In addition, postoperative pain can result in splinted breathing. Recurrent laryngeal nerve injury can predispose to aspiration of gastric contents. Other factors attributed to cause pulmonary complications include bronchial denervation and revascularization and impaired lymphatic drainage. Impaired preoperative pulmonary function has been identified as a risk factor for postoperative complications, and pulmonary function tests (spirometry and diffusion capacity) can identify patients at increased risk and allow risk stratification and optimization before surgery.[3,12-15] Details of pulmonary function testing are available in the chapter on "Perioperative Care for Major Pulmonary Resection."

- *Cardiac evaluation*: There is handling and retraction of the heart during mobilization of the esophagus and the gastric conduit. This is particularly significant in transhiatal esophagectomies, where the dissection is performed entirely transhiatally. This may cause arrhythmias and/or abnormal cardiac contractility. Preoperative history of effort tolerance, electrocardiogram (ECG), and resting 2D-ECHO are performed for all patients. Depending on the risk factors for coronary artery disease, further cardiac evaluation may be indicated.

- *Cardiopulmonary exercise testing (CPET)*: Studies have shown that anaerobic threshold and peak oxygen consumption achieved on CPET can be used to stratify patients at risk of major complications after elective surgery.[16,17] The role of CPET in patients undergoing esophagectomy is yet to be established. A study by Moyes in patients undergoing esophagogastric resections found a correlation between anaerobic threshold and cardiopulmonary complications; however, an exact cutoff of anaerobic threshold could not be determined, and the discriminatory ability was poor.[18] Nagamatsu determined that the maximum oxygen uptake of 800 mL/min/m^2 was adequate for patients undergoing esophagectomy.[19] In a study by Patel, the only independent predictor of major morbidity after esophagectomy was peak oxygen consumption of <17 mL/kg/min.[20] Other studies failed to find an association between anaerobic threshold or peak oxygen consumption and postoperative complications.[21,22] The role of CPET as a risk stratification tool in patients undergoing esophagectomy remains unclear and needs to be researched further.

- *Submaximal exercise tests*: The 6-minute walk test and the shuttle walk test have been proposed as alternatives for formal CPET. However, there is inadequate evidence to establish their role in preoperative risk assessment in patients undergoing esophagectomy.[23-25]

PRE-OPTIMIZATION AND PREHABILITATION[26]

As for all major surgeries, patients need to abstain from smoking and alcohol consumption for at least 4 weeks prior to surgery. Many of these patients have a combination of nutritional depletion and postchemotherapy debilitation and will need aggressive pulmonary rehabilitation and muscle strengthening before proceeding for major surgery. They are familiarized with spirometry, which they will need to perform in the postoperative period. Preoperative anemia should be corrected by iron supplementation.

RISK STRATIFICATION SCORES

Various scores have been proposed to predict patients at risk of postoperative complications after esophagectomy. However, most of these still need external validation. Tekkis proposed the O-POSSUM (Physiological and Operative Severity Score for the enumeration of Mortality and morbidity) model as a variant of the P-POSSUM model; however, subsequent studies have shown that the O-POSSUM has poor predictive and discriminatory properties.[27-31] Lagarde developed a nomogram based on preoperative risk factors to predict the severity of complications after esophagectomy.[32] Ferguson described a scoring system to predict pulmonary complications after esophagectomy.[12] There have been several other models described to predict complications after esophagectomy, none of which has been validated or adopted in general use.[33]

ANESTHESIA PLAN

The plan is general anesthesia with some form of regional anesthesia for perioperative analgesia. The degree of esophageal obstruction should be evaluated and care should be taken to prevent aspiration of gastric contents.

Perioperative Analgesia

The use of thoracic epidural analgesia (TEA) decreases pulmonary complications in patients undergoing major surgery; in esophagectomy patients, the use of TEA reduces pulmonary infections, chronic post-thoracotomy pain, and postoperative mortality.[34,35] TEA improves microcirculation in the gastric conduit and has also been shown to reduce anastomotic leak rates.[36,37] Standard guidelines for the management of thoracotomy pain recommend TEA as the first-line technique.[38] However, systemic hypotension is a recognized side effect of TEA. In one study, it was found that anastomotic dehiscence was related to the number of episodes of systemic hypotension.[39] It has also been shown that epidural local anesthetic boluses may reduce perfusion at the anastomotic end of the gastric conduit, although the clinical impact of this is unclear.[40,41]

An alternate technique for the management of thoracotomy pain, with comparable analgesia and less adverse effects, is paravertebral blockade.[42-45] However, paravertebral block will not be useful to treat the pain from the abdominal incision in an esophagectomy.

Erector spinae plane (ESP) block and serratus anterior plane (SAP) block have been described as newer techniques for thoracotomy pain. There is inadequate literature comparing these with standard techniques. The Enhanced Recovery After Surgery (ERAS) guidelines for patients undergoing esophagectomy recommend the use of TEA in the perioperative period.[26]

PATIENT POSITIONING

The patient is positioned in the left lateral position for thoracotomy and supine with the neck extended for the abdominal and cervical parts of the surgery. Care should be taken to prevent position-related pressure sores and nerve injuries.

AIRWAY MANAGEMENT

Minimally invasive esophagectomy requires right lung collapse for surgical exposure. Either double-lumen tubes or bronchial blockers can be used for lung isolation. Some surgeons use capnothorax to improve surgical access. For esophagectomy via open approach, lung isolation is not mandatory and many centers use low tidal volume ventilation as an alternative.

Ventilation Strategies

Patients undergoing esophagectomy are prone to respiratory complications, with the incidence of pulmonary morbidity as high as 25%.[4,12-15] The focus of intraoperative ventilation is to use strategies that minimize pulmonary trauma.

Large studies have looked at the role of lung-protective ventilation and the use of positive end-expiratory pressure (PEEP) in patients undergoing abdominal surgery. The

IMPROVE (Immediate Management of Patients with Ruptured Aneurysm: Open Versus Endovascular Repair) study showed that the use of lung-protective ventilation with modest levels of PEEP resulted in fewer pulmonary and extrapulmonary complications.[46] However, the PROVHILO (PROtective Ventilation using HIgh versus LOw positive end-expiratory pressure) study showed that high levels of PEEP offered no additional benefit but, in fact, led to hemodynamic instability.[47] In esophagectomy patients, randomized trials have shown that lung-protective ventilation reduces lung inflammation and pulmonary complications.[48,49] Current guidelines for the management of patients undergoing esophagectomy recommend the use of lung-protective strategies.[26]

Mode of Ventilation

Some small studies have suggested that pressure-controlled mode may offer some advantages over volume-controlled modes of ventilation during one-lung ventilation; however, the evidence is inconclusive.[50]

MAINTENANCE OF ANESTHESIA[51]

Volatile anesthetics have been shown to reduce inflammatory markers in lung fluid during one-lung ventilation; the clinical implication of this has not been determined. On the other hand, inhalational anesthetics may inhibit hypoxic pulmonary vasoconstriction (HPV), which is an important protective mechanism during one-lung ventilation—for this reason, the use of total intravenous anesthetics may be preferred. However, the impact of this at concentrations used in routine practice is unclear, especially since it has been proven that modern inhalational anesthetics have no effect on HPV at concentrations <1 MAC.

PERIOPERATIVE FLUID MANAGEMENT

Patients presenting for esophagectomy may be relatively hypovolemic due to dysphagia and vomiting. Esophagectomy is a prolonged surgery with significant fluid losses due to bleeding, lymphatic dissection, and evaporation from the exposed thoracic and abdominal cavities. These factors should be accounted for while planning fluid therapy. However, excessive intraoperative fluid administration can lead to bowel edema, impacting the quality of the anastomosis, and also increases pulmonary complications. Data from previous studies have established that a higher perioperative cumulative fluid balance is associated with increased pulmonary morbidity in esophagectomy patients.[3,52-55]

Over the last few years, the practice of fluid administration in major surgeries has moved from liberal to restrictive.

However, a recently published study in patients undergoing major abdominal surgery showed that a restrictive fluid regimen was associated with a significantly higher incidence of acute kidney injury and surgical site infections, with no impact on pulmonary complications or death.[56]

Another issue with the use of restrictive fluid strategies in esophagectomy patients is that they are based on goal-directed therapy using invasive arterial monitoring [pulse pressure variation (PPV)], cardiac output monitoring [stroke volume variation (SVV)], or esophageal Doppler (aortic blood flow). Studies looking at the reliability of dynamic indices such as PPV and SVV in patients with open thorax receiving low tidal volume ventilation have shown differing results.[57-61] Also, restrictive fluid regimens recommend the use of vasopressors to maintain perfusion pressure in normovolemic patients. In esophagectomy patients, the perfusion of the gastric conduit depends on the right gastroepiploic artery, and there may be concerns that the use of vasopressors may reduce the flow to the gastric conduit. Two small studies have, however, shown that the use of vasopressors in low doses actually improves blood flow in the gastric conduit.[40,41] The ERAS guidelines recommend "optimal" fluid therapy using balanced crystalloids aiming for a weight gain of not >2 kg/day.[26]

INTRAOPERATIVE MONITORING

Standard monitoring consists of electrocardiography, pulse oximetry, temperature, and invasive blood pressure. Arterial pressure monitoring provides beat-to-beat measurements and allows easy sampling to check adequacy of ventilation. Arterial lactate can be used as a marker of adequacy of perfusion. Central venous catheters may be used for central venous pressure monitoring and vasopressor infusions. As discussed earlier, dynamic indices of preload have limited value during the surgery.

EXTUBATION

For uncomplicated surgeries, if patients are warm, pain free, and hemodynamically stable, they can be extubated on table. Routine postoperative mechanical ventilation is not recommended and is reserved only for patients who have specific issues.[26]

USE OF PERIOPERATIVE STEROIDS AND OTHER ADJUNCTS

Two meta-analyses (consisting of small studies) have shown that the use of a single dose of preoperative corticosteroid may reduce inflammatory markers and improve clinical outcomes. However, further research is needed to establish this finding.[62,63] One study has shown that the use of ulinastatin (a protease inhibitor) decreased postoperative

complications and improved recurrence-free survival.[64] A meta-analysis looked at the use of sivelestat (neutrophil elastase inhibitor) in esophagectomy patients and found a decrease in acute lung injury with no impact on any other outcomes.[65] The confidence intervals for the relative risk were very wide, making this finding unreliable.

POSTOPERATIVE MANAGEMENT

Patients who are stable can be managed in a high-dependency unit. Routine transfer to an intensive care unit is not recommended.[26] Patients should be mobilized out of bed on the first postoperative day and encouraged to ambulate. They also need aggressive chest physiotherapy to minimize pulmonary complications. Early enteral feeding is recommended to promote peristalsis. The jejunum is the preferred route for feeding, and patients should aim to achieve their caloric target by the third postoperative day. If recovery is uncomplicated, the nasogastric tube and the urinary catheter should also be removed early. Venous thromboprophylaxis should be continued until the patient is fully mobilized. A multimodal analgesia regimen is used. Fluids should be administered judiciously with the aim of weight gain of not >2 kg/day.[26]

COMPLICATIONS AFTER ESOPHAGECTOMY

Pulmonary Complications

Pulmonary complications are the most frequent complications after esophagectomy occurring in up to 25% of patients.[2-4,12-15] These include pleural effusions, atelectasis, pneumonia, chylothorax, and acute respiratory failure. Potential risk factors for postoperative pulmonary complications include preexisting pulmonary disease, reduced preoperative spirometry and/or diffusion capacity, smoking, increased age, poor performance status, preoperative chemoradiation, and excessive fluid administration.[12-15,66] Aggressive chest physiotherapy is essential to minimize retention of secretions. This is aided by adequate analgesia. Vocal cord status should be checked postoperatively in all patients since vocal cord dysfunction may predispose the patients to aspiration and pneumonia.

The use of noninvasive ventilation and high-flow oxygen [THRIVE (Transnasal Humidified Rapid-Insufflation Ventilatory Exchange)] in these patients is controversial since these techniques may cause distension of the gastric conduit and tension on the anastomosis.[1] If these patients need re-intubation, it is advisable to use a rapid-sequence technique.[66]

Cardiac Complications

Atrial fibrillation (AF) is the most common arrhythmia after esophagectomy, occurring in up to 16% of patients.[67]

Advanced age, previous history of arrhythmias, coronary artery disease, and hypertension have been identified as risk factors for AF.[67,68] New-onset AF in the postoperative period should alert the clinician to the possibility of a pulmonary infection or an anastomotic leak. There is no role for prophylactic antiarrhythmics in patients undergoing esophagectomy, and the treatment of AF is as per standard guidelines. AF increases the risk of mortality by threefold.[67,68]

Surgical Complications[1,66]

Gastric conduit distension may occur in the postoperative period. This can predispose patients to regurgitation and aspiration, especially if the vocal cord function is impaired. In such cases, the gastric tube must be decompressed using the nasogastric tube. Prokinetic agents may be used to aid gastric emptying. The incidence of vocal cord palsy/paresis can be as high as 67% and predisposes to pulmonary complications.[69] In most cases, the vocal cord dysfunction can be managed by observation and dietary modification and does not need any surgical intervention.

Anastomotic leak and/or gastric conduit ischemia is one of the most dreaded complications after esophagectomy, with reported incidence varying from 15% to 37%.[1,66] Small leaks are usually managed conservatively with external drainage and antibiotics. Large leaks and extensive ischemia may present with full-blown sepsis and can be life-threatening. In these cases, disconnection of the esophagogastric anastomosis is indicated.

▌ REFERENCES

1. Howells P, Bieker M, Yeung J. Oesophageal cancer and the anaesthetist. BJA Educ. 2017;17:68-73.

2. McCulloch P, Ward J, Tekkis PP, ASCOT group of surgeons, British Oesophago-Gastric Cancer Group. Mortality and morbidity in gastro-oesophageal cancer surgery: initial results of ASCOT multicentre prospective cohort study. BMJ. 2003;327:1192-7.

3. Wei S, Tian J, Song X, Chen Y. Association of perioperative fluid balance and adverse surgical outcomes in esophageal cancer and esophagogastric junction cancer. Ann Thorac Surg. 2008;86:266-72.

4. Carney A, Dickinson M. Anesthesia for oesophagectomy. Anesthesiol Clin. 2015;33:143-63.

5. Navidi M, Phillips AW, Griffin SM, Duffield KE, Greystoke A, Sumpter K, et al. Cardiopulmonary fitness before and after neoadjuvant chemotherapy in patients with oesophago-gastric cancer. Br J Surg. 2018;105:900-6.

6. Jack S, West MA, Raw D, Marwood S, Ambler G, Cope TM, et al. The effect of neoadjuvant chemotherapy on physical fitness and survival in patients undergoing oesophagogastric cancer surgery. Eur J Surg Oncol. 2014;40:1313-20.

7. Thomson IG, Wallen MP, Hall A, Ferris R, Gotley DC, Barbour AP, et al. Neoadjuvant therapy reduces cardiopulmonary function in patients undergoing oesophagectomy. Int J Surg Lond Engl. 2018;53:86-92.

8. Sinclair R, Navidi M, Griffin SM, Sumpter K. The impact of neoadjuvant chemotherapy on cardiopulmonary physical fitness in gastro-oesophageal adenocarcinoma. Ann R Coll Surg Engl. 2016;98:396-400.

9. Miller KR, Bozeman MC. Nutrition therapy issues in esophageal cancer. Curr Gastroenterol Rep. 2012;14:356-66.

10. Mimatsu K, Fukino N, Ogasawara Y, Saino Y, Oida T. Effects of enteral immunonutrition in esophageal cancer. Gastrointest Tumors. 2018;4:61-71.

11. Mingliang W, Zhangyan K, Fangfang F, Huizhen W, Yongxiang L. Perioperative immunonutrition in esophageal cancer patients undergoing esophagectomy: the first meta-analysis of randomized clinical trials. Dis Esophagus. 2020. pii: doz111. doi: 10.1093/dote/doz111. [Epub ahead of print]

12. Ferguson MK, Durkin AE. Preoperative prediction of the risk of pulmonary complications after esophagectomy for cancer. J Thorac Cardiovasc Surg. 2002;123:661-9.

13. Ferguson MK, Celauro AD, Prachand V. Prediction of major pulmonary complications after esophagectomy. Ann Thorac Surg. 2011;91:1494-1500; discussion 1500-1.

14. Shirinzadeh A, Talebi Y. Pulmonary complications due to esophagectomy. J Cardiovasc Thorac Res. 2011;3:93-6.

15. Avendano CE, Flume PA, Silvestri GA, King LB, Reed CE. Pulmonary complications after esophagectomy. Ann Thorac Surg. 2002;73:922-6.

16. Older P, Hall A, Hader R. Cardiopulmonary exercise testing as a screening test for perioperative management of major surgery in the elderly. Chest. 1999;116:355-62.

17. Smith TB, Stonell C, Purkayastha S, Paraskevas P. Cardiopulmonary exercise testing as a risk assessment method in non cardio-pulmonary surgery: a systematic review. Anaesthesia. 2009;64:883-93.

18. Moyes L, McCaffer C, Carter R, Fullarton G, Mackay C, Forshaw M. Cardiopulmonary exercise testing as a predictor of complications in oesophagogastric cancer surgery. Ann R Coll Surg Engl. 2013;95:125-30.

19. Nagamatsu Y, Shima I, Yamana H, Fujita H, Shirouzu K, Ishitake T. Preoperative evaluation of cardiopulmonary reserve with the use of expired gas analysis during exercise testing in patients with squamous cell carcinoma of the thoracic esophagus. J Thorac Cardiovasc Surg. 2001;121:1064-8.

20. Patel N, Powell AG, Wheat JR, Brown C, Appadurai IR, Davies RG, et al. Cardiopulmonary fitness predicts postoperative major morbidity after esophagectomy for patients with cancer. Physiol Rep. 2019;7:e14174.

21. Forshaw MJ, Strauss DC, Davies AR, Wilson D, Lams B, Pearce A, et al. Is cardiopulmonary exercise testing a useful test before esophagectomy? Ann Thorac Surg. 2008;85:294-9.

22. Lam S, Alexandre L, Hardwick G, Hart AR. The association between preoperative cardiopulmonary exercise-test variables and short-term morbidity after esophagectomy: a hospital-based cohort study. Surgery. 2019;166:28-33.

23. Inoue T, Ito S, Kanda M, Niwa Y, Nagaya M, Nishida Y, et al. Preoperative six-minute walk distance as a predictor of postoperative complication in patients with esophageal cancer. Dis Esophagus. 2019. pii: doz050. doi: 10.1093/dote/doz050. [Epub ahead of print]

24. Murray P, Whiting P, Hutchinson SP, Ackroyd R, Stoddard CJ, Billings C. Preoperative shuttle walking testing and outcome after oesophagogastrectomy. Br J Anaesth. 2007;99:809-11.

25. Whibley J, Peters CJ, HallidayLJ, Chaudry AM, Allum WH. Poor performance in incremental shuttle walk and cardiopulmonary exercise testing predicts poor overall survival for patients undergoing esophago-gastric resection. Eur J Surg Oncol. 2018;44:594-9.

26. Low DE, Allum W, De Manzoni G, Ferri L, Immanuel A, Kuppusamy M, et al. Guidelines for perioperative care in esophagectomy: Enhanced Recovery After Surgery (ERAS®) Society Recommendations. World J Surg. 2019;43:299-330.

27. Tekkis PP, McCulloch P, Poloniecki JD, PrytherchDR, Kessaris N, Steger AC. Risk-adjusted prediction of operative mortality in oesophagogastric surgery with O-POSSUM. Br J Surg. 2004;91:288-95.

28. Lai F, Kwan TL, Yuen WC, Wai A, Siu YC, Shung E. Evaluation of various POSSUM models for predicting mortality in patients undergoing elective oesophagectomy for carcinoma. Br J Surg. 2007;94:1172-8.

29. Nagabhushan JS, Srinath S, Weir F, Angerson WJ, Sugden BA, Morran CG. Comparison of P-POSSUM and O-POSSUM in predicting mortality after oesophagogastric resections. Postgrad Med J. 2007;83:355-8.

30. Bosch DJ, Pultrum BB, de Bock GH, Oosterhuis JK, Rodgers MGG, Plukker JTM. Comparison of different risk-adjustment models in assessing short-term surgical outcome after transthoracic esophagectomy in patients with esophageal cancer. Am J Surg. 2011;202:303-9.

31. Morran CG. Comparison of P-POSSUM and O-POSSUM in predicting mortality after oesophagogastric resections. Postgrad Med J. 2007;83:355-8.

32. Lagarde SM, Reitsma JB, Maris A-KD, van Berge Henegouwen MI, Busch ORC, Obertop H, et al. Preoperative prediction of the occurrence and severity of complications after esophagectomy for cancer with use of a nomogram. Ann Thorac Surg. 2008;85:1938-45.

33. Warnell I, Chincholkar M, Eccles M. Predicting perioperative mortality after oesophagectomy: a systematic review of performance and methods of multivariate models. Br J Anaesth. 2015;114:32-43.

34. Ballantyne JC, Carr DB, deFerranti S, Suarez T, Lau J, Chalmers TC, et al. The comparative effects of postoperative analgesic therapies on pulmonary outcome: cumulative meta-analyses of randomized, controlled trials. Anesth Analg. 1998;86:598-612.

35. Sentürk M, Ozcan PE, Talu GK, Kiyan E, Camci E, Ozyalçin S, et al. The effects of three different analgesia techniques on long-term post-thoracotomy pain. Anesth Analg. 2002;94:11-5.

36. Richards ER, Kabir SI, McNaught C-E, MacFie J. Effect of thoracic epidural anaesthesia on splanchnic blood flow. Br J Surg. 2013;100:316-21.

37. Lázár G, Kaszaki J, Abrahám S, Horváth G, Wolfárd A, Szentpáli K, et al. Thoracic epidural anesthesia improves the gastric microcirculation during experimental gastric tube formation. Surgery. 2003;134:799-805.

38. Kehlet H, Wilkinson RC, Fischer HB, Camu F. PROSPECT: evidence-based, procedure-specific postoperative pain management. Best Pract Res Clin Anaesthesiol. 2007;21:149-59.

39. Fumagalli U, Melis A, Balazova J, Lascari V, Morenghi E, Rosati R. Intra-operative hypotensive episodes may be associated with post-operative esophageal anastomotic leak. Updat Surg. 2016;68:185-90.

40. Al-Rawi OY, Pennefather SH, Page RD, Dave I, Russell GN. The effect of thoracic epidural bupivacaine and an intravenous adrenaline infusion on gastric tube blood flow during esophagectomy. Anesth Analg. 2008;106:884-7.

41. Pathak D, Pennefather SH, Russell GN, Al Rawi O, Dave IC, Gilby S, et al. Phenylephrine infusion improves blood flow to the stomach during oesophagectomy in the presence of a thoracic epidural analgesia. Eur J Cardio-Thorac Surg. 2013;44:130-3.

42. Ding X, Jin S, Niu X, Ren H, Fu S, Li Q. A comparison of the analgesia efficacy and side effects of paravertebral compared with epidural blockade for thoracotomy: an updated meta-analysis. PLoS One. 2014;9:e96233.

43. Baidya DK, Khanna P, Maitra S. Analgesic efficacy and safety of thoracic paravertebral and epidural analgesia for thoracic surgery: a systematic review and meta-analysis. Interact Cardiovasc Thorac Surg. 2014;18:626-35.

44. Joshi GP, Bonnet F, Shah R, Wilkinson RC, Camu F, Fischer B, et al. A systematic review of randomized trials evaluating regional techniques for postthoracotomy analgesia. Anesth Analg. 2008;107:1026-40.

45. Yeung JHY, Gates S, Naidu BV, Wilson MJA, Gao Smith F. Paravertebral block versus thoracic epidural for patients undergoing thoracotomy. Cochrane Database Syst Rev. 2016;2:CD009121M.

46. Futier E, Constantin J-M, Paugam-Burtz C, Pascal J, Eurin M, Neuschwander A, et al. A trial of intraoperative low-tidal-volume ventilation in abdominal surgery. N Engl J Med. 2013;369:428-37.

47. The PROVE Network Investigators. High versus low positive end-expiratory pressure during general anaesthesia for open abdominal surgery (PROVHILO trial): a multicentre randomised controlled trial. Lancet. 2014;384:495-503.

48. Shen Y, Zhong M, Wu W, Wang H, Feng M, Tan L, et al. The impact of tidal volume on pulmonary complications following minimally invasive esophagectomy: a randomized and controlled study. J Thorac Cardiovasc Surg. 2013;146:1267-74.

49. Michelet P, D'Journo X-B, Roch A, Doddoli C, Marin V, Papazian L, et al. Protective ventilation influences systemic inflammation after esophagectomy: a randomized controlled study. Anesthesiology. 2006;105:911-9.

50. Kim KN, Kim DW, Jeong MA, Sin YH, Lee SK. Comparison of pressure-controlled ventilation with volume-controlled ventilation during one-lung ventilation: a systematic review and meta-analysis. BMC Anesthesiol. 2016;1:72.

51. Veelo DP, Geerts BF. Anaesthesia during oesophagectomy. J Thorac Dis. 2017;9:S705-12.

52. Kita T, Mammoto T, Kishi Y. Fluid management and postoperative respiratory disturbances in patients with transthoracic oesophagectomy for carcinoma. J Clin Anesth. 2002;14:252-6.

53. Glatz T, Kulemann B, Marjanovic G, Bregenzer S, Makowiec F, Hoeppner J. Postoperative fluid overload is a risk factor for adverse surgical outcome in patients undergoing oesophagectomy for esophageal cancer: a retrospective study in 335 patients. BMC Surg. 2017;17:6.

54. Eng OS, Arlow RL, Moore D, Chen C, Langenfeld JE, August DA, et al. Fluid administration and morbidity in transhiatal oesophagectomy. J Surg Res. 2016;200:91-7.

55. Casado D, López F, Martí R. Perioperative fluid management and major respiratory complications in patients undergoing oesophagectomy. Dis Esophagus. 2010;23:523-8.

56. Myles PS, Bellomo R, Corcoran T, Forbes A, Peyton P, Story D, et al. Restrictive versus liberal fluid therapy for major abdominal surgery. N Engl J Med. 2018;378:2263-74.

57. Suehiro K, Okutani R. Stroke volume variation as a predictor of fluid responsiveness in patients undergoing one-lung ventilation. J Cardiothorac Vasc Anesth. 2010;24:772-5.

58. Fu Q, Duan M, Zhao F, Mi W. Evaluation of stroke volume variation and pulse pressure variation as predictors of fluid responsiveness in patients undergoing protective one-lung ventilation. Drug Discov Ther. 2015;9:296-302.

59. Wyffels PA, Sergeant P, Wouters PF. The value of pulse pressure and stroke volume variation as predictors of fluid responsiveness during open chest surgery. Anaesthesia. 2010;65:704-9.

60. Veelo DP, van Berge Henegouwen MI, Ouwehand KS, Geerts BF, Anderegg MC, van Dieren S, et al. Effect of goal-directed therapy on outcome after esophageal surgery: a quality improvement study. PLoS One. 2017;12:e0172806.

61. Haas S, Eichhorn V, Hasbach T, Trepte C, Kutup A, Goetz AE, Reuter DA. Goal-directed fluid therapy using stroke volume variation does not result in pulmonary fluid overload in thoracic surgery requiring one-lung ventilation. Crit Care Res Pract. 2012;2012:687018.

62. Gao Q, Mok HP, Wang WP, Xiao-Feizuo, Chen LQ. Effect of perioperative glucocorticoid administration on postoperative complications following oesophagectomy: a meta-analysis. Oncol Lett. 2014;7:349-56.

63. Engelman E, Maeyens C. Effect of preoperative single-dose corticosteroid administration on postoperative morbidity following oesophagectomy. J Gastrointest Surg. 2010;14:788-804.

64. Zhang L, Wang N, Zhou S, Ye W, Yao Q, Jing G, Zhang M. Preventive effect of ulinastatin on postoperative complications, immunosuppression, and recurrence in oesophagectomy patients. World J Surg Oncol. 2013;11:84.

65. Wang ZQ, Chen LQ, Yuan Y, Wang WP, Niu ZX, Yang YS, et al. Effects of neutrophil elastase inhibitor in patients undergoing oesophagectomy: a systematic review and meta-analysis. World J Gastroenterol. 2015;21:3720-30.

66. Oxenberg J. (2018). Prevention and management of complications from oesophagectomy. [online] https://www.intechopen.com/books/esophageal-cancer-and-beyond/prevention-and-management-of-complications-from-esophagectomy. [Last accessed March, 2020]

67. Schizas D, Kosmopoulos M, Giannopoulos S, Giannopoulos S, Kokkinidis DG, Karampetsou N, et al. Meta-analysis of risk factors and complications associated with atrial fibrillation after oesophagectomy. Br J Surg. 2019;106:534-47.

68. Chen LT, Jiang CY. Impact of atrial arrhythmias after oesophagectomy on recovery: a meta-analysis. Medicine (Baltimore). 2018;97:e10948.

69. Nishimaki T, Suzuki T, Suzuki S, Kuwabara S, Hatakeyama K. Outcomes of extended radical oesophagectomy for thoracic esophageal cancer. J Am Coll Surg. 1998;186:306-12.

CHAPTER

Perioperative Myocardial Infarction

Virendra K Arya, Sunder L Negi, Rajeev Chauhan

INTRODUCTION

Perioperative myocardial infarction (POMI) is one of the very significant and frequently undetected problems after noncardiac surgery. This is evidently associated with morbidity and mortality in the perioperative period.[1] Mortality at 30 days was found around 11.6% in those who had a POMI as compared to 2.2% in those who did not.[2] In comparison with spontaneous myocardial infarction (MI), POMI usually does not manifest with characteristic symptoms of MI, such as chest pain, angina pectoris, or dyspnea, and is consequently overlooked in routine clinical practice.[3] The incidence of POMI is variable; it ranges from 0.3% to 36%.[4] Around 14% of POMI patients exhibit classic chest pain which is very low and only 53% of them show clinical signs or symptoms of ischemia.[5]

Over 290 million surgeries are done annually and an increasing number of surgical patients with elevated cardiovascular risk are resulting in, thus adopting policies to improve the early recognition and treatment, which may have the possibility to provide major medical benefits. An overlooked diagnosis eventually leads to a missed chance for treatment. Therefore, rapid and dependable recognition of POMI is a vital step in efforts targeting for better outcomes of this less valued perioperative complication. Electrocardiogram (ECG) is least sensitive;[6] thus, the detection and quantification of acute cardiomyocyte injury by measuring cardiac troponin (cTn) is decisive for the clinical diagnosis of POMI.[7] Due to silent nature of this pathology and high mortality rates in the perioperative period, the revised global definition of MI recommends a routine monitoring of modern cardiac biomarkers cTns in high-risk patients, both prior to and 48–72 hours after major surgery.[8] Most troponin elevations start within 24–48 hours after surgery and are ascribed to postoperative stress.[9]

Perioperative myocardial infarction is an event of myocardial ischemia happening during or in the days after noncardiac surgery. The joint task force [European Society of Cardiology, American College of Cardiology (ACC) Foundation, American Heart Association (AHA), and World Heart Federation] defines POMI as myocardial necrosis in a clinical setting consistent with acute MI, and the most common diagnostic criteria consist of an elevated troponin value with either an ischemic symptom or an ischemic electrocardiographic finding.[10] Prevention of a POMI is an important prerequisite for the enhancement of the overall postoperative outcome, and planning effective preventive measures will require fundamental understanding of the etiology of POMI.

PATHOPHYSIOLOGY OF PERIOPERATIVE MYOCARDIAL INFARCTION

Despite uncertainty about the leading pathophysiology of POMI, two different pathophysiologic mechanisms are proposed that may cause POMI:
1. Type 1 POMI is related to acute coronary thrombosis.
2. Type 2 POMI is related to myocardial oxygen demand–supply mismatch when in the setting of stable coronary artery disease (CAD), compromised myocardial oxygen supply is unable to match for increased oxygen demand due to perioperative stress.[11]

Acute Coronary Syndrome (Type 1 Perioperative Myocardial Infarction)

Plaque rupture on the intimal surface of a vessel is a complex process involving multiple cellular processes that stimulate plaque instability and physical processes that regulate the dispersal of stress on the plaque (**Flowchart 1**). During various kinds of vigorous physical activity and emotional stress, plaque rupture is more common.[12] A cascade of platelet aggregation and release of mediators including thromboxane A$_2$, serotonin, adenosine diphosphate, platelet-activating factor, thrombin, and oxygen-derived free radicals is triggered by the endothelial injury at the

Flowchart 1: Unstable coronary artery disease.

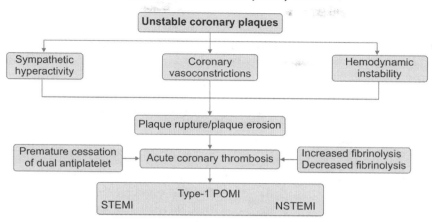

(NSTEMI: non-ST-elevation myocardial infarction; POMI: perioperative myocardial infarction; STEMI: ST-elevation myocardial infarction)

Flowchart 2: Severe but stable coronary artery disease.

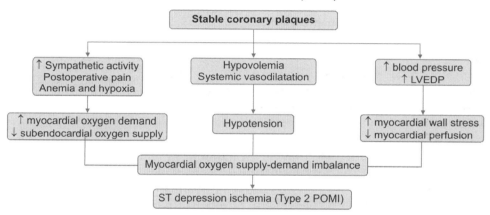

(LVEDP: left ventricular end-diastolic pressure; POMI: perioperative myocardial infarction; ↑: increase; ↓ decrease)

site of a plaque rupture. Platelet aggregation and activation of various inflammatory and noninflammatory mediators augment thrombus formation and lead to dynamic vasoconstriction distal to the thrombus. The collective effects of dynamic and physical blood vessel narrowing produce ischemia or infarction. This condition is further deteriorated by distal embolization of microthrombi and coronary spasm caused by local release of vasoconstrictors or systemic sympathetic stimulation.

During the perioperative period, stress response triggered by pain and tissue injury activates the sympathetic nervous system, hypothalamic pituitary axis, and renin angiotensin system, a combination of which leads to hypertension, tachycardia and increased plasma concentrations of catecholamines, and blood viscosity. These are accompanied by considerable increases in platelet aggregation and decreases in fibrinolytic activity, which favor thrombosis.[13] This combination of reduced fibrinolytic and increased prothrombotic activity could

trigger proliferation of clot and total blockade of the coronary artery by a mural thrombus overlying a small plaque erosion that might otherwise have been harmless.

Myocardial Oxygen Supply–Demand Imbalance (Type 2 Perioperative Myocardial Infarction)

The myocardial oxygen utilization is primarily determined by heart rate, myocardial contractility, and wall stress (**Flowchart 2**). A rise in heart rate shortens diastole and thus can decrease subendocardial perfusion. Coronary perfusion pressure may reduce as a result of systemic hypotension or increased left ventricular end-diastolic pressure (LVEDP). Ventricular relaxation is impaired with the onset of ischemia, which further compromises perfusion due to decreased subendocardial perfusion time and decreased diastolic compliance resulting in increased LVEDP. Tachycardia is the most common cause of postoperative oxygen supply–demand disparity.[14] Postoperative hypotension secondary to hypovolemia, bleeding, or systemic vasodilatation; hypertension due to elevated stress hormones or vasoconstriction; anemia, hypoxemia, and hypercarbia—these all worsen ischemia.[15] Stress-induced and ischemia-induced coronary vasoconstriction furthermore reduces coronary perfusion.[16] Moreover, systolic and/or diastolic dysfunction typical of patients with CAD is deteriorated by ischemia and volume overload, ensuing cardiac decompensation and type 2 POMI.[17]

PREVENTION

Preoperative Evaluation

Major adverse cardiac events in noncardiac surgery are responsible for 50% of perioperative mortality.[18] Primarily, two factors contribute to perioperative risk:

1. Type of surgery and degree of hemodynamic cardiac stress associated with surgery-specific techniques
2. Patient characteristics

The aim of the preoperative assessment is to recognize patients with high perioperative cardiac risk in noncardiac surgery. Risk stratification for POMI should be an essential part of preoperative assessment.

The Revised Cardiac Risk Index (RCRI) score is the most frequently used cardiovascular risk score. This is a simple, authenticated, and well-established tool for the evaluation of perioperative risk of major cardiac complications.[19] It has six prognosticators for major cardiac complications (**Table 1**). A patient with 0 or 1 prognosticator of risk would have a low risk. Patients with ≥2 prognosticators of risk would have high risk. Contemporary guidelines[20] advocate

the use of National Surgical Quality Improvement Program (NSQIP) risk calculator developed by the American College of Surgeons (ACS).[21]

The standard 12-lead ECG is an insensitive test of the risk for myocardial ischemia. It is normal in up to 50% of patients with CAD, and in conduction defects it renders the ECG uninterpretable for ischemia.[22] For patients with known CAD or other significant structural heart disease, preoperative resting 12-lead ECG is sensible, except for low-risk surgery. This may also be considered for asymptomatic patients undergoing high-risk surgery.[23]

A dependable predictor of perioperative and long-term cardiac events is the functional status of the patient and it can be realized during history taking. Effort tolerance is classified as excellent when metabolic equivalent of task (MET) is >10, good (7–10 METs), moderate (4–6 METs), poor (<4 METs), or unknown. Perioperative cardiac problems are increased in patients who have poor functional reserve evidenced by inability to perform 4 METs of work during routine activities. For patients with an excellent (>10 METs) functional capacity, it is sensible to forgo further exercise testing with cardiac imaging and proceed to even high-risk surgery.[24] Cardiopulmonary exercise testing is recommended for patients undergoing high-risk procedures in whom functional capacity is not known.[25] It is realistic for patients who are at a high risk for noncardiac surgery and have poor functional capacity (<4 METs) to undertake noninvasive pharmacological stress testing either with dobutamine stress echocardiogram (DSE) or with pharmacological stress myocardial perfusion imaging (MPI) if these tests will alter the management.[26]

MEDICATIONS

Beta-blocker

Beta-blockers are important drugs for cardiac prophylaxis and treatment following an acute coronary syndrome. β-blockers mainly safeguard the heart by controlling the maximum increase in heart rate secondary to stress response during the perioperative period, but at an added risk of perioperative hypotension. The Perioperative Ischemic Evaluation (POISE) trial reported a substantial decrease in the occurrence of MI postoperatively, but accompanied by an increase in overall mortality due to a significant increase in stroke.[27] For patients who are found at intermediate or high risk for myocardial ischemia during preoperative risk stratification tests, it may be rational to begin perioperative β-blockers.[28] Starting β-blockers <1 day before surgery is not only ineffective but may in fact be detrimental.[29] Patients already getting β-blockers should continue to take them. Earlier starting and titration of β-blockers few weeks before the surgery whether improves outcome remains unclear.[30]

Table 1: Revised Cardiac Risk Index (RCRI) components and expected cardiac risk.	
Components of RCRI	**Points assigned**
High-risk surgery (intraperitoneal, intrathoracic, or suprainguinal vascular procedure)	1
Ischemic heart disease	1
History of congestive heart failure	1
History of cerebrovascular disease	1
Diabetes mellitus requiring insulin	1
Creatinine > 2.0 mg/dL	1
RCRI score	**Risk of major cardiac events**
0	0.4%
1	1.0%
2	2.4%
≥3	5.4%

Aspirin

Aspirin is an integral part of primary and secondary cardiovascular prevention in the nonsurgical setting; however, the augmented bleeding risk complicates its perioperative utility.[31] The POISE-2 trial has shown that continuing or starting aspirin did not have protective effect for cardiac complications and death during perioperative period in patients undergoing noncardiac surgery.[32] Continuation of aspirin in a patient already taking may be considered and the risk of increased bleeding should be balanced against the cardiovascular benefit.[7]

Statins

Statin is a hydroxymethylglutaryl coenzyme A (HMG Co-A) reductase inhibitor and it has multiple effects that include lowering the cholesterol levels, plaque stabilization, and immunomodulation. It is suggested to continue an established therapy in the perioperative period[7,31] as withdrawal could increase the risk of cardiovascular complications.[33] Two meta-analyses reported less rate of cardiovascular complications after noncardiac surgery; however, excluding vascular surgery patients, no significant change in overall mortality was found.[33,34] Hence, proof regarding the benefit of newly initiated statin therapy is limited to vascular surgery, where it is advocated to initiate statin therapy, preferably >2 weeks before the surgery.[7] In this group of patients, even starting statins perioperatively is reasonable.[35]

Dual Antiplatelet Therapy

Dual antiplatelet therapy is a necessity following a spontaneous MI or postcoronary stenting.[36] Early stoppage for surgery is correlated with high risk of potentially lethal stent thrombosis.[37] Hence, recommendations are to delay elective surgery pending the end of the typical time course for dual antiplatelet therapy following percutaneous intervention.[7] Existing guidelines strongly recommend dual antiplatelet therapy to continue for at least 4 weeks post bare metal stent implantation and for at least a year after drug-eluting coronary stenting.[7] Using antithrombin, anticoagulants, or glycoprotein IIb/IIIa agents for the purpose of "Bridging" stent patients has not been shown successful.

Coronary Revascularization

Preoperative prophylactic coronary revascularization has not been shown to improve outcome despite the fact that it might look a tempting possibility.[38] Prophylactic preoperative coronary revascularization, mostly by coronary artery bypass graft (CABG) to optimize cardiac status, was associated with improved outcomes only in patients undergoing major vascular surgery.[39] Preoperative coronary artery revascularization showed a benefit only in the subgroup of patients with unprotected left main disease.[40]

Dual antiplatelet therapy increases the vulnerability for bleeding. Hence, this possibility must be balanced against the risk of in-stent thrombosis when early interruption of antiplatelet agents is required. Consequently, the AHA/ACC guideline in 2014 recommends that elective surgery be deferred and that urgent or emergency surgery has a multidisciplinary conversation and shared decision-making concerning the danger and advantage of continuing or stopping antiplatelet agents perioperatively.[30] Aspirin should not be stopped whenever possible.

Choice of Anesthetic Technique

Administering anesthesia to patients with known CAD or high risk is challenging. Induction of anesthesia in a patient with high risk undergoing noncardiac surgery should be smooth. In patients with normal left ventricular (LV) function, a combination of opioid and volatile agent or intravenous (IV) anesthetic agent is acceptable. Etomidate causes minimum hemodynamic changes. In patients with impaired LV function, etomidate is a drug of choice along with potent opioid like fentanyl or sufentanil. Systematic appraisal of volatile versus IV anesthesia showed similar effectiveness of both.[41] The use of neuraxial blocks, nerve blocks, and facial plan blocks instead of or supplementing general anesthesia and goal-directed volume therapy may possibly improve outcome.[42]

▌ INTENSIVE CARE UNIT MANAGEMENT

The diagnostic pathway in POMI in perioperative settings differs from that for patients exhibiting a classical MI. The occurrence of chest pain in POMI is very low.[43] Residual effects of anesthetics and analgesia often mask the chest pain, even if it is present. The initial ECG findings are normal in 10% of nonsurgical patients after MI. They are diagnostic only in 50% of cases. Though they are abnormal, they are not diagnostic in 40% of MI cases.[44] In intraoperative period under general anesthesia patient will not complain of chest pain but may have hypotension, arrhythmias, appearance of new heart murmur, desaturation episodes, and signs of congestive heart failure. If transesophageal echocardiography (TEE) is used in selected cases, new regional wall motion abnormalities (RWMAs) or mitral regurgitations could be earliest most sensitive and specific indicators of POMI. However, most of POMI occur during early postoperative period and are without symptoms.

Biomarkers

Latest cardiac biological markers are cTns that are quickly discharged into the circulation after myocyte injury. They are almost absolutely specific for myocardial tissue injury and also have very high sensitivity.[45] Hence, these are currently the biomarkers of choice to identify myocardial injury. The cTns are highly specific and sensitive cardiac markers for detection of POMI than the creatine kinase-MB (CK-MB) isoenzyme.[14] Creatine phosphokinase-MB (CPK-MB) concentrations may rise only 10–20 times of normal during infarction and return to normal within 72 hours while the cardiac troponins T (cTnT) and cardiac troponins I (cTnI) levels may rise more than 20 times above the reference range within 3 hours after onset of chest pain and may persist for up to 10–14 days. This may assist in late diagnosis of infarction. Postoperative increases in cTnT >0.1 ng/mL were associated with postoperative cardiac events within the first 6 months following noncardiac surgery; postoperative increases in cTnT >0.02 ng/mL suggested a 15-fold increase in 1-year mortality in elderly patients undergoing noncardiac surgery.[46] All-cause mortality likelihood within the first 6 months after vascular surgery was facilitated by routine cTnI measurements during the first 3 postoperative days of surgery.[47] Even small increases in serum concentrations of cTns in the perioperative period suggest clinically significant myocardial injury with short- and long-term effects on outcome. Hence, perioperative measurements in high-risk patients are suggested that may enable early initiation of suitable diagnostic and therapeutic actions, which may affect long-term cardiac outcome. To date, there are no decisive criteria or recommendations for the diagnosis of POMI in the surgical setting; however, any rise of cTns in thousands is very definitive sign of POMI even soon after cardiac surgery.

Electrocardiogram Monitoring

Perioperative myocardial infarction is frequently silent. The ECG mostly does not show specific ST-segment elevation or Q-waves and is often difficult to interpret.[14] Low incidence of chest pain makes the diagnosis of POMI more difficult. Residual anesthetics and analgesia often mask POMI-associated pain. As mentioned before the initial ECG findings are not specific of POMI in 60% of patients.[44] Thus, the diagnosis of POMI based exclusively on the classical triad leads to substantial underreporting of its true occurrence and probably obscure the etiology of POMI. Under these circumstances of the frequent absence of typical symptoms and ECG signs of acute POMI, the diagnosis of POMI has to depend greatly on changes in biochemical markers. The VISION (Vascular Events in Noncardiac Surgery Cohort Evaluation) study reported ECG changes only in 35% of all patients having POMI, signifying that ECG monitoring might not be sensitive enough to find POMIs.

The World Health Organization (WHO) recommends that at least two of the following three criteria must be fulfilled to diagnose MI:

1. Typical chest pain
2. Increased serum concentration of creatine kinase (CK)-MB isoenzyme
3. Typical electrocardiographic findings, including development of pathological Q-waves.[48] This definition provides adequate specificity but lacks high sensitivity.

A joint task force of the European Society of Cardiology and the ACC recommended that the definition of MI be broadened.[49] Either of the two following criteria meets the diagnosis of an acute, evolving, or a recent MI:

- Typical rise and gradual fall in cTnT and cTnI concentrations or more rapid rise and fall of CK-MB concentration in combination with at least one of the following:
  - Typical ischemic symptoms
  - Development of pathological Q-waves in the ECG
  - Electrocardiogram changes indicative of myocardial ischemia (ST-segment elevation or depression)
  - Coronary artery intervention
- Pathological findings of an acute MI.

Transesophageal Echocardiography

The use of TEE is now routine in the operating room for cardiac surgery but is less often used in noncardiac surgery. For trained and experienced anesthesiologists, TEE can be valuable in the early detection of myocardial ischemia.[50] The earliest manifestation of myocardial ischemia or infarction is the ventricular diastolic dysfunction followed by regional wall motion abnormalities and followed by ECG changes. The elective and emergency use of perioperative TEE in high-risk noncardiac patients is justifiable in the settings or in anticipation of refractory hemodynamic instability that is nonresponsive to attempted corrective therapy to determine the cause of hemodynamic instability, if expertise is readily available.

TREATMENT

Cardiovascular complications are very frequently encountered but underappreciated during the perioperative period and are the major contributors to morbidity and mortality in noncardiac surgery.[51] Devereaux et al. reported POMI incidence of 5.0% among patients aged 45 years or older undergoing noncardiac surgery.[2] POMI incidence rates of 0.25% for total hip arthroplasty and 0.18% for total knee arthroplasty have been reported.[52] A retrospective study by Li et al. showed an overall POMI incidence of 5.2 per 10,000 following noncardiac surgery.[53]

The basic principle for POMI management is to differentiate between type 1 POMI and type 2 POMI because the treatment recommendations for type 1 and type 2 POMI are different. Type 1 POMI implicates the rupture of atherosclerotic plaques and the formation of a thrombus. Hence, type 1 POMI has been shown to benefit from anticoagulation, platelet inhibition, and early coronary revascularization,[54] whereas these treatments may harm patients with type 2 POMI due to bleeding risks in perioperative settings and due to different etiology in type 2 POMI which is an imbalance between myocardial oxygen demand and supply.[55] Rapid correction of the underlying conditions such as volume replacement in the case of hypotension, heart rate control in case of tachycardia and blood transfusion in case of anemia would benefit type 2 POMI patients.[56]

All causes of increased heart rate, high or low blood pressure, anemia and pain must be treated aggressively. An understanding of the patient's baseline and postoperative myocardial and coronary physiology is essential for the treatment of tachycardia with concomitant hypotension which is often challenging. ST elevation or intractable cardiogenic shock is the only indication for emergency coronary intervention which involves coronary revascularization or glycoprotein IIb/IIIa antagonists in the immediate postoperative period.[57]

In pragmatic clinical practice, during postoperative period, the differential diagnosis between type 1 POMI and type 2 POMI is challenging. Present guidelines recommend some diagnostic clues such as type 1 POMI usually manifest with spontaneous symptom onset, associated with ECG changes, higher cTn rise and absence of conditions leading to increased myocardial oxygen consumption and decreased blood flow.[55] In real world of perioperative setting these are difficult to apply.[58] The best principles seem to be whether there are situations present that suggest type 2 MI[59] such as longer periods of tachycardia, hypotension, respiratory failure, or anemia.

Some of the basic principles to be followed in ICU care for the management of POMI irrespective of type are:

- Maintain hemodynamic stability which includes norepinephrine as the first line of drug for POMI-related cardiogenic shock. Vasopressin infusion up to 2.4 IU/h should be considered early if norepinephrine doses required are >0.1 µg/kg/min. Starting dose of vasopressin is 0.6 IU/h and boluses should be avoided as they are associated with intestinal ischemia.
- *Correction of volume status*: Small boluses of fluids 250 m at a time to correct hypovolemia as filling pressures may be already elevated due to cardiac dysfunction and larger volume may worsen pulmonary congestion and hypoxia. These boluses should be titrated with left

ventricular outflow tract velocity time integral (LVOT VTI) (indicator of LV stroke volume) and only should be repeated if improvement in LVOT VTI is seen.

- Drug of choice for POMI-related arrhythmias remains amiodarone and digoxin as second line in the setting of cardiogenic shock. In extreme cases of electric storm related to POMI, induction of complete atrioventricular (AV) block by loading doses of combination of amiodarone, digoxin, lignocaine, procainamide together and subsequent pacing with dual chamber paced, sensed and response mode (DDD) mode of pacer with heart rate of 70–80/min is effective. However, this therapy may necessitate back up of mechanical support such as intra-aortic balloon pump (IABP) or extracorporeal membrane oxygenation (ECMO) to maintain circulation.
- In cases of refractory cardiogenic shock due to POMI and structural complications of POMI such as ventricular septal defect (VSD) and ventricular rupture, some form of mechanical assist device is indicated such as IABP, ECMO or left ventricle/right ventricle assist device (LVAD/RVAD) or both, or Impala, etc. during resuscitative phase. The choice of device remains on the degree of shock, residual cardiac contractility and cardiorespiratory collapse. In cases of rising lactate, deteriorating renal functions and pulmonary edema, ECMO is preferred over IABP. Also, IABP cannot be used with patients who have grade 4 and 5 atheroma in descending aorta.
- Important question about thrombolysis for ST-elevation myocardial infarction (STEMI) in POMI within 30 minutes of diagnosis remains to be answered by shared decision-making between the various team members and patient relatives weighing the relative risks of bleeding versus thrombolysis or heparin use. Neurosurgical procedures demand not using any anticoagulation for at least 24–48 hours. Here only supportive therapy needs to be maintained in terms of cardiorespiratory support by ventilation, cardiac-assist devices, and drugs till definitive intervention can be done. In a high-risk bleeding case, ECMO with heparin-coated circuits can be used without any anticoagulations if flows are kept >3 L/min; however, circuit may need replacement after 5–7 days of use and fibrinogen levels and fibrinogen degradation product (FDP) levels need to be regularly monitored along with a transoxygenator gradient for any micro-thrombosis blocking oxygenator.
- One important question for patients who receive thrombolysis for STEMI or pulmonary embolism remains is when to start heparin as maintenance therapy. The answer to this lies in 12 hourly monitoring of activated partial thromboplastin time (APTT). When APTT comes back to 1.5–2 of normal value post thrombolysis, heparin infusion 1,000 IU/h should be started and titrated to

target APTT value without loading bolus till definite intervention is done.

- For ventilated and intubated patients sedation with ketofol (1,000 mg propofol + 100 mg ketamine) mixture at the rate of 20–30 µg/kg/min (1–1.5 mg/kg/h) of propofol usually gives 2–5 µg/kg/min of ketamine (analgesic dose) and is quite effective way of amnesia, analgesia, and sedation without much hemodynamic effects. Alternatively, dexmedetomidine 0.2–0.5 µg/kg/h alone or with propofol or with ketamine analgesic dose is good alternative.

- There is some evidence to suggest that a higher transfusion limit (such as Hb 100 g/dL) might result in better outcome for patients with acute coronary syndrome; however, the evidence is weak and moreover no survival benefit has been confirmed with higher transfusion thresholds in patients who are at risk of cardiovascular disease perioperatively.

- Some evidence suggests that mild hypothermia is associated with increased perioperative myocardial ischemia and cardiac events as compared to normothermia. Attention should be given to the normothermic temperature control of these patients in ICU.

- In any situation of POMI, the goal of ICU care remains supportive therapy and to move patients on first available opportunity to cardiac catheterization laboratory for definitive diagnosis and intervention. Choice of intervention percutaneous coronary intervention (PCI) versus CABG or type of stents is again based on shared decision-making among various teams and patient relatives considering all possible risk benefit ratios.

All these recommendations are derived from the treatment of spontaneous acute myocardial infarction (AMI); however, the robust guidelines for treatment of POMI are still lacking. More research needs to be done in future.

CONCLUSION

The identification of patients at the risk of POMI is one of the main purposes of preoperative evaluation. The early identification and management of perioperative myocardial ischemia/infarction is especially important to start secondary prevention early in order to prevent untoward cardiac complications. Patients who have sustained a POMI should have their subsequent management by multidisciplinary team consisting of intensivists, cardiologists, anesthetists, surgeons, pharmacologists, and nursing. Once medical and resuscitative therapy optimized, the timing of coronary angiography should be considered on the basis of early risk stratification. The pathophysiology involves in POMI and its management is quite different from medical acute MI settings. In future, more randomized controlled trials are required in this patient population for definitive management strategies.

REFERENCES

1. Devereaux PJ, Chan MT, Alonso-Coello P, Walsh M, Berwanger O, Villar JC, et al. Association between postoperative troponin levels and 30-day mortality among patients undergoing noncardiac surgery. JAMA. 2012;307(21):2295-304.

2. Devereaux PJ, Xavier D, Pogue J, Guyatt G, Sigamani A, Garutti I, et al. Characteristics and short-term prognosis of perioperative myocardial infarction in patients undergoing noncardiac surgery: a cohort study. Ann Intern Med. 2011;154(8):523-8.

3. van Waes JA, Nathoe HM, de Graaff JC, Kemperman H, de Borst GJ, Peelen LM, et al. Myocardial injury after noncardiac surgery and its association with short-term mortality. Circulation. 2013;127(23):2264-71.

4. Idris H, Lo S, Shugman IM, Saad Y, Hopkins AP, Mussap C, et al. Varying definitions for periprocedural myocardial infarction alter event rates and prognostic implications. J Am Heart Assoc. 2014;3(6):e001086.

5. Devereaux PJ, Goldman L, Yusuf S, Gilbert K, Leslie K, Guyatt GH. Surveillance and prevention of major perioperative ischemic cardiac events in patients undergoing noncardiac surgery: a review. CMAJ. 2005;173(7):779-88.

6. Botto F, Alonso-Coello P, Chan MT, Villar JC, Xavier D, Srinathan S, et al. Myocardial injury after noncardiac surgery: a large, international, prospective cohort study establishing diagnostic criteria, characteristics, predictors, and 30-day outcomes. Anesthesiology. 2014;120(3):564-78.

7. Kristensen SD, Knuuti J, Saraste A, Anker S, Bøtker HE, Hert SD, et al. 2014 ESC/ESA Guidelines on non-cardiac surgery: Cardiovascular assessment and management: The joint task force on non-cardiac surgery: Cardiovascular assessment and management of the European Society of Cardiology (ESC) and the European Society of Anaesthesiology (ESA). Eur Heart J. 2014;35(35):2383-431.

8. Thygesen K, Alpert JS, Jaffe AS, Simoons ML, Chaitman BR, White HD, et al. Third universal definition of myocardial infarction. J Am Coll Cardiol. 2012;60(16):1581-98.

9. Dawood MM, Gutpa DK, Southern J, Walia A, Atkinson JB, Eagle KA. Pathology of fatal perioperative myocardial infarction: Implications regarding pathophysiology and prevention. Int J Cardiol. 1996;57(1):37-44.

10. Thygesen K, Alpert JS, Jaffe AS, Simoons ML, Chaitman BR, White HD, et al. Third universal definition of myocardial infarction. Circulation. 2012;126(16):2020-35.

11. Thygesen K, Alpert JS, White HD; Joint ESC/ACCF/AHA/WHF Task Force for the Redefinition of Myocardial Infarction. Universal definition of myocardial infarction. J Am Coll Cardiol. 2007;50(22):2173-95.

12. Mittleman MA, Maclure M, Tofler GH, Sherwood JB, Goldberg RJ, Muller JE. Triggering of acute myocardial infarction by heavy physical exertion. Protection against triggering by regular

exertion. Determinants of myocardial infarction onset study investigators. N Engl J Med. 1993;329(23):1677-83

13. World Health Organization MONICA Project (monitoring trends and determinants in cardiovascular disease): a major international collaboration. WHO MONICA Project Principal Investigators. J Clin Epidemiol. 1988;41(2):105-14.

14. Landesberg G, Mosseri M, Zahger D, Wolf Y, Perouansky M, Anner H, et al. Myocardial infarction after vascular surgery: the role of prolonged stress-induced, ST depression-type ischemia. J Am Coll Cardiol. 2001;37(7):1839-45.

15. Nelson AH, Fleisher LA, Rosenbaum SH. Relationship between postoperative anemia and cardiac morbidity in high-risk vascular patients in the intensive care unit. Crit Care Med. 1993;21(6):860-6.

16. Sambuceti G, Marzilli M, Fedele S, Marini C, L'Abbate A. Paradoxical increase in microvascular resistance during tachycardia downstream from a severe stenosis in patients with coronary artery disease: reversal by angioplasty. Circulation. 2001;103(19):2352-60.

17. Landesberg G. The pathophysiology of perioperative myocardial infarction: facts and perspectives. J Cardiothorac Vasc Anesth. 2003;17(1):90-100.

18. Devereaux PJ, Goldman L, Cook DJ, Gilbert K, Leslie K, Guyatt GH. Perioperative cardiac events in patients undergoing noncardiac surgery: a review of the magnitude of the problem, the pathophysiology of the events and methods to estimate and communicate risk. CMAJ. 2005;173(6):627-34.

19. Lee TH, Marcantonio ER, Mangione CM, Thomas EJ, Polanczyk CA, Cook EF, et al. Derivation and prospective validation of a simple index for prediction of cardiac risk of major noncardiac surgery. Circulation. 1999;100(10):1043-9.

20. Fleisher LA, Fleischmann KE, Auerbach AD, Barnason SA, Beckman JA, Bozkurt B, et al. 2014 ACC/AHA guideline on perioperative cardiovascular evaluation and management of patients undergoing noncardiac surgery: a report of the American College of Cardiology/American Heart Association Task Force on practice guidelines. J Am Coll Cardiol. 2014;64(22):e77-137.

21. Gupta PK, Gupta H, Sundaram A, Kaushik M, Fang X, Miller WJ, et al. Development and validation of a risk calculator for prediction of cardiac risk after surgery. Circulation. 2011;124(4):381-7.

22. Payne CJ, Payne AR, Gibson SC, Jardine AG, Berry C, Kingsmore DB. Is there still a role for preoperative 12-lead electrocardiography. World J Surg. 2011;35(12):2611-6.

23. van Klei WA, Bryson GL, Yang H, Kalkman CJ, Wells GA, Beattie WS. The value of routine preoperative electrocardiography in predicting myocardial infarction after non-cardiac surgery. Ann Surg. 2007;246(2):165-70.

24. Tsiouris A, Horst HM, Paone G, Hodari A, Eichenhorn M, Rubinfeld I. Preoperative risk stratification for thoracic surgery using the American College of Surgeons National Surgical Quality Improvement Program data set: Functional status predicts morbidity and mortality. J Surg Res. 2012;177(1):1-6.

25. Hartley RA, Pichel AC, Grant SW, Hickey GL, Lancaster PS, Wisely NA. Preoperative cardiopulmonary exercise testing and

26. Morgan PB, Panomitros GE, Nelson AC, Smith DF, Solanki DR, Zornow MH. Low utility of dobutamine stress echocardiograms in the preoperative evaluation of patients scheduled for noncardiac surgery. Anesth Analg. 2002;95(3):512-6.

27. Devereaux PJ, Yang H, Yusuf S, Guyatt G, Leslie K, Villar JC, et al. Effects of extended-release metoprolol succinate in patients undergoing non-cardiac surgery (POISE trial): a randomised controlled trial. Lancet. 2008;371(9627):1839-47.

28. Boersma E, Poldermans D, Bax JJ, Steyerberg EW, Thomson IR, Banga JD, et al. Predictors of cardiac events after major vascular surgery: role of clinical characteristics, dobutamine echocardiography, and beta-blocker therapy. JAMA. 2001;285(14):1865-73.

29. Dai N, Xu D, Zhang J, Wei Y, Li W, Fan B, et al. Different β-blockers and initiation time in patients undergoing noncardiac surgery: a meta-analysis. Am J Med Sci. 2014;347(3):235-44.

30. Wijeysundera DN, Duncan D, Nkonde-Price C, Virani SS, Washam JB, Fleischmann KE, et al. Perioperative beta blockade in noncardiac surgery: A systematic review for the 2014 ACC/AHA guideline on perioperative cardiovascular evaluation and management of patients undergoing noncardiac surgery: A report of the American College of Cardiology/American Heart Association Task Force on practice guidelines. J Am Coll Cardiol. 2014;64(22):2406-25.

31. Montalescot G, Sechtem U, Achenbach S, Andreotti F, Arden C, Budaj A, et al. 2013 ESC guidelines on the management of stable coronary artery disease: the task force on the management of stable coronary artery disease of the European Society of Cardiology. Eur Heart J. 2013;34(38):2949-3003.

32. Junejo MA, Mason JM, Sheen AJ, Moore J, Foster P, Atkinson D, et al. Cardiopulmonary exercise testing for preoperative risk assessment before hepatic resection. Br J Surg. 2012;99(8): 1097-104.

33. Le Manach Y, Godet G, Coriat P, Martinon C, Bertrand M, Fléron MH, et al. The impact of postoperative discontinuation or continuation of chronic statin therapy on cardiac outcome after major vascular surgery. Anesth Analg. 2007;104(6):1326-33.

34. Winchester DE, Wen X, Xie L, Bavry AA. Evidence of pre-procedural statin therapy a meta-analysis of randomized trials. J Am Coll Cardiol. 2010;56(14):1099-109.

35. Durazzo AE, Machado FS, Ikeoka DT, De Bernoche C, Monachini MC, Puech-Leão P, et al. Reduction in cardiovascular events after vascular surgery with atorvastatin: a randomized trial. J Vasc Surg. 2004;39(5):967-75.

36. Winjns W, Kolh P, Danchin N, Di Mario C, Falk V, Folliguet T. Guidelines on myocardial revascularization. Rev Port Cardiol. 2010;29(9):1441-2.

37. Kałuza GL, Joseph J, Lee JR, Raizner ME, Raizner AE. Catastrophic outcomes of noncardiac surgery soon after coronary stenting. J Am Coll Cardiol. 2000;35(5):1288-94.

38. McFalls EO, Ward HB, Moritz TE, Goldman S, Krupski WC, Littooy F, et al. Coronary-artery revascularization before elective major vascular surgery. N Engl J Med. 2004;351(27):2795-804.

39. Kertai MD. Preoperative coronary revascularization in high-risk patients undergoing vascular surgery: a core review. Anesth Analg. 2008;106(3):751-8.

40. Garcia S, Moritz TE, Ward HB, Pierpont G, Goldman S, Larsen GC, et al. Usefulness of revascularization of patients with multivessel coronary artery disease before elective vascular surgery for abdominal aortic and peripheral occlusive disease. Am J Cardiol. 2008;102(7):809-13.

41. Lindholm EE, Aune E, Norén CB, Seljeflot I, Hayes T, Otterstad JE, et al. The anesthesia in abdominal aortic surgery (ABSENT) study: a prospective, randomized, controlled trial comparing troponin T release with fentanyl-sevoflurane and propofol-remifentanil anesthesia in major vascular surgery. Anesthesiology. 2013;119(4):802-12.

42. Kristensen SD, Knuuti J. New ESC/ESA guidelines on non-cardiac surgery: cardiovascular assessment and management. Eur Heart J. 2014;35(35):2344-5.

43. Ashton CM, Petersen JN, Wray NP, Kiefe CI, Dunn JK, Wu L, et al. The incidence of perioperative myocardial infarction in men undergoing noncardiac surgery. Ann Intern Med. 1993;118(7):504-10.

44. Zimetbaum PJ, Josephson ME. Use of the electrocardiogram in acute myocardial infarction. N Engl J Med. 2003;348(10):933-40.

45. Wu AH, Apple FS, Gibler WB, Jesse RL, Warshaw MM, Valdes R Jr. National academy of clinical biochemistry standards of laboratory practice: recommendations for the use of cardiac markers in coronary artery diseases. Clin Chem. 1999;45(7):1104-21.

46. Oscarsson A, Eintrei C, Anskär S, Engdahl O, Fagerström L, Blomqvist P, et al. Troponin T-values provide long-term prognosis in elderly patients undergoing non-cardiac surgery. Acta Anaesthesiol Scand. 2004;48(9):1071-9.

47. Kim LJ, Martinez EA, Faraday N, Dorman T, Fleisher LA, Perler BA, et al. Cardiac troponin I predicts short-term mortality in vascular surgery patients. Circulation. 2002;106(18):2366-71.

48. Tunstall-Pedoe H, Kuulasmaa K, Amouyel P, Arveiler D, Rajakangas AM, Pajak A. Myocardial infarction and coronary deaths in the World Health Organization MONICA Project. Registration procedures, event rates, and case-fatality rates in 38 populations from 21 countries in four continents. Circulation. 1994;90(1):583-612.

49. Myocardial infarction redefined—a consensus document of the Joint European Society of Cardiology/American College of Cardiology Committee for the redefinition of myocardial infarction. Eur Heart J. 2000;21(18):1502-13.

50. Harris SH. Hypotension, hypertension, perioperative myocardial ischemia and infarction. In: Benumof JL, Saidman LJ (Eds). Anesthesia and Perioperative Complications, 2nd edition. St Louis: Mosby; 1999. pp. 293-307.

51. Ollila A, Vikatmaa L, Virolainen J, Vikatmaa P, Leppäniemi A, Albäck A, et al. Perioperative myocardial infarction in non-cardiac surgery patients: a prospective observational study. Scand J Surg. 2017;106(2):180-6.

52. Menendez ME, Memtsoudis SG, Opperer M, Boettner F, Gonzalez Della Valle A. A nationwide analysis of risk factors for in-hospital myocardial infarction after total joint arthroplasty. Int Orthop. 2015;39(4):777-86.

53. Li SL, Wang DX, Wu XM, Li N, Xie YQ. Perioperative acute myocardial infarction increases mortality following noncardiac surgery. J Cardiothorac Vasc Anesth. 2013;27(6):1277-81.

54. Thygesen K, Alpert JS, Jaffe AS, Simoons ML, Chaitman BR, White HD, et al. Third universal definition of myocardial infarction. Eur Heart J. 2012;33(20):2551-67.

55. Gualandro DM, Calderaro D, Yu PC, Caramelli B. Acute myocardial infarction after noncardiac surgery. Arq Bras Cardiol. 2012;99(5):1060-7.

56. Gualandro DM, Campos CA, Calderaro D, Yu PC, Marques AC, Pastana AF, et al. Coronary plaque rupture in patients with myocardial infarction after noncardiac surgery: frequent and dangerous. Atherosclerosis. 2012;222(1):191-5.

57. Berger PB, Bellot V, Bell MR, Horlocker TT, Rihal CS, Hallett JW, et al. An immediate invasive strategy for the treatment of acute myocardial infarction early after noncardiac surgery. Am J Cardiol. 2001;87(9):1100-2, A6, A9.

58. Alpert JS, Thygesen KA, White HD, Jaffe AS. Diagnostic and therapeutic implications of type 2 myocardial infarction: Review and commentary. Am J Med. 2014;127(2):105-8.

59. Saaby L, Poulsen TS, Hosbond S, Larsen TB, Pyndt Diederichsen AC, Hallas J, et al. Classification of myocardial infarction: frequency and features of type 2 myocardial infarction. Am J Med. 2013;126(9):789-97.

Neurosciences

Perioperative Management of Intracranial Aneurysm

Shashi Srivastava, Devendra Gupta

INTRODUCTION

Spontaneous subarachnoid hemorrhage (SAH) and intracranial hemorrhage (ICH) are devastating diseases with significant morbidity and mortality and burden of the healthcare system. SAH patients are routinely admitted to an emergency department or an intensive care unit (ICU) and are cared for by a multidisciplinary team including neurosurgeons, neurointensivists, neuroanesthesiologists, and interventional neuroradiologists. The success of management in intensive care depends on understanding of the pathophysiology and clinical characteristics of disease and multisystemic care including management of delayed cerebral ischemia (DCI), hemodynamic management, glycemic management, dyselectrolemia, and prevention of rebleed to improve neurological outcomes.

Intracranial aneurysms are localized dilatations, formed within the circle of Willis at the vascular bifurcations where there is turbulent blood flow and a very high hemodynamic stress. These cerebral aneurysms vary in size from small (<5 mm), medium (6–25 mm) to large (>25 mm) and are classified as saccular or berry aneurysms and fusiform aneurysm.[1] Aneurysms most commonly occur in the anterior circulation (80–90%) involving the anterior communicating (ACom) artery in 30–35%, middle cerebral artery (MCA) in 20%, and posterior communicating (PCom) artery in 25% of cases. The incidence of posterior circulation aneurysms is low (5–15%)[2] (**Fig. 1**).

EPIDEMIOLOGY

Unruptured aneurysms are found in 3.2% of the adult population worldwide, detected incidentally on radiological evaluation. Aneurysmal rupture is the most common cause of spontaneous SAH (70–80%). The epidemiology of spontaneous SAH is quite variable in its presentation in patients of differing ethnicities and gender. The overall

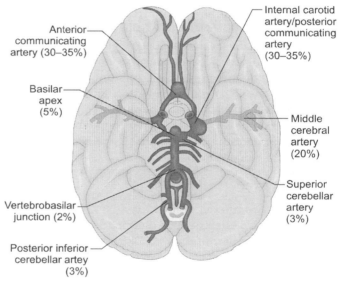

Fig. 1: Circle of Willis showing common sites of aneurysm.

incidence of SAH is approximately 9 per 10,000 persons/year with a fatality rate of around 50% with doubled rates in Japan and Finland and extreme lower rates in South and Central America.[3] Though the incidence is higher in women and increased with age, the gender distribution varied with age. At young ages, the incidence was higher in men, while after the age of 55 years, the incidence was higher in women. The incidence of SAH has probably decreased slightly over the past 45 years.[3] The risk of rupture is high for an aneurysm > 7 mm in size.[4] A small aneurysm may rupture with an increase in blood pressure.[5] According to the American Heart Association (AHA) recommendation, treatment of hypertension may reduce the risk of SAH.[5] Other risk factors are positive family history, oral contraceptives, cigarette smoking, alcohol intake, and certain other conditions such as autosomal dominant polycystic ovarian disease, coarctation of aorta, and connective tissue disorders.

COURSE AND PROGNOSIS

Subarachnoid hemorrhage, once diagnosed, needs prompt treatment because risk of rebleeding is very high within the first 12 hours of rupture. 70% of patients who do not succumb to initial rupture are at risk of DCI or cerebral vasospasm which is seen angiographically.[6] Approximately 20–40% of these patients develop DCI with neurological deficits.[7] Patients with a favorable neurological recovery suffer from severe cognitive dysfunction due to exposure of brain to subarachnoid blood, generalized cerebral edema, and cerebral vasospasm. Poor Hunt and Hess grade, aged patient, comorbidities, and rebleeding are associated with bad prognosis.

CLINICAL PRESENTATION

In 10–30% cases, sentinel headaches of mostly mild in severity may precede the aneurysm rupture by a few hours to a few months. Almost 80% of the patients experience sudden a very severe headache which is described by the patient "as the worst headache of my life" and may be associated with nausea, vomiting, meningismus, photophobia, seizures, and loss of consciousness. In some cases, focal neurological deficits in the form of third nerve palsy and hemiparesis may be present. Coma following SAH may point toward raised intracranial pressure (ICP), global ischemia, and brain tissue damage due to hematoma.

IMAGING AND DIAGNOSIS

Noncontrast computed tomography (NCCT) is the first-line diagnostic modality which detects >95% of SAH. SAH is detected best within the first few hours of bleeding. Diagnostic accuracy begins to decline once the hyperdense blood appears more similar to the surrounding cerebral cortex because of the normal flow of cerebrospinal fluid (CSF). It should be performed as soon as possible after the patient presents with headache, preferably within 48 hours. It detects hematoma, quantity of blood in brain, and hydrocephalus. The location of most density of blood suggests the site of lesion like clots in Sylvian fissure denote MCA and PCom aneurysm rupture, interhemispheric fissure bleed suggests ACom aneurysm, and prepontine hematoma is seen in basilar top and superior cerebellar artery aneurysm rupture. Computed tomography (CT) scan findings are often graded according to the Fisher scale, which remains the primary method to describe CT findings in regard to the amount of hematoma and risk of vasospasm, i.e., the higher the grade, the more likely to develop vasospasm (**Fig. 2**).

In patients with high suspicion of hemorrhage with negative NCCT, a lumbar puncture (LP) is the next diagnostic test. Characteristic findings on LP are xanthochromia and raised red blood cells (RBC) count of >1,00,000 mm³

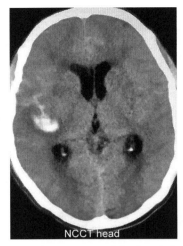

Fig. 2: Plain computed tomogram of the head showing a Sylvian subarachnoid hemorrhage with a hematoma and perifocal edema in the temporal lobe. There is a mild hydrocephalus with dilatation of the frontal horns and periventricular lucency. The gyri and sulci are obliterated indicating a diffuse edema.

and high protein. However, before the LP procedure, CT should be evaluated to rule out midline shift, obstructive hydrocephalus, and signs of raised ICP. Association of these may lead to transtentorial herniation after LP; moreover, sudden CSF drainage during LP decreases ICP thus increases transmural pressure (TMP)–ICP gradient and may precipitate rebleeding. Magnetic resonance imaging (MRI) is not useful in acute cases but useful after 5–7 days.

Once SAH is confirmed, the next step is to find out the cause of hemorrhage. The commonly used methods are CT angiography after contrast media injection (**Fig. 3**). Digital subtraction angiography (DSA) is generally used as the gold standard in detection of intracranial aneurysms and occult arteriovenous malformation (AVM) which are not detectable on other imaging modalities (**Figs. 4A and B**).[8-10] In the emergent setting, CT angiography is less invasive and less resource intensive than traditional angiography; it gives an idea about aneurysm wall calcification, thrombosis in the lumen of aneurysm, and its relation of aneurysm to bony structures. Three-dimensional (3D) rotational angiography (3DRA) depicts substantially small (≤3 mm) aneurysms, but with the problem of higher contrast load par acquisitioned run (18–24 vs. 6–8 mL), longer acquisition time (6–8 seconds), and increased patient radiation dose.[11] MR angiography can detect aneurysms of size 5 mm or more with high sensitivity with the added advantage of not requiring any contrast media and no exposure to radiation.

PREOPERATIVE GRADING OF SUBARACHNOID HEMORRHAGE

There are many grading systems to know the prognosis of the patient and assessment of the risk associated with surgery. The commonly used grading systems are modified

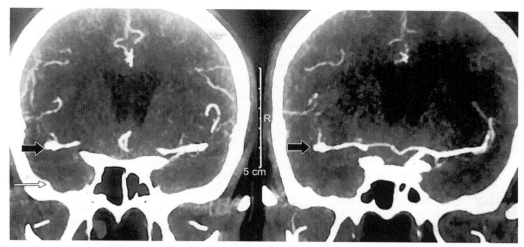

Fig. 3: A computed tomographic angiogram, coronal image, showing a middle cerebral artery aneurysm (arrow) arising from the middle cerebral artery bifurcation and pointing toward the temporal lobe. The two distal branches of the middle cerebral artery can be seen distal to the aneurysm.

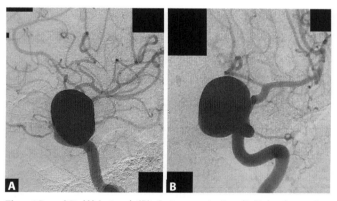

Figs. 4A and B: (A) Lateral; (B): Anteroposterior digital subtraction angiogram showing a giant paraclinoid aneurysm that initially presented with visual deficits and had ruptured causing a subarachnoid hemorrhage.

Table 1: Modified Hunt and Hess grading scale.[13]

Grade	Clinical description
Grade 0	Unruptured aneurysm
Grade 1	Asymptomatic or mild headache and slight nuchal rigidity
Grade 1a	No acute meningeal/brain reaction, but with fixed neurodeficit
Grade 2	Moderate-to-severe headache, nuchal rigidity, no neurological deficit other than cranial nerve (III, VI) palsy
Grade 3	Drowsiness, confusion, or mild focal deficit
Grade 4	Stupor, moderate-to-severe hemiparesis, possible early decerebrate rigidity, vegetative disturbance
Grade 5	Deep coma, decerebrate rigidity, moribund appearance

Hunt and Hess grade, World Federation of Neurological Surgeons (WFNS) grade, and Fisher grade.

The Hunt and Hess grading scale is the most commonly used; it includes 1–5 grades.[12] The Hunt and Hess grading was later on revised that included grade 0—unruptured aneurysm and grade 1a—no acute meningeal/brain reaction, but there is fixed neurodeficit (**Table 1**).[13] Morbidity and mortality risk increases with the increase of the Hunt and Hess grade.

In 1980, the WFNS grading was introduced based on the Glasgow Coma Scale (GCS) and motor deficit (**Table 2**).[14] In the WFNS grading important correlation with outcome is preoperative level of consciousness. A modified WFNS grading system has been proposed which required further validation.[15]

Delayed cerebral ischemia leading to permanent neurologic injury or death can occur as a complication of vasospasm, and the incidence and severity of vasospasm are related to the amount of blood in the subarachnoid space. The Fisher grading system was proposed, based on the extent of blood detected in the subarachnoid space in a CT scan (**Table 3**).[16]

Severe systemic diseases such as hypertension, diabetes, severe atherosclerosis, chronic pulmonary disease, and severe vasospasm on arteriography result in assignment of the patient to the next less favorable category.[13]

A comprehensive grading system combining factors that are independently and strongly associated with a long-term outcome was proposed. One point is assigned for Hunt and Hess grades IV and V, Fisher grades III and IV, patient age > 50 years, aneurysm size > 10 mm, and a giant (25 mm or larger) posterior circulation lesion.[17] Adding the total points results in a 5-point grading system (grade 0–5) that separates patients into groups with markedly different outcomes.[17] The AHA recommends that the initial rapid determination of the severity of SAH should be done by Hunt and Hess or

Table 2: WFNS grading.[14]

WFNS grade	GCS score	Motor deficit
Grade 1	GCS 15	No motor deficit
Grade II	GCS 14–13	No motor deficit
Grade III	GCS 14–13	Motor deficit present
Grade IV	GCS 12–7	Motor deficit present or absent
Grade V	GCS 6–3	Motor deficit present or absent

(GCS: Glasgow coma scale; WFNS: World Federation of Neurological Surgeons)

Table 3: Fisher grading system.[16]

Fisher grade	Description
Grade I	No blood detected
Grade II	Diffuse thin layer of subarachnoid blood <1 mm thick
Grade III	Localized clot or thick layer of subarachnoid blood ≥1 mm thick
Grade IV	Intracerebral or intraventricular blood with diffuse or no subarachnoid blood

WFNS grade which is the best indicator of recovery after SAH (class 1; level of evidence B).[5]

MANAGEMENT

Management of aneurysmal SAH can be divided into three distinct stages—immediate and preoperative management, intervention (clipping/coiling), and postoperative management.

Preoperative Concerns in an Intensive Care Unit

Aneurysmal SAH is a complex critical illness with multisystem complication in which the neurological outcome is directly affected by prompt and aggressive management by a multidisciplinary team of specialists. The initial neurological concerns of the management are decrease in the level of consciousness, risk of rebleed, DCI, hydrocephalus, and seizures. Other systemic concerns are cardiopulmonary dysfunction, dyselectrolemia, and poor glycemic control.

Rebleeding

The major risk of mortality following aneurysmal SAH occurs within the first 24 hours and is related to the risk of re-rupture of the aneurysm. The overall risk of rebleeding after SAH is 11% and mostly occurs on the first day (9–17%).[18] More than one-third of rebleeding takes place within the first 3 hours and almost half within 6 hours of the onset of symptom;[19] late rebleeding has a better outcome than early rebleeding;[20] chances of rebleeding are more in patients with sentinel headaches (severe headaches lasting >1 hour without SAH diagnosis), with initial loss of consciousness, worse neurological status on admission, longer time to aneurysm treatment, bigger size of aneurysm, and in hypertensive patient.[21,22] The AHA recommends that while awaiting surgery, blood pressure should be controlled to minimize the risk of stroke, rebleeding, and preservation of cerebral perfusion pressure within a normal range.[5] The general recommendation is to keep systolic blood pressure (SBP) < 160 mm Hg by administering short-acting, titratable intravenous agents such as labetalol/esmolol and nicardipine to control hypertension.

Antifibrinolytic therapy (<72 hours) with tranexamic acid or aminocaproic acid has been found to reduce the risk of early rebleeding which is thought to occur due to breakdown of fresh thrombus on the aneurysm wall (class IIa; level of evidence B).[5] Roos et al. in their Cochrane review showed no improvement in clinical outcome because the benefit of prevention in rebleed is offset by an increase in poor outcome caused by cerebral ischemia as a result of treatment with antifibrinolytics. Data do not support the routine use of antifibrinolytic drugs in the treatment of patients with aneurysmal SAH.[23]

Delayed Cerebral Ischemia and Early Brain Injury

Post SAH (>15 days), sometimes patients worsen neurologically due to early brain injury, cerebral ischemia, convulsions, hydrocephalus, systemic illness, and dyselectrolytemia.

Early brain injury was first described in 2004 by Kusaka et al.[24] and is recognized as an important denominator related to DCI and long-term morbidity and mortality after SAH. During the aneurysmal rupture, there is arterial bleeding under high pressure and blood is collected into the ventricles, subarachnoid space, and brain parenchyma leading to acute rise in ICP and decrease in cerebral perfusion pressure, resulting in global cerebral ischemia and loss of consciousness.[25]

About 30% of patients who survive early hemorrhage develop DCI which is an acute development of focal neurological symptoms such as hemiparesis, loss of speech, difficulty in performing skilled activity, or if there is a decrease in GCS by 2 points for >1 hour not explained by any other cause on clinical and radiological examination.[26] DCI is the major cause of poor outcome in patients who reach up to the stage of aneurysm treatment.[27]

Patients with minor aneurysmal bleed with or without loss of consciousness are still at a higher risk of DCI.[28,29]

Cerebral vasospasm (angiographic), which is conventionally related to DCI, starts at the 3rd day and reaches to peak in 1 week after aneurysm rupture. It starts resolving after 2 weeks.[30,31] Despite the popular belief, DCI may also develop in cerebral vessels without any vasospasm.[32]

Vasospasm appears as concentric narrowing. It can be either focal, segmental, or diffuse.[33] Imbalance of certain factors causing contraction and relaxation of the arteriolar smooth muscle is accountable for the development of vasospasm. Various studies have concentrated on the breakdown product of blood, oxyhemoglobin, which causes release of endothelin-1, an irritant to vascular endothelium leading to vasoconstriction. Elevated levels of endothelin have been found in plasma and CSF of patients with cerebral vasospasm.[34] Another factor which has been implicated in pathogenesis is nitric oxide (NO) which is a potent vasodilator. Decreased production and attenuated response of NO in the endothelium is one of the probable mechanisms of vasospasm.[35] Vasospasm and red cell agglutination at the microvascular level have also been associated with cerebral vasospasm.[36] Cortical spreading depolarization due to irritant molecules like glutamate, endothelins, and electrolyte changes also causes neuronal damage, edema, and injury.[37]

Microthrombosis is commonly seen after SAH.[38] There is activation of inflammatory pathways due to presence of blood in the subarachnoid area. This with some tissue factors leads to damage of endothelium and thrombus and microemboli development.[39]

Increased coagulation activity leading to cerebral infarction and poor prognosis has been found with DCI.[40]

Delayed cerebral ischemia ultimately results from cerebral vasospasm, cerebral ischemia, and thrombosis in microcirculation.

Diagnosis: Delayed cerebral ischemia is diagnosed on clinical suspicion. Certain factors such as hypoxia, dyselectrolytemia, fever, hydrocephalus, and seizures lately can lead to neurological symptoms like DCI and should be kept in mind during the treatment. Presence of radiologic vasospasm along with clinical evidence of cerebral ischemia does not exclude the role of other factors in DCI; in many such cases, neurological deficits could also be treated with induced hypertension. DCI is often difficult to diagnose in patients with cardiac events, pneumonia, and acute respiratory distress developed after the aneurysm ruptures. Clinically stable patients who are on sedation should be awakened to detect any new focal neurological deficits. As per the Neurocritical Care Guidelines on the management of SAH, "in sedated or poor-grade SAH patients, clinical deterioration may be difficult to assess, and transcranial Doppler (TCD), continuous electroencephalography (cEEG), brain tissue oxygen pressure (PtiO$_2$) monitoring, and/or cerebral microdialysis (CMD) are options for monitoring for vasospasm and DCI."[41]

Transcranial Doppler is a noninvasive modality for the diagnosis of cerebral vasospasm, which leads to high blood flow velocity. Mean velocity of 100–120, 120–200, and >200 cm/s is associated with mild, moderate, and severe angiographic vasospasm in the MCA, respectively. The Lindegaard ratio [LR; ratio of mean flow velocity (mFV) in ipsilateral MCA to extracranial internal carotid artery (ICA)] differentiates between increased flow velocity due to hyperemia and vasospasm. LR of <3 indicates hyperemia and >3 reflects vasospasm. Low Gosling's pulsatility index (PI) is an independent predictor of symptomatic vasospasm.[42] DCI should be assumed in case there is a rise in the MCA mFV of >50 cm/s during 24 hours or mean FVMCA of at least 200 cm/s or MCA/ICA ratio of >6 or both.[5]

Cerebral microdialysis has emerged as the more promising modality for detecting DCI than TCD and angiography. Cerebral ischemia results in increased levels of metabolites such as glutamate, glycerol, lactate/pyruvate ratio much before the clinical symptoms of DCI.[43] The basis of diagnosing DCI with microdialysis is brain tissue oxygen tension (P$_{bt}$O$_2$) of <20 mm Hg (*see* **Fig. 4**) or lactate/pyruvate ratio > 40, glucose <0.5 mM and secondly glutamate >40 mM or both.[44] Positron emission tomography and xenon-enhanced CT assess cerebral blood flow (CBF) quantitatively, which reduces in vasospasm. CBF < 25 mL/100 g/min or mean transit times (MTTs) > 6.5 seconds or both are in favor of vasospasm.[45] Diffusion-weighted MRI and CT perfusion can also detect early ischemia. Automated assessment of the papillary light reflex has been increasingly used as a reliable way of assessing papillary reactivity; the neurological pupil index (NPi) has been shown to decrease hours before clinical manifestation of ischemic injury and could be an early sign of clinical deterioration. NPi values range from 0 to 5, and 3 and more is considered normal.[46]

Pharmacological Prophylaxis

Calcium channel blockers: Vasospasm is known to occur due to constriction of vascular smooth muscle. Calcium channel blockers stop the entry of calcium through L-type voltage-gated calcium channels, thereby causing smooth muscle relaxation and reducing spasm. Dihydropyridines calcium channel blockers mostly act on arterial smooth muscles. Out of these, nimodipine specially is lipid soluble; therefore, it crosses the blood–brain barrier. Nimodipine perhaps is a neuroprotective, which acts by lessening the influx of calcium, after cerebral ischemia due to DCI. It also increases the endogenous fibrinolysis; therefore, it might reduce the occurrence of microemboli.[47] Nimodipine has been shown to improve long-term outcome in poor-grade patients too.[48] Therefore, SAH management guidelines recommend that after SAH, oral nimodipine 60 mg four times a day should be used in all the patients for 21 days (class I; level of evidence A).[5] Most centers prefer to start from the 3rd day.[5]

Magnesium: N-methyl D-aspartate (NMDA) receptor antagonist acts by inhibiting voltage-dependent calcium channels to inhibit smooth muscle contraction. Magnesium reduces glutamate release and has a neuroprotective role. Hypomagnesemia is seen in 38% of patients with SAH at admission and linked with poor WFNS grade.[49] Magnesium in the Aneurysmal Subarachnoid Hemorrhage (MASH) trial showed a nonsignificant reduction in DCI and 3 months' poor clinical outcomes among 283 patients who continuously received 14 days of intravenous magnesium infusion that started within 4 days of SAH.[50] Subsequently, the Intravenous Magnesium Sulfate for Aneurysmal Subarachnoid Hemorrhage (IMASH) trial and MASH2 trial did not show any improvement in the outcomes of patients who received magnesium therapy.[51] Currently, routine use of intravenous magnesium therapy is not recommended for the treatment of cerebral vasospasm.

Endothelin-1 receptor antagonists: Endothelin-1 is a potent cerebral vasoconstrictor and has been associated with vasospasm. Studies have shown that blockade of endothelin receptors (A and B) leads to improvement in cerebral vasospasm. Clazosentan, an endothelin A receptor antagonist, has been studied in various trials to reverse cerebral vasospasm in SAH.

Statins: Statins are anti-inflammatory agents, reduce oxidative stress, and inhibit thrombogenesis; they also increase NO synthase levels leading to relaxation of arterial smooth muscle and vasodilatation. Earlier trials with pravastatin and simvastatin showed some beneficial effects on cerebral vasospasm.[52,53] Subsequent trials did not show any effect on the incidence of vasospasm or on the long-term outcome. Simvastatin in the Aneurysmal Subarachnoid Hemorrhage (STASH) trial, which is a randomized, double-blind phase III trial, evaluated the effects of 40-mg simvastatin in acute SAH; there was no benefit in terms of long- or short-term outcome.[54]

Milrinone: Milrinone is a phosphodiesterase (PDE) III inhibitor and has been used intra-arterially as an infusion (8 mg over half hour) with a maximum dose of 24 mg to treat cerebral vasospasm. Infusion was continued for 14 days post SAH. Milrinone was found to be effective in reversal of vasospasm without causing hypotension.[55]

Papaverine: Papaverine causes strong vasodilatation of cerebral and coronary blood vessels by inhibiting cyclic adenosine monophosphate (cAMP). The disadvantage with papaverine has been its short duration of action which requires repeated infusions. Another problem with papaverine is increased ICP postinfusion, due to increased venous capacitance, leading to increased blood flow, hypotension, seizures, and transient neurological deficits. Due to these drawbacks, papaverine is no longer the drug of choice for intra-arterial infusions. It is administered in concentration of 0.3% at the rate of 3 mL/min into the affected vascular area. The maximum dose is 300 mg.

Treatment of Delayed Cerebral Ischemia and Vasospasm in a Critical Care Unit

Formerly, popular triple-H therapy, which included hypertension, hypervolemia, and hemodilution, aimed to increase CBF and improve rheology, has fallen out of favor over the years. The complications of triple-H therapy are heart failure, dyselectrolytemia, coagulopathy, and pulmonary edema due to fluid overload. It may also lead to rupture of aneurysm. There is no role of prophylaxis hypertensive therapy in aneurysmal SAH.[36]

The recent guidelines recommend maintenance of euvolemia for prevention of DCI. Hypertension should be induced in patients who develop DCI only if the cardiac condition permits it (class I; level of evidence B).[5] In the case of neurological deterioration, and other causes such as hydrocephalus or rebleeding being ruled out, rapid and aggressive hemodynamic management is required. Blood pressure is increased gradually by the use of noradrenaline. For this purpose, SBP is kept in the range of 160–200 mm Hg initially with the help of fluids or drugs. Cerebral perfusion pressure of 80–120 mm Hg is helpful in maintaining cerebral autoregulation and reduces the complications of hypervolemia.[56] There is no clear consensus on the blood pressure limits, although maximum SBP of 220 mm Hg and mean arterial pressure (MAP) of 140 mm Hg have been used after aneurysm clipping. For the treatment of vasospasm, some studies have used MAP of 20–30 mm Hg above the baseline value.[57] During the stay in ICU, low hemoglobin is a usual finding in 40–50% of patients with SAH.[58] Anemia has been found to be associated with increased morbidity due to cerebral infarction leading to disability and ultimately death.[59] In a normal patient, the effects of low hemoglobin (<6 g%) are not manifested due to intact cerebral autoregulation while in patients with poor-grade SAH, due to impaired autoregulation these effects may manifest even at higher hemoglobin concentration.[28] Optimal hemoglobin concentration in SAH patients is still debatable; nevertheless, studies have shown improved outcome with hemoglobin concentration >11 g.[60] Guidelines also favor keeping the high hemoglobin level. Though the optimal level is debatable, based on all the available data, the target hemoglobin in SAH patients should be kept >10 g%.

Neuroradiological intervention: Balloon angioplasty is not suggested before the development of angiographic spasm (class III; level of evidence B).[5] In patients with symptomatic cerebral vasospasm, cerebral angioplasty with and without selective intra-arterial vasodilator therapy is suggested, mainly in patients not responding to hypertensive therapy (class IIa; level of evidence B).[5]

Cardiac Dysfunctions

Myocardial injury occurs following SAH and is thought to be related to sympathetic stimulation and catecholamine discharge. Elevations of troponin I levels occur in approximately 35%, arrhythmias in 35%, and wall motion abnormalities on echocardiography in about 25% of patients with SAH.[61-64] The terms "neurogenic stress cardiomyopathy" and "stunned myocardium or neurogenic stunning" include chest pain, breathlessness, hypoxia, cardiogenic shock, and pulmonary edema, and raised cardiac markers clinically resemble closely takotsubo (stress) cardiomyopathy soon after SAH. This syndrome varies in severity and may lead to death in 12% of patients. The manifestations are usually transient lasting 1–3 days after which myocardial function returns to normal. In general, cardiac abnormalities are more common in patients who later develop DCI and have worse outcomes.[65] Management is only supportive that balances cardiac with the neurological goals.[66] However, severely impaired left ventricular function and DCI may require the use of inotropic agents such as dobutamine, levosimendan, milrinone, and even intra-aortic balloon pump to improve the cardiac function and CBF.[67-70]

Neurogenic Pulmonary Edema

Subarachnoid hemorrhage patients (2–8%) may develop neurogenic pulmonary edema (NPE) with mortality as high as 50%.[71] Abrupt increase in ICP causes excessive sympathetic activity and catecholamine surge, which causes intense pulmonary vasoconstriction with a concomitant increase in capillary permeability due to the release of inflammatory cytokinins, leading to pulmonary edema and impaired oxygenation. NPE may develop within few minutes to hours or as late as 12–24 hours after SAH. Clinically, the patient may present with dyspnea, tachypnea, tachycardia, and cyanosis with pink frothy sputum. Pulmonary edema may get worse by excessive fluid administration. X-ray chest will show bilateral diffuse alveolar infiltrates. Treatment of NPE is more of supportive. Maintain normovolemia, lung protective measures such as low tidal volume and positive end expiratory pressure (PEEP), and oxygen saturation by titration of inhaled oxygen. Avoid hypercapnia because this will increase ICP.

Hydrocephalus

Acute hydrocephalus is seen in 20% of patients after aneurysmal subarachnoid hemorrhage (aSAH). Poor Hunt and Hess grade, Fisher grade 4, distal posterior circulation aneurysms, female patients, and advancing age are some factors associated with hydrocephalus. The cause of hydrocephalus may be simple obstruction of aqueduct, third and fourth ventricles with blood clot in acute cases and scarring of arachnoid villi in chronic cases. Acute hydrocephalus associated with a decreased level of consciousness is managed by CSF diversion [external ventricular drainage (EVD) or lumbar drainage] (class I; level of evidence B).[5] EVD placement is generally associated with neurological recovery.[72-75] Hyperosmolar agents, mannitol and hypertonic saline, are usually considered when CSF diversion fails to reduce ICP. Chronic hydrocephalus requires placement of a ventricular shunt (class I; level of evidence C).[5]

Seizures

Early onset seizure-like activity may be seen in 26% of aSAH cases and late onset in 3–7%. Risk factors may be thick blood clots, rebleeding, intracerebral hematoma, MCA aneurysms, infarction, and poor grade; a short course of anticonvulsants may be given. However, long-term therapy is not recommended.[5] The recommendation is that prophylactic anticonvulsants may be considered in the acute SAH patients (class IIb; level of evidence B).[5] The routine use of anticonvulsants is not recommended for a long time; however, they may be continued in patients prone for delayed seizures such as previous history of seizures, intracerebral hematoma, uncontrollable hypertension, cerebral infarction, and MCA aneurysm (class IIb; level of evidence B).[5]

Dyselectrolemia

Both hyponatremia and hypernatremia are commonly seen after aSAH, but other electrolyte disorders can also be there.[5] Hyponatremia is most common and occurs in 10–30% of patients and hypernatremia in 19–20%.[76] Causes of hyponatremia include hypovolemia, a syndrome involving inappropriate secretion of antidiuretic hormone, glucocorticoid deficiency, and cerebral salt-wasting (CSW) syndrome in poor-grade patients wherein excessive secretion of atrial natriuretic peptide (ANP) and brain natriuretic peptide (BNP) causes loss of water and sodium from the body.[77,78] This condition should be differentiated from syndrome of inappropriate secretion of antidiuretic hormone (SIADH) which is associated with hyponatremia and water retention. CSW is treated with hypertonic saline and fludrocortisone (class IIa evidence) for prevention and treatment of hyponatremia.[5] CSW is usually found in patients of low clinical grade, with ruptured AComartery aneurysms, and it may be an independent risk factor for bad prognosis.[79] Hypertonic saline solution is effective in correcting hyponatremia; additionally, its use improves regional CBF, brain tissue oxygen, and pH status in patients with poor-grade aSAH.[80] Correction of hyponatremia should be slow to prevent osmotic demyelination. Hypernatremia develops less frequently than hyponatremia, related to hypothalamic dysfunction which induces central diabetes insipidus.[81]

Glycemic Management

Hyperglycemia, commonly observed in aSAH patients, is independently related to poor outcome.[82] According to AHA/American Society of Anesthesiologists (ASA) guidelines, glucose should be carefully managed. Hypoglycemia should be avoided during the critical care management of patients with SAH (class IIb, level B).[5] As per the Neurocritical Care Society, a serum glucose level of <80 mg/dL should be avoided (high quality of evidence, strong recommendation) and <200 mg/dL should be maintained (moderate quality of evidence).[83]

Deep Venous Thrombosis

Subarachnoid hemorrhage is a prothrombotic state that may lead to the development of deep venous thrombosis (DVT) and pulmonary embolism. The incidence of DVT in SAH ranges from 1.5% to 18%.[84,85] Poor-grade SAH patients appear to have the highest rates of DVT. The conventional methods for DVT prophylaxis in SAH patients include the use of mechanical methods such as sequential compression devices (SCDs) and medical treatments including unfractionated heparin, low molecular weight heparin, or nonheparinoid anticoagulant agents. The risk of ICH appears to be higher with low molecular weight heparin and the lowest risk is with SCDs.[86] The timing of DVT prophylaxis in relation to aneurysm occlusion is controversial, but typically prophylactic medications are withheld until the aneurysm has been either clipped or coiled.

Fever

Fever is a common problem in patients with aSAH. This is associated with amount of hemorrhage, vasospasm, and systemic inflammatory state triggered by blood and its byproducts.[87] Several retrospective or prospective observational studies showed that fever was significantly associated with mortality and poor neurological outcome.[88] Better functional outcome is seen with good control of fever.[89]

Perioperative Management

Surgical Clipping versus Endovascular Coiling

International Subarachnoid Aneurysm Trial (ISAT) included 2,143 patients with aSAH and compared surgical clipping

with endovascular treatment.[90] The results of ISAT showed the risk of death or dependency as 31% with surgical clipping compared to 24% in endovascular coiling. However, the risk of late rebleeding was more with endovascular (2–9%) as compared to 0.9% with clipping. Complete obliteration of aneurysm was there in the clipped group (81%) than in the coiling group (58%). The threat of death at 5 years was considerably less in the coiled group than in the clipping group.[91] ISAT included patients only with good-grade SAH and to address many concerns of this trial, another multicenter trial, ISAT II, was started to compare coiling versus surgery in non-ISAT aSAH.[92] With surgical clipping, there is complete sealing of neck and removal of any hematoma; therefore, it should be of choice in patients with large intraparenchymal hematoma (>50 mL), MCA aneurysms, and aneurysms with neck:dome ratio > 2. On the contrary, endovascular coiling does not have the risk of tissue damage and is combined with diagnostic angiography. Coiling may be desired in elderly patients with comorbidities, basilar top aneurysms, and high-grade SAH.[5] Substantial progress has been done in endovascular approaches to aneurysm treatment, starting from the Guglielmi Detachable Coils in the year 1991; later on, to mitigate the risk of coil-associated parent artery occlusion and thromboembolic complications, new techniques such as balloon-assisted coiling, stent-assisted coiling, and flow directors came into practice. The multinational trial ISAT II will bring forth the safety of these new devices.

Timing of Surgery

The brain is acutely swollen due to blood clots following SAH, so it was believed that late surgery seems to provide better operative conditions and decrease the incidence of postoperative vasospasm. Although delaying surgery allows brain swelling to lessen, both risk of rebleeding and vasospasm occur during the waiting period. In a cooperative study, no significant difference was found in the outcome between early (3 days or before) and late (after 10 days); however, results were worst between 7 and 10 days.[93] Later, data from North American centers showed the best results when surgery was done before 3 days.[94] The recent trend is for early surgery, to avoid chances of rebleeding and vasospasm.

Anesthetic Management

All the medications including nimodipine, which the patient is taking preoperatively, should be continued. Grade I and II patients can be given mild anxiolytic. Antacid prophylaxis should be administered in all the grades. Basic anesthetic goals are the same for both the surgical clipping and endovascular treatment of aneurysm. Though rare (<1% with modern anesthesia), aneurysmal rupture during induction of anesthesia is usually precipitated with acute hypertension during tracheal intubation and carries a high mortality rate of 75%.[95] Therefore, the main anesthetic goal at induction is to keep TMP low which is the driving force for the aneurysm to rupture and simultaneously to maintain of cerebral perfusion pressure to prevent cerebral ischemia (TMP = MAP – ICP). In patients with good clinical grade, hyperventilation should be avoided as this will lead to decrease in ICP, increase in TMP which causes rupture of aneurysm. MAP should be reduced to 20% below the preoperative level at the time of intubation with thiopentone sodium or propofol. Poor-grade patients have increased ICP and low cerebral perfusion pressure. Elevated ICP partially prevents aneurysm from rupture. These patients do not tolerate fall in blood pressure and require hyperventilation to reduce ICP. Patient comorbidities must guide the anesthetic plan.

Monitoring of the patient is done by routine monitors such as electrocardiogram (ECG), pulse oximetry, invasive blood pressure for the rapid measurement of blood pressure intraoperatively, and central venous pressure to guide fluid therapy. Neuromonitoring can be used during surgery to detect cerebral ischemia; somatosensory-evoked potentials (SSEPs) and motor-evoked potentials (MEPs) are helpful in detecting anterior and posterior circulation ischemia while brainstem auditory evoked potential (BAEP) and SSEP are helpful in detection of posterior circulation ischemia. Both SSEP and MEP are helpful in detecting ischemia during temporary clipping. Perioperative blood sugar monitoring is essential as both low and high blood glucose levels are associated with poor outcome; targeted blood glucose should be 110–180 mg/dL.[96]

The goals of the maintenance of anesthesia are stable hemodynamics, good brain relaxation, early smooth recovery, and use of neuromonitoring. The measures for intraoperative brain relaxation are head-up of 15–30°, lumbar drain, mild hypocapnea (30–35 mm Hg), 20% osmotic diuretic mannitol, or 3% hypertonic saline.

Induced hypotension for reducing the pressure within aneurysm sac and facilitate clipping is no longer in practice because it may lead to ischemia in an already injured brain. Temporary arterial clipping proximal to aneurysm will make it slack to facilitate perianeurysmal dissection and safe permanent clipping of aneurysm. It also controls bleeding in case of aneurysm rupture. However, there is always a threat of focal ischemia in the area supplied by the feeding artery. Temporary clipping may be applied safely for 10 minutes; longer time increases the chances of cerebral ischemia.[97] To increase the blood supply in the ischemic area through collaterals, MAP is maintained around 90 mm Hg. In case of expected prolonged temporary clipping time, induced hypertension or suppression of cerebral metabolic activity

with hypothermia/pharmacologic agents (barbiturates, propofol) helps to reduce cerebral ischemia. Transient flow arrest, using adenosine, is an option when it is difficult to put a temporary clip in wide-neck large aneurysms. Adenosine slows conduction through the atrioventricular (AV) node; therefore, it should not be used in patients with sick sinus syndrome/heart block, asthma, or coronary artery disease (CAD). External defibrillator pads should be placed in all the patients to treat asystole/severe prolonged bradycardia.[98] Adenosine is used in the incremental boluses of 6–12 mg to achieve 30 seconds of cardiac arrest.[99] Aneurysm rupture is a grave intraoperative complication. It may occur before the dissection (7%), during dissection (48%), or applying clip (45%).[100] In a hemodynamically stable patient, a short period of hypotension or even adenosine flow arrest can be provided to secure the aneurysm.

Neuroradiological procedures of aneurysm coiling, digital subtraction angiography, and intra-arterial therapy for cerebral vasospasm have different concerns such as transportation of these patients to radiology department, radiation exposure, keeping immobility, anticoagulation, management of intracranial complications, and rapid recovery. General anesthesia (GA) is preferred in patients with poor-grade SAH and in uncooperative and hemodynamically unstable patients; GA assures patients total immobility and respiratory control. Good intravenous line and anesthesia circuit long enough are required in all the cases. Hypothermia is common in a radiological suite and thus should be prevented. Arterial pressure can be measured directly from the femoral artery sheath through a transducer. Procedural complications can occur such as aneurysmal rupture, coil migration in the parent vessel causing occlusion, thromboembolism, and air embolism. Monitored anesthesia care (MAC) provides the advantage of repeated neurological assessment and prevents potential hemodynamic changes associated with intubation and emergence. To relieve anxiety and for analgesia, intravenous midazolam/fentanyl boluses/remifentanil 0.03–0.1 µg/kg/min, propofol infusion 25–75 µg/kg/min should be administered. Although propofol is fast acting, it has short half-life and rapid recovery but it may also induce respiratory depression. Highly selective α-2 agonist dexmedetomidine is a preferred drug, for providing sedation and analgesia without respiratory depression.

Postoperatively, patients are observed in a neurosurgical intensive care area. Recovery and extubation depend on the preoperative status and intraoperative events. Good clinical grade SAH patients can be successfully extubated on the table using standard extubation criteria. Poor preoperative SAH grade, prolonged temporary occlusion time, and severe intraoperative vasospasm are likely to need postoperative ventilation. These patients are likely to deteriorate necessitating vigorous monitoring in ICU. Patients should be provided with adequate postoperative analgesia. Paracetamol 1 g should be given by intravenous infusion, starting intraoperatively and continuing 6–8 hourly, to provide analgesia and to prevent and treat hyperthermia. Oxycodone 2–3 mg given intravenously can be used to supplement analgesia. Prophylaxis or treatment of DCI should continue in the postoperative period.

CONCLUSION

Patients with aneurysmal SAH may present with multiple neurological and systemic complications in the perioperative period; therefore, a thorough understanding of pathophysiology and management options is needed. The perioperative plan should be based on a patient's neurological status and focused on treating associated comorbidities including DCI, hemodynamic disturbance, fever, dyselectrolemia, and hyperglycemia to improve neurological outcomes. The same quality of care should be extended in the postoperative ICU. Timely management of complications improves the outcome of these patients.

REFERENCES

1. Zhou S, Dion PA, Rouleau GA. Genetics of intracranial aneurysms. Stroke. 2018;49(3):780-7.

2. Vega C, Kwoon JV, Lavine SD. Intracranial aneurysms: current evidence and clinical practice. Am Fam Physician. 2002;66(4):601-8.

3. de Rooij NK, Linn FH, van der Plas JA, Algra A, Rinkel GJ. Incidence of subarachnoid haemorrhage: a systematic review with emphasis on region, age, gender and time trends. J Neurol Neurosurg Psychiatry. 2007;78(12):1365-72.

4. Wiebers DO, Whisnant JP, Sundt TM Jr, O'Fallon WM. The significance of unruptured intracranial saccular aneurysms. J Neurosurg. 1987;66(1):23-9.

5. Connolly ES Jr, Rabinstein AA, Carhuapoma JR, Derdeyn CP, Dion J, Higashida RT, et al. Guidelines for the management of aneurysmal subarachnoid hemorrhage: a guideline for healthcare professionals from the American Heart Association/ American Stroke Association. Stroke. 2012;43(6):1711-37.

6. Biller J, Godersky JC, Adams HP Jr. Management of aneurysmal subarachnoid hemorrhage. Stroke. 1988;19(10):1300-5.

7. Treggiari-Venzi MM, Suter PM, Romand JA. Review of medical prevention of vasospasm after aneurysmal subarachnoid hemorrhage: a problem of neurointensive care. Neurosurgery. 2001;48(2):249-62.

8. Kouskouras C, Charitanti A, Giavroglou C, Foroglou N, Selviaridis P, Kontopoulos V, et al. Intracranial aneurysms: evaluation using CTA and MRA. Correlation with DSA and intraoperative findings. Neuroradiology. 2004;46(10):842-50.

9. Yoon DY, Lim KJ, Choi CS, Cho BM, Oh SM, Chang SK. Detection and characterization of intracranial aneurysms with 16-channel multidetector row CT angiography: a prospective comparison of volume-rendered images and digital subtraction angiography. AJNR Am J Neuroradiol. 2007;28(1):60-7.

10. Jayaraman MV, Mayo-Smith WW, Tung GA, Haas RA, Rogg JM, Mehta NR, et al. Detection of intracranial aneurysms: multi-detector row CT angiography compared with DSA. Radiology. 2004;230(2):510-8.

11. van Rooij WJ, Sprengers ME, de Gast AN, Peluso JP, Sluzewski M. 3D rotational angiography: the new gold standard in the detection of additional intracranial aneurysms. AJNR Am J Neuroradiol. 2008;29(5):976-9.

12. Hunt WE, Hess RM. Surgical risk as related to time of intervention in the repair of intracranial aneurysms. J Neurosurg. 1968;28(1):14-20.

13. Hunt WE, Kosnik EJ. Timing and perioperative care in intracranial aneurysm surgery. Clin Neurosurg. 1974;21:79-89.

14. Report of World Federation of Neurological Surgeons Committee on a Universal Subarachnoid Hemorrhage Grading Scale. J Neurosurg. 1988;68(6):985-6.

15. Sano H, Satoh A, Murayama Y, Kato Y, Origasa H, Inamasu J, et al. Modified World Federation of Neurosurgical Societies subarachnoid hemorrhage grading system. World Neurosurg. 2015;83(5):801-7.

16. Fisher CM, Kistler JP, Davis JM. Relation of cerebral vasospasm to subarachnoid hemorrhage visualized by computerized tomographic scanning. Neurosurgery. 1980;6(1):1-9.

17. Ogilvy CS, Carter BS. A proposed comprehensive grading system to predict outcome for surgical management of intracranial aneurysms. Neurosurgery. 1998;42(5):959-70.

18. Starke RM, Connolly ES Jr; Participants in the International Multi-Disciplinary Consensus Conference on the Critical Care Management of Subarachnoid Hemorrhage. Rebleeding after aneurysmal subarachnoid hemorrhage. Neurocrit Care. 2011;15(2):241-6.

19. Tanno Y, Homma M, Oinuma M, Kodama N, Ymamoto T. Rebleeding from ruptured intracranial aneurysms in North Eastern Province of Japan: a cooperative study. J Neurol Sci. 2007;258(1-2):11-6.

20. Cha KC, Kim JH, Kang HI, Moon BG, Lee SJ, Kim JS. Aneurysmal rebleeding: factors associated with clinical outcome in the rebleeding patients. J Korean Neurosurg Soc. 2010;47(2): 119-23.

21. Naidech AM, Janjua N, Kreiter KT, Ostapkovich ND, Fitzsimmons BF, Parra A, et al. Predictors and impact of aneurysm rebleeding after subarachnoid hemorrhage. Arch Neurol. 2005;62(3):410-6.

22. Ohkuma H, Tsurutani H, Suzuki S. Incidence and significance of early aneurysmal rebleeding before neurosurgical or neurological management. Stroke. 2001;32(5):1176-80.

23. Roos YB, Rinkel GJ, Vermeulen M, Algra A, van Gijn J. Antifibrinolytic therapy for aneurysmal subarachnoid haemorrhage. Cochrane Database Syst Rev. 2003;(2):CD001245.

24. Kusaka G, Ishikawa M, Nanda A, Granger DN, Zhang JH. Signaling pathways for early brain injury after subarachnoid hemorrhage. J Cereb Blood Flow Metab. 2004;24(8):916-25.

25. de Oliveira Manoel AL, Goffi A, Marotta TR, Schweizer TA, Abrahamson S, Macdonald RL. The critical care management of poor-grade subarachnoid haemorrhage. Crit Care. 2016;20:21.

26. Vergouwen MD, Vermeulen M, van Gijn J, Rinkel GJ, Wijdicks EF, Muizelaar JP, et al. Definition of delayed cerebral ischemia after aneurismal subarachnoid hemorrhage as an outcome event in clinical trials and observational studies: proposal of a multidisciplinary research group. Stroke. 2010;41(10):2391-5.

27. Jaeger M, Schuhmann MU, Soehle M, Meixensberger J. Continuous assessment of cerebrovascular autoregulation after traumatic brain injury using brain tissue oxygen pressure reactivity. Crit Care Med. 2006;34(6):1783-8.

28. Oddo M, Milby A, Chen I, Frangos S, MacMurtrie E, Maloney-Wilensky E, et al. Hemoglobin concentration and cerebral metabolism in patients with aneurysmal subarachnoid hemorrhage. Stroke. 2009;40(4):1275-81.

29. Hop JW, Rinkel GJ, Algra A, van Gijn J. Initial loss of consciousness and risk of delayed cerebral ischemia after aneurismal subarachnoid hemorrhage. Stroke. 1999;30(11):2268-71.

30. Weir B, Grace M, Hansen J, Rothberg C. Time course of vasospasm in man. J Neurosurg. 1978;48(2):173-8.

31. Rowland MJ, Hadjipavlou G, Kelly M, Westbrook J, Pattinson KT. Delayed cerebral ischaemia after subarachnoid haemorrhage: looking beyond vasospasm. Br J Anaesth. 2012;109(3):315-29.

32. Washington CW, Zipfel GJ; Participants in the International Multi-disciplinary Consensus Conference on the Critical Care Management of Subarachnoid Hemorrhage. Detection and monitoring of vasospasm and delayed cerebral ischemia: a review and assessment of the literature. Neurocrit Care. 2011;15(2):312-7.

33. Janjua N, Mayer SA. Cerebral vasospasm after subarachnoid hemorrhage. Curr Opin Crit Care. 2003;9(2):113-9.

34. Chow M, Dumont AS, Kassell NF. Endothelin receptor antagonists and cerebral vasospasm: an update. Neurosurgery. 2002;51(6):1333-42.

35. Inagawa T. Risk factors for cerebral vasospasm following aneurysmal subarachnoid hemorrhage: a review of the literature. World Neurosurg. 2016;85:56-76.

36. Dreier JP, Windmüller O, Petzold G, Lindauer U, Einhäupl KM, Dirnagl U. Ischemia triggered by red blood cell products in the subarachnoid space is inhibited by nimodipine administration or moderate volume expansion/hemodilution in rats. Neurosurgery. 2002;51(6):1457-67.

37. Macdonald RL. Delayed neurological deterioration after subarachnoid haemorrhage. Nat Rev Neurol. 2014;10(1):44-58.

38. Romano JG, Forteza AM, Concha M, Koch S, Heros RC, Morcos JJ, et al. Detection of microemboli by transcranial Doppler ultrasonography in aneurysmal subarachnoid hemorrhage. Neurosurgery. 2002;50(5):1026-31.

39. Stein SC, Browne KD, Chen XH, Smith DH, Graham DI. Thromboembolism and delayed cerebral ischemia after subarachnoid hemorrhage: an autopsy study. Neurosurgery. 2006;59(4):781-8.

40. Peltonen S, Juvela S, Kaste M, Lassila R. Hemostasis and fibrinolysis activation after subarachnoid hemorrhage. J Neurosurg. 1997;87(2):207-14.

41. Diringer MN, Bleck TP, Claude Hemphill J 3rd, Menon D, Shutter L, Vespa P, et al. Critical care management of patients following aneurysmal subarachnoid hemorrhage: recommendations from the Neurocritical Care Society's Multidisciplinary Consensus Conference. Neurocrit Care. 2011;15(2):211-40.

42. Rajajee V, Fletcher JJ, Pandey AS, Gemmete JJ, Chaudhary N, Jacobs TL, et al. Low pulsatility index on transcranial Doppler predicts symptomatic large-vessel vasospasm after aneurysmal subarachnoid hemorrhage. Neurosurgery. 2012;70(5):1195-206.

43. Sarrafzadeh AS, Sakowitz OW, Kiening KL, Benndorf G, Lanksch WR, Unterberg AW. Bedside microdialysis: a tool to monitor cerebral metabolism in subarachnoid hemorrhage patients? Crit Care Med. 2002;30(5):1062-70.

44. Hänggi D; Participants in the International Multi-Disciplinary Consensus Conference on the Critical Care Management of Subarachnoid Hemorrhage. Monitoring and detection of vasospasm II: EEG and invasive monitoring. Neurocrit Care. 2011;15(2):318-23.

45. Cremers CH, van der Schaaf IC, Wensink E, Greving JP, Rinkel GJ, Velthuis BK, et al. CT perfusion and delayed cerebral ischemia in aneurysmal subarachnoid hemorrhage: a systematic review and meta-analysis. J Cereb Blood Flow Metab. 2014;34(2):200-7.

46. Aoun SG, Stutzman SE, Vo PN, El Ahmadieh TY, Osman M, Neeley O, et al. Detection of delayed cerebral ischemia using objective pupillometry in patients with aneurysmal subarachnoid hemorrhage. J Neurosurg. 2019;11:1-6.

47. Vergouwen MD, Vermeulen M, de Haan RJ, Levi M, Roos YB. Dihydropyridine calcium antagonists increase fibrinolytic activity: a systematic review. J Cereb Blood Flow Metab. 2007;27(7):1293-308.

48. Petruk KC, West M, Mohr G, Weir BK, Benoit BG, Gentili F, et al. Nimodipine treatment in poor-grade aneurysm patients. Results of a multicenter double-blind placebo-controlled trial. J Neurosurg. 1988;68(4):505-17.

49. van den Bergh WM, Algra A, van der Sprenkel JW, Tulleken CA, Rinkel GJ. Hypomagnesemia after aneurysmal subarachnoid hemorrhage. Neurosurgery. 2003;52(2):276-82.

50. van den Bergh WM, Algra A, van Kooten F, Dirven CM, van Gijn J, Vermeulen M, et al. Magnesium sulfate in aneurysmal subarachnoid hemorrhage: a randomized controlled trial. Stroke. 2005;36(5):1011-5.

51. Dorhout Mees SM, Algra A, Vandertop WP, van Kooten F, Kuijsten HA, Boiten J, et al. Magnesium for aneurysmal subarachnoid haemorrhage (MASH-2): A randomised placebo-controlled trial. Lancet. 2012;380(9836):44-9.

52. Tseng MY, Czosnyka M, Richards H, Pickard JD, Kirkpatrick PJ. Effects of acute treatment with pravastatin on cerebral vasospasm, autoregulation, and delayed ischemic deficits after aneurysmal subarachnoid hemorrhage: a phase II randomized placebo-controlled trial. Stroke. 2005;36(8):1627-32.

53. Lynch JR, Wang H, McGirt MJ, Floyd J, Friedman AH, Coon AL, et al. Simvastatin reduces vasospasm after aneurysmal subarachnoid hemorrhage: results of a pilot randomized clinical trial. Stroke. 2005;36(9):2024-6.

54. Kirkpatrick PJ, Turner CL, Smith C, Hutchinson PJ, Murray GD; STASH Collaborators. Simvastatin in aneurysmal subarachnoid

haemorrhage (STASH): a multicentre randomised phase 3 trial. Lancet Neurol. 2014;13(7):666-75.

55. Fraticelli AT, Cholley BP, Losser MR, Saint Maurice JP, Payen D. Milrinone for the treatment of cerebral vasospasm after aneurysmal subarachnoid hemorrhage. Stroke. 2008;39(3): 893-8.

56. Touho H, Karasawa J, Ohnishi H, Shishido H, Yamada K, Shibamoto K. Evaluation of therapeutically induced hypertension in patients with delayed cerebral vasospasm by xenon-enhanced computed tomography. Neurol Med Chir (Tokyo). 1992;32(9):671-8.

57. Darby JM, Yonas H, Marks EC, Durham S, Snyder RW, Nemoto EM. Acute cerebral blood flow response to dopamine-induced hypertension after subarachnoid hemorrhage. J Neurosurg. 1994;80(5):857-64.

58. Kurtz P, Schmidt JM, Claassen J, Carrera E, Fernandez L, Helbok R, et al. Anemia is associated with metabolic distress and brain tissue hypoxia after subarachnoid hemorrhage. Neurocrit Care. 2010;13(1):10-6.

59. Kramer AH, Gurka MJ, Nathan B, Dumont AS, Kassell NF, Bleck TP. Complications associated with anemia and blood transfusion in patients with aneurysmal subarachnoid hemorrhage. Crit Care Med. 2008;36(7):2070-5.

60. Stevens RD, Naval NS, Mirski MA, Citerio G, Andrews PJ. Intensive care of aneurysmal subarachnoid hemorrhage: an international survey. Intensive Care Med. 2009;35(9):1556-66.

61. Hravnak M, Frangiskakis JM, Crago EA, Chang Y, Tanabe M, Gorcsan J 3rd, et al. Elevated cardiac troponin I and relationship to persistence of electrocardiographic and echocardiographic abnormalities after aneurysmal subarachnoid hemorrhage. Stroke. 2009;40(11):3478-84.

62. Deibert E, Barzilai B, Braverman AC, Edwards DF, Aiyagari V, Dacey R, et al. Clinical significance of elevated troponin I levels in patients with nontraumatic subarachnoid hemorrhage. J Neurosurg. 2003;98(4):741-6.

63. Wartenberg KE, Schmidt JM, Claassen J, Temes RE, Frontera JA, Ostapkovich N, et al. Impact of medical complications on outcome after subarachnoid hemorrhage. Crit Care Med. 2006;34(3):617-23;quiz 624.

64. Banki N, Kopelnik A, Tung P, Lawton MT, Gress D, Drew B, et al. Prospective analysis of prevalence, distribution, and rate of recovery of left ventricular systolic dysfunction in patients with subarachnoid hemorrhage. J Neurosurg. 2006;105(1):15-20.

65. Coghlan LA, Hindman BJ, Bayman EO, Banki NM, Gelb AW, Todd MM, et al. Independent associations between electrocardiographic abnormalities and outcomes in patients with aneurysmal subarachnoid hemorrhage: Findings from the intraoperative hypothermia aneurysm surgery trial. Stroke. 2009;40(2):412-8.

66. Lee VH, Oh JK, Mulvagh SL, Wijdicks EF. Mechanisms in neurogenic stress cardiomyopathy after aneurysmal subarachnoid hemorrhage. Neurocrit Care. 2006;5(3):243-9.

67. Levy ML, Rabb CH, Zelman V, Giannotta SL. Cardiac performance enhancement from dobutamine in patients refractory to hypervolemic therapy for cerebral vasospasm. J Neurosurg. 1993;79(4):494-9.

68. Busani S, Rinaldi L, Severino C, Cobelli M, Pasetto A, Girardis M. Levosimendan in cardiac failure after subarachnoid hemorrhage. J Trauma. 2010;68(5):E108-10.

69. Lannes M, Teitelbaum J, del Pilar Cortés M, Cardoso M, Angle M. Milrinone and homeostasis to treat cerebral vasospasm associated with subarachnoid hemorrhage: The Montreal Neurological Hospital Protocol. Neurocrit Care. 2012;16(3): 354-62.

70. Lazaridis C, Pradilla G, Nyquist PA, Tamargo RJ. Intra-aortic balloon pump counterpulsation in the setting of subarachnoid hemorrhage, cerebral vasospasm, and neurogenic stress cardiomyopathy. Case report and review of the literature. Neurocrit Care. 2010;13(1):101-8.

71. Busl KM, Bleck TP. Neurogenic pulmonary edema. Crit Care Med. 2015;43(8):1710-5.

72. Rajshekhar V, Harbaugh RE. Results of routine ventriculostomy with external ventricular drainage for acute hydrocephalus following subarachnoid haemorrhage. Acta Neurochir (Wien). 1992;115(1-2):8-14.

73. Ransom ER, Mocco J, Komotar RJ, Sahni D, Chang J, Hahn DK, et al. External ventricular drainage response in poor grade aneurysmal subarachnoid hemorrhage: effect on preoperative grading and prognosis. Neurocrit Care. 2007;6(3):174-80.

74. Milhorat TH. Acute hydrocephalus after aneurysmal subarachnoid hemorrhage. Neurosurgery. 1987;20(1):15-20.

75. Hasan D, Vermeulen M, Wijdicks EF, Hijdra A, van Gijn J. Management problems in acute hydrocephalus after subarachnoid hemorrhage. Stroke. 1989;20(6):747-53.

76. Qureshi AI, Suri MF, Sung GY, Straw RN, Yahia AM, Saad M, et al. Prognostic significance of hypernatremia and hyponatremia among patients with aneurysmal subarachnoid hemorrhage. Neurosurgery. 2002;50(4):749-56.

77. Kao L, Al-Lawati Z, Vavao J, Steinberg GK, Katznelson L. Prevalence and clinical demographics of cerebral salt wasting in patients with aneurysmal subarachnoid hemorrhage. Pituitary. 2009;12(4):347-51.

78. Hannon MJ, Behan LA, O'Brien MM, Tormey W, Ball SG, Javadpour M, et al. Hyponatremia following mild/moderate subarachnoid hemorrhage is due to SIAD and glucocorticoid deficiency and not cerebral salt wasting. J Clin Endocrinol Metab. 2014;99(1):291-8.

79. Sayama T, Inamura T, Matsushima T, Inoha S, Inoue T, Fukui M. High incidence of hyponatremia in patients with ruptured anterior communicating artery aneurysms. Neurol Res. 2000;22(2):151-5.

80. Al-Rawi PG, Tseng MY, Richards HK, Nortje J, Timofeev I, Matta BF, et al. Hypertonic saline in patients with poor-grade subarachnoid hemorrhage improves cerebral blood flow, brain tissue oxygen, and pH. Stroke. 2010;41(1):122-8.

81. Beseoglu K, Etminan N, Steiger HJ, Hänggi D. The relation of early hypernatremia with clinical outcome in patients suffering from aneurysmal subarachnoid hemorrhage. Clin Neurol Neurosurg. 2014;123:164-8.

82. Steiner T, Juvela S, Unterberg A, Jung C, Forsting M, Rinkel G, et al. European Stroke Organization guidelines for the

management of intracranial aneurysms and subarachnoid haemorrhage. Cerebrovasc Dis. 2013;35(2):93-112.

83. Dority JS, Oldham JS. Subarachnoid Hemorrhage: an update. Anesthesiol Clin. 2016;34(3):577-600.

84. Mack WJ, Ducruet AF, Hickman ZL, Kalyvas JT, Cleveland JR, Mocco J, et al. Doppler ultrasonography screening of poor-grade subarachnoid hemorrhage patients increases the diagnosis of deep venous thrombosis. Neurol Res. 2008;30(9):889-92.

85. Ray WZ, Strom RG, Blackburn SL, Ashley WW, Sicard GA, Rich KM. Incidence of deep venous thrombosis after subarachnoid hemorrhage. J Neurosurg. 2009;110(5):1010-4.

86. Collen JF, Jackson JL, Shorr AF, Moores LK. Prevention of venous thromboembolism in neurosurgery: a metaanalysis. Chest. 2008;134(2):237-49.

87. Dorhout Mees SM, Luitse MJ, van den Bergh WM, Rinkel GJ. Fever after aneurysmal subarachnoid hemorrhage: relation with extent of hydrocephalus and amount of extravasated blood. Stroke. 2008;39(7):2141-3.

88. Kramer CL, Pegoli M, Mandrekar J, Lanzino G, Rabinstein AA. Refining the association of fever with functional outcome in aneurysmal subarachnoid hemorrhage. Neurocrit Care. 2017;26(1):41-7.

89. Badjatia N, Fernandez L, Schmidt JM, Lee K, Claassen J, Connolly ES, et al. Impact of induced normothermia on outcome after subarachnoid hemorrhage: a case-control study. Neurosurgery. 2010;66(4):696-701.

90. Molyneux AJ, Kerr RS, Yu LM, Clarke M, Sneade M, Yarnold JA, et al. International subarachnoid aneurysm trial (ISAT) of neurosurgical clipping versus endovascular coiling in 2143 patients with ruptured intracranial aneurysms: a randomised comparison of effects on survival, dependency, seizures, rebleeding, subgroups, and aneurysm occlusion. Lancet. 2005;366(9488):809-17.

91. Molyneux AJ, Kerr RS, Birks J, Ramzi N, Yarnold J, Sneade M, et al. Risk of recurrent subarachnoid haemorrhage, death, or dependence and standardised mortality ratios after clipping

or coiling of an intracranial aneurysm in the International Subarachnoid Aneurysm Trial (ISAT): long-term follow-up. Lancet Neurol. 2009;8(5):427-33.

92. Darsaut TE, Jack AS, Kerr RS, Raymond J. International subarachnoid aneurysm trial - ISAT part II: study protocol for a randomized controlled trial. Trials. 2013;14:156.

93. Kassell NF, Torner JC, Haley EC Jr, Jane JA, Adams HP, Kongable GL. The International cooperative study on the timing of aneurysm surgery. Part 1: Overall management results. J Neurosurg. 1990;73(1):18-36.

94. Haley EC Jr, Kassell NF, Torner JC. The International cooperative study on the timing of aneurysm surgery. The North American experience. Stroke. 1992;23(2):205-14.

95. Hamid RKA, Hamid NA, Newfield P, Bendo AA. Anesthetic management of cerebral aneurysms and arteriovenous malformations. In: Newfield P, Cottrell JE (Eds). Handbook of Neuroanaesthesia. New Delhi: Wolters Kluwer (India) Pvt. Ltd; 2013.

96. Kramer AH, Roberts DJ, Zygun DA. Optimal glycemic control in neurocritical care patients: a systematic review and meta-analysis. Crit Care. 2012;16(5):R203.

97. Levine SD, Masri LS, Levy ML, Giannotta SL. Temporary occlusion of the middle cerebral artery in intracranial aneurysm surgery: time limitation and advantage of brain protection. J Neurosurg. 1997;87(6):817-24.

98. Bebawy JF, Gupta DK, Bendok BR, Hemmer LB, Zeeni C, Avram MJ, et al. Adenosine-induced flow arrest to facilitate intracranial aneurysm clip ligation: dose-response data and safety profile. Anesth Analg. 2010;110(5):1406-11.

99. Khan SA, McDonagh DL, Adogwa O, Gokhale S, Toche UN, Verla T, et al. Perioperative cardiac complications and 30-day mortality in patients undergoing intracranial aneurysmal surgery with adenosine-induced flow arrest: a retrospective comparative study. Neurosurgery. 2014;74(3):267-72.

100. Batjer H, Samson D. Intraoperative aneurysmal rupture: incidence, outcome, and suggestions for surgical management. Neurosurgery. 1986;18(6):701-7.

Perioperative Management of Brain Tumor Surgeries including Awake Craniotomy

Shwetal Goraksha, Joseph Monteiro

INTRODUCTION

In the United States, the incidence of tumors in the brain and the central nervous system (CNS), both benign and malignant, has an average annual age-adjusted incidence of 28.57 per 100,000 people.[1] The incidence of CNS tumors in India ranges from 5 to 10 per 100,000 people with an increasing trend and accounts for 2% of malignancies.[2] The principal aim of perioperative neurocritical care in these patients is preoperative assessment, prehabilitation, prediction, prevention, and detection followed by prompt treatment of perioperative complications. The more critical complications occur in the immediate postoperative period: cerebral edema, seizures, postoperative hemorrhage, and intracranial hypertension, and other complications such as thromboembolism or infections can occur later and can also vary from mild to severe. The protocoled management of alterations in homeostasis in this subset of patients with their existing comorbidities and medications will halt and/ or totally prevent the development of complications that may have the potential to alter brain function and generate collateral morbidity and adverse outcomes.

PATHOLOGY

Approximately 60% of supratentorial neoplasms are primary brain tumors, of which gliomas are the most common. These may vary from the benign pilocytic and well-differentiated astrocytomas to aggressive anaplastic astrocytomas and glioblastoma multiforme. Other common benign neoplasms include meningiomas and pituitary adenomas. Tumors in the posterior fossa are the most common lesions requiring surgical intervention. In children, posterior fossa tumors account for approximately 60% of all brain tumors. In the adult population, posterior fossa tumors are less frequent and include acoustic neuroma, metastases, mainly from the breast and lung, meningioma and hemangioblastoma, which may be associated with polycythemia and occult pheochromocytoma.

PREOPERATIVE MANAGEMENT

Besides the general assessment of the patients for anesthesia, a more specific neurological assessment includes an accurate evaluation of the lesion, its site, size, location, symptoms and signs of raised intracranial pressure (ICP), neurological deficits, medications, and associated comorbidities.

Enhanced recovery after surgery (ERAS) protocols are being incorporated in several institutions in neurosurgery. Prehabilitation involves preadmission counseling, evaluation and optimization of organ dysfunction, cessation of smoking, abstinence from alcohol if applicable, and nutritional support and micronutrient supplementation.[3]

Considerations of surgical approach, ease of surgical access, positioning of the patient, and the potential for hemorrhage are important factors that contribute, and the risk–benefit ratio of each is balanced before individualizing the plan for each patient.

Medications such as anticonvulsants and steroids are continued in the perioperative period. Patients with posterior fossa lesions, specially in the presence of raised ICP, are more sensitive to sedatives and analgesics and these drugs should be used with caution if given preoperatively. In a special situation like an "awake craniotomy," careful patient selection is the key; developing a good rapport with the patient, detailed explanation of the procedure, realistic expectations, importance of the patient realizing the importance of patient cooperation in the safety and the success of the procedure are imperative.

INTRAOPERATIVE MANAGEMENT

Intraoperative management of anesthesia for any brain tumor surgery requires a good understanding of basic neurophysiology and pathophysiology. Maintenance of optimal cerebral hemodynamics helps in good surgical exposure with minimal retraction damage and also avoids secondary damage due to various factors such as increased ICP, vasospasm, hypoxia, and hypercapnia.

The brain consumes almost 20% of the total body oxygen. The cerebral metabolic rate (CMR) is usually expressed as $CMRO_2$ (cerebral oxygen consumption 3–3.8 mL/100 g/min adults, 5 mL/100 g/min in children). The ICP (normal ICP is 10–15 mm Hg) can increase due to the tumor or the edema surrounding it or due to obstructive hydrocephalus, especially in infratentorial or ventricular tumors. The pressure–volume relationship between ICP, volume of cerebrospinal fluid (CSF), blood and brain tissue, and cerebral perfusion pressure (CPP) is defined by the Monroe Kellie hypothesis. This states that the cranial compartment is inelastic and the volume inside the cranium is fixed, and as the tumor increases in size, there is initial displacement of blood and CSF and increased reabsorption of CSF. However, once these mechanisms reach their limit, the ICP increases exponentially, resulting in decrease in CPP and cerebral ischemia, brain shifts, and herniation.

Cerebral perfusion pressure is derived as the difference between the mean arterial pressure (MAP) and the ICP (CPP = MAP – ICP), and maintenance of an adequate CPP is key to optimizing cerebral blood flow (CBF) and cerebral function. CBF should be maintained at minimum 50 mL/100 g/min and MAP between 50 and 150 mm Hg. CBF depends on various factors which include autoregulation, drugs, $CMRO_2$, temperature, and partial pressures of oxygen and carbon dioxide (PaO_2 and $PaCO_2$) **(Fig. 1; Table 1)**.

The basic principles of management of anesthesia for brain tumors include:

- Smooth and hemodynamically stable induction of anesthesia
- Maintenance of CPP (CPP > 70 mm Hg), oxygenation, and perioperative hemodynamics
- Allowing ease of surgical exposure with minimal retraction damage or secondary injury
- Facilitating neurophysiological monitoring
- Early awakening and early postoperative neurological assessment on emergence

In keeping with ERAS protocols, intraoperative monitoring, understanding steroid dosing and tapering, intraoperative hemodynamic stability and blood transfusion, seizure prophylaxis and an extubation protocol with anticipation of extubation difficulties are important.[3]

Premedication

It is necessary to maintain a balance between oversedation which leads to hypercapnia, hypoxia, and increased ICP which may lead to development of vasogenic edema, and agitation leading to increased sympathetic response which can also increase myocardial and oxygen consumption. Titrated doses of midazolam and fentanyl under controlled supervision can be used for sedation. If ICP is already raised and there is history of vomiting, premedication is avoided. However, mild sedation can also exacerbate or unmask focal neurological deficits in patients with intracranial lesions.

Steroids are used to reduce cerebral edema. Dexamethasone is used for supratentorial tumors, while in tumors involving cranial nerves or posterior fossa methyl

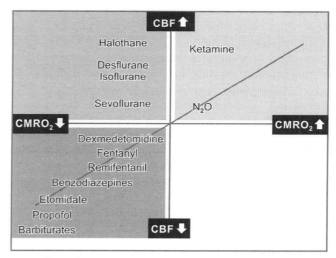

Fig. 1: Effect of anesthesia drugs on cerebral blood flow (CBF) and cerebral metabolic rate of oxygen ($CMRO_2$).
Source: Joseph Monteiro

Drugs	Cerebral blood flow	Cerebral metabolic rate of oxygen ($CMRO_2$)	Cerebral autoregulation	CO_2 reactivity	Intracranial pressure
Propofol	↓↓↓	↓↓↓	↔	↔	↓↓
Ketamine	↑↑↑	↑↑	↔	↔	↑↑
Etomidate	↓↓↓	↓↓	↔	↔	↓↓
Barbiturates	↓↓↓	↓↓↓	↔	↔	↓↓
Benzodiazepines	↓↓	↓	↔	↔	↓
Dexmedetomidine	↓↓	↓↓	↓	↓	↓
Opioids	↓	↑	↔	↔	↔

Table 1: Effect of anesthetic drugs on the cerebral metabolism.

↑ increases, ↓ decreases, ↔ no effect.

prednisolone is preferred, and in pituitary tumors, hydrocortisone is used. In patients on long-term steroid therapy, intraoperative hypotension should be anticipated due to adrenocortical suppression.

Therapeutic plasma levels of anticonvulsants should be checked preoperatively, and if starting intraoperatively, a loading dose should be given. Drugs commonly used intraoperatively are levetiracetam, fosphenytoin, phenytoin, and sodium valproate. Anticonvulsant agents such as phenytoin may decrease the duration of action of nondepolarizing muscle relaxants.

Monitoring

Minimal mandatory monitoring includes electrocardiogram, pulse oximetry, capnography, temperature, noninvasive blood pressure (BP), and urine output measurement. Arterial pressure monitoring should be ideally done for all craniotomies to closely monitor and control MAP and CPP. It should be measured at the circle of Willis level (approximately at the middle ear). It is recommended in patients with pre-existing cardiac disease and in surgeries where hemodynamic instability is anticipated; it also facilitates arterial blood gas and hematocrit estimation. In addition to large-bore intravenous (IV) access, central venous pressure monitoring is beneficial in patients with severe comorbidities, large vascular tumors, in sitting or semisitting positions [to aspirate air in case of venous air embolism (VAE)]. In the sitting position, transesophageal echocardiography (TEE) or precordial Doppler may also be used to detect air embolism by monitoring microbubbles in the circulation. Neuromuscular blockade should be monitored using a train-of-four (TOF) monitor. Since hypo- and hyperglycemia are both detrimental to the brain, blood glucose levels are monitored. Depth of anesthesia monitors such as bispectral index (BIS) or entropy can also help maintain an adequate plane of anesthesia. Intraoperative neuromonitoring (IONM) such as electroencephalography (EEG), electrocorticography (ECoG), brainstem auditory evoked potentials (BAEPs), somatosensory evoked potentials (SSEPs), and motor evoked potentials (MEPs) may also be required depending on the location of the tumor.

Induction and Maintenance of Anesthesia

Various drugs used for anesthesia may affect $CMRO_2$, CBF, CBF–metabolism coupling, ICP, autoregulation, vascular response to CO_2, and brain electrical activity. They act in a dose-dependent manner to decrease $CMRO_2$. IV drugs such as propofol and barbiturates are most potent as compared to inhalational agents. IV agents, except ketamine, decrease ICP, while inhalational agents increase ICP. Propofol

reduces cerebral blood volume (CBV), CBF, and ICP and preserves autoregulation and vascular reactivity; therefore, it may be the drug of choice for induction of anesthesia for neurosurgery. Inhalational agents cause cerebral vasodilation and therefore can increase ICP. Sevoflurane causes the least vasodilation as compared to desflurane and isoflurane and maintains autoregulation. Isoflurane impairs autoregulation, although this is reversible with hyperventilation.[4] Opioids such as fentanyl can be used for analgesia. Neuromuscular blockade with a nondepolarizing muscle relaxant is used before intubation and to maintain muscle relaxation throughout the surgery. It has minimal effect on cerebral hemodynamics. Mild hyperventilation ($PaCO_2$) at induction may be useful in decreasing raised ICP by causing cerebral vasoconstriction.

Laryngoscopy and tracheal intubation cause profound stimulation and are associated with increased BP, heart rate, and ICP. This can be prevented with opioids, fentanyl bolus or remifentanil infusion, short-acting beta-blockers, calcium channel blockers, or lignocaine.

Intraoperatively, sevoflurane allows for rapid changes in the depth of anesthesia and rapid emergence, facilitating early neurological examination. Propofol, in addition to the advantages mentioned earlier, may offer neuroprotection based on its effects on neuronal activity, similar to thiopentone, which is a result of a decrease in $CMRO_2$, and maintenance of CBF and helps in preventing further increase in glucose, which in turn may worsen cerebral ischemia.[5] However, it tends to decrease the BP if used in higher doses. Therefore, a balanced anesthesia with sevoflurane or desflurane [minimum alveolar concentration (MAC) > 1) and propofol is preferred. Nitrous oxide has detrimental effects on the cerebral vasculature and the brain tissue and is known to increase CBF, cerebral metabolism, and ICP. When used with inhalational agents, it causes a greater increase in CBF than an equipotent concentration of the latter alone. Similarly, autoregulation is altered to a greater extent with this combination than when used alone.[6]

Positioning

Ideal patient positioning balances surgical convenience and the risks related to the patient and is the joint responsibility of the surgeon and the anesthesiologist. The patient is positioned after induction of anesthesia and placement of arterial and venous lines.

Most neurosurgical patients get positioned with a three-pin holder (Mayfield clamp) to maintain and stabilize the position of the head. This "pinning or pin fixation" of the head is a nociceptive stimulus which can result in potentially hazardous hemodynamic consequences. It can be prevented by administration of additional doses of

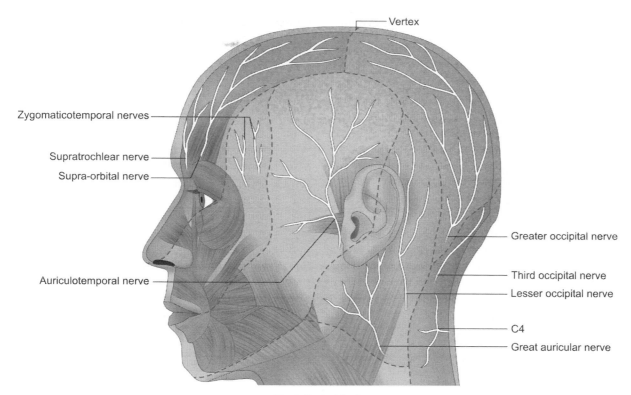

Fig. 2: Scalp block.
Source: JN Monteiro

fentanyl, propofol, or beta-blockers or by infiltration of the scalp with a local anesthetic agent or scalp block (**Fig. 2**).

Optimal patient positioning can reduce the ICP and brain swelling, thereby allowing ease of surgical access and avoiding secondary brain damage. Raised ICP is usually caused by increased intra-abdominal pressure, inadequate abdominal bolstering, excessive flexion or rotation of the head, and position of the head below the level of the heart. Elevation of the head about 15–20° (reverse Trendelenburg) helps decrease the ICP.

Supine

Supine is the most common position used in neurosurgery. All skin to metal contact should be prevented, arms positioned alongside the body or on arm boards, elbows and heels padded, and 15–20° angulation and flexion at the trunk–thigh–knee given, with a pillow placed under the knees to keep them flexed.

Prone

Prone position is used to approach the posterior fossa and suboccipital region. Access to the patient's airway is poor and complications such as pressure sores, vascular compression, brachial plexus injuries, air embolism, and blindness are common. This position increases the intra-abdominal pressure, decreases venous and increases

systemic and pulmonary vascular resistance, and can potentially cause hemodynamic instability. As a result of an improved ventilation–perfusion (V/Q) match, due to an increase in the perfusion of the lungs and positive pressure ventilation, oxygenation may improve. Precautions should be taken to ensure no disconnection in lines and inadvertent tracheal extubation. The head is kept in the neutral position while checking for any pressure on the eyes and nose, and adequate padding done to prevent pressure sores. The upper extremities are arranged along the body or abducted on padded arm boards without hyperextension to prevent brachial plexus injury. Postoperative visual loss is a rare but devastating complication, usually with prolonged surgery, steep reverse Trendelenburg position, hypotension, and blood loss with associated low hematocrit and low plasma oncotic pressures. This could be due to either (1) central retinal artery occlusion (CRAO) ischemia caused by orbital compression resulting in central retinal vessel compression; (2) ischemic optic neuropathy (ION) which may be anterior—due to hypoperfusion or occlusion of the anterior optic nerve, which is common in cardiac and vascular surgeries, or posterior—due to infarction of the optic nerve posterior to lamina cribrosa, common in spine surgeries; (3) cortical blindness caused by decreased perfusion of the occipital cortex by the posterior cerebral artery; or (4) posterior reversible encephalopathy syndrome

(PRES), caused by a severe hypertensive episode, cytotoxic drugs, or disease causing edema.

Lateral

Lateral position is used for a surgical approach to the temporal lobe, skull base, and posterior fossa. Risks include brachial plexus injuries, pressure palsies, and V/Q mismatch. In this position, the lower arm should be hanging or rested on a low padded arm board so as to prevent axillary artery compression and brachial plexus injury. A roll is placed under the upper chest to prevent ischemia and brachial plexus injury. The upper arm is positioned on the armrest anterior to the patient's body. The lower extremities should be slightly flexed, with a pillow placed between the legs. In the Park-bench position, an adaptation of lateral position, the upper arm is positioned along the lateral trunk.

Sitting

The sitting position is used for resection of tumors located in the posterior fossa. This position ensures good surgical access, less bleeding, and better ventilation, but is also associated with complications such as VAE, cerebral ischemia due to hemodynamic compromise, quadriplegia, tension pneumocephalus, and compressive neuropathy. Therefore, it should be used only in selected patients after a thorough preoperative assessment.

Postural hypotension due to decreased venous return is prevented by preloading the patient with adequate fluids, pneumatic compression stockings, and treating with IV fluid and vasopressors as required. The modified sitting or semisitting position provides better venous return and less hemodynamic instability. All the bony prominences are padded to prevent nerve injuries. Excessive neck flexion may result in quadriplegia, and a minimum distance between the chin and the nearest bone (at least 2 fingerbreadth) is recommended. This also ensures adequate jugular venous and CSF drainage and prevents postoperative macroglossia and facial edema.

Since the site of surgery is above the level of the heart, there is a risk of VAE, as air gets entrained through the exposed veins into the pulmonary circulation and may decrease cardiac output by creating an airlock. VAE is detected by a fall in end-tidal CO_2 ($ETCO_2$) > 2 mm Hg or with precordial Doppler and TEE. It is recommended to rule out a patent foramen ovale preoperatively with TEE or transthoracic echocardiography, as it is a source of paradoxical air embolism. The treatment for VAE is irrigation of the surgical site with saline, ventilating with 100% oxygen, aspirating air from the central venous catheter, giving a Trendelenburg tilt with a left lateral position, and cardiovascular support with administration of inotropes and vasopressors if required.

Lateral Oblique Semiprone

This position is used for posterior fossa and parieto-occipital surgery. Though the risk of VAE is lower, there is a chance of brachial plexus injury, pressure sores, and macroglossia. The principles of positioning are similar to those for lateral position, but the head may be placed on the table and the lower arm placed behind the body.[7]

Management of "Tight Brain"

Intraoperatively, patients who are symptomatic for raised ICP tend to pose problems of "tight brain" or "massive intraoperative brain swelling" at surgery. Ease of surgical exposure helps minimize retraction injury and cause further damage to the brain.

There are various methods to manage a bulging brain. These include smooth induction, adequate muscle relaxation, administration of IV lignocaine prior to intubation, and avoiding intubation in light planes of anesthesia **(Box 1)**.[5]

Intraoperative Hemodynamic Management

Optimal BP management helps in preventing major complications. If autoregulation is impaired, CBF becomes pressure-dependent. Any decrease in MAP will decrease CBF, while hypertension increases CBF and ICP. Induced hypotension to reduce blood loss is

---

Box 1: Intraoperative measures for management of tight brain.

- Mechanical
  - Adequate head-up position 15–30° to ensure blood and CSF drainage
  - Check for kinking of neck or tight endotracheal tube ties to ensure free jugular venous drainage
- Physiological
  - Mild hyperventilation—hypocapnia ($PaCO_2$ 30–35 mm Hg) causes vasoconstriction and decreases CBV. CBF decreases by 2–3% for each mm Hg fall in $PaCO_2$ up to 20 mm Hg. If hyperventilation is sustained, CBF and CBV return to baseline after 4 hours.
  - Hypoxemia is avoided.
- Pharmacological
  - Intravenous drugs, such as propofol, preferred to inhalation, as they decrease CBF and $CMRO_2$ to a greater extent and cause less cerebral vasodilation.
  - Osmotic diuretics—mannitol 0.5–2 mg/kg ± Furosemide. Mannitol, given 15–20 minutes before opening the dura, causes cerebral dehydration and decreases the ICP. Adverse effects of osmotic diuretics are dehydration, hyponatremia, hypokalemia, renal failure, transient increase in ICP before the diuresis sets in, and exaggeration of brain shifts.
- Surgical
  - Lumbar CSF drain
  - Direct puncture of the lateral ventricle

(CBF: cerebral blood flow; CBV: cerebral blood volume; $CMRO_2$: cerebral metabolic rate of oxygen; CSF: cerebrospinal fluid)

associated with significantly high neurological morbidity and minimal benefits. For control of BP intraoperatively, the choice of antihypertensives depends on their effects on cerebral circulation and ICP. Direct vasodilators, sodium nitroprusside, nitroglycerine, and calcium antagonists are avoided but beta-blockers and angiotensin-converting enzyme inhibitors are preferred.

Intraoperative Neuromonitoring

Intraoperative neuromonitoring is utilized to monitor neural pathways during surgery, detect intraoperative stress or damage, detect and define the level of lesions, and define abnormalities by detecting changes in cerebral hemodynamics, oxygenation, and neuronal function. It helps predict postoperative outcomes and decreases the incidence of postoperative neurological deficits (**Table 2**).

These techniques include EEG, ECoG, BAEP, SSEP, and MEP. Evoked potentials are easier to interpret than EEG; they are either present or absent, delayed, or have a normal or abnormal wave.[8]

Somatosensory Evoked Potentials

It is a test of the functional integrity of the pathway from the periphery via the posterior columns of the spinal cord, through to the cerebral cortex. It involves applying repeated electrical stimuli to a peripheral nerve, e.g., the posterior tibial nerve, and measuring the evoked response over the cerebral cortex using scalp electrodes. The time interval between electrical stimulation of the peripheral nerve and recording the evoked response over the cortex is defined as latency. An increase in latency, decrease in amplitude, or a complete loss of evoked response is indicative of surgical injury or ischemia unless proven otherwise. A 50% decrease in amplitude or a 10–15% increase in latency is a cause of serious concern. Anesthetic drugs (volatile agents, propofol, and benzodiazepines) affect SSEPs, but muscle relaxants do not affect SSEPs; narcotics and dexmedetomidine have the least effect. All other drugs have a dose-dependent increase in latency and decrease in amplitude, while nitrous oxide decreases amplitude without an effect on latency. Ketamine and etomidate increase the amplitude and can be used in cases where the SSEPs are suppressed due to use of other anesthetic agents.[9] Other factors that affect SSEP are hypotension and hypothermia.

Motor Evoked Potentials

Motor evoked potentials are elicited by directly stimulating the spinal cord by needle electrodes inserted by the surgeon in the epidural space. MEPs are less affected by inhalational anesthetic agents, but muscle relaxants have to be avoided.

Intraoperative Fluid Management

The perioperative fluid management in neurosurgical patients aims to restore intravascular volume, optimize hemodynamic parameters, and maintain tissue perfusion, integrity, and function. The goal is to minimize the risk of inadequate CPP and to maintain good neurosurgical conditions. During the perioperative period, these patients may receive diuretics such as mannitol and furosemide to reduce the ICP. Intraoperatively, administration of anesthetic drugs causes vasodilatation, severe blood loss may lead to depletion of the intravascular volume, and development of diabetes insipidus (DI) or syndrome of inappropriate antidiuretic hormone secretion (SIADH) may lead to hemodynamic instability. Fluid administration should be guided by the trends in the arterial BPs and central venous pressures (**Table 3**). It is important to maintain normovolemia and normotension during intracranial surgery. Fluids should be warmed to ensure normothermia during as well as at emergence from anesthesia.[10]

Hyperglycemia, which worsens the consequences of cerebral ischemia and hypo-osmolarity (target osmolarity 290–320 Osm/kg), which can increase cerebral edema, should be avoided. The use of hypotonic fluids can lead to tissue edema, which results in oxygen diffusion and CBF impairments.[11] Iso-osmolar fluids should be preferred for infusion intraoperatively such as 0.9% NaCl and balanced solutions such as Plasmalyte and Sterofundin. Newer 6% hydroxyethyl starch in a balanced solution (~310 Osm/kg) has no deleterious effects on coagulation. The hematocrit should be maintained above 28%. Hypo-osmolar fluids

Table 2: Effect of anesthetic agents on intraoperative neuromonitoring.

| Agents | SSEP | | MEP | BAEP | VEP |
	Amplitude	Latency			
Halothane (0.5–1)	↓	↑	+	–	+
Isoflurane (0.5–1)	↓	↑	+	–	+
Sevoflurane (>1.5)	↓	↑	+	–	+
Desflurane (>1.5)	↓	↑	+	–	+
Nitrous oxide (60–70%)	↓	–	+	–	+
Barbiturates	↓	↑	+	–	+
Propofol	↓	–	+	–	+
Ketamine	↑	–	–	–	+
Etomidate	↑	–	–	–	+
Opioids	↓	↑	–	–	–
Benzodiazepines	–	–	+	–	+
Dexmedetomidine	–	–	–	–	–
Muscle relaxants	–	–	+	–	+

↓ increase, ↑ decrease, – no effect, + has effect.

(BAEP: brainstem auditory evoked potential; SSEP: somatosensory evoked potential; MEP: motor evoked potential; VEP: visual evoked potential)

Table 3: Composition and properties of commonly used intravenous fluids.

	NaCl 0.9%	Ringer lactate	Plasmalyte	NaCl 0.45%	Dextrose 5%	Plasma
Na⁺ (mmol/L)	154	130	70	77	0	135–145
Cl⁻ (mmol/L)	154	109	49	77	0	95–105
K⁺ (mmol/L)	0	4	2.5	0	0	3.5–5.3
HCO₃⁻ (mmol/L)	0	28 (lactate)	13.5 (acetate)	0	0	24–32
Ca⁺⁺ (mmol/L)	0	1.4	0	0	0	0.8–1.2
Mg⁺⁺ (mmol/L)	0	0	0.75	0	0	0.8–1.2
Glucose	0	0	0	0	277.8 (50 g)	3.5–5.5
pH	4.5–7	6–7.5	6.5–8	4.5–7	3.5–5.5	7.35–7.45
Osmolarity (mOsm/L)	308	273	295	154	278	278–295

Table 4: Osmolarities of various solutions used in the treatment of raised intracranial pressure.

Hypertonic solution	Osmolarity (mOsm/kg)
Normal saline	308
3% hypertonic saline	1,026
7.5% hypertonic saline	2,567
20% hypertonic saline	6,844
30% hypertonic saline	10,267
10% mannitol	550
20% mannitol	1,100
25% mannitol	1,375

should be avoided as they may reduce the plasma osmolarity (**Table 4**). Small volumes of lactated Ringer's (measured osmolality 252–255 mOsm/kg) can be used without any detrimental physiological effects. In case of massive blood loss, isotonic fluids can be safely administered. Large volumes of 0.9% NaCl may result in hyperchloremic metabolic acidosis; therefore, a combination of isotonic crystalloids, colloids, and blood transfusion may be a better choice. Pentastarch has little effect on factor VIII in comparison to hetastarch infusion which in volumes >1 L leads to factor VIII depletion.[10] In patients undergoing pituitary surgery, DI can occur during the intraoperative and postoperative periods, and fluid balance needs close monitoring to avoid complications and disabling electrolyte imbalance and to avoid fluid overload. In cases where there is severe blood loss, it is important to maintain adequate fluid status without fluid overload.[12]

The ROSE concept was suggested by Malbrain et al. for patients with critical illness. It consists of four phases: (1) resuscitation (salvage or rescue treatment with fluids administered quickly as a bolus, (2) optimization (phase of ischemia and reperfusion which requires titrating of fluids to maintain cardiac output, (3) stabilization (fluid therapy only for normal maintenance and replacement), and (4) evacuation (fluid overload causes end-organ damage and requires late goal-directed fluid removal or deresuscitation to achieve negative fluid balance). It advocates restriction of fluids, which is consistent with the prevention of a "tight brain" in neurosurgery; however, it is conflicting with the aim of normovolemia and maintenance of adequate cerebral perfusion and oxygenation and adversely affects cerebral perfusion.[11,13]

AWAKE CRANIOTOMY

When the tumor is located in the eloquent areas of the brain (areas involving speech, language, and motor), surgery may be performed in an "awake" patient under local anesthesia, scalp block, and IV sedation. Cortical mapping and clinical monitoring aim to localize the eloquent area, minimize damage, and result in postoperative neurological dysfunction. In addition to excision of brain tumors in the eloquent areas, awake craniotomy is used for epilepsy surgery, deep brain stimulation, and, less commonly, mycotic aneurysms and arteriovenous malformations near critical brain areas (**Table 5; Box 2**).

Other advantages include a shorter hospitalization stay, reduced cost, and lesser incidence of postoperative complications such as nausea and vomiting.

Proper patient selection, and full anesthetic assessment and optimization of the patient's comorbidities, is important. Preoperative counseling is necessary to explain the procedure, the monitoring, and the risks involved.[14,15]

In addition to the routine monitors, depth of anesthesia monitors such as BIS, capnography with an oxygen mask, or nasal prongs should be used.

The patient is awake during the mapping procedure, and any alteration of speech, language, and motor function is communicated to the surgeon; resection takes place only after the cortex has been functionally mapped by this process. The rest of the surgery can be done under sedation or general anesthesia (**Box 3**).

Table 5: Contraindications for awake craniotomy.

Absolute contraindications	Relative contraindications
Patient refusal	Patient cough
Inability to lie still for any reason	Learning difficulties
Inability to cooperate—confusion	Inability to lay flat
	Patient anxiety
	Language barriers
	Obstructive sleep apnea
	Young age

Box 2: Adverse events during awake craniotomy.

Airway or respiratory compromise
- Hypoventilation
- Obstruction
- Hypoxemia
- Hypercapnia

Inadequate or excessive sedation

Failure of block—conversion to general anesthesia

Hemodynamic instability
- Hypotension
- Hypertension
- Bradycardia
- Tachycardia

Seizures—treated with cold saline irrigation and intravenous midazolam or propofol

Local anesthesia toxicity

Patient discomfort
- Position
- Fatigue

Nausea, vomiting

Box 3: Aims during extubation.

- Adequate oxygenation.
- Maintain MAP, CPP, ICP, and $CMRO_2$.
- Avoid coughing and repeated suctioning which may increase BP.
- Check adequate seizure prophylaxis and steroid cover.
- Control BP with antihypertensive drugs such as esmolol and labetalol
- Prevent postoperative nausea, vomiting, and shivering which increases oxygen consumption, ICP, and BP.
- Prevent and anticipate postcraniotomy pain.

(BP: blood pressure; $CMRO_2$: cerebral metabolic rate of oxygen; CPP: cerebral perfusion pressure; ICP: intracranial pressure; MAP: mean arterial pressure)

The preferred anesthetic technique varies, but all patients will receive antibiotics, steroids, and some IV analgesics such as paracetamol or nonsteroidal anti-inflammatory drugs (NSAIDs).

- *Local anesthesia/scalp block:* Six nerves blocked on both sides of the scalp—auriculotemporal, zygomaticotemporal, supraorbital, supratrochlear, greater occipital, and lesser occipital nerves, with approximately 40 mL of local anesthetics—bupivacaine, levobupivacaine, or ropivacaine ± adrenaline.
- *Monitored anesthesia care:* Monitoring vitals, administration of IV sedatives and analgesics, and providing psychological support. Drugs used for sedation are midazolam, fentanyl, and titrated infusions of remifentanil, propofol, and dexmedetomidine to maintain "conscious sedation." The infusion is stopped 15–20 minutes before testing so that the patient is fully awake during mapping.
- *Asleep awake asleep (AAA):* This technique consists of general anesthesia before and after brain mapping with or without involvement of an airway device (endotracheal tube or supraglottic device) at the start and end of the procedure. It has three phases. The first phase involves administration of propofol and a short-acting opioid such as fentanyl or remifentanil, with controlled ventilation. In the second phase, anesthetics are discontinued, patient is awakened, and functional and electrophysiological testing is performed. In the third phase, general anesthesia is again induced.

Postoperatively, after the scalp block has worn off, systemic pain relief with IV analgesia, paracetamol, and NSAIDS can be used.

POSTOPERATIVE MANAGEMENT

Ideally, early recovery and extubation help in immediate postoperative neurological examination of the patient and early diagnosis of complications. Patients who had a good preoperative level of consciousness with a Glasgow Coma Score (GCS) of >13, once they obey commands, maintain a patent airway with a gag reflex, and meet other general clinical extubation criteria such as adequate minute ventilation and stable hemodynamics, can be extubated. The aim is to achieve smooth emergence with minimal straining and coughing, which in turn increases ICP.

Postoperative pain can be pre-empted with a scalp nerve block, paracetamol, and minimal opioid use. Emergence hypertension should be treated with short-acting, titrated doses of esmolol or labetalol.

Patients who do not meet the above criteria of extubation and have preoperative morbid conditions or major intraoperative complications should be electively ventilated in the postoperative period; the decision should be a multidisciplinary effort.

In the intensive care unit, normovolemia and euglycemia should be maintained, and early initiation or enteral feeding ensures better outcomes. Ondansetron 0.15 mg/kg is given as prophylaxis for nausea and vomiting. Thromboembolic prophylaxis is by autocompression stockings and pumps, with early mobilization.

COMPLICATIONS

Delayed Emergence

Delayed emergence is usually multifactorial, due to drug, patient, surgical, or metabolic factors. These

Box 4: Risk factors for perioperative seizures.

- Anesthetic factors
  - Proconvulsant anesthetic agents (methohexital, enflurane)
  - Light anesthesia
  - Hypo-/hypercapnia
  - Hypoxemia
- Metabolic factors
  - Hypo-/hypernatremia
  - Hypoglycemia
  - Hypocalcemia
  - Uremia
  - Hypomagnesemia
- Neurological factors
  - Postcraniotomy hematoma
  - Poorly controlled epilepsy

include seizures, intracranial hematoma, brain edema or swelling, and tension pneumocephalus, which warrant a postoperative computed tomography (CT) scan to rule them out. Other causes are hypothermia, hypo- or hyperglycemia, hypoxemia, hypercapnia, metabolic acidosis, and hyponatremia.[16]

Emergence Agitation

Nearly 30% of the patients after elective craniotomy for brain tumors exhibited at least one episode of agitation during the early postoperative period. Emergence agitation is associated with the risk of self-extubation (**Box 4**). Independent predictors include male sex, history of long-term use of antidepressant drugs or benzodiazepines, frontal approach of the operation, method and duration of anesthesia, and presence of endotracheal intubation. Total intravenous anesthesia (TIVA), balanced anesthesia, and shorter duration are protective factors. The clarification and anticipation of risk factors could help identify the high-risk patients, facilitate the prevention and treatment of agitation, and prevent complications.[17]

Seizures

The risk for seizures in patients who are anesthetic, metabolic, or has neurosurgical risk factors, mentioned in **Box 4**, gets increased in the immediate few hours after surgery, with a potential to progress to status epilepticus. After excluding anesthetic and metabolic causes in the postoperative period, a surgical cause such as a hematoma should be excluded by the CT scan.

Seizures should be treated aggressively to avoid cerebral damage and to prevent progression to status epilepticus. Prolonged action of benzodiazepine, when administered after anesthetic/sedative drugs, may limit postictal neurological assessment. Propofol and thiopental in small doses rapidly and effectively terminate postoperative seizures; however, there is a risk of apnea, respiratory depression, airway compromise as well as hemodynamic instability due to myocardial depression and peripheral vasodilation leading to hypotension.[18]

Plasma levels of long-acting antiepileptic drugs should be checked and top-up doses administered as required. Persistent and recurrent seizures in the postoperative period require adjuvant therapy.

Fluid Abnormalities

The major concern of fluid management of neurosurgical patients is the prevention of brain swelling, which increases ICP, thus reducing CPP. The methods used to minimize intracranial interstitial water may produce hypovolemia and dyselectrolytemias (**Table 6**).[10]

SIADH is associated with ectopic neoplastic antidiuretic hormone (ADH) secretion or excessive hypothalamic–pituitary release of ADH secondary to neurologic surgery, neuropathologic states, pain, neuroendocrine abnormalities, and surgery in general. It is characterized by urinary sodium of >20 mmol/L, hyponatremia, hypervolemia, and hyposmolarity.

It is managed by free water restriction sufficient to reduce total body water by 0.5–1.0 L/day. The resultant reduction in the glomerular filtration rate enhances proximal tubular reabsorption of salt and water and stimulates aldosterone secretion. Demeclocycline and lithium antagonize the renal actions of ADH in refractory cases of SIADH.

Neurologic symptoms with profound hyponatremia serum Na^+ < 115–120 mEq/L require aggressive therapy; 3% hypertonic saline is indicated in patients who have seizures or who develop signs of water intoxication.

The administration of 3% hypertonic saline at a rate of 1–2 mL/kg/h to increase serum Na^+ by 1–2 mEq/L/h should be monitored every 1–2 hours to avoid overcorrection.

Cerebral salt wasting (CSW) syndrome is caused by the release of atrial natriuretic factor (ANF) in response to subarachnoid hemorrhage or injury. ANF increases renal sodium excretion causing a decrease in plasma volume. CSW syndrome is characterized by hyponatremia, hypovolemia, and urine sodium >50 mmol/L. The management involves rapid restoration of intravascular volume; the recommended fluid is 0.9% saline.

Diabetes insipidus is common following pituitary and hypothalamic lesions and other cerebral pathologies such as intracranial surgery and head trauma. It is characterized by polyuria, dehydration, hypernatremia, low urinary sodium, and low urinary specific gravity.

Management varies according to its cause—central or nephrogenic. Central DI requires exogenous replacement of ADH with either desmopressin (DDAVP) or aqueous vasopressin. DDAVP may be given either subcutaneously at

Table 6: Common dyselectrolytemias.

	Diabetes insipidus	SIADH	Cerebral salt wasting syndrome
Etiology	Decreased ADH	Increased ADH	Release of brain natriuretic factor
Serum Na⁺	Hypernatremia	Hyponatremia	Hyponatremia
Osmolality	Hyperosmolality	Hypo-osmolality	
Urine	Output > 3 mL/kg/h Specific gravity < 1.002 Na⁺ < 15 mEq/L	>20 mEq/L	>50 mEq/L
Urine osmolality vs. serum osmolality	Lower	Higher	Higher
Intravascular volume	Reduced	Normal/increased	Reduced

(ADH: antidiuretic hormone; SIADH: syndrome of inappropriate antidiuretic hormone secretion)

a dose of 1–4 µg every 12–24 hours or intranasally at a five times larger dose. Incomplete ADH deficits (partial DI) are effectively managed with chlorpropamide 250–750 mg/day, clofibrate 250–500 mg/6–8 hours or carbamazepine 400–100 mg/day. Nephrogenic DI is managed by restricting sodium and water intake and hydrochlorothiazide 50–100 mg/day.

Hemodilution

Hemodilution is characterized by low hematocrit in the presence of euvolemia or hypervolemic states. With a low hematocrit level, the blood viscosity is less, which may be useful in areas of ischemic brain with low flow states. Hematocrit can be lowered only to a point where the decreased oxygen-carrying capacity of the blood does not in itself compromise tissues. In the absence of a universal transfusion trigger, the decision to transfuse blood has to be individualized to each patient depending on the age, associated comorbidities, and the severity of the surgical procedure.

Thromboembolism

Prevention of deep venous and pulmonary thromboembolism requires prophylaxis in terms of autocompression stockings perioperatively.

Prophylactic anticoagulation entails the risk of hemorrhagic intracranial complications. A thromboprophylaxis protocol in the neurosurgical intensive care unit is useful in controlling the complications arising from deep venous thrombosis (DVT) and pulmonary embolism as well as avoiding the risk of intracerebral hematoma at the same time.[19]

Infections

Postoperative nosocomial infections may complicate the clinical course of postsurgical patients admitted in the neurological intensive care unit. A history of surgery; CSF leak; presence of cranial or extracranial infections such as otitis, sinusitis, or pneumonia; and a potentially immunocompromised state are the important risk factors.[20] A recent meta-analysis of 23 retrospective studies reported a cumulative rate of positive cultures of 8.8% per patient and 8.1% per external ventricular drainage.[21] Multidrug-resistant pathogens contribute to the complexity of management of nosocomial infections in the CNS. Continuous surveillance including systematic collection and analysis of the local epidemiological data, timely diagnosis, and prompt initiation of appropriate antimicrobial therapy is important to improve the outcome.[22]

CONCLUSION

There is a need for better understanding of multimodal pathways for optimizing perioperative care in patients undergoing elective neurosurgeries. Dedicated neurosurgical enhanced recovery pathways have the potential to reduce the length of stay and cost of hospitalization and improve functional outcomes and patient satisfaction after a well-conducted, protocolized, multidisciplinary approach to the perioperative care of patients undergoing neurosurgery for tumor excision.

REFERENCES

1. Ostrom QT, Gittleman H, Fulop J, Liu M, Blanda R, Kromer C, et al. CBTRUS statistical report: primary brain and central nervous system tumors in the United States in 2008-2012. Neuro Oncol. 2015;17(Suppl 4):iv1-62.

2. Yeole BB. Trends in the brain cancer incidence in India. Asian Pac J Cancer Prev. 2008;9:267-70.

3. Hagan KB, Bhavsar S, Raza SM, Arnold B, Arunkumar R, Dang A, et al. Enhanced recovery after surgery for oncological craniotomies. J Clin Neurosci. 2016;24:10-6.

4. Dinsmore J. Anaesthesia for elective neurosurgery. Brit J Anaesth. 2007;99:68-74.

5. Umamaheswara Rao GS. Anaesthetic management of supratentorial intracranial tumours. The Indian Anaesthetists' Forum October 2005(2). [online] Available from www.theiaforum.org [Last accessed March, 2020].

6. Hancock SM, Nathanson MH. Nitrous oxide or remifentanil for the at-risk brain. Anaesthesia. 2004;59:313-5.

7. Rozet I, Vavilala MS. Risks and benefits of patient positioning during neurosurgical care. Anesthesiol Clin. 2007;25(3):631-53, x.

8. Bithal PK. Anaesthetic considerations for evoked potentials monitoring. J Neuroanaesthesiol Crit Care. 2014;1:2-12.

9. Schubert A, Licina MG, Lineberry PJ. The effect of ketamine on human somatosensory evoked potentials and its modification by nitrous oxide. Anesthesiology. 1990;72:33-39.

10. Monteiro JN. Fluids and electrolyte management. In: Prabhakar H (Ed). Essentials of Neuroanesthesia, Ch. 49. San Diego: Academic Press; 2017. pp. 823-4.

11. Monteiro JN, Goraksha SU. 'ROSE concept' of fluid management: relevance in neuroanaesthesia and neurocritical care. J Neuroanaesthesiol Crit Care. 2017;4:10-6.

12. Ali Z, Prabhakar H. Fluid management during neurosurgical procedures. J Neuroanaesthesiol Crit Care. 2016;3(Suppl S1):35-40.

13. Malbrain ML, Marik PE, Witters I, Cordemans C, Kirkpatrick AW, Roberts DJ, et al. Fluid overload, de-resuscitation, and outcomes in critically ill or injured patients: a systematic review with suggestions for clinical practice. Anaesthesiol Intensive Ther 2014;46:361-80.

14. Burnand C, Sebastian J. Anaesthesia for awake craniotomy. Contin Educ Anaesth Crit Care Pain. 2014;14(1):6-11.

15. Rath GP, Mahajan C, Bithal PK. Anaesthesia for awake craniotomy. J Neuroanaesthesiol Crit Care. 2014;1(3):173-7.

16. Rhona CF, Sinclair B, Faliero RJ. Delayed recovery of consciousness after anaesthesia. Contin Educ Anaesth Crit Care Pain. 2006;6(3):114-8.

17. Chen L, Xu M, Li GY, Cai WX, Zhou JX. Incidence, risk factors and consequences of emergence agitation in adult patients after elective craniotomy for brain tumor: a prospective cohort study. PLoS One. 2014;9(12):e114239.

18. Smith M. Anesthesia for epilepsy surgery. In: Shorvon S, Perucca E, Fish D, Dodson E (Eds). The Treatment of Epilepsy. Oxford: Blackwell Science; 2004.

19. Nickele CM, Kamps TK, Medow JE. Safety of a DVT chemoprophylaxis protocol following traumatic brain injury: a single center quality improvement initiative. Neurocrit Care. 2013;18:184-92.

20. Beer R, Pfausler B, Scmutzhard E. Infectious intracranial complications in the neuro-ICU patient population. Curr Opin Crit Care. 2010;16:117-22.

21. Lozier AP, Sciacca RR, Romagnoli MF Connolly ES Jr. Venticulostomy related infections: a critical review of the literature. Neurosurgery. 2002;51(1):170-81.

22. Umamaheshwar Rao GS, Bansal S. Neurological critical care. In: Prabhakar H (Ed). Essentials of Neuroanesthesia. San Diego: Academic Press; 2017. pp. 602-3.

Perioperative Management of Spinal Surgeries

Devendra Gupta, Shashi Srivastava

INTRODUCTION

There have been dramatic advances in the field of spine surgery for the last few decades and these procedures not only increase in numbers but also in complexity. The steep rise in spine surgery is attributed to many transformations, including a rapidly aging population with degenerative spinal disease, minimally invasive technology, advanced surgical techniques and equipment, and a change in practice toward more instrumented spinal fusion procedures that were previously treated with a simple decompression.[1] Overall, a wide range of spinal procedures from short, almost bloodless outpatient procedures to extremely long reconstructive procedures requiring multiple transfusions are being performed. The type of surgery performed for various pathological disorder of spine includes trauma, tumor, deformity, and myelopathy (**Table 1**). Spinal surgery can be divided into categories based on the invasiveness of the procedure (**Table 2**).[2] Complex spine surgery is a high-risk procedure and is often quite morbid in nature.[3] The combination of prolonged surgery in the prone or lateral position with high blood loss in locations that can result in severe neurological injury or airway compromise and patients with more comorbidities frequently requires skillful preoperative optimization for better outcome. Very often postoperative course of the patient is stormy due to persistent blood loss associated unstable hemodynamic and transfusion related coagulopathies and lung injury; the vigilant care of the patient in ICU is essential. The

Table 1: Type of spinal disorder.		
Cervical spine	*Thoracic spine*	*Lumbosacral spine*

Cervical spine trauma:
• Atlas fracture
• Axis fracture
• Cervical subaxial fracture
Craniovertebral anomalies:
• Atlantoaxial dislocation
• Basilar invasion
Degenerative disorders:
• Cervical spondylosis
• Cervical myelopathy
• Cervical radiculopathy
Ossification of posterior longitudinal ligament
Paget's disease
Rheumatic arthritis
Ankylosing spondylitis
	Spinal deformity:
	Scoliosis and kyphosis (thoracic or thoracolumbar)
	Tumor:
	• *Primary tumors*
	  – *Intramedullary*: Ependymoma, astrocytoma, hemangiomas
	  – *Intradural–extramedullary*: Meningioma, schwannoma, neurofibroma, arachnoid cysts,
	  – *Extradural*: Chondroma, osteoma, osteoblastoma, osteoclastoma, sarcoma, lymphomas
	• *Metastatic tumor*
	Infection:
	• Intramedullary abscess
	• Subdural and epidural abscess
	• Osteomyelitis
	• Pott's spine
	Vascular malformations: Arteriovenous malformation
		Congenital disorder:
		• Spinal dysraphism including meningocele or meningomyelocele
		• Lumbosacral fracture
		Degenerative disorder:
		• Intervertebral disk herniation
		• Spondylolisthesis
		• Lumbar stenosis
		• Cauda equine syndrome
		Trauma
		Tumor*
		Vascular malformations*

*Same as thoracic spine.

Table 2: Classification of spinal surgery based on invasiveness.		
Complexity of surgery	*Predicted blood loss*	*Common type of procedure*
Minor	<100 mL	Anterior or posterior cervical diskectomy and fusion, lumbar diskectomy with or without fusion of ≤2 level
Major	100 and 1,000 mL	Anterior lumbar interbody instrumentation of <3 level
Complex	>1,000 mL	Kyphoscoliosis correction surgery, vascular tumor surgery, ≥3 levels fusion (anterior or posterior), and instrumentation

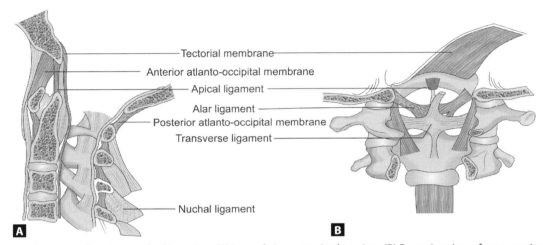

Figs. 1A and B: Anatomy of craniovertebral junction. (A) Lateral view—sagittal section; (B) Posterior view after removing posterior elements showing the ligamentous attachment.

pediatric group has specific indication of spine surgery with a different set of problems. There are substantial anatomic differences between the cervical and the thoracolumbar vertebral columns; consequently clinical presentation, critical concerns, and outcome differ considerably between thoracolumbar and cervical spine disorders.

CERVICAL SPINE

Anatomical Considerations

The cervical spine is made up of seven vertebrae. The first two, C1 and C2 (atlas and axis), are highly specialized and form the upper cervical vertebrae; and C3–C7 are more classic vertebrae, having a body, pedicles, laminae, and spinous processes, and facet joints form the lower cervical or subaxial spine. The cervical spine is much more mobile than the thoracolumbar regions of the spine. Unlike the other parts of the spine, the cervical spine has transverse foramina in each vertebra for the vertebral arteries that supply blood to the brain.

The craniovertebral junction (CVJ) or occipitoatlantoaxial (OAA) collectively refers to the posterior skull base (clivus, foramen magnum, and occiput), the atlas (C1), the axis (C2), supporting ligaments (cruciate, apical, alar, and cruciform ligaments), and membranes (anterior and posterior atlanto-

occipital membranes; tectorial membrane). The cruciate ligament is composed of transverse and cervical ligaments (**Figs. 1A and B**). Most of the cervical movements occur between the atlanto-occipital and the atlantoaxial joints. The mechanical properties of the atlanto-occipital joint are primarily determined by bony structures, whereas those of the altlanto-axial joint are by various ligaments and membranes. In the dorsal aspect of the dens there is a transverse groove over which passes the thick transverse ligament. Transverse ligament is attached between the two bony tubercles on the inner anterolateral aspect of atlas and effectively limit anterior translation and flexion of the altlanto-axial joint. *Alar ligaments* are two strong cords attached to the dorsolateral body of the dens.[4] These fibers extend laterally and rostrally. They are ventral and cranial to the transverse ligament. Normally, these do not allow >3 mm of translation between the dens and the anterior arch of the atlas (anterior atlas–dental interval).

COMMON SPINE DISORDERS

Surgery on the cervical spine is commonly performed to relieve compression of the spinal cord (myelopathy), a nerve root (radiculopathy) or to provide bony stabilization to prevent secondary neurological injury.

Cervical spondylosis is a nonspecific degenerative condition of the cervical spine that results into spinal stenosis and neural foraminal intrusion in the form of disk herniation (central and lateral), osteophytes hypertrophy, facet joint osteophytes, and hypertrophied of longitudinal ligament and ligamentum flavum. Radiculopathy is the most common symptoms which is defined as a neurological condition characterized by dysfunction of a cervical spinal nerve, the nerve roots, or both. The common symptoms are neck pain, pain at arm, radicular pain such as shooting pain that radiates from the shoulder to the arm, or hand, paresthesias, and/or muscle weakness in the nerve root distribution.

Cervical Spondylotic Myelopathy

Cervical spondylotic myelopathy (CSM) manifests itself following static or dynamic compression of the spinal cord resulting in spinal cord ischemia. CSM is the most common cause of myelopathy in adults >55 years of age, causing progressive disability and impairing the quality of life. The common signs and symptoms of CSM are pain in the neck, shoulder, subscapular area, paresthesia in upper limb, motor weakness in upper and lower limbs, gait disturbances, bladder and bowel dysfunctions, and spastic hyper-reflexia.

Cervical disk herniation most commonly occurs between C5–C6 and C6–C7 vertebral bodies causing symptoms at C6 and C7, respectively (**Fig. 2**). The most common symptoms are neck pain and radicular symptoms; however, patients may present with symptoms of cervical myelopathy if the disk herniation is central location. The primary treatment of the cervical disk herniation is medical management and 90% patient experience improvement with it. If the patient does not respond to medical therapy, surgical therapy is

indicated in the form of anterior cervical diskectomy and fusion (ACDF) with or without anterior cervical plating.

Craniovertebral junction anomalies are developmental disorders that affect the skeleton and enclosed neuraxis at the junction of cranium and cervical spine. There are three main issues in dealing with congenital CVJ anomalies, namely, Arnold–Chiari malformation (ACM), basilar invagination (BI), and atlantoaxial dislocation (AAD) (**Figs. 3A and B**). Clinical features of CVJ anomalies are due to compression of the brain stem and the spinal cord

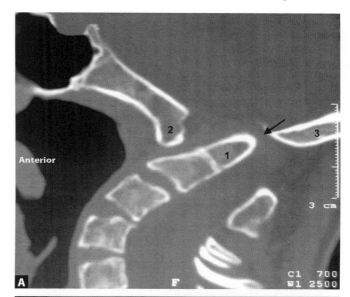
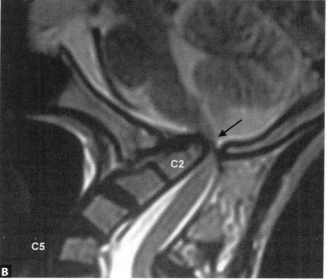

Figs. 3A and B: Craniovertebral junction (CVJ) anomaly: Sagittal view of (A) computerized tomography; (B) T2-weighted magnetic resonance image showing atlantoaxial dislocation, with basilar invagination, 1: Odontoid process of axis, 2: Anterior tubercle of atlas fused with clivus, 3: Occiput with occipital posterior arch of atlas. The arrow shows severe spinal cord compression and very narrow space available for the cord at the cervicomedullary junction.

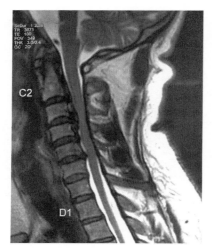

Fig. 2: T2-weighted magnetic resonance image—sagittal view showing severe cervical spondylosis with spinal cord compression at the C3–C4 and C5–C6 levels.

and may include recurrent occipital headaches, neck aches, bulbar palsy, and upper and lower motor neuron palsy. CVJ anomalies can also obstruct the flow of cerebrospinal fluid (CSF), causing syringomyelia (SM) and/or hydrocephalus.

RHEUMATOID ARTHRITIS

Rheumatoid arthritis (RA) is now known to be a chronic systemic inflammatory disorder characterized by deforming symmetrical polyarthritis of varying extent and severity, associated with synovitis of joint and tendon sheaths, articular cartilage loss, and erosion of juxta-articular bone.[5] The atlantoaxial joint is commonly affected in RA because of attenuation of the transverse ligament and erosion of the odontoid. This can lead to atlantoaxial instability in about 25% of patients suffering from RA. In the anterior subtype (80% of cases), the C1 vertebra moves forward on C2 because of destruction of the transverse ligament and there is a risk of spinal cord compression by the dens. In the posterior subtype (affecting 5% of cases of AAD) posterior destruction of the odontoid may cause backward movement of C1 on C2 and posterior atlantoaxial subluxation (AAS) is worsened by neck extension. Involvement of the cricoarytenoid joints may result in dyspnea, stridor, hoarseness, and occasionally severe upper airway obstruction.[6] Patients with cricoarytenoid RA may present with a mass in the larynx, which can cause significant destruction of the surrounding structures.[7] Patients with RA with myelopathy often have a very high morbidity and mortality; hence, early surgical stabilization is indicated. Visceral manifestations of the underlying disease need particular attention, especially when related to the cardiac (pericardial effusions, pericarditis, myocarditis, endocarditis, increased atherosclerosis, and coronary heart disease), the pulmonary (pleural effusion, pulmonary fibrosis, restriction lung disease, and pulmonary hypertension) or the hematological (anemia, chronic infection, and thrombocytosis) system.[8]

DOWN SYNDROME

Approximately 20% of the patients with Down syndrome have ligamentous laxity of the atlantoaxial joint. This condition may allow C1–C2 subluxation and predispose patients with Down syndrome to spinal cord injury. Hypoplasia, malformation, and absence of the odontoid process mar the causes that predisposed to the C1–C2 instabilty.[9] Cardiac abnormalities are common in Down syndrome such as atrial septal defect, atrioventricular septal defects, ventricular septal defects, patent ductus arteriosus, tetralogy of Fallot, and pulmonary vascular disease. Respiratory diseases (upper and lower) are frequent in this subset of the patients which include tracheal stenosis (subglottic), enlarged tongue, enlarged tonsils and adenoids,

obstructive sleep apnea (OSA), and small lower airway. Pulmonary vascular disease may also arise due to OSA, chronic hypoxemia due to repeated pulmonary infections, and hypoventilation due to muscle hypotonia.[10]

KLIPPEL–FEIL SYNDROME

Klippel–Feil syndrome (KFS) is a rare disease characterized by a classic triad comprising a short neck, a low posterior hairline, and restricted motion of the neck due to fused cervical vertebrae. KFS can be associated with a number of other anomalies, including renal dysfunction (64%), scoliosis (60%), deafness (30%), Sprengel's scapula deformity (25–35%), congenital heart disease (4.2–14%), mental deficiency, pulmonary disability, and cleft lip and palate.[11] Patients with KFS are also more likely to have cervical instability, increasing their risk of neurologic damage with minor trauma or during laryngoscopy, intubation, and positioning.[12]

ACHONDROPLASIA

Achondroplasia is a congenital disfiguring condition which is the most common form of short-limbed dwarfism. Defective cartilage formation is the hallmark of this condition, which results in a wide spectrum of skeletal abnormalities including spinal defects (**Figs. 4A and B**). AAD may concurrently exist in achondroplastic patients either de novo, following surgery (foramen magnum decompression) or due to odontoid abnormalities (os odontoideum).[13,14]

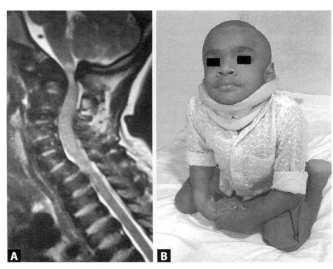

Figs. 4A and B: A case of a 16-year-old child with achondroplasia: (A) T1-weighted magnetic resonance image—sagittal view showing spinal cord compression at the craniovertebral junction and cervical spondylosis; (B) Short-statured child with short neck stabilized by the cervical collar.

ARNOLD–CHIARI MALFORMATION

Arnold–Chiari malformation is a developmental malformation characterized by downward displacement of cerebellar tonsils into spinal canal due to reduced capacity of the posterior fossa. ACM may be complicated by other malformations such as platybasia, BI, and occipitalization although SM is most commonly seen (**Fig. 5**).[15]

Syringomyelia is the development of a cystic cavity or syrinx within the spinal cord. About 10% of SM have communication with the 4th ventricle; however, in 50% of all cases, the communication of syrinx is caused by obstruction of CSF circulation from the basal posterior fossa to the caudal space without 4th ventricular communication. The most common example is ACM, which is also associated with communicating SM.[16] The most common form of presentation is central cord syndrome; this largely depends on the location of the syrinx. The most frequent symptom was segmental sensory loss (93%), followed by pyramidal signs (82%) and muscle atrophy (60%). Surgical options include removal of known causes, decompression, laminectomy, duraplasty, shunting, excision of syrinx, and a suboccipital craniotomy.

OSSIFIED POSTERIOR LONGITUDINAL LIGAMENT

Ossification of the posterior longitudinal ligament (OPLL) is a hyperostotic condition that results in ectopic calcification of the posterior longitudinal ligament. The most commonly involved vertebrae are C4–C5, followed by C5–C6 and C3–C4. Lower cervical vertebrae around the level of C4, C5, and C6 may impinge on the esophagus and distal trachea, where it is tethered at the level of cricoid, whereas the upper cervical spine may impinge more on the oropharynx, causing globus, stridor, or respiratory compromise. Patients with OPLL present with varying degrees of neurologic syndromes including both radiculopathy and myelopathy. The patients with OPLL are prone to spinal cord injury (central cord syndrome) and the risk factors include old age as well as the presence of a segmental type of OPLL and/or ossification of the anterior longitudinal ligament.[17] Patients with mild myelopathy/cord compression rarely require surgery, while those with moderate/severe myelopathy/cord compression often warrant anterior, posterior, or circumferential approaches.

ANKYLOSING SPONDYLITIS

Ankylosing spondylitis (AS) is an inflammatory rheumatism that may induce structural damage in the cervical spine. Microscopic changes include bone fragility[18] arising from decreased bone density, which has been shown to be related to persistent systemic inflammation and hypervascularization of the bone. Cervical spine surgery is associated with AS in two main situations—management of trauma[19] and correction of sagittal "chin-to-chest" deformity.[20] Both remain strategically and technically challenging. As with cervical spine fractures in the general population, traumatic fracture/dislocation in the patient with AS usually occurs in the lower cervical spine (C5 to T1). However, AS-related fractures are frequently more severe, with specific features compared to cervical fractures in the healthy population.[18] AS fractures are, for example, highly unstable because the anterior and the posterior elements are involved in a transverse or short oblique pattern that does not follow the classical three-column criteria for stability as seen in normal spines.[21]

KYPHOSCOLIOSIS

Kyphoscoliosis (KS) is a complex progressive type of spinal deformity which is characterized by anterior flexion, lateral bending, and rotation of vertebrae (**Figs. 6A and B**).[22] It is also associated with ribcage deformity. There may be secondary involvement of cardiovascular, respiratory, and neurological system due to which patients land up in problems postoperatively and may require ventilator support. KS is characterized by diminished chest wall compliance and impaired respiratory mechanics, leading to progressive hypoventilation, hypercapnia, chronic respiratory failure, pulmonary hypertension, cor pulmonale, and potentially right heart failure.[22] Severity of scoliosis is measured by Cobb's method, it consists of locating the superior and inferior end of vertebra then drawing intersecting perpendicular lines from superior surface of superior end vertebra and inferior surface of inferior end

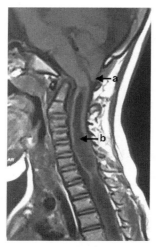

Fig. 5: T1-weighted magnetic resonance image—sagittal view showing (a) downward herniation of the cerebellar tonsils through the foramen magnum suggesting Arnold–Chiari malformation and (b) syrinx within the cervical cord from C2 downward.

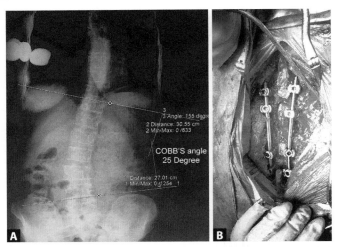

Figs. 6A and B: (A) Preoperative radiograph showing a left thoracolumbar curve between T11 and L4 with measured Cobb's angle of 25°; (B) A surgical view of the lumbar spine with rod reduction instruments attached to the pedicle screws.

Cobb's angle (°)	Clinical manifestation
<10	No symptoms
>25	Increase in pulmonary artery pressure
>40	Consider surgical intervention
>70	Significant decrease in lung volume
>100	Dyspnea on exertion
>120	Alveolar hypoventilation, chronic respiratory failure

Table 3: Severity of scoliosis and clinical implications.[23]

vertebra. Angle of deviation of these perpendicular lines from straight line is the angle of curve. Surgery is performed when Cobb's angle exceeds 50° in the thoracic spine and 40° in the lumbar spine **(Table 3)**.[23]

SPINAL CORD TUMORS

Spinal cord tumors may be primary tumors of the spinal cord or secondary to metastases. Primary tumors may be intramedullary (located inside the cord) or intradural extramedullary (IDEM) which are located within dura but outside the cord. Intramedullary tumors commonly are gliomas, ependymoma, astrocytoma, and hemangioblastomas. IDEM tumors are benign in nature such as meningiomas and peripheral nerve sheath tumors such as schwannomas and neurofibromas account for majority of these tumors, with almost half of them being located at the thoracic level. Metastatic tumors are very common spinal tumors and primarily arise from breast, lung, renal, gastric, or hematopoietic/lymphoid tissue; they reach bone through blood or direct extension of the tumor.

These tumors commonly occur at thoracic spine though occurrence at cervical spine causes more perioperative morbidity.

POTT'S SPINE

Spinal tuberculosis (TB) remains the most prevalent spinal infection worldwide and accounts for 1–3% of all TB cases and over 40% of all spine infections.[23] Characteristically, there is destruction of the intervertebral disk space and the adjacent vertebral bodies with collapse, and anterior wedging leading to kyphosis formation. Modern surgical management of spinal TB includes debridement of diseased vertebrae, decompression of the spinal cord, correction of deformities, stabilization of spine, and further protection of the spinal cord.

SURGICAL APPROACHES

Atlantoaxial subluxations, which are reducible or can be reduced with C1–C2 joint manipulation, are treated with foramen decompression and posterior fixation in prone position. Traditionally, an anterior approach (transoral odontoidectomy) to the CVJ is the treatment of choice in a variety of diseases affecting the CVJ, including BI, RA, or neoplastic processes. When both are indicated in a patient of AAD with BI, transoral odontoidectomy is done in supine position followed by posterior decompression and fixation in prone position as a single-stage procedure. Anterior cervical diskectomy or corpectomy and fusion approach is used in CSM, OPLL, and other compressive myelopathy of cervical spine in supine position. Most of the surgery in thoracolumbar spine for tumor or degenerative diseases is preferred to be done through posterior approaches in prone position.

Sometime, collapsed vertebral body of the thoracic spine due to tumour, osteoporosis, or infective disease like Potts spine is surgically treated by anterior and anterolateral decompression by thoraco-abdominal approach, and posteriorly costo-transversectomy and laminectomy; and for lumbar spine, anterior and antero-lateral posterior are all possible options **(Figs. 7A to C)**.

Preoperative Risk Assessment and Optimization

Surgery is mostly designed to relieve compression of the spinal cord or spinal nerve roots. Complication rates for complex adult cervical surgery (anterior approach, posterior approach, or combined) are unacceptably high and too often result in unacceptable patient impairment and disability. Though most of the thoracolumbar surgeries are simple but complex procedure such as correction

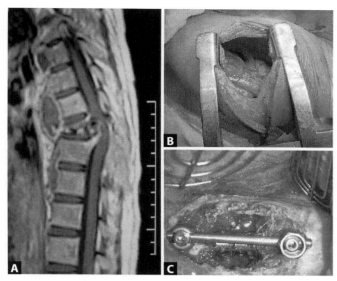

Figs. 7A to C: A case of a 56-year-old male with the diagnosis of Pott's spine at the T6 level. (A) T1-weighted magnetic resonance image—sagittal view showing vertebral body collapse of T6 vertebra with spinal cord compression. Intraoperative photographs showing (B) right thoracotomy done by skin incision parallel to rib in lateral position, transpleural with visible lung in the surgical field, and (C) insertion of implant after retraction of the lung.

surgery, the transthoracic or transabdominal approach needs special preoperative preparations. The complexity of procedures and associated comorbidities determine the appropriate preoperative testing, optimization, and anesthesia plans. A much systemic approach is required by a team consisting of anesthesiologists, surgeon, clinician, and supportive therapists which implement a series of preoperative interventions to expedite a better recovery after major spine surgery.

Cervical Instability

Clinical instability of the cervical spine is defined as the inability of the spine under physiological loads to maintain its normal pattern of intervertebral displacement which results in pain or deformity over a period of years. AAS is seen in Down syndrome, Morquio syndrome, RA, and infections of the head and neck (Grisel's syndrome). The adult lower cervical spine is considered to be unstable when one of the following conditions is there:

- All the anterior or all the posterior elements are destroyed
  or
- There is >3.5-mm horizontal displacement of one vertebra in relation to an adjacent one on a lateral X-ray
  or
- There is more than 11° of rotation of one vertebra to an adjacent one.

The basis of management in instability is immobilization or at least reduction of movement. A rigid cervical collar

is commonly used for this purpose. Though the purpose of the cervical collar is to maintain the cervical spine in a neutral position with as little displacement as possible, there is evidence that collars do not reliably achieve this, one study concluding "Full cervical immobilization is a myth."[24] Collars may actually promote paradoxical motion of vertebrae and risk cord compromise, especially at the cervicothoracic junction, and inappropriately sized or applied collars exaggerate vertebral malalignment. Active and forceful neck movement in patients emerging from sedation, head injured or agitated with a cervical collar may actually increase the risk of neurological deterioration.[24] Pressure sores related to collars or bed sores may occur in up to 44% of patients and can act as a source of sepsis and require skin grafting.[25] Extrication or rigid collars are inappropriate for prolonged use in ICU, exerting high cutaneous pressures and producing unacceptable rates of necrosis. Nonetheless, there is probably little doubt that rigid cervical collars seem a reasonable extrication and transfer adjunct when used with full spinal immobilization and lateral restraints. An alternative may be to transfer a cervical unstable patient to an ICU or diagnostic suits in a cervical collar, but have it removed at the earliest possible opportunity.[26] Patients of CVJ anomalies associated with BI show rapid clinical improvement after preoperative application of cervical traction.[27]

Pulmonary System

Cervical spinal cord is a crucial organ involving descending tracts in the dorsolateral columns containing descending reticulospinal pathways which are essential for respiratory muscle activity. Chronic compressive cervical spinal lesions such as cervical spondylotic myelopathy and cervical OPLL cause respiratory dysfunction due to injury to the segments from which the phrenic nerves originate, weakness of respiratory muscles, loss of intercostal muscular tone and probably due to spastic movement of the chest wall. The preoperative assessment of the patient's respiratory function and nutritional state by a spirometer, blood gas analysis, and albumin may predict a postoperative course. The simple measurements in the preoperative period such as an exercise program to improve lung capacity and function, micronebulization with mucolytic agents, tracheal stretch exercise, and chest physiotherapy are advised to reduce risk of postoperative ventilation and pulmonary complication.[28] Other than respiratory risk, smokers have a significantly higher pseudarthrosis and postoperative infection rate; therefore, abstinence from smoking is required prior to elective surgery.[29]

In CVJ anomalies, respiratory impairment is also due to compression of the respiratory center by dens and cord compression of the C1–C2 level. Further, impaired lower cranial nerve function results in a poor gag and cough reflex causing frequent aspiration and repeated pulmonary infection. Although the respiratory dysfunction is mild or subclinical, it assumes importance in view of the potential intraoperative or postoperative respiratory complications [such as atelectasis, respiratory failure, pneumonia, and acute respiratory distress syndrome (ARDS)] because of various anesthetic and surgical reasons.[30] However, many patients with severe compressive myelopathy have severe respiratory impairment may result in atelectasis and, over time, respiratory fatigue and failure. A weak or ineffective cough may lead to retained secretions and subsequent pneumonia. If patients with poor respiratory failure require mechanical ventilation, early tracheostomy is indicated.[31]

In KS, the severity of pulmonary function derangement is affected by Cobb's angle or more number of vertebra involved, cephalad site of curvature, and degree of loss seen in thoracic kyphosis. Additionally, the impairment of pulmonary function in kyphosis correlates with spinal mobility (especially forward flexion)[32] and is notable when the kyphosis angle is >55°.[33] Acute exacerbations, particularly respiratory tract infections, rapidly worsen these patients' respiratory conditions and precipitate acute respiratory failure (ARF), which usually requires ICU hospitalization and either noninvasive or invasive mechanical ventilation. Patients who have preexisting neuromuscular disease, severe restrictive lung disease with the vital capacity (VC) of <35% of predicted, obese patients, right ventricular failure, congenital heart defects, anterior thoracic spine surgery, and blood loss of 30 mL/kg should be counseled for postoperative mechanical ventilation. Patients with chronic obstructive pulmonary disease (COPD) are at increased risk for pleural effusion and pneumonia, and treatment with bronchodilators, antibiotics, intensive spirometry, and cessation of smoking and steroids can help to reduce the risk.[34] Anterior thoracic approaches requiring thoracotomy theoretically have a higher risk of pulmonary complications and may require postoperative ventilation in ICU; therefore, vigorous preoperative pulmonary preparation is needed.

Cardiovascular System

Large part of CSM patients also suffered from hypertension presuming that both CSM and hypertension are chronic progressive diseases that are associated with aging. CSM is associated with a 3.10-fold increase of arrhythmia risk compared to patients without cervical spondylosis, especially atrial fibrillation, and ventricular and supraventricular tachycardia.[35] CSM is also found to be associated with an increased risk of acute coronary syndrome. Autonomic nervous system stimulation could explain the related mechanism of these findings. Clinical evidence had shown that cervical spondylosis can cause sympathetic nerve irritation and associated sympathetic

symptoms.[35] Thus, electrocardiogram would be needed in those CSMs presented with sympathetic symptoms or those who had several identified risk markers of arrhythmia. Primary prevention with anticoagulations or antiarrhythmic medications for fatal arrhythmia or ischemia stroke would be beneficial. Cardiac manifestations such as cardiac valve thickening, dysfunction, and conduction abnormalities are common in patients of AADs associated with the mucopolysaccharidosis (MPS) such as Morquio syndrome.[36] The AS patients may also have similar cardiac concerns pertinent to the anesthetist which include aortic valve insufficiency, cardiac conduction defects, and pulmonary fibrosis. There is an increased risk of cardiovascular-related death for patients with RA as compared to the general population. Overall, individuals with RA have a higher risk of myocardial infarction which is similar to individuals with diabetes mellitus or a person 10 years older than the age of the patient. Traditional risk factors do not completely explain the risk for cardiovascular disease in patients with RA. Preoperative cardiac evaluation including echocardiography is recommended in all such cases.

Cardiac changes are due to mediastinal shifts following scoliotic curves and also secondary to chronic respiratory insufficiency leading to alteration in cardiovascular function. Mechanical compression on heart can affect its normal filling during exercise and even at rest. Echocardiography and stress testing can be done to know the myocardial functioning and pulmonary pressures. Chronic hypoxia leads to pulmonary hypertension which in turn leads to right heart strain and failure.[37] Presence of right-side heart failure suggests complete heart evaluation.[37] Patients with congenital heart defects are prone to have scoliosis; therefore, these patients should be screened for tetralogy of Fallot, atrial septal defects, and patent ductus arteriosus.[38]

Obesity

Obesity contributes to disk degeneration and low back pain and potentially increases the risk of developing operative pathology. Obese patients undergoing spine surgery have a higher risk of developing postoperative complications, particularly surgical site infection and venous thromboembolism.[39] Obesity is closely correlated with additional medical comorbidities, including hypertension, coronary artery disease, congestive heart failure, and diabetes mellitus. The operating team should discuss and plan all necessary arrangements in an operation room as there is a potential for increased operative times, difficulties with airway, anesthesia and operative positioning, higher blood loss, and postextubation complications.

Geriatric Population

Older patients frequently harbor multiple overlapping comorbidities that increase their susceptibility to the major risks and complications associated with spinal surgery, particularly when involving extensive instrumented fusions. A plan of surgery should be discussed by anesthesiologists with the surgical team considering age and comorbidity appropriate and avoid "too much" (instrumented fusions) as well as "too little" surgery where feasible.[40] These patients should receive preoperative cognitive screening in the form of a mini-mental status examination by neuropsychology.

Diabetes

Uncontrolled diabetes is a known risk factor of prolonged length of hospital stay, postoperative infection, and postoperative complications. Patients with hemoglobin A1c (HbA1c) >8% are referred to the endocrinologists for preoperative optimization. Preoperatively, patients are encouraged to achieve average blood glucose of <180 mg/dL. Surgery is scheduled no earlier than 2 weeks after the initial endocrinology consultation to allow for adequate time for effective blood glucose management.

Nutrition

Malnutrition is common in bedridden quadriplegic syndromic AAD children and is likely to place them at an increased risk of adverse surgical outcomes. As nutritional status is a potentially modifiable risk factor, optimizing a child's preoperative nutritional status sometime by putting a feeding gastric tube may potentially lead to improved short- and long-term outcomes. Signs of malnutrition in the form of albumin levels < 3.5 g/dL, serum total, lymphocyte count < 1,500 cells/mm^3, and transferrin levels <200 mg/dL are associated with increased complications. There is high prevalence of clinical and subclinical B$_{12}$ deficiency in the elderly CSM, and optimization of vitamin B$_{12}$ levels can improve surgical outcome.[41] Anemia is a common presentation in patients with spinal tumors and is associated with increased postoperative pulmonary complications, length of stay, and mortality. Therefore, hemoglobin < 10 g% should be investigated and corrected. All patients undergoing either major or complex elective spine surgery are screened for anemia and should be administered oral iron, an iron infusion, or erythropoietin to reach a target hemoglobin of 13 g/dL.

Thromboembolism

The prevalence of preoperative deep vein thrombosis (DVT) in patients with CSM was relatively high (4%). The risk factors for asymptomatic DVT in patients with CSM were old age, a longer duration with CSM, abnormal D-dimer levels, and a history of ischemic cardiovascular events. Anesthesiologists should consider vascular evaluation for patients with CSM when they have these risk factors.[42] There is high incidence of DVT and pulmonary embolism in severe cases of CVJ with quadriparesis and require prophylactic heparin and intermittent pneumatic compression preoperatively. Preoperatively in all patients with spinal tumor, a lower extremity Doppler ultrasound should also be considered, because of the increased risk for development of DVT and pulmonary embolism due to the paresis-induced prolonged immobilization or malignancy-related hypercoagulability.

Neurological Evaluation

Careful neurological evaluation should be done in the patient presenting for spine surgery. Though a thorough neurological evaluation has been done by a neurologist or neurosurgeon, anesthesiologists should also carefully examine and document the pre-existing neurological deficit for comparison in the postoperative period. Additional efforts should be made to examine and document the clinical examination of the nerve liable to position-related injury during surgery (ulnar, sciatic, etc.).

Evaluation of Airway

Airway evaluation of the patient for spine surgery is the same as for other surgical patients according to difficult airway guidelines; however, potential for difficulty in airway management should always be considered, particularly in those patients presenting for surgery of the upper thoracic or cervical spine. A careful assessment should be made for previous difficulty in intubation, restriction of neck movement, and the stability (discussed above) or otherwise of the cervical spine. A full clinical and radiological [lateral or flexion/extension plain films, computer-aided tomography, and magnetic resonance imaging (MRI)] assessment of the cervical spine is must preoperatively. Concerned anesthesiologists should plan an airway management accordingly.

Preparation of difficult airway should always be made when any high risk patient for spine surgery is in high dependency unit or ICU during preoperative preparatory phase. The MACOCHA score [Mallampati score III or IV, apnea syndrome (obstructive), cervical spine limitation, opening mouth 3 cm, coma, hypoxia and anesthesiologist nontrained] has been recently developed to identify patients with potentially difficult airway in the ICU.[43] This score considers not only patient-related anatomical difficulty but also physiological factors and operator experience.

Imaging

Patients who undergo spinal surgery typically have multiple preoperative imaging studies. Preoperative evaluation of images including plain radiographs, computed tomography (CT) scan, and MRI of surgical pathology can help anesthesiologists to predict intraoperative and postoperative complications. A systemic approach in analyzing radiology for "visualization" of actual bony and soft-tissue structures of cervical spine to assist in prediction of difficult airway may be of immense help to the anesthesiologist and crucially guide intraoperative and postoperative airway and ventilator management.

Intraoperative Concerns

Choice of the induction agent is guided primarily by the patient's condition and by consideration of the ease with which the trachea may be intubated. Preoxygenation is advisable in all patients. The use of succinylcholine is always a concern in patients with muscular dystrophies. A decision of awake fiberoptic intubation must be made on preoperative assessment and the patient must be counselled. Direct laryngoscopy with manual in-line stabilization or a hard collar is an accepted means of intubation for many patients provided this can be achieved without any neck movement. Difficult airway cart and presence of experience anestheiologists should always be assured. The anterior transthoracic approach for thoracic spine surgery may necessitate the use of a double-lumen endobronchial tube. Central venous access may be useful when anticipating blood loss, cardiac comorbidities or need of administering vasoactive drugs. Patients who are anticipated to require ICU stay postoperatively should have a central line inserted intraoperatively. An intra-arterial cannula is indicated for blood pressure monitoring and arterial blood gas analysis during major spine surgery and can be continued postoperatively. Extra care should be taken while positioning the patient in prone to compulsively avoid compression of eye, face, abdomen, and breast. Pressure points should be padded to avoid any nerve compression. With increasing numbers of adult spinal deformity surgery being performed, and with greater numbers of levels of fusion required, reported blood loss in the literature have ranged from <1 to 3 L or more.[44] Intraoperative blood management consists of the use of tranexamic acid (TXA), standardized transfusion parameters, and use of adjunctive devices (cell savage) to minimize blood loss. A substantial body of literature supports the intraoperative use of mechanical prophylaxis via pneumatic compression devices to prevent DVT during prolong spine surgery. Intraoperative cardiac arrest (CA) is rare during spine surgery and has the specific difficulties in the management associated with the prone position. Commonly reported etiologies of cardiac arrest were air embolism, hypovolemia, and dural traction leading to vasovagal response. In the majority of cases, extubation is performed in an operation room immediately after the surgery. In the patients with a pre-existing neuromuscular disorder, severe restrictive pulmonary dysfunction with a preoperative VC of <35% of predicted, difficult tracheal intubation, a congenital cardiac abnormality, right ventricular failure and obesity, the decision to provide a period of postoperative artificial ventilation should have been made preoperatively. Delayed tracheal extubation and postoperative ventilation should be considered in case of a prolonged procedure, cervical cord handling and risk of cord edema, surgical invasion of the thoracic cavity, blood loss >30 mL/kg, difficult tracheal intubation, risk of postoperative airway edema, and risk of airway obstruction.

Postoperative Care

Postoperative Airway Obstruction

One of the most potentially life-threatening complications is postoperative airway obstruction due to development of pharyngeal edema, wound hematoma, or vocal cord paralysis; less common causes include dislodgement of bone graft and fixation plate, posterior fusion of the spine in an overflexed position, CSF leak, or angioedema.[45] The incidence of hematomas after anterior cervical diskectomy and fusion surgery ranges from 0.6 to 0.7%, and risk factors include presence of diffuse idiopathic skeletal hyperostosis, presence of OPLL, therapeutic heparin use, longer operative time, and greater number of surgical levels. Risk factors for airway complications after anterior cervical procedures are operative duration >5 hours; blood loss greater than 300 mL; exposure of more than three vertebral levels; or surgery on C2, C3, or C4; and preoperative myelopathy and multilevel corpectomy.[46] Emergency intubation for airway obstruction from hematoma or edema can be challenging. Opening the neck at the bedside will relieve tracheal pressure from a rapidly expanding hematoma but may be less helpful for edema or a hematoma tracking cephalad. Awake or asleep intubation with a variety of airway devices, including direct laryngoscopy or video laryngoscopy, may be utilized depending on the situation and degree of airway compromise. Vocal cord palsy is a significant morbidity and should be considered early in the differential if patients exhibit respiratory distress after extubation during anterior cervical surgery. Consultation with an otolaryngologist can be helpful in diagnosing vocal cord dysfunction.[47]

Postoperative Fluid Therapy

Postoperative intravenous maintenance fluid therapy ensures adequate organ perfusion, prevents catabolism, and ensures electrolyte- and pH-balance. However, in many cases, postoperative patients with extensive intraoperative blood loss or long-segment surgery will require replacement fluid therapy and blood product transfusion in addition to maintenance therapy to compensate for preoperative and intraoperative losses, stress response to surgery, blood loss, and other bodily fluid loss. Special attention to the intraoperative blood loss and postoperative losses through drain output will be needed. Frequent arterial blood gas analysis to assess acid–base status and laboratory assessment of hematocrit, coagulation parameters, and electrolyte are required to guide resuscitation efforts.

Postoperative Pain Relief

Adequate postoperative pain management after spine surgery has been seen to correlate well with improved functional outcome, less infection, early ambulation, early discharge, and prevention of the development of chronic pain. Patients undergoing spinal surgery, particularly through a thoracic approach, may have a large incision extending over several dermatomes. A multimodal approach to analgesia is most effective, using a combination of simple primary analgesics [acetaminophen, nonsteroidal anti-inflammatory drugs (NSAIDs), etc.], opioids, clonidine, dexamethasone, gabapentin, pregabalin, and regional anesthesia techniques where appropriate. Opioid-based intravenous patient-controlled analgesia is a very effective form of postoperative analgesia in patients undergoing posterior spinal fusion.

Thromboembolism Prophylaxis

Postoperatively, patients may have prolonged periods of immobilization due to pain, CSF leakage, or disability secondary to neurogenic compression possibly leading to venous thromboembolism (VTE).[48] In addition to early mobilization, it is essential to start both mechanical and chemoprophylaxis postoperatively to minimize the risk of developing DVT or VTE.

All patients are started on VTE prophylaxis immediately postoperatively with sequential compression devices, followed by heparin 5,000 IU twice daily on postoperative day 2 unless contraindicated.

Postoperative Vision Loss

Perioperative visual loss (POVL) associated with spine surgery is a rare and disastrous complication. POVL is associated with male gender, obesity, increasing blood loss, and operative procedures duration >6 hours. The use of the Wilson frame has also been implicated.[49] Although the final common pathway is thought to be hypoperfusion of the optic nerve, there is no clear association with either intraoperative systemic hypotension or with the presence of peripheral vascular disease or diabetes. According to the American Society of Anesthesiologists Postoperative Visual Loss Registry, the most common causes of POVL in spine procedures are the two different forms of ischemic optic neuropathy—anterior ischemic optic neuropathy and posterior ischemic optic neuropathy, accounting for 89% of the cases.[50] Intraoperatively careful positioning with the head at the same level as the heart, meticulous hemostasis, and possibly staging prolonged procedures should be considered. In high-risk cases, an early ophthalmic opinion should be sought as soon as possible in the postoperative recovery unit. Initial management should include optimization of arterial pressure, oxygenation, and correction of anemia.[51]

Major complications are more likely to be associated with longer hospital stay and need for long ICU stay. These complications include pneumonia, respiratory failure, CA, shock, arrhythmia, stroke, prolonged use or need for reinsertion of chest tube, wound infection requiring debridement, diffuse intravascular coagulopathy, thromboembolic disease, and intraoperative injury to great vessels (e.g., vertebral artery injury during cervical spine surgery and inferior vena cava injury during thoracic spine surgery).

CONCLUSION

Effective preoperative evaluation and aggressive optimization is critical to mitigating risk and avoiding complications in complex spine surgery and ensures the provision of appropriate and successful management of patient for spine surgery. Thorough multispecialty preoperative and postoperative care reduces the likelihood of many complications.

REFERENCES

1. Deyo RA, Mirza SK, Martin BI, Kreuter W, Goodman DC, Jarvik JG. Trends, major medical complications, and charges associated with surgery for lumbar spinal stenosis in older adults. JAMA. 2010;303(13):1259-65.
2. Chakravarthy VB, Yokoi H, Coughlin DJ, Manlapaz MR, Krishnaney AA. Development and implementation of a comprehensive spine surgery enhanced recovery after surgery protocol: The Cleveland Clinic experience. Neurosurg Focus. 2019;46(4):E11.
3. Charosky S, Guigui P, Blamoutier A, Roussouly P, Chopin D; Study Group on Scoliosis. Complications and risk factors of primary adult scoliosis surgery: A multicenter study of 306 patients. Spine (Phila Pa 1976). 2012;37(8):693-700.
4. Offiah CE, Day E. The craniocervical junction: Embryology, anatomy, biomechanics and imaging in blunt trauma. Insights Imaging. 2017;8(1):29-47.
5. Furst DE, Breedveld FC, Kalden JR, Smolen JS, Burmester GR, Dougados M, et al. Updated consensus statement on biological agents for the treatment of rheumatoid arthritis and other immune mediated inflammatory diseases (May 2003). Ann Rheum Dis. 2003;62(Suppl 2):ii2-9.

6. Kolman J, Morris I. Cricoarytenoid arthritis: A cause of acute upper airway obstruction in rheumatoid arthritis. Can J Anaesth. 2002;49(7):729-32.

7. Chen JJ, Branstetter BF 4th, Myers EN. Cricoarytenoid rheumatoid arthritis: An important consideration in aggressive lesions of the larynx. AJNR Am J Neuroradiol. 2005;26(4):970-2.

8. Skues MA, Welchew EA. Anaesthesia and rheumatoid arthritis. Anaesthesia. 1993;48(11):989-97.

9. Kobel M, Creighton RE, Steward DJ. Anaesthetic considerations in Down's syndrome: Experience with 100 patients and a review of the literature. Can Anaesth Soc J. 1982;29(6):593-9.

10. Bhattarai B, Kulkarni AH, Kalingarayar S, Upadya MP. Anesthetic management of a child with Down's syndrome having atlanto axial instability. JNMA J Nepal Med Assoc. 2009;48(173):66-9.

11. Naguib M, Farag H, Ibrahim A el-W. Anaesthetic considerations in Klippel-Feil syndrome. Can Anaesth Soc J. 1986;33(1):66-70.

12. Dave N, Sharma RK, Andrade NN. Anaesthesia for retrognathia correction in a case of Klippel Feil syndrome. Indian J Anaesth. 2006;50(2):128-30.

13. Kaushal A, Haldar R, Ambesh P. Anesthesia for an achondroplastic individual with coexisting atlantoaxial dislocation. Anesth Essays Res. 2015;9(3):443-6.

14. Hammerschlag W, Ziv I, Wald U, Robin GC, Floman Y. Cervical instability in an achondroplastic infant. J Pediatr Orthop. 1988;8(4):481-4.

15. Di Lorenzo N, Cacciola F. Adult syringomyelia. Classification, pathogenesis and therapeutic approaches. J Neurosurg Sci. 2005;49(3):65-72.

16. Nelson RS, Urquhart AC, Faciszewski T. Diffuse idiopathic skeletal hyperostosis: A rare cause of dysphagia, airway obstruction, and dysphonia. J Am Coll Surg. 2006;202(6):938-42.

17. Onishi E, Sakamoto A, Murata S, Matsushita M. Risk factors for acute cervical spinal cord injury associated with ossification of the posterior longitudinal ligament. Spine (Phila Pa 1976). 2012;37(8):660-6.

18. Feldtkeller E, Vosse D, Geusens P, van der Linden S. Prevalence and annual incidence of vertebral fractures in patients with ankylosing spondylitis. Rheumatol Int. 2006;26(3):234-9.

19. Cornefjord M, Alemany M, Olerud C. Posterior fixation of subaxial cervical spine fractures in patients with ankylosing spondylitis. Eur Spine J. 2005;14(4):401-8.

20. Belanger TA, Milam RA 4th, Roh JS, Bohlman HH. Cervicothoracic extension osteotomy for chin-on-chest deformity in ankylosing spondylitis. J Bone Joint Surg Am. 2005;87(8):1732-8.

21. Argenson C, Lovet J, Sanouiller JL, de Peretti F. Traumatic rotatory displacement of the lower cervical spine. Spine (Phila Pa 1976). 1988;13(7):767-73.

22. Hines RL, Marschall KE. Stoelting's Anesthesia and Co-Existing Disease, 5th edition. Philadelphia: Churchill Livingstone; 2008. pp. 459-60.

23. Alam MS, Phan K, Karim R, Jonayed SA, Munir HK, Chakraborty S, et al. Surgery for spinal tuberculosis: A multi-center experience of 582 cases. J Spine Surg. 2015;1(1):65-71.

24. Hughes SJ. How effective is the Newport/Aspen collar? A prospective radiographic evaluation in healthy adult volunteers. J Trauma. 1998;45(2):374-8.

25. Watts D, Abrahams E, MacMillan C, Sanat J, Silver R, VanGorder S, et al. Insult after injury: Pressure ulcers in trauma patients. Orthop Nurs. 1998;17(4):84-91.

26. Morris CG, McCoy E. Cervical immobilisation collars in ICU: Friend or foe? Anaesthesia. 2003;58(11):1051-3.

27. Goel A. Cervical fusion as a protective response to craniovertebral junction instability: A novel concept. Neurospine. 2018;15(4):323-8.

28. Zhang Y, Tian L, Zhao X, Wu Z, Wang L, Shi L, et al. Effect of preoperative tracheal stretch exercise on anterior cervical spine surgery: A retrospective study. J Spinal Disord Tech. 2015;28(10):E565-70.

29. Jackson KL 2nd, Devine JG. The effects of smoking and smoking cessation on spine surgery: A systematic review of the literature. Global Spine J. 2016;6(7):695-701.

30. Rath GP, Bithal PK, Guleria R, Chaturvedi A, Kale SS, Gupta V, et al. A comparative study between preoperative and postoperative pulmonary functions and diaphragmatic movements in congenital craniovertebral junction anomalies. J Neurosurg Anesthesiol. 2006;18(4):256-61.

31. Jones TS, Burlew CC, Johnson JL, Jones E, Kornblith LZ, Biffl WL, et al. Predictors of the necessity for early tracheostomy in patients with acute cervical spinal cord injury: A 15-year experience. Am J Surg. 2015;209(2):363-8.

32. Mellin G, Harjula R. Lung function in relation to thoracic spinal mobility and kyphosis. Scand J Rehabil Med. 1987;19(2):89-92.

33. Harrison RA, Siminoski K, Vethanayagam D, Majumdar SR. Osteoporosis-related kyphosis and impairments in pulmonary function: A systematic review. J Bone Miner Res. 2007;22(3):447-57.

34. Smetana GW. Preoperative pulmonary evaluation. N Engl J Med. 1999;340(12):937-44.

35. Hong L, Kawaguchi Y. Anterior cervical discectomy and fusion to treat cervical spondylosis with sympathetic symptoms. J Spinal Disord Tech. 2011;24(1):11-4.

36. Braunlin EA, Harmatz PR, Scarpa M, Furlanetto B, Kampmann C, Loehr JP, et al. Cardiac disease in patients with mucopolysaccharidosis: Presentation, diagnosis and management. J Inherit Metab Dis. 2011;34(6):1183-97.

37. Davies G, Reid L. Effect of scoliosis on growth of alveoli and pulmonary arteries and on right ventricle. Arch Dis Child. 1971;46(249):623-32.

38. Kawakami N, Mimatsu K, Deguchi M, Kato F, Maki S. Scoliosis and congenital heart disease. Spine (Phila Pa 1976). 1995;20(11):1252-6.

39. Jackson KL 2nd, Devine JG. The effects of obesity on spine surgery: A systematic review of the literature. Global Spine J. 2016;6(4):394-400.

40. Epstein NE. Spine surgery in geriatric patients: Sometimes unnecessary, too much, or too little. Surg Neurol Int. 2011;2:188.

41. Nouri A, Patel K, Montejo J, Nasser R, Gimbel DA, Sciubba DM, et al. The role of vitamin B12 in the management and optimization of treatment in patients with degenerative cervical myelopathy. Global Spine J. 2019;9(3):331-7.

42. Liu L, Liu YB, Sun JM, Hou HF, Liang C, Li T, et al. Preoperative deep vein thrombosis in patients with cervical spondylotic myelopathy scheduled for spinal surgery. Medicine (Baltimore). 2016;95(44):e5269.

43. De Jong A, Molinari N, Terzi N, Mongardon N, Arnal JM, Guitton C, et al. Early identification of patients at risk for difficult intubation in the intensive care unit: Development and validation of the MACOCHA score in a multicenter cohort study. Am J Respir Crit Care Med. 2013;187(8):832-9.

44. Hu SS. Blood loss in adult spinal surgery. Eur Spine J. 2004;13(Suppl 1):S3-5.

45. Yoshida M, Neo M, Fujibayashi S, Nakamura T. Upper-airway obstruction after short posterior occipitocervical fusion in a flexed position. Spine (Phila Pa 1976). 2007;32(8):E267-70.

46. O'Neill KR, Neuman B, Peters C, Riew KD. Risk factors for postoperative retropharyngeal hematoma after anterior cervical spine surgery. Spine (Phila Pa 1976). 2014;39(4): E246-52.

47. Tan TP, Govindarajulu AP, Massicotte EM, Venkatraghavan L. Vocal cord palsy after anterior cervical spine surgery: A qualitative systematic review. Spine J. 2014;14(7):1332-42.

48. Schoenfeld AJ, Herzog JP, Dunn JC, Bader JO, Belmont PJ Jr. Patient-based and surgical characteristics associated with the acute development of deep venous thrombosis and pulmonary embolism after spine surgery. Spine (Phila Pa 1976). 2013;38(21):1892-8.

49. Postoperative Visual Loss Study Group. Risk factors associated with ischemic optic neuropathy after spinal fusion surgery. Anesthesiology. 2012;116(1):15-24.

50. Lee LA, Roth S, Posner KL, Cheney FW, Caplan RA, Newman NJ, et al. The American Society of Anesthesiologists Postoperative Visual Loss Registry: Analysis of 93 spine surgery cases with postoperative visual loss. Anesthesiology. 2006;105(4):652-9.

51. American Society of Anesthesiologists Task Force on Perioperative Visual Loss. Practice advisory for perioperative visual loss associated with spine surgery: An updated report by the American Society of Anesthesiologists Task Force on Perioperative Visual Loss. Anesthesiology. 2012;116(2):274-85.

Perioperative Management of Neurotrauma

Kapil Zirpe, Balkrishna Nimavat

Hippocratic aphorism: "No head injury is so serious that it should be despaired of, nor so trivial that it can be ignored."

INTRODUCTION

Traumatic brain injury (TBI) is increasingly being recognized as a public health problem with the substantial burden of disability and death occurring in low and middle income countries (LMICs). In high income countries, the incidence of TBI due to road traffic incidents has decreased after successful implementation of preventive measures such as legislations, safer roadway infrastructure, car safety measures and helmets; but still the burden of TBI in these countries remains high due to an increasing number of elderly patients with TBI due to a fall. Road traffic accidents remain the main cause of TBI in low and middle income countries like India[1]. In recent days treatment of TBI has changed drastically. Management of TBI now days mostly practiced from Brain Trauma Foundation guideline. Principle management objectives include reduction in intracranial hypertension and prevention of secondary injuries such as hypoxemia, hypotension, hyperthermia, and hypoglycemia. There is no guideline for intraoperative or anesthetic management for brain injury patient. Most of our recommendation or suggestions are based on TBI guidelines and physiological rationale rather than direct evidence. This chapter focuses on the perioperative management of neurotrauma patient.

PATHOPHYSIOLOGY RELATED TO BRAIN INJURY

- Monro–Kellie doctrine hypothesis is the pressure-volume relationship between components mentioning intracranial pressure, cerebrospinal fluid volume, blood, brain tissue and cerebral perfusion pressure (CPP). It states that cranial compartment is an inelastic area in which volume inside is fixed. When new volume is added to this, it would be compensated by reduction in other component or change in pressure. Initially curve is compensated by buffering capacity of another component but later it rises exponentially **(Fig. 1)**.
- Damage to brain can be broadly divided into direct or primary injury and indirect or secondary injury.
- Primary injury mainly is of vascular or mechanical.
  - *Mechanical:* When there is mass/lesion/hematoma/edema, it compresses the surrounding neuronal structure or vessels. Mechanical damage is directly related to size of hematoma or extend of injury. In severe brain injury it leads to brain herniation that required urgent intervention or surgical help.
  - *Vascular:* Compromised blood flow to brain tissue occurs as product of increase intracranial pressure compared to CPP. When this continues it leads to

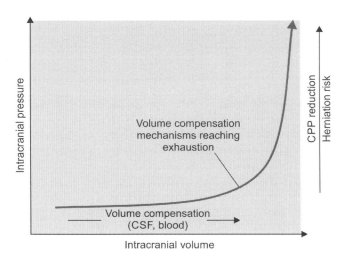

Fig. 1: Relationship between intracranial pressure and volume during brain injury. (CPP: cerebral perfusion pressure; CSF: cerebrospinal fluid)

ischemia of brain tissue and promotes cytotoxic edema. So high intracranial pressure and edema go hand by hand and leads to vicious cycle of cellular injury.

- Secondary insult happens by more of systemic problem. Low sugar level, low blood pressure, high temperature and low oxygen supply or impaired oxygen demand supply ratio responsible for secondary brain injury. Secondary insults responsible for increase metabolic waste products and formation of free radicals related brain injuries.[2]

MANAGEMENT OF BRAIN INJURY

The aims and objectives of perioperative neurosurgical patients' or TBI management are started with maintaining the vital parameters such as airway, breathing and blood pressure followed by assessment of neurological findings, monitoring of intracranial pressure and measures to reduce it. Optimizing the other system to prevent the secondary injuries and thus improving oxygen demand supply of neuronal tissue. On later stage prevent the secondary infection, and start physiotherapy and rehabilitation.[3]

Step 1: Initial Assessment/Preoperative Optimization/Stabilization of Vital Parameters Immediate Postoperative Period

Airway Control and Ventilation

- Hypoxemia is associated with poor outcome in TBI patients.
- *Caution while intubation [preoperative if low Glasgow coma scale (GCS) or hemodynamics unstable]:* Secure cervical spine—motor vehicle accident and GCS <8 more likely associated with cervical spine injury. In line neck stabilization should be carried out while intubation to prevent damage to neurovascular structure.
- *Consider difficult airway cart and chances of aspiration injury:* High ICP, full stomach, cervical injuries, facial trauma, lung trauma (decrease oxygen reserve) make the intubation more difficult.
- *Consider rapid sequence intubation and choice of muscle relaxant (preoperative):* Short acting agents such as rocuronium or succinylcholine should be preferred. Succinylcholine associated with increased intracranial pressure, but many studies discard the clinical significance of it. To blunt the autonomic response while laryngoscopy opioid group of drugs are preferable, i.e., fentanyl.
- *Adequate sedative and analgesic agent perioperatively:* Adequate sedation and muscle relaxation required to decrease patient ventilator dyssynchrony and thus

reducing coughing and high ICP. Adequate sedation will also lead to optimize demand of metabolic product such as oxygen to brain tissue.

- *Choice of sedative agent:* Ideal anesthetic drugs should not increase ICP and having least side effect on hemodynamics. Propofol can be used but should be used carefully in hypotensive patients. Ketamine is good choice in hypotensive trauma patient.
- *Ventilator strategy perioperatively:* Optimal amount of PEEP 5–10 mm Hg should be selected so that it will prevent the atelectasis and not damaging the brain by increasing ICP too. Hypoventilation and hyperventilation both should be avoided. In selected cases to reduce the ICP as bridge to decompressive surgery for transient period, hyperventilation can be allowing with targeting $PaCO_2$ of 25 mm Hg.[3]

Blood Pressure and Cerebral Perfusion Pressure

- *Source control and fluid assessment:* Extracranial source of hemorrhage should be searched first and controlled. Hypotension is associated with poor outcome in TBI patients.
- *Choice of fluid:* Hypotonic solutions should be avoided. Normal saline is the most common crystalloid used in such patients. If large volume resuscitation required than balanced crystalloid solutions may be a good alternative. Colloid (e.g., albumin) should be avoided in TBI patients.
- *Role of vasopressors and choice of vasopressors:* Data on choice of vasopressors in TBI is scarce but noradrenaline should be preferred as having more consistent effect on blood pressure and thus on improvement in CPP.
- *Target systolic blood pressure (SBP) and CPP:*
  - Maintaining SBP at ≥100 mm Hg (50–69 years old) or a ≥110 mm Hg (15–49 or over 70 years) decrease mortality and improve outcomes.
  - CPP value should be targeted between 60 and 70 mm Hg.
  - High value of CPP, i.e., >70 mm Hg by adding vasopressors or giving fluids having no extra advantage plus it can lead to more damage in term of acute lung damage.[3]

Step 2: Neurological Assessment

- Size and reactivity of pupil
- Assesses level of alertness
- Assesses ability to follow commands
- Assesses motor strength
- Assesses cerebellar function
- NIHSS in stroke patients (post-mechanical thrombectomy)
- Four score

- GCS score
- Ramsay score for sedated patient
- Monitor ICP

Red Alert Findings

Sign and symptoms of raised ICP/underlying brain pathology:

- New motor weakness/sensory changes compared to baseline
- Diplopia/pupillary changes (sluggish, irregular or dilated pupils)
- New facial asymmetry
- Changes in speech (receptive and expressive)
- Decline in level of consciousness
- New or worsening headache/headache that is not relieved by medicine/pharmacological measures
- Nausea/emesis
- Bradycardia with hypertension or other dysrhythmias (Cushing Response).

If any of above red alerts findings found in patients, advisable to do neuroimaging after discussion with involved neurosurgeon or neurologic team.

Indications of CT in TBI

CT scan brain should be carried out in all mild/moderate to severe TBI **(Table 1)**.

Factors that Affects Neurological Examinations Findings

- Seizure (convulsive and non-convulsive)
- Dyselectrolytemia (hyponatremia)
- Fever (hypo/hyperthermia)
- Hypoglycemia
- Dehydration
- Hospital psychosis/delirium
- Drug abuse or withdrawal
- Alcohol abuse or withdrawal
- Anesthesia especially in a previously neurologically compromised patient
- Medications (opioids, benzodiazepines)

Glasgow Coma Scale and Limitations

It is most widely used method of recording the level of consciousness in traumatic brain injury patients. A score of ≥13 indicates mild brain injury, 9–12 suggestive of moderate injury, and ≤8 as severe brain injury. Glasgow coma scale is a strong predictor of in-hospital mortality and need of any surgical intervention. Glasgow coma score of 3 associated with around 50% poor neurological outcome. GCS can be used in post-cardiac arrest patient and posterior circulation stroke apart from trauma, but its consistency is not that great. Limitations of GCS are interobserver variability, hemodynamic and respiratory parameters are not included, pupil charting or findings not considered. It is also difficult and unreliable to sum GCS score in sedated and ventilated patients as verbal score cannot be done.

FOUR Score

Full outline of unresponsiveness score (FOUR) includes brainstem response and respiratory part apart from motor and eye response. Four score is better in term of having less interobserver variability compared to GCS and better tool in severe consciousness problems such as locked in syndrome or vegetative states. FOUR score and GCS score both can be affected by sedative and paralytic agent, but FOUR score affected less as it includes pupillary findings instead of verbal score. It can be used in postcardiac arrest patient for neuroresponse and prognostication. The improvement in score of 2 suggestive of improvement and associated with better survival.

Rancho Los Amigos Scale

Traumatic brain injury patients and in patient having neurological insult having variable level of cognitive dysfunction. Rancho Los Amigos Scale (RLAS) used in brain injury patient to detect level of activity and cognitive function. It can be used with GCS in early phase, but not limited to early phase like GCS **(Table 2)**. Later two more level added to it to make scale more comprehensive and named RLAS-R (Revised). Limitation of RLAS is that scale having high interobserver variability.

Table 1: Indications (CT scan) for mild traumatic brain injury (TBI).[4]

High risk for neurosurgical interventions:	Moderate risk of brain injury on CT:
• Open or depressed skull fracture • Sign of basilar skull fracture • Vomiting more than 2 episodes • Age >65 years • Anticoagulant use	• Loss of consciousness more than 5 minutes • Amnesia more than 30 minutes • Dangerous mechanism includes: – Pedestrian hit by vehicle – Eject from motor vehicle – Fall from more than 3 feet height/five stairs

Table 2: Rancho Los Amigos Scale (RLAS).

Level	Response
1	No response and require total assistance
2	Generalized reflex response to pain plus required total assistance
3	Localized response to pain plus total assistance
4	Confused/agitated and required maximal assistance
5	Confused/nonagitated inappropriate verbalization
6	Confused/appropriate, inconsistent orientation to time and place
7	Appropriate, automatic and require standby assistance
8	Appropriate, purposeful and independent

Step 3: Monitoring of ICP and Measures to Reduce ICP

- It is evident that high ICP is associated with poor neurological outcome and associated with mortality. Even guideline suggests that ICP monitoring and guided change in plan reduce hospital mortality and short-term mortality. But there are evidences that ICP based management is not superior than conventional neuro-monitoring plus serial CT monitoring. There is also lack of data on group of population where ICP monitoring help. Timing of ICP monitoring is also not well defined. Risk benefit ratio should be considered when choosing this modality. It is common practice to use it in low GCS <8, having refractory ICP despite medical management, where neurological examination is not reliable, i.e., facial injury or spine injury. Contraindications of invasive ICP monitoring are bleeding disorder or local site infection or abscess. Limitation of invasive ICP is in localized elevation of intracranial pressure.
- *Three-tiered approach to control ICP:* Various measures or intervention in isolation or combined used to control intracranial pressure. They arranged in term of their size of effect, invasiveness and their risk-benefit. If patient is not responding to lower tier, i.e., ICP is refractory to measure it should be switched to higher tier intervention

(**Table 3**).[3,5,6] The staircase approach to ICP is given in **Table 4**.[2]

Sedation and Analgesia

Ideally, sedation free hours from sedation and avoiding deep sedation shown to reduce number of ventilator days and improve outcome, but these trials exclude patients having TBI or having neurological issues. Role of sedation in traumatic brain injury is to optimize the ventilation by decreasing patient ventilator dyssynchrony, reducing cerebral metabolic rate and thus decreasing intracranial pressure. There is limited evidence on which agent is better for TBI. Physician should use the agent based on patient's hemodynamic status and depends on severity of TBI. So, in nutshell, hemodynamically unstable patients' ketamine and fentanyl combination will be justifiable. For hemodynamically stable patients propofol or thiopentone with fentanyl should be considered. Thiopentone is not used as routine maintenance agent but considered as agent to induce burst suppression in refractory ICP.[3,7]

Osmotherapy

- *Osmotherapy:* Available agents are mannitol and hypertonic saline. Superiority of any one agent over other is still uncertain. Dose of mannitol is 1–1.5 g/kg over 30

Table 3: Three-tiered approach to control ICP.

Tier 1 (if ICP ≥20–25 mm Hg proceed to Tier 2)	Tier 2 (if ICP ≥20–25 mm Hg proceed to Tier 3)	Tier 3 (includes potential salvage therapies)
30° head elevation straightening of head prevention of hypoxemia, hypotension, hypoglycemia, hyperthermia	Hyperosmolar therapy should be given intermittently as needed (but not on a routine schedule)	Decompressive craniectomy
Sedation and analgesia in intubated patients	Neuromuscular paralytic agents, if patient is responder to test dose then continuous infusion	Barbiturate or propofol coma, if patient is responder to test dose
Intermittently ventricular drainage (continuous drainage not routinely indicated)		Hypothermia (only reserved for "rescue" or "salvage" therapy)

Table 4: Staircase approach to ICP.[2]

Therapy steps	Level of evidence	Treatment	Risk
8	Not reported	Surgical intervention such as decompressive craniectomy	Hematoma, meningitis, hydrocephalus
7	3	Barbiturate coma	Fall in blood pressure, increase chances of infection
6	3	Hypothermia	Infection, coagulopathy, electrolyte imbalance
5	3	Hyperventilation induced hypocapnia	Cerebral ischemia
4	3	Hypeosmolar therapy	Dyselectrolytemia, renal failure
3	Not reported	Ventricular fluid drainage by inserting external ventricular drain	Infection
2	3	Sedation	Fall in blood pressure
1	Not reported	Intubation with normocarbic ventilation	Exposure to medication, chances of VAP, patient-ventilatory dyssynchrony

minutes every 6 hourly and when needed to achieve the serum osmolarity of 320 mOsm/L. In patient of renal injury and dyselectrolytemia use of mannitol should be avoided. Hypertonic saline available in different concentration. In acute need, higher concentration with less volume should be selected, such as 23.4% over 15 min bolus dose. Maintenance management can be carried out by 2/3% saline as infusion to maintain sodium level of around 150–155 mEq/L. This target should be achieved over 1 to 2 days not faster. Many studies compared superiority of mannitol versus hypertonic saline in TBI. There is no significant difference in term of mortality and lowering ICP. Only difference they found is that hypertonic saline had lower ICP burden.[3,7]

Surgical management of neurocritical care patients: Decompressive craniectomy (DC) and indication of surgery in subdural hematoma (SDH)/extradural hematoma (EDH)

- In TBI, cerebral edema is considered as main complication and once all conventional treatment fails to reduce intracranial pressure DC is the therapeutic option. There is much debate about timing of surgery and type of surgery. Current evidence based on RCTs suggest that role of decompression craniectomy such as doing bifrontal craniectomy for mild to moderate ICP is not better than usual conventional medical management. While in case of severe and refractory case of intracranial pressure, doing decompression craniectomy, i.e., large frontotemporoparietal DC leads to mortality benefit, but with increase chances of disability.[3,7]

- *Role of decompression craniectomy in stroke:* For malignant MCA stroke surgical therapy reduce the mortality with expense of greater risk of mRS ≥4. Timing of surgery should be ≤48 hours from stroke symptoms.

- *Indication of surgery in IC bleed patients:* Younger age group, low GCS <6, large size >50 mL, IVH extension, infratentorial and patients with refractory ICP should benefit with DC with expansile duraplasty (ED). Timing of surgery should be early but not <4 hours as chances of rebleeding is higher in this phase.

- *Role of minimally invasive surgery (MIS):* It includes stereotactic aspiration of clot or endoscopic clot removal by burr hole ± thrombolytic agent. Data suggests MIS reduce surgical trauma, improve clot evacuation and trends toward positive outcome.

- Differences between SDH and EDH, and the indication of surgery are given in **Figure 2** and **Table 5**, respectively.[8]

Step 4: Advanced Tool to Monitor CPP

Every patient has its own range of autoregulation, so it is very important to individualized ICP and CPP. It can be done by need of downstream markers such as oxygenation need/demand supply and metabolic mismatch.

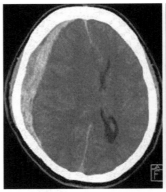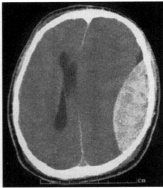

Figs. 2A and B: (A) Subdural hematoma (SDH); (B) Extradural hematoma (EDH).

Table 5: Differences between extradural hematoma (EDH) and subdural hematoma (SDH).

EDH	SDH
• Usually accidental injury • Middle meningeal artery • Lentiform by shape • Do not cross sutures	• Usually not accidental • Bridging veins and dural venous sinuses • Crescentic • Cross sutures
Indication of surgery: • Size >30 cm³ should go for surgical option irrespective to Glasgow Coma score. • Size <30 cm³ and with <15 mm thickness and with <5 mm midline shift in patients with a GCS score greater than 8 without focal deficit should be managed with nonoperative approach – Neuromonitoring and repeated neuroimaging required in this group of patients.	*Indication of surgery:* • Thickness >10 mm or midline shift >5 mm should be evacuated regardless of Glasgow coma score • Thickness <10 mm or <5 mm midline shift should be observed for Glasgow coma score, Drops 2 or more points from injury to admission, pupillary function is abnormal, or ICP >20 mm Hg should go for surgery.
Timing: Hematoma with Glasgow coma score <9 and patient with unequal pupil should go for surgical evacuation urgently. Craniotomy is better surgical option for complete evacuation of the hematoma.	*Timing:* "As soon as possible" *Methods:* Craniotomy with or without bone flap removal/duraplasty

- *Brain tissue oxygenation monitoring by measuring PbtO₂:* Brain tissue oxygen is considered as surrogate marker for cerebral blood flow. PbtO₂ is the product of 2 factors cerebral blood flow and arteriovenous oxygen tension difference. It can be used with ICP monitoring to tailored CPP threshold for patient. Normal PbtO₂ is around 25–35 mm Hg. Values below 20 mm Hg or fall in value <5–10 mm Hg give insight about need to intervene for reduction in ICP.

- *Measuring of global oxygenation by SjVO₂:* Specific catheter placed at the skull base measure difference between cerebral oxygen demand and supply.

Normal value of $SjVO_2$ is 60–75%. Value less than 50% considered as ischemia while value >75% give insight about hyperemia or infarct area. BTF guide to use $SjVO_2$ to manage ICP and related decision, but level of recommendation is low.

- *Cerebral metabolism monitoring by microdialysis catheter:* Microcatheter inserted into subcortical area of brain. Principle of microdialysis is based on glucose metabolism in aerobic and anaerobic environment. With the help of combination of value of glucose, lactate and pyruvate and ratio of them helps the physician to guide therapeutic strategies. Lactate/pyruvate ratio of >20–25 suggestive of severe ischemia and associated with poor outcome.
- *Transcranial Doppler ultrasound:* TCD monitoring can be useful in common injuries of brain, i.e., traumatic brain injury, stroke and subarachnoid injury. TCD is sensitive and specific to detect ICA and MCA occlusion. Advantage of TCD is its inexpensive, portable, repeatable and noninvasive nature. Limitation is its operator dependent, depends on skill of operator and in few of patients facing difficulty of inadequate transtemporal acoustic window.[9]
- Mean flow velocities and Lindegaard ratio by severity of vasospasm in subarachnoid hemorrhage (SAH) **(Table 6)**[9]:
- *Optic nerve sheath diameter (ONSD):* Optic nerve sheath diameter is a simple, noninvasive and sensitive tool to detect increased intracranial pressure. There are different cut-off values for ONSD, but >4 mm is suggestive of papilledema. Cut-off value of 5 mm or more is sensitive for CT findings of high intracranial pressure. ONSD findings also correlate well with modified Frisen scale used for severity of papilledema. Limitation of ONSD is it depends on observer skill and interobserver variation likely.[10]
- *Neuroelectrophysiology:* It consists of EEG and its variant or derivatives such as BIS (bispectral index), SSEP (somatosensory evoked potential test) and BAEP (brainstem auditory evoked potential test) **(Tables 7 and 8)**. BIS is the tool can be used perioperatively to guide the anesthetic about level of sedation and optimizing the dose of medication. SSEP and BAEP are more helpful for level or extent of brain damage, that will help in diagnose the disease and its progress. These modalities can be used as adjunctive to other tests to diagnose brain death too.[9]
- *EEG:* In critical care setting EEG is helpful particularly in patients who having suspected absence seizure or having altered mental status. Continuous EEG monitoring is also helpful in status epilepticus and in barbiturate coma to monitor suppression of activity and response to medication. EEG interpreted with imaging gives idea

Table 6: Severity of vasospasm in subarachnoid hemorrhage (SAH).

Vasospasm severity	Flow velocity mean cm/s	Lindegaard ratio
None	<120	<2
Mild	120–150	2–3
Moderate	>150–200	>3–6
Severe	>200	>6

Table 7: Index for bispectral monitoring device.[9]

Index range	Clinical state
>90–100	Awake
>60–90	Light to moderate sedation
>40–60	General anesthesia
20–40	Burst suppression
<20	Isoelectric electroencephalogram

Table 8: Brainstem auditory evoked potentials.[9]

Wave		Probable anatomical correlate
P1	I	Auditory portion of 8th cranial nerve
P2	II	Nerve at or around cochlear nucleus
P3	III	At the level of lower pons
P4	IV	Mid/upper pons level
P5	V	Lesion in lower midbrain

about which part of brain or area is damaged or affected by insult.[9]

Step 5: Other Modalities or Drugs

Anticonvulsant Therapy

Seizure episode in traumatic brain injury patient leads to neurological damage and associated with poor outcome. Phenytoin is effective in reducing early post-traumatic convulsion. For late seizure there is no role of prophylactic therapy. Levetiracetam is a safe and effective alternative to phenytoin for early posttraumatic convulsion in traumatic brain injury patients. Prolonged therapy such as more than 7 days should not be practiced routinely.[3,7]

Temperature Management

Role of therapeutic hypothermia in TBI remains controversial. Multiple RCTs and meta-analysis failed to show any morality benefit or positive neurological outcome. In contrary TH might increase risk of pneumonia and mortality in traumatic brain injury patient group.[3,7]

Role of Steroids

Corticosteroid was used in past with thought of reducing ICP, but CRASH trial result shows increase mortality in traumatic brain injury patients.[3,4,7]

Hemoglobin Resuscitation

Red blood cell transfusion threshold in critical care patient is <7 g/dL based on TRICC trial. In patient of cerebral ischemia liberal blood transfusion failed to show any benefit. There is no current guideline of optimal transfusion strategy in TBI. HEMOTION trial is ongoing which may give better insight.[3]

Antibiotic Therapy

Traumatic brain injury patients are more prone for hospital acquired infection as they have invasive lines, catheter and increase changes of lung infection (aspiration pneumonia). The risk of infection in EVD is higher than intracranial pressure monitoring devices. Data is insufficient to make any guidelines on antibiotic prophylaxis for neuro-procedures. Guidelines for using antibiotic coated catheter to reduce infection having low level of recommendation. For penetrating traumatic brain injury antibiotic can be used for 1–2 weeks.[3]

Role of Tracheostomy

There are conflicting data on early versus late tracheostomy in neurotrauma patient as definition of early tracheostomy varies in literature. But many trials show positive benefit on early tracheostomy in terms of reducing total ICU days and ventilatory days. Most of trials failed to show mortality benefit.[3,7]

Other Drugs

There is no evidence for a routine application of magnesium, statins, or progesterone in neurocritical care patients after aSAH (aneurysmal SAH) or TBI.[11]

Step 6: Supportive Care and ICU Bundle

Glycemic Control

Glucose containing fluid should be avoided. Both hyperglycemia and hypoglycemia are harmful to traumatic brain injury patient. Data showing plasma glucose level of < 140 mg/dL associated with improve neurological outcome, but we have to more vigilant for episodes of hypoglycemia.[3]

Nutrition

Enteral feeding should be preferred method in neurotrauma patients. Early nutrition, i.e., within 48 hours of ICU admission should be considered. If patient having high residual volume or intolerance can consider prokinetic agent such as metoclopramide. Target is to achieve basal caloric need by 5th day and at most by 7th day of injury.[3]

Other Considerations

- *Thromboprophylaxis:* Traumatic brain injury patient having high risk of deep vein thrombosis (DVT) and pulmonary embolism. This group of patients should receive at least one of the thromboprophylaxis measures such as mechanical thromboprophylaxis or pharmacological agents such as heparin/LMWH (low molecular heparin) or both can be started depending on perceived risk. Pharmacological agent can be start after 48 hours if neurosurgeon agrees or no risk of increase in bleed. Pharmacological agents reduced risk of DVT compared to mechanical prophylaxis. LMWH reduce risk of DVT compared to UFH (unfractionated heparin) with same rate of risk of bleeding. Combined treatment is better than isolated pharmacological treatment.
- Other care includes stress ulcer prophylaxis, bed sore care, eye and oral care, position change, speech therapy, proper suctioning of endotracheal or tracheostomy tube, physiotherapy and care of invasive lines and urine catheter.

Step 7: Identify Complications in Postoperative Neurosurgical Patients

- Trauma induced coagulopathy
- ARDS/negative pressure pulmonary edema
- Paroxysmal sympathetic hyperactivity/stress cardio-myopathy
- Hypothalamic-pituitary-adrenal dysfunction/SIADH/cerebral salt wasting/DI
- Hydrocephalus
- Heterotopic ossification
- Spasticity
- Chronic traumatic encephalopathy/post-traumatic headache and depression/cognitive impairment
- GI and GU complications
- Gastric ulceration and DVT
- Secondary infections, i.e., ventilator induced lung injury and infection, urinary tract infection, surgical site infection, meningitis, blood stream infection, bed sore skin and soft tissue infection.[12]

Step 8: Outcome Measures

Three tools commonly used to measure outcome after TBI are: (1) functional independence measure (FIM), (2) Glasgow outcome scale (GOS), and (3) disability rating scale (DRS).

Step 9: Prognostification

- Very difficult and complex
- Poor GCS score, increasing age, bilaterally absent pupillary light reflex having at least 70% positive predictive value of having poor prognostic outcome
- Hypotension SBP <90 mm Hg was found to have a 67% positive predictive value for poor outcome.

- Hypotension with hypoxia showing positive predictive value of 79%
- *CT findings associated with poor prognosis:* Absence or compressed basal cisterns, tSAH (traumatic SAH), presence and degree of midline shift (CT severity) and presence of abnormalities in initial CT
- The Abbreviated Injury Scale and Traumatic Coma Data Bank Computed Tomography are good objective tool to predict outcome in severe traumatic brain injury patient.[13]

REFERENCES

1. Gururaj G. Epidemiology of traumatic brain injuries: Indian scenario. NeurolRes. 2002 ;24:24-8.
2. Stocchetti N, Maas AI. Traumatic intracranial hypertension. N Engl J Med. 2014;370:2121-30.
3. Dash HH, Chavali S. Management of traumatic brain injury patients. Korean J Anesthesiol. 2018;71:12.
4. American College of Surgeons. ATLS, Advanced Trauma Life Support, Student Course Manual, 10th edition. 2018. Chicago, Illinois: ACS; 2018.
5. Surgical Critical Care Evidence-Based Medicine Guidelines Committee, 2019. Severe traumatic brain injury management. [Online] Available from http://www.surgicalcriticalcare.net/Guidelines.pdf. [Last accessed March, 2020].
6. American College of Surgeons. Best practices in the management of traumatic brain injury. Chicago, Illinois: ACS; 2015.
7. Carney N, Totten AM, O'Reilly C, Ullman JS, Hawryluk GW, Bell MJ, et al. Guidelines for the management of severe traumatic brain injury. Neurosurgery. 2017;80:6-15.
8. Bullock MR, Chesnut R, Ghajar J, Gordon D, Hartl R, Newell DW, et al. Surgical management of traumatic brain injury. Neurosurgery. 2006;58:16-24.
9. Harris C. Neuromonitoring indications and utility in the intensive care unit. Crit Care Nurse. 2014;34:30-40.
10. Nithya Raghunandan MJ, Nithyanandam S, Karat S. Role of ultrasonographic optic nerve sheath diameter in the diagnosis and follow-up of papilledema and its correlation with Frisén's severity grading. Indian J Ophthalmol. 2019;67:1310.
11. Siegemund M, Steiner LA. Postoperative care of the neurosurgical patient. Curr Opin Anesthesiol. 2015;28:487-93.
12. Wijayatilake DS, Sherren PB, Jigajinni SV. Systemic complications of traumatic brain injury. Curr Opin Anesthesiol. 2015;28:525-31.
13. Brain Trauma Foundation (USA), 2000. Early indicators of prognosis in severe traumatic brain injury. [Online] Available at: https://braintrauma.org/uploads/01/03/prognosis_guidelines.pdf. [Last accessed March, 2020].

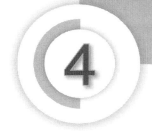

SECTION

4

Pediatrics

CHAPTER

25

Perioperative Management of Neonatal Developmental Defects

Neerja Bhardwaj, Anudeep Jafra

INTRODUCTION

According to the World Health Organization, 1 in 33 infants born has one or more associated congenital anomalies and will; therefore, require urgent or emergency surgical treatment in the neonatal period.[1] The various developmental defects which need surgical intervention during the neonatal period are mentioned in **Table 1**. The most common lesions encountered in clinical practice include esophageal atresia (EA) with or without tracheoesophageal fistula (TEF), congenital diaphragmatic hernia (CDH), pyloric stenosis (PS), abdominal wall defects (omphalocele, gastroschisis), intestinal obstruction [anorectal malformations (ARMs)] and neurodevelopmental lesions such as meningomyelocele (MMC) and hydrocephalus.

ESOPHAGEAL ATRESIA WITH OR WITHOUT TRACHEOESOPHAGEAL FISTULA

Esophageal atresia with or without TEF is one of the most challenging congenital anomalies for which a newborn undergoes surgery. The incidence is 1:2,500–3,000 live births with a male preponderance (25:3).[2] Out of these, 10–40% are preterm, about 50% have other associated congenital lesions, with 25% having undetected congenital heart disease (CHD).[3] Neonates with associated complex CHD, weight <2 kg, poor pulmonary compliance, large pericarinal fistula, and those undergoing thoracoscopic repair are at higher risk of complications.[4]

Embryogenesis

The primary mechanism of development of TEF remains unknown. During the 3rd week of intrauterine life, endodermal cells from the lateral aspect of the ventral diverticulum of the foregut form trachea and esophagus. Abnormalities in this process lead to the formation of TEF (**Fig. 1**).[5]

Prenatal and Postnatal Detection

Esophageal atresia and TEF are difficult to diagnose in the prenatal period because of the presence of nonspecific signs.[6] Prenatal ultrasonography (USG) showing polyhydramnios or absent/small gastric bubble raises the suspicion of their presence (predictive value 44–56%).

Post birth, presence of excessive salivation, choking on attempted feeds, and inability to pass the suction catheter beyond 9–10 cm makes one suspect the presence of TEF. Half of these neonates have associated congenital syndromes such as VACTERL (vertebral, anorectal, cardiac, TEF, renal and limb defects) and CHARGE (coloboma, heart defects, anal atresia, retarded growth, genital hypoplasia, ear anomalies).[7]

Pathophysiology

In TEF, the collected saliva and secretions in the upper esophageal pouch, as well as from the distal fistula, drool over and cause lung spillage. The pathophysiological effect of aspiration of gastric secretions is depicted in

Table 1: Common developmental defects in a neonate.	
Airway lesions	*Abdominal lesions*
Choanal atresia	Omphalocele
Pierre-Robin syndrome	Gastroschisis
Upper airway obstruction	Intestinal atresia
• Cystic hygroma	Pyloric stenosis
• Cleft lip and palate	Imperforate anus
	Exstrophy of the bladder
	Hirschsprung's disease
Thoracic lesions	*Neurosurgical lesions*
Tracheoesophageal fistula and atresia	Myelomeningocele
	Encephalocele
Congenital diaphragmatic hernia	Hydrocephalus
Eventration of the diaphragm	Spinal tumors
Lobar emphysema	Craniostenosis
Congenital heart lesions	

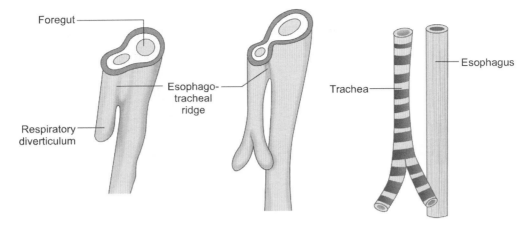

Fig. 1: Embryology of EA and TEF.

(EA: esophageal atresia; TEF: tracheoesophageal fistula)

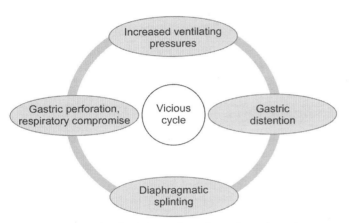

Fig. 2: Pathophysiology of esophageal atresia and tracheoesophageal fistula

Figure 2. Almost 30–40% of these neonates are preterm, and the presence of respiratory distress syndrome (RDS) may contribute to pulmonary impairment. An emergent ligation of the fistula may be required to minimize aspiration pneumonia and start early enteral feeds as well as in neonates with respiratory distress. Neonates with complex CHD could be ductal dependent (requiring a perioperative prostaglandin infusion—PGE1) or nondependent.

Classification of Tracheoesophageal Fistula

Several anatomical classifications are available to classify EA and TEF, but most frequently used are the Gross and Vogt classification (**Table 2**) with Vogt type 3B being the most common (80%).[3] Waterson introduced a classification based on birth weight (BW), presence of pneumonia, and associated congenital anomalies to prognosticate the outcome and determine surgical timing (**Table 3**).[8] Of

these, BW of <1,500 g and the presence of CHD produce significantly increased risk.

Various other classifications have been formulated to guide treatment and predict outcome and are of benefit in parental counseling. In 1994, an outcome-based classification (BW and presence of major CHD) was given by Spitz, revised in 2006, and is still in use.[9] The overall survival rate predicted by it is 86.4% and it aids to guide treatment, parental counseling, and compare the international outcomes (**Table 4**).

Okamoto identified BW as an important risk factor and used stepwise logistic regression analysis and operating receiver curve to statistically extrapolate the at-risk weight group (<2 kg with CHD, survival rate 27%; >2 kg without CHD, survival rate 100%).[10]

Preoperative Management

Once TEF is diagnosed, oral feeds are stopped immediately to prevent lung soiling. The neonate is nursed in a semiupright position. Continuous low-pressure suction of the upper pouch using the Replogle tube reduces spillage into the lungs. Neonates may present with dehydration, aspiration pneumonia, and acid-base abnormalities, especially if presenting late to the hospital. An intravenous (IV) line is placed, and the child is given maintenance fluids to ensure euvolemia and normoglycemia. If required, a central venous (CV) line can be placed for the optimization of fluid status. Correction of acid-base abnormalities in the first 24–72 hours of life before taking up for surgery is important. There may be respiratory acidosis due to aspiration pneumonitis, atelectasis, and elevation of the diaphragm (gastric distension) leading to shunting, hypercarbia, and hypoxia. Similarly, metabolic acidosis might occur due to severe

Table 2: Classification of esophageal atresia and tracheoesophageal fistula.

Type	Incidence (%)	Classification (Gross/Vogt)	Pictorial representation
Esophageal atresia without fistula	7	A/II	
Proximal TEF with distal esophageal atresia	2	B/III	
Proximal esophageal atresia with distal TEF	86	C/IIIb	
Esophageal atresia with proximal and distal fistula	<1	D/IIIa	
TEF without esophageal atresia	4	E/H type	

(TEF: tracheoesophageal fistula)

Table 3: Waterson's risk classification.

	Criteria	Management
A	Birth weight >2.5 kg and neonate's general condition is well	Immediate definitive surgery
B1	1.8–2.5 kg and general condition is well	Staged repair and gastrostomy first
B2	>2.5 kg with moderate pneumonia and congenital heart disease	Postpone surgery till stabilization
C1	<1.8 kg	
C2	1.8–2.5 kg with severe pneumonia and congenital heart disease	

Table 4: Spitz revised risk assessment.

Group I	>2.0 kg without cardiac disease	Low risk
Group II	<2.0 kg without cardiac disease	Moderate risk
Group III	>2.0 kg + major cardiac disease	Relatively high risk
Group IV	<2.0 kg + major cardiac disease	High risk

dehydration leading to shock. Prophylactic antibiotics need to be started as a prophylaxis to aspiration pneumonitis.[11]

Role of Mechanical Ventilation

Neonates may present with respiratory distress due to prematurity, aspiration of gastric contents, and cardiac pathology necessitating intubation and mechanical ventilation. Positive pressure ventilation (PPV) in the presence of distal fistula will cause the entry of gases into the stomach leading to gastric insufflation and increased diaphragmatic excursions, and regurgitation, thus worsening the already compromised ventilatory parameters.

Operative correction is a medical but not surgical emergency. But preterm neonates with severe respiratory compromise who require PPV may be considered as candidates for emergency surgery in view of increased gastric distention. Since the 1980s, advances in neonatal ventilation techniques, and modes of ventilation (pressure-limited and volume-targeted synchronized modes), and use of antenatal steroids and surfactant have allowed stabilization of a sick neonate before definitive surgery.

Thompson et al. published a single-center retrospective review in 2019, which included all the neonates with EA-TEF from 2008 to 2018.[12] The authors proposed to reassess the risk of preoperative PPV in this group of patients, and one of the outcomes studied was gastric perforation and perioperative death. The authors reported an overall mortality of 12.5%, which was found to be higher in cases where PPV using newer ventilation strategies ensued before fistula ligation (29% vs. 5%); none of the newborns had a gastric perforation. But all those neonates who were on mechanical ventilation were premature with life-threatening comorbidities.

Several studies have demonstrated short-term benefits linked to the use of synchronized ventilation in neonates, shown to improve oxygenation status and reduce the delivered tidal volumes (TV) and hence lesser gastric distention and volutrauma to lungs.[13] A recent Cochrane review analyzed trials comparing studies of synchronized versus nonsynchronized ventilation in neonates and reported reduced air leaks and duration of mechanical ventilation in the synchronized group. For premature neonates, flow-triggered ventilation is now the standard of care.[14]

Similarly, in neonatal intensive care units (NICU), volume-targeted modes of ventilation like pressure-regulated volume controlled, volume controlled ventilation, and volume guaranteed ventilation are a better choice in neonates. A recently published Cochrane review[15] and meta-analysis[16] demonstrated that there was a significant reduction in rates of death, bronchopulmonary dysplasia (BPD), intraventricular hemorrhage, incidence of hypocarbia and pneumothorax, and the number of ventilator days in volume-targeted approach.

Preoperative Investigations

Routine blood investigations which may be required include full blood count, coagulation studies, baseline biochemistry, and a blood group and cross-match. Chest roentgenogram [coiled nasogastric tube (NGT) in an upper pouch with the absent gas bubble], USG abdomen (for renal anomalies) and an echocardiogram (ECHO) are recommended for detection of coexistent cardiac anomalies and right-sided aortic arch.

Surgical Repair

Definitive surgery is the ultimate treatment modality. Usually, surgery is done 24–72 hours after birth, once the neonate stabilizes, as delay in surgery increases the risk of aspiration. Surgery can be an open or thoracoscopic procedure. Surgery could be a single-stage repair, which involves isolation and ligation of fistula and subsequent esophageal anastomoses. It can be a staged repair in case of a very long gap between the esophageal segments involving a first stage of isolation and ligation of fistula and a gastrostomy with esophagostomy and a second stage of definitive repair of esophageal anastomoses once the esophageal segments have sufficiently grown.

Airway and Ventilation Problems

Airway and ventilation problems are based on the size, location, and orientation of TEF, the respiratory status of the neonate, and the surgical plan (thoracotomy or thoracoscopy). Anesthesia management aims to avoid ventilating the fistula by keeping the endotracheal tube (ETT) below the fistula. If the fistula is close to the carina or in the mainstem bronchus, it will be difficult/impossible to place the ETT between carina and fistula as well as to ventilate both lungs. Moreover, the fistula can be very wide and at an angle to the trachea like mainstem bronchus. Because of this, the fistula may get intubated while trying to place ETT. Also, there may be excessive distension of the stomach if the tip of the ETT is above the fistula.

Monitoring

Standard ASA (American Society of Anesthesiologists) monitoring is recommended [ECG, noninvasive blood pressure (NIBP), SPO$_2$ (pre- and postductal), ETCO$_2$, and temperature]. Good peripheral lines are a must, and CV catheterization is not usually required. An arterial catheter may be useful because of the high possibility of hemodynamic fluctuations during lung retraction as well as for arterial blood gas (ABG) analysis. The target is to maintain blood pressure and perfusion.

Anesthesia Management

The neonate can be induced with either an inhalational or an IV anesthetic agent and maintained using opioids (fentanyl 0.5–1 µg/kg), intermittent doses of nondepolarizing muscle relaxants (NDMRs) (such as atracurium 0.5 mg/kg), and inhalational agents [sevoflurane or isoflurane 0.9–1 minimum alveolar concentration (MAC)].

There is still a controversy regarding whether the child should be intubated under spontaneous breathing or paralyzed with NDMRs. Intubation under spontaneous breathing creates a negative intrathoracic pressure which causes the gas to enter the lungs rather than the fistula. It also allows awakening of the neonate in the situation of difficulty in maintaining oxygenation. However, the use of spontaneous breathing has the drawback of producing coughing and a poor/suboptimal glottic view. Also, if

the child has an already poorly compliant lung, the gas exchange will not be optimal without PPV.

The use of muscle relaxants for intubation produces optimal intubating conditions without coughing and straining. But it has the possibility of causing stomach distension because the gases would find the path of least resistance, through fistula to stomach. Also, the surgical technique would ultimately require PPV.

The placement of an ETT is essentially a blind process with the possibility that it may enter the wide fistula. The proposed methods for the correct location of ETT vis-a-vis the fistula location include:
- Placing the ETT into the bronchus and then withdrawing it slowly while auscultating the left chest till breath sounds are heard. This enables the location of ETT below the fistula with minimal leak into the stomach.[17]
- Rotation of tube so that the bevel faces anteriorly away from the fistula.[18]
- Use of a cuffed ETT may cause occlusion of fistula.

In spite of this, there is the possibility of preferential intubation of fistula, difficult bilateral lung ventilation if the fistula is too low near the carina, and the occlusion/displacement of ETT during surgical manipulation.

Presurgery Bronchoscopy

Keeping in view the above possibilities, some surgeons prefer to do a rigid bronchoscopy before definitive repair to recognize the presence of two fistulas, delineate the airway anatomy, rule out associated airway anomalies, and identify the position and type of fistula (C type, H type).[19] It will also help in identifying the presence of a large pericarinal fistula which is likely to produce difficulty in ventilation for the anesthetist.[20] It can help in placing a Fogarty catheter for occluding the fistula and for identification of fistula during surgery.[21]

Ventilatory Management

Difficulty with ventilation is common during TEF repair and may be related to many factors—presence of preoperative aspiration, lateral decubitus position, and lung retraction/collapse during surgery. All these factors result in changes in lung compliance and so the difficulty in ventilation and oxygenation. During surgery, there may be episodes of hypercarbia, hypoxia, and inability to ventilate. Hypercarbia may be tolerated in most neonates with TEF; however, in those with CHD, it may result in a return to fetal circulation and changes in pulmonary vascular resistance. For hypoxia, these neonates may have to be maintained on higher inspired oxygen concentration (FiO$_2$) intraoperatively, although recommendations are to target SPO$_2$ of 85–95% at a lower FiO$_2$, especially in preterm infants.

Postoperative Management

Postoperative (PO) pain can be managed using opioids, epidural catheters, intercostal block, local anesthetic (LA) infiltration, and paravertebral block. Commonly used LAs in neonates include 0.5% bupivacaine and 0.2% ropivacaine. LA in neonates has greater volume of distribution, which counteracts the increased potential for toxicity due to increased free, nonprotein bound fraction. While giving continuous infusion of LA, attention should be paid to immature metabolism systems.[22]

Some neonates get extubated on the operating table; others may need PO ventilation based on their prematurity, preoperative and intraoperative respiratory status, ease and duration of surgery as well as surgical need. In some centers, elective PO ventilation for 24–48 hours is mandatory in all operated TEFs.

Postoperative Complications (Early and Late)

All neonates, whether extubated or not, should be kept in NICU PO. *The early complications include* injury to the recurrent laryngeal nerve, an overlooked fistula, a recurrent fistula, anastomotic leaks,[23] and strictures.[24] Anastomotic leaks occur in 15–20% of cases PO with major leaks presenting within 48 hours postsurgery leading to life-threatening complications. Minor leaks heal spontaneously but can lead to the formation of strictures (incidence 30–40%), managed by repeated endoscopic dilatations. If a postsurgical repair infant presents with recurrent respiratory infections or symptoms (cyanosis, coughing, choking), the possibility of a recurrent fistula should be kept in mind (incidence 5–14%).

Late complications include tracheomalacia (11–33%),[25] dysphagia (21–84%), gastric dysmotility and gastric esophageal reflux disease (35–58%),[26] hyperbronchial reactivity and asthma, and scoliosis or chest wall deformities due to the post-thoracotomy syndrome.[27]

▌CONGENITAL DIAPHRAGMATIC HERNIA

Congenital diaphragmatic hernia results due to a developmental defect in the diaphragm with an incidence of 1:2,500 to 1:3,500 live births. It results due to failure of the pleural and peritoneal canals to close during the 8th week of gestation, with subsequent herniation of the abdominal contents into the thorax, thereby resulting in pulmonary hypoplasia owing to compression of the developing lungs by the viscera. The defect usually occurs on the left side (85–90%) but can occur on the right side or bilaterally and may be associated with other anomalies. In 70–80% cases, the defect comprises the posterolateral (Bochdalek) region of the diaphragm, but the anterior (Morgagni; 25–30%) or central regions (2–5%) can also be involved. Children with CDH may have associated lung, vascular, and cardiac abnormalities [lung hypoplasia and pulmonary hypertension (PHT)], which can lead to high mortality.

Embryology

At 8 weeks of gestation, the common pleuroperitoneal cavity is divided into two compartments—the pleural cavity and the peritoneal cavity via the pleuroperitoneal membrane. The posterolateral portion of the membrane is the last to develop, with the right side closing before the left. At approximately the 9th gestational week, the gut, which was in the yolk sac, migrates to the peritoneal cavity. If this migration occurs before the pleuroperitoneal membrane closes off the pleural cavity, the stomach, spleen, liver, and bowel can migrate into the pleural cavity and compress the developing lungs. Also, the contralateral lung is affected and may be hypoplastic.[28]

Prediction of Outcome and Prognosis

The antenatal detection of CDH and prediction of the worst outcome can be the basis for parental counseling or the decision to perform surgery during fetal life. The presence of associated cardiac and skeletal anomalies has a poorer prognosis and requires fetal ECHO or amniocentesis to rule out chromosomal defects. ECHO can identify concomitant CHD, assess the right and left heart function, and estimate the degree of PHT.

In case of isolated CDH, antenatal predictors assessed include detection of the intrathoracic liver, lung-to-head circumference ratio (LHR), size of the diaphragmatic defect, lung-to-transverse thorax ratio, MRI-determined fetal lung volume and cardiac axis, or presence of pleural and pericardial effusion. Out of these, only LHR and liver position are reliable in predicting the outcome.[28-31] The European CDH registry data revealed that irrespective of gestation, the LHR increases in fetuses with left- or right-sided CDH, while the change in the observed and the expected LHR in normal fetuses was minimal.[32] The outcome is poor if the observed LHR is <25% of the expected. In a retrospective study, the presence of liver in the thorax had a worse prognosis (45% survival vs. 95% if the liver was in the abdomen). A fetal LHR <1.0 and liver herniation are factors for a poor outcome and indication for fetal intervention.[29]

EUROCAT (European Registration of Congenital Anomalies and Twins)[33] program is an initiative of the European communities for surveillance of congenital anomalies. It recommends routine antenatal USG scanning for congenital anomalies; MRI (if the results of USG are equivocal), USG assessment of lung size by observed/expected LHR and assessment of liver herniation as predictors of survival, antenatal counseling, genetic consultation and amniocentesis, termination of pregnancy for those with poor prognosis, and fetal surgery in selected cases.

Various strategies have been tried to reduce the morbidity and mortality of CDH. Surfactant administration has been tried to improve the lung maturity. However, it failed to reduce the need for extracorporeal membrane oxygenation (ECMO) and development of BPD and also did not improve survival. Corticosteroids, both prenatal and postnatal, have also not shown any beneficial effect on the outcome. Fetal surgery for repair of CDH thought to help in lung development and improved outcome increases chances of fetal death. Surgical or fetoscopic occlusion of the fetal lung to allow gradual distension of the hypoplastic lung with fetal lung fluid has also failed to improve survival.[34]

Pulmonary Development

During fetal life, major airways develop by 16 weeks, and by 24 weeks of gestation canalization of the major airways with the formation of the air-blood barrier ensues followed by a period of differentiation and further growth of the air columns. At 36 weeks of gestation, most of the lung growth is complete, along with the continued production of surfactant. In CDH, the abdominal organs enter into the thorax, leading to mediastinal shift and hampered lung growth. Lung hypoplasia is associated with a reduction in lung tissue and airway smooth muscle dysregulation. Also, lung volumes of both the ipsilateral and the contralateral lungs are decreased. Pulmonary hypoplasia increases pulmonary vascular resistance (PVR), with subsequent right heart failure leading to hypoxia and acidosis. Abnormally developed pulmonary vasculature leads to persistent pulmonary hypertension of the newborn (PPHN) and pulmonary vasculature hyper-reactivity leading to persistent fetal circulation and mortality.[35]

Clinical Presentation

A neonate presenting with respiratory distress at birth or within the first few hours of life with cyanosis and poor feeding suggests a high suspicion of CDH. There is a resultant decrease in air entry on the affected side (with audible bowel sounds) along with a flat or scaphoid abdomen. With Bochdalek hernia, the radiograph shows the absence of the diaphragm and presence of bowel loops in the chest, with a paucity of loops in the abdomen, the tip of the NGT in the chest (if the stomach is herniated), and mediastinal shift. In right-sided CDH, a radioopaque space-occupying solid shadow (liver) replaces the lung tissue in the lower chest.[28]

Neonates who present with respiratory distress at birth have high chances of having associated CHD and have lower Apgar score at birth and lower postductal saturation. Research studies have shown that neonates with a sustained alveolar-to-arterial gradient of >600 mm Hg and oxygenation index >40 up to 6–8 hours post birth have higher mortality. Also, infants with $PaO_2 < 80$ mm Hg, who cannot sustain a preductal value of at least 100, have severe pulmonary hypoplasia incompatible with life.[28]

Postnatal Resuscitation and Management

If CDH has been diagnosed antenatally, the patient should be referred to a center with NICU and surgical facilities. Emergent neonatal resuscitation is done immediately at birth to achieve cardiopulmonary stability and prevent the development of hypercapnia and hypoxemia, which leads to PPHN. To achieve this, immediate endotracheal intubation is done, and mechanical ventilation is initiated, avoiding bag-mask ventilation to prevent gastrointestinal distension with further compression of the hypoplastic lungs.[34] Gastric decompression with NGT drainage is instituted, CV access and monitoring are established, and fluid management is optimized before surgery. ECHO is performed to identify structural abnormalities of the heart and assess heart function and response to therapy as well as the severity of PHT. Preductal and postductal oxygen saturations should be monitored to assess the degree of ductal shunting because of PHT.[36] For advanced hemodynamic monitoring, invasive arterial and venous access needs to be obtained for advanced invasive monitoring.

Critical Care Management

In the past, CDH was considered a surgical emergency. However, now the child's respiratory and cardiovascular problems are first stabilized, and then the child is operated. It includes ventilatory management, treatment of PHT, and use of ECMO.

Ventilation Strategies

The most important part of the management of a neonate with CDH is ventilatory support. In the past, the belief was that the creation of chemical and ventilatory alkalosis (pH >7.55, PCO_2 <20) could lead to a reduction in PVR and right-to-left shunt.[36] Since this could be achieved only with high peak inspiratory pressures (PIP), it led to an increased risk of barotrauma and high mortality. It was Wung et al. who came up with the concept of "permissive hypercapnia" in the management of infants with PHT (non-CDH infants). In their study, the authors could avoid barotrauma by limiting the PIP.[37] Also, based on adult Acute Respiratory Distress Network Trial (ARDSNET), mortality could be reduced by minimizing ventilator-induced lung injury (VILI).[38] Based on these, the lung-protective approach is thought to be the best technique to reduce mortality and morbidity as it allows the growth of lung parenchymal vasculature.

The principles of ventilation are to keep peak airway pressures limited to 25 cm H_2O or less and PIP limited to 28 cm H_2O, with positive end-expiratory pressure (PEEP) between 2 and 5 cm H_2O. The target preductal saturation range is 85–95% and postductal saturation ≥70%, allowing $PaCO_2$ levels up to 60 and 65 mm Hg.[39] If the pH is <7.25, $PaCO_2$ is >65 mm Hg, and preductal saturation is <80–85% with an FiO_2 of 60%, then alternative forms of ventilatory support such as high-frequency oscillatory ventilation (HFOV), inhaled nitric oxide (iNO), and ECMO are indicated.[40]

High-frequency oscillatory ventilation has mainly been studied in non-CDH neonates with variable outcomes in terms of mortality. The *V*entilation in *I*nfants with *C*ongenital diaphragmatic hernia: An *I*nternational randomized clinical (VICI) trial was done to determine the optimal initial ventilation mode in patients with CDH.[41] This study found no significant difference in the combined mortality or BPD in neonates ventilated by conventional or HFOV groups. However, neonates in the conventional ventilation group showed shorter ventilation times and lesser need for ECMO. The ventilator settings for HFOV should be a mean airway pressure of 13–15 mm Hg and a pressure delta ranging from 30 to 40 cm H_2O based on the extent of chest rise established on chest radiographs (8 ribs).

Management of Pulmonary Hypertension

Various therapeutic modalities to manage reversible PHT have been tried alone or in combination including iNO, sildenafil, prostacyclins, prostaglandins, and nonspecific endothelin inhibitors.

Inhaled nitric oxide is a direct pulmonary vasodilator (5–20 parts per million) and improves oxygenation and lessens the requirement for ECMO in newborns with PPHN.[42] The literature lacks conclusive evidence on the role of iNO in reducing the requirement for ECMO or death in CDH patients. In patients who are nonresponsive to iNO or have rebound PPHN, oral or IV sildenafil can be considered. It is a selective cyclic guanosine monophosphate (cGMP) phosphodiesterase-5 inhibitor and enhances iNO-mediated vasodilatation leading to improved oxygenation in refractive cases of CDH.[40] Milrinone is a phosphodiesterase-3 inhibitor which acts on the PVR and cardiac function and has shown some efficacy in neonates with PPHN by improving pulmonary vasodilatation.[40] Prostaglandin and prostacyclin help to relax the vascular smooth muscle cells and maintain the patency of ductus arteriosus

(DA), through cyclic adenosine monophosphate (cAMP) formation. Prostaglandin E1 is considered in unstable hemodynamic patients who have ECHO-proven right ventricular dysfunction associated with hypotension and poor tissue perfusion. Epoprostenol is an intravenously administered analog of PGI2 whereas iloprost is an inhaled analog.[42]

Extracorporeal Membrane Oxygenation

In patients with labile physiology and low preductal saturations despite the use of maximum ventilatory support, inotropic support, and pulmonary vasodilation, ECMO may be considered. However, ECMO as a "rescue therapy" for neonates with severe CDH remains debatable. ECMO is beneficial in neonates with severe respiratory failure associated with reversible lung disease. Indications for ECMO include a low oxygenation index, rising lactates despite maximum ventilation and treatment for PPHN and inotropic support, and associated severe hypoxemia and hypercapnia. In CDH, it is difficult to identify those neonates with severe disease who have reversible lung disease, compared to those who are irreversible from the beginning.[35] A meta-analysis of randomized trials as well as a Cochrane review has failed to show benefit of ECMO in neonates with CDH.[43] The morbidity induced by ECMO in those who survive included intracranial infarct or bleed, major bleeding, seizures, infection, and neurodevelopmental problems in addition to being costly. Two centers compared the outcome of patients using HFOV versus ECMO as rescue and found no difference in overall survival rate between the two groups.[44] The ideal length of time on ECMO in patients with CDH is debated. The other dilemma is the timing of repair in those on ECMO. Surgical repair on ECMO can be associated with a higher incidence of bleeding. Therefore, repair has traditionally been performed after decannulation from ECMO.

Surgical Repair

The surgical repair is delayed until the child is physiologically stable and the PHT has improved. The surgical procedure may be an open abdominal or a thoracoscopic repair. The outcome is similar for both the surgical procedures. However, some studies have shown a higher recurrence rate with thoracoscopic procedures. Usually, the laparoscopic approach is used for the less common Morgagni hernia. For Bochdalek hernia, thoracoscopy is the favored approach.

CO_2 insufflation is used during both laparoscopy and thoracoscopy for CDH repair.[33] Lung collapse with insufflation impairs the respiratory capacity for oxygenation and excretion of CO_2 leading to increased end-tidal CO_2 levels and acidosis. Presence of PPHN, lung hypoplasia, and pulmonary vasculature hyperactivity in CDH interferes with washout of increased CO_2 levels. Acidosis may increase shunting and worsen any PHT with deleterious effects on systemic perfusion pressures, ventilation, and oxygenation. The limits of "intraoperative permissive hypercapnia" in CDH have not been established. High-frequency ventilation is another modality available for intraoperative management of CO_2 load during thoracoscopy.[35]

Anesthesia Management

The aim of anesthesia management should be to avoid hypoxia, hypercarbia, hyperthermia, and acidosis and to prevent reversal of shunt. One should also prevent gut distension due to PPV and nitrous-oxide (N_2O). N_2O can lead to hypoxia as infants with CDH have high FiO_2 requirement. Hypothermia should be avoided to prevent vasoconstriction, increase in oxygen consumption, and development of PHT. If not already intubated, neonates should undergo modified rapid-sequence intubation. Induction of anesthesia is via inhalational or IV agents with assisted/controlled ventilation avoiding high inflation pressures to reduce the risk of aspiration of gastric contents owing to the incompetence of lower esophageal sphincter. N_2O is avoided to prevent its diffusion into bowel lumen, thereby compromising lung expansion if the bowel is in the chest. Invasive monitoring may be required if the child is in respiratory or cardiovascular distress. Cannulation of the right radial artery provides continuous blood pressure measurement and assessment of blood gases. Preductal and postductal oxygen saturation allows early detection of right-to-left shunting.

PYLORIC STENOSIS

Pyloric stenosis is one of the common gastrointestinal entities seen in neonates with an incidence of 1:500 live births and a male preponderance. The child becomes symptomatic at 2–6 weeks of life, and the condition is due to hypertrophy of the muscular layer of the pylorus.[27] On examination, it feels like an olive-shaped mass on the right of the midline in the epigastrium and ultrasound could be used for diagnosis. The presentation is in the form of persistent vomiting, with loss of water, hydrogen, chloride, sodium, and potassium leading to metabolic derangements. To maintain a normal serum pH, the kidneys excrete potassium in place of hydrogen. With severe sodium depletion, the kidneys secrete potassium and hydrogen in place of sodium resulting in a picture of hypokalemia, hypochloremia, and alkalosis. In continuum to electrolyte loss, kidneys secrete acidic urine and metabolic alkalosis becomes more severe finally leading to metabolic acidosis from dehydration and hypoperfusion.[28]

Anesthesia Management

The first step before surgery in these neonates involves correction of dehydration and electrolyte loss because an alkalotic child postoperatively can develop hypoxia by hypoventilating to correct the alkalotic state. If the chloride is >90 mEq/L and urine-specific gravity is <1.020, i.e., the dehydration and electrolyte disturbance is mild to moderate, a balanced electrolyte solution is administered at the rate of 10 mL/kg/h. In case of severe dehydration and electrolyte imbalance, i.e., chloride <90 mEq/L, sodium <120 mEq/L and no urine output, volume expansion with isotonic saline or colloid are required till the urine output is established.

Gastric decompression is initially done with the placement of NGT. Anesthesia induction is by the IV route with intubation using the rapid sequence to avoid aspiration risk. The surgery is done either via laparotomy or laparoscopy. Monitoring is routine with special attention to hemodynamics. Adequate muscle relaxation is required to prevent injury to duodenal mucosa during pyloromyotomy. Intraoperative pain is managed with fentanyl 0.5–1 μg/kg or paracetamol 7.5 mg/kg. The surgical incision site can be infiltrated with bupivacaine 0.25%. Postoperatively, the neonate may be drowsy and may need PO ventilation, owing to hypokalemia potentiating the effect of NDMR. Hypokalemia may also lead to the development of cardiac dysrhythmias.

OMPHALOCELE AND GASTROSCHISIS

These are abdominal wall defects detectable during fetal USG in as early as the first trimester. Omphalocele has an incidence of 1:6,000 births and results due to failure of the gut to migrate from the yolk sac to the abdomen during gestation.[45] There is external herniation of abdominal viscera into the base of the umbilical cord, with the presence of sac (amnion/peritoneum) on the contents. These neonates are usually preterm and have a high incidence of associated cardiac, gastrointestinal (malrotation, Meckel's diverticulum, and intestinal atresia), genitourinary (exstrophy of the bladder), metabolic, and chromosomal abnormalities. Cardiac and thoracic defects are more common in neonates with epigastric omphalocele, whereas cloacal abnormalities and exstrophy of the bladder are more frequent with hypogastric omphalocele.[28]

Gastroschisis is the result of occlusion of the omphalo-mesenteric artery during gestation and results in herniation of viscera through the lateral abdominal defect with the absence of covering sac.[46] It has an incidence of 1:15,000 live births and is associated with a low incidence of associated anomalies but a higher incidence of intestinal atresia.

Anesthesia Management

The main aim is to prevent infection and to minimize fluid and heat loss. The fluid and heat loss prevention necessitate covering the exposed viscera with sterile saline-soaked dressings and wrapping them with plastic wrap. Initial management would involve giving fluids at 10–15 mL/kg/h along with a cover of antimicrobials to prevent infection.[47]

In spite of the urgency of surgery, efforts should be made to evaluate the neonate for associated anomalies and to correct fluid and electrolyte imbalance. Intraoperatively, efforts should be made to prevent heat loss and hypothermia as well as provide volume resuscitation if needed. The closure of the defect without increasing intra-abdominal pressure (IAP) may be a challenge even if the child is relaxed with muscle relaxants. This increased IAP may lead to ventilatory compromise and decreased organ perfusion. There may also be bowel edema, anuria, and hypotension because of this increased pressure. Suspicion arises if the oxygen saturation falls as shown by a pulse oximeter in the lower limb owing to congestion of lower extremities due to obstructed venous return. One can also measure intragastric pressure, CV pressure, and cardiac index to decide if primary closure will be possible. If closure is not possible immediately, then a staged procedure may be appropriate, i.e., extraperitoneal encasement of the bowel in a synthetic mesh or a plastic pouch and then attempting a gradual, staged reduction, spread over few days, till the abdomen is closed without compromising the perfusion and ventilation. One should be vigilant about the fluid and heat loss, both intra- and postoperatively.

MENINGOMYELOCELE AND HYDROCEPHALUS

Meningomyelocele and hydrocephalus are two of the most common congenital malformations of the central nervous system (CNS). During the first 4 weeks of gestation, there is a fusion of neural tube. Failure of fusion leads to herniation of meninges (meningocele) or meninges with neural elements (MMC) usually at the lumbar level of the spinal cord. A neural tube defect in cranium leads to herniation of meninges with or without neural tissue in the cranium (encephalocele). The incidence of MMC is 0.4–1/1,000 live births,[48] with male preponderance, usually accompanied by Arnold-Chiari type II malformation and hydrocephalus.[49] It is one of the leading causes of infantile paralysis with life-long disability.

The condition of myelodysplasia leads to exposure of CNS tissue with the risk of infection, and if the closure is delayed, it can lead to progressive neural damage and decreased motor function. Preoperative evaluation includes screening for other associated congenital anomalies. These neonates are also at risk of latex allergy.

Anesthetic Considerations

There may be associated CHD which needs to be identified before anesthesia. Airway management may be difficult, especially with a large head due to hydrocephalus and encephalocele. Avoid succinylcholine in patients with neurological manifestations and deficits. The neuroplaque needs to be protected. There is a risk of hypothermia as well as fluid and heat loss from the exposed neuroplaque due to poor autonomic control below the lesion. Given other comorbidities, the perioperative challenges include respiratory complications such as apneic episodes, hypoventilation, bronchospasm, and breath-holding due to derangements of the medullary respiratory center.[47] Also of concern is the presence of Chiari malformations, which can lead to bradycardia, hypotension, tachycardia, and brain stem compression and coning.

Concerns include prone surgical positioning. Avoid extreme head flexion as it can lead to brain stem compression and displacement of the ETT. Improper positioning can lead to venous congestion of face, head, and tongue and also increased IAP which can lead to vena cava compression and increased surgical bleeding.

These neonates during the intraoperative period may also present with unexplained hypotension which can occur due to a sudden loss of cerebrospinal fluid (CSF) from the sac leading to the increased gradient between cranial and spinal CSF fluid pressures resulting in brain herniation. Postoperatively, these infants are nursed in prone position to avoid pressure over the surgical site.

ANORECTAL MALFORMATION

Anorectal malformations encompass a wide spectrum of congenital malformations involving the anorectal and urogenital systems. ARM is one of the most common congenital malformations with an incidence of 1:4,000–5,000 live births with male preponderance.[50] It is also one of the leading causes of intestinal obstruction in neonates. The cause is not clear but implicated to genetic and environmental factors and drug exposure. The defect usually occurs at 5–7 weeks of fetal development where the anus and rectum do not develop properly, and 20–80% cases of ARM are associated with other congenital anomalies including vertebral anomalies (hemivertebrae, absent vertebrae, or tethered cord), kidney and urinary tract anomalies (duplication of urinary tract, horseshoe kidney, renal agenesis, hypospadias, vesicoureteral reflux), gastrointestinal tract abnormalities (tracheal and esophageal defects, duodenal atresia, Hirschsprung's disease), CHD (atrial septal defect, ventricular septal defect, patent ductus arteriosus), and chromosomal abnormalities (Down syndrome). The prognosis is related to the presence of other associated congenital lesions and along with low BW, there is a delay in seeking medical care and sepsis. Morbidity and mortality are higher due to the presence of other associated conditions such as hypothermia, hypoglycemia, poor immunity, and sepsis.

Imperforate anus mostly is not noticed until birth; literature reveals cases wherein antenatal diagnosis or suspicion has been made at 12 weeks of gestation, wherein the findings reveal bowel dilatation.[51] Most of the neonates are either diagnosed at birth or later on with signs and symptoms of intestinal obstruction. In cases of delayed presentation, the neonates may present with intestinal obstruction leading to increased intraluminal pressure, which exceeds capillary and venous pressures in the bowel wall eventually leading to bowel ischemia and decreased lymphatic drainage. All these lead to gut perforation and bacterial translocation leading to sepsis and multisystem derangement. These neonates would also present with electrolyte disturbances in the form of hyponatremia, hypokalemia, hypoglycemia, and metabolic acidosis. Acute intestinal obstruction with a distended abdomen can lead to compromised respiration, which is the result of restricted diaphragmatic movement and decreased functional residual capacity in the supine position.

Hence, these neonates should be kept in an NICU and optimized before taking up for surgery. Resuscitation will include correction of hypovolemia, hypoglycemia, hypothermia, acid-base and electrolyte abnormalities, and respiratory and ventilatory support. Immediate decompression should be done with NGT, followed by colostomy; definitive surgery could follow later. A presurgery evaluation will require investigations in the form of hematocrit, serum electrolytes, and ABG analysis; also the newborn should be evaluated for the presence of other associated anomalies and hydration status (capillary refill, NIBP).

Once a stabilized newborn is taken up for diversion colostomy, anesthetic induction follows a thorough suction via NGT.[52] At least two peripheral IV lines should be secured. Rapid-sequence intubation using IV induction agents (thiopentone and propofol) and a depolarizing muscle relaxant, succinylcholine (2 mg/kg), to prevent aspiration should be done. Fluid resuscitation should be continued. The ongoing losses during laparotomy would require resuscitation fluids as high as 8-10 ml/kg/hr. Blood transfusion should be done when the loss exceeds 10% of the total blood volume or hemoglobin goes below 12 g/dL. Ventilation should be done using pressure control ventilation using lower pressures to prevent barotrauma.

Postoperatively, the neonates should be kept in an NICU irrespective of whether they are intubated or extubated. PO analgesia includes use of epidural catheters

(0.1–0.3 mL/kg/h of 0.1% bupivacaine or ropivacaine for 48 hours), though regional techniques should be avoided in case of severe abdominal sepsis. Other modalities include opioid infusion in neonates who are mechanically ventilated either using morphine or fentanyl and use of IV paracetamol (maximum recommended dose in preterm neonates 25 mg/kg/day and in term neonates 30 mg/kg/day).

CONCLUSION

Neonatal congenital lesions requiring surgical repair pose a great challenge for the pediatric surgeon as well as the anesthetist. Most of the conditions pose as medical emergencies and require a multidisciplinary approach for stabilization. Thorough knowledge regarding the individual conditions, associated congenital pathologies, and optimization is required for a fruitful outcome. With the advent of newer technology for monitoring and newer modes of mechanical ventilation, the neonatal outcomes post surgical repair are on improving trends. In developing countries, emphasis is required in improving the peripheral healthcare system, NICU and surgical techniques, and early and safe transfer of sick neonates, leading to improved neonatal outcomes.

REFERENCES

1. Hines MH. Neonatal cardiovascular physiology. Semin Pediatr Surg. 2013;22(4):174-8.
2. Pinheiro PF, Simões e Silva AC, Pereira RM. Current knowledge on esophageal atresia. World J Gastroenterol. 2012;18(28):3662-72.
3. Spitz L. Oesophageal atresia. Orphanet J Rare Dis. 2007;2:24.
4. Krosnar S, Baxter A. Thoracoscopic repair of esophageal atresia with tracheoesophageal fistula: anesthetic and intensive care management of a series of eight neonates. Paediatr Anaesth. 2005;15(7):541-6.
5. Sañudo JR, Domenech-Mateu JM. The laryngeal primordium and epithelial lamina. A new interpretation. J Anat. 1990;171:207-22.
6. Houben CH, Curry JI. Current status of prenatal diagnosis, operative management and outcome of esophageal atresia/tracheo-esophageal fistula. Prenat Diagn. 2008;28(7):667-75.
7. Crabbe DC. Isolated tracheo-oesophageal fistula. Paediatr Respir Rev. 2003;4(1):74-8.
8. Niramis R, Tangkhabuanbut P, Anuntkosol M, Buranakitjaroen V, Tongsin A, Mahatharadol V. Clinical outcomes of esophageal atresia: comparison between the Waterston and the Spitz classifications. Ann Acad Med Singapore. 2013;42(6):297-300.
9. Spitz L, Kiely EM, Morecroft JA, Drake DP. Oesophageal atresia: at-risk groups for the 1990s. J Pediatr Surg. 1994;29:723-5.
10. Okamoto T, Takamizawa S, Arai H, Bitoh Y, Nakao M, Yokoi A, et al. Esophageal atresia: prognostic classification revisited. Surgery. 2009;145:675-81.

11. Broemling N, Campbell F. Anesthetic management of congenital tracheoesophageal fistula. Paediatr Anaesth. 2011;21:1092-9.

12. Thompson A, Thakkar H, Khan H, Yardley IE. Not all neonates with oesophageal atresia and tracheoesophageal fistula are a surgical emergency. J Pediatr Surg. 2019;54:244-6.

13. Cleary JP, Bernstein G, Mannino FL, Heldt GP. Improved oxygenation during synchronized intermittent mandatory ventilation in neonates with respiratory distress syndrome: A randomized, crossover study. J Pediatr. 1995;126:407-11.

14. Greenough A, Rossor TE, Sundaresan A, Murthy V, Milner AD. Synchronized mechanical ventilation for respiratory support in newborn infants. Cochrane Database Syst Rev. 2016;9:CD000456.

15. Klingenberg C, Wheeler KI, McCallion N, Morley CJ, Davis PG. Volume-targeted versus pressure-limited ventilation in neonates. Cochrane Database Syst Rev. 2017;10:CD003666.

16. Peng W, Zhu H, Shi H, Liu E. Volume-targeted ventilation is more suitable than pressure-limited ventilation for preterm infants: a systematic review and meta-analysis. Arch Dis Child Fetal Neonatal Ed. 2014;99:F158-65.

17. Salem MR, Wong AY, Lin YH, Firor HV, Bennett EJ. Prevention of gastric distention during anesthesia for newborns with tracheoesophageal fistulas. Anesthesiology. 1973;38:82-3.

18. Andropoulos DB, Rowe RW, Betts JM. Anaesthetic and surgical airway management during tracheo-oesophageal fistula repair. Paediatr Anaesth. 1998;8:313-9.

19. Kosloske AM, Jewell PF, Cartwright KC. Crucial bronchoscopic findings in esophageal atresia and tracheoesophageal fistula. J Pediatr Surg. 1988;23:466-70.

20. Shoshany G, Vatzian A, Ilivitzki A, Smolkin T, Hakim F, Makhoul IR. Near-missed upper tracheoesophageal fistula in esophageal atresia. Eur J Pediatr. 2009;168:1281-4.

21. Filston HC, Chitwood WR Jr, Schkolne B, Blackmon LR. The Fogarty balloon catheter as an aid to management of the infant with esophageal atresia and tracheoesophageal fistula complicated by severe RDS or pneumonia. J Pediatr Surg. 1982;17:149-51.

22. Bosenberg A, Flick RP. Regional anesthesia in neonates and infants. Clin Perinatol. 2013;40:525-38.

23. Chittmittrapap S, Spitz L, Kiely EM, Brereton RJ. Anastomotic leakage following surgery for esophageal atresia. J Pediatr Surg. 1992;27:29-32.

24. Chittmittrapap S, Spitz L, Kiely EM, Brereton RJ. Anastomotic stricture following repair of esophageal atresia. J Pediatr Surg. 1990;25:508-11.

25. Tsai JY, Berkery L, Wesson DE, Redo SF, Spigland NA. Esophageal atresia and tracheoesophageal fistula: surgical experience over two decades. Ann Thorac Surg. 1997;64:778-84.

26. Parker AF, Christie DL, Cahill JL. Incidence and significance of gastroesophageal reflux following repair of esophageal atresia and tracheoesophageal fistula and the need for anti-reflux procedures. J Pediatr Surg. 1979;14:5-8.

27. Kovesi T, Rubin S. Long-term complications of congenital esophageal atresia and/or tracheoesophageal fistula. Chest. 2004;126:915-25.

28. Liu LM, Pang LM. Neonatal surgical emergencies. Anesthesiol Clin North Am. 2001;19:265-86.

29. Rollins MD. Recent advances in the management of congenital diaphragmatic hernia. Curr Opin Pediatr. 2012;24:379-85.

30. Bösenberg AT, Brown RA. Management of congenital diaphragmatic hernia. Curr Opin Anaesthesiol. 2008;21:323-31.

31. Aspelund G, Fisher JC, Simpson LL, Stolar CJ. Prenatal lung-head ratio: threshold to predict outcome for congenital diaphragmatic hernia. J Matern Fetal Neonatal Med. 2012;25:1011-6.

32. Jani J, Nicolaides KH, Keller RL, Benachi A, Peralta CF, Favre R, et al. Observed to expected lung area to head circumference ratio in the prediction of survival in fetuses with isolated diaphragmatic hernia. Ultrasound Obstet Gynecol. 2007;30:67-71.

33. Lanzoni M, Morris J, Garne E, Loane M, Kinsner-Ovaskainen A. European Monitoring of Congenital Anomalies: JRC-EUROCAT Report on Statistical Monitoring of Congenital Anomalies (2006-2015). Luxembourg: Luxembourg Publications Office of the European Union; 2017.

34. Kotecha S, Barbato A, Bush A, Claus F, Davenport M, Delacourt C, et al. Congenital diaphragmatic hernia. Eur Respir J. 2012;39:820-9.

35. McHoney M. Congenital diaphragmatic hernia, management in the newborn. Pediatr Surg Int. 2015;31:1005-13.

36. Fox WW, Duara S. Persistent pulmonary hypertension in the neonate: diagnosis and management. J Pediatr. 1983;103:505-14.

37. Wung JT, James LS, Kilchevsky E, James E. Management of infants with severe respiratory failure and persistence of the fetal circulation, without hyperventilation. Pediatrics. 1985;76:488-94.

38. Brower RG, Matthay MA, Morris A, Schoenfeld D, Thompson BT, Wheeler A. Ventilation with lower tidal volumes as compared with traditional tidal volumes for acute lung injury and the acute respiratory distress syndrome. N Engl J Med. 2000;342:1301-8.

39. Boloker J, Bateman DA, Wung JT, Stolar CJ. Congenital diaphragmatic hernia in 120 infants treated consecutively with permissive hypercapnea/spontaneous respiration/elective repair. J Pediatr Surg. 2002;37:357-66.

40. Puligandla PS, Grabowski J, Austin M, Hedrick H, Renaud E, Arnold M, et al. Management of congenital diaphragmatic hernia: a systematic review from the APSA outcomes and evidence-based practice committee. J Pediatr Surg. 2015;50:1958-70.

41. van den Hout L, Tibboel D, Vijfhuize S, te Beest H, Hop W, Reiss I. The VICI-trial: high frequency oscillation versus conventional mechanical ventilation in newborns with congenital diaphragmatic hernia: an international multicentre randomized controlled trial. BMC Pediatr. 2011;11:98.

42. Shiyanagi S, Okazaki T, Shoji H, Shimizu T, Tanaka T, Takeda S, et al. Management of pulmonary hypertension in congenital diaphragmatic hernia: nitric oxide with prostaglandin-E1 versus nitric oxide alone. Pediatr Surg Int. 2008;24:1101-4.

43. Mugford M, Elbourne D, Field D. Extracorporeal membrane oxygenation for severe respiratory failure in newborn infants. Cochrane Database Syst Rev. 2008;CD001340.

44. Azarow K, Messineo A, Pearl R, Filler R, Barker G, Bohn D. Congenital diaphragmatic hernia—a tale of two cities: the Toronto experience. J Pediatr Surg. 1997;32:395-400.

45. Rankin J, Dillon E, Wright C. Congenital anterior abdominal wall defects in the north of England, 1986-1996: Occurrence and outcome. Prenat Diagn. 1999;19:662-8.

46. Hoyme HE, Higginbottom MC, Jones KL. The vascular pathogenesis of gastroschisis: intrauterine interruption of the omphalomesenteric artery. J Pediatr. 1981;98:228-31.

47. Brett CM, Davis PJ, Bikhazi G. Anesthesia for neonates and premature infants. In: Motoyama EK, Davis PJ (Eds). Smith's Anesthesia for Infants and Children, 7th edition. Philadelphia: Elsevier; 2005. pp. 521-70.

48. Adzick NS. Fetal myelomeningocele: natural history, pathophysiology, and in-utero intervention. Semin Fetal Neonatal Med. 2010;15:9-14.

49. McLone DG, Knepper PA. The cause of Chiari II malformation: a unified theory. Pediatr Neurosci. 1989;15:1-12.

50. de Buys Roessingh AS, Mueller C, Wiesenauer C, Bensoussan AL, Beaunoyer M. Anorectal malformation and Down's syndrome in monozygotic twins. J Pediatr Surg. 2009;44:e13-16.

51. Mirza B, Ijaz L, Saleem M, Sharif M, Sheikh A. Anorectal malformations in neonates. Afr J Paediatr Surg. 2011;8:151-4.

52. Pena A, Migotto-Krieger M, Levitt MA. Colostomy in anorectal malformations: a procedure with serious but preventable complications. J Pediatr Surg. 2006;41:748-56.

Perioperative Management of Pediatric Major Abdominal Cancer

Jeson Rajan Doctor, Nayana Amin

▮ INTRODUCTION

Children are a unique subset of patients. They have a different anatomy and physiology as compared to adults. In this chapter, we have emphasized the perioperative management of common abdominal cancer surgeries, namely neuroblastoma, Wilms' tumor, and hepatoblastoma, in their order of occurrence in children. Each of these surgeries has its unique set of challenges and management which is discussed in the subsequent text.

▮ NEUROBLASTOMA

Introduction and Background

Neuroblastoma is the most frequently diagnosed neoplasm in children.[1] It composes of 7–10% of childhood cancers.[2] The median age at diagnosis is 17 months to 2 years.[1-3] It arises anywhere within the sympathetic nervous system, infiltrates local structures, and surrounds nerves and vessels, e.g., celiac trunk. The site of origin could be adrenal and abdomen (65%), thoracic (20%), cervical (1–5%), and pelvic (2–3%) in decreasing order of frequency.[2] It may metastasize to bone marrow, liver, and regional lymph nodes.[4] Pulmonary and intracranial metastases are less common.

Neuroblastoma has unpredictable behaviors because it is associated with contrasting patterns from life-threatening progression or maturation to ganglioneuroma and even spontaneous regression (approximately 10%).[1] High-risk neuroblastoma continues to have poor long-term survival (<40%).

Symptomatology

The symptoms depend on the site of the mass, symptoms of catecholamine excess, and symptoms of paraneoplastic syndrome. Metastatic sites may present with symptoms of advanced disease.[5]

Symptoms Based on Anatomic Site

The most common presentation for an abdominal neuroblastoma is an abdominal mass.[5] It may just be an incidental finding "incidentaloma." Cervical neuroblastoma may present with Horner's syndrome—ptosis, miosis, and anhidrosis. Paravertebral neuroblastoma may present with cord compression and intraspinal extension and paralysis.

Symptoms Based on Catecholamine Excess

Hypertension, tachycardia, and palpitations are common symptoms of catecholamine-secreting tumors. The incidence of hypertension in neuroblastoma varies from 35 to 1–5%.[3] The child may also present with complications such as hypertensive encephalopathy, cardiogenic shock, coagulopathy, renal failure, and metabolic acidosis due to catecholamine excess. These children may be vasoconstricted with a decreased blood volume.[4]

Symptoms of Paraneoplastic Syndrome

The child may present with watery diarrhea because of VIPoma—vasoactive intestinal polypeptide (VIP) secretion by the tumor. He/she may also present with immune-mediated nystagmus or dancing eyes cerebellar opsoclonus–myoclonus syndrome (OMS) with cerebellar ataxia with or without rhythmic jerky movements of limbs.

Symptoms of Metastatic Disease

The child may be visibly unwell with poor nutrition, irritability, and failure to thrive. There may be bone pain due to marrow involvement. Metastasis to the orbit may present with periorbital ecchymosis (Raccoon eyes) and proptosis. There may be a sudden increase in the size of the mass with abdominal pain in case of bleeding and spontaneous hemorrhage into the tumor.[5]

Diagnostic Evaluation and Investigations Related to the Tumor

For Diagnosis

- Imaging-guided biopsy and histopathology
- Urinary increased catecholamines and vanillylmandelic acid (VMA) in cases of secretory tumors[5]
- Serum ferritin and lactate dehydrogenase (LDH) may be elevated.

For Staging of Disease

- Ultrasound, CT scan with 3-D CT reconstruction for resectability and spread
- Magnetic resonance imaging (MRI)—for intraspinal extension
- Metaiodobenzylguanidine (MIBG) scan —MIBG resembles norepinephrine and is selectively concentrated in the sympathetic nervous system
- Bone marrow aspiration and biopsy for detection of bone marrow metastasis from two separate sites with a total of four samples[5]
- X-ray and bone scan
- Routine blood investigations—complete blood count (CBC), renal function test (RFT), and liver function test (LFT) for general condition of the patient
- 2D ECHO—in secretory tumors, left ventricular (LV) hypertrophy may be present. It is recommended as baseline for patients receiving doxorubicin- and daunorubicin-based chemotherapy.

Treatment Modalities[5]

- *Surgery:* In low- and intermediate-risk groups, the goal of surgery is complete resection when possible. In high-risk groups and highly *infiltrative* tumors, the goal is gross total resection to decrease the tumor load.
- *Chemotherapy:* It consists of three phases: induction, consolidation, and maintenance. Combination chemotherapy with rapid COJEC regime is recommended for neuroblastoma. This includes therapy with cisplatin (C), vincristine (O), carboplatin (J), etoposide (E), and cyclophosphamide (C). The incidence of doxorubicin- and daunorubicin-induced myocardial dysfunction ranges from 2 to 32%.[3] Retinoids have also been found to have a promising role.
- *Radiotherapy:* The utility of radiotherapy is controversial in view of long-term side effects. When used in intraspinal tumors, it can cause vertebral damage, growth arrest, and scoliosis.
- *Immunotherapy:* Diganglioside is being tried.
- *Opsoclonus–myoclonus syndrome:* Adrenocorticotropic hormone (ACTH) and corticosteroids are known to be beneficial in paraneoplastic syndromes with OMS.

▌WILMS' TUMOR

Introduction and Background

Wilms' tumor or nephroblastoma was described by Max Wilms, a German anatomist and surgeon. It accounts for 6% of pediatric oncological diseases and is the most common renal neoplasm affecting children. Ninety percent of the cases occur before the age of 8 years with the mean age of presentation as 3.5 years. It has good prognosis if diagnosed in time with cure rates as high as 85–90%.[6] The incidence of intracaval extension is between 4 and 10% and that of intracardiac extension is about 1%.[7,8]

Wilms' tumor is sporadic in its incidence in a majority of cases. Familial incidence is less common (1.5%) due to mutations. It may occur as a part of genetic syndromes in 10% of cases.

Symptomatology

Majority of the cases present as an asymptomatic abdominal mass. It may be associated with abdominal pain, anorexia, nausea, and vomiting.[6] Hypertension may be an associated finding in 50–60% of cases with renin-secreting tumors causing LV hypertrophy and volume contraction.[6,9] Hematuria may be an associated finding in 30% of cases. Coagulopathy may be present in 10% of patients due to acquired Von Willebrand's disease. Apart from these, the child may have features of other syndromic associations. Bilateral disease may occur in 6% of children presenting with Wilms' tumor.[6]

Diagnostic Evaluation and Investigations Related to the Tumor

An ultrasound examination and a biopsy in the same sitting are essential for diagnosis of Wilms' tumor. A preoperative contrast-enhanced CT scan of the thorax, abdomen, and pelvis is helpful to delineate the extent of disease, local lymphatic spread, renal vein, and inferior vena cava (IVC) tumor thrombus, status of contralateral kidney for presence of bilateral disease, and liver and lung metastases. It also helps to differentiate it from an adrenal neuroblastoma which is its closest differential diagnosis.

Treatment Modalities

The treatment modalities for Wilms' tumor are surgery and chemotherapy.

- *Surgery:* It may be performed as an upfront treatment option (primary radical nephrectomy) or may be done following chemotherapy (delayed radical nephrectomy). Following chemotherapy, the common surgeries done are radical nephrectomy with cavotomy, bilateral partial

Table 1: Various chemotherapeutic drugs and their side effects of perioperative relevance.[6]

Chemotherapy drugs	Side effects of perioperative relevance
Vincristine	Peripheral neuropathy, syndrome of inappropriate antidiuretic hormone secretion (SIADH), convulsions
Actinomycin-D	Myelosuppression, severe diarrhea, fulminant hepatic failure and hepatic impairment
Doxorubicin	Cardiac dysfunction and decreased cardiac contractility in cumulative doses of 200 mg/m^2
Carboplatin	Myelosuppression, peripheral neuropathy, nephrotoxicity, hepatotoxicity
Etoposide	Anaphylaxis, myelosuppression
Cyclophosphamide	SIADH, myocardial necrosis, hemorrhagic cystitis, myelosuppression

nephrectomy, or nephron-sparing nephrectomy. The problems related to surgery and Wilms' tumor are discussed subsequently.

- *Chemotherapy:* The indications for starting chemotherapy prior to surgery are bilateral disease, unresectable tumors, and tumor thrombus in the IVC with or without intra-atrial extension. Chemotherapy is given for 6–8 weeks followed by reassessment for feasibility for surgical excision. Chemotherapy leads to a decrease in the size of the tumor increasing the chances of more complete surgical resections and surgical complications. Surgery, however, has to be done to remove the tumor; otherwise, there is a likelihood of an increase in the chemotherapy and radiotherapy-resistant tumor.

The commonly used drugs and their side effects are mentioned in **Table 1**.

HEPATOBLASTOMA

Introduction and Background

Hepatoblastoma is the third most common intra-abdominal malignancy in children after adrenal neuroblastoma and Wilms' tumor. It comprises only 1% of all pediatric malignancies, and approximately 70–80% of hepatic tumors are malignant.[10] The primary treatment modality is complete surgical resection. In unresectable tumors, pre-operative neoadjuvant chemotherapy (NACT) may make it resectable. In chemo-responsive but unresectable tumors, liver transplant may be an option.[11]

Improvements in the understanding of liver anatomy, patient selection, and also surgical and anesthetic techniques have contributed to a reduction in quoted perioperative mortality to around 3%.[12,13]

Symptomatology

The most common presenting symptom of hepatoblastoma is abdominal distention and a palpable abdominal mass.

Weight loss, anorexia, and fever are also commonly present. Less commonly, there may be obstructive symptoms such as ascites (secondary to occlusion of the portal or hepatic veins), gastrointestinal bleeding, or splenomegaly from portal hypertension, portal vein occlusion, and jaundice with scleral icterus and pruritus from obstruction of the biliary tree.

Diagnostic Evaluation and Investigations Related to the Tumor

Serum alpha-fetoprotein (AFP) is elevated in 60–70% of the cases of hepatoblastoma and is a reliable diagnostic and prognostic tumor marker. Liver enzymes and bilirubin are usually within normal limits. Abdominal ultrasound and CT scan (plain, contrast + spiral CT) of thorax and abdomen are useful for staging the disease (number of liver segments involved), assessing resectability (proximity to IVC, portal and hepatic veins), evaluating response to chemotherapy, calculation of future liver remnant (FLR) and CT volumetric assessment.[10,14-16] A CT scan of the thorax may also help in diagnosing pulmonary metastasis.

Treatment Modalities

The treatment modalities available for hepatoblastoma are surgery and chemotherapy.

- *Surgery:* This is the primary treatment modality for treatment of hepatoblastoma. It may be performed as an upfront treatment option or may be done following chemotherapy. The right lobe of the liver consists of segments 5, 6, 7, and 8 whereas the left lobe consists of segments 1, 2, 3, and 4.[17] The liver has an excellent capacity to regenerate following more aggressive resections. Up to 70–80% of the liver can therefore be resected safely.[10,18] Children specially have a residual liver which is normal (unlike adults in whom it may be cirrhotic) making extended resections possible without the chances of development of liver failure.
- *Chemotherapy:* NACT is often given with the aim of making unresectable or borderline tumors resectable. The chemotherapy given is PLADO which includes cisplatin and Adriamycin or SuperPLADO which includes alternating dose of cisplatin with a combination of carboplatin and Adriamycin.[19] Other regimes with Vincristine (VCR), 5-fluorouracil (5-FU), and cisplatin combinations may be given in patients with cardiac dysfunction who cannot be given Adriamycin-based chemotherapy.
- *Other modalities:* Like transarterial chemoembolization (TACE), transarterial radioembolization (TARE) has been used to decrease the size of the tumor by giving higher doses of chemotherapy or radioactive particles with

lower systemic effects.[10] Portal vein embolization (PVE) is helpful in allowing preferential hypertrophy of the normal liver, thereby increasing the FLR. These strategies have been applied mainly in patients with a nonresectable, advanced tumor load and a liver remnant that was predicted to be too small for resection.[13] Other modalities such as radiofrequency ablation and cryoablation are useful in adults where the residual liver is diseased, but their role in children has not been documented.

Perioperative Optimization and Management

Preoperative Evaluation

History and examination of any child with intra-abdominal tumors will essentially be the same.

History: The routine preoperative evaluation with regards to history, birth history, immunizations, upper respiratory tract infection symptoms, any medications, allergies, etc., should be elicited. Symptoms for catecholamine-secreting tumors should be inquired in children diagnosed with neuroblastoma or suprarenal masses.

Examination: Special attention should be paid to the general condition and nutritional status of a child with intra-abdominal tumors. Chest condition should be assessed in children with large tumors causing abdominal distension. Chemotherapy-induced side effects with relevance to the perioperative period should be checked and documented (**Table 1**). Look for syndromic features such as macroglossia and hypotonia. Venous cannulation may be difficult, especially in children who have received chemotherapy. Blood pressure charting should be done for children with an age- and weight-appropriate cuff. About 50–60% of the children with Wilms' tumor may be hypertensive. Antihypertensive medications should be started and blood pressure should be optimized according to the child's age. The cardiovascular system should also be examined for the presence of murmurs, failure, gallops, etc. Other signs of paraneoplastic syndromes such as OMS and Horner's syndrome are discussed earlier, and pressure effects of the tumor on the surrounding structures should also be checked.

Investigations:

- *CBC:* Hemoglobin may be low in cases of nutritional deficiency or hematuria. Patients may be neutropenic if they have received chemotherapy.
- *Renal function test:* Serum creatinine and electrolytes should be checked. In children with Wilms' tumor, estimation of glomerular filtration rate (GFR) of the remaining/other kidney may also be required.

- *Liver function test:* In case of patients receiving hepatotoxic drugs for chemotherapy, the liver function should be assessed. It also indicates the function of the remaining normal liver and serves as a baseline. Serum bilirubin and liver enzymes are usually normal in cases of hepatoblastoma. The Child Pugh and other scoring systems may be used to assess the risk status of the patient but are more useful in adults than children.[12]
- *Coagulation profile:* It is useful for baseline synthetic function and to rule out underlying coagulopathy prior to major surgery. It may also be needed in cases of associated acquired von Willebrand disease.
- *2D ECHO:* It is recommended in hypertensive patients on treatment, catecholamine-secreting tumors, syndromic children, poor nutritional status, huge abdominal masses, patients who have received doxorubicin, or patients with an IVC tumor thrombus to check for its extension into the right atrium. It is preferable to have a baseline ECHO in all infants with intra-abdominal tumors and in all patients undergoing major liver resections.
- Imaging done for evaluation of tumor should be checked for the size and extent of resections. The IVC, liver, and lungs may also be seen in the imaging to check for metastasis. It is important to rule out intraspinal extensions in children with neuroblastoma. The FLR and CT volumetric analysis should also be checked in children coming for liver resections.

Intraoperative Management and Anesthetic Concerns

Anesthesia Management

The child should be premedicated to avoid parental separation anxiety. Alternatively, parental presence during inhalational induction with sevoflurane is a popular technique. Problems specific to pediatric anesthesia are beyond the scope of this chapter. Adequate preoxygenation in propped-up position will help in prolonging the apnea time during endotracheal intubation in children with large intra-abdominal tumors. Intubation with pediatric microcuffed endotracheal tubes with controlled ventilation is recommended. Care should be taken that the cuff of the endotracheal tube is just beyond the vocal cords so as to avoid inadvertent endobronchial migration of the tube during upper abdominal retraction. Two wide-bore intravenous (IV) access should be secured in all cases where major blood is anticipated.

Secreting tumors and hypertensive children may be volume contracted and may have hypotension following induction of general anesthesia. Intraoperative monitoring should be done with ECG, capnography, pulse oximetry, and blood pressure and hourly urine output. Temperature and blood sugars should also be monitored. Invasive arterial blood pressure monitoring and central venous pressure (CVP) monitoring may be recommended for large tumors, major anticipated blood loss, cardiac dysfunction, fluid shifts due to extensive lymph node clearance, and inferior vena cavotomy for tumor thrombus excision. In children undergoing surgery for neuroblastoma excision, invasive arterial blood pressure monitoring should always be done in view of the hemodynamic changes that may occur due to extensive resections and catecholamine release due to tumor handling. Intraoperative monitoring of arterial blood gases is also recommended. Capillary refill time can be used to assess the tissue perfusion.

The position is usually supine for abdominal tumors with midline or transverse incisions depending on the location and extent of the mass. Thoracic epidural analgesia at the T6-T9 level is recommended after discussing the extent of surgical incision, provided there is no metastatic involvement of the spine and no intraspinal extension of the mass.[20] The risk–benefit ratio of epidural is to be assessed with coagulopathy, hypotension, and bleeding. Intraoperative analgesia is managed with IV fentanyl and epidural bolus and infusion of levobupivacaine taking care not to exceed the toxic dose. Anesthesia is maintained with oxygen and nitrous oxide (N_2O) (50:50) with low flows and an inhalational agent with closed circuit on controlled ventilation and a muscle relaxant. During liver resections, N_2O should be avoided keeping in mind a theoretical risk of venous air embolism and bowel distention.

Fluid therapy: A balanced crystalloid such as Ringers lactate with or without dextrose (1–2%) should be used as maintenance fluid depending on the blood sugars. 4% or 5% albumin may be tried in cases due to extensive dissection and retroperitoneal handling for maintaining the intravascular volume and oncotic pressure. Blood loss should be assessed and replaced with packed cells, fresh frozen plasma, cryoprecipitate, and platelets.

Intraoperative Goals and Monitoring
- Adequate hydration and maintenance of intravascular volume
- Maintaining hemodynamics to minimize blood loss. Avoid hypotension and maintain blood volume and mean arterial pressure to avoid ischemic injury to residual normal liver and kidney. Monitoring of CVP during liver resections is currently debatable and not recommended by a number of clinicians.[21,22] A low CVP during liver surgery is associated with a reduction in estimated blood loss; however, it does not translate into an improvement in postoperative morbidity.[22]
- Correction of blood loss and coagulopathy with blood and blood products

- Hourly urine output monitoring and maintaining urine output of 0.5–1 mL/kg
- Blood glucose monitoring and maintaining normoglycemia
- *Thermoregulation:* Maintenance of normothermia is essential with the use of forced air warmers with blankets and fluid warmers.
- *Analgesia:* Opioids and epidural analgesia with local anesthetics may be used intraoperatively. The risk–benefit ratio of paracetamol (PCM) and nonsteroidal anti-inflammatory drugs (NSAIDs) should be weighted. NSAIDs should be avoided in children undergoing nephrectomy, massive blood loss, or if there is hypotension not responding to fluids. Following major hepatectomies, PCM is contraindicated if there is major blood loss or poor residual liver function.

Intraoperative Problems and Management During Neuroblastoma Resection

- Neuroblastomas are known to invade the tunica adventitia of large blood vessels so dissection should be meticulous and care is to be taken to avert major disasters and blood loss.[23] There can be a sudden and torrential blood loss due to injury to a major vessel during dissection.
- Extensive retroperitoneal dissection can cause major fluid shifts requiring adequate replacement of the intravascular compartment.
- Handling of tumor can cause surges in blood pressure if the tumor is a secretory tumor. The incidence of this is rare, <3%.[3,24] Managing the hemodynamics may be challenging and may require the use of vasopressors after resection of the tumor.
- Patients with adrenalectomies may need steroid supplementation, but this needs to be individualized after discussion with an endocrinologist.
- Watch for intraoperative hyperthermia.

Intraoperative Problems and Management During Excision of Renal Tumors

- *Extensive transabdominal retroperitoneal dissection:* Maintain intravascular blood volume, replace blood loss, and maintain fluid and glucose balance.
- *Low intraoperative urinary output:* Rule out all the causes including mechanical and surgical causes.
- IVC compression during retroperitoneal dissection may decrease the preload to the heart and cause hypotension.
- *IVC cavotomy with supra- or infrahepatic cross-clamping for excision of tumor thrombus:* This may cause hypotension due to a decrease in the preload to the heart, hepatic and intestinal congestion, tumor

embolization, and sudden torrential blood loss during dissection. In large thrombi extending up to the right atrium, cardiopulmonary bypass may be needed for removal of the tumor thrombus.[8]

- *Paraneoplastic phenomenon:* In cases of hypertensive patients, maintaining intraoperative blood pressure to preoperative values is recommended. Acquired coagulopathy with massive blood loss may warrant aggressive correction of coagulopathy.
- *Nephron-sparing nephrectomy or partial nephrectomy:* In cases of bilateral Wilms' tumor, blood loss should be replaced as these surgeries are known to have blood loss.
- *Avoidance of capsular rupture and tumor spillage:* This is known to increase the likelihood of recurrence.
- *Increased intra-abdominal pressure and ventilation problems:* Huge tumors may cause compromised ventilation with high peak pressures. They usually resolve after removal of the mass.

Intraoperative Problems and Management During Hepatectomies

The goals of surgery are to achieve:
- Adequate oncological clearance
- Preservation of enough healthy liver to avoid liver failure and allow regeneration
- Minimize blood loss

A right hepatectomy is more challenging than a left hepatectomy.

The changes in intraoperative hemodynamics at various time points during the surgery are as follows:
- Inflow control with hepatic pedicle which may be complete or partial (selective). It reduces bleeding but decreases cardiac output (CO) due to a decrease in the preload and increase in systemic vascular resistance (SVR).[12]
- Total vascular occlusion includes clamping of portal vessels with supra- and intrahepatic IVC occlusion. This results in approximately 40–60% reduction in venous return and CO (due to a decrease in preload to the heart) and the SVR increases by 80%. It is associated with an increase in heart rate by 50%.[12]
- The liver can tolerate up to 60 minutes of continuous occlusion and 120 minutes of intermittent occlusion.[18,25]
- The fall in preload can be minimized by adequately correcting volume deficit and aiming for a higher CVP (approximately 14 cm of H_2O).
- Handling and mobilization of the liver may lead to tenting or kinking of the IVC and may also lead to hypotension and tachycardia secondary to a drop in the cardiac preload.

- Vasoactive agents and vasopressors may be used if necessary.
- A test clamp prior to formally applying clamps is essential to identify whether the patient will tolerate the procedure of clamping and resection.[18] Intermittent clamping is better than continuous clamping.
- If the child is intolerant to test clamping and develops severe hypotension, a venovenous bypass may be necessary to bypass the liver and maintain the cardiac preload.
- Renal injury may be a concern, so maintenance of mean arterial pressure and intravascular volume is essential.
- Blood loss may be minimized by adequate inflow and outflow control. In addition, newer equipment such as ultrasonic cutting and coagulation [CUSA (Cavitron ultrasonic surgical aspirator)], Ligasure™, harmonic scalpel, endoscopic staplers, and pressurized water jets may be used.
- The use of intraoperative cell salvage in malignancy is contraindicated for the fear for transfusing malignant cells back into the circulation. Aprotinin and tranexamic acid may be tried in reducing blood loss.

Intraoperative Complications

- *Massive blood loss and coagulopathy:* This should be managed with blood and blood products. A thromboelastography (TEG) may be helpful in identifying the cause for coagulopathy and correcting the same.
- *Air embolism:* Transesophageal echo (TEE) and esophageal Doppler are useful in diagnosis apart from a drop in end-tidal CO_2 ($ETCO_2$). N_2O should be avoided. This may be a complication of right hepatectomy with IVC cavotomy.
- Damage to portal vein, hepatic artery, and hepatic duct during the surgical dissection.

Patients should be extubated only after they are hemodynamically stable, normothermic, and the gas exchange parameters and investigations are normalized.

Postoperative Intensive Care Management

Postoperative Problems and Concerns Following Neuroblastoma Resection

Major blood loss may lead to hypotension,[24] coagulopathy, acute renal failure (ARF), and ischemic bowel and must be addressed in an intensive care setting.[23]

Management of intravascular fluid status, vasopressors, and hemodynamics is important for the first 24–48 hours as some of them are known to have a turbulent perioperative course.

*Postoperative Problems and Concerns Following Wilms'
Tumor Excision*

- Major blood loss, hemodynamic instability, and
  coagulopathy
- Hypothermia and requirement for postoperative
  ventilation
- Decreased urine output, renal failure, and requirement
  of dialysis including becoming dialysis-dependent
- Hyperkalemia
- Tumor thrombus with embolization into the pulmonary
  circulation and pulmonary embolism
- *Hypertension*: Renin levels may fall post resection
  in renin-secreting tumors, but blood pressure may
  take a month to normalize. Antihypertensives can be
  discontinued after 1–3 weeks' postsurgery.
- Postoperative analgesia should be continued with
  epidural analgesia.[6]

*Postoperative Problems and Concerns Following
Liver Resections*

Postoperatively: Monitor coagulation parameters, TEG,
hemodynamics, urine output (renal function), sugars, and
liver profile (to rule out liver failure).

Postoperative problems:[12]

- *Postoperative liver dysfunction and liver failure:* It
  starts approximately 72 hours after surgery. The
  predisposing factors are previously diseased liver,
  low volume liver remnant, liver ischemia, massive
  blood loss, and reperfusion injury due to free radicals.
  The proposed methods to avoid this are ischemic
  preconditioning, infusion of NAC intraoperatively
  and postoperatively, avoiding hypotension, careful
  case selection, and minimizing blood loss. The patient
  may present with encephalopathy, deteriorating liver
  function, and persistent increase of liver enzymes. The
  goals of treatment are management of hypoglycemia,
  management of salt and water retention (due to secondary
  hyperaldosteronism) along with therapies such as
  proton-pump inhibitors, enteral feeding, lactulose,
  NAC infusion, and correction of dyselectrolytemia and
  coagulation abnormality.
- *Bleeding and coagulation abnormalities:* There may
  be a cause for concern while considering removal of
  the epidural catheter on post-operative days 4–5 if the
  international normalized ratio (INR) is >1.4.[18]
- Renal dysfunction
- Sepsis and infections—adequate coverage with
  antibiotics is essential.
- Respiratory failure

REFERENCES

1. Mullassery D, Losty PD. Neuroblastoma. Paediatrics Child Health. 2016;26(2):68-72.
2. Brouwers FM, Eisenhofer G, Lenders JW, Pacak K. Emergencies caused by pheochromocytoma, neuroblastoma, or ganglioneuroma. Endocrinol Metab Clin North Am. 2006;35(4):699-724.
3. Kain ZN, Shamberger RS, Holzman RS. Anesthetic management of children with neuroblastoma. J Clin Anesth. 1993;5(6): 486-91.
4. Farman JV. Neuroblastomas and anaesthesia. Br J Anaesth. 1965;37:866-70.
5. Shohet JM, Nuchtern JG. Clinical presentation, diagnosis, and staging evaluation of neuroblastoma. [online] Available from https://www.uptodate.com/contents/clinical-presentation-diagnosis-and-staging-evaluation-of-neuroblastoma. [Last accessed February, 2020].
6. Whyte SD, Mark Ansermino J. Anesthetic considerations in the management of Wilms' tumor. Paediatr Anaesth. 2006;16(5):504-13.
7. Abraham M, Samuel M, Mathew M. Wilms tumour with intracardiac extension—multimodal approach to a challenging case. Indian J Anaesth. 2016;60(3):216-8.
8. Abdullah Y, Karpelowsky J, Davidson A, Thomas J, Brooks A, Hewitson J, et al. Management of nine cases of Wilms' tumour with intracardiac extension—A single centre experience. J Pediatr Surg. 2013;48(2):394-9.
9. Charlton GA, Sedgwick J, Sutton DN. Anaesthetic management of renin secreting nephroblastoma. Br J Anaesth. 1992;69(2): 206-9.
10. Herzog CE, Andrassy RJ, Eftekhari F. Childhood cancers: Hepatoblastoma. Oncologist. 2000;5(6):445-53.
11. Towu E, Kiely E, Pierro A, Spitz L. Outcome and complications after resection of hepatoblastoma. J Pediatr Surg. 2004;39(2):199-202.
12. Hartog A, Mills G. Anaesthesia for hepatic resection surgery. Contin Educ Anaesth Crit Care Pain. 2009;9(1):1-5.
13. Clavien PA, Petrowsky H, DeOliveira ML, Graf R. Strategies for safer liver surgery and partial liver transplantation. N Engl J Med. 2007;356(15):1545-59.
14. Shoup M, Gonen M, D'Angelica M, Jarnagin WR, DeMatteo RP, Schwartz LH, et al. Volumetric analysis predicts hepatic dysfunction in patients undergoing major liver resection. J Gastrointest Surg. 2003;7(3):325-30.
15. Vauthey JN, Chaoui A, Do KA, Bilimoria MM, Fenstermacher MJ, Charnsangavej C, et al. Standardized measurement of the future liver remnant prior to extended liver resection: Methodology and clinical associations. Surgery. 2000;127(5):512-9.
16. Shirabe K, Shimada M, Gion T, Hasegawa H, Takenaka K, Utsunomiya T, et al. Postoperative liver failure after major hepatic resection for hepatocellular carcinoma in the modern era with special reference to remnant liver volume. J Am Coll Surg. 1999;188(3):304-9.
17. Belgihiti J, Clavien PA, Gadzijev E, Garden JO, Lau WY, Makuuchi M, et al. The Brisbane 2000 terminology of liver anatomy and resections. HPB. 2000;2(3):333-9.

18. Loveland JA, Krog F, Beale P. A review of paediatric liver resections in Johannesburg: experiences and preferred technique. S Afr Med J. 2012;102(11 Pt 2):881-3.

19. Manuprasad A, Radhakrishnan V, Sunil BJ, Ramakrishnan AS, Ganesan TS, Ganesan P, et al. Hepatoblastoma: 16-years' experience from a tertiary cancer centre in India. J Pediatr Hematol Oncol. 2018;3(1):13-6.

20. Tzimas P, Prout J, Papadopoulos G, Mallett SV. Epidural anaesthesia and analgesia for liver resection. Anaesthesia. 2013;68(6):628-35.

21. Lentschener C, Ozier Y. Anaesthesia for elective liver resection: Some points should be revisited. Eur J Anaesthesiol. 2002;19(11):780-8.

22. Hughes MJ, Ventham NT, Harrison EM, Wigmore SJ. Central venous pressure and liver resection: A systematic review and meta-analysis. HPB (Oxford). 2015;17(10):863-71.

23. Joyner BD, Kopell BH. Neuroblastoma treatment and management. [online] Available from https://emedicine.medscape.com/article/439263-treatment. [Last accessed March, 2020].

24. Haberkern CM, Coles PG, Morray JP, Kennard SC, Sawin RS. Intraoperative hypertension during surgical excision of neuroblastoma. Case report and review of 20 years' experience. Anesth Analg. 1992;75(5):854-8.

25. Mogane P, Motshabi-Chakane P. Anaesthetic considerations for liver resections in paediatric patients. South Afr J Anaesth Analg. 2013;19(6):290-4.

Neonatal Postoperative Critical Care

Swetha RD

INTRODUCTION

A surgical neonate is defined as a neonate who is either:

- Born at >37 weeks of gestation (term neonate) and is <29 days at the day of surgery or
- Born at <37 weeks of gestation (preterm neonate) and is <50 full weeks postconception at the time of operation.[1]

Care of a surgical neonate starts with a comprehensive care from womb. A detailed history and physical examination in collaboration with investigations predict the postoperative outcome. It is important to support the neonate well to tolerate the impact of surgery with respect to multiple parameters like ventilation, hydration, nutrition, metabolic, and blood parameters, and also address other associated comorbid conditions to improve outcome.

Intensive care in surgical neonate supports potentially failing or failed systems to address the acute problem by some form of surgery. The delivery of this care varies between centers intra- and interstates. The care involves support for immature organ system and to attain adequate nutrition for a good neurodevelopmental outcome.

MANAGEMENT OF POSTOPERATIVE NEONATE

It starts with the coordination triad **(Fig. 1)**. All surgical neonates should be given the right to be transferred in utero to a tertiary center with the facilities available for surgical and intensive care. There is a need for the well coordination between the surgeon and the neonatology team for the perioperative care with a family-centered approach. An empathetic approach with detailed information to patients' family about multiple stages the neonate progresses helps in early preparedness for postoperative care.[2]

Temperature Stability

Frequent handling of babies, invasive and noninvasive procedures, transportation, operation theater temperatures,

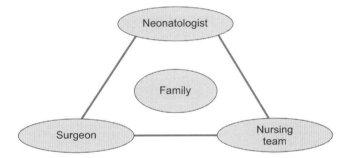

Fig. 1: Family centric approach to neonate in perioperative period

painting with cold solutions like betadine or chlorhexidine, and many other factors lead to hypothermia and associated complications. These can be minimized by:

- In utero transfer to tertiary center
- Preheated transport incubators or polythene sheets for inter- and intrahospital transports
- Optimizing theater temperature with heaters, use of Bair Hugger therapy
- Bedside neonatal intensive care unit (NICU) surgery model[3]
- Prewarmed intravenous fluids, intraoperative wash, and surgical mops

Airway Stability and Ideal Neonate Positioning

- Many postoperative babies need a specific neck position for care [example: neck flexion in tracheoesophageal fistula (TEF) to avoid tension at anastomotic site].
- Some studies preferred prone nursing in ventilated neonates, though clear evidence is lacking. Head raise allow expansion of lungs but may cause pooling of basal secretions.
- Preterm baby's head should lie in midline position to prevent the head position on jugular venous drainage at

least the first 3 days to decrease risk of germinal matrix hemorrhage.[4]

- Surgical neonates have increased gastric reflux and are multifactorial. This delays establishment of enteral feeds and is at risk of respiratory complications. Body positioning can be considered an effective nonpharmacological strategy for both acid and nonacid gastroesophageal reflux. Prone and left lateral positions are effective, whereas supine and right lateral positioning seem to play a worsening effect.[5]

The ideal body position in neonate should be to optimize diaphragmatic and lung functions without complicating surgical issues.

Ventilation

Noninvasive ventilation is the preferred mode in neonates. However, most surgical neonates need invasive ventilation due to various reasons like:

- Multiple system involvement
- Abdominal defects
- Associated cardiac anomalies
- Thoracic surgeries
- Analgesia/sedation [functional residual capacity (FRC) may be reduced with anesthesia. Abdominal distention leads to distress]
- Few mandatory ventilatory situations like postoperative paralysis in TEF to avoid tension at anastomotic site, higher analgesia causing respiratory depression.[6]

Neonates may have hyperventilation, hypoventilation, or periodic breathing as a response to pain, gastric reflux, sepsis, secretions, and aspiration pneumonia or as a part of primary etiology. They should be optimally supported to prevent under- and overventilation. Invasive ventilation when necessary is done with low-tidal volumes, relatively high positive end-expiratory pressure (PEEP) and low peak inspiratory pressure (PIP). The use of optimal PEEP prevents atelectasis. Most lungs have regions of atelectasis with overlapping normal lung regions causing an inhomogeneity. Hence, low pressures may cause more alveoli to collapse and high pressures may cause overdistention of normal regions. Hence, no strategy is ideal for any condition, as ventilation is controlled by variable factors.

Choice of ventilator mode depends on equipment availability, patient condition, and physician comfort, as there is no single ideal mode of ventilation. Volume-controlled and volume guarantee modes offer greater advantage. Patient-triggered modes like synchronized intermittent mandatory ventilation (SIMV), assist/control ventilation/synchronized intermittent positive pressure ventilation (AC/SIPPV), and pressure support ventilation (PSV) are associated with decreased air leaks and decreased duration of ventilation.

General guidelines for adequate ventilation while minimizing complications are:[7]

- *Minimize ventilation duration*
- *Lowest inspiratory oxygen concentration (FiO₂)* to minimize oxygen toxicity, to start with 30–50% and increase further to reach target saturations. The target saturation for NICU is currently 91–95% in the preductal region.[8] High FiO_2 of 90–100% may be needed in cardiac anomalies and in conditions like persistent pulmonary hypertension of newborn (PPHN), congenital diaphragmatic hernia (CDH), large congenital lobar emphysema, and thymic cyst.
- *Maintain some spontaneous respiratory efforts*—to prevent disuse atrophy of respiratory muscles while synchronizing with ventilator.
- *Permissive hypercapnia*: Permissive hypercapnia (PHC) or controlled ventilation is a strategy that minimizes baro-/volutrauma by allowing relatively high levels of arterial CO_2 (55–65 mm Hg), provided the arterial pH does not fall below a preset minimal value (7.2). Though practiced in many units to minimize lung damage by avoiding high ventilation settings, PHC by itself may cause chronic lung disease and unintended neurologic consequences. Hence, further studies are needed for appropriate levels of acceptance of PCO_2.[9,10]
- *Low-tidal volumes ventilation*: 4–6 mL/kg with upper limit of 8 mL/kg. Higher tidal volumes >8 mL may cause volutrauma and low ≤3 mL cause atelectrauma.
- *Peak inspiratory pressure*: Start with 12–16 cm H_2O and increase to 20–25 cm H_2O based on lung compliance. Ideally, PIP should be just enough to chest rise, audible breath sounds, and adequate tidal volume delivery. PIP depends on age, size, and condition of infant.
- *Peak end-expiratory pressure*: Maintain FRC and oxygen adequacy by optimizing mean arterial pressure (MAP). Start with 5–6 cm H_2O. Increase PEEP, if FiO_2 >40%, to open up atelectatic lung.

In surgical neonate, systemic inflammatory response system (SIRS) and abdominal distention may cause collapse and needs higher PEEP. Inadvertent higher PEEP leads to overdistention, hypercarbia, air leaks, decreases venous return, and compromises perfusion.

- *Inspiratory time (Ti) (0.3–0.5 second)*: A Ti as long as 3–5 time constants (a measure of how rapidly gas can get in and out of the lungs) allows relatively complete inspiration. Selection of Ti should reflect the infant's time constants. Small preterm infants have very short time constants and should be ventilated with Ti of 0.35 second or less. Larger infants or those with increased airway resistance have longer time constants and require longer Ti up to 0.5 second.[11]

- Hence, poor compliance conditions need shorter constants 0.25–0.35. Example is hyaline membrane disease (mostly a preterm condition).
- Higher airway resistance conditions need longer constants 0.4–0.5 second. Examples are bronchopulmonary dysplasia, meconium aspiration syndrome, pulmonary hypoplasia in CDH, and aspiration pneumonia in TEF (mostly term baby issues).
- *Respiratory rate*—as physiological as possible to avoid asynchrony and respiratory alkalosis. Start at 40–60 breaths per minute. Set higher rates in conditions with shorter time constants, lower rates in longer constants.
- *Appropriate humidification*—to maintain mucociliary clearance, secretion liquefaction, reduce tube occlusion, to avoid increase in dead space or breathing resistance

Parameters to be monitored clinically are:

- Patient comfort and synchrony—change the mode and settings accordingly
- Perfusion, heart rate, color, and heart sounds—high PEEP decreases venous return hence reduces pressures. Muffled heart sounds indicate air leaks and warrant insertion of drain.
- Chest rise, retractions, increased work of breathing, and lower saturations indicate hypoventilation. Optimize the ventilator settings.

Circulation

Neonatal circulation has an unique physiology of evolving from fetal circulation after birth. The physiology gets more complex, dynamic, and diverse with an underlying disease. *Several factors contribute to this imbalance:*

- Limited sympathetic innervation in preterm myocardium
- Myocardium functioning near limits of physiological capacity
- Variable sensitivity of catecholamine receptors with gestation (α- > β-receptors in early gestation)

Assessment of Cardiovascular Stability

End organ function is the key factor for assessment of cardiovascular stability. Blood pressure, though most commonly used surrogate, is unreliable in situations like extreme prematurity.

Hence, a concurrent assessment of other clinical indicators is needed like:

- *Heart rate*: Tachycardia manifests with fever, pain, sepsis, medications like caffeine and it exaggerates myocardial depression. Hence, the source of tachycardia has to be addressed early with close monitoring.[6]
- *Hypotension*: Systolic hypotension mostly indicates decreased cardiac output and diastolic hypotension

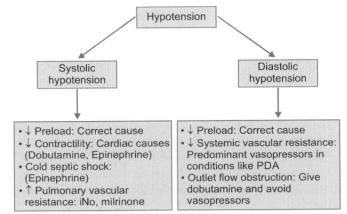

Fig. 2: Postoperative hypotension in neonates: type, pathophysiology and management

indicates decreased preload or increased systemic vascular resistance.

Conditions with decreased preload are blood loss, 3rd space leaks, aspirates and drains, abdominal wall defects, sepsis, increased mean airway pressure, air leaks, and dropping venous return. Cardiac contractility is mostly affected secondary to anesthesia, SIRS, or sedation. Inotropes improve contractility but may compromise on splanchnic blood flow.

- Patient color, capillary refill time, and pulse volume
- *End-organ perfusion*: Urine output, poor activity (level of consciousness), metabolic acidosis, and increased lactate

Management Stratergies[12]

- Preventable strategies like sedation for pain, permissive hypercapnia, and reduced MAP minimize medications with adverse effects like caffeine and narcotics
- Vasoactive medications are mainly categorized into three groups:
  1. *Vasopressors activity*—dopamine, norepinephrine, vasopressin, terlipressin, and methylene blue
  2. *Inotropic activity*—dobutamine, milrinone, and levosimendan
  3. *Others*—epinephrine (has mixed actions), hydrocortisone, and dopexamine

Choice of ionotropes has been discussed in **Figure 2**.

Fluid Management and Renal Support

Neonates are vulnerable for both dehydration and overload as concentrating and diuretic phases need maturation. Minimizing the fluid and electrolyte imbalance with close monitoring of electrolytes and sugars preoperatively is the key factor to reduce postoperative complications. Neonates are also susceptible for syndrome of inappropriate antidiuretic hormone secretion (SIADH) and fluid restriction may be needed.

- Glucose infusion rate of 4–6 µg/kg/min should be maintained to prevent hypoglycemia and protein breakdown. Glucose rate may be increased based on increased demand like intrauterine growth retardation (IUGR), sepsis, and others to avoid hypoglycemic episodes. Avoid high-glucose concentration fluids and boluses to prevent rebound hypoglycemia.
- Fluid requirements are balanced based on weight, electrolytes, clinical condition (patent ductus arteriosus, bronchopulmonary dysplasia, and abdominal wall defects), input output charts and weight check. Ensure adequate intravascular volume for renal perfusion.
- *Electrolytes correction*: Neonates are susceptible to electrolyte imbalances due to variable pathology over the maturing physiology.
  - Hyponatremia may be due to excess loss in preterms, abdominal wall defects, drainage tubes, ileus, third space leaks in necrotizing enterocolitis (NEC), secondary to SIADH (dilutional), medications and others. Hypernatremia may be due to excessive fluid restriction, increased sodium supplementation, medications like bicarbonate, aminoglycosides, decreased production of antidiuretic hormone and others. Hence, fluid management with maintenance of sodium (start with 2–3 mEq/kg/day) and treating of the underlying pathology is essential.
  - Hypokalemia is one the most common treatable causes of ileus. Normal maintenance of daily potassium is 1–2 mEq/kg/day and should be optimized to prevent feed intolerance.
  - Preterm babies born to diabetic mothers and IUGR babies may need calcium maintenance as well.
- *Blood gas analysis*: Periodic blood gas analysis is an essential monitoring key in a sick neonate.
  - Arterial is preferred over venous gas (as venous indicates local perfusion and is also altered by various factors). It is ideal to secure an arterial line for blood pressure monitoring and frequent sampling in any surgical neonate.
  - Blood gas is used to monitor the increasing metabolic acidosis (in sepsis, decreased perfusion, anemia, blood loss) and guides for treating the underlying cause and supporting with inotropes.
  - Blood gas also shows the ventilation and oxygenation status of a ventilated neonate and guides for further modifications on ventilation strategies.

Hematological Support

- Most babies are anemic due to:
  - Decreased erythropoiesis (prematurity, SIRS, and drugs like antibiotics leading to myelosuppression) or

Table 1: Packed red blood cell transfusion guidelines in <32 weeks' preterm neonates.

Postnatal age	Hemoglobin threshold in ventilated patients	Hemoglobin threshold in patient on oxygen support	Hemoglobin threshold in patient without oxygen support
1st day	<12	<12	<10
2–7 days	<12	<10	<10
8-14 days	<10	<9.5	<7.5–8.5
≥15 days	<10	<8.5	<7.5

Table 2: Packed red blood cell transfusion guidelines in term babies.

Condition	Hemoglobin
Severe pulmonary disease	<12
Moderate pulmonary disease	<10
Severe cardiac disease	<12
Major surgery	<10
Asymptomatic anemia	<7

Moderate and severe pulmonary disease is based on collaborative information of neonate clinical and comorbid conditions.

  - Increased loss (blood loss and frequent sampling)
  - Leukodepleted irradiated packed red blood cells (PRBCs) are preferred to correct anemia **(Tables 1 and 2)**.
- Coagulation profile may be impaired in surgical neonates due to SIRS, drugs, and altered gut flora and needs correction with vitamin K and fresh frozen plasma.

Asepsis

Most surgical neonates are aseptic to begin with. With repeated medical procedures, the risk of sepsis is increased. Sepsis is one of the most common postsurgical complications in a surgical neonate.

The all or none approach is essential to prevent nosocomial infections. For example, a procedure with strict aseptic steps but improper maintenance results in infection. Hence, the concept of bundles—a set of evidence-based processes to be implemented.[13]

World Health Organization (WHO) recommends the Aseptic Non-Touch Technique (ANTT) practices.

- To identify the key part (equipment part that must be sterile) and key site (that patient area to be protected from microorganisms)
- Use standard cleaning techniques for procedures:
  CDC (Center for Disease Control and Prevention) and United Kingdom have guidelines for skin preparation before cannulation and central lines for adults and children over 2 months of age with chlorhexidine

gluconate 2% in 70% isopropyl alcohol. However, there are no specific guidelines for infants <2 months.[14,15] There are no specific guidelines for an ideal antiseptic in NICU.[16]

Practices in few units are:

- **>27 weeks**: Use 1% chlorhexidine solution. Allow to dry for 30 seconds. Wash off excess solution after the procedure with sterile water or saline to prevent chemical burns. Some studies have shown the topical application of chlorhexidine and its systemic absorption in neonates though clinical significance is not clear. Few in vitro studies have shown its genotoxic and cytotoxic on human lymphocytes.
- **≤27 weeks**: Use povidone–iodine 10% solution. Allow to dry for 1 minute then wash off all solution with sterile water or saline before the procedure. Wash excess povidone–iodine, as iodine can be absorbed through their immature nonkeratinized skin.[17]
- *Routine environmental cleaning*: Decontaminate the working surface area with 70% alcohol solution prior to equipment set-up.[18]
- Catheter site care with transparent semipermeable dressing for central venous catheters
- *Tube changing*: Every 96 hours for daily fluids and continuous infusion medications (unless a change of shorter duration is ordered), every 24 hourly for total parenteral nutrition (TPN), and a new set for each blood transfusion
- *Hand hygiene*: The cornerstone in prevention of neonatal infections is hand hygiene.
- Hand hygiene once thought "handwashing with soap" has taken an evolution with the introduction of alcohol-based hand rubs and chlorhexidine. Many studies have proven that the alcohol-based hand rub is superior over povidone–iodine scrub and thorough hand wash of 2 minutes with soap and water.[19]
- *Fungal prophylaxis*: Fungal infections are third most common infection in NICU. The risk is:
  - Increased with prematurity, low birth weight (LBW), use of >2 antibiotics, H2 blockers, TPN, lack of enteral feds, gastrointestinal surgery, and central venous catheters.
  - For neonates <1,000 g or ≤27 weeks, IV fluconazole 3 mg/kg has to be administered twice a week till removal of all IV lines.
  - For neonates 1,000–1,500 g, prophylaxis is based on unit protocol.
- Use of emollients (oils) to maintain skin integrity.
- *Prevention of ventilator-associated pneumonia (VAP)*: VAP is defined by CDC as new and persistent radiographic infiltrates and worsening gas exchange in infants who are ventilated for at least 48 hours and who exhibit at least three of the following criteria:
  - Temperature instability with no other recognized cause
  - Leukopenia
  - Change in the characteristic of respiratory secretions
  - Respiratory distress
  - Bradycardia or tachycardia
  - *VAP prevention bundle*:[20]
    ◆ Head end elevation to 30–45°
    ◆ Re-enforcement of hand hygiene
    ◆ Sterile handling of respiratory equipment and suction
    ◆ Change ventilator circuit, if malfunctioning or visibly soiled
    ◆ Mouth care with normal saline and suction of oropharyngeal secretions
    ◆ Intubation, reintubation, and endotracheal suction strictly as per protocol
    ◆ Sedation vacation for sedated babies
    ◆ Daily evaluation for extubation readiness
- Treatment of infections with appropriate antibiotics as per unit flora and sensitivity pattern, with supportive care of immunoglobulins, probiotics, and bovine lactoferrin, as required.

Pain and Discomfort Management

Neonates experience acute pain with diagnostic and therapeutic interventions and controlling pain is beneficial in improving physiologic, behavioral, and hormonal outcome.

- Reduce painful events by cluster care, minimizing procedures, Kangaroo care, facilitated tucking, nonnutritive sucking, sucrose and other sweeteners, and use of noninvasive therapeutic approaches for analgesia (e.g., transdermal patches, iontophoresis, and compressed air injectors).
- Unstable or ventilated cases are frequently managed by narcotics (morphine, fentanyl, and others) **(Table 3)**. Currently, there are no studies for the safety and efficacy of postoperative morphine analgesia in preterm neonates.[21]
- Outpatient surgery/minor surgeries are treated with acetaminophen with local anesthetic infiltration (example—circumcision).
- Lower extremity/abdominal/thoracic surgeries are to be managed by systemic analgesia along with regional analgesia techniques for pain relief after surgery under general anesthesia.[21]

Table 3: Drugs used in neonatal intensive care unit for pain management and its advantages and disadvantages.

Drug	Advantages	Disadvantages
Morphine	• Term hypoxic–ischemic encephalopathy • Postsurgery • Ventilator synchrony • Potent pain relief • Sedation • Muscle relaxation • Inexpensive	• Hypotension • Longer ventilator support • Feed intolerance • Constipation • Urinary retention • CNS depression • Tolerance and dependence
Fentanyl	• Preterm and term • Shorter half life • Fast acting • Less hypotension • Reduced effects on gastrointestinal motility/urinary retention	• Less sedation • Respiratory depression • Short half life • Chest wall rigidity • Quick tolerance and dependence

(CNS: central nervous system)

Nutrition

Nutrition is the most vital factor influencing growth and long-term neurodevelopmental outcome. Parenteral nutrition can be used as the sole source of nutrition for those who cannot be fed. Minimal enteral nutrition can be initiated with the parenteral nutrition.

Energy in parenteral nutrition is provided by carbohydrate and lipid to ensure proper utilization of protein. In parenteral nutrition, carbohydrates constitute 60–75% and lipids constitute 25–40% of nonprotein calorie in kcal. Start glucose infusion rates of 4–6 µg/kg/min to maximum of 12.5 µg/kg/min, amino acids at 1.5 mg/kg/min and increase to 12 mg/kg/min, and lipids at 1–2 g/kg/day and increase to 3–3.5 g/kg/day (can be started at higher values based on unit protocols). Other components like electrolytes, minerals, trace elements, and vitamins to be supplemented. Parenteral nutrition can be provided with ready-to-use solutions, prepare with lamellar flow based on patient needs or partial parenteral nutrition.[22,23]

- *Indications of parenteral nutrition*:
  - *Absolute indications*:
    - ◆ Functional immaturity as in ≤30 weeks, ≤1.25-kg weight
    - ◆ Intestinal failure like pseudo-obstruction, short bowel syndrome, postgastrointestinal surgeries, congenital gastrointestinal defects, and NEC
  - *Relative indications*:
    - ◆ >30 weeks of age, >1.25 kg not expected to reach ≥75% of nutrition in 3–5 days
    - ◆ Severe IUGR associated with absent or decreased end diastolic flow on umbilical artery Doppler
    - ◆ Intractable diarrhea or vomiting
    - ◆ Malabsorption syndromes
- Establishing feeds in gastrointestinal surgeries poses a challenge as compared to other surgeries since multiple factors affect bowel motility and its ability to tolerate feeds.[24] Prevent aversion for oral feeding by minimal feeds by mouth or with pacifiers.
  - General strategies for feed establishment:
    - ◆ Bowel rest (duration is based on severity of gut inflammation, longer in NEC, and other major abdominal/colonic surgery patients) and continuous decompression of stomach
    - ◆ To start minimal enteral nutrition 10 mL/kg/day (as per unit protocols)
    - ◆ Volume and color of gastric aspirates reflect gastric motility. Dark green large volume indicates decreased gastric motility (conditions like gastroschisis and duodenal atresia have specific patterns though). Aspirates have to be replaced with intravenous normal saline with potassium chloride.
    - ◆ *Intestinal rehabilitation*: Freshly expressed mother's milk is the feed of choice. Complex patients may need either a hydrolyzed (for high stoma output and large resections), lactose-free, or a feed containing fat as medium chain triglycerides (for cholestasis). Continuous feeds may be preferred over intermittent, if motility is affected and mandated in jejunal feeding.

Postoperative Complications

Preoperative physiology and stability of the neonates predicts the risk of postoperative complications. The most common risk factors are postconceptual age <40 weeks, presence of cardiac anomalies, hyaline membrane disease, preoperative ICU status, NEC, and fluid status.[25]

The common complications are technical (25%), gastrointestinal (22%), respiratory (21%), and first 48 hours being the most critical period.[26]

- Prematurity, IUGR, perinatal asphyxia, sepsis, hemodynamic instability, TPN-related metabolic derangements and cholestasis, associated comorbid conditions like cardiac, and syndromes pose the primary complications.

- Abdominal surgeries present with immediate complications like anastomotic leaks (in TEF and NEC), abdominal compartment syndrome (in abdominal wall defects), inferior vena cava compression, gastroesophageal reflux and pylorospasm. Long-term complications are short bowel syndrome and malabsorption, strictures liver failure secondary to prolonged parenteral nutrition and others.
- *Respiratory complications*: The most important are pneumothorax, pneumonia (secondary to aspiration or gastric reflux), and atelectasis. Babies may develop chronic lung disease, if the primary pathology is lung as in congenital diaphragmatic hernia.

Other Supportive Care

- Careful maintenance of catheters in situ like feeding tube in TEF surgery to keep the anastomotic site patent, urinary catheter in posterior urethral valve ablation to maintain lumen integrity in urethra.
- Barium studies to check anastomotic leak postsurgery.

Parent Training

Minor/major surgeries terminology is just for assessing the risk and outcome for professionals. For parents, it is operating on a hand-sized life. Hence, family-centered care is essential to tide over the crisis. Parents are to be involved in the daily care of neonate, feeding, medications, and surgical site care. They are trained for the stoma care and danger signs to watch for.

A detailed discharge plan has to be made, as most surgeries are multiphasic and need corrective surgeries. Parents are also trained about early stimulation and a close follow-up on neurodevelopmental outcome. Enrollment into projects like smile project for other associated comorbid conditions would help them socially and emotionally.

Long-term Care

- Reaching enteral autonomy may take as long as 2–5 years in few abdominal surgeries.
- Short bowel syndrome and intestinal failure and chronic lung disease are associated with significant failure to thrive, developmental delay, and neurological deficits. Early stimulation with maximizing early supplementation is advised.

REFERENCES

1. Bucher BT, Duggan EM, Grubb PH, France DJ, Lally KP, Blakely ML, et al. Does the American College of Surgeons National Surgical Quality Improvement Program pediatric provide actionable quality improvement data for surgical neonates? J Pediatr Surg. 2016;51(9):1440-4.
2. Gephart SM, McGrath JM. Family-centered care of the surgical neonate. Newborn Infant Nurs Rev. 2012;12(1):5-7.
3. Kumar Sinha S, Neogi S. Bedside neonatal intensive care unit surgery—myth or reality! J Neonatal Surg. 2013;2(2):20.
4. Rocha G, Soares P, Gonçalves A, Silva AI, Almeida D, Figueiredo S, et al. Respiratory care for the ventilated neonate. Can Respir J. 2018;2018:7472964.
5. Corvaglia L, Martini S, Aceti A, Arcuri S, Rossini R, Faldella G. Nonpharmacological management of gastroesophageal reflux in preterm infants. Biomed Res Int. 2013;2013:141967.
6. Lister P, Ramaiah R, Peters M. Surgical neonates. London, UK: NHS, Great Ormond Street Hospital for Children; 2005 (Updated 2007). pp. 1-9.
7. Agarwal R, Deorari A, Paul V, Sankar MJ, Sachdeva A. AIIMS protocol in neonatology, 2nd edition. New Delhi: Noble Vision Medical Books Publishers; 2019.
8. Stevens TP, Finer NN, Carlo WA, Szilagyi PG, Phelps DL, Walsh MC, et al. Respiratory outcomes of the surfactant positive pressure and oximetry randomized trial (SUPPORT). J Pediatr. 2014;165(2):240-9.e4.
9. Logan JW. First, do no harm. Consequences of permissive hypercapnia in the neonate. Respir Care. 2018;63(8):1070-2.
10. Varughese M, Patole S, Shama A, Whitehall J. Permissive hypercapnia in neonates: the case of the good, the bad, and the ugly. Pediatr Pulmonol. 2002;33(1):56-64.
11. Al Hazzani FN, Al Hussein K, Al Alaiyan S, Al Saedi S, Al Faleh K, Al Harbi F, et al. Mechanical ventilation in newborn infants: Clinical practice guidelines of the Saudi Neonatology Society. J Clin Neonatol. 2017;6(2):57-63.
12. Giesinger RE, McNamara PJ. Hemodynamic instability in the critically ill neonate: An approach to cardiovascular support based on disease pathophysiology. Semin Perinatol. 2016;40(3):174-88.
13. Wasserman S, Messina A; International Society for Infectious Diseases. (2018). Bundles in infection prevention and safety. In: Bearman G (Ed). Guide to Infection Control in Hospital. [online] Available from https://isid.org/wp-content/uploads/2018/02/ISID_InfectionGuide_Chapter16.pdf. [Last accessed March, 2020].
14. O'Grady NP, Alexander M, Burns LA, Dellinger EP, Garland J, Heard SO, et al. Guidelines for the prevention of intravascular catheter-related infections. Am J Infect Control. 2011;39(4 Suppl 1):S1-34.
15. Loveday HP, Wilson JA, Pratt RJ, Golsorkhi M, Tingle A, Bak A, et al. epic3: national evidence-based guidelines for preventing healthcare-associated infections in NHS hospitals in England. J Hosp Infect. 2014;86 (Suppl 1):S1-70.
16. Sathiyamurthy S, Banerjee J, Godambe SV. Antiseptic use in the neonatal intensive care unit—a dilemma in clinical practice: An evidence based review. World J Clin Pediatr. 2016;5(2):159-71.
17. Government of Western Australia North Metropolitan Health Service. (2018). Aseptic Technique in the NICU; Clinical Practice

Guideline coverage includes NICU KEMH, NICU PCH and NETS WA. [online] Available from https://www.kemh.health.wa.gov.au/~/media/Files/Hospitals/WNHS/For%20health%20professionals/Clinical%20guidelines/NEO/WNHS.NEO.AsepticTechniqueintheNICU.pdf. [Last accessed March, 2020].

18. Ramasethu J. Prevention and treatment of neonatal nosocomial infections. Matern Health Neonatol Perinatol. 2017;3:5.

19. Sharma VS, Dutta S, Taneja N, Narang A. Comparing hand hygiene measures in a neonatal ICU: a randomized crossover trial. Indian Pediatr. 2013;50(10):917-21.

20. Azab SF, Sherbiny HS, Saleh SH, Elsaeed WF, Elshafiey MM, Siam AG, et al. Reducing ventilator-associated pneumonia in neonatal intensive care unit using "VAP prevention Bundle": a cohort study. BMC Infect Dis. 2015;15:314.

21. Hall RW, Anand KJ. Pain management in newborns. Clin Perinatol. 2014;41(4):895-924.

22. ElHassan NO, Kaiser JR. Parenteral Nutrition in the Neonatal Intensive Care Unit. Neo Reviews. 2011;12(3):e130-e140.

23. Radbone L. (2019). East of England Perinatal Networks Clinical Guideline: Parenteral Feeding of Infants on the Neonatal Unit. [online] Available from TPN--Parenteral-Feeding--of-Infants-on-the-Neonatal-Unit.-regional-network.pdf. [Last accessed March, 2020].

24. Penman G, Tavener K, Hickey A. Neonatal feeding: care and outcomes following gastrointestinal surgery. Infant. 2017;13(2):61-4.

25. Michelet D, Brasher C, Kaddour HB, Diallo T, Abdat R, Malbezin S, et al. Postoperative complications following neonatal and infant surgery: Common events and predictive factors. Anaesth Crit Care Pain Med. 2017;36(3):163-9.

26. Catré D, Lopes MF, Madrigal A, Oliveiros B, Cabrita AS, Viana JS, et al. Predictors of major postoperative complications in neonatal surgery. Rev Col Bras Cir. 2013;40(5):363-9.

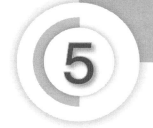

SECTION

5

Obstetrics and Gynecology

CHAPTER

28

Perioperative Management of Postpartum Obstetric Hemorrhage

Sapna Ravindranath, Bharathram Vasudevan

INTRODUCTION

Obstetric hemorrhage is one of the leading causes of maternal mortality and morbidity. Although the rate of maternal mortality attributed to obstetric hemorrhage varies widely, there has been an increasing trend to 3–11% of all maternal deaths[1,2] in developed countries and >30% in Asia and Africa.[3] Postpartum hemorrhage (PPH) is defined as blood loss > 500 mL and >1,000 mL within the first 24 hours following vaginal and cesarean delivery, respectively. Estimation of blood loss (EBL) by visual inspection is highly inaccurate compared to quantitative measurement of blood loss.[4,5] It is further classified as primary occurring within the first 24 hours following childbirth and secondary if occurring after 24 hours up to 6 weeks postpartum.[6,7] Obstetric hemorrhage is also one of the most common reasons for admission to an intensive care unit (ICU), the reasons for admission being acute blood loss, anemia coagulopathy, and multiorgan dysfunction.[8]

The risk factors for PPH are listed in **Table 1**.

PATHOPHYSIOLOGY

Mechanism of Hemostasis after Delivery

Hemostasis after delivery and prevention of excess bleeding depend on a complex interplay between mechanical factors in the uterine myometrium driven by neurohumoral factors and the coagulation system in the third stage of labor. The third stage of labor starts with delivery of the baby and ends with placental delivery. Myometrial contraction in this period is stimulated by two neurohumoral factors—oxytocin and prostaglandins. Oxytocin acts on myometrial oxytocin receptors and causes contractions. Prostaglandins PGE2 and PGF2α are potent uterotonics and are locally secreted in large amounts by the placenta, fetal membranes, and decidua. The ensuing intense myometrial contractions and retractions cause the placenta to shear off.[9] The formation of a retroplacental hematoma at the placental site has been postulated, but this has not been found in a study of the third stage of labor using ultrasonographic imaging.[10] The myometrial fibers compress the spiral arterioles supplying the placental bed and cause hemostasis. The critical role played by interlacing myometrial fibers in prevention of excess hemorrhage is emphasized by the term "living ligatures."

Pregnancy is a hypercoagulable state with an increase in fibrinogen and clotting factors and a decrease in anticlotting factors. The decidua is a known source of tissue factor and plasminogen activator inhibitor (PAI).[11] These factors, in addition to other clotting factors, platelets and von Willebrand factor (vWF), play a role in hemostasis after placental separation. Blood levels of fibrinolytic factors are high in the immediate puerperium which probably prevents clot formation in the rest of the body while a local pro-inflammatory state promotes coagulation in the placental bed.

Table 1: Risk factors for postpartum hemorrhage.		
Maternal	*Uterine*	*Other*
Advanced maternal age	Placenta previa	Fetal macrosomia
Multiparity	Morbidly adherent placenta	Prolonged labor
Obesity	Placental abruption	Augmented labor
Anemia	Uterine rupture	History of significant postpartum hemorrhage
Pre-eclampsia	Chorioamnionitis	Disseminated intravascular coagulation

Mechanism of Major Obstetric Hemorrhage

Excessive obstetric hemorrhage occurs due to a disruption of one or more factors involved in normal hemostasis in the peripartum period. The exact mechanism varies depending upon the etiology. The most common cause of primary PPH is uterine atony which contributes to 75–80% of the cases.[12] Uterine atony refers to failure of the normal myometrial contraction in the third stage of labor and immediate puerperium. Risk factors for uterine atony include conditions where the uterus is overdistended, thereby leading to impaired actin–myosin interactions and impaired contractility. These include polyhydramnios, multiple gestation, high parity, and macrosomia.[12] Induction of labor or prolonged labor can lead to desensitization of oxytocin receptors which can lead to atony. In many patients, the cause for such myometrial dysfunction is unknown, thereby making PPH unpredictable but it is responsive to administration of uterotonic agents.

Retained products and abnormal placentation contribute to uterine atony in a smaller percentage of patients, but the PPH associated with these conditions is usually severe and requires operative interventions leading to significant morbidity and mortality. Retained products could be the entire placenta/placental bits or a succenturiate lobe. These conditions cause mechanical impediment to uterine contraction and cause atony. Abnormal placentation mainly includes placenta previa and morbidly adherent placenta. Placenta previa is abnormal low implantation of the placenta in the lower uterine segment near or across the cervical os. Placenta previa can present as painless antepartum hemorrhage as well as lead to excessive PPH after delivery. The lower uterine segment has a different arrangement of myometrial fibers and does not contract easily leading to uterine atony and high risk for PPH. A morbidly adherent placenta includes placenta accreta (placenta attached to myometrium), increta (partial invasion of myometrium by placenta), and percreta (placenta traverses the myometrium and extends to the serosal surface or other organs). Previous cesarean deliveries and gynecological procedures are the main risk factors for a morbidly adherent placenta. The placenta accreta spectrum poses a high risk of retained placenta and severe PPH.[13]

Genital trauma during delivery such as vaginal, cervical, or perineal lacerations can lead to PPH. Uterine rupture is a rare cause of antepartum hemorrhage in the setting of trial of labor after a previous cesarean section or due to prolonged obstructed labor which is extremely rare in developed settings.

Postpartum hemorrhage can also result from congenital or acquired coagulopathies and bleeding diatheses due to platelet dysfunction. Women with hemophilia and von Willebrand disease are at a high risk of PPH.[14]

Conversely, PPH itself can lead to a picture of consumption/dilutional coagulopathy which leads to a vicious cycle and disseminated intravascular coagulation (DIC), if uncorrected. Acquired coagulopathy during pregnancy can result from HELLP (hemolysis, elevated liver enzymes and low platelet count) syndrome or severe preeclampsia.

Placental abruption and amniotic fluid embolism are rare causes of DIC in the peripartum period. Placental abruption is due to detachment of the placenta before the delivery of the fetus. The separation occurs due to rupture of maternal blood vessels and bleeding between the decidual and placental interface and causes antepartum hemorrhage. Uteroplacental insufficiency and decidual hypoxia are associated with placental abruption. This can in turn lead to expression of vascular endothelial growth factor (VEGF) which acts on the decidual endothelial cells to produce tissue factor and generation of thrombin.[15] Decidual bleeding in turn exposes tissue thromboplastin and generation of thrombin. Thrombin is a potent uterotonic agent and leads to release of inflammatory cytokines. The activation of coagulation cascade can lead to DIC and major hemorrhage in the peripartum period.[16] Additionally, bleeding into the myometrium can lead to Couvelaire uterus and subsequent severe atony in the postpartum period.

Different components of the above-mentioned pathophysiological processes may coexist at any one time in patients with PPH. The 4Ts mnemonic has been widely used to remember the etiology and pathogenesis of PPH. It includes Tone (uterine atony), Tissue (retained products, placental abnormalities), Trauma, and Thrombin (coagulopathy). This provides an easy tool to remember and rule out causes in any case of PPH.

Secondary PPH is less common and refers to hemorrhage occurring later than 24 hours after delivery up to 6 weeks in the postpartum period. This is most commonly related to infection, retained products, subinvolution of the placental site and rarely due to bleeding diatheses, vascular malformations, dehiscence of cesarean incision, etc.[17]

The physiological consequence of any PPH is a state of hypovolemic shock which leads to tachycardia, hypotension, decreased urine output, and ultimately circulatory collapse and death, if left uncorrected. The stage of shock depends on the amount of blood loss. In some patients, concealed bleeding can occur within the uterine cavity and the patient can be in a worse stage than evident from the amount of external bleeding. Therefore, it is really important to recognize PPH early and identify the exact cause to take corrective actions (**Flowchart 1**).

Postpartum Hemorrhage Safety Bundle

Institutional Preparedness

Standardized protocols for the management of PPH have been shown to improve maternal morbidity. Based on these

Flowchart 1: Pathophysiology of PPH.

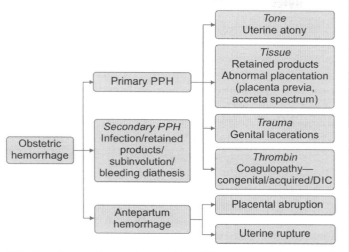

(DIC: disseminated intravascular coagulation; PPH: postpartum hemorrhage)

results, a consensus bundle on obstetric hemorrhage was released by the Council on Patient Safety in Women's Health Care in collaboration with other professional societies through the national partnership for maternal safety (NPMS) initiative.[5]

The bundle consists of 13 elements (**Box 1**) under four main domains:
1. Readiness
2. Recognition and prevention
3. Response
4. Reporting and systems learning

The actual method of implementation of different components of the bundle must be individualized to each institution depending upon the available resources and standardized across different areas in the same institution

Readiness of Every Unit

A readily accessible hemorrhage cart should be present in labor and delivery, antepartum and postpartum floors. The contents of the cart should be determined by a multidisciplinary team of obstetrician, anesthesiologist, and nursing and pharmacy providers. Examples of contents of the hemorrhage cart have been published.[18] Medications used in the management of hemorrhage should be easily available and accessible without waiting for pharmacy approval/delivery, and the kit should be designed in conjunction with pharmacy. The drug tray of the anesthesia cart is an ideal location to keep the medication kit in labor and delivery area.[19] Examples of medications to be kept include oxytocin (bags and vials), 15-methyl PGF2α ampules, methylergonovine ampule, tranexamic acid (TXA) bag, and misoprostol tablets.

A PPH response team for emergency management should be formulated and must include obstetrician, anesthesiologist, nurses, support staff, pharmacists, laboratory personnel, and blood bank staff with clearly defined roles and responsibilities. Complicated patients would require involvement of gynecology-oncologists, interventional radiologists, and critical care physicians who should be available.

Massive transfusion protocols and emergency transfusion protocols (for O-negative/un-crossmatched blood) should be in place and designed specific to the institution in collaboration with the blood bank.[18] The staff should be aware of activation methods which should not be complicated. Automated delivery of blood products in the prespecified ratio should continue until massive transfusion protocol (MTP) is deactivated.

Antenatal Risk Assessment, Laboratory Testing, and Optimization

Even though a large proportion of PPH occurs in low-risk patients, identifying those with known risk factors for PPH can help prenatal optimization, improve readiness, and help early recognition and response from the care team. Risk assessment should start in the prenatal period and repeated on admission to labor and delivery with continued assessment during the intrapartum and postpartum periods. It also helps to involve the anesthesia team early in patients with known risk factors in the prenatal period. Preanesthesia clinic referral for medium- and high-risk patients can provide an opportunity for the consulting anesthesiologist to review history and perform physical examination, counsel patients on anesthetic/analgesia modalities, and identify patients needing further consultations and interventions to optimize before admission for delivery.[20] Various risk assessment tools have been established to identify patients with medium and high risk for PPH. The California Maternal Quality Care Collaborative toolkit provides one such risk stratification tool (**Box 2**) which has been externally validated in a study.[21]

The identification of such risk factors can guide management and dictate further testing/consultations or transfer of care to a different facility. The planning and timing of elective delivery for specific conditions such as placenta previa/accrete or prior cesarean section depend on delineation of those risk factors in the prenatal period. Ultrasonographic localization of the placental location is extremely important in patients with previous cesarean sections. Ultrasound forms the main modality for

---

Box 2: Risk stratification.

Risk factors—prenatal/on admission
- *Low risk*
  - No previous uterine surgery
  - Singleton pregnancy
  - ≤4 vaginal births
  - No known bleeding diathesis
  - No history of PPH
- *Medium risk—type and screen on admission*
  - Previous cesarean section or uterine surgery
  - >4 vaginal births
  - Multiple gestation
  - History of PPH
  - Chorioamnionitis
  - Large fibroids
- *High risk—type and crossmatch on admission*
  - Placenta previa
  - Suspected placenta accreta spectrum
  - HCt < 30 and other risk factors
  - Platelets < 100,000
  - Known coagulopathy
  - Active bleeding
  - Two or more medium risk factors

Intrapartum risk factors
- Prolonged second stage
- Prolonged oxytocin use > 24 hours
- Active bleeding
- Chorioamnionitis
- Magnesium sulfate use

Third stage/postpartum risk factors
- Vacuum- or forceps-assisted birth
- Urgent/emergent cesarean section
- Retained placenta

(CMQCC: California Maternal Quality Care Collaborative; HCt: hematocrit; PPH: postpartum hemorrhage)

(*Source*: Modified from CMQCC Obstetric Hemorrhage Toolkit.[33])

---

identification of the placenta accreta spectrum. Magnetic resonance imaging (MRI) is useful to identify a morbidly adherent placenta if ultrasound is inconclusive. Though MRI was shown to be highly sensitive and specific, it could also be misleading and lead to incorrect diagnosis in some patients.[22,23] Therefore, careful correlation is necessary in doubtful cases. Prenatal oral or iron therapy is useful in high-risk patients to optimize hemoglobin levels. Erythropoietin use can be beneficial, especially in patients who refuse transfusion. A blood product acceptance checklist form can be routinely used on admission to the labor floor and signed by the parturient.[24] For patients who accept selective products, the form can come in handy in emergency situations to identify which product to use for resuscitation. Patients with a history of known or suspected bleeding disorders should have hematology consultation and workup in the third trimester. Recommendations for prophylactic treatment of inherited bleeding disorders have been published.[14] Suspected placenta accreta spectrum, coagulopathy, prepregnancy body mass index (BMI) > 50, significant comorbid conditions such as cardiac disease, and patients who refuse transfusion are conditions that would warrant transfer to a facility with a higher level of care equipped to handle such patients including availability of services such as ICU and interventional radiology.

Risk assessment should be dynamic and continue periodically during the intrapartum and postpartum periods to identify new risk factors that may arise during the peripartum period.

Recognition of Peripartum Hemorrhage

Blood Loss Measurement

The American College of Obstetricians and Gynecologists (ACOG) practice guidelines define PPH as cumulative blood loss > 1,000 mL or blood loss accompanied by signs or symptoms of hypovolemia within 24 hours of delivery.[6] Traditionally, visual estimation has been the most commonly used method to quantify blood loss. Visual estimation has been shown to be very poor at accurately quantifying blood loss in PPH and can underestimate the amount by up to 50%. Accuracy can be improved by using calibrated drapes and containers. The gravimetric method is more accurate at measuring blood loss.[25] It involves subtracting the dry weight of absorbent material from the weight of material after soakage with blood and weighing clots. The volume of blood loss (in mL) is assumed to be equal to the weight in grams. Use of under-buttock calibrated vaginal delivery drapes has been shown to be more accurate than the indirect gravimetric method of weighing blood-soaked chux pads/gauzes.[26] Estimating the cumulative amount of blood loss during the birthing process is the most crucial step in recognizing PPH. The safety bundle emphasizes the use of quantitative measurements whenever feasible.

Hemodynamic Evaluation

Hemodynamic monitoring of heart rate (HR) and blood pressure (BP), along with urine output, has been used traditionally to classify the severity of hemorrhagic shock. While tachycardia, hypotension, and decreased urine output are seen in severe stages of shock, physiologic compensation can mask the degree of blood loss in early stages. It has been shown in trauma literature that mortality rates can be high even with normal vital signs in the early stages of hemorrhagic shock. Hypotension [systolic BP (SBP) < 90 mm Hg] is seen only in late stages.[27] Using these traditional parameters can, therefore, delay the recognition of PPH. A shock index, which is the ratio of HR to SBP, has been proposed to identify the early stages of shock. The shock index has been shown to be more sensitive than either parameter alone and an index of >1.1 is associated with higher mortality in a study of trauma patients.[28] Thus, a shock index of >1.1 can be used to identify patients with significant blood loss when BP values are still in the normal range.

Laboratory Testing

Serial hemoglobin and hematocrit measurements can be useful to guide transfusion in patients with significant blood loss. The values can, however, lag behind in the setting of active hemorrhage. Coagulation testing can guide transfusion and should include fibrinogen levels in addition to prothrombin time, partial thromboplastin time, and international normalized ratio (INR). Fibrinogen levels are increased in pregnancy, and hypofibrinogenemia < 200 mg/dL is predictive of severe hemorrhage and needs replacement.[29] Newer advances include the use of thromboelastography (TEG) and rotational thromboelastometry (ROTEM) to rapidly identify specific deficiencies in the setting of ongoing blood loss and guide replacement.[30] For instance, one study reported decrease in fibrinogen thromboelastometry (FIBTEM) values measured by ROTEM which correlated with hypofibrinogenemia in PPH and was helpful in early identification.[31] When using these modalities, it is prudent to remember that the normal values for pregnant women are different from the general population due to changes associated with pregnancy and the test results should be interpreted accordingly.

Response to Peripartum Hemorrhage

The NPMS bundle advocates staged management of PPH which helps to initiate a stepwise response to blood loss and maternal warning signs.[5] A stagewise emergency management protocol with a checklist should be created by each institution and used in all parturients to facilitate early recognition and management of PPH. Several samples of such protocols have been tested in different areas and have been shown to improve care of patients with PPH. One such example is given in **Table 2** which demonstrates stepwise escalation of care depending upon the stage.

Role of an Anesthesiologist

Preanesthetic Consultation

An antenatal preanesthetic consultation with an obstetric anesthesiologist is essential for patients who are thought to be at high risk for PPH. This includes patients with placenta previa, morbidly adherent placenta (accreta, percreta, increta), morbid obesity, twin gestation, and bleeding disorders. This consultation is typically done in the late second trimester or early third trimester. It allows for preoperative evaluation, physical examination, review of diagnostic studies, and multidisciplinary consultation with the hematologist and cardiologist as necessary. The anesthesiologist should discuss various anesthetic plans including risks, benefits, possible use of invasive monitors, central venous access, transfusion of blood products, and admission to an ICU. The patients should be counseled about the need to deliver at a tertiary medical center.

Patients with placenta previa and morbidly adherent placenta are frequently admitted to the hospital in the third trimester. All patients who are admitted with vaginal bleeding and/or develop risk factors for PPH should be evaluated by an anesthesia provider. It is important to establish at least one large-bore intravenous (IV) access and resuscitate with nondextrose-containing balanced salt solution (e.g., lactated Ringer's, normal saline). At least 1–2 units of crossmatched blood should be available at labor and delivery unit for patients with a morbidly adherent placenta. Hemoglobin measurement may be needed after every episode of vaginal bleed. The American Association of Blood Banks (AABB) recommends testing for serum antibodies every 72 hours in pregnant women because of the small risk for developing a new alloantibody during pregnancy.[35]

Intraoperative Management

The choice of the anesthetic technique depends on the indication and urgency for delivery or surgical intervention, obstetric history, and the timing and severity of PPH.

Postpartum Hemorrhage after a Vaginal Delivery

The anesthesia provider, when notified, should do a brief assessment of history, risk factors, vital signs, amount of blood loss, and necessity of surgical intervention. It is

Table 2: Example of a staged emergency obstetric hemorrhage management protocol.

Stage	Definition	Interventions
0	<500 mL EBL—vaginal delivery <1,000 mL EBL—cesarean	Routine care—active management third stage of labor
1	>500 mL EBL—vaginal >1,000 mL—EBL cesarean Vital signs normal	Obstetrician assessment for etiology—4Ts Anesthesiologist at bedside Wide-bore IV access, IV fluids, urinary catheter Fundal massage Escalate uterotonics—oxytocin. Consider additional agents (methergine, hemabate, misoprostol) Type, screen, and crossmatch blood
2	1,000–1,500 mL EBL or >2 uterotonics Continued bleeding Vital signs normal	Notify the entire obstetric hemorrhage emergency response team Two 16G or 18G IVs Stat labs—Hb, fibrinogen, coagulation profile Additional uterotonics, consider tranexamic acid Obtain 2 units PRBC, FFP—transfuse based on clinical signs Consider balloon tamponade for uterine atony Rule out other etiology—consider moving to OR
3	EBL > 1,500 mL or >2 RBC transfused or coagulopathy or hemodynamically unstable/abnormal labs/oliguria	Mobilize additional help Move to OR MTP activation Anesthesia—conversion to GA if needed, consider arterial /central venous access Continue uterotonics—repeat as indicated, TXA Achieve hemostasis based on etiology Possible interventions—Bakri balloon, B-lynch suture/compression suture, uterine artery ligation, hysterectomy Notify IR for possible embolization Postoperative ICU care
4	Cardiovascular collapse—massive hemorrhage Profound shock	Mobilize help ACLS if indicated Simultaneous aggressive transfusion Immediate surgical hemostasis—hysterectomy

(ACLS: advanced cardiac life support; ACOG: American College of Obstetricians and Gynecologists; EBL: estimation of blood loss; FFP: fresh frozen plasma; GA: general anesthesia; IR: interventional radiology; IV: intravenous; MTP: massive transfusion protocol; PRBC: packed red blood cell; TXA: tranexamic acid)

(*Source*: Adapted from ACOG District II obstetric hemorrhage bundle.[34])

critical to establish a large-bore IV access and optimize hemodynamics with fluids and vasopressors. Continuous monitoring of HR, pulse oximetry, and frequent BP monitoring are essential. In the presence of functioning epidural, local anesthetic bolus through the epidural catheter should suffice for laceration repairs. If there is no epidural catheter in situ, local anesthetic infiltration by an obstetrician and moderate sedation with small doses of benzodiazepine, narcotic, and/or ketamine can be provided for a laceration repair. If PPH is significant (>1,000 mL blood loss) requiring major surgical intervention and in the absence of an epidural catheter, the decision to provide neuraxial block versus general anesthesia can be based on the amount of blood loss, hemodynamic status, coagulations abnormalities, and comorbidities of the patient. In patients requiring general anesthesia for surgical intervention, rapid-sequence induction should be performed with cricoid pressure to reduce the risk of aspiration. Ramping and availability of video laryngoscope may be necessary in obese and in patients with suspected difficult intubation. Propofol can cause hypotension in hypovolemic patients. Ketamine and etomidate preserve hemodynamic stability and are better choices in unstable patients. Succinylcholine should achieve quick vocal cord paralysis for intubation. Maintenance of general anesthesia can be provided by 0.5 minimum alveolar concentration (MAC) of sevoflurane in 50% of nitrous oxide and narcotics.

Postpartum Hemorrhage during a Cesarean Delivery

In patients with risk factors for PPH, large-bore IV access and invasive monitors should be considered. Patients should receive isotonic crystalloid bolus preferably with lactated Ringer's prior to induction of anesthesia. If severe intraoperative hemorrhage is anticipated, availability of resources including fluid warmers, ultrasound machine, central venous access kit, arterial access kit, blood products, massive transfusion protocol, rapid infuser, autologous blood salvage, and thromboelastogram devices should be ensured.[20] Arterial line allows for beat-to-beat monitoring of BP and quick sampling of blood. Pulse pressure variation may assist with estimation of intravascular fluid status.[36] Central venous line allows for rapid transfusion of blood products and vasoactive medications. Additional invasive monitors such as transesophageal echocardiogram and pulmonary artery catheter can be placed to analyze cardiac function and guide appropriate therapy with fluids and inotropes. Blood transfusion should be initiated based on clinical signs and hematocrit testing. If uterine atony is the cause, appropriate uterotonic agents need to be administered (**Box 1**). It is prudent to start phenylephrine infusion in the beginning and escalate to norepinephrine, epinephrine, and vasopressin. Inotropes including milrinone, dopamine, and dobutamine should be readily available. Severe hemorrhage leading to DIC and massive blood transfusion ultimately results in multiorgan dysfunction requiring continued mechanical ventilation and extracorporeal membrane oxygenation.

Postpartum Hemorrhage with Abnormal Placentation

Patients with placenta previa and morbidly adherent placenta are at increased risk of significant PPH. The chances of hysterectomy are as high as 80% in patients with morbidly adherent placenta and requiring admission in 40% of these patients to an ICU.[37] Practitioners should consider risk stratification and access to resources when planning such high-risk cases. This includes referral to tertiary hospital, preoperative planning, and multidisciplinary care for cesarean delivery and hysterectomy in an operating room setting.[38,39] Preoperative planning entails preanesthetic consultation and availability of necessary resources (equipment, invasive monitoring, vasoactive medications, uterotonics, massive transfusion and obstetric hemorrhage protocols, and multidisciplinary team). In patients without active bleeding, it is prudent to administer neuraxial anesthesia (spinal or combined spinal–epidural anesthetic) until the delivery to avoid in utero exposure of fetus to inhalational agents and associated neurobehavioral effects.[40,41] After the fetal delivery, conversion to general anesthesia is considered for anticipated hemodynamic instability and complicated hysterectomy. Epidural anesthesia was associated with more stable BP after delivery and lower transfusion rates with similar hematocrit measurements on the day after surgery in a randomized controlled trial comparing epidural with general anesthesia

for cesarean delivery in women with placenta previa in the absence of active bleeding. There were no differences with operative times, estimated blood loss, urine output, and Apgar scores in the two groups.[42]

Medical Management

Uterotonic Agents

Routine active management of the third stage of labor is the single-most effective strategy to prevent PPH. This includes three components—oxytocin administration, uterine massage, and cord traction. Of these, prophylactic oxytocin administration as IV infusion or intramuscular injection is the most effective agent to prevent uterine atony. Several regimens for oxytocin administration have been described. Each unit should develop and follow a routine protocol for oxytocin administration. In patients who develop PPH, additional uterotonics can be used in addition to escalating the dose of oxytocin. Methylergonovine (methergine), 15-methyl PGF2α (hemabate, carboprost), and misoprostol (Cytotec, PGE1) are the options. The choice usually depends on balancing the patient's comorbidities with the side effect profile of agents.[43] An overview of the different uterotonics is provided in **Table 3**.

Blood Transfusion Strategies

Blood product administration is a critical component in the management of severe PPH. The exact transfusion triggers have not been delineated very well. Transfusion can be guided by laboratory values or clinical parameters in acute hemorrhage. In case of massive hemorrhage, it is prudent to initiate a MTP. MTP components vary depending on the institution. Most centers use a fresh frozen plasma (FFP):packed red blood cell (PRBC) ratio of 1:1 during transfusion for PPH. All members of the obstetric hemorrhage team, especially anesthesiologists, must be familiar with their institution-specific MTP. Emergency transfusion of un-crossmatched/O-negative blood may be needed in case of life-threatening hemorrhage. The risk of hemolytic reaction with such transfusions is low compared to the potential benefits in such cases. The general targets of transfusion are Hb 7–8 g/dL, INR < 1.5, and platelet > 50,000. Fibrinogen level < 200 mg/dL is a known predictor of severe PPH, and efforts should be taken to replete it. The amount of fibrinogen present in FFP is low and the transfusion of cryoprecipitate/fibrinogen concentrate might be essential. Point-of-care coagulation testing modalities such as TEG and ROTEM have been used successfully to guide transfusions. It is important to develop PPH-specific protocols when using such modalities to guide transfusion. Intraoperative cell salvage can be safely used in obstetric patients, provided routine precautions are taken

Table 3: Uterotonic agents.

Drug	Dose/route	Repeat doses	Side effects/contraindications
Oxytocin	30U in 500 mL bag IV infusion (300–600 mL/hour)	Continuous infusion	Hypotension from rapid IV push Nausea/vomiting/ hyponatremia
Methylergonovine	0.2 mg IM	Every 2–4 hours	Contraindicated in hypertension/preeclampsia Can cause nausea/vomiting/hypertension
15-methyl PGF2α	0.25 mg IM or intramyometrial	Every 15–90 minutes. Max 8 doses—2 mg	Contraindication—asthma. Relative contraindication—hypertension, cardiac, hepatic, pulmonary disease Can cause bronchospasm, nausea, vomiting, diarrhea, fever, chills
Misoprostol	600–1,000 µg PO/rectal/sublingual	–	Nausea, vomiting, diarrhea, fever, headache

(ACOG: American College of Obstetricians and Gynecologists; IM: intramuscular; IV: intravenous)
(*Source*: Modified from ACOG practice bulletin number 183, October 2017—Postpartum hemorrhage[6])

for Rh isoimmunization. Some patients who refuse blood transfusions agree to cell salvage, and this can be potentially lifesaving in such patients.[44-46]

Pharmacological Hemostasis

Tranexamic acid is an antifibrinolytic agent which prevents plasmin formation and subsequent fibrin/clot breakdown. TXA can be considered in patients with ongoing PPH despite uterotonic agents. It has been studied in various surgical populations and is associated with decreased blood loss and need for blood transfusion. Studies in PPH have resulted in similar results of decreased blood loss and transfusion with the use of TXA. The World Maternal Antifibrinolytic (WOMAN) trial showed a decrease in death due to PPH in the TXA group when TXA was administered within 3 hours of childbirth with no increase in thromboembolic complications.[47] TXA can be a valuable adjunct in routine management to prevent PPH in patients who refuse blood transfusion.

Desmopressin (DDAVP) is used prophylactically in parturient with known von Willebrand disease or hemophilia A to prevent excessive hemorrhage. The role of DDAVP is unclear in severe PPH patients with suspected platelet dysfunction but no known coagulopathy.[44]

Recombinant factor VII has been used in the management of severe PPH but is associated with a high risk of thromboembolic complications.[48] It should, therefore, be reserved only to cases of life-threatening hemorrhage with ongoing hemorrhage despite optimizing all factors and utilization of all other modalities.

Fibrinogen concentrate (RiaSTAP) is currently approved in the United States for the treatment of severe hypofibrinogenemia during PPH.[49]

Fibrinogen concentrate use is not beneficial unless fibrinogen levels are <200 mg/dL.[50] Fibrinogen concentrate can be prepared and administered within 15 minutes when the cryoprecipitate is not readily available.[51]

Surgical Hemostasis

Uterus-conserving techniques include uterine packing, balloon tamponade, B-lynch compression sutures, uterine artery ligation, and embolization. Bakri balloon when inflated with saline or sterile water causes direct compression of the bleeding sites. Uterine packing, aortic compression, and balloon tamponade are temporizing measures to reduce bleeding before definitive treatment.[52] Hysterectomy is the definitive treatment for severe and persistent PPH.

Postoperative Care

Many patients with severe PPH require care in an ICU before and after surgical intervention, especially those requiring mechanical ventilation, massive transfusion, and patients in DIC. Stable patients with no active bleeding may be cared in a non-ICU setting. The goals in the postoperative period include close monitoring with frequent laboratory testing, continued resuscitation, and early recognition and management of further bleeding or other complications. Patients with severe PPH and shock may develop multiorgan complications such as acute respiratory distress syndrome, acute renal or liver failure, Sheehan's syndrome (pituitary necrosis), DIC, dilutional coagulopathy, and other complications related to massive transfusion. One study of PPH patients in an ICU identified that DIC was the major cause of mortality in such patients and late-onset DIC was associated with poor outcomes.[53]

REFERENCES

1. Clark SL, Belfort MA, Dildy GA, Herbst MA, Meyers JA, Hankins GD. Maternal death in the 21st century: causes, prevention, and relationship to cesarean delivery. Am J Obstet Gynecol. 2008;199(1):36.e1-5;discussion 91-2. e7-11.

2. Cantwell R, Clutton-Brock T, Cooper G, Dawson A, Drife J, Garrod D, et al. Saving mothers' lives: Reviewing maternal deaths to make motherhood safer: 2006-2008. The eighth report of the confidential enquiries into maternal deaths in the United Kingdom. BJOG. 2011;118(Suppl 1):1-203.

3. Khan KS, Wojdyla D, Say L, Gülmezoglu AM, Van Look PF. WHO analysis of causes of maternal death: A systematic review. Lancet. 2006;367(9516):1066-74.

4. Hancock A, Weeks AD, Lavender DT. Is accurate and reliable blood loss estimation the 'crucial step' in early detection of postpartum haemorrhage: An integrative review of the literature. BMC Pregnancy Childbirth. 2015;15:230.

5. Main EK, Goffman D, Scavone BM, Low LK, Bingham D, Fontaine PL, et al. National partnership for maternal safety: Consensus bundle on obstetric hemorrhage. Obstet Gynecol. 2015;126(1):155-62.

6. Committee on Practice Bulletins-Obstetrics. Practice bulletin No. 183: Postpartum hemorrhage. Obstet Gynecol. 2017;130(4):e168-86.

7. Cunningham FG, Leveno KJ, Bloom SL, Spong CY, Dashe JS, Hoffman BL, et al. Obstetrical hemorrhage. In: Williams Obstetrics, 24th edition. New York, NY: McGraw-Hill Education; 2013.

8. O'Brien D, Babiker E, O'Sullivan O, Conroy R, McAuliffe F, Geary M, et al. Prediction of peripartum hysterectomy and end organ dysfunction in major obstetric haemorrhage. Eur J Obstet Gynecol Reprod Biol. 2010;153(2):165-9.

9. Khan RU, El-Refaey H. Pathophysiology of postpartum haemorrhage and third stage of labor. In: Arulkumaran A, Karoshi M, Keith LG, Lalonde AB, B-Lynch C (Eds). A Comprehensive Textbook of Postpartum Haemorrhage, 2nd edition. London: Sapiens Publishing; 2012. pp. 94-100.

10. Herman A, Weinraub Z, Bukovsky I, Arieli S, Zabow P, Caspi E, et al. Dynamic ultrasonographic imaging of the third stage of labor: New perspectives into third-stage mechanisms. Am J Obstet Gynecol. 1993;168(5):1496-9.

11. Lockwood CJ, Krikun G, Schatz F. The decidua regulates hemostasis in human endometrium. Semin Reprod Endocrinol. 1999;17(1):45-51.

12. Bateman BT, Berman MF, Riley LE, Leffert LR. The epidemiology of postpartum hemorrhage in a large, nationwide sample of deliveries. Anesth Analg. 2010;110(5):1368-73.

13. Booker W, Moroz L. Abnormal placentation. Semin Perinatol. 2019;43(1):51-9.

14. Abdul-Kadir R, McLintock C, Ducloy AS, El-Refaey H, England A, Federici AB, et al. Evaluation and management of postpartum hemorrhage: Consensus from an international expert panel. Transfusion. 2014;54(7):1756-68.

15. Krikun G, Huang ST, Schatz F, Salafia C, Stocco C, Lockwood CJ. Thrombin activation of endometrial endothelial cells: A possible role in intrauterine growth restriction. Thromb Haemost. 2007;97(2):245-53.

16. Cunningham FG, Nelson DB. Disseminated intravascular coagulation syndromes in obstetrics. Obstet Gynecol. 2015;126(5):999-1011.

17. Dossou M, Debost-Legrand A, Déchelotte P, Lémery D, Vendittelli F. Severe secondary postpartum hemorrhage: A historical cohort. Birth. 2015;42(2):149-55.

18. Spiegelman J, Sheen JJ, Goffman D. Readiness: Utilizing bundles and simulation. Semin Perinatol. 2019;43(1):5-10.

19. Rosenbaum T, Mhyre JM. The anesthesiologist's role in the national partnership for maternal safety's hemorrhage bundle: A review article. Clin Obstet Gynecol. 2017;60(2):384-93.

20. Ring L, Landau R. Postpartum hemorrhage: Anesthesia management. Semin Perinatol. 2019;43(1):35-43.

21. Dilla AJ, Waters JH, Yazer MH. Clinical validation of risk stratification criteria for peripartum hemorrhage. Obstet Gynecol. 2013;122(1):120-6.

22. Einerson BD, Rodriguez CE, Kennedy AM, Woodward PJ, Donnelly MA, Silver RM. Magnetic resonance imaging is often misleading when used as an adjunct to ultrasound in the management of placenta accreta spectrum disorders. Am J Obstet Gynecol. 2018;218(6):618.e1-618.e7.

23. Familiari A, Liberati M, Lim P, Pagani G, Cali G, Buca D, et al. Diagnostic accuracy of magnetic resonance imaging in detecting the severity of abnormal invasive placenta: A systematic review and meta-analysis. Acta Obstet Gynecol Scand. 2018;97(5):507-20.

24. Fleischer A, Meirowitz N. Care bundles for management of obstetrical hemorrhage. Semin Perinatol. 2016;40(2):99-108.

25. Andrikopoulou M, D'Alton ME. Postpartum hemorrhage: Early identification challenges. Semin Perinatol. 2019;43(1):11-7.

26. Ambardekar S, Shochet T, Bracken H, Coyaji K, Winikoff B. Calibrated delivery drape versus indirect gravimetric technique for the measurement of blood loss after delivery: A randomized trial. BMC Pregnancy Childbirth. 2014;14:276.

27. Parks JK, Elliott AC, Gentilello LM, Shafi S. Systemic hypotension is a late marker of shock after trauma: A validation study of advanced trauma life support principles in a large national sample. Am J Surg. 2006;192(6):727-31.

28. Vandromme MJ, Griffin RL, Kerby JD, McGwin G Jr, Rue LW 3rd, Weinberg JA. Identifying risk for massive transfusion in the relatively normotensive patient: Utility of the prehospital shock index. J Trauma. 2011;70(2):384-90.

29. Ducloy-Bouthors AS, Susen S, Wong CA, Butwick A, Vallet B, Lockhart E. Medical advances in the treatment of postpartum hemorrhage. Anesth Analg. 2014;119(5):1140-7.

30. de Lange NM, Lancé MD, de Groot R, Beckers EA, Henskens YM, Scheepers HC. Obstetric hemorrhage and coagulation: An update. Thromboelastography, thromboelastometry, and conventional coagulation tests in the diagnosis and prediction of postpartum hemorrhage. Obstet Gynecol Surv. 2012;67(7):426-35.

31. Huissoud C, Carrabin N, Benchaib M, Fontaine O, Levrat A, Massignon D, et al. Coagulation assessment by rotation

thrombelastometry in normal pregnancy. Thromb Haemost. 2009;101(4):755-61.

32. Obstetric Hemorrhage (+AIM). (2015). Council on Patient Safety in Women's Health Care. [online] Available from https://safehealthcareforeverywoman.org/patient-safety-bundles/obstetric-hemorrhage/. [Last accessed March, 2020].

33. OB Hem Task Force. (2015). OB Hem Risk Factor Assessment. California Maternal Quality Care Collaborative. [online] Available from https://www.cmqcc.org/resource/ob-hem-risk-factor-assessment. [Last accessed March, 2020].

34. The American College of Obstetricians and Gynecologists. Obstetric Hemorrhage. [online] Available from https://www.acog.org/About-ACOG/ACOG-Districts/District-II/SMI-OB-Hemorrhage. [Last accessed March, 2020].

35. Banayan JM, Hofer JE, Scavone BM. Antepartum and postpartum hemorrhage. In: Chestnut D, Wong C, Tsen L, Ngan Kee WD, Beilin Y, Mhyre J, Bateman BT, Nathan N (Eds). Chestnut's Obstetric Anesthesia, 6th edition. Philadelphia, PA: Elsevier; 2019. p. 913.

36. Yang X, Du B. Does pulse pressure variation predict fluid responsiveness in critically ill patients? A systematic review and meta-analysis. Crit Care. 2014;18(6):650.

37. Farquhar CM, Li Z, Lensen S, McLintock C, Pollock W, Peek MJ, et al. Incidence, risk factors and perinatal outcomes for placenta accreta in Australia and New Zealand: A case-control study. BMJ Open. 2017;7(10):e017713.

38. Panigrahi AK, Yeaton-Massey A, Bakhtary S, Andrews J, Lyell DJ, Butwick AJ, et al. A standardized approach for transfusion medicine support in patients with morbidly adherent placenta. Anesth Analg. 2017;125(2):603-8.

39. Grant TR, Ellinas EH, Kula AO, Muravyeva MY. Risk-stratification, resource availability, and choice of surgical location for the management of parturients with abnormal placentation: A survey of United States-based obstetric anesthesiologists. Int J Obstet Anesth. 2018;34:56-66.

40. Taylor NJ, Russell R. Anaesthesia for abnormally invasive placenta: A single-institution case series. Int J Obstet Anesth. 2017;30:10-5.

41. De Tina A, Palanisamy A. General anesthesia during the third trimester: Any link to neurocognitive outcomes? Anesthesiol Clin. 2017;35(1):69-80.

42. Hong JY, Jee YS, Yoon HJ, Kim SM. Comparison of general and epidural anesthesia in elective cesarean section for placenta previa totalis: Maternal hemodynamics, blood loss and neonatal outcome. Int J Obstet Anesth. 2003;12(1):12-6.

43. Pacheco LD, Saade GR, Hankins GDV. Medical management of postpartum hemorrhage: An update. Semin Perinatol. 2019;43(1):22-6.

44. Papazian J, Kacmar RM. Obstetric hemorrhage: Prevention, Recognition, and treatment. Adv Anesth. 2017;35(1):65-93.

45. Kogutt BK, Vaught AJ. Postpartum hemorrhage: Blood product management and massive transfusion. Semin Perinatol. 2019;43(1):44-50.

46. Butwick AJ, Goodnough LT. Transfusion and coagulation management in major obstetric hemorrhage. Curr Opin Anaesthesiol. 2015;28(3):275-84.

47. WOMAN Trial Collaborators. Effect of early tranexamic acid administration on mortality, hysterectomy, and other morbidities in women with post-partum haemorrhage (WOMAN): An international, randomised, double-blind, placebo-controlled trial. Lancet. 2017;389(10084):2105-16.

48. Murakami M, Kobayashi T, Kubo T, Hata T, Takeda S, Masuzaki H. Experience with recombinant activated factor VII for severe postpartum hemorrhage in Japan, investigated by Perinatology Committee, Japan Society of Obstetrics and Gynecology. J Obstet Gynaecol Res. 2015;41(8):1161-8.

49. Bell SF, Rayment R, Collins PW, Collis RE. The use of fibrinogen concentrate to correct hypofibrinogenaemia rapidly during obstetric haemorrhage. Int J Obstet Anesth. 2010;19(2):218-23.

50. Collins PW, Cannings-John R, Bruynseels D, Mallaiah S, Dick J, Elton C, et al. Viscoelastometric-guided early fibrinogen concentrate replacement during postpartum haemorrhage: OBS2, a double-blind randomized controlled trial. Br J Anaesth. 2017;119(3):411-21.

51. Levy JH, Welsby I, Goodnough LT. Fibrinogen as a therapeutic target for bleeding: A review of critical levels and replacement therapy. Transfusion. 2014;54(5):1388-405.

52. American College of Obstetricians and Gynecologists. ACOG practice bulletin: Clinical management guidelines for obstetrician-gynecologists number 76, October 2006: Postpartum hemorrhage. Obstet Gynecol. 2006;108(4):1039-47.

53. Krishna H, Chava M, Jasmine N, Shetty N. Patients with postpartum hemorrhage admitted in intensive care unit: Patient condition, interventions, and outcome. J Anaesthesiol Clin Pharmacol. 2011;27(2):192-4.

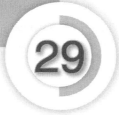
Perioperative Management of Major Gynecological Cancer

Rakesh Garg, Mahima Gupta

INTRODUCTION

Surgery forms the mainstay of treatment modalities for gynecological cancers which are potentially curable. Oncology patients undergoing surgery are nutritionally impaired, immunocompromised, and prone to infection and delayed wound healing and may have organ dysfunction due to pre-existing comorbidities and as a complication of neoadjuvant chemotherapy. This enhances the need for monitoring these postoperative patients in high-dependency unit (HDU) or critical care units.

The needs of patients after major gynecological oncosurgical interventions are varied and require not only early recognition but also its intensive management. Also, the patient requires intensive monitoring to identify these concerns and thus needs a well-equipped critical care unit with trained manpower. Equally important is to avoid occurrence of these complications and thus the need of preoperative optimization and intraoperative optimal management. Thus, reorganization of an optimal perioperative individualized care is of utmost importance after gynecological oncological surgeries.

Critical care management of gynecological oncological surgeries includes various components such as monitoring, airway and breathing, circulation and hemodynamics, coagulation, electrolyte and fluid imbalance, stress ulcer prophylaxis, thromboprophylaxis, and surgical complications like due to chemotherapeutic agents used during hyperthermic intraperitoneal chemotherapy (HIPEC).[1] A large number of critical care issues can arise and have to be addressed while caring for these patients requiring a good tertiary care setup. Some of these critical care issues are being addressed here in this chapter with an aim to understand various concerns and to maintain physiology of the patient and thus an uneventful recovery.

NEED FOR DEDICATED CRITICAL CARE FOR GYNECOLOGICAL CANCER SURGERIES

The gynecological oncological surgeries usually are extensive surgical interventions and alter body physiology. Timely and appropriately management in a controlled environment shall improve the overall outcome after the surgical intervention. Hence, management of these patients in dedicated critical care unit or similar monitoring unit shall be helpful. Dedicated care units allow for the multimodal management of patients after major surgery for improving uneventful and better functional recovery.[2] These include various components such as early postoperative rehabilitation, optimal analgesia with use of regional blocks, early feeding and nutrition, optimal fluid management, and judicious consideration for needs of tubes and drains. In addition, appropriate counseling and patient education remain equally important.[3,4] These concepts appear to be very apt for gynecological cancer surgeries as well. Nevertheless, the appropriate preoperative assessment and optimization of associated comorbidities shall also affect the overall postoperative outcome through proper planning.[4]

ENHANCED RECOVERY AFTER SURGERY FOR GYNECOLOGICAL CANCER SURGERIES

Enhanced recovery after surgery (ERAS) protocols have shown to be beneficial with regards to various perioperative recovery characteristics including decreased length of hospital stay and economic benefits along with better patient satisfaction.[4,5] ERAS is primarily related to protocolized perioperative care leading to avoidance of unnecessary variation in patient management and thus leading to better outcome with reduced costs. It aims at maintenance of physiology of the body in the perioperative period and attenuation of surgical stress, which finally leads to early and better mobilization even after major gynecological cancer surgeries. Various components of ERAS include nutritional optimization, avoidance of mechanical bowel preparation, thromboembolism prophylaxis, optimal fluid therapy with limited preoperative fasting and early postoperative oral intake, early removal of drains and tubes (including nasogastric tube, Foleys drain, and surgical drains), prevention of bowel ileus, optimal analgesia, management of nausea and vomiting, early ambulation, and patient counseling and education.[2,4,5] Overall improved perioperative outcome is primarily due to maintenance of body physiology being better maintained by components of ERAS.

BOWEL PREPARATION

Conventionally, mechanical and antibiotic bowel preparation was followed for major abdominal procedures, particularly if bowel resection was being contemplated.[6] This was in anticipation to prevent the risk of infection and bowel anastomosis dehiscence. However, it has been shown in a Cochrane review that use of mechanical bowel preparation does not improve the chances of such complications.[7] So, the use of bowel preparation is required in selected population such as low rectal anastomosis, significant tumor burden, with ascites and low serum albumin.[6] The use of mechanical bowel preparation needs to be avoided unless specifically indicated. The use of antibiotic prophylaxis should be as per institutional antibiotic policy and if suggested, then it should administer 1 hour before surgical incision.

THROMBOEMBOLISM IN GYNECOLOGICAL CANCER PATIENTS

The risk of thrombosis and embolism is higher in cancer patients, especially in patients undergoing gynecological cancer surgeries. The incidence varied from 7 to 45% with a fatal pulmonary embolism being 1%.[2,8] The factors include female gender, type of surgery, duration and extent of surgical intervention, length of hospital stay, ambulation, venous stasis due to compression by tumor masses, previous history of thrombosis, and anticancer treatments (surgery, chemotherapy, hormone therapy, molecularly targeted-therapy, and irradiation).[9-11] The risk is seen higher in major abdominal or pelvic surgery.[6] The cancer-related factors are release of tissue factors from cancer cells, which are procoagulant; release of inflammatory cytokines, monocytes, macrophages, platelet, and endothelial cells; and decreases in protein C and protein S levels.[2,8]

The use of deep vein thrombosis prophylaxis needs to be started timely and use of scoring, such as Caprini Risk Assessment score, shall be useful.[12] The use of screening tools using ultrasound and serum markers is useful as well to identify the thrombosis occurrence. The finding of presence of deep venous thrombosis is a strong surrogate evidence for possible occurrence of pulmonary embolism.[2] It is suggested to start thromboprophylaxis for gynecological cancer patients undergoing cancer surgeries preoperatively and continued for 7–10 days in the postoperative period. In high-risk cases with propensity of thrombosis and embolism, thromboprophylaxis may be continued for even 4 weeks. These groups of patients include patients with residual tumor, history of thrombosis and embolism, and obesity.[8,13] Delayed thrombosis up to 21 days after surgery has also been reported with an incidence of up to 40% and thus needs of thromboprophylaxis.[13]

The modality of perioperative thromboprophylaxis includes a combination of mechanical and pharmacological methods. Mechanical methods of thromboprophylaxis include graduated compression stockings, intermittent pneumatic calf compression devices, mechanical foot pumps, etc. These devices prevent the occurrence of thrombosis by preventing venous stasis or actively pump blood and thus avoid stasis in the deep venous system. These modalities are not efficacious when used alone but should be used in combination with pharmacological methods. The agents for pharmacological prophylaxis include unfractionated heparin (UFH), low-molecular-weight heparin (LMWH), fondaparinux, and vitamin-K antagonists such as warfarin.[11,14,15]

GYNECOLOGICAL ONCOSURGERY IN PATIENTS WITH PRE-EXISTING THROMBOSIS

Due to increased risk of thrombosis, patients of gynecological cancer may present with thrombosis preoperatively itself. The perioperative management for such patients remains challenging. Based on the patient's assessment, the extent of thrombosis, and the urgency of surgery, a plan needs to be individualized. Patients require appropriate anticoagulation prior to surgery itself and at times may require rescheduling of the surgery.[8] It is essential to anticoagulate these patients but carries the risk of increased bleeding in the perioperative period. On the other hand, avoiding anticoagulation carries the risk of embolism.[16] In view of urgency of surgery, placement of inferior vena caval filter may be advocated. This prevents pelvic and lower limb thrombus to emboli to central circulation.[8]

AMBULATION AND PHYSIOTHERAPY

Early mobilization of patient in the postoperative period improves body physiology and early recovery and hence steps needs to be taken to mobilize as early as possible in the postoperative period preferably within 24 hours of surgery. Patient should be encouraged to stand or stay in the sitting position and walk at the earliest. The respiratory physiotherapy such as deep breathing exercise and incentive spirometry also aids in early recovery and prevents respiratory morbidity such as pneumonia.[17] Early ambulation improves muscle tone and prevents lung atelectasis, especially in the bases, and thus improves pulmonary function, tissues perfusion, and oxygenation. Also, it involves a lesser risk of stress-induced insulin resistance.[18-20] This also mandates an optimal analgesia to allow early optimal ambulation. Early ambulation after surgery has been reported to have many beneficial effects on patient's overall outcome.[21] Patient education and its initiation for mobilization need to be started in the preoperative period itself. Good patient motivation and optimal analgesia remain the key for early mobilization after surgery.

ANALGESIA

Postoperative analgesia is often challenging in these surgeries as the procedures are extensive. Use of multimodal analgesic technique provides better analgesia. More recently, in cancer surgeries, opioid-sparing techniques such as the use of regional blocks have been found to improve outcome without added side effects of opioids that sometimes may lead to delayed recovery. Patients are often on prophylactic doses of LMWH, so the timing of regional anesthesia should be timed accordingly. This also requires adequate monitoring of pain score appropriately to titrate the analgesic requirement of the patient. The cancer patients may have pre-existing pain and thus needs to be optimized and continues in the perioperative period as well. Nonsteroidal anti-inflammatory drugs (NSAIDs) should be avoided as they can further compromise the renal function in case the patient develops nephrotoxicity due to the chemotherapeutic agent. The role of preventive analgesia also needs to be emphasized as initializing pain management before the noxious stimulus and peripheral and central receptors are blocked and thus appears to provide better analgesia.[5,8] Uncontrolled pain in postoperative period impacts the patient's quality of life and also affects early ambulation, feeding, respiratory physiotherapy, risk of thrombosis, etc. These may lead to increased catabolic stress response and increased length of stay.[6,8,22] The role of multimodal pain management including regional blocks has shown to provide better perioperative pain relief.[6]

DRAINS, TUBES, AND CATHETERS

The urine output monitoring is an important monitoring tool, especially after a major gynecological oncological surgery, and Foley catheterization provides an appropriate and accurate monitoring of urine output.[8] However, Foley catheter used for postoperative bladder drainage may be removed early, preferably within <24 hours. Early removal decreases the catheter-related complications such as infection and thus reduces the length of hospital stay.[6] The conventional indication for the insertion of the nasogastric tube was to decompress the stomach for reducing the complications related to regurgitation and aspiration, reducing the risk of nausea and vomiting, and promoting early bowel activity.[6] However, these indications have been refuted with recent evidences and are not associated for any of these beneficial benefits as thought conventionally.[8,23,24] Avoidance of nasogastric tube or its early removal, in case if it is indicated, also improves the recovery of the patient in the postoperative period. The routine use of peritoneal drains in gynecological surgeries with abdominal or pelvic surgery has not been shown to have a positive effect on the overall outcome.[25] The utility of surgical drains and its early removal have been found useful with lesser morbidity and anastomotic leakage rates. Also, the avoidance of drains for blood drain to avoid its intra-abdominal collection has been improved with meticulous dissection and hemostasis surgical techniques.[6,8]

NAUSEA AND VOMITING

Postoperative nausea and vomiting after gynecological oncological surgeries has adverse effect on the overall outcome. It not only delays the discharge but is also a reason for readmission after discharge. It is associated with various ill effects such as delayed wound healing, electrolyte imbalance, pain, risk of bleeding, and increased length of hospital stay.[8] Nausea and vomiting may be related to various anesthetic and surgical-related factors. These include the use of drugs such as opioids, female gender, history of smoking, and history of motion sickness.[6,15] Nausea and vomiting needs to be controlled as it leads to delayed recovery and poorer outcome, especially in gynecological cancer surgeries.[5,8] A multimodal approach using more than one antiemetics including $5HT_3$ antagonists, D_2 receptor antagonists, prokinetic agents, dexamethasone, and, more recently, NK_1 antagonists is desirable.

TEMPERATURE REGULATION

Hypothermia is reported to occur in major surgical interventions due to large exposures like in laparotomies for extended duration.[8] Hypothermia has been associated with increased risk of wound infection, dehiscence, impaired coagulation, cardiac events, and impaired oxygen transportation. These all lead to delayed postanesthetic recovery.[26,27] This may continue in the postoperative period as well due to major fluid shifts and resuscitation with fluid and blood products. It is suggested to use Bair Hugger and fluid warmers to maintain normothermia.

FASTING, FLUID, AND ORAL INTAKE

Restriction of prolonged preoperative fasting has been found to be useful. Patients may be allowed fluid intake even up to 2 hours prior to surgeries. Also, addition of carbohydrate loading 2 hours prior to surgery is useful. The fluid management in perioperative period should be goal-directed and overzealous fluid administration delays recovery and affects the surgical outcome by causing edema in body tissues leading to organ dysfunction.[6,8] Proper fluid administration reduces the number of postoperative complications and hospital stay, helps in the early return of peristaltic movements and flatus, and reduces the number of episodes of nausea, vomiting, and postoperative pain.[8,28]

Conventionally, patients were not allowed orally postoperatively due to the concern of abdominal distension, ileus, bowel obstruction, and prolonged length of stay. However, recent evidence is contrary to it. It has been found that early feeding after surgeries reduces morbidity without increasing bowel ileus or obstruction rates and improves patient satisfaction.[6] The beneficial effect of early feeding is via activation of cephalic-vagal pathway which in turn stimulates intestinal myoelectric activity of the gastrointestinal µ-opioid receptors leading to better bowel movement. Feeding orally in sitting position also facilitates bowel activity by eliciting the gastrocolic reflex.[8] The oral intake may be initiated on the day of surgery, if possible, and intravenous fluid therapy may be tapered subsequently. The oral intake may consist of protein-rich drinks as well to build the protein loss and for better recovery of the patient.

The surgical stress response triggers the endocrine responses and the sympathetic nervous system including hypothalamic-pituitary-adrenal (HPA) axis activation with secretion of cortisol and increase in peripheral insulin resistance. The control of blood glucose levels in the range of 180–200 mg/dL is desirable to avoid adverse effect of hyperglycemia such as infection, increased length of stay, and postoperative mortality.[29] A tight control regimen for glucose may lead to episodes of hypoglycemia.

MAINTENANCE OF HEMODYNAMICS

Major gynecological procedures are associated with major fluid shift. The surgical intervention such as cytoreductive surgeries (CRSs) along with procedures such as HIPEC procedures can lead to massive fluid shifts due to tissue trauma, altered capillary permeability, inflammation, damage to endothelium and glycocalyx, bleeding, and loss of plasma proteins during ascitic fluid drainage. Also,

hemodynamic fluctuations may happen due to ascitic fluid removal during surgery like in cases of advanced ovarian carcinoma. This fluid is rich in proteins (exidroma), out of which 50–70% is albumin, 30–40% globulins, and 0.3–4.5% fibrinogen.[30] The manifestations of such fluid shifts affect hemodynamics not only in the intraoperative period but also continue in the postoperative period.[31] HIPEC procedure usually results in a hypermetabolic state with peripheral vasodilation, with accompanying decrease in stroke volume and increase in the heart rate to balance the increased demand of high cardiac output. This phenomenon necessitates vasopressor requirement even after optimal fluid resuscitation to maintain adequate tissue perfusion. Aggressive monitoring in the intensive care unit using dynamic hemodynamic indices should be done to guide the fluid therapy or the vasopressor requirement. Monitoring of drain and urine output, and noninvasive cardiac monitoring with FlowTrac are advisable.[32] A urine output of at least 1–2 mL/kg/h should be maintained post-HIPEC.[32] Lactate is a surrogate marker for tissue perfusion, and it is advisable to follow its trend rather than a single constant value. Crystalloids are the first choice of fluid for resuscitation and albumin infusion should be considered a good option for patients developing hypoalbuminemia as it restores the protein levels, maintains the oncotic pressure, and assists in intravascular volume optimization. Routine use of low-dose dopamine and furosemide is not recommended. Excessive fluid administration can cause tissue edema, fluid overload, and abdominal and cardiac complications. Neoadjuvant chemotherapy comprising of cisplatin can cause autonomic dysfunction. Autonomic disturbances can lead to hypotension, requiring vasopressors mandating HDU monitoring.[33] While chemotherapeutic agents such as docetaxel and paclitaxel may cause cardiac dysfunction requiring intraoperative invasive monitoring and also in the intensive care, taxanes can lead to prolonged QT interval and in these patients, drugs such as dexmedetomidine, glycopyrrolate, atropine, and caution should be excised with drugs such as ondansetron, metoclopramide, and dexamethasone.

COAGULATION

Coagulation abnormalities can occur perioperatively in CRS with HIPEC. Patients are prone to coagulation abnormalities due to preoperative chemotherapy and hypoalbuminemia due to ascitic drainage and nutritional deficiencies.[34] Excessive volume resuscitation can cause dilution of platelets and coagulation factors leading to functional decrease in platelet count and deranged coagulation profile. Fresh frozen plasma (FFP) transfusions may be required to correct these parameters if there is an evidence of bleeding postoperatively, which can manifest as hemodynamic instability, hemorrhagic fluid, or fresh blood from surgical drains and abdominal distension with associated hypertension. The coagulation profile usually takes at least 5 days to normalize.[35] Coagulation profile is most commonly monitored using prothrombin time (PT), activated partial thromboplastin time (aPTT), or international normalized ratio (INR). Other point-of-care techniques such as thromboelastography (TEG or ROTEM) or activated coagulation time (ACT) can be used.[31,32]

BREATHING AND RESPIRATION

The respiratory status may also be affected in gynecological procedures in view of extensive prolonged duration of surgery, massive fluid shifts, and heated chemotherapy, which can lead to peritoneal inflammation and systemic inflammatory response. During CRS, diaphragmatic stripping of the tumor and its resection with or without reconstruction take place and may affect the breathing system. These patients should be monitored for the development of pleural effusion, hemothorax, and pneumothorax, the management of which should be done appropriately. Bedside lung ultrasound has proven a boon for the intensivists.[36] The risk of basal atelectasis and lung collapse due to pre-existing ascites and pleural effusion predisposing the patients to postoperative pulmonary complications such as pneumonia also remain. A detailed history, clinical examination, chest imaging, preoperative drainage of ascites, and pleural effusion may be undertaken if it improves the physical condition of the patient. Incentive spirometry and deep breathing exercises are recommended to negate the effects of lung collapse and general anesthesia postoperatively. Even during the HIPEC procedure, there is an increase in intra-abdominal pressure leading to intraoperative basal atelectasis and increased airway pressures. Continuous positive pressure ventilation (CPAP) and high-flow nasal cannula (HFNC) can be used for the recruitment of lung areas and prevention of respiratory complications.[35,36] Active management of postoperative atelectasis to prevent pneumonia and sepsis is required as their patients are prone to rapidly develop infections. Optimal pain control after upper abdomen surgeries is the cornerstone for prevention of postoperative pulmonary complications (PPCs). Pain contributes to restricted diaphragmatic movements, reduced lung expansion, and mobility.[37] Hyperthermia during intraperitoneal chemotherapy can lead to ventilator-induced acute lung injury and pulmonary edema. Vigorous respiratory toilet, including the use of incentive spirometry and patient positioning, is an integral part of postoperative care. If acute respiratory distress occurs, pulmonary embolus, myocardial infarction, or congestive heart failure should be considered.

ELECTROLYTE AND METABOLIC IMBALANCE

Significant electrolyte imbalance can occur after HIPEC, considering the extensive nature of the surgery, fluid loss, effect of the dialysate carrying the chemotherapeutic agent, and the agent itself. The lactates have to be monitored serially. There is a propensity for lactate levels to rise since HIPEC simulates an aseptic vasodilatory shock state. Baseline electrolyte profile is necessary for comparison perioperatively. There can be hyponatremia, hyperglycemia, and metabolic acidosis (especially if oxaliplatin is used in 5% dextrose).[31] Cisplatin and oxaliplatin can cause hyponatremia, hypocalcemia, hypokalemia, and renal magnesium wasting leading to QT prolongation.

STRESS ULCER THROMBOPROPHYLAXIS

Patients can develop stress ulcers owing to long hours of fasting, prolonged surgery, hypotension, use of vasopressors analgesics such as corticosteroids and NSAIDs, and delayed start of feeds postoperatively. Stress ulcer prophylaxis with proton pump inhibitor or H_2 receptor antagonists is advisable.

OVERVIEW OF INTRAOPERATIVE MANAGEMENT

A well-planned intraoperative management is desirable for gynecological oncological procedures. The surgical intervention may be of varied extent and duration. The inclusion of prehabilitation concept has beneficial effect on the operative outcome. The choice of anesthetic technique depends on the type and the extent of surgeries. Usually, practice shall be a combination of general anesthesia along with the regional block. The use of regional block could be central neuraxial block or a plane block. These have opioid-sparing effect and provide better analgesia. Apart from routine monitoring, additional monitoring such as use of cardiac output monitors shall depend on patient comorbidity and extent of surgeries. The blood loss should be appropriately monitored and replaced adequately. The risk of blood transfusion and its impact on immunomodulation and cancer recurrence remain a concern. The need of postoperative ventilation depends on intraoperative condition and at time may be required in cases of massive blood loss.

SURGICAL COMPLICATIONS

Most common complications related to the procedure were wound disruption/infection, gastrointestinal fistula, genitourinary fistula, and ileus/small bowel obstruction. Mortality is rare and age associated with more risk in patients

>65 years of age. Sepsis, adult respiratory distress syndrome, heart failure, pulmonary embolus, and multiorgan system failure are typical terminal events. Complications relating to prior medical problems and those seen with more commonly performed gynecologic procedures may also occur. CRS is associated with intra-abdominal sepsis, anastomotic leaks, intestinal perforation, bile leaks, pancreatitis, infections, intestinal fistula, renal failure, ureteric or diaphragmatic injury, bleeding, and sepsis.[38,39] Surgical complications due to pelvic exenteration procedures are related to small bowel obstruction which can eventually culminate into source of sepsis. Risk factors for acute kidney injury in major noncardiac surgeries include chronic renal dysfunction, preoperative hypoalbuminemia, increased body mass index, surgical time >600 minutes and hyperglycemia during surgery, transfusion of blood products, and blood loss. All these concerns require vigilance and repeated assessment for early detection and management.

Prolonged position-related neurological complications may be seen after surgeries. Postoperative period requires identification and timely management of these complications to prevent permanent neurological deficit.

To conclude, the gynecological oncological surgical interventions are challenging. A meticulous planning is required for perioperative period for an uneventful outcome. A critical care backup is essential to combat any untoward event and also to monitor these patients for early detection and management.

■ REFERENCES

1. Solanki SL, Mukherjee S, Agarwal V, Thota RS, Balakrishnan K, Shah SB, et al. Society of Onco-Anaesthesia and Perioperative Care consensus guidelines for perioperative management of patients for cytoreductive surgery and hyperthermic intraperitoneal chemotherapy (CRS-HIPEC). Indian J Anaesth. 2019;63(12):972-87.

2. Uyeda MGBK, Girão MJBC, Carbone EDSM, Fonseca MCM, Takaki MR, Sartori MGF. Fast-track protocol or perioperative care in gynaecological surgeries: cross-sectional study. Taiwane J Obstet gynecol. 2019;58(3):359-63.

3. Powell R, Scott NW, Manyande A, Bruce J, Vögele C, Byrne-Davis LM, et al. Psychological preparation and postoperative outcomes for adults undergoing surgery under general anaesthesia. Cochrane Database Syst Rev. 2016;5:CD008646.

4. Dahabreh IJ, Steele DW, Shah N, Trikalinos TA. Oral mechanical bowel preparation for colorectal surgery: systematic review and meta-analysis. Dis Colon Rectum. 2015;58(7):698-707.

5. Nelson G, Bakkum-Gamez J, Kalogera E, Glaser G, Altman A, Meyer LA, et al. Guidelines for perioperative in gynecologic/oncology: Enhanced recovery after surgery (ERAS) society recommendations-2019 update. Int J Gynecol Cancer. 2019;29(4):651-68.

6. Carter J. Fast-track surgery in gynecology and gynaecologic oncology: a review of a rolling clinical audit. ISRN Surgery. 2012;368014:1-19.

7. Guenaga KK, Matos D, Wille-Jørgensen P. Mechanical bowel preparation for elective colorectal surgery. Cochrane Database Syst Rev. 2011;(9):CD001544.

8. Gadducci A, Cosio S, Spiriti N, Genazzani AR. The perioperative management of patients with gynecological cancer undergoing major surgery: a debated clinical challenge. Crit Rev Oncol Hematol. 2010;73(2):126-40.

9. Levitan N, Dowlati A, Remick SC, Tahsildar HI, Sivinski LD, Beyth R, et al. Rates of initial and recurrent thromboembolic disease among patients with malignancy versus those without malignancy. Risk analysis using Medicare claims data. Medicine (Baltimore). 1999;78(5):285-91.

10. Einstein MH, Pritts EA, Hartenbach EM. Venous thrombo-embolism prevention in gynecologic cancer surgery: a systematic review. Gynecol Oncol. 2007;105(3):813-9.

11. Von Tempelhoff GF, Heilmann L. Antithrombotic therapy in gynecologic surgery and gynecologic oncology. Hematol Oncol Clin North Am. 2000;14(5):1151-69.

12. Caprini JA. Thrombosis risk assessment as a guide to quality patient care. Dis Mon. 2005;51(2-3):70-8.

13. Agnelli G, Bolis G, Capussotti L, Scarpa RM, Tonelli F, Bonizzoni E, et al. A clinical outcome-based prospective study on venous thromboembolism after cancer surgery: the @RISTOS project. Ann Surg. 2006;243(1):89-95.

14. De Cicco M. The prothrombotic state in cancer: pathogenic mechanisms. Crit Rev Oncol Hematol. 2004;50(3):187-96.

15. Oates-Whitehead RM, D'Angelo A, Mol B. Anticoagulant and aspirin prophylaxis for preventing thromboembolism after major gynaecological surgery. Cochrane Database Syst Rev. 2003;(4):CD003679.

16. Clarke-Pearson DL. Prevention of venous thromboembolism in gynecologic surgery patients. Curr Opin Obstet Gynecol. 1993;5(1):73-9.

17. Kehlet H. Multimodal approach to control postoperative pathophysiology and rehabilitation. Br J Anaesth. 1997;78(5):606-17.

18. Kalogera E, Dowdy SC. Enhanced recovery pathway in gynecologic surgery: improving outcomes through evidence based medicine. Obstet Gynecol Clin North Am. 2016;43(3):551-73.

19. Kehlet H, Wilmore DW. Evidence-based surgical care and the evolution of fast-track surgery. Ann Surg. 2008;248(2):189-98.

20. Wren SM, Martin M, Yoon JK, Bech F. Postoperative pneumonia-prevention program for the inpatient surgical ward. J Am Coll Surg. 2010;210(4):491-5.

21. Marx C, Rasmussen T, Jakobson DH, Ottosen C, Lundvall L, Ottesen B, et al. The effect of accelerated rehabilitation on recovery after surgery for ovarian malignancy. Acta Obs Gyn Scand. 2006;85(4):488-92.

22. Power I, Barratt S. Analgesic agents for the postoperative period: nonopioids. Surg Clin North Am. 1999;79(2):275-95.

23. Cheatham ML, Chapman WC, Key SP, Sawyers JL. A meta-analysis of selective versus routine nasogastric decompression after elective laparotomy. Ann Surg. 1995;221(5):469-78.

24. Nelson R, Edwards S, Tse B. Prophylactic nasogastric decompression after abdominal surgery. Cochrane Database Syst Rev. 2007;(3):CD004929.

25. Lopes AD, Hall JR, Monaghan JM. Drainage following radical hysterectomy and pelvic lymphadenectomy: dogma or need? Obstet Gynecol. 1995;86(6):960-3.

26. Kurtz A, Sessler I, Lenhardt R. Perioperative normothermia to reduce the incidence of surgical wound infection and shorten hospitalization. N Eng J Med. 1996;334(19):1209-15.

27. Lenhardt R, Marker E, Goll V, Tschernich H, Kurz A, Sessler DI, et al. Mild intraoperative hypothermia prolongs postanesthestic recovery. Anesthesiology. 1997;87(6):1318-23.

28. Jia FJ, Yan QY, Sun Q, Tuxun T, Liu H, Shao L. Liberal versus restrictive fluid management in abdominal surgery: A meta-analysis. Surg Today. 2017;47(3):344-56.

29. Al-Niaimi AN, Ahmed M, Burish N, Chackmakchy SA, Seo S, Rose S, et al. Intensive postoperative glucose control reduces the surgical site infection rates in gynecologic oncology patients. Gynecol Oncol. 2015;136(1):71-6.

30. Vorgios G, Iavazzo C, Mavromatis J, Leontara J, Katsoulis M, Kalinoglou N, et al. Determination of the necessary total protein substitution requirements in patients with advanced stage ovarian cancer and ascites, undergoing debulking surgery. Correlation with plasma proteins. Ann Surg Oncol. 2006;14(6):1919-23.

31. Raspe C, Flother L, Schenider R, Bucher M, Piso P. Best practice for perioperative management of patients with cytoreductive surgery and HIPEC. Eur J Surg Oncol. 2017;43(6):1013-27.

32. Garg R. Cytoreductive surgery and hyperthermic intraperitoneal chemotherapy: Fluid and temperature remain the culprit! Indian J Anaesth. 2018;62(3):162-5.

33. Lacerda AM. Chemotherapy and anesthesia. Rev Bras Anestesiol. 2001;51(3):250-70.

34. Gupta N, Kumar V, Garg R, Bharati SJ, Mishra S, Bhatnagar S. Anesthetic implications in hyperthermic intraperitoneal chemotherapy. J Anaesthesiol Clin Pharmacol. 2019;35(1):3-11.

35. Padmakumar AV. Intensive care management of patients after cytoreductive surgery and HIPEC—A concise review. Indian J Surg Oncol. 2016;7(2):244-8.

36. Ahmed S, Oropello MJ. Critical care issues in Oncological Surgery patients. Crit Care Clin. 2010;26(1):93-106.

37. Restrepo RD, Braveman J. Current challenges in the recognition, prevention and treatment of perioperative pulmonary atelectasis. Expert Rev Respir Med. 2015;9(1):97-107.

38. Verwaal VJ, van Ruth S, de Bree E, van Sloothen GW, van Tinteren H, Boot H, et al. Randomized trial of cytoreduction and hyperthermic intraperitoneal chemotherapy versus systemic chemotherapy and palliative surgery in patients with peritoneal carcinomatosis of colorectal cancer. J Clin Oncol. 2003;21(20):3737-43.

39. Jaehne J. Cytoreductive procedures-strategies to reduce postoperative morbidity and management of surgical complications with special emphasis on anastomotic leaks. J Surg Oncol. 2009;100(4):302-5.

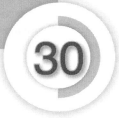

30

Perioperative Management of Patients with Pre-eclampsia and Eclampsia

Gauri Saroj, Sonali Saraf, Dilip R Karnad

CASE HISTORY

A 26-year-old primigravida was detected to have hypertension with a blood pressure (BP) of 150/100 mm Hg during a routine antenatal visit during the 25th week of pregnancy. She was started on oral methyldopa in a dose of 250 mg twice daily. BP was controlled for the first 4 weeks and then it gradually started increasing despite an increase in the dose of methyldopa and addition of oral labetalol. Urine examination showed absence of proteinuria. Baseline blood tests showed that serum creatinine was 0.5 mg/dL, uric acid 3.2 mg/dL, hemoglobin 12 g/dL, total leukocyte count 9,600/μL, platelet count 3,10,000/μL, serum glutamic oxaloacetic transaminase (SGOT) 38 IU/mL, and serum glutamic pyruvic transaminase (SGPT) 43 IU/mL. An obstetric ultrasonography (29th week of gestation by date) of a single live fetus with intrauterine growth retardation with fetal size corresponding to 26 weeks.

During the 31st week of pregnancy, she came to the emergency room with a history of severe headache and blurring of vision. BP had increased to 170/112 mm Hg, heart rate 100 bpm, and other vital signs were normal. Systemic examination was unremarkable and fundus examination showed no papilledema. She was admitted to a general room in the hospital for observation.

Laboratory tests showed: Hb 11.4 g/dL, white blood cell (WBC) count 9,600/μL, platelets 118,000/μL, SGOT 49 IU/mL, SGPT 38 IU/mL, serum albumin 3.2 g/dL, normal liver function tests, creatinine 1.0 mg/dL, urine protein ++, serum uric acid 5.9 mg/dL.

HYPERTENSION IN PREGNANCY: DEFINITIONS

The American College of Obstetrics and Gynecology has published definitions for various hypertensive disorders in pregnancy.[1]

Chronic hypertension is hypertension that predates pregnancy or is detected before 20 weeks of gestation.

Gestational hypertension or pregnancy-induced hypertension is BP elevation after 20 weeks of pregnancy in the absence of preeclampsia.

Preeclampsia is defined as BP ≥ 140/90 mm Hg on two occasions 4 hours apart after 20 weeks of gestation in a woman with previously normal BP, and *proteinuria* is defined as >300 mg/24 hours, or protein/creatinine ratio > 0.3, or dipstick reading of 1+ or higher. In the absence of proteinuria, it may be diagnosed if hypertension is accompanied by platelet count <100,000/μL or creatinine > 1.1 mg/dL or liver transaminases >2 times normal.

Severe preeclampsia is defined by the presence of any one of the following:

- Systolic BP > 160 mm Hg or diastolic BP > 110 mm Hg on two occasions 4 hours apart while the patient is on bed rest
- Platelet count > 1,00,000/μL, impaired liver function, persistent right upper quadrant pain or epigastric pain not explained by an alternative diagnosis
- Progressive renal insufficiency with serum creatinine > 1.1 mg/dL or doubling of serum creatinine
- Pulmonary edema
- New onset of cerebral or visual disturbance.

Superimposed preeclampsia is diagnosed if a chronic hypertensive woman develops preeclampsia. In the initial stages, the classical criteria for diagnosis of preeclampsia may not be met. Features that should arouse suspicion of evolving preeclampsia include sudden increase in BP that was previously well controlled and increase in proteinuria. Rapid weight gain, increased nondependent edema, and rising serum uric acid are other warning signs.

Eclampsia is defined as the presence of new-onset grand mal seizures in a woman with preeclampsia. It can occur before, during, or after labor.

Based on the clinical course and laboratory tests, this patient had gestational hypertension at 25 weeks. Subsequently, when seen in the 31st week of pregnancy, she met the criteria for diagnosis of preeclampsia when she was admitted to the hospital (hypertension with BP > 160/110 mm Hg, visual disturbances, and proteinuria). The plan of treatment was to treat the hypertension under observation in hospital and keep a close watch for new-onset organ involvement or development of features of severe preeclampsia or eclampsia. If the pregnancy could be safely continued for a few more weeks, this would improve fetal maturation and survival. Fetal well-being too could be closely monitored during the hospital stay.

PATHOPHYSIOLOGY OF PREECLAMPSIA

Hypertension affects 10% of pregnant women, and preeclampsia complicates around 5–7% of all pregnant women.[2,3] It is responsible for over 70,000 maternal deaths and 500,000 fetal deaths worldwide every year.[3] Of the 71,792 estimated maternal deaths in India in 2013, hypertensive disorders were responsible for 6,043 deaths.[4] Preeclampsia and its complications account for nearly 50% of all obstetric admissions to the ICU.[5-7]

Preeclampsia is a multisystem disease characterized by impaired organ perfusion resulting from vasospasm and activation of the coagulation system.[1,3,8] It is more common in primigravida or the first pregnancy with a particular partner. Other risk factors include a positive family history, preexisting hypertension, diabetes mellitus, multiple pregnancy, increasing maternal age, autoimmune diseases, increased interval between pregnancies, chronic kidney disease, and obesity.[1,3]

The pathogenesis of preeclampsia appears to result from abnormal placenta formation.[1,3] Failure of the second phase of trophoblast invasion results in the lack of destruction of the muscularis layer of the spiral arterioles, impairing vasodilation and resulting in placental ischemia. The ischemic placenta releases vasoactive and angiogenic substances that cause systemic endothelial injury and systemic organ dysfunction in the mother.[1,3] As pregnancy progresses, placental ischemia worsens and the mother becomes hypertensive and hypovolemic and may develop renal dysfunction.[3,8] There is disordered prostaglandin metabolism resulting in platelet dysfunction, endothelial damage, and further vasoconstriction. Abnormalities in the renin-angiotensin system, release of cytokines, and altered sympathetic nervous system function also contribute to the pathogenesis of preeclampsia.[3,8]

The characteristic renal lesion of preeclampsia is caused by glomeruloendotheliosis that results in a reduced glomerular filtration rate and increased glomerular permeability that manifests as proteinuria.[9] Cardiovascular changes in preeclamptic patients are complex. Increased systemic vascular resistance, reduced intravascular volume, and reduction in cardiac output accompany hypertension, as disease severity progresses. Left ventricular function tends to deteriorate with worsening preload and afterload such that overzealous fluid resuscitation can precipitate pulmonary edema. The propensity to pulmonary edema is further exacerbated by reduction in colloid oncotic pressure and increased capillary permeability.[1,3,8]

Eclampsia is an extreme complication of preeclampsia and is defined by the occurrence of seizures in the absence of other neurologic disorders. Up to 40% of seizures occur following delivery. Convulsions are believed to result from severe intracranial vasospasm, local ischemia, intracranial hypertension, and endothelial dysfunction associated with vasogenic and cytotoxic edema. Seizures tend to be self-limiting, and status epilepticus is unusual.[1,6,10]

CLINICAL FEATURES

Preeclampsia is a serious complication of pregnancy; its onset is insidious and some symptoms such as pedal edema resemble "normal" effects of pregnancy. Moreover, in a pregnant lady with chronic hypertension, recognition of the onset of superimposed preeclampsia is difficult, yet important, as the management drastically changes.[1]

Common clinical features include edema on the feet and hands and puffiness around the eyes. Headache usually correlates with the severity of hypertension. Nausea or vomiting is significant when the onset is sudden and after midpregnancy. Abdominal pain in the epigastrium and right hypochondrium or shoulder pain could be the only symptom of severe preeclampsia. Sudden weight gain, shortness of breath, anxiety, decreased urine output, and visual changes require prompt and detailed assessment.[1,10-12] The diagnosis of preeclampsia is confirmed by the presence of hypertension and proteinuria. Severe preeclampsia is confirmed by the presence of BP > 160/110 mm Hg, thrombocytopenia, elevated liver transaminases, increase in serum creatinine, deranged coagulation tests, and new onset of neurological symptoms including hyper-reflexia. Severe hypertension along with altered mental status and laboratory abnormalities suggesting severe preeclampsia are indications for hospital admission, usually in the ICU as life-threatening complications can develop within few hours.[1,10-14]

BIOMARKERS

Biomarkers for the prediction of preeclampsia are being studied.[1,2] Promising biomarkers include angiogenic factors such as soluble fms-like tyrosine kinase-1 (sFlt-1), placental growth factor (PlGF), and soluble endoglin.[1-3] Detecting elevated levels of these early in the second trimester could predict onset of preeclampsia and help distinguish preeclampsia from other hypertensive-proteinuric disorders; however, this requires further investigation.[1,2] Current evidence suggests that a combination of these biomarkers along with uterine artery Doppler studies may provide the best predictive accuracy for the identification of early onset preeclampsia.[1,3]

DIAGNOSIS/DIFFERENTIAL DIAGNOSIS

Severe preeclampsia is diagnosed by the presence of BP > 160/110 mm Hg, thrombocytopenia, elevated serum transaminases, right upper quadrant or epigastric pain, progressive renal insufficiency, pulmonary edema, and new-onset cerebral or visual disturbances.

Some pregnant women present with a specific constellation of laboratory findings—hemolysis, elevated liver enzymes, and low platelet count—the "HELLP syndrome." The HELLP syndrome is often considered a variant or subtype of preeclampsia since most women with this syndrome also have coexisting hypertension and proteinuria.[10,11,14]

The HELLP syndrome is also closely mimicked by thrombotic thrombocytopenic purpura (TTP).[10-15] The two can be differentiated by an elevated serum lactate dehydrogenase level, often in the absence of preeclampsia in TTP. Neurologic abnormalities and acute renal failure are often seen in TTP and the hemolytic uremic syndrome (HUS).[10,15] ADAMTS13 (a Disintegrin and Metalloproteinase with Thrombospondin motifs, member 13) deficiency in blood is diagnostic of TTP.

Acute fatty liver of pregnancy (AFLP) too could mimic HELLP syndrome. Anorexia, nausea, and vomiting are common clinical features of AFLP. Low-grade fever may be present. Unlike HELLP, AFLP is associated with more serious liver dysfunction, hypoglycemia, elevations in serum ammonia, and disseminated intravascular coagulation (DIC). Mild DIC may also complicate HELLP or preeclampsia. Acute kidney injury is more common in AFLP as compared to HELLP syndrome or preeclampsia.[11-13]

Other hypertensive-proteinuric disorders that mimic preeclampsia include systemic lupus erythematosus (SLE) and other rheumatological disorders and acute or chronic glomerulonephritis.[11,13] Flares of SLE are associated with hypocomplementemia and increased titers of anti-dsDNA antibodies. Complement levels are usually normal or increased in preeclampsia.

Eclampsia with seizures and coma should be differentiated from hypertensive intracranial hemorrhage, subarachnoid hemorrhage due to ruptured berry aneurysm,

> **Box 1:** Five-step approach to critical care in pregnancy.
> - Step 1: Is this a medical disorder or obstetric disorder?
> - Step 2: Is there failure of multiple organ systems?
> - Step 3: Is there a risk to the mother or fetus if pregnancy is continued?
> - Step 4: Early delivery—vaginal or cesarean section? General or neuraxial anesthesia?
> - Step 5: What needs to be done to optimize the patient for delivery?

central nervous system (CNS) lupus, cerebral venous sinus thrombosis, cerebral malaria, and acute viral hepatitis E infection with hypoglycemia. A general dictum is that seizure after 20 weeks of pregnancy should be managed as eclampsia till another diagnosis is found.[10]

Antiphospholipid syndrome can present in pregnancy with hypertension, proteinuria, and thrombocytopenia and thrombotic manifestations. Laboratory evidence of antiphospholipid antibodies should be looked for in an appropriate setting.

MANAGEMENT

A systematic approach is important in the management of a critically ill obstetric patient in the ICU. This has been discussed in detail in a recent review.[11] This involves five steps (**Box 1**). An assessment and management plan involves close interaction between many specialties such as obstetrics, anesthesia, intensive care, and neonatology.

Step 1: Is this a Medical Disorder or an Obstetric Disorder?

Many medical disorders may mimic preeclampsia and must be looked for. SLE may flare up in pregnancy leading to hypertension, lupus nephritis, immune thrombocytopenia, and seizures, mimicking eclampsia. Presence of malar rash, arthritis, and oral ulcers should be looked for and the diagnosis confirmed by detecting appropriate autoantibodies. Similarly, diagnosing superimposed preeclampsia is very difficult in pregnant patients with chronic kidney disease because of overlap of clinical features such as hypertension, proteinuria, and rising creatinine.[11]

Step 2: Is There Failure of Multiple Organ Systems?

Most patients with critical illness in pregnancy have multiple organ failure. Physiological changes in pregnancy may make it difficult to identify organ dysfunction. For example, serum creatinine of 1.2 mg/dL may be normal in a nonpregnant patient but serum creatinine decreases by >50% in pregnancy, and this value could imply acute kidney injury in pregnancy. Moreover, AFLP or the HELLP syndrome may occur with increased frequency in preeclampsia. The extent of involvement of specific organs could help identify the presence of these disorders.[11-13]

Step 3: Is there a Risk to the Mother or Fetus if Pregnancy is Continued?

Severe preeclampsia and eclampsia are usually indications for urgent termination of pregnancy. The organ dysfunction often progresses rapidly and may be fatal for the mother necessitating prompt delivery. On the other hand, continuation of pregnancy till 37 weeks may be considered in a mother who appears to be improving with initial management. Fetal well-being should be monitored carefully in such cases. Ultrasonographic assessment of the biophysical profile is often used to assess fetal well-being. Growth restriction due to placental insufficiency and prematurity contributes to a poor fetal outcome. Fetal risk of early delivery versus continuing pregnancy in an unfavorable uterine environment needs to be carefully balanced by frequent evaluation by the obstetrician and a neonatologist. The need for prolonged neonatal intensive care and prognosis should be discussed in detail with the patient and her family.[11-13]

Step 4: Early Delivery—Vaginal or Cesarean Section? General or Neuraxial Anesthesia?

By and large, urgent cesarean section under general anesthesia is the preferred mode of delivery and is discussed in more detail in the following text.[11]

Step 5: What Needs to be done to Optimize the Patient for Delivery?

Optimization usually means initial maternal resuscitation, medications to optimize BP and fluid balance, correction of thrombocytopenia and coagulation abnormalities, treatment of seizures, and care of airway and breathing where appropriate. Two doses of intravenous (IV) betamethasone or dexamethasone (12 mg) are administered 12 hours apart to improve fetal lung maturation if the gestational age is between 24 and 34 weeks. IV magnesium sulfate ($MgSO_4$) is also commonly used for its dual effect of tocolysis and fetal neuroprotection in pregnancies of <32 weeks.[11-13]

Three days later, this patient had a seizure. She was immediately transferred to the ICU.

Critical Care Management

Early diagnosis and management of preeclampsia, eclampsia, and HELLP syndrome are critical with involvement of a multidisciplinary team that includes

> **Box 2:** Points to remember when intubating a critically ill obstetric patient.[12]
>
> - Perform a rapid and complete airway assessment
> - Have a low threshold for calling for help
> - Neutralize gastric acid
> - Optimize patient positioning and displace the uterus laterally to prevent aortocaval compression
> - Choose the most appropriate laryngoscopic device
> - Have difficult airway equipment readily available
> - Select a smaller diameter endotracheal tube as there may be airway edema
> - Preoxygenation for at least 3 minutes with 100% oxygen
> - Have a back-up plan should intubation with standard laryngoscopic technique prove difficult or impossible
> - After intubation, consider spontaneous ventilation modes as positive-pressure ventilation may worsen the effects of aortocaval compression on venous return.

obstetrics, maternal–fetal medicine, critical care, anesthesia, and neonatology.[11-13]

While traditionally the mortality from eclampsia has been high, death is now uncommon due to neurological complications, and much of the mortality is attributable to other complications including hepatic failure, hemorrhage, acute kidney injury, or severe sepsis. Initial evaluation and resuscitation of the obstetric patient should focus on airway, breathing, and circulation. A good understanding of the physiological and anatomical changes in pregnancy is important to optimally evaluate and manage the critically ill obstetric patient.[11-13]

Airway and Breathing

If the patient is maintaining airway in lateral position and the SpO_2 is >95% with a nonrebreathing mask, after thorough suctioning one can wait for tracheal intubation. Keep in mind that a difficult intubation is 4 times more likely in the obstetric population and failed intubation is 10 times more likely; all obstetric patients should be considered as having potential difficult airways (**Box 2**).[11-13]

Circulation

Two large-bore IV canulae (16G or 18G) should be placed to administer IV fluids. A Foley catheter should be inserted to monitor urine output. Judicious fluid administration is needed to optimize preload and at the same time to avoid pulmonary edema. Central venous pressure monitoring may be required in certain cases. Uterine displacement should be considered part of the initial airway, breathing, and circulation (ABC) evaluation in the hemodynamically unstable obstetric patient. A wedge or doubled-up pillow can be placed under the patient's right hip to facilitate inclination to her left.[11-13]

An invasive arterial line for close and accurate monitoring of BP may be needed. The goal of antihypertensive treatment is prevention of potential complications such as stroke (intracerebral hemorrhage), cardiac failure, and placental abruption while maintaining a pressure that is adequate to maintain uteroplacental perfusion. A slow but steady reduction of BP to between 140–160 mm Hg systolic and 90–110 mm Hg diastolic is usually optimal. Avoid large precipitous drops in BP as this may compromise uteroplacental perfusion.[1,11-13]

The drugs commonly used in the acute setting for BP control are as follows:[1,11-13]

Labetalol: 20 mg IV gradually over 2 minutes followed by a continuous IV infusion of 1–2 mg/min can be used. If BP remains >160/110 mm Hg after 10 minutes, another bolus of 40 mg is given IV over 2 minutes. The cumulative maximum dose is 300 mg.

Hydralazine: 5 mg IV gradually over 1–2 minutes. Adequate reduction of BP is less predictable than with IV labetalol. If BP remains above the target level at 20 minutes, repeat the IV dose of 5 or 10 mg administered over 2 minutes. Repeat the doses if target levels are not achieved or the maximum dose is 30 mg.

Nifedipine extended release: 10–20 mg orally. If target BP is not achieved in 1–2 hours, another dose can be administered. A sublingual dose of 5–10 mg can be used, but this often results in a precipitous drop in the BP that could compromise uteroplacental blood flow.

Nicardipine (parenteral): The initial dose is 5 mg/h IV by an infusion pump and can be increased to a maximum of 15 mg/h. Rapid titration is avoided to minimize the risk of overshooting dose.

In general, one should switch over to another class of agent if target BP is not achieved with a single antihypertensive drug.

Fetal Monitoring

Fetal monitoring is an essential aspect of the management of the critically ill obstetric patient and should be performed by an obstetric nurse in the ICU at least every 4–8 hours while the patient is critically ill and more frequently should their condition deteriorate.[11-13] Continuous fetal monitoring is appropriate in the most serious situations. Ultrasonographic assessment of the biophysical profile may be done frequently. Senior obstetric and midwifery staff need to be notified early of the critically ill obstetric patient as delivery of the fetus may be required to rescue a deteriorating situation. The obstetric anesthesiologist should assess the patient. IV dexamethasone or betamethasone is administered for fetal lung maturity.[11-13]

■ LABORATORY INVESTIGATIONS

The usual laboratory investigations in a patient with severe preeclampsia include complete blood count to look for anemia and thrombocytopenia; serum haptoglobin level and lactate dehydrogenase to look for hemolysis, and a blood smear to test for schistocytes (microangiopathic hemolytic anemia). Bilirubin, aspartate transaminase, and alanine transaminase could identify liver involvement in preeclampsia, HELLP syndrome, or AFLP.[11-13] Renal function tests and electrolyte, including urine routine examination and microscopy to assess acute kidney injury, prothrombin time, activated thrombin time, fibrinogen level, and fibrin degradation products to diagnose subclinical DIC, are recommended. Blood grouping and cross-matching are done as postpartum hemorrhage (PPH) may occur. Fetal ultrasound is done to study Doppler velocimetry of the umbilical, cerebral, and uterine arteries; estimation of fetal weight; assessment of fetal well-being; and examination of the placenta.[11-13]

Treatment and Prevention of Seizures

Eclampsia often results in recurrent seizure activity that, if uncontrolled, could lead to neuronal damage, rhabdomyolysis, metabolic acidosis, aspiration pneumonitis, neurogenic pulmonary edema, and respiratory failure.[11-13] $MgSO_4$ is the drug of choice for prevention of seizures in severe preeclampsia. The Magpie Trial Collaborative group published a landmark randomized trial in 2002 that found that women allocated to $MgSO_4$ had 58% less risk of an eclamptic seizure than those randomized to placebo.[16] A standard regime for treatment with IV $MgSO_4$ is given in **Box 3**.

During magnesium treatment, it is important to watch for the clinical manifestations of magnesium toxicity (**Table 1**). Specific treatment modalities for severe hypermagnesemia with toxicity include IV administration of 10 mL of 10% calcium gluconate in the patient with cardiorespiratory compromise and aggressive fluid therapy and loop diuretics to enhance renal magnesium excretion. Hemodialysis could be considered to rapidly reduce the serum magnesium level in patients with severe respiratory or cardiovascular compromise.

Box 3: A standard prophylactic and therapeutic regime for parenteral magnesium sulfate.

- Loading dose of 4–6 g over 15 minutes intravenously or 5 g in each buttock intramuscularly
- Maintenance infusion of 1–2 g/h or 5 g by intramuscular injection every 4 hours
- Monitoring of magnesium levels
- Target serum concentration of magnesium: 2–3.5 mmol/L (4.8–8.4 mg/dL)
- Plan for hastened delivery within the next 24 hours
- Most centers continue $MgSO_4$ therapy for at least 24 hours postpartum.

Table 1: Clinical manifestations of hypermagnesemia.

Magnesium level	Clinical features
2–3.5 mmol/L (4.8–8.4 mg/dL)	Nausea, flushing, headache, lethargy, drowsiness, and diminished deep tendon reflexes
3.5–5 mmol/L (8.4–12 mg/dL)	Somnolence, hypocalcemia, absent deep tendon reflexes, hypotension, bradycardia, and ECG changes
>5 mmol/L (>12 mg/dL)	Muscle paralysis, respiratory failure, respiratory paralysis, complete heart block, and cardiac arrest

Intravenous $MgSO_4$ has also proven to be the agent of choice to prevent recurrent seizures in eclamptic patients who have already had a seizure. The international Eclampsia Trial Collaborative Group study randomly allocated 1,687 patients with eclampsia to two treatment groups—one group received $MgSO_4$ or diazepam and the other received $MgSO_4$ or phenytoin.[17] This study showed that patients treated with $MgSO_4$ had a 52% lower incidence of recurrent convulsions than patients receiving diazepam and a 67% lower incidence than those receiving phenytoin.[17]

If seizures recur while on $MgSO_4$ infusion, IV phenytoin or levetiracetam may be added. Magnetic resonance (MR) imaging of the brain and MR venogram should be done in all the cases of eclampsia to rule out intracranial hemorrhage, posterior reversible edema syndrome (PRES), or cerebral venous thrombosis.[10]

After initial stabilization measures, the obstetrician discussed the situation with the family and explained about the likelihood of possible deterioration of the mother's condition if pregnancy was continued. The problems related to premature delivery were also discussed and the neonatologist explained the need for prolonged neonatal intensive care that the baby would need. The anesthesiologist who had seen the patient earlier explained the risks related to urgent lower segment cesarean section (LSCS) in a critically ill pregnant patient with eclampsia.

Selection of an Appropriate Treatment Plan

Delivery or termination of pregnancy is the cure for severe preeclampsia or eclampsia. The prime objectives in this situation are to forestall convulsion, prevent intracranial hemorrhage and serious damage to vital organs, and ultimately to deliver a healthy infant if possible.[1,10-13]

Obstetric management of mild preeclampsia consists of expectant management (<34 weeks)—bed rest and sedation, antihypertensive therapy, and close monitoring of weight and urine output. The aim is to continue the pregnancy till 37 weeks if maternal and fetal well-being is not compromised. With development of some features

of severe preeclampsia, IV $MgSO_4$ is started for seizure prophylaxis with monitoring of deep tendon reflexes.[1,10-13] Aggressive management in severe preeclampsia consists of induction of labor and delivery within 48–72 hours. If time permits, two doses of IV corticosteroids are administered to the parturient to promote fetal lung maturity, especially if the gestation is <34 weeks.[10-13] The indications for immediate delivery are an uncontrolled hypertension >160/110 mm Hg, worsening oliguria and renal dysfunction, hepatic dysfunction, imminent eclampsia, seizures, pulmonary edema, or fetal distress.[11,13]

Proper counseling of the patient and family about the risks and benefits of emergency surgery is needed. Complications such as eclampsia, cerebral edema, subarachnoid hemorrhage, pulmonary edema, left ventricular failure, renal failure, and intraoperative bleeding due to deranged liver function, coagulopathy and low platelets, risk of atonic PPH, and requirement of blood and blood products need to be explained prior to them. Fetal outcome may depend on the fetal organ maturity, and the need for delivery in a well-equipped setup with good neonatal intensive care is preferable.

Careful preanesthetic assessment is required for airway edema and compromise, aspiration prophylaxis, auscultation of lungs for pulmonary edema, fluid balance with correction of hemoconcentration, hemodynamic status, left uterine displacement causing uterine vascular hypotension, liver and renal function, and coagulation status.[11-13]

Perioperative Management: Anesthesia Issues

Neuraxial anesthesia is the technique of choice in the absence of any contraindications. Preeclamptic patients may benefit from epidural labor analgesia if normal delivery is planned. Maternal pain during labor induces a stressful condition with release of catecholamines, cortisol, and adrenocorticotropic hormone (ACTH), all of which reduce the uterine perfusion and can adversely affect fetal well-being. Maternal hyperglycemia, with poor insulin release, lipolysis, and increased levels of fatty acids, causes fetal acidosis and increased fetal oxygen requirements. Analgesia during labor mitigates all these deleterious effects and thus improves overall maternal satisfaction and fetal well-being.[18,19] It will also help in expansion of intravascular volume due to vasodilatation caused by sympatholysis and thus can help prevention of fluid extravasation in third space. If the platelet count is >75,000/μL with no other coagulation abnormality, the likelihood of major complications is minimal. Titrated epidural, single shot spinal, and combined spinal-epidural anesthesia are equally safe. The incidence of hypotension after neuraxial anesthesia in preeclamptic patients is low and can be managed easily with titrated doses of IV ephedrine (3–5 mg) or phenylephrine (50–100 μg) bolus.[19]

Though neuraxial anesthesia is the choice for cesarean section, general anesthesia may be required in patients with coagulopathy, pulmonary edema, eclampsia, and in extreme emergency where the baby has to be delivered as soon as possible.[18,19] The patient may not be adequately starving, increasing the chances of aspiration. Rapid-sequence induction with cricoid pressure may be required in these cases. An anesthesia checklist should confirm the presence of fully functioning suction. It should be possible to place the operation table in a head-down position if needed, to prevent aspiration if regurgitation occurs. The intubation trolley should include smaller sized endotracheal tubes, good working laryngoscopes with proper blades, and intubating aids such as airways, bougie, difficult airway equipment.[12,18,19] Respiratory reserve may be poor due to pregnancy, and hence adequate preoxygenation is a must. The achievement of rapid and smooth induction is of utmost importance, which may be challenging in these patients. The degree of safety with available anesthetic techniques may vary in different patients so the technique should be individualized, and adequate monitoring is mandatory.[19]

The pressor response to laryngoscopy with general anesthesia can lead to a dangerously high surge in BP that may cause intracranial hemorrhage in these parturients. Fentanyl, alfentanil, remifentanil, esmolol, lignocaine, and $MgSO_4$ may be used to blunt the hypertensive response, but one should choose a familiar drug in this situation. Neonatal resuscitation facilities must be available as all opioids rapidly cross the placenta. Respiratory depression by remifentanil is usually brief as it is rapidly metabolized by the neonate. As preeclamptic patients are usually on $MgSO_4$, this may enhance the action of muscle relaxants, so appropriate neuromuscular monitoring is required. Maintenance of anesthesia is done by inhalational agents, usually isoflurane.[1,19]

Routine IV fluids (lactated Ringer's solution) should be administered at 60–100 mL/h due to contracted intravascular volume unless unusual fluid loss from vomiting, diarrhea, or diaphoresis or excessive blood loss at delivery occur. Invasive hemodynamic monitoring is usually required to prevent the serious complication of fluid overload, pulmonary edema. Infusion of large fluid volumes increases the risk of pulmonary and cerebral edema. Tocolytics such as oxytocin administered after baby delivery can also lead to sudden expansion of intravascular blood volume due to autotransfusion during uterine contraction.[20,21] A reduced dose of oxytocin is preferable and the ergot alkaloid methylergometrine is contraindicated as it will worsen hypertension. The prostaglandin PG-F2 analog, carboprost, also requires caution as it can cause

rise in BP and pulmonary edema after its use in PPH in preeclamptics.[22] IV furosemide can be used to prevent fluid overload during surgery. During recovery from anesthesia, extreme caution is required to prevent hypertension, aspiration, and acute pulmonary edema.

Postoperative Care

A stable preeclamptic patient may be recovered bedside. Medications can be given orally postoperatively for BP control when the patient is permitted oral intake. Strict monitoring of respiratory rate, BP, urine output, and oxygen saturation is mandatory. Severe preeclamptics should be managed in the ICU. $MgSO_4$ infusion needs to be continued in the postoperative period for 48 hours if the patient has had eclamptic convulsions.[11,13] Convulsions can occur for the first time in the first week after delivery. Patients with preeclampsia are predisposed to PPH due to uterine atony and may need surgical intervention.[13] Coexisting coagulation disturbances due to DIC or thrombocytopenia should also be treated with appropriate blood products. Liver enzymes gradually normalize over the next few days in patients with HELLP syndrome, although thrombocytopenia may worsen in the first 24 hours after delivery. Women with preeclampsia may need oral antihypertensive drugs for up to 6 weeks postpartum. Some women continue to develop chronic hypertension needing lifelong medication.

▌ REFERENCES

1. American College of Obstetricians and Gynecologists; Task Force on Hypertension in Pregnancy. Hypertension in pregnancy. Report of the American College of Obstetricians and Gynecologists' Task Force on Hypertension in Pregnancy. Obstet Gynecol. 2013;122(5):1122-31.
2. Duhig KE, Myers J, Seed PT, Sparkes J, Lowe J, Hunter RM, et al. Placental growth factor testing to assess women with suspected pre-eclampsia: a multicenter, pragmatic, stepped-wedge cluster-randomised controlled trial. Lancet. 2019;393(10183):1807-18.
3. Rana S, Lemoine E, Granger JP, Karumanchi SA. Preeclampsia: pathophysiology, challenges, and perspectives. Circ Res. 2019;124(7):1094-112.
4. Kassebaum NJ, Bertozzi-Villa A, Coggeshall MS, Shackelford KA, Steiner C, Heuton KR, et al. Global, regional, and national levels and causes of maternal mortality during 1990-2013: a systematic analysis for the Global Burden of Disease Study 2013. Lancet. 2014;384(9947):980-1004.
5. Karnad DR, Guntupalli KK. Critical illness and pregnancy: review of a global problem. Crit Care Clin. 2004;20(4):555-76, vii.
6. Munnur U, Karnad DR, Bandi VD, Lapsia V, Suresh MS, Ramshesh P, et al. Critically ill obstetric patients in an American and an Indian public hospital: comparison of case-mix, organ dysfunction, intensive care requirements, and outcomes. Intensive Care Med. 2005;31(8):1087-94.

7. Karnad DR, Lapsia V, Krishnan A, Salvi VS. Prognostic factors in obstetric patients admitted to an Indian intensive care unit. Crit Care Med. 2004;32(6):1294-9.

8. Dildy GA, Belfort MA. Complications of preeclampsia. In: Belfort M, Saade G, Foley MR, Phelan JP, Dildy GA (Eds). Critical Care Obstetrics, 5th edition. Oxford, England: Wiley-Blackwell; 2010. pp. 438-645.

9. Chaiworapongsa T, Chaemsaithong P, Yeo L, Romero R. Pre-eclampsia part 1: Current understanding of its pathophysiology. Nat Rev Nephrol. 2014;10(8):466-80.

10. Karnad DR, Guntupalli KK. Neurologic disorders in pregnancy. Crit Care Med. 2005;33(Suppl 10):S362-71.

11. Guntupalli KK, Karnad DR, Bandi V, Hall N, Belfort M. Critical illness in pregnancy: Part II: Common medical conditions complicating pregnancy and puerperium. Chest. 2015;148(5):1333-45.

12. Casey E, Hayes N, Ross A. Obstetric critical care: Clinical problems. Belgium: European Society of Intensive Care Medicine, Patient Centred Acute Care Training; 2013. pp. 5-30.

13. Munnur U, Karnad DR, Yeomans ER, Guntupalli KK. Critical care in pregnancy. In: Powrie RO, Greene MF, Camann W (Eds). De Swiet's Medical Disorders in Obstetric Practice, 5th edition. Chichester, England: Blackwell Publishing; 2010. pp. 583-97.

14. Sibai BM. Diagnosis, controversies, and management of the syndrome of hemolysis, elevated liver enzymes, and low platelet count. Obstet Gynecol. 2004;103(5 Pt 1):981-91.

15. Martin JN Jr, Bailey AP, Rehberg JF, Owens MT, Keiser SD, May WL. Thrombotic thrombocytopenic purpura in 166 pregnancies: 1955-2006. Am J Obstet Gynecol. 2008;199(2):98-104.

16. Altman D, Carroli G, Duley L, Farrell B, Moodley J, Neilson J, et al. Do women with pre-eclampsia, and their babies, benefit from magnesium sulphate? The Magpie Trial: a randomised placebo-controlled trial. Lancet. 2002;359(9321):1877-90.

17. Which anticonvulsant for women with eclampsia? Evidence from the Collaborative Eclampsia Trial. Lancet. 1995;345(8963):1455-63.

18. American Society of Anesthesiologists Task Force on Obstetric Anesthesia. Practice guidelines for obstetric anesthesia: An updated report by the American Society of Anesthesiologists Task Force on Obstetric Anesthesia. Anesthesiology. 2007;106(4):843-63.

19. Singh J, Kaur M, Kulshrestha A, Bajwa SJS. Recent advances in pre-eclampsia management: an anesthesiologist's perspective. Anaesth Pain Intensive Care. 2014;18(2):209-14.

20. Sibai BM, Mabie BC, Harvey CJ, Gonzalez AR. Pulmonary edema in severe preeclampsia-eclampsia: analysis of thirty-seven consecutive cases. Am J Obstet Gynecol. 1987;156(5):1174-9.

21. Upadya M, Rao ST. Hypertensive disorders in pregnancy. Indian J Anaesth. 2018;62(9):675-81.

22. Leslie D, Collis RE. Hypertension in pregnancy. BJA Educ. 2016;16(1):33-7.

31

Perioperative Management of Nonobstetric Major Surgeries in Pregnant Patient

Rupesh Yadav, Amlendu Yadav, Usha Yadav

INTRODUCTION

Nonobstetric major surgeries can be required in any stage of pregnancy depending on the urgency and emergency of the presentation. Frequency of nonobstetric surgeries conducted in pregnant women ranges between 0.75% and 2%.[1,2] These numbers are likely to be an underestimation, because pregnancy may be unrecognized at the time of surgery and the increasing numbers of laparoscopic and fetal procedures. Nonobstetric surgeries are commonly performed for acute abdominal disease (most commonly appendicitis and cholecystitis), ovarian disorders (torsion), trauma and malignancies.[3]

Anesthesia plans must consider the needs of mother and the fetus. Anesthetic techniques need to be modified to accommodate pregnancy-induced physiologic changes in the mother and the presence of the fetus.

PRINCIPLES OF PERIOPERATIVE MANAGEMENT

Anesthetic techniques used in pregnant patient must not affect the uteroplacental perfusion and maintain adequate blood flow and oxygenation to the fetus to:

- Minimum alteration in maternal physiologic parameters
- Optimize uteroplacental perfusion during any surgical procedure in mother and fetus
- Optimize oxygenation of maternal blood
- By avoidance of use of any contraindicated drug in pregnancy
- Prevent any premature uterine contraction/activity
- Prevent five "H", that is, hypotension, hypoxemia, hypovolemia, hydrogen ion (acidosis), and hypercarbia
- Prevent five "T", that is, tamponade, tension, thrombosis, trauma, and pneumothorax.

MATERNAL PHYSIOLOGICAL ADAPTION IN PREGNANCY

Understanding the physiological changes in pregnancy would help us provide the correct anesthetic techniques.

Cardiovascular Changes

The cardiovascular system undergoes significant physiological changes and this leads to major complications during pregnancy.[4] Maternal blood volume increases to 15–20% by 6 weeks and between 30% and 50% by 34 weeks. Systemic vascular resistance (SVR) will decrease by 33% by the time of 6 weeks of pregnancy and remains at that level until delivery. The cardiac output will rise 30% by 6 weeks of pregnancy, where it will rise to as high as 8–9 L/min in the third trimester of pregnancy. The maternal heart rate generally sees its highest increase in the third trimester, rising to approximately 15–20% above baseline. At the same time, maternal hematocrit will usually fall from 39% to 35% at term (**Table 1**). This fall in hematocrit is further worsened by concurrent iron, macronutrient and multivitamin deficiency.

Arrhythmias are common during pregnancy and they rarely require treatment unless they are symptomatic. Mechanism underlying arrhythmias are due to atrial stretching arising from increased intravascular volume which results in disturbances in cardiac conduction pathways and increased levels of estragon which further lowers the threshold for arrhythmias.[5] During the second trimester, compression of inferior vena cava (IVC) by the gravid uterus reduces the venous return and cardiac output by approximately 30%; therefore, hypotension occurs in the supine position following a neuraxial or general anesthesia. It is essential to displace the uterus laterally during any operation performed after 18–20 weeks' gestation to prevent IVC compression and prevent supine hypotension syndrome.

Table 1: Maternal adaption to pregnancy.

Physiological changes	% of change
Cardiovascular system	
Cardiac output	↑30–40
Heart rate	↑20–25
Systemic vascular resistance	↓15–20
Blood pressure	↑5–15
Central venous pressure	↔
Hematological system	
Blood volume	↑30–40
Plasma volume	↑20–25
RBC volume	↑15–20
Hemoglobin	↓10–20
Coagulation factors	↑
Respiratory system	
Tidal volume	↑30–35
Respiratory rate	↑10–15
Functional residual capacity	↓20–25
Oxygen consumption	↑15–20
Metabolic changes	
pH	↑
pO_2	↑
pCO_2	↓
HCO_3	↓

(HCO_3: bicarbonate; pCO_2: partial pressure of carbon dioxide; pO_2: partial pressure of oxygen: RBC: red blood cell)

Hematological Changes

Blood volume expands in the first trimester, increases 30–45% by end of third trimester, whereas red blood cell (RBC) volume increases by 15–20%, and thus results in dilutional anemia. Pregnancy is associated with benign leukocytosis. That is commonly seen in pregnancy and hence it is an unreliable indicator of infection. Pregnancy is a hypercoagulable state, associated with increases in fibrinogen; factors VII, VIII, X, and XII; and fibrin degradation products (FDPs). During the postoperative period, pregnant surgical patients are at higher risk for thromboembolic complications; thromboembolism prophylaxis is recommended in postoperative period including both mechanical and pharmacological alone or in combination is better.

Respiratory System Changes

In order to meet the oxygen demand of growing fetus, minute ventilation of mother rises 40% in the first trimester and mother maintains this increase throughout the duration of pregnancy. The expiratory reserve volume (ERV) of mother decreases as the uterus displaces abdominal contents cephalad. It is decreased as much as by one-third while mother is in sitting position.[6] The reduction in ERV is the most significant when performing general anesthesia on late-term pregnant patients. The ERV is used as an oxygen reserve to ensure that the mother maintains adequate blood oxygen saturation despite potentially prolonged apnea period. On an average, nonpregnant patient consumes approximately 3 mL/kg/min of oxygen, while the average pregnant mother in their third trimester consumes approximately 4 mL/kg/min, which may be rising to as high as 15 mL/kg/min when in labor.[7] The ERV in a nonpregnant patient is approximately 1.3 L, while in the third trimester; it is approximately 0.8 L only. Nonpregnant patient may maintain blood oxygen saturation as long as 6 minutes after adequate preoxygenation, while a pregnant patient in labor may begin to desaturate as early as within 1 minute of induction of general anesthesia.

Higher minute ventilation results in chronic respiratory alkalosis with a $PaCO_2$ of 28–32 mm Hg, a slightly alkaline pH (approximately 7.44), and decreased levels of bicarbonate and buffer base. Despite the increased oxygen consumption in pregnancy, PaO_2 usually increases only slightly or remains within the normal range.

Airway Changes

The airway of mother undergoes significant change during pregnancy. The weight gain acquired during pregnancy can result in increased neck girth and size of oropharyngeal structures, airway edema resulting from reduced oncotic pressure, and increase in extracellular fluid results in engorgement of soft tissues in the mouth and pharynx. Pilkington examined the airway in 242 pregnant women and found that from 12–38 weeks of gestational age, the incidence of class IV airways increased by 34%.[8] These changes may lead to difficulty in mask ventilation and intubation of the pregnant patient.

Gastrointestinal System

Aspiration of gastric contents is uncommon, but can have a disastrous consequence of inducing general anesthesia prior to placement of the endotracheal tube (ETT). Gastroesophageal reflux is observed in many women during pregnancy. This is due to the upward displacement of the stomach and displacement of the intra-abdominal esophagus into the thorax. The risk for gastroesophageal reflux is increased due to incompetence of the lower esophageal sphincter and distortion of gastric and pyloric anatomy during pregnancy. Though gastric emptying remains unchanged, overall intestinal transit time gets prolonged.[8]

Renal System

There is a 20–25% increase in renal blood flow and up to 50% increase in glomerular filtration rate (GFR) during pregnancy. Laboratory measurements of kidney function, including serum creatinine, urea, and uric acid also decrease during pregnancy due to increase in blood volume and increase in GFR.

EFFECTS OF ANESTHETICS ON FETAL OUTCOME

Fetal Development and Teratogenicity

During the early embryonic period, the human brain and central nervous system (CNS) develop from a small set of embryonic cells to a more complex and efficient network of over 100 billion neurons. The neural development begins early with proliferation of neural stem cell, followed by migration and further differentiation into a specialized neuron by 4 weeks' gestation in pregnancy.

The United States Food and Drug Administration (FDA) (2016)[9] issued a warning that "repeated or lengthy use (>3 hours) of general anesthetic and sedation drugs during surgeries or procedures in children younger than 3 years or in pregnant women during their third trimester may affect the development of children's brains." The agents implicated are of two major classes of anesthetic agents:
1. Gamma-amino butyric acid (GABA) receptor agonists
2. N-methyl D-aspartate (NMDA) antagonists

Gamma-amino butyric acid agonists are drugs that enhance activity at the GABA receptors resulting in sedation, decreased anxiety and muscle relaxation. The GABA receptor agonists are inhalational anesthetics (Isoflurane, sevoflurane and desflurane), benzodiazepines (such as midazolam), and the other sedative-hypnotic agent such as propofol. The NMDA antagonist class of drugs such as ketamine are anesthetic agents that inhibit or antagonize the NMDA receptor and subsequently cause a dissociative anesthesia.

The human embryo is the most vulnerable during the first trimester to the teratogenic effects of various drugs including anesthetic and nonanesthetic drugs. Apart from the teratogenic effects, many of these drugs can cause premature labor, abortion and growth retardation. Fortunately, most of the anesthetic and sedative agents are free from teratogenic effects, but they should be used with caution as they lack human studies **(Table 2)**.

Category A: Controlled studies showed absence of risk
Category B: Without evidences of human risk
Category C: The risk cannot be ruled out
Category D: Positive evidence of risk
Category X: Contraindicated in pregnancy

Table 2: The United States Food and Drug Administration (FDA) classification of anesthetic drugs.

Drug	FDA category
Morphine/pethidine/fentanyl	B (small doses)/D (high doses)
Sufentanil/remifentanil	C
Thiopentone sodium	C
Propofol	B
Succinylcholine	C
Rocuronium	C
Bupivacaine	C
Lignocaine	B
Butorphanol/nalbuphine	C (small doses)/D (high doses)

The *teratogenicity* depends on the dose administered, and the timing of exposure with respect to development, and the route of administration of any drug given during pregnancy can potentially jeopardize the development of the fetus. Until now, no anesthetic drug has been proven to be clearly hazardous to the human fetus. It should also be noted that no animal model perfectly simulates human gestation and it is unethical to perform a randomized trial on pregnant patients in this regard. Hence, definitive evidence seems elusive.

PLACENTAL TRANSFER OF ANESTHETIC DRUGS

The placental drug transfer depends on various factors. The highly lipid soluble drugs are rapidly transferred, but may result in trapping of the drug in the placenta.

Broadly, three types of drug transfer across the human placenta are recognized during pregnancy:[10]
1. *Complete transfer (type 1 drugs):* For example, thiopentone sodium
   a. These types of drugs will transfer rapidly across the placenta with pharmacologically significant concentrations equilibrating in maternal and fetal blood rapidly.
2. *Exceeding transfer (type 2 drugs):* For example, ketamine
   a. These drugs cross the placenta quickly and reach higher concentrations in fetal blood as compared with maternal blood.
3. *Incomplete transfer (type 3 drugs):* For example, succinylcholine
   a. These type of drugs are unable to cross the placenta completely, resulting in higher concentrations in maternal blood as compared with fetal blood.

The underlying principles of drug transfer across placenta includes: (i) simple diffusion, e.g., paracetamol, midazolam; (ii) facilitated diffusion, e.g., glucocorticoids, cephalosporins; (iii) active transport, e.g., dopamine, norepinephrine; or (iv) pinocytosis.

Induction Agents

Thiopentone sodium is the most commonly used induction agent in pregnant patients. It is a highly lipid-soluble weak acid, which is 61% unionized at plasma pH and 75% bound to plasma albumin. Thiopentone rapidly crosses the placenta because of lipid solubility but is quickly cleared by the neonate after delivery.[11] Propofol is lipid soluble drug, which crosses the placenta easily. It has been associated with neurobehavioral effects and transient depression of Apgar scores in the neonates.

Nitrous Oxide

Nitrous oxide has been shown to be a weak teratogen in rat studies. These effects are seen only after a prolonged exposure to high concentrations of nitrous oxide, which is very rare in clinical anesthesia in humans. Nitrous oxide's use in anesthesia has decreased recently and is being replaced by air or any other anesthetic gas. Nitrous oxide also crosses the placenta rapidly. Diffusion hypoxia may occur in neonates exposed to nitrous oxide. Diffusion hypoxia with nitrous oxide is prevented by use of supplemental oxygen.

Inhalation Agents

Volatile anesthetic agents are highly lipid soluble and they readily cross the placenta. Uterine perfusion was maintained at 1.0–1.5 minimum alveolar concentration (MAC) of halothane or isoflurane; however, higher concentrations may (e.g., 2.0 MAC) results in marked maternal hypotension, reduced uteroplacental blood flow, fetal hypoxia, and fetal acidosis.

Neuromuscular Blocking Agents

Neuromuscular blocking drugs are large and highly ionized molecules. These are poorly lipid soluble drugs, so they cross the placenta very slowly and pose no significant clinical problems to the neonate during pregnancy and delivery.[12]

Opioids

Almost all opioids cross the placenta and therefore cause fetal respiratory depression. Pethidine was commonly used during labor; it is 50% protein-bound and crosses the placenta readily. Peak action of pethidine in fetus usually occurs 2–3 hours after a maternal intramuscular (IM) dose. This is the time when neonatal respiratory depression is most likely to occur. This effect may last up to 72 hours or more after delivery due to the prolonged half-life of both pethidine and its metabolite, normeperidine, in the neonate. Morphine is less protein-bound, therefore, readily crosses the placenta. Fentanyl is a lipid-soluble drug, which crosses the placenta rapidly. The remifentanil also crosses the placenta. It undergoes rapid hydrolysis by nonspecific blood and tissue esterase. Its use for labor analgesia has not been associated with adverse neonatal effects during pregnancy and post delivery period.

Local Anesthetic Agents

Local anesthetics drugs are weak bases and have relatively low degrees of ionization at physiological pH. The long-acting local anesthetic such as bupivacaine and ropivacaine are highly lipid soluble with high degree of protein binding. Systemic absorption of local anesthetic occurs through the large epidural venous plexuses with subsequent transfer across the placenta by simple diffusion. The lipid solubility of lignocaine is less than bupivacaine but has a lower degree of protein binding, so it will also cross the placenta well. During fetal acidosis, the local anesthetics can accumulate in the fetus leading to "ion trapping". Low pH in the fetus produces an increased proportion of ionized drug, which is then unable to cross the placenta leading to "ion trapping".

Anticholinergics

Transfer of anticholinergic drugs across the placenta is simulate to the transfer of these drugs across the blood–brain barrier (BBB). Glycopyrrolate is fully ionized, therefore, poorly transferred across the placenta. Atropine is lipid soluble, which is readily transferred through the placenta.

Neostigmine

Neostigmine is a small molecule, which is able to cross the placenta more rapidly than glycopyrrolate. Fetal bradycardia has been reported when neostigmine is used with glycopyrrolate to reverse nondepolarizing neuromuscular blockers in pregnancy.[12,13] Therefore, for general anesthesia in pregnancy where the baby is remained in utero, it is advisable to use neostigmine with atropine rather than with glycopyrrolate.

Benzodiazepines

The benzodiazepines, such as midazolam and lorazepam, are lipid soluble and unionized drugs, so they are readily transferred across the placenta.

Vasoactive Drugs

Sympathomimetic drugs like ephedrine and phenylephrine are often used to treat maternal hypotension following

Flowchart 1: Timing of nonobstetric surgery during pregnancy.

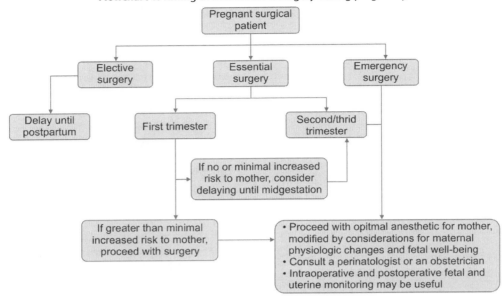

regional anesthesia. The ephedrine increases maternal arterial pressure mainly by increasing cardiac output (CO) via cardiac β-1 receptors, with a smaller contribution from vasoconstriction via α-1 receptor agonistic action. It has minimal effects on uteroplacental blood flow. The ephedrine crosses the placenta and has been shown to be associated with a decrease in umbilical arterial pH, stimulating an increase in fetal metabolic rate.

The phenylephrine increases maternal arterial pressure by vasoconstriction through its direct effect on α-1 receptors. It acts as an α-1 receptor agonist. It prevents maternal hypotension without causing fetal acidosis, when combined with rapid crystalloid infusion immediately after spinal anesthetic injection.[14]

TIMING OF SURGERY

The elective surgery should have been avoided during pregnancy. Any surgical procedure should be avoided especially during the first trimester, which is the period of organogenesis. The second trimester is the best time to perform elective surgical procedures if required during pregnancy, because the risk for preterm labor is lowest at that time. Mazze and Kallen, in 1989, looked at 5,405 surgeries during 2 million pregnancies in Sweden and found no increase in teratogenicity but an increase in premature birth.[2] A multidisciplinary team-involving surgeons, anesthesiologists, obstetricians and perinatologists should be involved in the decision on proceeding with surgery. The second trimester is chosen most often for semielective surgery, which cannot be postponed. The urgent and emergency surgery should not be delayed

because secondary complications may increase the risk to the mother and/or fetus. High risk of uterine irritability and preterm labor is seen during later stages of pregnancy. The conditions associated with a particularly high risk are lower abdominal and pelvic inflammatory conditions, such as acute appendicitis with peritonitis **(Flowchart 1)**.

An interim update has been nonobstetric surgery in pregnant patients has been released by the American College of Obstetricians and Gynecologists' (ACOGs) Committee on Obstetric Practice and the American Society of Anesthesiologists (ASA). Their opinion is given in **Box 1**.

PREOPERATIVE PREPARATION

The pregnant woman requiring surgery needs counseling regarding the anesthetic risks and safety to the fetus and pregnancy in addition to standard preoperative assessment. Good counseling is often effective for anxious patient. The problems, which are specific to pregnant women, should be considered in preoperative period, including risks of aspiration, difficult intubation, thromboembolism, and the well-being of the fetus before and during the delivery. The standard adult fasting guidelines, i.e., 6–8 hours for solid food, depending on the type of food ingested (e.g., fat content) are applicable to these patients. Longer period of 8 hours may be considered with intravenous (IV) fluids **(Box 2)**.

- *Aspiration prophylaxis*: Although the gastric emptying time is normal in pregnancy, but the risk of aspiration is still higher due to reduced gastric barrier pressure and lower esophageal sphincter tone because of progesterone effect. Prophylaxis against aspiration pneumonitis should

Box 1: General principles of nonobstetric surgery during pregnancy (Committee on Obstetric Practice American Society of Anesthesiologists), 2019.[15]

- A pregnant woman should never be denied medically necessary surgery or have that surgery delayed regardless of trimester because this can adversely affect the pregnant woman and her fetus
- Elective surgery should be postponed until after delivery
- No currently used anesthetic agents have been shown to have any teratogenic effects in humans when using standard concentrations at any gestational age
- There is no evidence that in utero human exposure to anesthetic or sedative drugs has any effect on the developing fetal brain; and there are no animal data to support an effect with limited exposures less than 3 hours in duration
- Given the potential for preterm delivery with some nonobstetric procedures during pregnancy, corticosteroid administration for fetal benefit should be considered for patients with fetuses at viable premature gestational ages, and patients should be monitored in the perioperative period for signs or symptoms of preterm labor
- Fetal heart rate monitoring may assist in maternal positioning and cardiorespiratory management and may influence a decision to deliver the fetus
- Pregnant women undergoing nonobstetric surgery should be screened for venous thromboembolism risk and should have the appropriate perioperative prophylaxis administered
- Surgery should be done at an institution with neonatal and pediatric services
- An obstetric care provider with cesarean delivery privileges should be readily available
- A qualified individual should be readily available to interpret fetal heart rate patterns.

Box 2: Anesthetic considerations.

- Postpone surgery until postpartum, if possible
- Counsel the patient preoperatively
- Obtain obstetric consultation and discuss the use of perioperative tocolytics
- Use aspiration prophylaxis
- Maintain uterine displacement perioperatively
- Monitor and maintain oxygenation, CO_2, normotension, and euglycemia
- Consider use of fetal heart monitoring intraoperatively
- No outcome difference in anesthetic technique (regional or general)
- No outcome difference shown between anesthetic agents
- Monitor uterine contractions and fetal heart tones postoperatively.

be administered from 16 weeks' gestation onwards with H_2 receptor antagonists and nonparticulate antacids.

- *Antibiotic prophylaxis*: The need for antibiotic prophylaxis depends on the specific procedure and the underlying risk factors and comorbidity. However, attention should be paid in selecting antibiotics with good safety profile in pregnancy.
- *Prophylactic glucocorticoids*: Administration of a course of antenatal glucocorticoids for maturation of lung 24–48 hours before surgery between 24 and 34 weeks' period of gestation can reduce perinatal morbidity/mortality, if preterm birth occurs. This should be considered seriously.

- *Thromboprophylaxis*: Pregnancy is a hypercoagulable state. Mechanical and/or pharmacologic thromboprophylaxis must be provided for all pregnant patients undergoing surgery during and after surgery. This hypercoagulable state persists even after surgery.
- *Prophylactic tocolytics*: The routine administration of prophylactic perioperative tocolytic therapy has no proven benefit and should be avoided. Minimal uterine manipulation reduces the risk of development of uterine contractions and preterm labor.

CHOICE OF ANESTHESIA

The maternal indications and the type of surgery should guide the choice of anesthesia. No study has conclusively found an association between improved fetal outcome and any specific anesthetic technique. However, local or regional anesthesia is preferred whenever feasible, because it permits the administration of less number of drugs with no clinical evidence of teratogenesis during pregnancy.

PREVENTION OF AORTOCAVAL COMPRESSION

After 18–20 weeks of gestation, the pregnant patient should be transported on her left side and the uterus should be displaced leftward with the use of wedge when she is positioned on the operating table.

MONITORING DURING ANESTHESIA

Maternal Monitoring

The maternal monitoring should include blood pressure measurement [noninvasive blood pressure (NIBP), capnography [end-tidal CO_2 ($EtCO_2$)], electrocardiography (ECG), pulse oximetry (SpO_2), temperature monitoring, and the use of a peripheral nerve stimulator (PNS).

Fetal Monitoring

The ASA/ACOG joint statement[15] recommends the use of intraoperative monitoring when the fetus is viable, an obstetrician is present and available to intervene surgically, and the nonobstetric surgery is amenable to both intraoperative monitoring and interruption if an emergency delivery is necessary.

ANESTHETIC TECHNIQUE

Regardless of the anesthetic technique, adequate precautionary measures should be taken to prevent hypoxemia, hypotension, acidosis, and hyperventilation. Preoxygenation should precede the induction of anesthesia.

The rapid sequence induction consisting of the application of cricoid pressure has been the standard practice for the induction of general anesthesia during pregnancy; some experts have argued against that it is unnecessary in fasted pregnant women undergoing elective surgery.[16] Anesthetic drugs commonly used are safe during pregnancy, which include thiopentone sodium, propofol, morphine, fentanyl, succinylcholine, and nondepolarizing muscle relaxants. The general anesthesia is preferably maintained with a high concentration of oxygen, a muscle relaxant, an opioid, and a moderate concentration of a volatile halogenated agent. The recent evidence does not support avoidance of nitrous oxide during pregnancy, particularly after the sixth week of gestation although it is increasingly being replaced by air at many places.[17] Hyperventilation should be avoided in order to maintain normocapnia with continuous capnography monitoring.

Hypotension following spinal and epidural blockade should be avoided, this can be prevented by using rapid administration of crystalloid before spinal anesthesia and administration of vasopressors. Maternal hypotension should be treated aggressively.

SPECIFIC SURGERY CONSIDERATIONS

Laparoscopy

The creation of pneumoperitoneum causes upward displacement of the diaphragm, which reduces the patient's functional residual capacity (FRC), thereby increases the peak airway pressure, increases ventilation–perfusion mismatch, and decreases thoracic cavity compliance. This may lead to significant hypoxia and difficulty with ventilation in pregnant patients. The Society of American Gastrointestinal and Endoscopic Surgeons (SAGES) Guidelines for the use of laparoscopy during pregnancy states that CO_2 insufflation pressures of 10–15 mm Hg can be safely used for laparoscopy.[18] However, the level of insufflation needs be adjusted to the patient's physiology, hemodynamics and period of gestation. They also recommend intraoperative maternal $EtCO_2$ monitoring to avoid maternal hypercapnia and ensure eucarbia.

POSTOPERATIVE MANAGEMENT

Ensure adequate recovery of residual effects of anesthetic drugs before shifting the pregnant patient. Fetal monitoring [Fetal heart rate (FHR)] and uterine contractions has to be monitored in postoperative period as described earlier. Adequate analgesia should be ensured with systemic or neuraxial opioids, acetaminophen, or neural blockade. Early ambulation and adequate hydration has to be maintained. Prophylaxis against venous thrombosis should be considered, especially if patients are immobilized.

Critical Care Management of Postoperative Pregnant Patient

Pregnant patient might require intensive care management for various reasons, including:

- *Pregnancy-related conditions:* Hemorrhage, hypertensive disorders of pregnancy, amniotic fluid embolism, complex cardiac diseases, acute fatty liver, aspiration syndromes, infections, ovarian hyperstimulation syndrome, tocolytic-induced pulmonary edema, etc.
- *Surgical/medical condition not related to pregnancy:* Trauma, sepsis, asthma, diabetes, autoimmune diseases, etc.

Management of obstetric hemorrhage and hypertensive disorders of pregnancy is dealt separately in the textbook.

MANAGEMENT OF SEPSIS

Initial Assessment

Management of sepsis and septic shock is as per surviving sepsis guidelines. Initial evaluation and resuscitation of the obstetric patient is similar to a nonpregnant patient and follows the same protocol wherein airway (A), breathing (B) and circulation (C) are focused upon. Uterine displacement should be considered a part of the initial ABC evaluation in any hemodynamically unstable obstetric patient. Choice of antibiotics should be dictated by patient's clinical condition and antibiotics should be chosen to reduce fetal teratogenicity. Fluid resuscitation in pregnant patient should be guided by dynamic parameters of fluid assessment.

Vasopressors

In those cases, where fluid therapy alone is unable to achieve an MAP above 60–65 mm Hg, vasopressors are commonly used.

The vasopressor of choice in septic shock is norepinephrine. Norepinephrine increases blood pressure primarily by increasing SVR; obstetricians in past have traditionally expressed concern regarding the potential adverse effects of vasopressors on uteroplacental perfusion but fluid resuscitation and restoration of maternal organ perfusion pressure by vasopressors is essential for fetal survival and well-being.

Vasopressin is a peptide hormone synthesized in the hypothalamus and stored in the posterior pituitary gland. Evidence regarding the use of vasopressin during septic shock in pregnant women is very weak and not yet available in the robust form. Theoretically, it may activate uterine V1a receptors, leading to uterine contractions. Extreme caution is advised and recommended if this agent is used during pregnancy (**Table 3**).

Table 3: Summaries of commonly used vasopressors in critical illness.

Medication	FDA pregnancy category	Comments
Norepinephrine	C	Uterine vessels are very sensitive to norepinephrine vasoconstriction because they are rich in alpha-adrenergic receptors. This agent used after adequate volume resuscitation with continuous electronic FHR monitoring. Recent evidence suggests that norepinephrine is the vasopressor of choice in pregnancy as well as sepsis
Dopamine	C	Clinicians more familiar with the use of dopamine as a vasopressor in sepsis during pregnancy. Dopamine associated more with tachyarrhythmia than norepinephrine. It is after adequate fluid resuscitation and with continuous electronic FHR monitoring. It may also be considered in maternal bradycardia
Vasopressin	C	Low doses used for the treatment of diabetes not associated with fetal harm. No data exist on its use as a continuous infusion in pregnancy. The vasopressin may lead to activation of V1a receptors and uterine contractions therefore, extreme caution is recommended if used during pregnancy. Continuous electronic FHR monitoring is highly desirable
Epinephrine	C	Used with caution. Associated with tachyarrhythmias. Used in persistent hypotension despite norepinephrine and maternal bradycardia
Dobutamine	B	Low ejection fraction and low cardiac output state. Persistent hypoperfusion despite adequate fluid resuscitation. State of septic cardiomyopathy

(FHR: fetal heart rate)

VENOUS THROMBOPROPHYLAXIS

The obstetric critically ill pregnant patient has four times higher risk of developing deep vein thrombosis compared to other critically ill patients. The risk of venous thromboprophylaxis also persists after delivery for few more weeks afterwards. Pharmacological thromboprophylaxis [low molecular weight heparin (LMWH)] can be achieved with both unfractionated and LMWHs. Mechanical compression devices such as sequential compression device, graded stockings and pneumatic compression devices should be used alone and/or in combination to pharmacological thromboprophylaxis especially in high risk patients.

SUMMARY

- The incidence of nonobstetric surgeries in obstetric patient is steadily raising.
- Maternal and fetal physiological changes in pregnancy should be considered while anesthetizing the pregnant patient.
- Choice and technique of anesthesia depends on the type of surgery and indication of surgery.
- Second trimester is ideal for elective surgical procedures in pregnant women.
- No anesthetic drug is found to be a teratogen in routinely used clinical doses.
- Avoid maternal hypotension, hypoxia and acidosis during surgery and anesthesia.
- Management of sepsis and septic shock in pregnant women is similar to nonpregnant women; maintenance of uteroplacental perfusion is the key.
- Mechanical and pharmacological thromboprophylaxis either alone or in combination should be considered in high-risk pregnant patient undergoing surgery and intensive care unit care.

REFERENCES

1. Goodman S. Anesthesia for nonobstetric surgery in the pregnant patient. Semin Perinatol. 2002;26:136-45.
2. Mazze RI, Källén B. Reproductive outcome after anesthesia and operation during pregnancy: a registry study of 5405 cases. Am J Obstet Gynecol. 1989;161:1178-85.
3. Crowhurst JA. Anaesthesia for non-obstetric surgery during pregnancy. Acta Anaesthesiol Belg. 2002;53:295-7.
4. Creanga AA, Berg CJ, Ko JY, Farr SL, Tong VT, Bruce FC, et al. Maternal mortality and morbidity in the United States: where are we now? J Women Health. 2014;23:3-9.
5. Cox JL, Gardner MJ. Treatment of cardiac arrhythmias during pregnancy. Prog Cardiovasc Dis. 1993;36:137-78.
6. McAuliffe F, Kametas N, Costello J, Rafferty GF, Greenough A, Nicolaides K. Respiratory function in singleton and twin pregnancy. BJOG. 2002;109:765-9.
7. Pernoll M, Metcalfe J, Schlenker TL, Welch JE, Matsumoto JA. Oxygen consumption at rest and during exercise in pregnancy. Respir Physiol. 1975;25:285-93.
8. Macfie AG, Magides AD, Richmond MN, Reilly CS. Gastric emptying in pregnancy. Br J Anaesth. 1991;67:54-7.
9. Olutoye OA, Baker BW, Belfort MA, Olutoye OO. Food and Drug Administration warning on anesthesia and brain development:

implications for obstetric and fetal surgery. Am J Obstet Gynecol. 2018;218:98-102.

10. Pacifici GM, Nottoli R. Placental transfer of drugs administered to the mother, Clin Pharmacokinet. 1995;28:235-69.

11. Valtonen M, Kanto J, Rosenberg P. Comparison of propofol and thiopentone for induction of anaesthesia for elective caesarean section. Anaesthesia. 1989;44:758-62.

12. Reynolds F. Drug transfer across the term placenta, Trophoblast Res, 1998, 12: 239-55.

13. Clark RB, Brown MA, Lattin DL. Neostigmine, atropine and glycopyrrolate: does neostigmine cross the placenta?, Anesthesiology, 1996;84:450-2.

14. Kee WDN, Khaw KS, Ng F. Prevention of hypotension during spinal anesthesia for caesarean delivery: an effective technique using combination phenylephrine infusion and crystalloid cohydration. Anesthesiology, 2005;103:744-50.

15. ACOG Committee Opinion No. 775: Nonobstetric surgery during pregnancy. Obstet Gynecol. 2019;133:e285-6.

16. de Souza DG, Doar LH, Mehta SH, Tiouririne M. Aspiration prophylaxis and rapid sequence induction for elective caesarean delivery: time to reassess old dogma? Anesth Analg 2010;110:1503-5.

17. Sanders RD, Weimann J, Maze M. Biologic effects of nitrous oxide: a mechanistic and toxicologic review. Anesthesiology. 2008;109:707-22.

18. Pearl JP, Price RR, Tonkin AE, Richardson WS, Stefanidis D. SAGES guidelines for the use of laparoscopy during pregnancy. Surg Endosc. 2017;31:3767-82.

SECTION

6

Gastrointestinal

Perioperative Management of Pancreatic, Gastric and Retroperitoneal Mass Surgeries

Riddhi Joshi, Martin Jose Thomas, Vandana Agarwal

INTRODUCTION

Major abdominal surgeries can be either elective, open, laparoscopic, or emergency surgeries. The magnitude of stress response to surgery depends on the complexity of the intra-abdominal surgery. Major abdominal surgeries are associated with increased morbidity and mortality. Over the years with improved medical care and access to health care, increased number of elderly patients and those with multiple comorbidities are presenting for surgery. This further increases their perioperative risks for complications.

SURGICAL STRESS RESPONSE

Definition

The stress response consists of hormonal and metabolic changes occurring as a result of tissue injury.[1]
- Endocrine response causes activation of hypothalamic–pituitary–adrenal axis (HPA) which in turn causes the release of the following hormones:
  - *Anterior pituitary*: Increased secretion of adreno-corticotropic hormone (ACTH) from anterior pituitary stimulates the adrenal cortex, thus increasing the secretion of cortisol. Feedback mechanism becomes ineffective after surgery so that increased cortisol levels are unable to inhibit ACTH.
  - Cortisol promotes protein breakdown, increased lipolysis, and inhibits glucose uptake by cells, thereby accelerating gluconeogenesis in the liver. Anti-inflammatory effect interferes with the synthesis of inflammatory mediators, particularly prostaglandins.
  - Release of growth hormone stimulates protein synthesis, inhibits glucose uptake by cells, promotes lipolysis, and thus stimulates glycogenolysis.
  - *Posterior pituitary*: Increased antidiuretic hormone (ADH) production promotes water retention and the production of concentrated urine.
  - Insulin secretion is decreased due to alpha-adrenergic inhibition of beta-cell secretion as a result there is increased insulin resistance which is proportional to the magnitude of surgery and can persist for days to weeks after surgery. Perioperative hyperglycemia is associated with increased risk of postoperative infection.

Net effect is the increased secretion of catabolic hormones.
- *Carbohydrate metabolism*: Increased blood glucose concentration is a result of increased glycogenolysis and gluconeogenesis, and decreased peripheral utilization of glucose mediated by catecholamines and cortisol. Perioperative hyperglycemia is associated with adverse outcomes in diabetics and nondiabetics.[2]
- *Protein metabolism*: Catabolism stimulated by cortisol leading to skeletal muscle breakdown.
- *Fat metabolism*: Increased lipolytic activity (stimulated by cortisol, catecholamines, and grown hormone) leading to increased mobilization of triglycerides to form glycerol and fatty acids.
  1. Sympathetic nervous system activation by the hypothalamus causes increased secretion of catecholamines from adrenal medulla, and norepinephrine is released from presynaptic nerve terminal causing tachycardia and hypertension. There is activation of renin–angiotensin–aldosterone system leading to salt and water retention.
  2. Surgical trauma causes hematological and immunological response. Cytokines are released from injured tissue, which act locally and systemically depending on the magnitude of surgery. Major cytokines are interleukin 1 (IL-1), tumor necrosis factor alpha (TNF-α), IL-6, and many others. Activated cytokines in response to surgery produce systemic inflammatory effects known as the acute phase response.

In addition to various patient and surgical factors, magnitude of stress response following surgery affects the postoperative recovery. Enhanced recovery after surgery (ERAS) pathway incorporates various elements, which optimize patients preoperatively and attenuate the perioperative stress response; thus, hastening the entire recovery process and shortening the postoperative stay.

Various interventions can be done preoperatively to optimize modifiable risk factors.

PREOPERATIVE MANAGEMENT

Prehabilitation

It comprises several components to optimize preoperative function in order to improve postoperative outcomes. There is some evidence to show that this has a positive impact on length of stay, postoperative pain, and postoperative complications.[3] This is a multidisciplinary approach by surgeons, anesthetists, physicians, physiotherapists, nutritionists, and psychologists and it includes the following:

- *Medical optimization*: Smoking cessation, reduction in alcohol intake, weight optimization (for elective procedures, may not be feasible for time-sensitive procedures, e.g., cancer surgery), management of anemia, and optimization of medical conditions.
- Pulmonary rehabilitation for patients undergoing upper abdominal surgery. Physical exercise program aids in patient's recovery by preconditioning. Improved physical fitness helps them withstand perioperative stress better and improves early postoperative mobilization.
- *Nutritional support*: Poor nutritional status is associated with poor postoperative outcomes. Formal assessment of risk should be done and patients at risk of malnutrition or malnourished patients should receive nutritional support preoperatively.
- *Psychological support*: Surgery-related stress and anxiety produce immunological dysregulation acting via the same pathway that produces the surgical stress response.[4] This includes preoperative counseling regarding surgery and perioperative experience and expectations from the patient in the postoperative period.

Preadmission Risk Stratification Systems

The incidence of complications is greater in the high-risk population. Risk stratification systems include American Society of Anesthesiologists (ASA) classification, POSSUM (Physiological and Operative Severity Score for the enUmeration of Mortality and Morbidity) scores, cardiovascular risk calculator, and assessment of functional capacity using metabolic equivalents (METs)/cardiopulmonary exercise test (CPET).[5] These risk stratification systems help in optimally caring for the patient postoperatively, e.g., in intensive care unit (ICU) or high-dependency unit (HDU) for longer than usual period, if indicated.

Preoperative Carbohydrate Loading

Clear fluids should be allowed until 2 hours prior to induction of anesthesia and solids should be allowed until 6 hours prior to induction. Preoperative oral carbohydrate loading increases insulin sensitivity and reduces insulin resistance in the perioperative period, also increasing anabolism. Clinically, this has shown more impact (in terms of reduced length of stay) in major surgeries including major abdominal surgeries compared to minor surgeries.[6,7] Preoperative hydration until 2 hours before surgery helps maintain euvolemia.

No/Selective Bowel Preparation

Bowel preparation is not routinely recommended for pancreatic, gastric, and retroperitoneal surgeries. Bowel preparation adds to dyselectrolytemia, dehydration, and fluid imbalance.

Antibiotic Prophylaxis

Antibiotic should be administered within 30 minutes before incision. Redosing is recommended if the duration of procedure exceeds two half-lives of the drug or there is excessive blood loss during procedure.[8]

Thromboprophylaxis

Abdominal surgery is associated with moderate-to-high risk for postoperative thromboembolism and pharmacological prophylaxis is recommended. It should be initiated 12 hours prior to surgery and continued up to 4 weeks postoperatively. Mechanical measures may provide additional benefits, especially in patients with other risks such as malignancies.[9]

INTRAOPERATIVE AND POSTOPERATIVE MANAGEMENT

- *Analgesia*:
  - *Epidural*: Continuous epidural analgesia provides superior pain relief postoperatively compared to parenteral opioids in open abdominal surgery. Epidural analgesia is also associated with earlier return of bowel function and reduced respiratory complications. Although there is data to show improved outcomes with epidural analgesia in gastrectomy, the guidelines for epidural use in pancreatic resections are extrapolated from data from other upper abdominal surgeries.[9,10]

- *Wound catheters and abdominal fascial blocks*: There are some studies which suggest these modalities show improved pain relief and have opioid-sparing effects, but these studies are mainly limited to lower abdominal surgeries. The subcostal transversus abdominal plane (TAP) block shows promise in upper abdominal surgeries based on the dermatomes covered for analgesia.[11]
- *Multimodal opioid-sparing analgesia* to reduce opioid-related complications.

- *Preventing and treating postoperative nausea and vomiting (PONV)*: It is essential for risk stratification and multimodal approach to the management of PONV. All patients with one to two risk factors should receive a combination of antiemetics for prophylaxis. Patients with two to three risk factors should receive two to three antiemetics along with total intravenous anesthesia (TIVA) for prophylaxis. Opioid-sparing analgesia further contributes to reducing PONV.[5]

- *Anesthetic protocol and depth of anesthesia*: Monitoring depth of anesthesia can be done using either end-tidal anesthetic concentration or bispectral index (BIS). Depth should be monitored not only for prevention of awareness but also to titrate anesthetic to minimize complications. An end-tidal minimum alveolar concentration (MAC) of 0.7–1.3 or BIS of 40–60 aims to prevent awareness as well as reduce complications and facilitate early recovery from anesthesia.[5]

- *Neuromuscular blockade*: Most surgeries only require moderate neuromuscular blockade, which can further be complemented with adequate anesthetic depth and analgesia. Neuromuscular function should always be monitored when neuromuscular blockers are used. Quantitative methods such as peripheral nerve stimulator are preferred to qualitative clinical methods. This facilitates optimum return of neuromuscular function at the end of the surgery, especially in countries where sugammadex is not available.[5]

- *Prevention of hypothermia*: Hypothermia should be prevented as it increases the risk of surgical site infection, bleeding, and coagulopathy. Multimodal strategies such as forced air warmer, fluid warmers, and/or circulating water garments can be used. Active warming devices are recommended in all procedures lasting >30 minutes.[12]

- *Surgical techniques*: Minimally invasive surgery causing less wound trauma and tissue handling. Transverse incisions are associated with less postoperative opioid use and lower incidence of wound dehiscence, although there is no reduction in postoperative pulmonary complications or hospital stay compared to vertical incisions. Laparoscopic surgery is recommended when feasible and where expertise is available.[13]

- *Nasogastric intubation*: Routine nasogastric decompression following elective laparotomy should be avoided and if inserted should be removed when no longer needed.

- *Perioperative hemodynamic management*: Crystalloid-balanced isotonic solutions should be used. Predicted response to fluid is determined by the position of the patient on the Frank–Starling curve, with the steep portion indicating increases in stroke volume (SV) with increase in preload, thus indicating "fluid responsiveness." A volume of 250 mL colloid or crystalloid may be used for a fluid challenge, but even smaller volumes (100 mL) can be used. 10% or greater increase in SV indicates fluid responsiveness. The passive leg raising maneuver transfers about 300 mL of venous blood into the right atrium, similar to a fluid bolus, and can be used after surgery to determine fluid responsiveness.[14]

The RELIEF (Restrictive versus Liberal Fluid Therapy in Major Abdominal Surgery) trial compared liberal versus restrictive fluid therapy for intra- and postoperative management of major abdominal surgery. Some of the key findings in the study were that the restrictive group had a higher risk of acute kidney injury (AKI) and was not associated with a higher rate of disability-free survival compared to a liberal regimen. These findings suggest that a modestly liberal regimen of fluid administration may be safer than a restrictive regimen targeting zero balance. However, over resuscitation is also associated with complications, and thus judicious fluid management and goal-directed therapy is recommended.[15]

The INPRESS (Intraoperative Noradrenaline to Control Arterial Pressure) trial compared individualized blood pressure targeting to standard blood pressure management intraoperatively. The key finding was that management targeting individualized blood pressure was associated with significantly reduced risk of postoperative organ dysfunction. The individualized strategy targeted systolic blood pressure (SBP) within 10% of baseline using a continuous infusion of epinephrine. A baseline infusion of 4 mL/kg/h of lactated Ringer was given to both groups and additional fluid was given based on a hemodynamic algorithm.[16]

Individualized hemodynamic management with modestly liberal fluid strategy targeting SBP within 10% of baseline and using vasopressors when needed is recommended.

Enhanced recovery programs make the transition to oral diet at the earliest. Therefore, fluids should be discontinued in the postoperative period if oral feeding is established.

- *Prevention and treatment of postoperative ileus*: A multimodal approach to prevention of postoperative ileus is recommended. Minimally invasive surgery, opioid-sparing analgesia, early mobilization, early feeding, and early removal of nasogastric tubes are associated with reduced ileus. Laxatives and motility agents may be used to stimulate bowel movement, but robust evidence is lacking for their routine use.[5]

- *Early mobilization*: Exercise and mobilization should begin early in the postoperative period. Standardized protocols are recommended with involvement of nurses and physiotherapists. Early mobilization is associated with reduced complications, improved muscle function, and outcomes.[5]

While the above general principles apply to most major abdominal surgeries, some surgery specific management is outlined below.

PERIOPERATIVE MANAGEMENT OF PANCREATIC SURGERIES

- *Preoperative biliary drainage*: Recent evidence suggests that routine preoperative biliary drainage is not beneficial and may be associated with greater morbidity.[6,17]
- *Preoperative bowel preparation*: Preoperative bowel preparation is not routinely recommended and may be associated with fluid and electrolyte imbalances. Recent data have not found any beneficial effect in patients undergoing pancreaticoduodenectomy.[10,18]
- *Somatostatin analogs*: The rationale for use of octreotide is to reduce pancreatic secretions and thus reduce pancreatic fistulas. But based on available data, octreotide use is not recommended routinely because the presumed effects have not shown any clinical benefits.[10]
- *Perianastomotic drains*: There is no adequate evidence to suggest no drains in pancreatic surgery, but removing drains early after 72 hours is recommended in patients at low risk of pancreatic fistula.[10]
- *Early postoperative feeding*: Early oral feeding with escalation based on patient tolerance is recommended. If oral diet is not tolerated or patients develop complications, enteral nutrition is preferred to parenteral nutrition, and transition to oral nutrition should be initiated as early as possible.[10]
- *Delayed gastric emptying (DGE)*: It is a common complication following pancreatic resection. Patient may require reinsertion/prolonged nasogastric tube, nasojejunal tube for feeding, and/or total parenteral nutrition (TPN) depending on the duration of nutritional compromise secondary to DGE.[10]

PERIOPERATIVE MANAGEMENT OF GASTRIC RESECTIONS

- *Preoperative nutrition optimization*: Gastric outlet obstruction due to mechanical effects of tumor contributes to malnutrition and cachexia in patients with gastric cancer. Nausea, vomiting, dysphagia, and early satiety are common symptoms of gastric cancer.[19] Thus, identifying and managing malnutrition preoperatively is essential to improve patient outcomes. Enteral supplements or nasogastric or nasojejunal feeds may be commenced preoperatively to improve nutritional status. If there is gastric outlet obstruction due to the tumor, TPN may be warranted if enteral nutrition cannot be established. There is insufficient evidence to support the use of immunonutrition in patients undergoing gastric resections, but there is emerging evidence that indicates preoperative oral immune-enhanced formulas may be associated with reduced postoperative complication.[9,20]

- *Preoperative carbohydrates*: If a patient does not have obstruction, then solids should be allowed until 6 hours before surgery and clear fluids until 2 hours before surgery. Although data from patients undergoing gastric resection is lacking, extrapolation from patients undergoing other major gastrointestinal procedures suggests that complex carbohydrate drink 2 hours prior to surgery reduces thirst, hunger, anxiety, length of hospital stay, and postoperative insulin resistance.[21,22] Therefore, oral carbohydrate drinks should be given 2 hours before surgery in nondiabetic patients. The presence of gastric outlet obstruction secondary to tumors may preclude preoperative carbohydrate loading or clear fluids and perhaps be harmful.

- *Gastric outlet obstruction and anesthesia concerns*: Patients with gastric tumors may be at risk for gastric outlet obstruction and can have passive regurgitation and aspiration under anesthesia. Preoperative assessment of all patients with gastric cancer for symptoms of gastric outlet obstruction and adequate precautions such as preoperative decompression with nasogastric tube and/or rapid sequence induction may be appropriate.[23]

- *Surgical access*: Laparoscopic-assisted distal and total gastrectomy is associated with better outcomes compared to open approaches, especially in early gastric cancer.[9]

- *Perianastomotic drains*: Routine use of perianastomotic drains in gastric resections is not beneficial and may be associated with increased postoperative complications.[9]

- *Early postoperative diet*: Postgastrectomy patients should be allowed oral diet as tolerated from postoperative day (POD) 1. No adverse outcomes have been reported from early introduction of oral diet in total gastrectomy patients. These patients are at high risk of malnourishment. Nutritional support in the form of oral supplements and enteral feeding via nasogastric or nasojejunal tube may be required in patients who are unable to meet 60% of daily nutritional requirements by POD 6. Parenteral nutrition should only be considered if enteral feeding fails beyond 7 days.[9]

MANAGEMENT OF RETROPERITONEAL TUMORS

Retroperitoneal tumors can be both benign and malignant and consist of lipomas, teratomas, schwannomas, lymphomas, and sarcomas. Discussion of all tumors is beyond the scope of this text. Perioperative management of retroperitoneal sarcomas is summarized in the text; this can be extrapolated to other retroperitoneal tumors.

- *Preoperative imaging* should be thoroughly reviewed to determine the extent of the tumor and structures involved such as major vessels, kidneys, or spleen. Patient should be counseled and preoperative preparation should be in place anticipating resection of involved organs.
- *Retroperitoneal tumors* can cause several problems related to their large size.[24]
  - Increased abdominal pressure leading to vascular congestion
  - Compression of abdominal aorta and increased cardiac afterload
  - Compression of gastrointestinal tract causing malnutrition
  - Pressure on the diaphragm reducing respiratory compliance
- *Preoperative bowel preparation* may be done in anticipation of bowel resection.
- *Anticipation of massive hemorrhage* and adequate provision of blood and blood products, as well as vascular access (peripheral and central venous cannulas, arterial line, and cardiac output monitoring).
- *Fluid management* can be challenging associated with major fluid shifts in the retroperitoneum, massive hemorrhage, and/or nephrectomy.[25] They may require elective postoperative ventilation.
- Other general principles are applicable to gastrointestinal surgery as mentioned above.

REFERENCES

1. Desborough JP. The stress response to trauma and surgery. Br J Anaesth. 2000;85(1):109-17.
2. Kotagal M, Symons RG, Hirsch IB, Umpierrez GE, Dellinger EP, Farrokhi ET, et al. Perioperative hyperglycemia and risk of adverse events among patients with and without diabetes. Ann Surg. 2015;261(1):97-103.
3. Santa Mina D, Clarke H, AG, Ritvo P, Leung YW, Matthew Katz J, et al. Effect of total-body prehabilitation on postoperative outcomes: a systematic review and meta-analysis. Physiotherapy. 2014;100(3):196-207.
4. Kiecolt-Glaser JK, Page GG, Marucha PT, MacCallum RC, Glaser R. Psychological influences on surgical recovery. Perspectives from psychoneuroimmunology. Am Psychol. 1998;53(11):1209-18.
5. Feldheiser A, Aziz O, Baldini G, Cox BPBW, Fearon KCH, Feldman LS, et al. Enhanced Recovery After Surgery (ERAS) for gastrointestinal surgery, part 2: consensus statement for anaesthesia practice. Acta Anaesthesiol Scand. 2016;60(3):289-334.
6. Smith MD, McCall J, Plank L, Herbison GP, Soop M, Nygren J. Preoperative carbohydrate treatment for enhancing recovery after elective surgery. Cochrane Database Syst Rev. 2014;(8):CD009161.
7. Awad S, Varadhan KK, Ljungqvist O, Lobo DN. A meta-analysis of randomised controlled trials on preoperative oral carbohydrate treatment in elective surgery. Clin Nutr Edinb Scotl. 2013;32(1):34-44.
8. Bratzler DW, Dellinger EP, Olsen KM, Perl TM, Auwaerter PG, Bolon MK, et al. Clinical practice guidelines for antimicrobial prophylaxis in surgery. Am J Health-Syst Pharm. 2013;70(3):195-283.
9. Mortensen K, Nilsson M, Slim K, Schäfer M, Mariette C, Braga M, et al. Consensus guidelines for enhanced recovery after gastrectomy: Enhanced Recovery After Surgery (ERAS®) Society recommendations. Br J Surg. 2014;101(10):1209-29.
10. Lassen K, Coolsen MME, Slim K, Carli F, de Aguilar-Nascimento JE, Schäfer M, et al. Guidelines for perioperative care for pancreaticoduodenectomy: Enhanced Recovery After Surgery (ERAS®) Society recommendations. Clin Nutr Edinb Scotl. 2012;31(6):817-30.
11. Lee THW, Barrington MJ, Tran TMN, Wong D, Hebbard PD. Comparison of extent of sensory block following posterior and subcostal approaches to ultrasound-guided transversus abdominis plane block. Anaesth Intensive Care. 2010;38(3):452-60.
12. Esnaola NF, Cole DJ. Perioperative normothermia during major surgery: Is it important? Adv Surg. 2011;45:249-63.
13. Brown SR, Goodfellow PB. Transverse verses midline incisions for abdominal surgery. Cochrane Database Syst Rev. 2005;(4):CD005199.
14. Miller TE, Myles PS. Perioperative fluid therapy for major surgery. Anesthesiology. 2019;130(5):825-32.
15. Myles PS, Bellomo R, Corcoran T, Forbes A, Peyton P, Story D, et al. Restrictive versus liberal fluid therapy for major abdominal surgery. N Engl J Med. 2018;378(24):2263-74.
16. Futier E, Lefrant J-Y, Guinot P-G, Godet T, Lorne E, Cuvillon P, et al. Effect of individualized vs standard blood pressure management strategies on postoperative organ dysfunction among high-risk patients undergoing major surgery: A randomized clinical trial. JAMA. 2017;318(14):1346-57.
17. van der Gaag NA, Rauws EAJ, van Eijck CHJ, Bruno MJ, van der Harst E, Kubben FJGM, et al. Preoperative biliary drainage for cancer of the head of the pancreas. N Engl J Med. 2010;362(2):129-37.
18. Lavu H, Kennedy EP, Mazo R, Stewart RJ, Greenleaf C, Grenda DR, et al. Preoperative mechanical bowel preparation does not offer a benefit for patients who undergo pancreaticoduodenectomy. Surgery. 2010;148(2):278-84.

19. Donohoe CL, Ryan AM, Reynolds JV. Cancer cachexia: mechanisms and clinical implications. Gastroenterol Res Pract. 2011;2011:601434.

20. Okamoto Y, Okano K, Izuishi K, Usuki H, Wakabayashi H, Suzuki Y. Attenuation of the systemic inflammatory response and infectious complications after gastrectomy with preoperative oral arginine and ω-3 fatty acids supplemented immunonutrition. World J Surg. 2009;33(9):1815-21.

21. Ljungqvist O. Modulating postoperative insulin resistance by preoperative carbohydrate loading. Tight Glycemic Control Bench Bed Back. 2009;23(4):401-9.

22. Hausel J, Nygren J, Lagerkranser M, Hellström PM, Hammarqvist F, Almström C, et al. A carbohydrate-rich drink reduces preoperative discomfort in elective surgery patients. Anesth Analg. 2001;93(5):1344-50.

23. Wallace C, McGuire B. Rapid sequence induction: its place in modern anaesthesia. Contin Educ Anaesth Crit Care Pain. 2013;14(3):130-5.

24. Feng D, Xu F, Wang M, Gu X, Ma Z. Anesthetic management of a patient with giant retroperitoneal liposarcoma: case report with literature review. Int J Clin Exp Med. 2015;8(10):19530-4.

25. Tseng W. (2018). Surgical resection of retroperitoneal sarcoma. [online] Available from: https://www.uptodate.com/contents/surgical-resection-of-retroperitoneal-sarcoma/print/. [Last accessed March, 2020].

Perioperative Management of Major Liver Resections

Sohan Lal Solanki, Anuja Jain

INTRODUCTION

Hepatic resection has become routine in management of various conditions of liver. Liver being a complex and an important organ having important physiological function, its resection is associated with high postoperative morbidity and mortality. With evolving knowledge and advances in anesthesia, surgical technique, and postoperative care, outcomes have improved remarkably. Even with reduction in morbidity and mortality, liver resection (LR) patients still encounter various anesthesia and surgical complications. LRs are considered to be having >5% risk of cardiac event in the perioperative period, as classified by the European Society of Anesthesia (ESA) and European Society of Cardiology (ESC). With all of this, it becomes mandatory that we have in-depth knowledge of LR extending from preoperative, intraoperative to postoperative period.[1]

ANATOMY AND PHYSIOLOGY

Based on the distribution of vessels and bile duct, liver is divided into two lobar segments and eight Couinaud segments. The Brisbane 2000 Nomenclature was given to the types of resection done depending on the surgical segments of liver **(Table 1)**.

Liver performs various functions:
- Metabolism of glucose, fat, protein, hormones, toxins
- Excretion of bile, toxins, drugs, various waste products
- Production of albumin, coagulation factors, protein C, and protein S
- Immunological—Kupffer cells which remove bacteria from portal circulation, formation of immune factors
- Storehouse of blood, vitamin, and glycogen
- Removing senescent red cells.

INDICATIONS OF HEPATIC RESECTION

Malignancy is the most common reason for LR. The tumor can be either primary, metastatic, or recurrence. The most common primary liver malignancy is hepatocellular carcinoma (HCC) which is the sixth most common among all malignancies.[3] It can be inherited in the form of hemochromatosis or acquired after chronic liver disease

Anatomical term	Couinaud segments	Term for HRS	Major or minor resection
Right hemi liver	5, 6, 7, 8	Right hemihepatectomy or right hemihepatectomy	Major
Left hemi liver	2, 3, 4 (±1)	Left hemihepatectomy or left hemihepatectomy	Major
Right anterior section	5, 8	Right anterior sectionectomy	Minor
Right posterior section	6, 7	Right posterior sectionectomy	Minor
Left medial section	4	Left medial sectionectomy or resection segment 4 or segmentectomy 4	Minor
Left lateral section	2, 3	Left lateral sectionectomy or bisegmentectomy 2, 3	Minor
–	4, 5, 6, 7, 8, (±1)	Right trisectionectomy or extended right hemihepatectomy or extended right hepatectomy	Major
–	2, 3, 4, 5, 8, (±1)	Left trisectionectomy or extended left hemihepatectomy or extended left hepatectomy	Major

Table 1: Brisbane consensus nomenclature 2000 for describing hepatic resection surgery based on liver segmental and sectorial anatomy.[2]

(HRS: hepatorenal syndrome)

(CLD) such as hepatitis C, alcoholic cirrhosis, and metabolic syndromes.[4] Patients of hepatitis C, hepatitis B, alcoholic liver cirrhosis, or nonalcoholic steatohepatitis should be under evaluation every 6 months for serum markers (alpha fetoprotein) and imaging like ultrasonography for early diagnosis.[5] Metastasis to liver can occur from various solid organs. Hepatic resection is also an integral part of surgery for cholangiocarcinoma which requires extended cholecystectomy. Other indications are benign conditions such as hemangiomas, simple cysts, focal nodular hyperplasia, and trauma.

SCORING SYSTEM TO SELECT PATIENTS

Patients having cirrhosis of liver have to be evaluated and classified according to the Child–Turcotte–Pugh (CTP) classification or model for end-stage liver disease (MELD). These scoring systems are a tool for assessing the feasibility of surgery in patients with CLD. Of these scoring systems, CTP correlates better with postoperative morbidity.[6] Although MELD is used to predict the survival of patients on waiting list for surgery, along with CTP it gives a good estimate of perioperative risk.[7] A study done on 79 patients to compare various scoring systems concluded that CTP scoring is the best general mortality indicator; however, integrated MELD (iMELD) is the best indicator specifically for operative mortality.[8] CTP class A and B patients have increased mortality as compared to normal patients. Child–Pugh C patients are mostly a contraindication to surgery (**Tables 2 and 3**).

Indocyanine green (ICG) clearance is also used to predict mortality in the postoperative period in patients undergoing LR. The normal value is 10%. For safe resections, this should at least be 14–17%. Limited hepatectomies can be done at 40% and minor at 22%.[10]

To ensure least postoperative morbidity and mortality, it is required to find out the future liver remnant (FLR). For optimum functioning, the volume of residual liver should at least be 20–30% in a patient with normal liver and in patients with CLD the remnant liver should at least be 40–50%; below this critical volume, the patient might land into posthepatectomy liver failure.[11] The liver has a unique capability of regeneration which helps in extended resection. Although regeneration ensures adequate functioning, it is limited in diseased liver and in patients where portal flow is affected. There are various tools available to assess FLR in the form of biochemical test, magnetic resonance imaging, or scintigraphic techniques. A combination of two or more techniques gives more accurate result.[12]

SYSTEMIC CHANGES OF CHRONIC LIVER DISEASE

Cardiac

Parenchymal disease of liver is a state of hyperdynamic circulation attributed to systemic vasodilatation and reduction in peripheral vascular resistance. This can be explained by excessive production of nitric oxide (NO) by endothelial NO synthase.[13] This endothelial dysfunction has

Table 2: Child–Pugh–Turcotte score.[9]

Child–Pugh score			
Factor	1 point	2 points	3 points
Total bilirubin (μmol/L)	<34	34–50	>50
Serum albumin (g/L)	>35	28–35	<28
PT in seconds*	<4	4–6	>6
INR	<1.7	1.7–2.2	<2.2
Ascites	None	Mild	Moderate to severe
Hepatic encephalopathy	None	Grades I–II (or suppressed with medication)	Grades III–IV (or refractory)
	Class A	Class B	Class C
Total points	5–6	7–9	10–15
1-year survival	100%	80%	45%

(INR: international normalized ratio; PT: prothrombin time)
*Frequently INR is used as substitute

Table 3: Model for end-stage liver disease (MELD).[8]

MELD score = 9.57 × log e (creatinine mg/dl) +3.78 × log e (total bilirubin mg/dl) + 11.2 × log e (INR) + 6.43					
MELD score	≤9	10–19	20–29	30–39	≥40
Hospitalized patient	4%	27%	76%	83%	100%
Outpatient cirrhotic	2%	6%	50%		

prognostic and predictive value for adverse outcome and mortality in advanced liver disease.[14] Systemic vasodilatation because of NO results in peripheral pooling of blood and relative systemic hypovolemia. All this causes activation of the renin angiotensin system (RAS) and retention of salt and water which in turn leads to increase in cardiac output (CO) eventually leading to pathophysiological changes in the form of cardiac hypertrophy. Cirrhotic patients have elevated CO, increased heart rate, and reduced mean arterial pressure (MAP). All these lead to development of cirrhotic cardiomyopathy. With onset of cardiomyopathy, functioning of heart reduces resulting in decreased CO. Cardiac hypertrophy in turn leads to diastolic dysfunction diagnosed and graded echocardiographically by calculating E/A and E/e' ratio.[15] Systemic vasodilatation causes substantial damage to various organs by causing hepatorenal syndrome (HRS), hepatopulmonary syndrome (HPS), esophageal varices, ascites, and encephalitis.

Gastrointestinal System

Intrahepatic changes in CLD cause an increase in resistance to blood flow. This elevated resistance presents as portal hypertension (PH) which prevents blood flow through liver resulting in collateral formation. In addition to this, extrahepatic splanchnic vasodilatation leads to elevated blood flow through portal vein exacerbating PH. Combination of PH and sodium and water retention as a consequence of activation of the renin angiotensin aldosterone system (RAAS) results in formation of ascites. Around 50% of cirrhotic patients are complicated by ascites in a span of 10 years, and this is a marker of poor prognosis.[16]

Renal

Hepatorenal syndrome is impairment in renal function which occurs in a patient of advanced liver disease in the absence of any other cause of renal compromise. The exact pathophysiology of HRS is unknown. There are four postulations which in combination lead to HRS:[17]

1. NO-induced splanchnic vasodilatation causing reduced blood flow to kidney contributing activation of RAAS further reducing renal perfusion by vasoconstriction in renal afferent vessels
2. Stimulation of the sympathetic renal system also causing vasoconstriction in afferent vessels
3. Compromised functioning of heart because of cirrhotic cardiomyopathy causing reduced CO and blood flow to kidney
4. Various vasoactive cytokines causing vasodilatation of renal vessels.

The following are the major and minor diagnostic criteria for HRS of which minor is not necessary:[18]

Major criteria:
- Presence of cirrhosis and ascites
- Acute kidney injury with creatinine >1.5 mg/dL
- No improvement even after expansion of plasma volume by albumin 1 g/kg body weight and withholding diuretic for 2 days
- Absence of shock
- No recent use of nephrotoxic drugs such as amino-glycosides, iodinated contrast, or nonsteroidal anti-inflammatory drugs (NSAIDs)
- No signs of structural kidney injury (absence of microhematuria >50 red blood cells/high power field or proteinuria >500 mg/day) or normal renal ultrasound.

Minor criteria:
- <0.5 mL/day urine volume
- Urine sodium <10 mmol/day
- Urine osmolality > plasma osmolality
- Red blood cells in urine <130 mmol/L.

Hepatorenal syndrome can be type I or type II depending upon the duration of progression of renal compromise and rise in the serum creatinine level. Type I is rapidly progressive with doubling or increase in the creatinine level by 2.5 mg/dL within 2 weeks and have poor prognosis.[19] Type II is slowly progressive as compared to type I with creatinine >1.5 mg/dL and have better prognosis. Although classified as type I or II, treatment of both remain the same. In addition to this, renal compromise in a CLD patient can be attributed to the pre-existing renal parenchymal disease or prerenal or drug-induced failure.[20]

Pulmonary

Hepatopulmonary syndrome is characterized by:[21]
- Liver disease
- Intrapulmonary vasodilatation
- Alveolar–arterial oxygen gradient >15 mm Hg or >20 mm Hg in a patient >65 years and saturation on pulse oximetry <96%.

All this is because of dilatation of capillary and precapillary vessels leading to intrapulmonary shunting. They present with platypnea, orthodeoxia, dyspnea, cyanosis, and clubbing. On imaging, the X-ray can be normal or can show increased interstitial marking; diffusion capacity decreased as depicted in the pulmonary function test (PFT) and arterial blood gas shows changing levels of partial pressure of oxygen. Diagnosis of HPS can be done by microbubble contrast-enhanced transthoracic ECHO and 99m technetium radiolabeled macroaggregated albumin perfusion scan (MAA scan).[22]

Patients with CLD can also present with portopulmonary hypertension (PPHTN) differentiated from HPS by the presence of intrapulmonary vasoconstriction leading to right heart failure. PPHTN is present in about 5% of CLD defined by PH of >15 mm Hg and[22]

- Mean pressure in the pulmonary artery of 25 mm Hg at rest, >30 mm Hg with exercise
- Pulmonary artery occlusion pressure (POAP) <15 mm Hg
- Pulmonary vascular resistance (PVR) > 240 dynes/s/cm^{-5}

All this is further complicated by the presence of pleural effusion (PE) and ascites which lead to upward shift of diaphragm. PE in turn leads to reduction in lung volumes and capacities. PPHTN generally happens due to imbalance of vascular mediators leading to vasoconstriction, smooth muscle proliferation, microvascular thrombosis, and endothelial damage with remodeling.

Patients present with:
- Dyspnea on exertion, easy fatiguability, abdominal distention, syncope, and chest pain
- Edema of periphery, elevated jugular venous pressure, pulsatile liver, loud P2, and increased split in S2.

Primary pulmonary hypertension is diagnosed by:
- ECG—right axis deviation, right bundle branch block
- X-ray chest—cardiomegaly
- PFT may be normal but occasionally there may be reduced diffusion capacity.
- Transthoracic ECHO and Doppler has right ventricular systolic pressure >40 mm Hg.
- Right heart catheterization gives confirmatory diagnosis.

Anesthesia management is very challenging in these patients. It is advisable to use invasive pressure monitoring along with CO and transesophageal echocardiography to ensure maintenance of hemodynamics of the patient. Any compromise in hemodynamics can be detrimental to the patient.

Coagulation

The liver has a significant role in hemostasis as it synthesizes almost all procoagulant factors, anticoagulant factors, and components of the fibrinolytic system. PH leads to hypersplenism which causes destruction of platelets. Impaired formation of thrombopoietin also leads to thrombocytopenia. These changes are mentioned in **Box 1**.

With imbalance in pro- and anticoagulation factors, patients of CLD are in a state of "rebalanced hemostasis." This condition of rebalanced hemostasis can be compared to a see-saw where a patient swings between a state of thrombosis and bleeding most of the time maintaining a balance between both.[23] In fact, posthepatectomy patients are considered as hypercoagulable as these patients are in a prothrombotic state as they have malignancy, received chemotherapy, or have raised acute-phase reactants,

> **Box 1:** Coagulation factors in chronic liver disease.
>
> *Procoagulant factors:*
> - Increased factor VIII
> - Decreased levels of proteins C and S and antithrombin
> - Low levels of plasminogen
> - Elevated von Willebrand factor (vWF) as compensation of platelet dysfunction
>
> *Anticoagulant factors:*
> - Thrombocytopenia
> - Platelet function defect
> - Vitamin K deficiency
> - Decreased levels of factors II, V, VII, IX, X, and XI
> - Dysfibrinogenemia
> - Decreased plasmin inhibitor, factor XIII
> - Increased tissue plasminogen activator

decreased production of clotting factors, dilution due to fluids in the perioperative period, immobility, and long duration of surgery.[24] Bleeding from varices is commonly attributed to local factors rather than changes in hemostasis. Routine coagulation tests in the form of prothrombin time (PT), international normalized ratio (INR), and partial thromboplastin time (PTT) are not good predictors of bleeding; thromboelastography (TEG) rather remains a better choice.[25]

Preoperative Evaluation

Complete blood count, kidney function test, and coagulation profile along with liver function tests should be done. It should be remembered that the serum albumin level and coagulation factors depict the functional status of liver rather than alanine aminotransferase (ALT) and aspartate aminotransferase (AST) which signify integrity of the hepatocellular system. Along with PT, PTT and INR, TEG, if available, is the best predictor for coagulation status.

Depending upon the functional status, CTP scoring, and cardiac changes, electrocardiogram and echocardiography should be done. Cardiopulmonary exercise testing (CPET) is helpful in predicting postoperative morbidity in patients with advanced liver disease undergoing a vascular repair or major resection. CPET helps in anticipating complications in these patients. Oxygen consumption at an anaerobic threshold of <10.2 mL/kg/min indicates toward increased morbidity in the postoperative period.[26]

Preoperative Optimization

In patients with known liver disease, preoperative management aims at identifying the cause and optimizing the liver function by improving the nutritional status, correction of coagulopathy with blood products, and treating subtle or overt hepatic encephalopathy (HE), PH, and ascites.[27]

Nutritional Status

Hepatocellular carcinoma is the second most common cause of mortality due to cancer in the world.[28] 70–90% patients of HCC have cirrhosis secondary to hepatitis B or C or alcoholic liver disease and of these 50–90% patients suffer from malnutrition.[5] Although morbidity and mortality after hepatic resections have improved, it still remains high. One of the important modifiable factors is nutrition. Also, successful resection is dependent on regeneration of the remnant hepatic tissue by hyperplasia which in turn depends on the pathology of liver and systemic condition which in turn is dependent on the nutritional status. To ensure good outcome, nutritional evaluation and optimization in the preoperative period are of paramount importance. Subjective Global Assessment (SGA) is used for categorizing the patients as well nourished, moderately, or severely malnourished. The European Society for Clinical Nutrition and Metabolism (ESPEN) has formulated guidelines specifically for LR which elaborates on nutritional management of these patients extending from preoperative, intraoperative to postoperative period **(Box 2)**.[29]

The Enhanced Recovery After Surgery (ERAS) Society gives a strong recommendation with a high level of evidence for preoperative nutrition development. They suggest postponing surgery for at least 2 weeks in severely malnourished patients to build nutrition.[30]

The role of immunonutrition for patients undergoing hepatic resection to be started preoperatively is under evaluation although initial research shows a promising role.[31]

Albumin synthesized in the liver performs a very important role by maintaining oncotic pressure hence maintaining intravascular volume. Other functions of albumin are early recovery by wear and tear of wound, retaining muscle mass so maintaining respiratory muscle strength. Routine use of intravenous albumin is not recommended in patients unless liver functions are severely depressed. Along with a high protein diet, patients should be supplemented with fat-soluble vitamins and trace elements as deficiency of these is also known in these patients which might also increase the risk of infection or cause impaired wound healing. If patients are unable to take orally, feeding through the nasogastric tube is recommended. Patients of HE should be given a high lipid and carbohydrate diet to reduce the progression. Currently, the evidence recommends use of enteral nutrition as compared to parenteral. In conclusion, nutrition is one of the important parameters to be evaluated and optimized preoperatively. A dietician should be consulted and should be a part of team till the patient is discharged from the hospital.

Physical Status

Physical rehabilitation done preoperatively improves outcomes in patients of hepatic resection. With the advent of the era of ERAS, the importance of preoperative exercise has been further established. Debette-Gratien et al. did a pilot study in patients awaiting liver transplant by implementing adapted physical activity (APA) monitoring oxygen consumption. They observed that APA significantly improved a distance of 6-minute walk, strength test of knee extensor muscles, and anaerobic threshold value.[32] Although this was for patients awaiting liver transplant and the implementation time for APA was 12 weeks, which is not feasible in cancer patients, addition of chest physiotherapy, deep breathing exercises, and incentive spirometry will be effective by improving the quality of life.

Renal

Nephrotoxic drugs (like NSAIDs, aminoglycosides, contrast) and acidosis should be avoided perioperatively. Intravascular volume should be maintained and close monitoring should be kept on urine output and renal functions in these patients. Patients of type I HRS might benefit from albumin administration and vasopressor drugs such as terlipressin.

Ascites

For the management of ascites in these patients, sodium and water restriction should first be instituted followed by starting diuretics in the form of spironolactone. Finally, for those not responding to above, paracentesis is the option as this improves pulmonary function. Caution while paracentesis should be taken as rapid removal can lead to paracentesis-induced circulatory dysfunction.

Box 2: ESPEN guidelines adopted for hepatic surgery.[29]

Preoperative:
- Assess nutritional status. Indicators of severe risk—weight loss in last 6 months >10–15%, body mass index <18.5%, albumin <3 g/dL
- All patients with severe risk factors—delay the surgery to build up nutrition at least for 7–14 days.
- Wherever possible, avoid nutrition by the parenteral route.
- All patients should be provided extra nutritional support, if needed.
- Nil by mouth before surgery for solids 6 hours and clear liquids for 2 hours.

Intraoperative
- If postoperatively, prolong nil by mouth state is anticipated then it is recommended to insert a naso-gastric or naso-jejunal tube for enteral feed

Postoperative
- Restart oral/enteral feed within 24 hours.
- Reassess nutritional status frequently.

(ESPEN: European Society for Clinical Nutrition and Metabolism)

Hematological and Coagulation Disorders

Patients being in a rebalanced state of hemostasis, all the markers of coagulation are surrogate. TEG by measuring the viscoelastic properties of blood clotting provides precise information. With unavailability of TEG, optimization should be based on the available investigations. Prophylactic transfusion of platelet is recommended only if the platelet count is <50,000/mm^3.

Injection of vitamin K should be given preoperatively even though synthetic impairment of liver cannot be corrected but deranged INR due to malabsorption can be. Fresh frozen plasma (FFP) can be used (if INR > 1.7), but it should be remembered that coagulation factors have a very short half-life.[33]

Fluid and Electrolyte Abnormality

Close monitoring of fluid and electrolyte is recommended. With preserved liver functions, this balance is maintained. Hyponatremia in a cirrhotic patient signifies water overload due to reduced clearance. As a treatment, restriction of oral fluids is advised. Sodium correction is not given till the patient becomes symptomatic and levels drop below 125 mmol/L. Restricting fluid and sodium intake also prevents from postoperative ascites' formation. Hypokalemia, if present, should be corrected as this can precipitate and worsen HE. Potassium correction also restores the sodium value.

Counseling

A team of doctors involved in perioperative care of the patients should explain in detail about the surgery and potential perioperative complications. These include possibility of liver failure, pulmonary, cardiac and renal dysfunction, infection, and possibility of bile injury and leak necessitating exploration for hepaticojejunostomy or bile-enteric anastomosis. Depending on the extent of lesion, the probability of inoperability should be communicated.

Portal Vein Embolization

Portal vein embolization (PVE) is considered the technique for preoperative preparation in patients with small FLR.[34] Indication of PVE is where 70–75% of liver has to be removed in normal patients and 60–65% in cirrhotic patients. Post PVE, hypertrophy of the rest of the liver is one of the assessment factors for postoperative regeneration of liver. Transarterial chemoembolization (TACE) also accelerates hypertrophy of the rest of liver. Recurrence-free survival is also higher in a patient who underwent PVE. No or minimum hypertrophy warns us about the poor outcome in the postoperative period and should preferably not undergo resection.

ERAS

Various studies have been conducted on ERAS for liver surgery and have concluded that ERAS is safe and decreases complications and postoperative hospital stay. Qi et al. in their randomized controlled trial (RCT) found that ERAS significantly improved the synthetic function of liver and there was no difference in the rate of re-exploration as compared to patients in whom ERAS was not followed.[35] The recommendation from ERAS is given in **Box 3**.

Intraoperative

Goal

The goal of intraoperative management is to maintain hepatic blood flow and balance between demand and supply of oxygen and also to avoid hypotension, hypoxia, hypovolemia, hypothermia, and acidosis.

Monitoring

Standard anesthesia monitoring (pulse oximeter, electrocardiogram, noninvasive blood pressure monitor,

---

Box 3: Recommendation from the ERAS Society for liver surgery.[35]

Preoperative
- Preoperative counseling
- Perioperative nutrition
- 6-hour fasting for solids, carbohydrate loading prior evening and 2 hours before anesthesia
- No oral bowel preparation
- Avoid long-acting anxiolytics. Short-acting anxiolytics can be used to give regional anesthesia just before induction.
- Antithrombotic prophylaxis—low molecular weight heparin (LMWH) or unfractionated heparin 2–12 hours before surgery

Intraoperative
- Antimicrobial prophylaxis 1 hour prior to surgery
- Skin preparation with 2% chlorhexidine
- No nasogastric tube
- Minimally invasive technique, especially for left lateral sections and anterior section
- Incision according to patient's and surgeon's discretion. To avoid Mercedes type of incision
- Maintaining temperature perioperatively
- Maintaining low CVP <5 cm H$_2$O
- Using balanced salt solution

Postoperative
- Encourage oral feed. Enteral or parenteral feed for a malnourished patient
- Glycemic control
- Prevention of delayed gastric emptying
- Early mobilization
- Adequate pain relief
- Prevent postoperative nausea and vomiting
- To perform routine audits to improve outcome

(CVP: central venous pressure; ERAS: enhanced recovery after surgery)

temperature, and urinary catheter) should be routinely used along with hemodynamic monitoring, such as arterial blood pressure and central venous pressure (CVP), and agent gas monitoring. Fluid should be guided according to dynamic parameters such as pulse pressure variation (PPV) or stroke volume variation (SVV). TEG is used to guide blood and blood products. Arterial blood gas analysis done intermittently helps to analyze and correct the imbalance of acid and base. CO monitoring is reserved for patients with compromised functioning of heart. Transesophageal echocardiography is a novel technique for hemodynamic monitoring and guiding fluid therapy.

Choice of Anesthesia

General anesthesia with epidural analgesia (EA) can be used if the epidural is not contraindicated. There are reservations for use of epidural in liver patients; also the ERAS society advocates against the use of epidural as there are concerns about coagulation abnormality and hypotension causing organ dysfunction. Analysis of literature suggests to decide about epidural depending on the individual patient profile (liver function, platelet count, volume of liver left post-resection). In patients where EA is used and bleeding is a concern, a viscoelastic method in the form of TEG can be a guide about the coagulation status of patients. Various studies have found that epidural has better efficacy for pain relief for the first 2 days postsurgery after which there is no difference. Alternative methods for analgesia have also been suggested in the form of patient control analgesia (PCA) with opioids, intrathecal morphine, or abdominal wall catheters (AWC) in the form of transverses abdominis or rectus abdominis depending on the type of incision. In using opioids, respiratory depression in the postoperative period is always a concern. So either opioids should not be given or used cautiously in obese, elderly, and patients with obstructive sleep apnea AWC can be inserted either before surgery under ultrasonography guidance or after surgery before closure under direct vision. When inserted before incision, this might get displaced and will have to be replaced after surgery. The advantages of AWC are that it is opioid sparing and is as efficacious as EA, but accurate placement and frequent dosing are a concern.[36]

Anesthesia Drugs

The choice of drugs depends on the pharmacokinetic properties of drug such as distribution, protein binding, metabolism, and excretion. In opioids, fentanyl is safer than morphine as the later forms a long-acting active metabolite. Short-acting benzodiazepines such as midazolam are comparatively safer. In HE patients or severely compromised liver function, benzodiazepines are contraindicated which tend to precipitate or exacerbate HE. Propofol is the choice

for induction as this has rapid distribution but might cause vasodilatation and reduction in blood flow to liver (to be used in reduced dose, titrated to effect). Atracurium and cisatracurium have Hoffman elimination and are safer. Sevoflurane and desflurane are least metabolized in the liver and so are preferred. At minimum alveolar concentration (MAC) 1 both sevoflurane and desflurane do not affect liver and renal functions.

Fluid, Blood, and Blood Products

Excessive fluid administration causes increased morbidity in patients undergoing abdominal surgery. Fluid administration should be PPV/SPV-guided maintaining an optimum balance between adequate fluid administration and low CVP. Literature suggests the use of PPV or SVV as a guide to fluid therapy maintaining a target >13%.[37] The prerequisites for the use of PPV or SVV are no spontaneous breathing and the patient should be mechanically ventilated at 6–8 mL/kg ideal body weight.[38] A recent study which included 3,000 patients to compare between restrictive and liberal fluid in major abdominal surgery found that patients with restricted fluid therapy had no advantage of disability-free survival over liberal fluid; rather there was an increased incidence of acute kidney injury. However, the limitation of this study was that it controlled the fluid administration only for the first 24 hours after which there was no control.[39] Maintaining low CVP helps in reducing blood loss though a low CVP for minimizing loss is debatable as increase in CVP can be due to other factors such as surgical traction. Also, in normal liver, maintaining low CVP will not be helpful. Further, many studies have found no correlation between reduction in CVP and blood loss.[40] The perfect method of lowering CVP is also debatable. Acute normovolemic hemodilution is one of the techniques to reduce loss. The choice of fluid is always a balanced salt solution. Colloid is to be used only for replacing blood loss. Blood is to be transfused according to the maximum allowable blood loss formula, but blood transfusion should be started well before the allowable blood loss threshold is reached if more blood loss is expected. Blood products guided according to TEG is the most preferred technique. Hyperlactatemia is common in patients of LR due to inability of the liver to metabolize lactate. So, nonlactate-containing balanced salt solution should be used preferably.

Ventilation

Assist-control mode is to be used with tidal volume 6–8 mL/kg ideal body weight. Positive end-expiratory pressure (PEEP) is to be kept minimum at 5 cm H_2O as an increase in this increases CVP. The respiratory rate according to end-tidal CO_2 is to maintain this between 40 and 45 mm Hg.

Extubation

The decision of postoperative ventilation should be based upon the preoperative status of the patient, comorbidities, volume of LR, and intraoperative blood loss as prolonged ventilation in the postoperative period leads to pulmonary complications which increases morbidity **(Box 4)**.[41]

Fluid and Electrolyte Management

Fluid therapy has always been the most debatable topic. The post-resection phase of liver is associated with a large amount of fluid shifts and vasodilatation. The choice of fluid and the rate of infusion are best decided according to the clinical condition of the patient. Excessive fluid leads to various complications by causing an interstitial

---

Box 4: Postoperative care.

- Monitoring of vital parameters—ABP, MAP, HR, SpO_2, RR
- Intake output charting, fluid electrolyte management
- Drains
- Sugar monitoring, glycemic control
- Blood investigations—complete blood count (CBC), liver function tests (LFT), arterial blood gas (ABG), coagulation profile, electrolytes
- Pain relief
- Systemic examination—CVS, RS, CNS, GI
- Thromboprophylaxis
- Antibiotic prophylaxis
- Nutrition
- Complications—posthepatectomy liver failure (PHLF), coagulopathy, bile leak, bleeding, deranged LFT, pulmonary complication, infection

(ABP: arterial blood pressure; CNS: central nervous system; CVS: cardiovascular system; GI: gastrointestinal; HR: heart rate; MAP: mean arterial pressure; RR: respiratory rate; RS: respiratory system)

---

accumulation of fluid, reducing tissue perfusion, and various pulmonary complications and interferes with wound healing.[42] According to ERAS, it is advisable to shift to oral fluids as soon as possible. Encourage the patient to take orally. The American Society for Enhanced Recovery (ASER) suggests to use the intraoperative strategy of fluid management postoperatively also. The guidelines of ASER are depicted in **Flowchart 1**. Traditionally, urine output was considered as a parameter for adequate tissue perfusion but it has been proved that stress-induced perioperative release of vasopressin is the factor for reduced urine output.[43] Now it is not considered as a marker of kidney injury, especially when other parameters of hemodynamic management are normal. A urine output of 0.5 mL/kg is acceptable and <0.3 mL/kg is taken as oliguria.[44] Balanced salt solution is preferred over colloid. It is only in a condition where the liver function is severely compromised that colloid in the form of albumin is preferred.

Electrolyte Abnormality

The most commonly encountered abnormalities post-hepatic resection are hyperlactatemia and hypophosphatemia. Lactate is utilized by the liver for gluconeogenesis. In the postoperative period due to compromised liver function, this is not possible leading to accumulation of lactate. Hence, it is advised to use lactate-free fluids in these patients. Regenerating liver utilizes phosphate which causes hypophosphatemia, but recent evidence suggests excessive excretion by phosphaturic agents as one of the reasons for reduction in phosphate levels. This decrease in phosphate leads to disturbed energy metabolism, arrhythmias, respiratory failure, and insulin

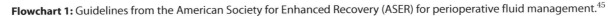

Flowchart 1: Guidelines from the American Society for Enhanced Recovery (ASER) for perioperative fluid management.[45]

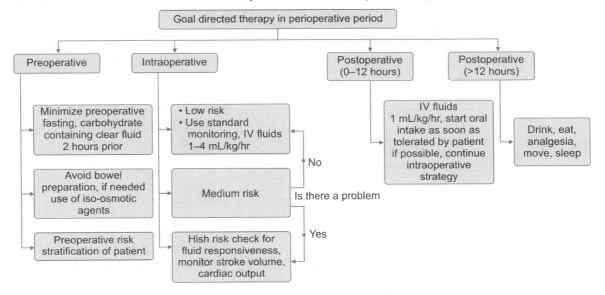

resistance and may exacerbate HE and neuromuscular and hematologic dysfunction.[46] Replacement can be done orally or intravenously by potassium phosphate depending upon the value of phosphate (normal phosphate level 0.80–1.45 mmol/L or 2.5–4.5 mg/dL). Brown et al. suggested that an intravenous correction rate of 7.5 mmol/h is safe.[47] Hyponatremia is seen in patients having either ascites or cirrhosis from the preoperative period. Correction should be done in symptomatic patients only. Hypokalemia and hypomagnesemia are known in these patients and should be corrected routinely. Patients who have received multiple blood transfusions have hyperkalemia which should be corrected promptly.

Pain Relief

The plan for this has to be formulated from the preoperative period and continued postoperatively. Multimodal analgesia is important. A combination of EA, AWC, and PCA with opioids and intravenous drugs are to be used. NSAIDs are to be used cautiously and best avoided in cirrhotic patients, old age, renal compromise, massive blood loss, and transfusion.

Thromboprophylaxis

As mentioned previously, these patients are in a state of rebalanced hemostasis shifting more toward a hypercoagulable state. Considering this, venous thromboembolism (VTE) prophylaxis should be received by all patients starting from the preoperative period in the form of pneumatic compression devices, with addition of early mobilization and pharmacologic therapy in postoperative period. Even though patients have a raised PT/INR, they may still be hypercoagulable with increased chances of VTE. De Pietri et al. found a higher chance of VTE in patients who did not receive prophylaxis in the postoperative period.[48] A study retrospectively analyzing a patient who had undergone major hepatectomy and received pharmacologic VTE did not have increased rate of blood transfusion; rather a decrease in VTE was seen.[24]

Glycemic Control

Both hypo- and hyperglycemia are known in patients of hepatic resection. Hyperglycemia occurs in response to stress-dysregulated metabolism of sugar in liver. Hypoglycemia occurs due to inability of the liver to synthesize glucose and also reduced stores of glycogen. Both these conditions are temporary and recover with improvement in liver functions. A regular monitoring of sugar is important with infusion of insulin according to a sliding scale.

Nutrition

The postoperative period in these patients is a phase of catabolism with imbalance in glucose and electrolyte and increased demand by regenerating liver. A plan for nutritional management is important for adequate recovery. Patients should be started on enteral feed as soon as possible. An evaluation of studies comparing enteral to parenteral feed concluded that enteral feed is safer as there is a less chance of infection and has better recovery.[49] Patients with a normal liver in the preoperative phase usually do not require any special intervention, but cirrhotic patients have greater requirement and benefit from early nutritional intervention. One of these interventions is addition of branched chain amino acids (BCAA) and other agents which increase immune response. So, the nutrition plan should be made for all patients in the postoperative period depending on the requirement of the individual patient and specific intervention such as BCAA in certain patients.

Complications

Coagulopathy

Derangement in PT, INR, platelet count, and fibrinogen levels is common in the postoperative period showing a rise in PT/INR and decrease in platelet and fibrinogen. These changes depend on the preoperative status of liver function and extent of resection. This takes about 24 hours to manifest and peaks in 2–5 days. De Pietri et al. found a higher chance of VTE in patients who did not receive prophylaxis in the postoperative period.[48] A raised PT/INR is self-limiting and usually does not need prophylactic FFP. Although many centers prefer prophylactic transfusion in patients with high risk of bleeding but platelets should be transfused only in patients with counts <30,000/mm^3 with active bleeding. Unnecessary transfusion of platelet leads to formation of antibody. TEG is the best guide to decide the component to be transfused. With unavailability of TEG FFP, recombinant factor VII and vitamin K should be used to correct coagulation derangement and prevent bleeding.

Infection

Around 25% of patients suffer from infection after LR. These infections are either abdominal (surgical site infection) or pulmonary. Recognition and source control along with antibiotics remain the mainstay of treatment. The risk factors for infection include age >60 years, obese, diabetes mellitus, massive blood loss, duration of surgery >180 minutes, cirrhosis, and major hepatic resection. For prevention of infection, early mobilization and enteral feed, antiseptic measures while caring for the patient, early removal of the urinary catheter and central line, chest physiotherapy, and incentive spirometry are recommended.

Hemorrhage

Although postoperative hemorrhage is blamed for raised PT/INR, it is known that posthepatectomy patients are hypercoagulable. A watch on drain and vitals helps in early recognition and treatment. CT abdomen can also help in diagnosis. TEG helps to rule out any coagulation abnormality. Blood and blood products, embolization of the bleeding vessel, and, if needed, exploration of the abdomen are the treatment options available.

Bile Leak

The incidence of bile leak reported in the literature is 3.6–12%.[50] Although this complication is rare, it is very serious and results in intra-abdominal sepsis which can lead to mortality. Various methods have been used to prevent bile leak after resection such as checking the patency of the system by intraoperative cholangiography, injection of air with ultrasonography guidance, bile leak test, and using fibrin glue.[51] Bile leak test involves introducing a catheter in the common hepatic duct and injecting ICG or fat emulsion and checking patency. There can be probability of leak after these tests also. Bile leak leads to fistula and results in collection in subhepatic and subphrenic areas or generalized peritonitis. The patient may present with fever, tachycardia, hypotension, and increase in drain and leukocytosis. Imaging should be done to reach a diagnosis, and a percutaneous biliary drainage guided by interventional radiology or endoscopic biliary stenting should be done.[52] Some patients might need exploratory laparotomy with hepaticojejunostomy.[53]

Posthepatectomy Liver Failure

Definition of posthepatectomy liver failure (PHLF) as given by the International Study Group of Liver Surgery (ISGLS): A postoperatively acquired deterioration in the ability of the liver (in patients with normal and abnormal liver function) to maintain its synthetic, excretory, and detoxifying functions, characterized by an increased INR (or need of clotting factors to maintain normal INR) and hyperbilirubinemia (according to the normal cutoff levels defined by the local laboratory) on or after postoperative day 5. If INR or serum bilirubin concentration is increased preoperatively, PHLF is defined by an increasing INR (decreasing PT) and increasing serum bilirubin concentration on or after postoperative day 5 (compared with the values of the previous day).[54] As per this definition, PHLF is graded as A, B, and C (**Box 5**).

Pathophysiology

There are several hypotheses which have been put forward for PHLF. In a patient with normal functioning liver in the preoperative period, posthepatectomy regeneration usually starts in the first 2 weeks and takes 3 months for completion. A sudden increase in portal pressure due to reduction in vascular volume leading to sheer stress on endothelium is one of the factors.[55] This results in necrosis of endothelium and oxidative damage. Also, excessive formation and release of inflammatory mediators may cause damage to cells.

Risk Factors for Posthepatectomy Liver Failure

The risk factors are as listed below:
- *Patient related:*
  - Age of patient >65 years
  - Metabolic factors such as insulin
  - Sepsis causing impairment of cytokines and disruption of hepatocytes
  - Miscellaneous—renal or cardiac compromise, thrombocytopenia.
- *Liver related:*
  - Hepatic steatosis
  - Postchemotherapy.
- Child–Turcotte–Pugh class B or C
- *Surgery related:*
  - Intraoperative blood loss and blood transfusion—blood loss >1,000 mL
  - Intraoperative vascular resections or IVC repair
  - FLR volume <20%.

Prevention: All preventive strategies are recommended to minimize liver damage and maintain liver function. These are listed as follows:
- Surgical techniques to ensure adequate FLR like PVE or two-staged hepatectomy or ischemic preconditioning
- Pharmacologic therapy such as somatostatin has an antioxidant property which is still under experiment
- Anesthesia techniques—preoperative optimization such as nutrition build-up, maintenance of low CVP, techniques to reduce blood loss minimizing transfusion
- Postoperative—prevent malnutrition, antimicrobial therapy, early recognition and treatment of complications such as bile leak or hemorrhage.

Management: The principles of management are the same as those of acute liver failure. The basic management of all grades of PHLF is similar. Diagnosis of complication of hepatectomy in the form of hemorrhage, infection, bile leak and initiation of treatment of the same is of

---

Box 5: Grades of posthepatectomy liver failure.[54]

- *Grade A*: PHLF resulting in abnormal laboratory parameters but requiring no change in the clinical management of the patient
- *Grade B*: PHLF resulting in a deviation from the regular clinical management but manageable without invasive treatment
- *Grade C*: PHLF resulting in a deviation from the regular clinical management and requiring invasive treatment

Table 4: Grades of PHLF.[54]

	Grade of PHLF A	B	C
LFT	INR <1.5	INR 1.5–2	INR >2
Renal	UO >0.5 mL/kg/h	UO <0.5 mL/kg/h	UO <0.5 mL/kg/h might need RRT
	BUN <150 mg/dL	BUN <150 mg/dL	BUN >150 mg/dL
	No symptoms of uremia	No symptoms of uremia	No symptoms of uremia
Respiratory	SO_2 >90% with or without O_2	SO_2 <90% with oxygen	Severe refractory hypoxemia SO_2 <85% even with high FiO_2
Other investigations	Not required	Culture—blood, urine, sputum	Culture—blood, urine, sputum
Imaging	Not required	• Abdomen • USG/CT/CXR • Brain CT	• Abdomen • USG/CXR/CT chest • Brain CT • ICP monitoring

(BUN: blood urea nitrogen; CXR: chest X-ray; ICP: intracranial pressure; INR: international normalized ratio; LFT: liver function tests; PHLF: posthepatectomy liver failure; UO: urine output)

primary importance in the form of appropriate antibiotics, drainage/stenting of biliary leaks, or exploration. Supportive treatment by maintaining mean arterial pressure (MAP) between 65 and 90 mm Hg, hematocrit ≥30%, saturation 93%, urine output >0.5 mL/kg/h, platelet ≥50,000/mm³, INR ≤1.5, enteral nutrition of at least 2,000 kcal/day, and treatment of HE is also recommended.[56] According to the grade of PHLF, management of patients is mentioned in **Table 4**.[54]

Hepatic Encephalopathy

Hepatic encephalopathy is reversible impairment of brain functions in patients with CLD. Compromised functioning of liver leads to accumulation of ammonia and mercaptans resulting in HE. Ammonia in brain is converted into glutamine which in turn causes edema. Ammonia is one of the factors which causes encephalopathy though no direct correlation is seen between levels of ammonia and grade of encephalopathy. This is precipitated by certain factors such as constipation, infections, alkalosis, sedative drugs such as benzodiazepine or morphine, dehydration, vomiting, diarrhea, excessive protein intake, hyponatremia, and diuretics. All the above factors should be avoided perioperatively **(Table 5)**.[57]

Pulmonary Complications

Atelectasis: It is a common complication after major abdominal surgery. This is due to airway secretion, inadequate pain relief interfering with deep breathing and coughing, and changes in lung compliance causing impaired regional ventilation and sub-diaphragmatic collection. This usually recovers with ensuring pain relief, mobilization, deep breathing exercises, spirometry, and chest physiotherapy. Those who still remain hypoxemic may need noninvasive ventilation (NIV) and continuous positive

Table 5: West Haven criteria of grading hepatic encephalopathy.[57]

Grade	Features
0	No abnormalities detected
I	Trivial lack of awareness, euphoria or anxiety, shortened attention span, impairment of addition or subtraction
II	Lethargy or apathy, disorientation to time, obvious personality change, inappropriate behavior
III	Somnolence to semistupor, responsive to stimuli, confused gross disorientation, bizarre behavior
IV	Coma, unable to test mental state

airway pressure (CPAP). Sometimes, it might need flexible bronchoscopy for bronchial lavage.

Pneumonia: Although uncommon, pneumonia may occur within 5 days of surgery. The patient presents with fever, hypoxemia, tachypnea, and leukocytosis. Antibiotic should be upgraded according to the culture sensitivity of sputum.

Pleural effusion: PE is common on the right side because of the surgical manipulation which is generally mild to moderate which resolves spontaneously. In some, PE might be due to hypoalbuminemia. Mild effusion does not require any intervention. Those which are symptomatic have to be drained. PE presenting 7–10 days after surgery may be reactionary to subdiaphragmatic collection and indicates toward infection. Collection has to be ascertained radiologically and drained. The patient should be evaluated for the reason of collection.

Pulmonary edema: This can be attributed to transfusion related to lung injury (TRALI) in many cases. In some, fluid overload can be the reason. Ensuring adequate dieresis and NIV with CPAP generally is adequate.

Future

Many new therapies are under evaluation for HCC. Novel chemotherapy in the form of sorafenib and intra-arterial 5-fluorouracil with interferon therapy are promising for advanced cancers.[58] With advanced tumors receiving chemotherapy, one can expect a larger number of patients with advanced disease for surgery.

A newer concept of "bridging liver resection (LR)" has been demonstrated by Belghiti et al. This LR could be a bridge to transplantation where the waiting list for the same is long. Belghiti et al. had concluded that bridging LR does not change survival as does not increase the risk as well.

Laparoscopic resection has shown to be advantageous in multiple ways by reducing postoperative morbidity as this is less invasive. Even patients with CLD with severe cirrhosis undergoing LR have been found to have lesser complications in the postoperative period.[59]

Experiments are underway for potential targets for liver regeneration to prevent any postoperative liver dysfunction. These are hepatic progenitor cells and cellular therapy and molecular targets such as von Willebrand factor (vWF).[60]

Liver Support System

Various devices with the goal of supporting liver as a bridge to transplantation or regeneration are under evaluation. Those which have found clinical application are the Single-Pass Albumin Dialysis System, Molecular Adsorbent Recirculating System™ (MARS™), and Fractionated Plasma Separation and Adsorption System (Prometheus™). All these systems only replace the detoxification function of liver. Replacement of other functions is still under development. The survival benefit of the already present system is still under evaluation.

■ REFERENCES

1. Kristensen SD, Knuuti J, Saraste A, Anker S, Bøtker HE, Hert SD, et al. 2014 ESC/ESA Guidelines on non-cardiac surgery: Cardiovascular assessment and management: The Joint Task Force on non-cardiac surgery: Cardiovascular assessment and management of the European Society of Cardiology (ESC) and the European Society of Anaesthesiology (ESA). Eur Heart J. 2014;35(35):2383-431.
2. Pang YY. The Brisbane 2000 terminology of liver anatomy and resections. HPB 2000; 2:333-39. HPB (Oxford). 2002;4(2):99-100.
3. Ferlay J, Shin HR, Bray F, Forman D, Mathers C, Parkin DM. Estimates of worldwide burden of cancer in 2008: GLOBOCAN 2008. Int J Cancer. 2010;127(12):2893-917.
4. Clavien PA, Petrowsky H, DeOliveira ML, Graf R. Strategies for safer liver surgery and partial liver transplantation. N Engl J Med. 2007;356(15):1545-59.
5. Poon D, Anderson BO, Chen LT, Tanaka K, Lau WY, Van Cutsem E, et al. Management of hepatocellular carcinoma in Asia: Consensus statement from the Asian Oncology Summit 2009. Lancet Oncol. 2009;10(11):1111-8.
6. Suman A, Carey WD. Assessing the risk of surgery in patients with liver disease. Cleve Clin J Med. 2006;73(4):398-404.
7. Cho HC, Jung HY, Sinn DH, Choi MS, Koh KC, Paik SW, et al. Mortality after surgery in patients with liver cirrhosis: Comparison of Child-Turcotte-Pugh, MELD and MELDNa score. Eur J Gastroenterol Hepatol. 2011;23(1):51-9.
8. Kim DH, Kim SH, Kim KS, Lee WJ, Kim NK, Noh SH, et al. Predictors of mortality in cirrhotic patients undergoing extrahepatic surgery: Comparison of Child-Turcotte-Pugh and model for end-stage liver disease-based indices. ANZ J Surg. 2014;84(11):832-6.
9. Pugh RN, Murray-Lyon IM, Dawson JL, Pietroni MC, Wlliams R. Transection of the esophagus in bleeding oesophageal varices. Br J Surg. 1973;60(8):646-9.
10. Ishizawa T, Hasegawa K, Aoki T, Takahashi M, Inoue Y, Sano K, et al. Neither multiple tumors nor portal hypertension are surgical contraindications for hepatocellular carcinoma. Gastroenterology. 2008;134(7):1908-16.
11. Ferrero A, Viganò L, Polastri R, Muratore A, Eminefendic H, Regge D, et al. Postoperative liver dysfunction and future remnant liver: Where is the limit? Results of a prospective study. World J Surg. 2007;31(8):1643-51.
12. Morise Z, Kawabe N, Tomishige H, Nagata H, Kawase J, Arakawa S, et al. Recent advances in liver resection for hepatocellular carcinoma. Front Surg. 2014;1:21.
13. Mookerjee RP, Vairappan B, Jalan R. The puzzle of endothelial nitric oxide synthase dysfunction in portal hypertension: The missing piece? Hepatology. 2007;46(3):943-6.
14. Vairappan B. Endothelial dysfunction in cirrhosis: Role of inflammation and oxidative stress. World J Hepatol. 2015;7(3):443-59.
15. Ruiz-del-Árbol L, Serradilla R. Cirrhotic cardiomyopathy. World J Gastroenterol. 2015;21(41):11502-21.
16. Planas R, Montoliu S, Ballesté B, Rivera M, Miquel M, Masnou H, et al. Natural history of patients hospitalized for management of cirrhotic ascites. Clin Gatroenterol Hepatol. 2006;4(11): 1385-94.
17. Ruiz-del-Arbol L, Monescillo A, Arocena C, Valer P, Ginès P, Moreira V, et al. Circulatory function and hepatorenal syndrome in cirrhosis. Hepatology. 2005;42(2):439-47.
18. Acevedo JG, Cramp ME. Hepatorenal syndrome: Update on diagnosis and therapy. World J Hepatol. 2017;9(6):293-9.
19. Salerno F, Gerbes A, Ginès P, Wong F, Arroyo V. Diagnosis, prevention and treatment of hepatorenal syndrome in cirrhosis. Gut. 2007;56(9):1310-8.
20. Ginès P, Schrier RW. Renal failure in cirrhosis. N Engl J Med. 2009;361(13):1279-90.
21. Fuhrmann V, Krowka M. Hepatopulmonary syndrome. J Hepatol. 2018;69(3):744-5.
22. Aldenkortt F, Aldenkortt M, Caviezel L, Waeber JL, Weber A, Schiffer E. Portopulmonary hypertension and hepatopulmonary syndrome. World J Gastroenterol. 2014;20(25):8072-81.

23. Weeder PD, Porte RJ, Lisman T. Hemostasis in liver disease: Implications of new concepts for perioperative management. Transfus Med Rev. 2014;28(3):107-13.

24. Reddy SK, Turley RS, Barbas AS, Steel JL, Tsung A, Marsh JW, et al. Post-operative pharmacologic thromboprophylaxis after major hepatectomy: Does peripheral venous thromboembolism prevention outweigh bleeding risks? J Gastrointest Surg. 2011;15(9):1602-10.

25. Stravitz RT. Potential applications of thromboelastography in patients with acute and chronic liver disease. Gastroenterol Hepatol (N Y). 2012;8(8):513-20.

26. Kasivisvanathan R, Abbassi-Ghadi N, McLeod AD, Oliver A, Rao Baikady R, Jhanji S, et al. Cardiopulmonary exercise testing for predicting postoperative morbidity in patients undergoing hepatic resection surgery. HPB (Oxford). 2015;17(7): 637-43.

27. Chang PE, Wong GW, Li JW, Lui HF, Chow WC, Tan CK. Epidemiology and clinical evolution of liver cirrhosis in Singapore. Ann Acad Med Singapore. 2015;44(6):218-25.

28. Tang A, Hallouch O, Chernyak V, Kamaya A, Sirlin CB. Epidemiology of hepatocellular carcinoma: Target population for surveillance and diagnosis. Abdom Radiol (NY). 2018;43(1):13-25.

29. Weimann A, Braga M, Carli F, Higashiguchi T, Hübner M, Klek S, et al. ESPEN guideline: Clinical nutrition in surgery. Clin Nutr. 2017;36(3):623-50.

30. Melloul E, Hübner M, Scott M, Snowden C, Prentis J, Dejong CH, et al. Guidelines for perioperative care for liver surgery: Enhanced recovery after surgery (ERAS) society recommendations. World J Surg. 2016;40(10):2425-40.

31. Mikagi K, Kawahara R, Kinoshita H, Aoyagi S. Effect of preoperative immunonutrition in patients undergoing hepatectomy; a randomized controlled trial. Kurume Med J. 2011;58(1):1-8.

32. Debette-Gratien M, Tabouret T, Antonini MT, Dalmay F, Carrier P, Legros R, et al. Personalized adapted physical activity before liver transplantation: Acceptability and results. Transplantation. 2014;99(1):145-50.

33. Holland LL, Brooks JP. Toward rational fresh frozen plasma transfusion: The effect of plasma transfusion on coagulation test results. Am J Clin Pathol. 2006;126(1):133-9.

34. Makuuchi M, Sano K. The surgical approach to HCC: Our progress and results in Japan. Liver Transpl. 2004;10(2 Suppl 1):S46-52.

35. Qi S, Chen G, Cao P, Hu J, He G, Luo J, et al. Safety and efficacy of enhanced recovery after surgery (ERAS) programs in patients undergoing hepatectomy: A prospective randomized controlled trial. J Clin Lab Anal. 2018:32(6):e22434.

36. Agarwal V, Divatia JV. Enhanced recovery after surgery in liver resection: Current concepts and controversies. Korean J Anesthesiol. 2019;72(2):119-29.

37. Marik PE, Cavallazzi R, Vasu T, Hirani A. Dynamic changes in arterial waveform derived variables and fluid responsiveness in mechanically ventilated patients: A systematic review of the literature. Crit Care Med. 2009;37(9):2642-7.

38. Choi SS, Kim SH, Kim YK. Fluid management in living donor hepatectomy: Recent issues and perspectives. World J Gastroenterol. 2015;21(45):12757-66.

39. Myles PS, Bellomo R, Corcoran T, Forbes A, Peyton P, Story D, et al. Restrictive versus liberal fluid therapy for major abdominal surgery. N Engl J Med. 2018;378(24):2263-74.

40. Kim YK, Chin JH, Kang SJ, Jun IG, Song JG, Jeong SM, et al. Association between central venous pressure and blood loss during hepatic resection in 984 living donors. Acta Anaesthesiol Scand. 2009;53(5):601-6.

41. Choudhuri AH, Chandra S, Aggarwal G, Uppal R. Predictors of postoperative pulmonary complications after liver resection: Results from a tertiary care intensive care unit. Indian J Crit Care Med. 2014;18(6):358-62.

42. Grocott MP, Mythen MG, Gan TJ. Perioperative fluid management and clinical outcomes in adults. Anesth Analg. 2005;100(4):1093-106.

43. Cochrane JP, Forsling ML, Gow NM, Le Quesne LP. Arginine vasopressin release following surgical operations. Br J Surg. 1981;68(3):209-13

44. Kunst G, Ostermann M. Intraoperative permissive oliguria— How much is too much? Br J Anaesth. 2017;119(6):1075-77.

45. Thiele RH, Raghunathan K, Brudney CS, Lobo DN, Martin D, Senagore A, et al. American Society for Enhanced Recovery (ASER) and Perioperative Quality Initiative (POQI) joint consensus statement on perioperative fluid management within an enhanced recovery pathway for colorectal surgery. Perioper Med (Lond). 2016;5:24.

46. Geerse DA, Bindels AJ, Kuiper MA, Roos AN, Spronk PE, Schultz MJ. Treatment of hypophosphatemia in the intensive care unit: A review. Crit Care. 2010;14(4):R147.

47. Brown KA, Dickerson RN, Morgan LM, Alexander KH, Minard G, Brown RO. A new graduated dosing regimen for phosphorus replacement in patients receiving nutrition support. JPEN J Parenter Enteral Nutr. 2006;30(3):209-14.

48. De Pietri L, Montalti R, Begliomini B, Scaglioni G, Marconi G, Reggiani A, et al. Thromboelastographic changes in liver and pancreatic cancer surgery: Hypercoagulability, hypocoagulability or normocoagulability? Eur J Anaesthesiol. 2010;27(7):608-16.

49. Richter B, Schmandra TC, Golling M, Bechstein WO. Nutritional support after open liver resection: A systemic review. Dig Surg. 2006;23(3):139-45.

50. Capussotti L, Ferrero A, Viganò L, Sgotto E, Muratore A, Polastri R. Bile leakage and liver resection: Where is the risk? Arch Surg. 2006;141(7):690-4.

51. Wang HQ, Yang J, Yang JY, Yan LN. Bile leakage test in liver resection: A systematic review and meta-analysis. World J Gastroenterol. 2013;19(45):8420-6.

52. Bhattacharjya S, Puleston J, Davidson BR, Dooley JS. Outcome of early endoscopic biliary drainage in the management of bile leaks after hepatic resection. Gastrointest Endosc. 2003;57(4):526-30.

53. Ahmad F, Saunders RN, Lloyd GM, Lloyd DM, Robertson GS. An algorithm for the management of bile leak following laparoscopic cholecystectomy. Ann R Coll Surg Engl. 2007;89(1):51-6.

54. Rahbari NN, Garden OJ, Padbury R, Brooke-Smith M, Crawford M, Adam R, et al. Posthepatectomy liver failure: A definition and grading by the International Study Group of Liver Surgery (ISGLS). Surgery. 2011;149(5):713-24.

55. Matsumoto K, Yoshitomi H, Rossant J, Zaret KS. Liver organogenesis promoted by endothelial cells prior to vascular function. Science. 2001;294(5542):559-63.

56. Ray S, Mehta NN, Golhar A, Nundy S. Post hepatectomy liver failure—A comprehensive review of current concepts and controversies. Ann Med Surg (Lond). 2018;34:4-10.

57. Dharel N, Bajaj JS. Definition and nomenclature of hepatic encephalopathy. J Clin Exp Hepatol. 2015;5(Suppl 1):S37-41.

58. Nagano H, Wada H, Kobayashi S, Marubashi S, Eguchi H, Tanemura M, et al. Long-term outcome of combined interferon-α and 5-fluorouracil treatment for advanced hepatocellular carcinoma with major portal vein thrombosis. Oncology. 2011;80(1-2):63-9.

59. Morise Z, Sugioka A, Kawabe N, Umemoto S, Nagata H, Ohshima H, et al. Pure laparoscopic hepatectomy for hepatocellular carcinoma patients with severe liver cirrhosis. Asian J Endosc Surg. 2011;4(3):143-6.

60. Pereyra D, Starlinger P. Shaping the future of liver surgery: Implementation of experimental insights into liver regeneration. Eur Surg. 2018;50(3):132-6.

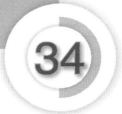

CHAPTER

34

Perioperative Management of Colorectal Surgeries

Lalita Gouri Mitra, Kelika Prakash

INTRODUCTION

Colorectal surgeries are one of the common surgeries in geriatric population and are associated with a length of stay of about 8 days for open surgery and 5 days for laparoscopic surgery, high costs, and high rate of surgical site infection (SSI).[1,2] Moreover, the incidence of perioperative nausea and vomiting (PONV) may approach as high as 80% in high-risk patients (Apfel Score)—female sex, previous PONV or motion sickness, nonsmokers, and use of opioids.[3,4] Enhanced recovery after surgery (ERAS), enhanced recovery programs (ERPs), or "fast-track" programs[4] are sets of standardized perioperative procedures and practices that have become an important focus of perioperative management after colorectal surgery, vascular surgery, thoracic surgery, and radical cystectomy. These programs, initiated by Professor Henrik Kehlet in the 1990s, attempt to modify the physiological and psychological responses to major surgery and have been shown to lead to a reduction in complications and hospital stay, improvements in cardiopulmonary function, earlier return of bowel function, and earlier resumption of normal activities. ERAS protocols emphasize an interdisciplinary approach between anesthesiologists and surgeons, and the key principles of the ERAS protocol include preoperative counseling, preoperative nutrition, avoidance of perioperative fasting and carbohydrate loading up to 2 hours preoperatively, standardized anesthetic and analgesic regimens (epidural and nonopioid analgesia), and early mobilization.[5] Indeed, the application of ERAS protocols has led to a decrease in the length of hospital stay (LOS) and incidence of postoperative complications worldwide.[5,6] This chapter will describe the ERAS recommendations provided by the American Society of Colon and Rectal Surgeons and Society of American Gastrointestinal and Endoscopic Surgeons 2019 for colorectal surgeries.

PREOPERATIVE INTERVENTIONS

A Preoperative Discussion of Milestones and Discharge Criteria

Specific discharge criteria after surgery have been formulated and state that patients are fit for discharge when there is tolerance of oral intake, recovery of lower gastrointestinal (GI) function, adequate pain control with oral analgesia, ability to mobilize, ability to perform self-care, no evidence of complications or untreated medical problems, adequate postdischarge support, and patient willingness to leave the hospital.[6-9] Though the level of evidence to support this intervention is low and compliance is variable, setting specific discharge criteria and communication with the patient preoperatively does seem to reduce LOS in some studies.

Ileostomy Education, Marking, and Counseling on Dehydration Avoidance

Making stomas is an independent risk factor for prolonged LOS.[10] In addition, dehydration is the most common cause for readmission following ileostomies.[11] Preoperative evaluation and marking of the stoma site as well as preoperative counseling on the importance of avoiding dehydration have been found to improve the quality of life and reduce hospital LOS and costs.[11-13]

Preadmission Nutrition and Bowel Preparation

Clear Liquid Diet to be Continued < 2 Hours before General Anesthesia

Ingestion of clear fluids up to 2–4 hours is associated with smaller gastric volumes and higher pH at the time of surgery.[14]

Carbohydrate Loading should be Encouraged before Surgery in Nondiabetic Patients

Carbohydrate loading before surgery in terms of providing a carbohydrate-rich diet reduces the perioperative catabolic state and decreases protein breakdown and insulin resistance. Though it has not been associated with a reduced LOS, carbohydrate loading 2 hours prior to surgery does reduce thirst, PONV, and anxiety.[15-17]

Mechanical Bowel Preparation Plus Oral Antibiotic Bowel Preparation (OBP) before Colorectal Surgery is Associated with Reduced Complication Rates

Till 2013, mechanical bowel preparation (MBP) was not recommended routinely for colorectal surgery. The American College of Surgeons-National Surgical Quality Improvement Program (ACS-NSQIP) study ($n = 5,729$) focused on the use of MBP and oral antibiotics (OAB) prior to left-sided elective colorectal surgery which showed that MBP and OAB were associated with reduction in the SSI rate and anastomotic leak without any increase in *Clostridium difficile* occurrences with the use of OAB. The same group did a Network Meta-analysis [$n = 8,458$; 38 randomized-controlled trials (RCTs)] which included both right and left colonic and rectal surgery and compared all four strategies—MBP + OAB, MBP alone, OAB alone, and no preparation. This study showed that MBP with OAB was associated with the lowest risk of SSI and was unable to demonstrate a statistically significant difference in anastomotic leak rates between the four approaches. A significant limitation of this study was that there were only three studies comparing MBP with OAB versus OAB alone.[18,19] The SELECT trial ($n = 485$), conducted by Abis et al., was a large multicenter RCT on the role of MBP with OAB for left-sided colectomies. A superiority study design, it was not able to show a statistically significant difference in anastomotic leak but on multivariate analysis it was able to show that MBP with OAB was associated with a reduction in infectious complications. There was a reduced load of Proteobacteria, Enterobacteriaceae, and *Escherichia coli* on microbial analysis and MBP with OAB was neither associated with an increase in multidrug-resistant organisms nor *C. difficile* infection.[18-20] ERAS 2013 and 2018 guidelines recommend to avoid the use of MBP in colonic surgery except for rectal surgery where a diverting stoma is often created and there may be residual stool in the diverted colon. This has been suggested as there is widespread universal use of prophylaxis systemic antibiotics, and omitting MBP avoids preoperative dehydration, electrolyte disturbance, and discomfort with no clinical gain for the patient.[21]

Prehabilitation of Patients and the Use of Preset Orders

Prehabilitation is defined as "A process in the continuum of care that occurs between the time of diagnosis and the beginning of acute treatment (surgery, chemotherapy, radiotherapy) and includes physical, nutritional, and psychological assessments that establish a baseline functional level, identify impairments, and provide interventions that promote physical and psychological health to reduce the incidence and/or severity of future impairments." Prehabilitation includes interventions to improve the functional capacity of the patients and includes medical interventions such as stoppage of smoking, preoperative exercise such as aerobic exercises and strength training, nutritional enhancement, and psychological support.[22-24] A follow-up RCT used multimodal structured prehabilitation protocols, which included aerobic and resistance exercises, protein supplementation, and relaxation strategies and demonstrated a positive impact on the preoperative physiologic reserve with >80% of patients who received the multimodal prehabilitation program returning to baseline values of functional walking capacity by 8 weeks. Only 40% of patients who did not receive prehabilitation returned to baseline values.[23] One RCT using a 4-week prehabilitation program showed an association between increase in preoperative aerobic capacity and reduction in complications (51% reduction in postoperative medical complications).[24] Both prehabilitation and the use of a preset order have not been conclusively found to reduce LOS or improve postoperative morbidity and are currently a weak recommendation.[25] From a metabolic and nutritional point of view, it is important to integrate nutrition into the overall management of the patient and avoid long periods of preoperative fasting. A systematic nutritional risk screening (NRS) has to be considered in all patients on hospital admission, and nutritional care protocols must include a detailed nutritional and medical history that includes body composition assessment, a nutrition intervention plan, good documentation, and resistance exercise whenever possible. Since preoperative serum albumin is a prognostic factor for complications after surgery and is associated with impaired nutritional status, it can be considered to define surgical patients at severe nutritional risk by the presence of at least one of the following criteria:

- Weight loss >10–15% within 6 months
- Body mass index (BMI) < 18.5 kg/m^2
- Subjective global assessment (SGA) grade C or NRS > 5
- Preoperative serum albumin < 30 g/L (no hepatic or renal dysfunction)

"Metabolic conditioning" of the patient focuses on prevention and treatment of insulin resistance, giving preoperative carbohydrates, preventing hypoglycemia, and reducing stress-induced inflammation. A new concept of "immunonutrition" and "ecoimmunonutrition" by using pre- and probiotics aims at the microbiome in the gut and the enhancement of mucosal immunity.[22]

INTRAOPERATIVE MEASURES

Prevention of Surgical Site Infections

A multimodal approach and implementation of an SSI bundle to prevent SSIs are necessary. Measures start from the preoperative state and continue till the postoperative period. There is considerable heterogeneity in the SSI bundle between various hospitals. Nevertheless, common features include antibiotic prophylaxis within 1 hour of incision, skin preparation with chlorhexidine-alcohol-based solutions, hair removal with the use of clippers immediately before surgery, maintenance of normothermia, and glycemic control.[26] Other measures that have been included in SSI bundles are chlorhexidine shower, use of a wound protector, gown and glove change before fascial closure, use of a dedicated wound closure tray, etc.

Anesthesia Management

With the aim of a clear-headed recovery, short-to-intermediate-acting anesthetic agents are commonly used. Patients are usually anxious before surgery and thus anxiolytic drugs are required. According to the American Geriatrics Society, the use of benzodiazepines should be avoided in elderly patients with a risk of delirium, cognitive impairment, and falls.[27] Gabapentanoids in the lowest dose could be an alternative in this group of patients. Propofol in combination with short-acting opioids such as fentanyl, remifentanil, and alfentanil is a good induction regimen. Tracheal intubation can be facilitated by using intermediate-acting nondepolarizing neuromuscular blocking agents (NMBAs). Both total intravenous anesthesia (TIVA) and inhalational anesthetic agents can be used for maintenance of anesthesia. Short-acting opioids should be used if and when required (NMBA). The use of cerebral function monitors such as bispectral index (BIS) monitors facilitates titration of anesthesia. It is also recommended that neuromuscular monitoring should be used to confirm full reversal of NMBAs.[28]

Perioperative Analgesia

Management of pain must include a multimodal approach with the aim of minimizing opioid consumption. All medications must be given as part of a routine regimen rather than an as-and-when approach.[28] A round-the-clock combination of paracetamol, nonsteroidal anti-inflammatory drugs (NSAIDs) such as ketorolac and diclofenac sodium, and oral gabapentin has been found to decrease postoperative opioid consumption. Infusions of lignocaine and dexmedetomidine started intraoperatively have also been found to have an opioid-sparing effect.[29,30] Abdominal wall blocks such as the transversus abdominis plane (TAP) block reduce opioid consumption in patients undergoing minimally invasive surgery.[31] Other modalities include port site infiltration and the use of subcostal and rectus sheath block (if areas above the umbilicus need to be covered). In addition, it is well established that the use of the thoracic epidural analgesia (TEA) at the level of T6 to T12 for open colorectal surgeries helps control postoperative pain and is now the gold standard. TEA should be provided with a combination of local anesthetics and opioids rather than either one alone.[32,33] Hydrophilic opioids or lipophilic opioids can be used epidurally. Other adjuvants, for example, α-2 agonists such as clonidine and adrenaline, can also be considered. Epidural analgesia has been found to reduce postoperative pulmonary complications and thromboembolic episodes and aid in early mobilization.[34] For laparoscopic colorectal surgeries, however, the benefits of TEA are outweighed by its side effects of urinary retention and hypotension.[35] Thus, in this group of patients the use of TEA should be limited to patients at high risk of postoperative pulmonary complications like those with preoperative cardiovascular diseases.[36]

Perioperative Nausea and Vomiting Prophylaxis

Perioperative nausea and vomiting is one of the most common ailments severely affecting patient recovery. All patients should be evaluated for the risk of PONV.[37] A commonly used score is the Apfel score. Patients at high risk for PONV (Apfel score > 2) should be premedicated intraoperatively with a combination of two antiemetics intraoperatively, for example, dexamethasone–ondansetron.[38] Other intraoperative modifications include the use of TIVA instead of inhalational agents. Gabapentin has also been found to reduce the incidence of PONV.

Intraoperative Fluid Management

Excessive fluid administration intraoperatively leads to bowel congestion, anastomotic leakage, increased pulmonary complications, and LOS. Traditionally, insensible losses have been thought to be as high as 8 mL/kg/h during open abdominal surgeries. It has been now estimated that during colorectal surgeries, insensible fluid loss does not exceed 1 mL/kg/h which remains true even if the bowel is completely exteriorized.[39] Moreover, fluid loading prior to or in response to hypotension due to TEA is not effective. This is because TEA leads to a state of relative hypovolemia. Hence, hypotension due to TEA must be treated with vasopressors and not fluids after ensuring that the patient is euvolemic. Intraoperative balanced salt solutions (crystalloids) are the fluid of choice at a maintenance rate of 1.5–2 mL/kg/h.[40] Fluids should be administered with the aim of restricting weight gain to <2.5 kg/day.[41]

Surgical Measures

Minimally invasive surgery facilitates early recovery, reduces postoperative pulmonary complications and LOS, and should be offered whenever possible to all patients.[42,43] Other surgical measures which form a part of the ERAS protocol include avoiding of routine use of unnecessary drains and nasogastric tubes.[44,45]

▐ POSTOPERATIVE MEASURES

Postoperative measures include:
- Early patient mobilization
- Preventing ileus
- Ideal time of removal of the urinary catheter
- Postoperative fluid management

Early Patient Mobilization

Definitions of early mobilization vary from mobilization of the patient in any form within 24 hours to mobilizing a patient for 8 hours a day from postoperative day 2.[46] Even though the quality of evidence is low, the recommendation is strong that if patients are mobilized early and progressively, it is associated with a shorter LOS, as physical activity reduces deconditioning associated with prolonged bed rest. It is well established that prolonged immobility causes loss and weakness of skeletal muscle causing decreased exercise capacity, insulin resistance, lung atelectasis, and thromboembolic disease. Early mobilization also shortens time to flatus postoperatively.

Prevention of Ileus

Feeding patients early (<24 hours) postoperatively after elective colorectal surgery accelerates GI recovery and decreases LOS and rate of complications and mortality.[47] Blood loss during open laparotomy is related to failure of early feeding, and one must be aware that the risk of vomiting increases with early feeding.

Sham feeding (i.e., chewing sugar-free gum for ≥10 minutes—three to four times a day) was first proposed in 2002 and now there is strong recommendation based on high-quality evidence that it is safe and is associated with reduction in the LOS.[48]

Alvimopan 12 mg reverses opioid-induced increased GI transit time and constipation. A Cochrane review of nine studies affirmed that alvimopan was safe and efficacious in treating postoperative ileus in open laparotomy and hand-assisted colectomy but does not have a benefit after laparoscopic colorectal resection.[49,50]

Ideal Time of Removal of the Urinary Catheter

Patients undergoing low rectal resections have a higher risk of urinary tract infection (UTI) with prolonged catheter in situ. Male patients and those with extensive pelvic dissection and increased intraoperative intravenous fluids (>2 L) should remain catheterized for a longer period of time. However, there is a strong recommendation with moderate quality evidence to attempt to remove urinary catheters within 48 hours of mid-rectal and lower-rectal resections. Patients who undergo colectomy and upper rectal surgery should be made catheter free on postoperative day 1.[51]

Postoperative Fluid Management

It is strongly recommended based on moderate-quality evidence that intravenous fluids should be discontinued in the early postoperative period once the patient moves out of the recovery room and clear fluids >1.7 L/day of water should be started enterally. Weight gain > 1–2 kg should be avoided for which daily postoperative weight should be monitored. Intravenous fluids should be administered only when there is a clinical indication. Signs, symptoms, and cause of hypovolemia and hypotension should be looked into and measure fluid responsiveness as studies show that only 46% of critically ill patients are fluid responsive.[52]

Intensive Care Unit Stay

Postoperative complications occur in up to one-third of patients undergoing colorectal procedures, common being wound infection or organ space infection, and GI motility complications, including ileus and bowel obstruction. Recently, failure to rescue or death following a major postoperative complication has been increasingly favored as a quality indicator of surgical care, and a high (>50%) failure-to-rescue rate has been found in patients who had colectomy for colon cancer with the following complications—coma, cardiac arrest, failure of vascular graft prosthesis, anastomotic leak, renal failure, pulmonary embolism, and progressive renal insufficiency. Scores such as the POSSUM (Physiological and Operative Severity Score for the enUmeration of Mortality and Morbidity) and its modification such as the p-POSSUM (Portsmouth POSSUM) have been developed to predict postoperative morbidity and mortality in patients undergoing general surgery. They utilize 12 physiological factors and 6 operative factors in a mathematical equation. The p-POSSUM score is a reliable predictor of postoperative morbidity in both elderly and young patients. One of the clear benefits of implementation of ERAS protocols is a significant decrease in LOS with an average hospital LOS ranging from 3 to 5 days. A large multicenter study involving

2,438 patients undergoing elective colectomy reported a decrease in LOS after implementation of ERAS protocols though the complication rate remained the same.[53] Certain studies have also reported that complications such as the duration of ileus were reduced after ERAS protocols were implemented.[54]

▌REFERENCES

1. Kang CY, Chaudhry OO, Halabi WJ, Nguyen V, Carmichael JC, Stamos MJ, et al. Outcomes of laparoscopic colorectal surgery: Data from the nationwide inpatient sample 2009. Am J Surg. 2012;204(6):952-7.

2. Thiele RH, Rea KM, Turrentine FE, Friel CM, Hassinger TE, McMurry TL, et al. Standardization of care: Impact of an enhanced recovery protocol on length of stay, complications, and direct costs after colorectal surgery. J Am Coll Surg. 2015;220(4):430-43.

3. Apfel CC, Korttila K, Abdalla M, Kerger H, Turan A, Vedder I, et al. A factorial trial of six interventions for the prevention of postoperative nausea and vomiting. N Engl J Med. 2004;350(24):2441-51.

4. Eberhart LH, Mauch M, Morin AM, Wulf H, Geldner G. Impact of a multimodal anti-emetic prophylaxis on patient satisfaction in high-risk patients for postoperative nausea and vomiting. Anaesthesia. 2002;57(10):1022-7.

5. Carmichael JC, Keller DS, Baldini G, Bordeianou L, Weiss E, Lee L, et al. Clinical practice guidelines for enhanced recovery after colon and rectal surgery from the American Society of Colon and Rectal Surgeons and Society of American Gastrointestinal and Endoscopic Surgeons. Dis Colon Rectum. 2017;60(8):761-84.

6. Currie AC, Malietzis G, Jenkins JT, Yamada T, Ashrafian H, Athanasiou T, et al. Network meta-analysis of protocol-driven care and laparoscopic surgery for colorectal cancer. Br J Surg. 2016;103(13):1783-94.

7. Fiore JF Jr, Browning L, Bialocerkowski A, Gruen RL, Faragher IG, Denehy L. Hospital discharge criteria following colorectal surgery: A systematic review. Colorectal Dis. 2012;14(3):270-81.

8. Gustafsson UO, Scott MJ, Schwenk W, Demartines N, Roulin D, Francis N, et al. Guidelines for perioperative care in elective colonic surgery: Enhanced Recovery After Surgery (ERAS®) Society recommendations. Clin Nutr. 2012;31(6):783-800.

9. Adamina M, Kehlet H, Tomlinson GA, Senagore AJ, Delaney CP. Enhanced recovery pathways optimize health outcomes and resource utilization: A meta-analysis of randomized controlled trials in colorectal surgery. Surgery. 2011;149(6):830-40.

10. Delaney CP, Zutshi M, Senagore AJ, Remzi FH, Hammel J, Fazio VW. Prospective, randomized, controlled trial between a pathway of controlled rehabilitation with early ambulation and diet and traditional postoperative care after laparotomy and intestinal resection. Dis Colon Rectum. 2003;46(7):851-9.

11. Messaris E, Sehgal R, Deiling S, Koltun WA, Stewart D, McKenna K, et al. Dehydration is the most common indication for readmission after diverting ileostomy creation. Dis Colon Rectum. 2012;55(2):175-80.

12. Millan M, Tegido M, Biondo S, García-Granero E. Preoperative stoma siting and education by stoma therapists of colorectal cancer patients: A descriptive study in twelve Spanish colorectal surgical units. Colorectal Dis. 2010;12(7 Online):e88-92.

13. Younis J, Salerno G, Fanto D, Hadjipavlou M, Chellar D, Trickett JP. Focused preoperative patient stoma education, prior to ileostomy formation after anterior resection, contributes to a reduction in delayed discharge within the enhanced recovery programme. Int J Colorectal Dis. 2012;27(1):43-7.

14. Smith I, Kranke P, Murat I, Smith A, O'Sullivan G, Søreide E, et al. Perioperative fasting in adults and children: Guidelines from the European Society of Anaesthesiology. Eur J Anaesthesiol. 2011;28(8):556-69.

15. Smith MD, McCall J, Plank L, Herbison GP, Soop M, Nygren J. Preoperative carbohydrate treatment for enhancing recovery after elective surgery. Cochrane Database Syst Rev. 2014;(8):CD009161.

16. Awad S, Varadhan KK, Ljungqvist O, Lobo DN. A meta-analysis of randomized controlled trials on preoperative oral carbohydrate treatment in elective surgery. Clin Nutr. 2013;32(1):34-44.

17. Amer MA, Smith MD, Herbison GP, Plank LD, McCall JL. Network meta-analysis of the effect of preoperative carbohydrate loading on recovery after elective surgery. Br J Surg. 2017;104(3):187-97.

18. Toh JW, Harlaar J, Di Re A, Pathmanathan N, El Khoury T, Ctercteko G. Understanding the role of mechanical bowel preparation and oral antibiotics prior to elective colorectal surgery. Ann Laparosc Endosc Surg. 2019;4:47-9.

19. Toneva GD, Deierhoi RJ, Morris M, Richman J, Cannon JA, Altom LK, et al. Oral antibiotic bowel preparation reduces length of stay and readmissions after colorectal surgery. J Am Coll Surg. 2013;216(4):756-62.

20. Mik M, Berut M, Trzcinski R, Dziki L, Buczynski J, Dziki A. Preoperative oral antibiotics reduce infections after colorectal cancer surgery. Langenbecks Arch Surg. 2016;401(8):1153-62.

21. Abis GSA, Stockmann HBAC, Bonjer HJ, van Veenendaal N, van Doorn-Schepens MLM, Budding AE, et al. Randomized clinical trial of selective decontamination of the digestive tract in elective colorectal cancer surgery (SELECT trial). Br J Surg. 2019;106(4):355-63.

22. Gustafsson UO, Scott MJ, Hubner M, Nygren J, Demartines N, Francis N, et al. Guidelines for perioperative care in elective colorectal surgery: Enhanced Recovery After Surgery (ERAS®) Society Recommendations: 2018. World J Surg. 2019;43(3):659-95.

23. Le Roy B, Selvy M, Slim K. The concept of prehabilitation: What the surgeon needs to know? J Visc Surg. 2016;153(2):109-12.

24. Gillis C, Li C, Lee L, Awasthi R, Augustin B, Gamsa A, et al. Prehabilitation versus rehabilitation: A randomized control trial in patients undergoing colorectal resection for cancer. Anesthesiology. 2014;121(5):937-47.

25. Barberan-Garcia A, Ubré M, Roca J, Lacy AM, Burgos F, Risco R, et al. Personalised prehabilitation in high-risk patients undergoing elective major abdominal surgery: A randomized blinded controlled trial. Ann Surg. 2018;267(1):50-6.

26. Tanner J, Padley W, Assadian O, Leaper D, Kiernan M, Edmiston C. Do surgical care bundles reduce the risk of surgical site infections in patients undergoing colorectal surgery? A systematic review and cohort meta-analysis of 8,515 patients. Surgery. 2015;158(1):66-77.

27. The American Geriatrics Society 2015 Beers Criteria Update Expert Panel. American Geriatrics Society 2015 updated beers criteria for potentially inappropriate medication use in older adults. J Am Geriatr Soc. 2015;63(11):2227-46.

28. Khoo CK, Vickery CJ, Forsyth N, Venall NS, Eyre-Brook IA. A prospective randomized controlled trial of multimodal perioperative management protocol in patients undergoing elective colorectal resection for cancer. Ann Surg. 2007;245(6):867-72.

29. Kranke P, Jokinen J, Pace NL, Schnabel A, Hollmann MW, Hahnekamp K, et al. Continuous intravenous perioperative lidocaine infusion for postoperative pain and recovery. Cochrane Database Syst Rev. 2015;(7):CD009642.

30. Cheung CW, Qiu Q, Ying AC, Choi SW, Law WL, Irwin MG. The effects of intra-operative dexmedetomidine on postoperative pain, side-effects and recovery in colorectal surgery. Anaesthesia. 2014;69(11):1214-21.

31. Keller DS, Ermlich BO, Delaney CP. Demonstrating the benefits of transversus abdominis plane blocks on patient outcomes in laparoscopic colorectal surgery: Review of 200 consecutive cases. J Am Coll Surg. 2014;219(6):1143-8.

32. Werawatganon T, Charuluxanun S. Patient controlled intravenous opioid analgesia versus continuous epidural analgesia for pain after intra-abdominal surgery. Cochrane Database Syst Rev. 2005;(1):CD004088.

33. Block BM, Liu SS, Rowlingson AJ, Cowan AR, Cowan JA Jr, Wu CL. Efficacy of postoperative epidural analgesia: A meta-analysis. JAMA. 2003;290(18):2455-63.

34. Pöpping DM, Elia N, Marret E, Remy C, Tramèr MR. Protective effects of epidural analgesia on pulmonary complications after abdominal and thoracic surgery: A meta-analysis. Arch Surg. 2008;143(10):990-1000.

35. Liu H, Hu X, Duan X, Wu J. Thoracic epidural analgesia (TEA) vs. patient controlled analgesia (PCA) in laparoscopic colectomy: A meta-analysis. Hepatogastroenterology. 2014;61(133):1213-9.

36. Levy BF, Scott MJ, Fawcett W, Fry C, Rockall TA. Randomized clinical trial of epidural, spinal or patient-controlled analgesia for patients undergoing laparoscopic colorectal surgery. Br J Surg. 2011;98(8):1068-78.

37. Kappen TH, Vergouwe Y, van Wolfswinkel L, Kalkman CJ, Moons KG, van Klei WA. Impact of adding therapeutic recommendations to risk assessments from a prediction model for postoperative nausea and vomiting. Br J Anaesth. 2015;114(2):252-60.

38. Gan TJ, Diemunsch P, Habib AS, Kovac A, Kranke P, Meyer TA, et al. Consensus guidelines for the management of postoperative nausea and vomiting. Anesth Analg. 2014;118(1):85-113.

39. Holte K, Foss NB, Svensén C, Lund C, Madsen JL, Kehlet H. Epidural anesthesia, hypotension, and changes in intravascular volume. Anesthesiology. 2004;100(2):281-6.

40. Navarro LH, Bloomstone JA, Auler JO Jr, Cannesson M, Rocca GD, Gan TJ, et al. Perioperative fluid therapy: A statement from the International Fluid Optimization Group. Perioper Med (Lond). 2015;4:3.

41. Brandstrup B, Tønnesen H, Beier-Holgersen R, Hjortsø E, Ørding H, Lindorff-Larsen K, et al. Effects of intravenous fluid restriction on postoperative complications: Comparison of two perioperative fluid regimens: A randomized assessor-blinded multicenter trial. Ann Surg. 2003;238(5):641-8.

42. Hewett PJ, Allardyce RA, Bagshaw PF, Frampton CM, Frizelle FA, Rieger NA, et al. Short-term outcomes of the Australasian randomized clinical study comparing laparoscopic and conventional open surgical treatments for colon cancer: The ALCCaS trial. Ann Surg. 2008; 248(5):728-38.

43. Veldkamp R, Kuhry E, Hop WC, Jeekel J, Kazemier G, Bonjer HJ, et al. Laparoscopic surgery versus open surgery for colon cancer: Short-term outcomes of a randomised trial. Lancet Oncol. 2005;6(7):477-84.

44. Brown SR, Seow-Choen F, Eu KW, Heah SM, Tang CL. A prospective randomised study of drains in infra-peritoneal rectal anastomoses. Tech Coloproctol. 2001;5(2):89-92.

45. Vlug MS, Wind J, Hollmann MW, Ubbink DT, Cense HA, Engel AF, et al. Laparoscopy in combination with fast track multimodal management is the best perioperative strategy in patients undergoing colonic surgery: A randomized clinical trial (LAFA-study). Ann Surg. 2011;254(6):868-75.

46. Feroci F, Lenzi E, Baraghini M, Garzi A, Vannucchi A, Cantafio S, et al. Fast-track colorectal surgery: Protocol adherence influences postoperative outcomes. Int J Colorectal Dis. 2013;28(1):103-9.

47. Boelens PG, Heesakkers FF, Luyer MD, van Barneveld KW, de Hingh IH, Nieuwenhuijzen GA, et al. Reduction of postoperative ileus by early enteral nutrition in patients undergoing major rectal surgery: Prospective, randomized, controlled trial. Ann Surg. 2014;259(4):649-55.

48. Alfonsi P, Slim K, Chauvin M, Mariani P, Faucheron JL, Fletcher D, et al. French guidelines for enhanced recovery after elective colorectal surgery. J Visc Surg. 2014;151(1):65-79.

49. McNicol ED, Boyce D, Schumann R, Carr DB. Mu-opioid antagonists for opioid-induced bowel dysfunction. Cochrane Database Syst Rev. 2008;(2):CD006332.

50. Barletta JF, Asgeirsson T, El-Badawi KI, Senagore AJ. Introduction of alvimopan into an enhanced recovery protocol for colectomy offers benefit in open but not laparoscopic colectomy. J Laparoendosc Adv Surg Tech A. 2011;21(10):887-91.

51. Lee SY, Kang SB, Kim DW, Oh HK, Ihn MH. Risk factors and preventive measures for acute urinary retention after rectal cancer surgery. World J Surg. 2015;39(1):275-82.

52. Thiel SW, Kollef MH, Isakow W. Non-invasive stroke volume measurement and passive leg raising predict volume responsiveness in medical ICU patients: An observational cohort study. Crit Care. 2009;13(4):R111.

53. Hedrick TL, Thiele RH, Hassinger TE, Donovan J, Reines HD, Damico E Jr, et al. Multicenter observational study examining the implementation of enhanced recovery within the virginia surgical quality collaborative in patients undergoing elective colectomy. J Am Coll Surg. 2019;229(4):374-82,e3.

54. Bednarski BK, Nickerson TP, You YN, Messick CA, Speer B, Gottumukkala V, et al. Randomized clinical trial of accelerated enhanced recovery after minimally invasive colorectal cancer surgery (RecoverMI trial). Br J Surg. 2019;106(10):1311-8.

Perioperative Management of Peritoneal Surface Malignancies for Cytoreductive Surgeries and Hyperthermic Intraperitoneal Chemotherapy

Sohan Lal Solanki, Shivacharan Patel, Reshma P Ambulkar

INTRODUCTION

Cancer is a debilitating disease. Incidence of cancer is increasing worldwide and morbidity and mortality of cancers are causing an increasing financial burden on all the countries in the world. Cancer treatment has evolved considerably in recent years. Difficult to treat cancers have been treated with advancement in treatment modality. In the past 20 years, treatment of peritoneal metastatic cancer has gained increasing interest.

Cytoreductive surgery (CRS) and hyperthermic intraperitoneal chemotherapy (HIPEC) are an important invention in the treatment of peritoneal surface malignancies. Primary peritoneal surface malignancies are malignant peritoneal mesothelioma and pseudomyxoma peritonei and secondary peritoneal surface malignancies comprise peritoneal metastases from different primaries such as colorectal, ovarian, and gastric cancers.

This complex surgery has improved the survival of patients and given a new ray of hope for terminal ill cancer patients.[1] But the survival of patients is dependent on multiple factors such as selection of patients, primary diagnosis, extent of disease, expertise of surgeon, chemotherapy and response to preoperative chemotherapy, and many others. Many studies are being done conducted across the world regarding the management of CRS and HIPEC.

Cytoreductive surgery and HIPEC require special surgical skill for the complex resection of peritoneal tumor. Management of patients for such complex surgeries requires a teamwork of doctors including surgeons, anesthetists, critical care specialists, chest medicine specialists, and allied healthcare workers including nursing team, nutrition experts, and physiotherapists.

BACKGROUND

Cytoreductive surgery and HIPEC provide a promising therapeutic option for highly selected patients with peritoneal carcinomatosis, arising from different malignancies such as colorectal cancer, gastric cancer, ovarian cancer, or peritoneal mesothelioma with improvement of both patient survival and quality of life. Before the introduction of CRS and HIPEC, patients with peritoneal malignancies were regarded as incurable and were given palliative chemotherapy.

Dr Paul Sugarbaker first described this approach for pseudomyxoma peritonei arising from appendix. He showed that CRS and HIPEC increased the survival and quality of life.[2] Verwaal et al. subsequently reported results from a randomized trial that compared systemic chemotherapy versus CRS with HIPEC and showed that, at the end of 8 years follow-up, a near twofold (13 months vs. 22 months) survival benefit was achieved in the arm receiving HIPEC. In the CRS and HIPEC group, those who underwent complete cytoreduction showed a median survival of 43 months.[3]

RATIONALE

Hyperthermic intraperitoneal chemotherapy involves perfusion of abdominal organs with cytotoxic chemotherapy drugs at a higher than normal body temperature. Intraperitoneal administration of anticancer drugs gives high response rates. It also has many pharmacokinetic advantages. This is because the peritoneal plasma barrier provides dose intensive therapy. There is higher concentration of anticancer drugs in direct contact with tumor cells with reduced systemic concentration and lower systemic toxicity. Heat at 42.5°C is cytotoxic in vitro. It is also shown that hyperthermia at 42°C enhances the antitumor effects of agents such as oxaliplatin, mitomycin, doxorubicin, and cisplatin by augmenting cytotoxicity and increasing the penetration of drugs into tissue. This has led to the development of new novel locoregional treatment called HIPEC.

The tumor volume reduction is the most important factor in achieving tumor response to chemotherapy and has been reported for ovarian cancer. Combination works as CRS is used to treat macroscopic disease and HIPEC to treat microscopic residual disease with a single procedure. Intraperitoneal chemotherapy penetrates by only 2–5 mm in peritoneal carcinomatosis, even when combined with heat. Hence, curative CRS should aim at maximum reduction of tumor volume. Only pseudomyxoma peritonei has shown long-term survival rate even without a significant reduction in tumor volume.

TECHNIQUE

Cytoreductive surgery and HIPEC comprise of three phases. First phase involves removal of all visible metastatic abdominal and pelvic disease with peritonectomy. It is a long duration surgery phase, where all the peritoneal deposits and the main tumor bulk are removed. It is followed by HIPEC, where chemotherapy agents are infused in the peritoneal cavity at 42°C for 60–120 minutes.

The chemotherapy agents are mixed with a fluid, like dialysate and heated to 42°C temperature in a specialized machine and it is introduced into peritoneal cavity via inlet channel. Outlet channel removes the fluid from the abdominal cavity back to the machine to be reheated and recirculated. The chemotherapy agent removes the microscopic metastatic tissues in the peritoneal cavity. It is followed by reconstruction phase wherein anastomosis of bowel is done and abdomen is closed **(Figs. 1 to 3)**.

CHALLENGES

Cytoreductive surgery with HIPEC is a long and complex procedure with significant blood and fluid loss during debulking. Hemodynamic, hematological, and metabolic alterations occur before and during the HIPEC phase and even in the early postoperative period with resultant significant morbidity and mortality.[2,4,5] During HIPEC, hyperthermic perfusion of chemotherapy causes large fluid shifts and hyperthermia-induced cardiovascular changes in the body. The patients are transfused large quantity of cold fluids intravenously during HIPEC for active cooling leading to changes in the fluid status of the patient and changes in the cardiovascular system. There is increase in heart rate, mean arterial pressure, and cardiac output during HIPEC.

The chemotherapy agents are cytotoxic and some of the agents like adriamycin are cardiotoxic. Even though the systemic absorption from the peritoneum is less compared to intravenous infusion, some systemic changes are expected after HIPEC due to chemotherapy agents. The chemotherapy drugs may also cause systemic inflammatory effects leading to cardiovascular instability of patients in the intraoperative period. There are changes in the tissue oxygenation, oxygen consumption, and electrolytes, which require serial blood gas analysis in the intraoperative as well as in the postoperative period. Thus, the patients need intense monitoring in the intraoperative and postoperative phases.

Despite most of the reported patients are with no comorbidities, the morbidity and mortality range from 12% to 65% in these procedures. For a good clinical outcome, it is imperative to have a well-coordinated team of anesthesiologist, surgeons and intensivists, and other ancillary services. The Society of Onco-Anaesthesia and Perioperative Care (SOPAC) came out with a 2019 consensus guideline recently for perioperative management of CRS-HIPEC.[6] In this consensus guideline, Solanki et al.[6] mentioned about preoperative, intraoperative, and

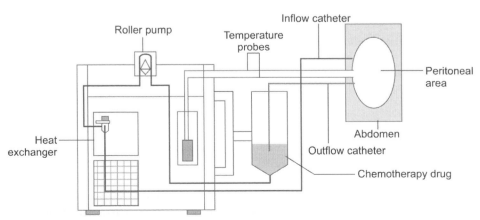

Fig. 1: A schematic diagram of hyperthermic chemotherapy perfusion into the abdomen.

postoperative management of CRS and HIPEC and level of consensus among expert's committee for perioperative management of CRS and HIPEC.

PREOPERATIVE WORKUP

All routine blood investigations and 12-lead electrocardiogram to be done for all the patients. Resting two-dimensional (2D) echocardiogram to know the heart function since there is a lot of hemodynamic variations in the intraoperative and postoperative period. Cardiac stress test might be indicated in patients with coronary artery disease or poor effort tolerance. Any underlying renal or hepatic dysfunction is a high risk for perioperative morbidity and mortality.[7]

Nutrition and physiotherapy play an important role in the reduction of morbidity and mortality after CRS and

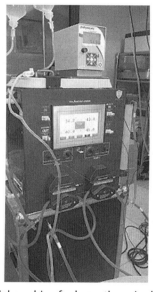

Fig. 2: A special machine for hyperthermic chemotherapy perfusion in abdomen.

HIPEC. Preoperative oral or enteral nutrition should be started in all malnourished patients to improve nutrition status. Preoperative physiotherapy and physical exercise should be started to help in enhanced recovery after surgery. Incentive spirometry helps as well. Patients undergo diaphragmatic stripping in some selected cases. In such cases, pulmonary rehabilitation plays a crucial role in preventing postoperative pulmonary complications.

INTRAOPERATIVE MANAGEMENT

Monitors and Preparation

Intraoperative monitoring should consist of regular ASA monitors such as electrocardiogram, end-tidal carbon dioxide monitor, noninvasive blood pressure monitor, pulse oximetry along with invasive arterial line, and cardiac output monitor. Central venous catheter must be inserted for central venous pressure monitoring, vasopressor administration, and fluid administration. Large-bore intravenous cannula may be secured for rapid infusion of intravenous fluids, blood, and blood products. Rapid fluid infuser must be kept standby in case of sudden blood loss.

Induction of Anesthesia

General anesthesia is the standard of care for prolonged and complex surgery such as CRS and HIPEC. Epidural placement for intraoperative and postoperative analgesia can be considered. It helps in early recovery and mobilization of patient in the postoperative period. Decreased pain can also help in chest physiotherapy and rehabilitation. Opioid such as fentanyl along with propofol or etomidate is used as induction anesthetics. Long-acting muscle relaxant such as vecuronium or rocuronium can be used. Rapid sequence induction may be indicated in patients with large peritoneal deposits and associated ascites causing increased intra-abdominal pressure which can lead to

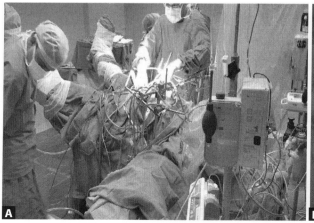
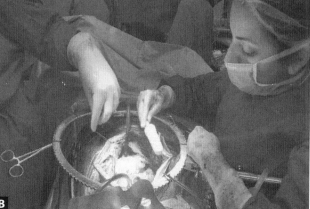

Figs. 3A and B: Clinical images showing hyperthermic chemotherapy perfusion in abdomen.

aspiration of gastric contents.[6] Endotracheal intubation is preferred over supraglottic airway devices since patient may require postoperative ventilation and chances of aspiration are higher with supraglottic airway devices. Total intravenous anesthesia or volatile anesthetics can be used for maintenance of anesthesia throughout the surgery.[6]

Hemodynamic Monitoring

Advanced hemodynamic monitoring is important as hemodynamic variation is tremendous during intraoperative and postoperative period. Arterial line along with arterial pressure-based cardiac output monitoring (stroke volume, stroke volume index, cardiac output, and cardiac index) is very useful to assess hemodynamics of patient throughout the surgery. Continuous central venous pressure monitoring also helps in knowing the volume status of the patient.[6]

With serial arterial and venous blood gases, lactate and mixed central venous oxygen saturation ($ScvO_2$) levels can be determined and oxygen delivery (DO_2) and oxygen consumption (VO_2) can be calculated to assess perfusion status of the body. Regular arterial blood gas is vital to monitor lactates, oxygenation, and base excess.

Monitoring of electrolytes is equally important. Hyperkalemia or hypokalemia can occur intraoperatively and cause fatal arrhythmias. Blood sugars may vary in the intraoperative period and should be monitored even in nondiabetic patients.[8] Ionized calcium should also be monitored.

Urine Output Monitoring

Urine output is an important indicator of renal perfusion. Maintaining adequate urine output thereby maintaining adequate renal perfusion is important to prevent acute kidney injury, which is common in CRS and HIPEC due to hypotension, chemotherapy drugs, and others. Minimum urine output of 0.5 mL/kg has to be maintained throughout the CRS phase. Urine output must be kept higher during the HIPEC phase at >2 mL/kg and 1–2 mL/kg during the reconstructive phase in order to enhance the excretion of chemotherapy drugs which are systemically absorbed during HIPEC phase.[6] Use of diuretics to increase urine output is not recommended. Euvolemia should be maintained to ensure adequate renal perfusion.[6]

Temperature Management

Temperature monitoring is vital. Hypothermia causes coagulation abnormalities. Temperature is to be maintained at normal level throughout the procedure. Core body temperature monitoring is recommended. Warming blanket and fluid warmers help in temperature regulation. Prolonged cytoreduction part of surgery can lead to hypothermia.

During HIPEC, body temperature increases above normal temperature.[9] Maximum temperature is reached around 60 minutes of perfusion of chemotherapy drugs at 42°C.[10] Higher perfusion temperature was related to more pronounced changes in serum glucose, sodium, and lactate.[11] Infusion of cold crystalloid solutions intravenously, cooling through forced air blanket or cooling mattress, and cooling patient with cold saline bottles in axilla and head neck areas can be done. If core body temperature continues to increase despite all measure and temperature goes beyond 39°C, temperature of perfusate can be decreased.[6] Hyperthermia is harmful for the patient. It causes tachycardia, increases metabolism, and can cause convulsions and coagulation abnormalities. Passive patient cooling (switching off warming devices) prior to beginning of HIPEC helps in controlling the temperature.[6]

Fluid Management

Intraoperative fluid management is very crucial. There is increased amount of fluid shifts, blood loss, and electrolyte disturbances during the surgery. Crystalloids may be started at 3–4 mL/kg for maintenance. Goal-directed fluid therapy must be advocated based on pulse pressure variation or stroke volume variation. Balanced solutions such as Ringer's lactate and acetate-containing solutions are used. Colloids in the form of albumin can be used as well. Other starch-based colloids are not recommended. Kajdi et al. found administration on hydroxyethyl starch-containing solutions had negative impact on renal function.[7] Massive blood loss might occur in a few cases and massive blood transfusion protocol has to be followed.

Use of vasopressors to maintain adequate blood pressure is recommended. Fluid overload can be prevented by early use of vasopressors. Noradrenaline is the vasopressor of choice. Fluid overload can lead to increase in bowel edema, anastomotic leak, pulmonary edema, and increases morbidity and mortality.

Coagulation Monitoring

Coagulation abnormality is very common during CRS and HIPEC due to increased blood loss, hypothermia, hyperthermia, and chemotherapy agents. This can occur during the surgery or in the postoperative period. Massive blood loss can cause dilutional coagulopathy. Monitoring of coagulation is important. Routine prothrombin time (PT), international normalized ratio (INR), and activated partial thromboplastin time (aPTT) are regularly tested during the surgery and in the postoperative period.[6] Thromboelastogram (TEG) or rotational thromboelastometry (ROTEM) can also be used to give better information about coagulation deficiencies. TEG or ROTEM gives better information than conventional tests such as PT and INR.[6] Correction according to TEG or ROTEM will help in determination of exact requirement of blood products and decrease unnecessary transfusion to the patients.

Extubation after the Surgery

Extubation after the surgery is dependent on the patient preoperative condition, nutritional status, cardiac, pulmonary or other major comorbidities, patient vitals, lactate levels, intraoperative blood loss, and the extent and duration of surgery. Extubation of trachea can be done in operating room in hemodynamically stable patients, patients with no major comorbidities, low volume [low peritoneal carcinomatosis index (PCI)] diseases, and not very prolonged surgeries. If the patient is hemodynamically unstable, extubation can be deferred. Patient can be shifted sedated and ventilated to the intensive care unit (ICU) and extubated after the hemodynamic parameters are normalized.[6]

POSTOPERATIVE MANAGEMENT

Patients who are shifted, intubated to ICU after the surgery have to be monitored. Advance hemodynamic monitoring must be continued. Extubation must be planned after adequate washout of anesthesia and adequate reversal of muscle relaxation. Patients can be extubated after they meet criteria of extubation. Patients who are hemodynamically stable, obeying commands, adequate oxygenation and breathing efforts with rapid shallow breathing index < 105, low lactate levels, and normal postoperative investigations can be extubated.

After extubation, patients can be switched to noninvasive ventilation (NIV) or high-flow nasal cannula in high-risk patients for postoperative respiratory failure. NIV provides support to patient efforts and prevents basal atelectasis. Patients can be gradually weaned from NIV or high-flow nasal cannula.

Prolonged ventilation in unstable patients who cannot be extubated can lead to ventilator-associated pneumonia. Hence, early tracheostomy along with early weaning must be attempted in such cases.

Regular surgical site prophylactic antibiotics are indicated prior to surgical incision and they are continued in the postoperative period also. Duration of antibiotic treatment is dependent on the condition of the patient. Increased bowel handling can lead to bacterial translocation and can cause bacteremia and sepsis. Patients with postoperative sepsis have to be managed aggressively. Anaerobic coverage may be added in bowel surgeries with risk of bowel perforation.

Postoperative complications can be divided into nonsurgical and surgical complications:

- *Nonsurgical complications*:
  - Acute respiratory failure
  - Postoperative hypovolemia
  - Postoperative hypotension
  - Septic shock
  - Reintubation
  - Acute blood loss anemia
  - Pulmonary embolism
  - Acute renal failure
  - Tracheostomy
  - Dilutional coagulopathy
  - Hypoalbuminemia
  - Arrhythmias
  - Catheter-related bloodstream infections
  - Intensive care unit delirium.
- *Surgical complications*:
  - Anastomotic leaks
  - Anastomotic leaks requiring re-exploration
  - Intra-abdominal abscess
  - Intra-abdominal abscess requiring drainage
  - Surgical bleeding
  - Deep wound infection
  - *Abdominal sepsis*: Anastomotic leak, abscess, and deep wound infection
  - Bacteremia
  - Postoperative parenteral nutrition.

Hemodynamic variation, electrolyte disturbances, blood sugar variations, and coagulopathies are common in postoperative period. Goal-directed therapy through invasive blood pressure monitoring, serial arterial blood gas and lactate measurement is recommended.

Blood and blood components have to be transfused in case of coagulation abnormalities. TEG or ROTEM is useful as well to decide the blood product which has to be transfused such as platelets or cryoprecipitate or fresh frozen plasma.

Complete blood count, serum electrolytes, renal function, and liver functions are to be serially monitored every day. Renal dysfunction is common in the postoperative period. Sequential organ failure assessment (SOFA) scores can be used to assess organ dysfunction.

Postoperative nutrition is very crucial. Parenteral nutrition or enteral nutrition has to be started as early as possible. Enteral nutrition may not be started in selected cases such as gastrectomy, small bowel resection, multiple anastomoses, and others. In such patients, parenteral nutrition is recommended as early as possible. Enteral nutrition may be started in other selective cases. Enteral nutrition can be given through oral or nasogastric tube or nasojejunal tube. Some practice combination of parenteral and enteral nutrition. Nutritionist plays an important role in the formulation of diet, as patients undergoing CRS and HIPEC require more calories and proteins compared to other surgeries since the postoperative stress and catabolism are higher. The length of ICU stay influences the start of feeding.[12]

Chest physiotherapy and rehabilitation are vital in the recovery of patients. Regular physiotherapy with early mobilization is very important. Patients can be mobilized on the postoperative day one if the vitals are stable. Spirometry helps in lung expansion and regular clearing of secretion is important to avoid development of postoperative respiratory complications, especially with patients who have undergone diaphragmatic stripping or opening of diaphragm. Pain control is very crucial, so that patient performs chest physiotherapy adequately.

Postoperative deep vein thrombosis (DVT) prophylaxis is very important in CRS and HIPEC as patients may be immobilized for prolonged period of time postsurgery. The risk of DVT is also higher in cancer patients. Low-molecular-weight heparin or unfractionated heparin must be started as early as possible in the postoperative period. Early mobilization also decreases the risk of DVT. Calf pumps or antiembolism stockings must be used in the intraoperative as well as postoperative period too.

Fagotti et al. in their study found the incidence of major complications to be 34.8%,[13] the most common was bleeding. Dominique et al. conducted a multicentric, cohort study and found that the PCI and the center at which the surgery was conducted as the two factors which increased morbidity and mortality.[12,14] Shen et al. found a morbidity and mortality of 41.8% and 5.5%, respectively.[15] Hagendoorn et al. found morbidity rate of 47% in their study.[16] Reoperation rate was 47% in morbid patients in a study conducted by Malfroy et al.[17] Patients have to be monitored and complications have to be identified at the earliest and treated. Re-exploration for surgical complications can complicate the postoperative course and increase in morbidity and mortality of the patients. Readmission rate in a study by Wallet et al. was found to be 44%.[18]

Simkens et al. found that serious postoperative complications requiring intervention as the only significant risk factor for early recurrence of cancer which was independent of the extent of peritoneal disease. This signifies the importance of minimizing the risk of postoperative complications. Early recurrence decreases overall survival after CRS and HIPEC procedure.[19]

PAIN MANAGEMENT

Pain control post-CRS and HIPEC is very crucial for the recovery of patient from surgery. Abdominal incision is large for the surgery. Epidural placement prior to induction of anesthesia helps in providing analgesia intraoperatively and postoperatively.[20] Addition of opioid along with local anesthetic enhances pain control. If epidural placement is contraindicated in a patient, postoperatively patient-controlled analgesia (PCA) with opioid such as fentanyl must be provided.[6] Inadequate pain control in the postoperative

period will lead to increase in postoperative complications, morbidity, and increase in hospital stay.

MORBIDITY AND MORTALITY

Newton et al. reviewed factors contributing to morbidity and mortality of patients undergoing CRS and HIPEC.[21] They found for a variety of cancer types, the rate of grade III-IV morbidity range was 22–34% and mortality from 0.8% to 4.1%. Mortality range for colorectal cancer, pseudomyxoma peritonei, and diffuse malignant peritoneal mesothelioma was 2–4%. Gastric cancer had a higher mortality rate (3.9% and 6.5% in two different studies) and ovarian cancer had least mortality (0.8%).

- *Patient factors*:
  - *With strong association with morbidity*:
    - Age
    - Hypoalbuminemia
    - Performance status
  - *With weak association with morbidity*:
    - Obesity.
- *Operative factors*:
  - *With strong association with morbidity*:
    - Peritoneal carcinomatosis index
    - Bowel resection
    - Diaphragmatic involvement
    - Distal pancreatectomy
    - Surgeon experience.
  - *With weak association with morbidity*:
    - Hepatobiliary procedures
    - Urologic procedures
    - Preoperative bevacizumab.

OTHER VARIATIONS OF CHEMOPERFUSION
Hyperthermic Intrathoracic Chemotherapy

Pleural malignancies may be of different origin such as malignant pleural mesothelioma, advanced thymoma with pleural dissemination, or spread from pseudomyxoma peritonei. It is difficult to achieve local control of these tumors due to diffuse and invasive local behavior of these malignant tumors.[22] Pleural metastases from abdominal tumor such as pseudomyxoma peritonei is believed to be due to diaphragmatic perforation during surgery for abdomen or transdiaphragmatic spread of the disease through lymphatic lacunae.[23]

The standard treatment of pleural malignancy is controversial.[24] Most of the patients are given palliative chemotherapy. There is no standard treatment regimen with a curative intent.[25,26] Multimodal therapy with induction chemotherapy, surgical resection, adjuvant chemotherapy, and even radiotherapy can reduce local recurrence and improve patient outcome.[27-29] Yellin A et al. studied hyperthermic pleural perfusion of cisplatin from

November 1994 to September 1998 and concluded that it was safe, easily feasible, and relatively safe.[30] Recently, CRS along with intraoperative hyperthermic intrathoracic chemotherapy (HITHOC) perfusion has been advocated to reduce local tumor spread and treat cancer.[31-33]

Hyperthermic Intrathoracic Chemotherapy Procedure

Cytoreductive surgery is performed with pleurectomy, decortication, or extrapleural pneumonectomy. The aim of cytoreduction is to remove all the macroscopic tumor deposits. The microscopic deposits pose a serious threat for local recurrence. Hence, local intracavitatory application of chemotherapy agent provides high local dose of drug and lesser systemic side effects.[34,35] Regional hyperthermia further increases the penetration of the drug. In case of pseudomyxoma peritonei, if the diaphragmatic stripping is done during CRS, it should not be closed during HIPEC to allow flow of chemotherapeutic agent to flow into the thoracic cavity and hence increasing the cytotoxic activity in the pleural cavity.[23] For pleural spread of peritoneal carcinomatosis, a complete removal of peritoneal metastasis and pleural metastasis is achieved by opening the diaphragm during abdominal surgery and a hyperthermic thoracoabdominal chemotherapy (HITAC) infusion is given.[36]

Efficacy of Hyperthermic Intrathoracic Chemotherapy

Zhou H et al. did a review of all the HITHOC/HITAC studies from all over the world. They selected 27 articles for systematic review and five were studied with randomized control. Results from meta-analysis showed significantly longer survival of patients treated with HITHOC therapy compared to patients treated without HITHOC therapy. HITHOC therapy was favored due to increase in 1-year survival rate, tumor-free survival rate, or Karnofsky performance status score.[37]

Complications of Hyperthermic Intrathoracic Chemotherapy

Complications of HITHOC are similar to complications associated with HIPEC such as thrombocytopenia, bleeding, and systemic inflammation. Some of the complications are exclusive for HITHOC such as pulmonary emboli, chest pain, dyspnea, bronchopleural fistula, pneumothorax, empyema, and air leak.[36]

Management of Hyperthermic Intrathoracic Chemotherapy

All the patients should be extensively worked up before CRS and HITHOC. Patients are prone for bleeding intraoperatively and hence sufficient blood and blood products must be arranged. Patients must be evaluated for cardiorespiratory function. Evaluation of heart by

12-lead electrocardiogram and 2D echocardiography and stress test is advised. Respiratory function can be assessed by pulmonary function tests, diffusion capacity of lung, and effort tolerance. Respiratory physician and cardiologist must be closely involved along with the surgeon and anesthesiologist for perioperative care. Preoperative chest physiotherapy should be advocated and patients must be adequately counseled regarding the surgery and postoperative pain management.[6,36]

The main anesthesia challenge during surgery is blood and fluid loss which is dependent on the disease load of cancer. Fluid administration must be based on stroke volume and delta stroke volume as increased fluid administration intraoperatively can lead to pulmonary edema. Pulse pressure variation and stroke volume variation are not reliable during thoracotomy procedures.[6] Maintenance of normal temperature throughout the procedure is important. Chemotherapy in the intrathoracic cavity causes increased fluid load and may lead to increased airway pressures, increased intrathoracic pressures, mediastinal shift, and decreased functional residual capacity.

Extubation after HITHOC procedures is not extensively studied. Extubation in postoperative unit is preferred in view of large fluid shifts and reduction of pulmonary lung volumes postsurgery. Hemodynamic monitoring to be continued in the postoperative period until the patient is hemodynamically stable. There should be consideration for reduction of postoperative lung volume after lung resection. Patient temperature should be monitored in the postoperative period too. Coagulopathy is a major concern after this procedure due to hyperthermia, major blood loss, and inflammation. Postoperative pain management should be adequate for the patient to do spirometry and chest physiotherapy, which are shown to reduce postoperative pulmonary complications.

Pressurized Intraperitoneal Aerosol Chemotherapy

Patients with low disease load (with no peritoneal metastasis) are treated with systemic chemotherapy and surgery. Patients with higher disease load with peritoneal metastasis are treated with systemic chemotherapy and CRS with HIPEC along with postoperative systemic chemotherapy.[38]

Pressurized intraperitoneal aerosol chemotherapy (PIPAC) is a new form of delivery of chemotherapy drugs in gaseous form under pressure within closed abdominal cavity which is created with laparoscopy technique. Aerosol is created with the help of nebulizer which is connected to an intravenous high pressure injector. Various chemotherapeutic agents are used for PIPAC such as doxorubicin for ovarian, gastric cancers, which is followed by cisplatin. Oxaliplatin is also used for colorectal and appendiceal cancers. The therapeutic capnoperitoneum which is created during the procedure is maintained for 30 minutes at a temperature of 37°C.[39] This chemotherapeutic agent dosage is 5–20 times less than that required for liquid intravenous chemotherapy while the target tissue drug concentration is doubled.[40]

Indications of Pressurized Intraperitoneal Aerosol Chemotherapy

Alyami M et al. conducted 437 PIPAC procedures in 147 consecutive patients who had unresectable peritoneal metastasis. After repeated PIPAC procedures, the disease burden reduced significantly and 26 patients were scheduled for CRS and HIPEC leading to complete removal of disease burden. They concluded that PIPAC can be instituted to patients with a PCI of up to 39 and also in symptomatic (pain, ascites, diarrhea, constipation) patients and PIPAC can be repeated up to six times in the same patient. Improvement in PCI and complete disappearance of symptoms are expected in >60% of patients treated with PIPAC. 7% 30-day mortality was observed.[41]

In 2019, review article on PIPAC procedures by Nowacki M et al. concluded that repeated PIPAC procedures were safe and feasible and can be considered as a treatment option for refractory peritoneal metastasis of various origins.[42]

Horvath P et al. did a case series of two patients in solid organ transplant patients and concluded that PIPAC can be used as an effective therapy for peritoneal metastasis in recipients of solid organ transplants. It can prove useful in liver transplant and combined kidney-pancreas transplant patients with both metachronous and synchronous peritoneal metastasis. It causes no measurable hepatorenal toxicity and does not necessitate interruption of immunosuppressive therapy.[39]

Conduct of Pressurized Intraperitoneal Aerosol Chemotherapy

Pressurized intraperitoneal aerosol chemotherapy requires general anesthesia. It is a short-duration procedure. Standard ASA monitors along with invasive arterial are indicated for intraoperative monitoring. After general anesthesia, pneumoperitoneum is created laparoscopically. The intra-abdominal pressure is maintained between 12 and 15 mm Hg. The chemotherapy agent is converted to aerosol form by nebulizer which is connected to a high-pressure injector. PIPAC is given for duration of 30 minutes at 37°C. After the procedure is done, the aerosol is exsufflated with a special filter. Patients can be extubated in the operation room and shifted to postanesthesia recovery unit for monitoring. Hemodynamic instability is unusual during the procedure as there is no much fluid shift/blood loss occurs.[43]

Electrostatic Precipitation of Chemotherapy Drugs

Willaert et al. did a study on adding electrostatic field during PIPAC. Addition of electrostatic field increases charged droplet precipitation and tissue penetration. They found that the procedure was well-tolerated and safe.[44]

Occupational Safety

Chemotherapy drugs in the aerosolized form pose occupational exposure to the doctors and operation room personnel during PIPAC. Chemotherapy drugs can get absorbed into the body through inhalation, skin contact, skin absorption, ingestion, or injection. Chemotherapy agents have several adverse effects such as hair loss, headache, acute irritation and hypersensitivity, congenital malformations in pregnant women, fetal loss, low birth weight, infertility, and risk of other cancers such as leukemia.[45] Hence, sufficient safety measures have to be in place during PIPAC.

Safe Conduct of Pressurized Intraperitoneal Aerosol Chemotherapy for Occupational Safety

Some safety measures have to be in place for safe conduct of PIPAC procedure. An N95 mask with a tight seal around the nose and mouth must be worn by all operation theater (OT) personnel.[43,46] The injection and nebulizer which produce aerosol must be remote controlled and should be controlled from outside operation room. No personnel should stay inside operation room and patient should be monitored remotely. The whole system of capnoperitoneum must be airtight with no leaks. Aerosol after the PIPAC procedure should be exsufflated into air waste system of the hospital. There should be no capno flow during the PIPAC procedure to prevent any leaks or increase in pressure.

Safety of PIPAC procedure has been studied by many researchers. Delhorme JB did a study with 26 samples from surgeons and coworkers after PIPAC procedure in nonlaminar flow operation room. They also collected air samples. All the air samples were negative and only one out of 26 samples from surgeon's glove was positive for chemotherapy agent. They concluded that when the procedure is done in approved security condition, even without laminar flow, PIPAC seems harmless.[47] Paul Ametsbichler also studied the air samples after PIPAC procedure and found low air contamination. They concluded that PIPAC has low occupational risk, but adequate safety and cleaning standards must be adopted.[35]

CONCLUSION

CRS and HIPEC is a complex surgery. It involves crucial perioperative management of patient, from preoperative period to postoperative recovery. It requires expertise and team work of several specialties like as oncology, surgery, anesthesia, critical care, pain management, nutrition and physiotherapy. Future remains bright in the treatment of peritoneal surface malignancies with evolving treatment strategies.

REFERENCES

1. Glehen O, Mohamed F, Gilly FN. Peritoneal carcinomatosis from digestive tract cancer: new management by cytoreductive surgery and intraperitoneal chemohyperthermia. Lancet Oncol. 2004;5:219-28.

2. Sugarbaker PH, Ryan DP. Cytoreductive surgery plus hyperthermic perioperative chemotherapy to treat peritoneal metastases from colorectal cancer: standard of care or an experimental approach? Lancet Oncol. 2012;13:e362-9.

3. Verwaal VJ, van Ruth S, de Bree E, van Sloothen GW, van Tinteren H, Boot H, et al. Randomized trial of cytoreduction and hyperthermic intraperitoneal chemotherapy versus systemic chemotherapy and palliative surgery in patients with peritoneal carcinomatosis of colorectal cancer. J Clin Oncol. 2003;21:3737-43.

4. Franko J, Ibrahim Z, Gusani NJ, Holtzman MP, Bartlett DL, Zeh HJ. Cytoreductive surgery and hyperthermic intraperitoneal chemoperfusion versus systemic chemotherapy alone for colorectal peritoneal carcinomatosis. Cancer. 2010;116: 3756-62.

5. Schmidt C, Creutzenberg M, Piso P, Hobbhahn J, Bucher M. Peri-operative anaesthetic management of cytoreductive surgery with hyperthermic intraperitoneal chemotherapy. Anaesthesia. 2008;63:389-95.

6. Solanki SL, Mukherjee S, Agarwal V, Thota RS, Balakrishnan K, Shah SB, et al. Society of Onco-Anaesthesia and Perioperative Care consensus guidelines for perioperative management of patients for cytoreductive surgery and hyperthermic intraperitoneal chemotherapy (CRS-HIPEC). Indian J Anaesth. 2019;63:972-87.

7. Kajdi ME, Beck-Schimmer B, Held U, Kofmehl R, Lehmann K, Ganter MT. Anaesthesia in patients undergoing cytoreductive surgery with hyperthermic intraperitoneal chemotherapy: retrospective analysis of a single centre three-year experience. World J Surg Oncol. 2014;12:136.

8. Stewart CL, Gleisner A, Halpern A, Ibrahim-Zada I, Luna RA, Pearlman N, et al. Implications of hyperthermic intraperitoneal chemotherapy perfusion-related hyperglycemia. Ann Surg Oncol. 2018;25:655-9.

9. Kamal JM, Elshaikh SM, Nabil D, Mohamad AM. The perioperative course and anesthetic challenge for cytoreductive surgery with hyperthermic intraperitoneal chemotherapy. Egypt J Anaesth. 2013;29:311-8.

10. Kanakoudis F, Petrou A, Michaloudis D, Chortaria G, Konstantinidou A. Anaesthesia for intra-peritoneal perfusion of hyperthermic chemotherapy. Haemodynamic changes, oxygen consumption and delivery. Anaesthesia. 1996;51:1033-6.

11. Ceelen W, De Somer F, Van Nieuwenhove Y, Vande Putte D, Pattyn P. Effect of perfusion temperature on glucose and

12. Arakelian E, Gunningberg L, Larsson J, Norlén K, Mahteme H. Factors influencing early postoperative recovery after cytoreductive surgery and hyperthermic intraperitoneal chemotherapy. Eur J Surg Oncol. 2011;37:897-903.

13. Fagotti A, Costantini B, Vizzielli G, Perelli F, Ercoli A, Gallotta V, et al. HIPEC in recurrent ovarian cancer patients: Morbidity-related treatment and long-term analysis of clinical outcome. Gynecol Oncol. 2011;122:221-5.

14. Elias D, Gilly F, Boutitie F, Quenet F, Bereder JM, Mansvelt B, et al. Peritoneal colorectal carcinomatosis treated with surgery and perioperative intraperitoneal chemotherapy: retrospective analysis of 523 patients from a multicentric French study. J Clin Oncol. 2009;28:63-8.

15. Shen P, Stewart JH, Levine EA. The role of cytoreductive surgery and hyperthermic intraperitoneal chemotherapy for metastatic colorectal cancer with peritoneal surface disease. Curr Probl Cancer. 2009;33:154-67.

16. Hagendoorn J, van Lammeren G, Boerma D, van der Beek E, Wiezer MJ, van Ramshorst B. Cytoreductive surgery and hyperthermic intraperitoneal chemotherapy for peritoneal carcinomatosis from colorectal and gastrointestinal origin shows acceptable morbidity and high survival. Eur J Surg Oncol. 2009;35:833-7.

17. Malfroy S, Wallet F, Maucort-Boulch D, Chardonnal L, Sens N, Friggeri A, et al. Complications after cytoreductive surgery with hyperthermic intraperitoneal chemotherapy for treatment of peritoneal carcinomatosis: risk factors for ICU admission and morbidity prognostic score. Surg Oncol. 2016;25:6-15.

18. Wallet F, Maucort Boulch D, Malfroy S, Ledochowski S, Bernet C, Kepenekian V, et al. No impact on long-term survival of prolonged ICU stay and re-admission for patients undergoing cytoreductive surgery with HIPEC. Eur J Surg Oncol. 2016;42:855-60.

19. Simkens GA, van Oudheusden TR, Luyer MD, Nienhuijs SW, Nieuwenhuijzen GA, Rutten HJ, et al. Serious postoperative complications affect early recurrence after cytoreductive surgery and HIPEC for colorectal peritoneal carcinomatosis. Ann Surg Oncol. 2015;22:2656-62.

20. Piccioni F, Casiraghi C, Fumagalli L, Kusamura S, Baratti D, Deraco M, et al. Epidural analgesia for cytoreductive surgery with peritonectomy and heated intraperitoneal chemotherapy. Int J Surg. 2015;16:99-106.

21. Newton DA, Bartlett KB, Karakousis CG. Cytoreductive surgery and hyperthermic intraperitoneal chemotherapy: a review of factors contributing to morbidity and mortality. J Gastroinest Oncol. 2016;7:99-111.

22. Sugarbaker DJ, Flores RM, Jaklitsch MT, Richards WG, Strauss GM, Corson JM, et al. Resection margins, extrapleural nodal status, and cell type determine postoperative long-term survival in trimodality therapy of malignant pleural mesothelioma: results in 183 patients. J Thorac Cardiovasc Surg. 1999;117:54-63.

23. Chua TC, Yan TD, Yap ZL, Horton MD, Fermanis GG, Morris DL. Thoracic cytoreductive surgery and intraoperative

hyperthermic intrathoracic chemotherapy for pseudomyxoma peritonei. J Surg Oncol. 2009;99:292-5.

24. Ried M, Potzger T, Braune N, Diez C, Neu R, Sziklavari Z, et al. Local and systemic exposure of cisplatin during hyperthermic intrathoracic chemotherapy perfusion after pleurectomy and decortication for treatment of pleural malignancies. J Surg Oncol. 2013;107:735-40.

25. Muers MF, Stephens RJ, Fisher P, Darlison L, Higgs CM, Lowry E, et al. Active symptom control with or without chemotherapy in the treatment of patients with malignant pleural mesothelioma (MS01): a multicentre randomised trial. Lancet. 2008;371: 1685-94.

26. Ruffini E, Van Raemdonck D, Detterbeck F, Rocco G, Thomas P, Venuta F, et al. Management of thymic tumors: a survey of current practice among members of the European Society of Thoracic Surgeons. J Thorac Oncol. 2011;6:614-23.

27. Zauderer MG, Krug LM. The evolution of multimodality therapy for malignant pleural mesothelioma. Curr Treat Options Oncol. 2011;12:163-72.

28. Rena O, Mineo O, Casadio C. Multimodal treatment for stage IVA thymoma: a proposable strategy. Lung Cancer. 2012;76:89-92.

29. Treasure T, Waller D, Tan C, Entwisle J, O'Brien M, O'Byrne K, et al. The mesothelioma and radical surgery randomized controlled trial: the Mars feasibility study. J Thorac Oncol. 2009;4: 1254-8.

30. Yellin A, Simansky DA, Paley M, Refaely Y. Hyperthermic pleural perfusion with cisplatin: early clinical experience. Cancer. 2001;92:2197-203.

31. de Bree E, van Ruth S, Baas P, Rutgers EJ, van Zandwijk N, Witkamp AJ, et al. Cytoreductive surgery and intraoperative hyperthermic intrathoracic chemotherapy in patients with malignant pleural mesothelioma or pleural metastases of thymoma. Chest. 2002;121:480-7.

32. Tilleman TR, Richards WG, Zellos L, Johnson BE, Jaklitsch MT, Mueller J, et al. Extrapleural pneumonectomy followed by intracavitary intraoperative hyperthermic cisplatin with pharmacologic cytoprotection for treatment of malignant pleural mesothelioma: a phase II prospective study. J Thorac Cardiovasc Surg. 2009;138:405-11.

33. Ried M, Potzger T, Braune N, Neu R, Zausig Y, Schalke B, et al. Cytoreductive surgery and hyperthermic intrathoracic chemotherapy perfusion for malignant pleural tumours: perioperative management and clinical experience. Eur J Cardiothorac Surg. 2013;43:801-7.

34. Flores M. Surgical options in malignant pleural mesothelioma: extrapleural pneumonectomy or pleurectomy/decortication. Semin Thorac Cardiovasc Surg. 2009;21:149-53.

35. Ametsbichler P, Böhlandt A, Nowak D, Schierl R. Occupational exposure to cisplatin/oxaliplatin during Pressurized Intraperitoneal Aerosol Chemotherapy (PIPAC)? Eur J Surg Oncol. 2018;44:1793-9.

36. Solanki SL, Bajaj JS, Rahman F, Saklani AP. Perioperative management of cytoreductive surgery and hyperthermic intraoperative thoraco-abdominal chemotherapy (HITAC) for pseudomyxoma peritonei. Indian J Anaesth. 2019;63:134-7.

37. Zhou H, Wu W, Tang X, Zhou J, Shen Y. Effect of hyperthermic intrathoracic chemotherapy (HITHOC) on the malignant pleural effusion: a systematic review and meta-analysis. Medicine (Baltimore). 2017;96:e5532.

38. Macrì A, Fortugno A, Saladino E. Rationale and techniques of cytoreductive surgery and peritoneal chemohyperthermia. World J Gastrointest Oncol. 2011;3:169-74.

39. Horvath P, Yurttas C, Struller F, Bösmüller H, Lauer UM, Nadalin S, et al. Pressurized intraperitoneal aerosol chemotherapy (PIPAC) for peritoneal metastases in solid organ graft recipients: first experience. Ann Transplant. 2019;24:30-5.

40. Solass W, Kerb R, Mürdter T, Giger-Pabst U, Strumberg D, Tempfer C, et al. Intraperitoneal chemotherapy of peritoneal carcinomatosis using pressurized aerosol as an alternative to liquid solution: first evidence for efficacy. Ann Surg Oncol. 2014;21:553-9.

41. Alyami M, Mercier F, Siebert M, Bonnot PE, Laplace N, Villeneuve L, et al. Unresectable peritoneal metastasis treated by pressurized intraperitoneal aerosol chemotherapy (PIPAC) leading to cytoreductive surgery and hyperthermic intraperitoneal chemotherapy. Eur J Surg Oncol. 2019. [Online ahead of print].

42. Nowacki M, Alyami M, Villeneuve L, Mercier F, Hubner M, Willaert W, et al. Multicenter comprehensive methodological and technical analysis of 832 pressurized intraperitoneal aerosol chemotherapy (PIPAC) interventions performed in 349 patients for peritoneal carcinomatosis treatment: an international survey study. Eur J Surg Oncol. 2018;44:991-6.

43. Solanki SL, Kumar PP, DeSouza A, Saklani AP. Perioperative concerns and management of pressurised intraperitoneal aerosolised chemotherapy: report of two cases. Indian J Anaesth. 2018;62:225-8.

44. Willaert W, Van de Sande L, Van Daele E, Van De Putte D, Van Nieuwenhove Y, Pattyn P, et al. Safety and preliminary efficacy of electrostatic precipitation during pressurized intraperitoneal aerosol chemotherapy (PIPAC) for unresectable carcinomatosis. Eur J Surg Oncol. 2019;45:2302-9.

45. Solass W, Giger-Pabst U, Zieren J, Reymond MA. Pressurized intraperitoneal aerosol chemotherapy (PIPAC): occupational health and safety aspects. Ann Surg Oncol. 2013;20:3504-11.

46. Graversen M, Detlefsen S, Bjerregaard JK, Fristrup CW, Pfeiffer P, Mortensen MB. Prospective, single-center implementation and response evaluation of pressurized intraperitoneal aerosol chemotherapy (PIPAC) for peritoneal metastasis. Ther Adv Med Oncol. 2018;10:1758835918777036.

47. Delhorme JB, Klipfel A, D'Antonio F, Greget MC, Diemunsch P, Rohr S, et al. Occupational safety of pressurized intraperitoneal aerosol chemotherapy (PIPAC) in an operating room without laminar airflow. J Visc Surg. 2019;156:485-8.

36

Perioperative Management of Blunt Trauma Abdomen

Neha Singh, Parnandi Bhaskar Rao

INTRODUCTION

Abdominal injury is one of the leading causes of death in trauma patients. Blunt abdominal trauma (BAT) is more common than penetrating trauma and road traffic accidents are the foremost causes. Out of all etiologies, fall from height, fall of an object over the body, and direct assaults are commonly associated with BAT.[1]

EPIDEMIOLOGY

Trauma is a major public health problem worldwide. It affects all age groups leading to high morbidity and mortality. In India, motor vehicle accidents, fall from height, and sports and industrial accidents are the major causes of blunt trauma.[2,3] Out of all abdominal organs, the most frequently injured are the spleen (40–55%), liver (35–45%), and small bowel (5–10%).[4] In addition, retroperitoneal hematoma is found in 15% of the cases undergoing laparotomy surgery for blunt trauma.[5]

PATHOPHYSIOLOGY

The mechanism of blunt trauma includes tensile injuries and shear injuries. Tensile injuries occur due to direct compression or stretching of the tissue while shear injuries are secondary to a force at the point of attachment of an organ during abrupt acceleration or deceleration. The direction of impact decides the organs involved during tensile injuries; e.g., impact from the front often leads to liver, spleen, and pancreas injury whereas flank impact causes injury to the kidneys. The kidneys, spleen, large bowel, and small bowel are the ones at risk for shear injuries.[6,7]

EVALUATION

Initial evaluation and resuscitation of any trauma patient involves primary survey, resuscitation, and secondary survey.[8] As the name suggests, primary survey includes hand-in-hand identification and resuscitation of immediate life-threatening injuries pertaining to airway, breathing, and circulation. Therefore, it includes maintenance of a patent Airway with cervical spine protection, optimization of Breathing and ventilation, attainment of hemodynamic stability by assessing different aspects of the Circulatory system, stabilization of any Disability, and Exposure without causing hypothermia (ABCDE).

A brief history must include mechanism of injury, type of vehicle if road traffic accident, speed, and air bag status which helps us to understand the mechanism of injury and identify potential injuries. Resuscitation and primary survey must proceed simultaneously. One must secure two large intravenous (IV) cannulae to start fluid resuscitation and send the sample for investigations, blood grouping, and cross matching. Nasal or oral nasogastric tube and urinary catheter may be used according to the patient's condition for gastric and bladder decompression.

The initial clinical assessment may be misleading, but important clinical findings include pain, tenderness, and abdominal distension. BAT can cause damage to the internal organs, internal bleeding, contusions, and injuries to the bowel, spleen, liver, and intestines. These may also be associated with extra-abdominal injuries such as extremities. In cases of peritonitis, abdominal rigidity, guarding and rebound tenderness may often be found. Most importantly, the mere absence of all of the discussed symptoms does not rule out abdominal injury.

ASSESSMENT OF THE ABDOMEN

A thorough but quick evaluation of the abdomen is of essence.

Inspection: Examine anterior and posterior abdomen for discoloration (**Fig. 1**), fullness in the flanks, which may indicate significant injury. Ecchymosis at flanks (Grey

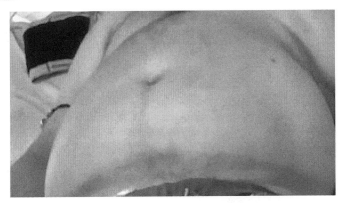

Fig. 1: Abdominal discoloration.

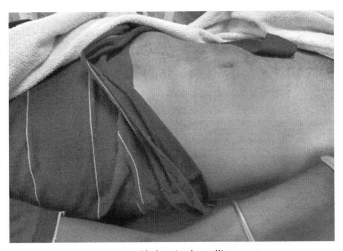

Fig. 2: Abdominal swelling.

Turner's sign) or at the periumbilical area (Cullen's sign) is suggestive of retroperitoneal hemorrhage. External genitalia and back should also be examined carefully. Blood at urethral meatus, swelling (**Fig. 2**), or laceration may be suggestive of pelvic fracture. Consider retrograde urethrogram to rule out urethral injury, and a suprapubic catheter may be considered for established cases.

Palpation: Localized and generalized tenderness if associated with guarding or rigidity is suggestive of peritonitis.

Percussion: Evidence of free fluid (fluid thrill, shifting dullness, etc.) suggests intra-abdominal hemorrhage.

Auscultation: Absent bowel sounds and peristalsis will suggest paralytic ileus or peritonitis.

Per-rectal or pervaginal examination: Fullness in the rectovaginal and rectovesical pouches indicates pelvic collection signifying rectal or vaginal injury.

We need to rule out other associated injuries such as head injury, thoracic injury, and bone fractures. Continuous

reassessment of the mental status for neurological injuries is a must.

Secondary survey includes head-to-toe extensive examination again after immediate threats to life have been identified and managed.

INVESTIGATIONS

Laboratory investigations include complete blood count, leukocyte count (not very specific), liver function tests (raised transaminases in liver injury), pancreatic enzymes (occasionally useful and normal range will not rule out pancreatic injury), serial hematocrit (can help to identify ongoing bleeding), urine analysis (microscopic hematuria suggests abdominal injury while gross hematuria suggests renal injury), coagulation profile, blood type, screen and crossmatch (according to the severity and duration of the injury), and arterial blood gas analysis (for oxygenation, ventilation, base deficit, lactate, electrolyte, and hematocrit). Drugs and alcohol screening is to be done in patients with altered consciousness or history of intake.[9]

Radiological Investigation[9]

- *Plain X-ray of abdomen:* It is not a very useful investigation. Free gas under diaphragm suggests perforation of hollow viscera while ground-glass appearance suggests free fluid.
- *Plain X-ray of chest:* It may help to detect rib fracture, hemothorax, pneumothorax and rupture of diaphragm.
- *Ultrasound:* It detects intraperitoneal and retroperitoneal collection of blood or fluid.

It is a useful investigation to observe a trauma victim under conservative management.[10] A low-frequency probe is used for better penetration.

FAST (Focused Assessment with Sonography for Trauma) Standard four views include:[7]
1. Right upper quadrant (RUQ)
2. Left upper quadrant (LUQ)
3. Subxiphoid/pericardial view
4. Suprapubic/pelvic view

Extended FAST (e-FAST): Extended FAST includes the above four views along with lung examination. A high-frequency probe is used for better resolution of pleura.
1. *RUQ:* Evaluate for free fluid in Morison's pouch/hepatorenal space (most dependent), the lower pole of the kidney, and the space below the diaphragm on the right.
2. *LUQ/perisplenic space:* Check the diaphragm, spleen, and signs of free fluid in the left hemithorax, splenorenal recess, and subphrenic area.
3. *Subxiphoid view or cardiac view:* Both the anterior and the posterior pericardium evaluation for collection.

4. *Suprapubic (bladder):* Fluid in the pelvic region flows to the microvesicular area in the male patient and the pouch of Douglas in the female patient as they are the most dependent areas of the pelvis.

5. *Lungs:* Pleura sliding back and forth is normal which is absent in pneumothorax. It is called seashore sign in M-mode. In cases of pneumothorax, the pleura sliding sign is absent and the M-mode will show a stratosphere sign or bar code sign.

A systematic review of observational studies of ultrasound in blunt abdominal and thoracic trauma (34 studies; 8,635 patients) reported overall sensitivity to be 0.74 (95% CI 0.65 to 0.81) and specificity to be 0.96 (95% CI 0.94 to 0.98). The authors concluded that the accuracy of ultrasound varied by the location of injury and patient's age (sensitivity and specificity were lower in children).[11]

Another systematic review including 22 prospective studies described the FAST examination as the most accurate bedside test for evaluating intra-abdominal injury compared to other modalities [adjusted likelihood ratio (LR) 30; 95% CI 20–46%] while a negative FAST examination substantially decreases the likelihood of injury (adjusted LR 0.26; 95% CI 0.19–0.34%).[4] The Sonography Outcomes Assessment Program (SOAP) study shows a reduction in time to surgery by an average of 109 minutes (a 64% reduction, 95% CI 48–76%), computerized tomography (CT) use [odds ratio (OR) 0.16, 95% CI 0.07–0.32%], hospital stay by 27% (95% CI 1–46%), complications (OR 0.16, 95% CI 0.07–0.32%), and cost by using FAST. They suggested the use of ultrasound as a triage tool to expedite definitive care.[12] Apart from several advantages of the use of ultrasound in BAT, few limitations include the following:

- Injury to diaphragm, solid parenchyma, and retro-peritoneum is not well appreciated.
- Obesity, bowel gas, and subcutaneous air may lead to a number of artifacts.
- Cannot reliably exclude clinically significant injuries, low sensitivity in comparison to CT, particularly for nonhypotensive patients[13,14]
- Does not appear to improve diagnostic yield following negative CT[15]
- Fluid differentiation is not possible. Blood cannot be distinguished from ascites.
- Subcapsular injuries cannot be detected.
- Insensitive for detecting bowel injury
- *CT scan:* It is the most useful investigation for evaluation of retroperitoneal structures such as kidneys and pancreas. It helps to grade the severity of the injury in hemodynamically stable patients, and the sensitivity and specificity of multidetector helical CT (MDCT) for identifying significant intra-abdominal pathology are

high (97–98% and 97–99%, respectively).[16,17] In patients with suspected blunt abdominal trauma who have a negative abdominal-pelvis MDCT, the rate of missed injury has been reported to be extremely low (<0.06%) with a negative LR of 0.034 (0.017–0.068).[17] Various other advantages of CT scan are as follows:

- It better defines organ injury and potential for nonoperative management (NOM) of splenic and liver injuries[18,19]
- It detects not only the presence but also the source and amount of hemoperitoneum. Active bleeding is often detectable.
- Retroperitoneum and vertebral column can be assessed in conjunction with intra-abdominal structures.
- Additional imaging can be performed when needed (e.g., head, cervical spine, chest, and pelvis).
- Patients with negative imaging are at low risk for clinically significant injuries.

Disadvantages of CT scan include the following:

- It remains an insensitive test for mesenteric, bowel, and pancreatic duct injuries.[20,21]
- IV contrast is used as oral contrast; it rarely adds to diagnostic accuracy and may delay imaging.[22,23]
- Relatively high cost
- Cannot be used in unstable patients[24]
- Radiation exposure

Diagnostic Peritoneal Lavage[9]

Introduced by Root et al. in 1965, diagnostic peritoneal lavage (DPL) was one of the most sensitive investigations in the case of blunt abdominal injury.[25] Aspiration of intraperitoneal fluid is done by placing a small catheter through a small incision below the umbilicus. Exploratory laparotomy is indicated if the aspirate is found to contain 10 mL of gross blood or bile. In case of negative aspiration, 1 L of fluid is introduced in the abdomen and the patient is rolled from side to side. The aspirate is collected and sent for analysis. The laboratory criteria for a positive DPL are:

- >100,000 red blood cells/mm^3
- >500 white blood cells/mm^3
- Presence of bacteria, bile, or food particles

Patients found to have significant free intra-abdominal fluid according to FAST examination (or DPL) and hemodynamic instability should undergo urgent surgery. European guidelines recommend multislice spiral CT scanning if patients are hemodynamically stable.[26] The incidence of complications is lower for open DPL compared with the closed technique, but closed DPL can be performed more rapidly.[27]

With an emerging role of NOM and selective embolization for abdominal injuries, DPL is mostly replaced by ultrasound and MDCT scanning. It may be useful in case of a hypotensive patient with equivocal results on FAST examination and limited resource setting with absence of imaging modalities.[28]

For unstable patients, one may perform e-FAST or DPL, both of which are associated with a high rate of false negatives and false positives.[29,30]

MANAGEMENT

After initial resuscitation, blunt abdominal injury patients may be divided into two groups—hemodynamically stable and hemodynamically compromised. Hypotensive patients require aggressive fluid resuscitation using crystalloids and colloids, but colloids are not associated with an improvement in survival and are considerably more expensive than crystalloids.[31]

Hemodynamically unstable patients require blood transfusion. The universal group is O Rh-negative blood which can be considered in all profusely bleeding patients with unknown grouping. Often, O Rh-positive blood is preferred in males and women past childbearing age due to the lack of Rh D antibodies.

A hemodynamically stable patient may be sent for CT scan or kept for a close monitoring according to general condition and repeated clinical examination. Stable patients with positive CT scan findings may go for NOM using embolization therapy.[32] The response rate to NOM was 90%

in patients with traumatic liver injury.[33] Hemodynamically unstable patients with FAST positive are candidates for surgical exploration (**Flowchart 1**). Similarly, patients with signs of peritonitis, ongoing bleed, or worsening clinical signs might require an immediate laparotomy. In addition to these, various complications such as sepsis and delayed splenic rupture are also to be managed with time. Various other indications of laparotomy are diaphragmatic injury, injury to solid organs, mesenteric tear, large amounts of free fluid inside abdomen, and failed NOM or embolization.[34]

Perioperative Management

In the perioperative period, evaluation and resuscitation must run simultaneously. Airway management could be challenging in the presence of facial trauma, secretions, blood, and tissue edema. Manual in-line stabilization should be followed starting from induction till securing the endotracheal intubation.

No single anesthetic drug is proven to be superior to others in a hemodynamically compromised trauma patient. Both thiopentone and propofol may further precipitate hypotension and cause negative inotropic effects. Etomidate, although offers better hemodynamics, may still cause inhibition of catecholamine release and adrenocortical suppression. Ketamine, being a sympathomimetic drug, was often used in trauma patients with small incremental doses with propofol. Anesthesia can be maintained by using lower concentrations of volatile anesthetics along with analgesics and muscle relaxants.

Flowchart 1: Algorithm for the approach for Blunt Trauma Abdomen.

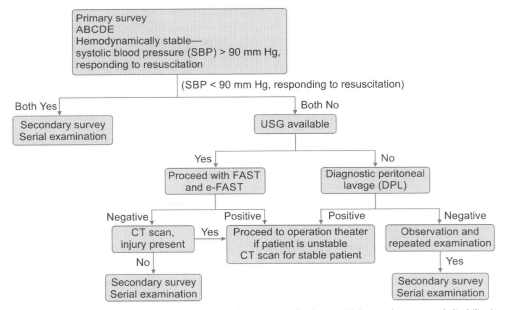

(ABCDEs: airway maintenance with cervical spine protection, breathing and ventilation, circulation with hemorrhage control, disability (neurologic evaluation) exposure and environmental control; CT: computerized tomography; FAST: focused assessment with sonography for trauma; USG: ultrasonography)

The concept of damage control surgery (DCS) and damage control resuscitation (DCR) came into practice as a measure to avoid the lethal triad of trauma (acidosis, hypothermia, and coagulopathy).[35] DCS was originally described by Rotondo and colleagues in 1993 as a three-phase technique.[36] This was later modified by Johnson and Schwab[37] to include a fourth, pretheater phase:

- *Phase 0 (DC 0):* It includes emergency department DCR along with rapid transport and triage for treatment. Rapid-sequence induction (RSI) of anesthesia and intubation with early rewarming are also the key elements.
- *Phase 1 (DC 1):* Main goals include controlling hemorrhage, limiting contamination, and maintaining optimal blood flow to vital organs during limited operative time.
- *Phase 2 (DC 2):* Balanced fluid resuscitation in the intensive care unit (ICU) and warming the patient.
- *Phase 3 (DC 3):* Definitive repair of injuries later according to the patient's condition.
- *Phase 4 (DC 4):* Delayed complex reconstructive surgery, which is delayed until after complete recovery from the associated injuries.

Appropriate patient selection for DCS is very crucial. Severity of injury may favor to opt for DCS along with physiological derangements including significant bleeding requiring massive transfusion (10 units of packed red blood cells), severe metabolic acidosis (pH of 7.30), hypothermia (temperature 35.8°C), operative time of 90 minutes, coagulopathy either on laboratory results or seen as "nonsurgical" bleeding, or lactate >5 mmol/L.[38,39]

Damage control laparotomy focuses on controlling hemorrhage and contamination as well as leaving the abdomen open to prevent abdominal compartment syndrome.[40] The damage control approach of trauma laparotomy has shown reduced mortality.[41]

Damage control resuscitation begins in the prehospital/emergency department phase with goals of continued fluid resuscitation,[42] permissive hypotension,[43] temperature maintenance, limitation of crystalloids and early use of blood and blood products, early use of tranexamic acid, DCS and measures which will help to normalize tissue oxygen delivery and resolve acidosis and coagulopathy.[44]

COMPLICATIONS

Various complications include inadequate resuscitation, missed abdominal injuries leading to delayed diagnosis, intra-abdominal sepsis, and delayed splenic rupture. Presence of chronic disease, hemoglobin level, delay before treatment, and abnormal pelvic-abdominal ultrasound may be few contributing factors.[1] The most common postoperative complication is surgical site infections due to bowel injury or late presentation.[45]

Other complications include small bowel obstruction, pulmonary infection, intra-abdominal abscesses, pancreatitis, and pancreatic fistula.[46] Temporary abdominal wall closure and abdominal vacuum dressing system were used for abdominal wound infection and dehiscence.[47]

PROGNOSIS

The risk factors for mortality in patients with BAT that require laparotomy include—hemodynamic instability as an indication for laparotomy,[1] presence of solid organ injury,[1] multiple intra-abdominal injuries,[1] necessity of damage control laparotomy,[1] severe head injury, severe chest trauma, pelvic or femoral fractures, and low trauma index. Good prognostic factors found were direct abdominal trauma, pain or peritonitis as surgical indication, and the finding of isolated hollow viscera injury during surgery.[48] Berg et al. have also found the presence of comorbid injuries and age >55 years as independent risk factors for mortality.[49]

SUMMARY

Blunt trauma abdomen is a common ailment in the current medical practice. A number of risk factors play an important role in the overall outcome of these patients independently. Associated injuries and medical illness, nature of injury, and availability of resources and personnel at the earliest are some of the determining factors. A systematic approach with particular attention to details during assessment and resuscitation is of essence. DCR and DCSs are a few principles well accepted globally with established better outcome and reduced mortality. The key to safe anesthesia management is to use small incremental doses of different agents with vigilant monitoring. Any of the available management algorithms may be followed but must be tailored to the specifics setup with specific skill and resources available. Improved motor vehicle safety, rapid emergency transport, and rapid intervention should help to reduce the mortality and morbidity associated with this major public health problem.

REFERENCES

1. Gad MA, Saber A, Farrag S, Shams ME, Ellabban GM. Incidence, patterns, and factors predicting mortality of abdominal injuries in trauma patients. N Am J Med Sci. 2012;4(3):129-34.
2. Maske AN, Deshmukh SN. Traumatic abdominal injuries: Our experience at rural tertiary care center. Int Surg J. 2016;3(2): 543-8.
3. Kulkarni S, Kanase V, Kanase N, Varute P. Blunt trauma to abdomen in rural setup: A multiple case study. Int J Sci Study. 2015;3(4):16-9.
4. Nishijima DK, Simel DL, Wisner DH, Holmes JF. Does this adult patient have a blunt intra-abdominal injury? JAMA. 2012;307(14):1517-27.

5. American College of Surgeons Committee on Trauma. ATLS Advanced Trauma Life Support for Doctors Manuals for Coordinators and Faculty, 9th edition. Chicago, IL: American College of Surgeons; 2015.

6. Davis JJ, Cohn I Jr, Nance FC. Diagnosis and management of blunt abdominal trauma. Ann Surg. 1976;183(6):672-8.

7. Marx JA, Isenhour JL. Abdominal trauma. In: Marx JA (Ed). Emergency Medicine Concepts and Clinical Practice, 6th edition. Philadelphia: Elsevier; 2006.

8. Smith J, Caldwell E, D'Amours S, Jalaludin B, Sugrue M. Abdominal trauma: A disease in evolution. ANZ J Surg. 2005;75(9):790-4.

9. Schwartz SI, Brunicardi FC (Eds). Swartz's Principles of Surgery, 9th edition. New York: McGraw-Hill Medical, c201; 1928. pp. 135-96.

10. Soyuncu S, Cete Y, Bozan H, Kartal M, Akyol AJ. Accuracy of physical and ultrasonographic examinations by emergency physicians for the early diagnosis of intraabdominal haemorrhage in blunt abdominal trauma. Injury. 2007;38(5):564-9.

11. Stengel D, Leisterer J, Ferrada P, Ekkernkamp A, Mutze S, Hoenning A. Point-of-care ultrasonography for diagnosing thoracoabdominal injuries in patients with blunt trauma. Cochrane Database Syst Rev. 2018;12:CD012669.

12. Melniker LA, Leibner E, McKenney MG, Lopez P, Briggs WM, Mancuso CA. Randomized controlled clinical trial of point-of-care, limited ultrasonography for trauma in the emergency department: The first sonography outcomes assessment program trial. Ann Emerg Med. 2006;48(3):227-35.

13. Natarajan B, Gupta PK, Cemaj S, Sorensen M, Hatzoudis GI, Forse RA. FAST scan: Is it worth doing in hemodynamically stable blunt trauma patients? Surgery. 2010;148(4):695-701.

14. Carter JW, Falco MH, Chopko MS, Flynn WJ Jr, Wiles Iii CE, Guo WA. Do we really rely on fast for decision-making in the management of blunt abdominal trauma? Injury. 2015;46(5):817-21.

15. Schneck E, Koch C, Borgards M, Reichert M, Hecker A, Heiß C, et al. Impact of abdominal follow-up sonography in trauma patients without abdominal parenchymal organ lesion or free intraabdominal fluid in whole-body computed tomography. Rofo. 2017;189(2):128-36.

16. Peitzman AB, Makaroun MS, Slasky BS, Ritter P. Prospective study of computed tomography in initial management of blunt abdominal trauma. J Trauma. 1986;26(7):585-92.

17. Holmes JF, McGahan JP, Wisner DH. Rate of intra-abdominal injury after a normal abdominal computed tomographic scan in adults with blunt trauma. Am J Emerg Med. 2012;30(4):574-9.

18. Haan JM, Biffl W, Knudson MM, Davis KA, Oka T, Majercik S, et al. Splenic embolization revisited: A multicenter review. J Trauma. 2004;56(3):542-7.

19. Mele TS, Stewart K, Marokus B, O'Keefe GE. Evaluation of a diagnostic protocol using screening diagnostic peritoneal lavage with selective use of abdominal computed tomography in blunt abdominal trauma. J Trauma. 1999;46(5):847-52.

20. Bhagvan S, Turai M, Holden A, Ng A, Civil I. Predicting hollow viscus injury in blunt abdominal trauma with computed tomography. World J Surg. 2013;37(1):123-6.

21. Steenburg SD, Petersen MJ, Shen C, Lin H. Multi-detector CT of blunt mesenteric injuries: Usefulness of imaging findings for predicting surgically significant bowel injuries. Abdom Imaging. 2015;40(5):1026-33.

22. Allen TL, Mueller MT, Bonk RT, Harker CP, Duffy OH, Stevens MH. Computed tomographic scanning without oral contrast solution for blunt bowel and mesenteric injuries in abdominal trauma. J Trauma. 2004;56(2):314-22.

23. Stafford RE, McGonigal MD, Weigelt JA, Johnson TJ. Oral contrast solution and computed tomography for blunt abdominal trauma: A randomized study. Arch Surg. 1999;134(6):622-7.

24. Neal MD, Peitzman AB, Forsythe RM, Marshall GT, Rosengart MR, Alarcon LH, et al. Over reliance on computed tomography imaging in patients with severe abdominal injury: Is the delay worth the risk? J Trauma. 2011;70(2):278-84.

25. Root HD, Hauser CW, McKinley CR, Lafave JW, Mendiola RP Jr. Diagnostic peritoneal lavage. Surgery. 1965;57:633-7.

26. Rossaint R, Bouillon B, Cerny V, Coats TJ, Duranteau J, Fernández-Mondéjar E, et al. The European guideline on management of major bleeding and coagulopathy following trauma: Fourth edition. Crit Care. 2016;20:100.

27. Cué JI, Miller FB, Cryer HM 3rd, Malangoni MA, Richardson JD. A prospective, randomized comparison between open and closed peritoneal lavage techniques. J Trauma. 1990;30(7):880-3.

28. Whitehouse JS, Weigelt JA. Diagnostic peritoneal lavage: A review of indications, technique, and interpretation. Scand J Trauma Resusc Emerg Med. 2009;17:13.

29. Sarychev LP, Sarychev YV, Pustovoyt HL, Sukhomlin SA, Suprunenko SM. Management of the patients with blunt renal trauma: 20 years of clinical experience. Wiad. Lek. 2018;71(3 pt 2):719-22.

30. Wortman JR, Uyeda JW, Fulwadhva UP, Sodickson AD. Dual-Energy CT for abdominal and pelvic trauma. Radiographics. 2018;38(2):586-602.

31. Jabaley C, Dudaryk R. Fluid resuscitation for trauma patients: Crystalloids versus colloids. Curr Anesthesiol Rep. 2014;4:216-24.

32. Alarhayem AQ, Myers JG, Dent D, Lamus D, Lopera J, Liao L, et al. "Blush at first sight": Significance of computed tomographic and angiographic discrepancy in patients with blunt abdominal trauma. Am J Surg. 2015;210(6):1104-11.

33. Inukai K, Uehara S, Furuta Y, Miura M. Nonoperative management of blunt liver injury in hemodynamically stable versus unstable patients: A retrospective study. Emerg Radiol. 2018;25(6):647-52.

34. Dharap SB, Noronha J, Kumar V. Laparotomy for blunt abdominal trauma-some uncommon indications. J Emerg Trauma Shock. 2016;9(1):32-6.

35. Lamb CM, MacGoey P, Navarro AP, Brooks AJ. Damage control surgery in the era of damage control resuscitation. Br J Anaesth. 2014;113(2):242-9.

36. Rotondo MF, Schwab CW, McGonigal MD, Phillips GR 3rd, Fruchterman TM, Kauder DR, et al. 'Damage control': An approach for improved survival in exsanguinating penetrating abdominal injury. J Trauma. 1993;35(3):375-83.

37. Johnson JW, Gracias VH, Schwab CW, Reilly PM, Kauder DR, Shapiro MB, et al. Evolution in damage control for exsanguinating penetrating abdominal injury. J Trauma. 2001;51(2):261-71.

38. Shapiro MB, Jenkins DH, Schwab CW, Rotondo MF. Damage control: Collective review. J Trauma. 2000;49(5):969-78.

39. Midwinter MJ. Damage control surgery in the era of damage control resuscitation. J R Army Med Corps. 2009;155(4):323-6.

40. Schreiber MA. Damage control surgery. Crit Care Clin. 2004;20(1):101-18.

41. Groven S, Gaarder C, Eken T, Skaga NO, Naess PA. Abdominal injuries in a major Scandinavian trauma center—Performance assessment over an 8 year period. J Trauma Manag Outcomes. 2014;8:9.

42. Bickell WH, Wall MJ Jr, Pepe PE, Martin RR, Ginger VF, Allen MK, et al. Immediate versus delayed fluid resuscitation for hypotensive patients with penetrating torso injuries. N Engl J Med. 1994;331(17):1105-9.

43. Dutton RP. Low-pressure resuscitation from hemorrhagic shock. Int Anesthesiol Clin. 2002;40(3):19-30.

44. Hodgetts TJ, Mahoney PF, Kirkman E. Damage control resuscitation. J R Army Med Corps. 2007;153(4):299-300.

45. Mehta N, Babu S, Venugopal K. An experience with blunt abdominal trauma: Evaluation, management and outcome. Clin Pract. 2014;4(2):599.

46. Wu CL, Chou MC. Surgical management of blunt abdominal trauma. Gaoxiong Yi Xue Ke Xue Za Zhi. 1993;9(9):540-52.

47. Howdieshell TR, Yeh KA, Hawkins ML, Cué JI. Temporary abdominal wall closure in trauma patients: Indications, technique, and results. World J Surg. 1995;19(1):154-8.

48. Pimentel SK, Sawczyn GV, Mazepa MM, da Rosa FG, Nars A, Collaço IA. Risk factors for mortality in blunt abdominal trauma with surgical approach. Rev Col Bras Cir. 2015;42(4):259-64.

49. Berg RJ, Okoye O, Teixeira PG, Inaba K, Demetriades D. The double jeopardy of blunt thoracoabdominal trauma. Arch Surg. 2012;147(6):498-504.

Perioperative Management of Emergency Laparotomy and Damage Control Surgeries

Praveen Kumar G, Deepak Govil

INTRODUCTION

Acute abdomen refers to pain abdomen associated with tenderness. On detailed clinical examination, most of these patients will have a surgical cause for the symptoms and might require emergency surgical intervention. Multiple causes for acute abdomen exist and an array of them requires emergency laparotomy. Various clinical conditions, which might require emergency laparotomy, are enumerated in **Box 1**. The prime objective of emergency surgical intervention is to prevent loss of life by limiting contamination, control bleeding, and to improve vital organ perfusion.

TIMING OF EMERGENCY SURGERY

Timing of emergency laparotomy is cornerstone for improved outcomes. Delaying the surgery, might spread the contamination, causes rupture of abscess, worsen hemorrhagic shock, worsen the progression of bowel ischemia and gangrene, impair organ perfusion, and eventually might lead to adverse impact on outcomes.[1] Triage of trauma patients in protocol driven across most institutions in the world. But in nontrauma settings, timing of emergency surgery is not well defined and more often than not, it is based on individual's interpretation of surgical disease. To establish uniform criteria for ideal timing of emergency surgery, the study group of world association of emergency surgery has defined five different categories of emergency surgeries based on immediate threat to life or limb.[1] Albeit, the timings have been defined for all emergency surgeries, it can be easily applied for laparotomies. The five categories are described in **Table 1**. Each category is identified by a color code similar to that of triage color code in trauma settings.

Detailed description of operative steps of laparotomy is beyond the scope of this chapter.

Box 1: Indications for emergency laparotomy.

- Gastrointestinal perforation
- Acute mesenteric ischemia with bowel gangrene
- Small and large bowel obstruction
- Toxic megacolon
- Intra-abdominal abscess with peritonitis
- Aneurysmal rupture
- Penetrating abdominal trauma
- Solid organ injury with hemoperitoneum and hemodynamic instability
- Abdominal compartment syndrome
- Ruptured ectopic pregnancy

Table 1: Timing of emergency surgery.

Timing	Characteristics
Immediate	• Patient has severe physiological derangement due to underlying illness and threat to life is extremely high and imminent • Intra-abdominal hemorrhage is the most frequent cause
Within an hour of diagnosis	• Patients have moderate physiological derangement in terms of sepsis and organ dysfunction • Though there is no imminent threat to life, there is an imminent threat to tissues • Acute mesenteric ischemia, strangulated or incarcerated hernias, bowel perforation leading to peritonitis are the frequent pathologies falling in this category
Within 6 hours of diagnosis	• Involves pathologies which have the potential to worsen if not treated with urgent surgical intervention • Localized peritonitis, abscess are the frequent indications for surgery within 6 hours of diagnosis
Within 24 hours of diagnosis	• Needs surgical intervention • Patient should remain on clinical treatment, with evidence that medical management will not lead to clinical deterioration • Acute appendicitis is frequent example
Within 24–48 hours	Those indications where intervention is needed to prevent morbidity

RISK FACTORS AND OUTCOMES FOR EMERGENCY LAPAROTOMY

Emergency laparotomy, though being a common procedure, is associated with multiple short-term and long-term complications. Elderly age, higher preoperative comorbid conditions, urgency of surgical intervention, need for perioperative critical care, underlying abdominal sepsis, need for small bowel resection, and skills of the operating surgeon are factors independently associated with poor outcomes following emergency laparotomy.[2] With increase in elderly population and better healthcare facilities, more elderly patients with multiple comorbid conditions undergo emergency surgeries. Among the various scoring systems, fitness score[3] and Reiss index,[4] best predicted the outcomes in elderly patients undergoing emergency surgery and should be used whenever possible. The organizational analysis of National Emergency Laparotomy Audit (NELA) showed that intraoperative consultant derived care, perioperative geriatric consult in elderly patients, and presence of perioperative care pathways improved survival after emergency laparotomy.[5] The audit also showed that risk model including age, physiological variables, American Society of Anesthesiologists (ASA) physical status classification, blood pressure, and heart rate predicted mortality better than other variables.[6] NELA is the first database in the world which is prospectively maintained for emergency laparotomies. It claims to have reduced perioperative mortality and length of stay in hospital.[7-10] Likewise, the National Surgical Quality Improvement Program (NSQIP) database of United States of America is also a nationally-validated risk-adjusted, outcome-based program to measure and improve quality of surgical care, but not only for emergency laparotomy, although many studies used these data for reporting emergency laparotomy outcomes and reported 14% mortality at 30 day, and it was higher among the elderly and those with preexisting comorbidities.[11]

Internationally, mortality and morbidity are different in different countries and it is higher in resource poor countries[12] but it is still not standard care pathway internationally. NELA perhaps can guide more and more countries to adopt its model for better care, quality assurance, and improvement after emergency laparotomies.

Enhanced recovery after surgery (ERAS) is a multifaceted approach to the pre-, intra-, and postoperative management of patients undergoing surgery and shown to improve the outcomes, reduced length of stay, and cost of treatment after elective surgeries especially in colorectal and other surgeries.[13-15] Major burden of emergency laparotomy are gastrointestinal surgery and these patients may get benefitted by implementing ERAS in these subset of patient. Few retrospective studies[16-18] have shown improved outcomes in terms of decreased length of stay, time to return to gastrointestinal functions, and postoperative complications in ERAS group as compared to traditional care in emergency laparotomy. One prospective study which compared outcomes after implementing ERAS protocol in emergency and elective colonic resections has shown no difference in postoperative complications and readmissions at 30 days, although there were increased length of stay for emergency laparotomy.[19] Although, all the components of ERAS are not possible to implement in emergency laparotomy like in bowel obstruction or perforation, fasting is unavoidable and carbohydrate loading is not possible. Epidural analgesia may not be possible in septic, unstable or anticoagulated patients. Studies and literature suggests that, even if all the aspects of ERAS were not possible, some essential components of ERAS confer some of the benefits shown in the elective setting, without a significant difference in mortality and readmission rate.

COMPLICATIONS AFTER EMERGENCY LAPAROTOMY

Multiple complications occur after emergency laparotomy. Most of the complications are associated with the underlying pathology for which the patient has undergone the procedure. In the short term, pulmonary and cardiovascular complications, wound dehiscence, intra-abdominal infections, surgical site infections, fistula formations, abdominal compartment syndrome, postoperative ileus, and anastomotic leaks can frequently complicate the postoperative course of the disease. Aggressive steps should be taken to prevent, identify, and treat these complications. A multicentric study involving 1,139 patients showed 30 days mortality of 20.2% and 1 year mortality of 34%. Majority (64%) of complications within 30 days of emergency laparotomy occur more than 72 hours after surgery and the majority (60%) of patients who die within 30 days of surgery survive the first 72 postoperative hours. In their study Clavien Dindo classification grade ≥ 3 complication rate [reoperation, intensive care unit (ICU) stay, or death] was 47%. Pulmonary complications can be affected by surgical and anesthetic techniques. Epidural analgesia, which is recommended in ERAS protocol, decreases the risk of respiratory complications but in emergency laparotomy it is not always possible to put epidural.[20] Defunctioning stoma (colostomy or ileostomy) after midline laparotomy and procedures are frequently performed during emergency laparotomy. The role of the stoma care team is very important and it includes intraoperatively assessment and marking of the location of the proposed stoma; and postoperatively education and counseling of the nursing care team, patient, and family about proper care. Infection, retraction or prolapse, necrosis, stenosis, skin ulceration, and bleeding are some of the complications that can happen after stoma formation. It is shown in a nationwide study that stoma formed as part of emergency laparotomy developed more complications as compared to elective setting.

DAMAGE CONTROL SURGERY

The damage control resuscitation (DCR) revolves around the concept that rapid control of hemorrhage in severely injured trauma patients is the cornerstone of trauma care. Damage control surgery (DCS) is integral to control of hemorrhage. Many patients do not have the physiological reserve to withstand the stress of prolonged definitive surgery in the setting of massive trauma. During the surgical intervention, trauma patients progressively deteriorate because of hypothermia, acidosis, and coagulopathy. This triad is called as lethal triad of death of trauma. DCS evolved as a method to halt the lethal triad, by rapid control of bleeding and resuscitation, allowing the stabilization of physiological parameters and leaving the definitive repair once the patient is stabilized. Though principles of damage control evolved from care of trauma victims, it is been used in nontraumatic abdominal emergencies as well.[21] DCS not only involves damage control laparotomy, but is been used in nonabdominal conditions as well, including thoracic and musculoskeletal surgeries.

Evolution of Damage Control Surgery

Damage control laparotomy as a concept was first described by Joseph Hogarth Pringle in 1908, where he described the concept of perihepatic packing in hepatic trauma patients. Albeit, the patient died in the postoperative period, postmortem examination revealed no signs of further bleeding or peritonitis due to packing and he was convinced that the patient survived the initial perioperative period because of the technique applied.[22] In the decades that followed, minimal handling of liver during acute trauma, either by arterial ligation, sutures or mere packing evolved and many patients survived the acute phase. In patients with coagulopathy at the onset of surgery, Stones et al. popularized the technique of truncated laparotomy, with constituted control of bleeding and packing of the abdomen with packs, followed by reexploration and definitive correction after correction of coagulopathy. This approach resulted in better outcomes in patients deemed to have lethal coagulopathy.[23] This concept was further popularized by Rotondo and his colleagues, in patients with penetrating abdominal trauma. In direct comparison with definitive laparotomy, damage control was associated with better survival, especially in patients with major vascular injuries and multivisceral injuries.[24] It is after this study that the name damage control evolved. The name damage control originated from American Navy, where it describes the ability of the ship to adsorb the damage and maintain its integrity for the mission. Rapid assessment of the ship is done and necessary repairs are carried out, just to return the ship safely to the port where detailed assessment and repairs can be carried.[25]

Indications for Damage Control Surgery

Not every trauma patient should be subjected to DCS. Liberal use of damage control concept might lead to inclusion of those set of patients who might benefit from definitive surgery at the onset. So, appropriate patient selection is of paramount importance for better outcomes. No single physiological parameter has been shown to accurately assess the need for DCS and DCR, although temperature, acidosis, lactate levels, markers of coagulopathy, number of blood, and blood products transfused have been assessed as objective markers. Factors which ought to be considered before initiating DCR and DCS are enumerated in **Box 2**.[25,26] There is emerging evidence that early hemostatic resuscitation with use of blood and blood products has reduced the incidence of lethal triad of trauma and thereby need for DCS and definitive repair can be attempted at the onset.[27] Because of this emerging evidence, the need for initiating DCS should be individualized.

Stages of Damage Control Surgery

The traditional approach to DCS involves three-legged approach.[26,28]

Step 1: Immediate exploratory laparotomy for control of hemorrhage and decontamination.

Methods to control bleeding include abdominal organ packing, ligation of bleeding vessels, balloon tamponade, and even vascular shunts when appropriate.

Minimum handling of tissues is done and the abdomen is packed, followed by simple temporary closure. The closure should be simple to prevent evisceration, drainage

---

Box 2: Factors to be considered for initiating damage control surgery (DCS).

- Evidence of hypoperfusion (high lactates and metabolic acidosis—pH < 7.20)
- Marked coagulopathy
- Evidence of bleeding for nontrauma site
- Estimated blood loss of more than 4 liters during the procedure
- Need for massive blood and blood products transfusion
- Severe hypothermia (core body temperature < 35°C)
- Expected duration of definitive surgery more than 90 minutes
- Hemodynamic instability
- High energy torso trauma and multiple penetrating injuries
- Major vascular injuries of abdominal vessels
- Multivisceral injuries of abdomen
- Injuries involving more than one region of the body with varying resuscitation priorities
- Nontrauma settings: Critically ill surgical patients

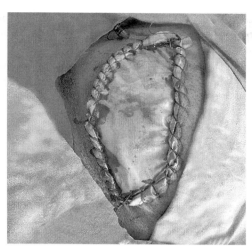

Fig. 1: Open abdomen with edges closed with sterile plastic bag similar to Bogota bag to prevent evisceration and contamination.

Table 2: Complications of damage control laparotomy.	
Immediate and short-term complications	**Long-term complications**
• Intra-abdominal infections • Wound infections and abscess • Enteroenteral and enterocutaneous fistulas • Abdominal compartment syndrome • Fluid losses through open abdomen	• Fistulas • Abdominal wall hernias • Intra-abdominal adhesions leading to bowel obstruction • Recurrent hospitalizations for fistula care

of fluids, and prevent development of intra-abdominal hypertension and abdominal compartment syndrome **(Fig. 1)**. In patients who are perceived to have high risk for abdominal compartment syndrome, open surgical abdomen with vacuum drainage should be considered.

Step 2: Continuation of resuscitative efforts to restore physiological milieu and correct acidosis, hypothermia, and coagulopathy. Judicious use of intravenous fluids and blood products, based on hemodynamic parameters, early initiation of enteral nutrition, and appropriate broad spectrum antibiotic strategy should be a part of this period.

Step 3: Once the patient's physiological reserve is achieved, patient is shifted back to operating room for pack removal and definitive surgery.

Though the three legged approach is routine followed, four and five staged DCS have also been described.[29]

Risks and Complications of Damage Control Surgery

Damage control surgery has been shown to improve survival and long-term outcomes in trauma patients. Albeit useful, liberal use of DCS in all patients will deny those patients with a good physiological reserve, benefits of definitive repair at the onset, and expose them to unwarranted complications. Multiple complications have been reported in literature with DCS, especially damage control laparotomy,[30,31] and are summarized in **Table 2**.

Damage Control Surgery in Nontrauma Settings

The principles of damage control have been extended to critically ill nontrauma patients with poor physiological reserve, who needs stabilization before and after limited

surgical intervention. The physiological derangement in trauma patients is because of hemorrhage, whereas in nontrauma patients it could be because of sepsis and bleeding. As discussed previously, multiple physiological parameters have been tested for DCS in trauma settings, especially the lethal triad of trauma. In the settings of septic shock, the timing of presentation could vary, underlying pathology leading to shock varies and the presurgery resuscitation is not uniform or standardized. Staged laparotomy based on the lethal triad in nontrauma settings, did not improve survival in nontrauma settings. In a multivariate analysis, none of the three parameters of lethal triad were associated with better outcomes when used a physiological marker for DCS in nontraumatic abdominal emergencies.[32] In the logistic regression analysis, preoperative presence of septic shock, hypoperfusion with high lactates (>3 mmol/L), patients with multiple comorbidities, age > 70, and male gender were the patients who benefited the most from limited rapid source controlling laparotomy.[32]

POSTOPERATIVE CHALLENGES AFTER EMERGENCY LAPAROTOMY

All high-risk patients should be admitted to the ICU. Challenges in the postoperative period include continuation of resuscitation, optimization of hemodynamics, fluid management, and maintaining distal organ perfusion, administration of appropriate broad-spectrum antibiotics, prevention of hypothermia, coagulopathy and acidosis, management of drain outputs, surgical site and open abdomen, initiation of early nutrition support, adequate pain relief and early mobilization and rehabilitation, and prevent hospital acquired infections. Many of the patients might require multiple surgeries affecting resuscitation and stabilization.

Unlike elective surgery, a patient postemergency laparotomy might have cardiovascular, respiratory and gastrointestinal derangements for a longer duration, and thereby complicates fluid administration. Moreover, patients might also have nasogastric losses, fluid losses from stoma high stoma output and open abdomen. Goal-directed fluid administration and hemodynamic optimization targeting flows such as stroke volume, cardiac output, and tissue perfusion have been shown to improve outcomes and reduce adverse events in the perioperative period.[33] In patients undergoing DCS, every attempt should be made to prevent the triangle of death. Assessment for enteral feed tolerance should be done frequently and enteral feeding should be initiated at the earliest to prevent gut mucosal atrophy and prevent bacterial translocation. Presence of postoperative ileus and nonfunctioning stoma are not absolute contraindications for enteral feeding, and trophic feeding should be considered after due consultation with surgical team. All patients who do not meet their calorie requirements for over 5 days should be considered for supplemental parenteral nutrition.

Early postoperative mobilization not only improves pulmonary functions, but also reduces the incidence of thromboembolic complications and should be aggressively pursued. Every other aspect of critical care should be continued in all patients postemergency laparotomy.

CONCLUSION

Patient selection and timing of surgical intervention is the key for successful outcome for both emergency laparotomy and DCS, in both trauma and nontrauma settings. Integral to the successful outcomes is the preoperative and postoperative resuscitation and the same should be perceived and done aggressively.

REFERENCES

1. Kluger Y, Ben-Ishay O, Sartelli M, Ansaloni L, Abbas AE, Agresta F, et al. World society of emergency surgery study group initiative on Timing of Acute Care Surgery classification (TACS). World J Emerg Surg. 2013;8:1-6.

2. Barrow E, Anderson ID, Varley S, Pichel AC, Peden CJ, Saunders DI, et al. Current UK practice in emergency laparotomy. Ann R Coll Surg Engl. 2013;95:599-603.

3. Playforth MJ, Smith GMR, Evans M, Pollock AV. Pre-operative assessment of fitness score. Br J Surg. 1987;74:890-2.

4. Reiss R, Deutsch A, Nudelman I. Surgical problems in octogenarians: epidemiological analysis of 1,083 consecutive admissions. World J Surg. 1992;16:1017-20.

5. Oliver CM, Bassett MG, Poulton TE, Anderson ID, Murray DM, Grocott MP, et al. Organisational factors and mortality after an emergency laparotomy: multilevel analysis of 39903 National Emergency Laparotomy Audit patients. Br J Anaesth. 2018;121:1346-56.

6. Eugene N, Oliver CM, Bassett MG, Poulton TE, Kuryba A, Johnston C, et al. Development and internal validation of a novel risk adjustment model for adult patients undergoing emergency laparotomy surgery: the National Emergency Laparotomy Audit risk model. Br J Anaesth. 2018;121:739-48.

7. NELA. (2015). First Patient Audit Report. [online] Available from: https://www.nela.org.uk/All-Patient-Reports#pt. [Last accessed March, 2020].

8. NELA. (2016). Second Patient Audit Report. [online] Available from: https://www.nela.org.uk/Second-Patient-Report-of-the-National-Emergency-Laparotomy-Audit. [Last accessed March, 2020].

9. NELA. (2017). Third Patient Audit Report. [online] Available from: https://www.nela.org.uk/Third-Patient-Audit-Report#pt. [Last accessed March, 2020].

10. NELA. (2018). Fourth Patient Audit Report. [online] Available from: https:// www.nela.org.uk/Fourth-Patient-Audit-Report#pt. [Last accessed March, 2020].

11. Al-Temimi MH, Griffee M, Enniss TM, Preston R, Vargo D, Overton S, et al. When is death inevitable after emergency laparotomy? Analysis of the American College of Surgeons National Surgical Quality improvement program database. J Am Coll Surg. 2012;215:503-11.

12. Gebremedhn EG, Agegnehu AF, Anderson BB. Outcome assessment of emergency laparotomies and associated factors in low resource setting. A case series. Ann Med Surg (Lond). 2018;36:178-84.

13. Zhuang C-L, Ye X-Z, Zhang X-D, Chen B-C, Yu Z. Enhanced recovery after surgery programs versus traditional care for colorectal surgery: a meta-analysis of randomized controlled trials. Dis Colon Rectum. 2013;56:667-78.

14. Roulin D, Donadini A, Gander S, Griesser A-C, Blanc C, Hübner M, et al. Cost-effectiveness of the implementation of an enhanced recovery protocol for colorectal surgery. Br J Surg. 2013;100:1108-14.

15. Visioni A, Shah R, Gabriel E, Attwood K, Kukar M, Nurkin S. Enhanced recovery after surgery for noncolorectal surgery: a systematic review and meta-analysis of major abdominal surgery. Ann Surg. 2018;267:57-65.

16. Lohsiriwat V. Enhanced recovery after surgery vs conventional care in emergency colorectal surgery. World J Gastroenterol. 2014;20:13950-5.

17. Shida D, Tagawa K, Inada K, Nasu K, Seyama Y, Maeshiro T, et al. Modified enhanced recovery after surgery (ERAS) protocols for patients with obstructive colorectal cancer. BMC Surg. 2017;17:18.

18. Shang Y, Guo C, Zhang D. Modified enhanced recovery after surgery protocols are beneficial for postoperative recovery for patients undergoing emergency surgery for obstructive colorectal cancer: a propensity score matching analysis. Medicine. 2018;97:e12348.

19. Roulin D, Blanc C, Muradbegovic M, Hahnloser D, Demartines N, Hubner M. Enhanced recovery pathway for urgent colectomy. World J Surg. 2014;38:2153-9.

20. Tengberg LT, Cihoric M, Foss NB, Bay-Nielsen M, Gögenur I, Henriksen R, et al. Complications after emergency laparotomy beyond the immediate postoperative period: a retrospective, observational cohort study of 1139 patients. Anaesthesia. 2017;72(3):309-16.

21. Weber DG, Bendinelli C, Balogh ZJ. Damage control surgery for abdominal emergencies. Br J Surg. 2014;101:109-18.

22. Wood JR, Lorrain WB, Newlands JB. Glasgow Royal Infirmary. Lancet. 1828;10(264):796.

23. Stone HH, Strom PR, Mullins RJ. Management of the major coagulopathy with onset during laparotomy. Ann Surg. 1983;197:532-5.

24. Rotondo MF, Schwab CW, McGonigal MD, Phillips GR, Fruchterman TM, Kauder DR, et al. 'Damage control': an approach for improved survival in exsanguinating penetrating abdominal injury. J Trauma. 1993;35(3):375-82.

25. Lee JC, Peitzman AB. Damage-control laparotomy. Curr Opin Crit Care. 2006;12(4):346-50.

26. Rotondo MF, Zonies DH. The damage control sequence and underlying logic. Surg Clin North Am. 1997;77(4):761-77.

27. Cotton BA, Reddy N, Hatch QM, Lefebvre E, Wade CE, Kozar RA, et al. Improvement in survival in 390 damage control. Ann Surg. 2013;254:1-15.

28. Godat L, Kobayashi L, Costantini T, Coimbra R. Abdominal damage control surgery and reconstruction: world society of emergency surgery position paper. World J Emerg Surg. 2013;8:1-7.

29. MacGoey P, Lamb CM, Navarro AP, Brooks AJ. Damage control: the modern paradigm. Trauma. 2016;18:165-77.

30. Brenner M, Bochicchio G, Bochicchio K, Ilahi O, Rodriguez E, Henry S, et al. Long-term impact of damage control lapaortomy: a prospective study. Arch Surg. 2011;146:395-9.

31. Miller RS, Morris JA, Diaz JJ, Herring MB, May AK, Rotondo MF, et al. Complications after 344 damage-control open celiotomies. J Trauma. 2005;59:1365-74.

32. Becher RD, Peitzman AB, Sperry JL, Gallaher JR, Neff LP, Sun Y, et al. Damage control operations in non-trauma patients: defining criteria for the staged rapid source control laparotomy in emergency general surgery. World J Emerg Surg. 2016;11:10.

33. Foss NB, Kehlet H. Perioperative haemodynamics and vasoconstriction: time for reconsideration. Br J Anaesth. 2019;123(2):100-103.

Perioperative Management of Intra-abdominal Hypertension and Abdominal Compartment Syndrome

Malini P Joshi, Shilpushp Bhosale, Atul Prabhakar Kulkarni

INTRODUCTION

Intra-abdominal hypertension (IAH) occurs when increased abdominal pressure causes decreased perfusion of the kidneys and other abdominal organs, with progressive difficulty in mechanical ventilation and/or hemodynamic compromise. These effects can progress to abdominal compartment syndrome (ACS), a cascade of ischemia and multiple organ dysfunction. Thus, ACS is a medical emergency, where increased intra-abdominal pressure (IAP) causes severe organ dysfunction and carries a very high mortality rate. It is important to recognize the risk factors and clinical signs of ACS to reduce the morbidity and mortality. We have to understand that IAH and ACS are two distinct clinical conditions occurring over a spectrum of elevated abdominal pressure and should not be used interchangeably.[1,2]

Intra-abdominal pressure depends on abdominal compliance which is determined by the elasticity of the abdominal wall and the diaphragm and the character of the abdominal contents.

A rapid increase in visceral edema and intra-abdominal volume due to injury to abdominal organs, or other disease processes such as trauma, burns, aortic rupture, and pancreatitis requiring large volume crystalloid resuscitation could be a cause for IAH and should warrant screening for IAH.[3,4] ACS primarily affects patients who are already very sick, have received massive intravenous fluid resuscitation in presence of capillary leak, and have a positive fluid balance. ACS remains under recognized because the organ dysfunction may be incorrectly attributed to progression of the primary illness.

Though the incidence of IAH and ACS was extremely high earlier when aggressive intravenous fluid resuscitation was widely practiced, there is a significant decrease in ACS with increasing awareness nowadays.[5] Early recognition is necessary so that interventions such as sedation, fluid removal, or decompression of bowel, etc., to decrease IAP can be undertaken. However, the clinical benefit of such therapies remains uncertain and surgical decompression remains the standard treatment once ACS is established.[2,6,7]

DEFINITION

Fietsam et al. initially coined the term ACS when he described raised IAP in patients having undergone aortic aneurysm surgery. Patients manifested with an increase in the peak inspiratory pressures, central venous pressure (CVP), and a decrease in urinary output.[8]

In 1872, the German physician Schatz used a balloon tube and manometer to measure pressure within the uterus while Wendt measured it through the rectum a year later; however, Odebrecht first measured it within the urinary bladder in 1875.[9] Emerson described that cardiovascular collapse was due to distension of the abdomen leading to overloading the resistance in the splanchnic circulation and further stated that relief of the laboring heart was seen after draining of ascitic fluid.[9]

The World Society on Abdominal Compartment Syndrome (WSACS) which was founded in 2004 came up with the consensus definitions in 2013 and stated that:[2]

- Intra-abdominal pressure is the steady-state pressure concealed within the abdominal cavity and IAH is defined as a sustained increase in IAP equal to or above 12 mm Hg.
- Abdominal compartment syndrome is defined by a sustained IAP above 20 mm Hg [with or without abdominal perfusion pressure (APP) <60 mm Hg] with new onset or progressive organ failure.
  Intra-abdominal hypertension is graded as Grade I (12–15 mm Hg), Grade II (16–20 mm Hg), Grade III (21–25 mm Hg), and Grade IV (>25 mm Hg).[6]

Primary IAH or ACS is said to be associated with injury or disease in the abdominal pelvic region that frequently requires early surgical or interventional radiological intervention, while secondary IAH or ACS refers to conditions that do not originate in the abdominopelvic region.[10] Recurrent IAH or ACS refers to the condition in which IAH or ACS redevelops following treated primary or secondary IAH or ACS.[11]

Normal IAP has been described up to 5–7 mm Hg but it has been observed that the morbidly obese and pregnant patients may have chronically high IAP (10–15 mm Hg) without adverse effects.[12] For critically ill patients, pressures more than 12 mm Hg are considered to represent IAH, and pressures more than 20 mm Hg with new organ dysfunction is termed as ACS.

The abdominal perfusion pressure (APP) is the difference between mean arterial pressure and intra-abdominal pressure (APP = MAP – IAP) and has been suggested as a target for management of IAH. APP has been demonstrated to be superior to MAP and IAP in predicting patient survival from IAH and ACS.[13] A target APP of at least 60 mm Hg is correlated with improved survival from IAH and ACS.[11]

This suggests that higher systemic blood pressure may maintain abdominal organ perfusion when IAP is increased. Abdominal wall compliance initially limits the extent of rise in IAP. Once a critical abdominal girth is reached, the abdominal wall compliance decreases abruptly leading to rapid rise of IAP and ACS, if untreated. Hence in practice due to individual variations in blood pressure and abdominal wall compliance, ACS is better defined as IAH-induced new organ dysfunction without a strict IAP threshold.[14]

Pediatric-specific Consensus Definitions

Intra-abdominal pressure in critically ill children is approximately 4–10 mm Hg. IAH is defined by a sustained or repeated pathological elevation in IAP more than 10 mm Hg, while ACS is defined as a sustained elevated IAP of greater than 16 mm Hg associated with new or worsening organ dysfunction that can be attributed to elevated IAP. Omphalocele and gastroschisis have been described to be associated with increased IAP in pediatric population.

INCIDENCE OF IAH/ACS

Though it is evident that IAH/ACS is independently associated with worse outcomes in medical or surgical patients, the incidence of IAH and ACS is not well characterized due to multiple factors such as underdiagnosis, lack of awareness, or most of the times simply inability to measure the IAP. Most of the times the organ dysfunction is falsely considered as primary disease process.

The incidence of IAH/ACS is rapidly declining from a high incidence in the old literature that suggested IAH incidence between 32 and 56%, and ACS incidence of about 2 to 10%.[6] The incidence of ACS in trauma patients seems to be approximately 14%.[15]

PATHOPHYSIOLOGY OF IAH/ACS

It has been observed that ACS can develop both in nonsurgical and surgical patients. Conditions, such as obesity, significant positive fluid balance, prolonged mechanical ventilation, massive blood transfusion, high organ failure scores, or end-stage liver disease, predispose patients for ACS. Mechanisms for increased IAP and end-organ dysfunction are conditions that decrease abdominal wall compliance, or increase intraluminal contents (such as abdominal collections of fluid, air, or blood) or capillary leak syndromes.

A two hit theory has been proposed for the development of ACS, which suggests that massive volume resuscitation after a "first hit" from any cause (i.e. burns, trauma, pancreatitis, hemorrhagic or septic shock) can lead to increased IAP, and the "second hit" probably results from the effects of capillary leak, ischemia-reperfusion injury with shock, and the release of cytokines combined with massive increases in total extracellular volume.[16,17]

With the development of ACS, there is direct compression of intestinal tract and collapse of portacaval system causing secondary effects such as thrombosis or bowel wall edema with translocation of bacterial products and fluid accumulation and further impairment of oxygen delivery.

Other contributory factor is the erroneous assessment of fluid responsiveness in IAH as decreased intrathoracic compliance may cause false elevation in pulse pressure ventilation (PPV) with ventilation or can cause IVC diameter to be less due to compression from increased abdominal pressure prompting the clinician to administer excessive fluids. The effects on different organ systems caused by IAH/ACS have been shown in **Figure 1**.

Acute IAH may lead to an increase in intracranial pressure (ICP), secondary to increase in pleural pressure.[18] Compression of the inferior vena cava and aorta can cause decrease in the preload and can increase afterload with subsequent reduction in the stroke volume (SV) and cardiac output (CO). Decrease in the extrathoracic compliance can lead to increase in shunt fraction, dead space, and transalveolar pressures. It can also cause hypoperfusion of the splanchnic-hepatic circulation as well as decrease in the renal filtration gradient.[19]

- Changes in IAP have a greater effect on renal function and filtration than changes in MAP.
- Glomerular filtration gradient (GFG) is the difference between glomerular filtration pressure and proximal tubular pressure (i.e., GFP – PTP). The PTP is equal to IAP and the GFP is equal to mean arterial pressure minus intra-abdominal pressure (MAP – IAP). Thus, the GFG can be defined as MAP – 2 (IAP). Hence, raised IAP can cause inadequate filtration gradient and decreased urine output.

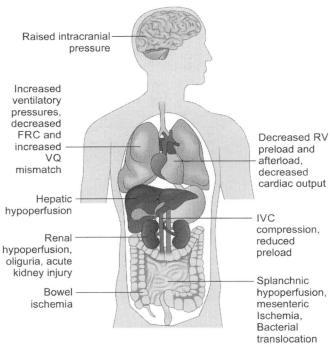

Fig. 1: The end organ effects in abdominal compartment syndrome. (FRC: functional residual capacity; IVC: inferior vena cava; RV: right ventricular)

RISK FACTORS

Understanding the risk factors and the conditions that lead to IAH and ACS is extremely important. The WSACS has suggested that IAP monitoring should be done if two or more risk factors as described by it are present. Previous studies have reported morbid obesity, sepsis, paralytic ileus, and massive fluid resuscitation as risk factors for the development of IAH/ACS.[20,21]

Risk factors for development of IAH/ACS have been enumerated below:[2]

- *Diminished abdominal wall compliance*:
  - Abdominal surgery
  - Major trauma, burns
  - Prone positioning
- *Increased intra-luminal contents*:
  - Gastroparesis/gastric distention/ileus
  - Colonic pseudo-obstruction
  - Volvulus
- *Increased intra-abdominal contents*:
  - Acute pancreatitis
  - Hemoperitoneum or intra-abdominal infection/abscess
  - Intra-abdominal or retroperitoneal tumors
  - Liver dysfunction/cirrhosis with ascites
  - Peritoneal dialysis
- *Others*:
  - Capillary leak/fluid resuscitation
  - Damage control laparotomy

- Increased APACHE-II (Acute Physiology And Chronic Health Evaluation II) or SOFA (Sequential Organ Failure Assessment) score
- Massive transfusion and fluid resuscitation or positive fluid balance
- Mechanical ventilation
- Obesity or increased body mass index
- Peritonitis
- Septic shock

DIAGNOSIS OF ABDOMINAL COMPARTMENT SYNDROME

Primary ACS occurs due to direct effects of any intra-abdominal pathology whereas secondary ACS occurs due to injuries not related to intra-abdominal pathology.

Since treatment can improve organ dysfunction, it is important that the diagnosis be considered in the appropriate clinical situation without delay. Definitive diagnosis of ACS requires measurement of the IAP. This is particularly important for patients who have trauma, have undergone liver transplant, bowel obstruction, pancreatitis, or peritonitis because these conditions are known to be associated with ACS.[20,21]

The key to recognizing ACS in a critically ill patient is demonstrating elevated IAP. The clinical importance of any IAP must be assessed in view of the baseline steady-state IAP for the individual patient. Clinical examination of the abdomen is a poor predictor of ACS, even though patients with ACS have a tender and distended abdomen.[22,23]

Attempts to estimate IAP or diagnose IAH based on changes in abdominal circumference are extremely unreliable. Physical examination has extremely poor sensitivity and accuracy for identifying elevated IAP, even by experienced clinicians.[24] Oliguria, high peak inspiratory pressures, and hemodynamic instability are also common indicators of ACS. Other findings may include severe metabolic acidosis, mesenteric ischemia, paralytic ileus, and raised ICP. Imaging, unfortunately, is not very helpful in the diagnosis of ACS. Chest X-ray may show elevated hemidiaphragm, with decreased lung volumes and atelectasis; CT scan may show nonspecific findings such as bowel wall thickening, or bilateral inguinal herniation or infiltration of the retroperitoneal space, compression of the inferior vena cava and renal vessels.

MEASUREMENT OF INTRA-ABDOMINAL PRESSURE (FIG. 2)

The basic premise in measuring the IAP is a consideration that abdomen with its contents is fluidic in character and behaves in accordance with Pascal's law; hence, the pressure measured at one point in the abdomen can

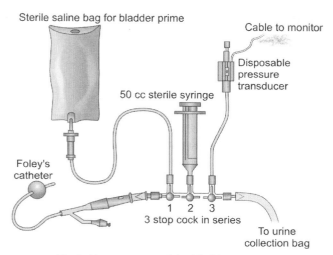

Fig. 2: Measurement of the bladder pressure.

represent pressure throughout the abdomen. The IAP is therefore defined as the steady-state pressure concealed within the abdominal cavity. In clinical practice, the IAP is always measured indirectly by measuring the intravesical bladder pressure through a Foley catheter and this has been shown to correlate well with directly-measured IAP.[10] It has to be noted that IAP increases with inspiration due to the diaphragmatic contraction and decreases with expiration. Other methods of measuring IAP are attaching a manometer to abdominal drains, measuring intra-gastric pressure via a nasogastric tube or measuring pressure from IVC via catheter placed into femoral vein. These methods have been tried but are not considered reliable.[25,26]

Intra-abdominal pressure can be directly measured with an intraperitoneal catheter attached to a pressure transducer or during CO_2 insufflation in laparoscopic surgery, where IAP is measured directly with the Veress needle. Different indirect methods for estimating IAP are used clinically because direct measurements are considered to be too invasive.[27] These techniques include rectal, gastric, inferior vena caval, and urinary bladder pressure measurements. Only gastric and bladder pressures are used clinically.[28] The IAP can also be measured via a balloon-tipped gastric catheter.[29] Several other methods for continuous IAP measurement via the stomach, peritoneal cavity (using air-chamber or piezoresistive membranes), and bladder have been validated. Although these techniques seem promising, further clinical validation needs to be done before their general use can be recommended. Bladder pressure is the standard method for the measurement of IAP. It is simple, minimally invasive, reliable, and accurate. To avoid variation in the measurement techniques, WSACS consensus guidelines suggest that the standard way for intermittent IAP measurements is through the bladder catheter with a maximal instillation volume of 25 mL sterile saline into the bladder for priming. IAP expressed in mm Hg

is measured at end of exhalation in the supine position, after ensuring no abdominal muscle contractions, and the transducer zeroed at the level of midaxillary line at the iliac crest.

For children the standard reference for intermittent IAP measurement through the bladder catheter is using 1 mL/kg of instillation volume since the instillation volume is important (minimum 3 mL to maximum 25 mL sterile saline). Studies have found that 1 mL/kg is reliable for IAP values when compared with higher volumes. Serial measurement of IAP via this method does not appear to lead to increased rates of catheter-associated urinary tract infections.[30]

Intermittent measurement of IAP every 4–6 hours is recommended when patients are at risk of developing IAH or ACS while, continuous measurement is preferred in impending or diagnosed IAH/ACS requiring abdominal decompression. APP is also used as a resuscitation endpoint. Recently continuous intra-abdominal pressure measurement commercial kits with Foley manometer are available and used.[31] When an intermittent method is used, measurements should be obtained at least every 4–6 hours, and in patients with evolving organ dysfunction, this frequency should be increased to hourly measurements.

Intra-abdominal pressure measurement should be continued until the risk factors for IAH are resolved with no organ dysfunction, and IAP is maintained below 10–12 mm Hg for at least 24–48 hours.

Although WSACS consensus guidelines recommend IAP measurement be performed in sedated patients, where muscle contractions are absent, in awake patients, attention should be paid to adequate pain relief during supine positioning and that no muscle contractions are present, especially in chronic obstructive pulmonary disease (COPD) patients, who have forced expiration, which may lead to erroneous readings.

MANAGEMENT OF IAH AND ACS

Management of IAH is essentially supportive care unless ACS mandates abdominal decompression. Procedures such as escharotomy release to relieve mechanical limitations due to burn eschars, and percutaneous ascitic drainage can be done in exceptional cases. Supportive care is generally aimed at reduction of intra-abdominal volume and measures to improve abdominal wall compliance.

Simple measures commonly practiced are nasogastric and rectal drainage in patients with bowel distension. Percutaneous drainage of ascites or intra-abdominal collections (e.g., hemoperitoneum, intra-abdominal or retroperitoneal abscess, etc.) is also performed.[32]

It is believed that percutaneous drainage can improve APP and organ dysfunction and may avoid the need for decompression laparotomy. Certain risk factors that may predict failure of percutaneous drainage are less than 1 liter of fluid drained or <9 mm Hg decrease in APP in the first 4 hours after catheter placement, suggesting that these patients need emergent open abdominal decompression.

Fluid management remains a major concern as it must be tailored to maintain adequate APPs while simultaneously avoiding volume overload. There is no evidence regarding particular type of fluid use. However, both hypertonic saline and colloid as resuscitative fluids have shown to reduce IAPs when compared with isotonic fluid. Also there is no evidence regarding the use of diuretics.

Other supporting measures for improving abdominal wall compliance can be adequate pain control, sedation, or muscle paralysis, if necessary.[33] Maintaining adequate ventilatory support is critical since this condition is associated with high airway pressures. Use of low tidal volume with permissive hypercapnia may be necessary. Optimization of positive end-expiratory pressure (PEEP) may improve oxygenation by reducing the ventilation–perfusion mismatch.

In extreme cases continuous renal replacement therapies (RRTs) with ultrafiltration may be used to decrease IAP.[34]

Special concern is for patients with concurrent intracranial hypertension and IAH.

In patients with trauma with refractory intracranial hypertension despite both maximal medical therapy and decompressive craniectomy, therapeutic decompressive laparotomy may need to be performed for reduction in intracranial hypertension.

In postoperative patients, an IAP of above 25 mm Hg with low urinary output and adequate blood volume may be an indication for re-exploration and abdominal decompression.[8]

The WSACS recommendations and suggestions for the management of IAH/ACS have been summarized here.[1,2]

- Measure IAP when known risk for IAH/ACS is present in critically ill or injured patient [GRADE 1C].
- Use of trans-bladder technique as the standard IAP measurement technique [UNGRADED].
- Use protocolized monitoring and management of IAP [GRADE 1C]
- Use protocols to avoid sustained IAH among critically ill or injured patients [GRADE 1C].
- Consider decompressive laparotomy in overt ACS in critically ill adults with ACS [GRADE 1D].
- In patients having open abdominal wounds, conscious and protocolized efforts be made to obtain an early or at least same-hospital-stay abdominal fascial closure [GRADE 1D].
- In critically ill/injured patients with open abdominal wounds, strategies utilizing negative pressure wound therapy be used [GRADE 1C].

Suggestions:

- Ensure optimal pain and anxiety relief for critically ill or injured patients [GRADE 2D].
- Brief trials of neuromuscular blockade as a temporary measure for treatment of IAH/ACS [GRADE 2D].
- Contribution of body position to elevated IAP be considered in patients at risk of ACS [GRADE 2D].
- Nasogastric or rectal tubes can be liberally used for enteral decompression when the stomach or colon are dilated in the presence of IAH/ACS [GRADE 1D].
- Neostigmine be used for the treatment of established colonic ileus not responding to other measures [GRADE 2D].
- Protocol to avoid a positive cumulative fluid balance in the critically ill or injured patient with, or at risk of IAH/ACS after the acute resuscitation has been completed [GRADE 2C].
- Increased ratio of plasma/packed red blood cells for resuscitation of massive hemorrhage [GRADE 2D].
- Percutaneous catheter drainage (PCD) to remove fluid (in the setting of obvious intraperitoneal fluid) in those with IAH/ACS when this is technically possible compared to nonintervention [GRADE 2C].
- Prophylactic use of the "open abdomen" in patients undergoing laparotomy for trauma [GRADE 2D].
- Bioprosthetic meshes should not be routinely used in the closure of the open abdomen [GRADE 2D].

The WSACS 2013 consensus statement management algorithm has been shown in **Flowchart 1**.[2]

Surgical Decompression

When surgical decompression is undertaken, the abdomen can be managed by temporary closure or open abdomen technique.

Temporary closure technique may help provide easy re-exploration, minimize fluid losses, and reduce fascial retraction. This can be achieved by techniques such as Wittmann patch which consists of two sheets of Velcro material sewn to the fascial edges after a plastic drape is placed over the viscera or by applying negative pressure wound therapy.

Since mortality among patients who developed ACS is extremely high, ranging from 40 to 100%, it is fairly evident that the only appropriate management is "open abdomen".

Open abdomen is a surgical strategy where the incisional defect in the abdominal wall is purposefully left temporarily unrepaired to relieve pressure.[35] However, a temporary cover with towels, sponges, a prosthetic patch or a translucent cover is left in place to avoid evisceration and heat or fluid losses from the abdominal defect.

Flowchart 1: Algorithm for management of IAH/ACS.[2]

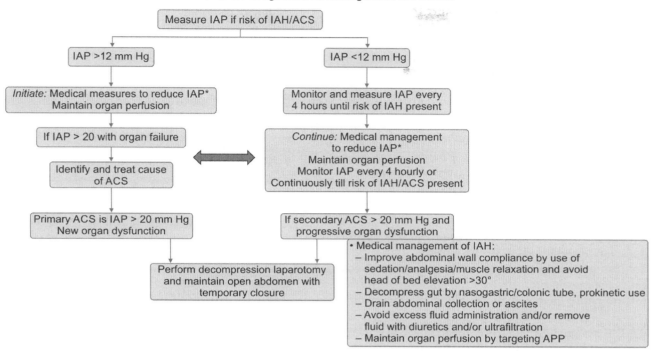

(ACS: abdominal compartment syndrome; IAP: intra-abdominal pressure; IAH: intra-abdominal hypertension; APP: abdominal perfusion pressure)

Just as there is no consensus on optimal timing of IAP measurement, there is no consensus on timing of decompression. Even though IAH is not an independent predictor of multiorgan failure, decompressing the abdomen prior to the development of ACS is becoming increasingly common and may improve survival. There is no consensus regarding at what level of IAP for surgical decompression should be done, some suggest surgical decompression be considered when the IAP is 20 mm Hg or greater, regardless of signs of ACS.

The WSACS suggests that surgical decompression not be delayed until the development of ACS (Grade 2C). Surgical decompression can be performed in the operating room if the patient is medically stable for transfer or at the bedside in the ICU. Surgical decompression also gives the ability to drain infection, debride necrotic material, repair intestinal injury, etc. as deemed necessary.

It should be understood that elevated IAP causes severe reduction of venous return leading to hypotension, increased airway pressures, renal failure, and with impaired mesenteric venous return that can lead to congestive intestinal ischemia. As volume is restored during resuscitation and the compromised bowel is reperfused, free-radical mucosal damage with capillary leak may occur. With this increased mucosal permeability, comes increasing bowel wall edema. There is also a systemic efflux of cytokines that may contribute to multiorgan failures. Elevated cardiac filling pressure that may occur

during resuscitation has also been implicated in worsening intestinal edema through inhibition of lymphatic outflow via the cistern chyli.

In such patients right ventricular end-diastolic volume index (RVEDVI) may be the most accurate predictor of intravascular volume since CVP and pulmonary artery occlusion pressure (PAOP) are less reliable. Additionally, clearance of lactate can be used as a marker of adequacy of fluid resuscitation.

There is a risk of reperfusion syndrome characterized by severe hemodynamic compromise due to the secondary effects after decompression possibly due to release of products of anaerobic metabolism and acidosis.

General measures such as volume resuscitation, reversal of coagulopathy, and correction of acidosis remain standard of care for all surgical patients.

Another important aspect is to note that abdominal decompression can result in immediate improvement in lung compliance necessitating need to read just the ventilator settings accordingly and also need to rapidly resuscitate the patient when decompression is performed.

Careful attention to maintenance of temperature and to the insensible heat loss is equally important in open abdomen since it is an independent predictor of mortality especially in patients with trauma.

Following decompression, open abdomen can be maintained using temporary abdominal closure techniques such as negative pressure systems or gauze/adhesive dressings which allow dressing and inspection of abdominal contents regularly.[36] Use of a negative pressure system helps to control and quantify fluid losses. Other conditions where the abdomen is left open are damage control surgery in trauma, severe septic abdomen, burns, etc.[37] Although damage control surgery has significantly reduced the incidence of ACS in trauma patients, decompression laparotomy for major burns has not been able to demonstrate mortality benefit probably because the inherent mortality in major burns patient is extremely high.[38] A few retrospective studies have shown reduction in mortality with decompressive laparotomy in burns patients with ACS. There is enough evidence to suggest that delay in surgical decompression after development of ACS can significantly increase the risk of mortality in both trauma and nonsurgical patients. It is hypothesized that surgical decompression improves visceral perfusion and with negative pressure peritoneal cover can reduce transmission of inflammatory mediators to the bloodstream as well as bacterial translocation, thereby preventing a septic cascade and organ dysfunction. Open abdomen, however, can lead to persistent hypercatabolic state and severe protein loss via peritoneal fluid, enterocutaneous or intestinal fistulae, retraction of the abdominal wall, or development of ventral hernias, etc. Hence, continued monitoring is necessary even after surgical decompression.

After resolution of ACS the open abdomen can be definitively closed with a primary fascial closure or use of skin grafts if lateralization of the abdominal wall occurs.[39-41]

In the postoperative period it has to be noted that patients with open abdomen will have increased fluid, electrolyte, and protein requirements because of large volume losses of these substrates through their open abdominal wound. Failure to recognize these losses in calculations of nitrogen balance and caloric needs will lead to severe underfeeding. Nearly 2–4 g of nitrogen is lost per liter of abdominal fluid output depending on the type of temporary abdominal closure.

Utmost care needs to be taken for preventing infection which is very commonly seen such as wound infection, a deep abdominal abscess, or an intestinal fistula.

It has shown that patients with epidural anesthesia can significantly decrease IAP with increased APP without hemodynamic compromise.

CONCLUSION

Although, ACS incidence has decreased over the last few years, it is associated with a high mortality and morbidity and poor outcomes. Early recognition of the risk factors and disease process remains the key for prevention of ACS since its treatment is difficult. Surgical decompression and open abdomen technique has become a common lifesaving procedure in the management of ACS. It is also important to attempt closure of the fascial defect as soon as clinically feasible.

REFERENCES

1. Kirkpatrick AW, De Waele JJ, De Laet I, De Keulenaer BL, D'Amours S, Bjoerck M, et al. WSACS—The Abdominal Compartment Society. A Society dedicated to the study of the physiology and pathophysiology of the abdominal compartment and its interactions with all organ systems. Anaesthesiol Intensive Ther. 2015;47:191.

2. Kirkpatrick AW, Roberts DJ, De Waele J, Jaeschke R, Malbrain ML, De Keulenaer B, et al. Intra-abdominal hypertension and the abdominal compartment syndrome: updated consensus definitions and clinical practice guidelines from the World Society of the Abdominal Compartment Syndrome. Intensive Care Med. 2013;39:1190-206.

3. Caldwell CB, Ricotta JJ. Changes in visceral blood flow with elevated intraabdominal pressure. J Surg Res. 1987;43:14-20.

4. Rubenstein C, Bietz G, Davenport DL, Winkler M, Endean ED. Abdominal compartment syndrome associated with endovascular and open repair of ruptured abdominal aortic aneurysms. J Vasc Surg. 2015;61:648-54.

5. Daugherty EL, Liang H, Taichman D, Hansen-Flaschen J, Fuchs BD. Abdominal compartment syndrome is common in medical intensive care unit patients receiving large-volume resuscitation. J Intensive Care Med. 2007;22(5):294-9.

6. Malbrain ML, Chiumello D, Cesana BM, Reintam Blaser A, Starkopf J, Sugrue M, et al. A systematic review and individual patient data meta-analysis on intra-abdominal hypertension in critically ill patients: the wake-up project. World initiative on Abdominal Hypertension Epidemiology, a Unifying Project (WAKE-Up!). Minerva Anestesiol. 2014;80:293-306.

7. Mentula P, Hienonen P, Kemppainen E, Puolakkainen P, Leppäniemi A. Surgical decompression for abdominal compartment syndrome in severe acute pancreatitis. Arch Surg. 2010;145:764-9.

8. Fietsam JR, Villalba M, Glover JL, Clark K. Intra-abdominal compartment syndrome as a complication of ruptured abdominal aortic aneurysm repair. Am Surg. 1989;55(6):396-402.

9. Emerson H. Intra-abdominal pressures. Arch Intern Med. 1911;7:754-84.

10. Balogh Z, McKinley BA, Holcomb JB, Miller CC, Cocanour CS, Kozar RA, et al. Both primary and secondary abdominal compartment syndrome can be predicted early and are harbingers of multiple organ failure. J Trauma. 2003;54:848-61.

11. Papavramidis TS, Marinis AD, Pliakos I, Kesisoglou I, Papavramidou N. Abdominal compartment syndrome–Intra-abdominal hypertension: Defining, diagnosing, and managing. J Emerg Trauma Shock. 2011;4:279.

12. Sanchez NC, Tenofsky PL, Dort JM, Shen LY. What is normal intra-abdominal pressure?/Discussion. Am Surg. 2001;67:243.

13. Cheatham ML, White MW, Sagraves SG, Johnson JL, Block EF. Abdominal perfusion pressure: a superior parameter in the assessment of intra-abdominal hypertension. J Trauma. 2000;49:621-7.

14. Malbrain M, Roberts DJ, De Laet I, De Waele JJ, Sugrue M, Schachtrupp A, et al. The role of abdominal compliance, the neglected parameter in critically ill patients—a consensus review of 16. Part 1: definitions and pathophysiology. Anaesthesiol Intensive Ther. 2014;46:392-405.

15. Madigan MC, Kemp CD, Johnson JC, Cotton BA. Secondary abdominal compartment syndrome after severe extremity injury: are early, aggressive fluid resuscitation strategies to blame? J Trauma. 2008;64:280-5.

16. Saggi BH, Sugerman HJ, Ivatury RR, Bloomfield GL. Abdominal compartment syndrome. J Trauma. 1998;45:597-609.

17. Trikudanathan G, Vege SS. Current concepts of the role of abdominal compartment syndrome in acute pancreatitis–an opportunity or merely an epiphenomenon. Pancreatology. 2014;14:238-43.

18. Deeren DH, Dits H, Malbrain ML. Correlation between intra-abdominal and intracranial pressure in nontraumatic brain injury. Intensive Care Med. 2005;31:1577-81.

19. Dalfino L, Tullo L, Donadio I, Malcangi V, Brienza N. Intra-abdominal hypertension and acute renal failure in critically ill patients. Intensive Care Med. 2008;34:707-13.

20. Kim IB, Prowle J, Baldwin I, Bellomo R. Incidence, risk factors and outcome associations of intra-abdominal hypertension in critically ill patients. Anaesth Intensive Care. 2012;40:79-89.

21. Ke L, Ni HB, Sun JK, Tong ZH, Li WQ, Li N, et al. Risk factors and outcome of intra-abdominal hypertension in patients with severe acute pancreatitis. World J Surg. 2012;36:171-8.

22. Sugrue M, De Waele J, De Keulenaer BL, Roberts DJ, Malbrain ML. A user's guide to intra-abdominal pressure measurement. Anaesthesiol Intensive Ther. 2015;47:241-51.

23. Kirkpatrick AW, Brenneman FD, McLean RF, Rapanos T, Boulanger BR. Is clinical examination an accurate indicator of raised intra-abdominal pressure in critically injured patients?. Can J Surg. 2000;43:207.

24. Castillo M, Lis RJ, Ulrich H, Rivera G, Hanf C, Kvetan V. Clinical estimate compared to intra-abdominal pressure measurement. Crit Care Med. 1998;26:78A.

25. De Keulenaer BL, Regli A, Dabrowski W, Kaloiani V, Bodnar Z, Cea JI, et al. Does femoral venous pressure measurement correlate well with intrabladder pressure measurement? A multicenter observational trial. Intensive Care Med. 2011;37:1620.

26. Sugrue M, Buist MD, Lee A, Sanchez DJ, Hillman KM. Intra-abdominal pressure measurement using a modified nasogastric tube: description and validation of a new technique. Intensive Care Med. 1994;20:588-90.

27. Risin E, Kessel B, Ashkenazi I, Lieberman N, Alfici R. A new technique of direct intra-abdominal pressure measurement: a preliminary study. Am J Surg. 2006;191:235-7.

28. Malbrain ML. Different techniques to measure intra-abdominal pressure (IAP): time for a critical re-appraisal. In: Pinsky MR, Brochard L, Mancebo J (Eds). Applied Physiology in Intensive Care Medicine. Berlin, Heidelberg: Springer; 2006. pp. 105-19.

29. Engum SA, Kogon B, Jensen E, Isch J, Balanoff C, Grosfeld JL. Gastric tonometry and direct intraabdominal pressure monitoring in abdominal compartment syndrome. J Pediatr Surg. 2002;37:214-8.

30. Desie N, Willems A, Dits H, Van Regenmortel N, Schoonheydt K, Van De Vyvere M, et al. Intra-abdominal pressure measurement using the Foley Manometer does not increase the risk for urinary tract infection in critically ill patients. Ann Intensive Care. 2012;2(S1):S10.

31. Balogh Z, Jones F, D'Amours S, Parr M, Sugrue M. Continuous intra-abdominal pressure measurement technique. Am J Surg. 2004;188:679-84.

32. Ouellet JF, Leppaniemi A, Ball CG, Cheatham ML, D'Amours S, Kirkpatrick AW. Alternatives to formal abdominal decompression. Am Surg. 2011;77:s51-7.

33. Hoste E, Verholen E, De Waele JJ. The effect of neuromuscular blockers in patients with intra-abdominal hypertension. Intensive Care Med. 2007;33:1811-4.

34. Dabrowski W, Kotlinska-Hasiec E, Schneditz D, Zaluska W, Rzecki Z, De Keulenaer B. Adjust fluid volume excess in septic shock patients reduces intra-abdominal pressure. Clin Nephrol. 2014;82:41-50.

35. De Waele JJ, Hoste EA, Malbrain ML. Decompressive laparotomy for abdominal compartment syndrome–a critical analysis. Crit Care. 2006;10:R51.

36. Quyn AJ, Johnston C, Hall D, Chambers A, Arapova N, Ogston S, et al. The open abdomen and temporary abdominal closure systems–historical evolution and systematic review. Colorectal Dis. 2012;14:e429-38.

37. Rotondo MF, Schwab CW, McGonigal MD, Fruchterman TM, Kauder DR, Latenser BA, et al. 'Damage control': an approach for improved survival in exsanguinating penetrating abdominal injury. J Trauma. 1993;35:375-82.

38. Strang SG, Van Lieshout EM, Breederveld RS, Van Waes OJ. A systematic review on intra-abdominal pressure in severely burned patients. Burns. 2014;40:9-16.

39. Regner JL, Kobayashi L, Coimbra R. Surgical strategies for management of the open abdomen. World J Surg. 2012;36:497-510.

40. Chiara O, Cimbanassi S, Biffl W, Leppaniemi A, Henry S, Scalea TM, et al. International consensus conference on open abdomen in trauma. J Trauma Acute Care Surg. 2016;80(1):173-83.

41. Acosta S, Bjarnason T, Petersson U, Pålsson B, Wanhainen A, Svensson M, et al. Multicentre prospective study of fascial closure rate after open abdomen with vacuum and mesh-mediated fascial traction. British Journal of Surgery. 2011;98:735-43.

Genitourinary

Perioperative Management of Bladder and Prostate Cancer Surgeries

Shagun Bhatia Shah, Uma Hariharan

SCIENTIFIC RATIONALE

The incidence and prevalence of bladder and prostate cancers are on the rise, especially associated with tobacco use.[1] There exists a cafeteria choice for prostate cancer surgery techniques ranging from the traditional open radical prostatectomy, transurethral resection of prostate (TURP), minimally invasive robot-assisted laparoscopic prostatectomy (RALP) to the totally noninvasive high-intensity focused ultrasound (HIFU).[1-3] The latter is most successful for prostate glands weighing 25 g or lesser. TURP preceding HIFU by 2–3 months is reserved for larger glands to downsize the gland to 20–25 g.[3] Analgesic requirement varies inversely with the invasiveness of the surgical technique. Extreme head-low position entailing unique positioning requirements exists for RALP and robotic cystoprostatectomy.[2] HIFU necessitates either a right lateral position or lithotomy, depending on the ablating device used. Transurethral resection of bladder tumor (TURBT) is the ideal procedure for nonmuscle invasive urinary bladder tumors. Open radical cystoprostatectomy (RCP) with urinary diversion with pelvic lymph node dissection is currently the gold standard for muscle-invasive, nonmetastatic bladder carcinoma.[4] It is a major and prolonged surgery with a 64% complication rate, performed in supine position.[5] That only about a third of these patients receive neoadjuvant chemotherapy (NACT), despite "level one" evidence of NACT being beneficial, is attributed to the fact that the average age at the time of diagnosis is 73 years and possibly because of the fear that NACT may delay surgery.[6]

The enhanced recovery after surgery (ERAS) pathway is a multimodal concept with 22 elements that can potentially lead to a significantly reduced length of hospital stay and complications without increasing the readmission rate.[7-9] Initially applied to colorectal surgery, ERAS in urology merits wider implementation and the current body of evidence shows encouraging results. Perioperative surgical

home (PSH), fast track surgery (FTS), and collaborative care pathway surgery (CCPS) are similar concepts. The preoperative, intraoperative, and postoperative periods need to be seamlessly linked to provide continuity in care culminating in better clinical outcomes and a positive patient experience.

Perioperative concerns involve considerations common to all robotic surgeries as well as those specific to each surgery, including open surgeries, apart from patient-specific issues. Anesthesiologists have to tailor their technique according to the surgical requirements and, at the same time, give top priority to patient safety.

This chapter provides deep insight into the nitty-gritty of perioperative care in patients with urinary bladder and prostate cancers.

PREOPERATIVE OPTIMIZATION OF THE PATIENTS

Availability of Standard Operating Procedures and Time Management

Before commencing surgery, the duration of surgery should be standardized to 2 hours for robot-assisted radical prostatectomy, 5 hours for robotic/open RCP with ileal conduit, and 8 hours for radical cystectomy/cystoprostatectomy with robot-assisted neobladder formation. Ideally, two robotic operation theaters (OTs) need to be assigned for urological malignancies—one OT reserved exclusively for radical RCP with neobladder and the second one for up to three RALPs in a working day. Alternatively, RALP cases may be taken up in batches of 2–3 per OT in case an RCP is not scheduled. Real-time feedback on cancelled/added/rescheduled cases should be readily available. Patients need to be wheeled to the OT with minimal waiting period for the patient and without wastage of OT time.[8,9]

Presurgical Care

Patients need to be educated on the available modes of surgery (open/laparoscopic/robot-assisted/HIFU) as well as alternative surgical options (neobladder/ileal conduit after RCP) to make an intelligent informed choice.[8,9]

A written informed consent after disclosing possible complications including conversion to open surgery in case of minimally invasive surgery is imperative.

A detailed discussion of infection prevention strategies with the patient goes a long way in losing good surgical results to postoperative infection.

Preanesthetic Care

Prehabilitation

A triage scheme should be applied in the preanesthetic checkup (PAC) clinic to identify patients requiring prehabilitation. Availability of a cardiopulmonary exercise testing (CPET) machine may prove useful as a point-of-care assessment tool for cardiopulmonary reserves, especially for patients undergoing surgery in steep Trendelenburg (ST) position.

Usually, a PAC checkup is performed 1–7 days before surgery and a patient may require 1–4 weeks of prehabilitation to address comorbidities such as uncontrolled diabetes, hypertension, hypothyroidism with optimization of medication, and improvement of nutritional status.[10] Echocardiography for determination of left ventricular ejection fraction is usually prescribed by the cardiologist, because of the age factor, associated hypertension, and postchemotherapy status of many patients. Anticoagulants need to be discontinued as per an institutional protocol based on national and international guidelines.

Screening

Screening for obstructive sleep apnea is important in view of the airway edema expected in ST position. Inspection for glaucoma and raised intracranial pressure (ICP) is vital since the physiological changes due to steep head-low position like raised ICP and intraocular pressure (IOP) can prove detrimental in these patients.

Carbohydrate Drink

Around 400 mL or 50 g of a clear maltodextrin drink should be offered to the patients 2 hours before surgery. Four hundred milliliters of ONS400 (Fresenius Kabi; Germany) supply 50 g carbohydrate, all of which is maltodextrin, and supply 200 calories of energy.[11] Ensure that clear/Gatorade thirst quencher (both manufactured by Pepsico) containing 43/21 g of carbohydrate, respectively, none of which is a maltodextrin, is being administered with questionable utility. Carbohydrate preloading is known to reduce thirst and insulin resistance and promotes maintenance of lean body mass and muscle power.[7-9,11,12]

Communication

A centralized electronic patient record system with updated patient information should be accessible to all stakeholders (clinicians including the surgeons, anesthesiologists, internal medicine physicians; nursing staff; physiotherapist; nutritionist) starting from the admission center, preoperative clinic, operation theater, postanesthesia care unit, and postoperative ward right until discharge of the patient and even during follow-up visits or emergency admissions in the casualty.[8,9,13,14]

Team member and team leader identification goes a long way in streamlining the process by allocation of responsibilities and maintaining answerability.

A designated anesthesia technician should be assigned for each case. The cleaning staff, OT technician, and scrub nurse should commence cleaning the instruments and set up the OT as soon as the incision is closed in preparation for the fresh case.

Robot and Instruments on the Day of Surgery

There should be standardization of equipment and instruments across all surgeons. The requisite minimum number of instrument trays/sets should be readily available to avoid the need for processing/sterilization of equipment in between two cases. It should be ensured that all trays are complete and in working order. A tray with requisite instruments should be available in case there is conversion to open surgery during a difficult robotic/laparoscopic surgery.[9]

Pain, Postoperative Nausea Vomiting, and Venous Thromboembolism Prophylaxis

A multimodal pain management program should be available and activated prior to the surgical incision to provide preemptive analgesia exemplified by intravenous (IV) paracetamol 1 g before docking of the robotic arms or surgical incision.

The postoperative nausea vomiting (PONV) prevention protocol should also be initiated preoperatively with a ranitidine tablet (150 mg) along with a 5-HT3 antagonist (granisetron tablet 2 mg) taken the night before surgery and on the morning of surgery with sips of water.[8,9,15-17]

Venous thromboembolism (VTE) prophylaxis acquires special importance as cancer, especially prostatic carcinoma, results in a hypercoagulable state. A compression ultrasound or venous Doppler study of the lower limb in the elderly or immobile patient subsets can reveal asymptomatic deep vein thrombosis. Prostatic surgery entails blood loss and robotic surgery too necessitates an international normalized ratio (INR) < 1.5; hence, anticoagulants need to be discontinued before surgery. Sequential compression stockings and other mechanical methods should be applied intraoperatively.[8,9,13-17] Pressure point padding prevents bedsores and nerve injury.

The antibiotic dose should be administered within 1 hour before surgery.

INTRAOPERATIVE CONTINUATION OF OPTIMIZATION PROTOCOL

Safety Checklist

Intraoperative time-out should be performed meticulously. The surgical and anesthetist safety checklist should be signed by the respective surgeon and anesthetist on paper or in the Computerized Patient Record System (CPRS).

Regional Anesthesia

A thoracic epidural catheter placed at the T9-11 level for cystectomy patients augments intraoperative analgesia diminishing opioid requirements and provides excellent postoperative analgesia which is superior to IV opioids.[9,12,14] It hastens functional recovery and decreases the incidence and severity of cardiopulmonary complications. Open radical prostatectomy and TURP procedures are generally performed under subarachnoid block which provides effective analgesia continuing into the early postoperative period. Obturator nerve block supplementation is desirable in TURBT patients with tumors located on the lateral walls of the urinary bladder to avoid catastrophic bladder perforation in wake of a strong obturator jerk.

Goal-directed Fluid Therapy

An arterial line and central venous pressure (CVP) line should be placed in all open cystectomy patients. Goal-directed fluid therapy keeping stroke volume variation (SVV), pulse pressure variation, CVP or pleth variability index as the goal should be employed in all surgeries, whether open or minimally invasive. Arterial blood gas analysis for serum lactate levels[14] sheds light on tissue perfusion.

Special Perils of Robotic Surgery in Steep Trendelenburg Position

Both robotic cystoprostatectomy and RALP are performed under general anesthesia, in ST position **(Figs. 1 and 2)**.

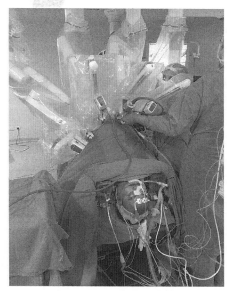

Fig. 1: Steep Trendelenburg position for robot-assisted laparoscopic surgery (anteroposterior view) with the robotic arms docked in position.

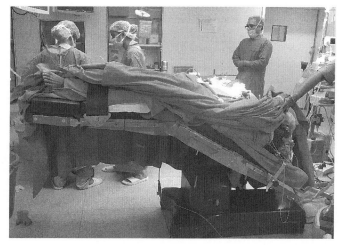

Fig. 2: Steep Trendelenburg position for robot-assisted laparoscopic surgery (lateral view).

The perils of ST position are attributed to drastic changes in physiology such as doubling of CVP, pulmonary artery pressure, pulmonary capillary wedge pressure, 25% rise in mean arterial pressure, and a 65% increase in right and left ventricular stroke work. Systemic vascular resistance is initially increased and then normalized whereas the heart rate stroke volume and cardiac output remain largely unchanged. Patients with compromised systolic function may be pushed into acute failure.

Patients with obstructive coronary disease may experience demand ischemia.[18]

Total lung capacity and compliance are reduced and both peak and plateau airway pressures witness a steep rise. A 15 mm Hg pneumoperitoneum may translate into a 9 mm Hg rise in intrathoracic pressure. Cephalad shifting of the diaphragm results in a 50% fall in the functional residual capacity and may result in endotracheal tube (ETT) shift into the right bronchus signaled by a sudden increase in airway pressure and fall in arterial oxygen saturation. Lung volume approaches closing capacity and may produce atelectasis and increase in shunt fraction. Minute ventilation must increase to offset hypercarbia. The ventilator rate is more amenable to a rise since increasing the tidal volume may further increase the already high airway pressures. Application of positive end expiratory pressure (PEEP) is akin to a double-edged sword. A 5 mm Hg PEEP increases functional residual capacity, elevating lung volumes above the closing capacity, diminishing the atelectasis, and improving lung compliance and arterial oxygenation.

On the flip side, pneumoperitoneum with addition of PEEP may abruptly drop the cardiac output.[19]

Volume-controlled ventilation (VCV) keeping peak airway pressure <30 mm Hg suffices in most patients. The surgeon is requested to keep the capnoperitoneum pressure <12 mm Hg. In many patients, the ventilator strategy needs to be changed to a pressure-controlled ventilation mode to avoid barotraumas since the airway pressures tend to increase with advent of pneumoperitoneum and increase further if ST position is required for the surgery. In such situations, it is vital to remember to reduce set control pressure/switchover to VCV once the patient is supine again, otherwise abruptly mammoth volumes sometimes exceeding 15 mL/kg may be inadvertently delivered to the patient. Only a few such breaths may cause substantial volutrauma.

A rise in ICP is also observed in the ST position and can be noninvasively monitored intraoperatively using serial sonographic evaluation of optic nerve sheath diameter (ONSD). A 5 mm ONSD corresponds to a 20 mm Hg ICP.[20]

A rise in systemic blood pressure, CVP, and airway pressure all contribute to a rise in IOP. In one study, patients reached elevated IOP levels averaging 13 mm Hg above baseline, comparable to glaucoma which was time- and end-tidal CO_2 ($EtCO_2$)-dependent.[21]

Any downward gravitational shift of the patient can prove catastrophic during robotic surgery in ST position. The "combination approach" for positioning of patients in ST position seems ideal, since it employs multiple mechanisms such as mechanical restraints as well as friction and anatomical concavities of the body to achieve complete immobilization. It necessitates placement of a horizontal linen sheet in the lumbar anatomical concavity. The hip and torso of the patient are positioned on a hypoallergenic warming gel pad with a large coefficient of friction. Two additional hypoallergenic gel pads are squeezed in between the shoulder and the shoulder-brace bilaterally and the latter are placed more medially (flush with the head).[2]

A Glitch book should be placed in a handy position and used if problems with docking of robot arise. The Da Vinci Xi robot is more user-friendly and its laser targeting system simplifies positioning the robot. Pointing the camera at the target anatomy makes the Xi position the boom into optimal configuration for surgery.[22]

Intraoperative measures to prevent postoperative cognitive dysfunction (fluid restriction, 8 mg dexamethasone, 10–20 mg furosemide and/or mannitol) must be employed.

Maintaining adequate depth of anesthesia by utilizing a depth of anesthesia monitor (bispectral index or entropy) and keeping the neuromuscular blockade intensity <10 PTCs (post-titanic count) with a peripheral nerve stimulator (PNS) to avoid patient movement with robot docked are desirable. Fluid chasing and slight head-up position after dedocking and supination aid in avoiding hypotension and reducing airway edema, respectively. Sign-out in safety checklist should only be done after the final instrument and swab count coincides with the initial count.

High-intensity Focused Ultrasound

High-intensity focused ultrasound noninvasively, and without introduction of surgical instruments, produces coagulative necrosis of diseased prostatic tissue. ALBATHERM™ (EDAP-TMS, S.A., Lyons, France) is the most commonly employed device for delivering HIFU for carcinoma prostate. The patient is placed in the right lateral position, and a rectal probe with an inbuilt ultrasound imaging transducer (7.5 MHz) and HIFU therapy transducer (2 MHz) is introduced per rectum **(Fig. 3)**. HIFU therapy

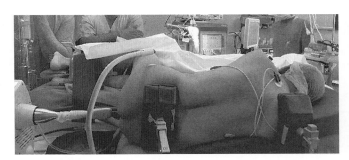

Fig. 3: Rectal probe in situ for high intensity focused ultrasound (HIFU) therapy.

is divisible into three sequential parts: Imaging, planning, and actual treatment. The area to be ablated is targeted by a focused high-intensity ultrasound beam emitted by the probe. A cooling balloon engulfs the probe and protects the rectal mucosa from thermal burns. The 45–85°C temperature attained at the target site by HIFU causes prostatic tissue ablation due to direct heating within the cancerous lesion coupled with the mechanical effects of acoustic cavitations.[3,23,24] The critical dimension of prostate that determines treatability is the prostatic height which should be <35 mm since the focal length of the HIFU lens is 4 cm. The purpose of anesthesia is to prevent motion artifacts as the pain is usually mild [3–5 on the visual analog scale (VAS) score]. The duration of HIFU procedure is 1–4 hours depending on the prostatic size and the slightest movement like that associated with coughing or sighing can move the gland, compromise precision, and injure adjacent healthy tissue or nerves.[24] In this eventuality, the HIFU planning needs to be repeated to ensure removal of the entire diseased tissue and prevent nerve injury. HIFU for prostatic lesions necessitates general anesthesia or neuraxial blocks supplemented with dexmedetomidine or propofol sedation. HIFU is radiation free, spares the intervening tissue, and has provision for different strategies such as whole gland, nerve sparing, and hemi-ablation.

POSTOPERATIVE CRITICAL CARE MANAGEMENT IN AN INTENSIVE CARE UNIT OR RECOVERY ROOM

Prostate and bladder cancer surgeries can be fraught with complications due to extensive and radical nature of the procedure, blood loss, opening-up of prostatic venous sinuses, positioning-related problems, bowel handling, and pain. These can lead to delayed extubation, shock, hypothermia, coagulopathy, and neuropathies. The goal is to maintain normothermia, normotension, and normocarbia. Extubation must be cautious after excluding airway edema or residual neuromuscular weakness. Postoperative issues can be compounded by the patient's preexisting comorbidities, causing prolonged intensive care unit (ICU) stays.

After a quick dressing, the patient must be handed over to the OT anesthesiologist for reversal and subsequent handover to the surgical intensive care unit (SICU) anesthesiologist for timely detection and management of any SICU complications. Aldrete discharge criteria need to be met for discharge to ward and a postanesthetic scoring system (PASS) score >13 merits discharge home from the ward.[25] The discharge order should contain prescription analgesics based on the severity of postoperative pain.

[VAS 1–3: diclofenac 50 mg 8 hourly; VAS 4–6: tramadol 50 mg SOS and 6 hourly; VAS 7–10: fentanyl 50 µg SOS]. For PONV, IV ondansetron 4–8 mg and/or IV dexamethasone 4–8 mg are beneficial. Oral alvimopan (µ-opioid receptor antagonist) 12 mg single dose before surgery and 12 hourly for 7 postoperative days or till the first bowel movement has been shown to reduce the incidence of postoperative ileus in patients undergoing radical cystectomy.[26-28] In compliance with the ERAS protocol, use of morphine and opioids needs to be minimized or avoided altogether in favor of alternative multimodal analgesia. Removal of the nasogastric tube and early enteral feed are the objectives.

Patient status update and follow up are accomplished on following lines:

- The perioperative checklist must be completed timely by the surgeon and anesthesiologist, along with real-time, next-patient status update with information on potential delays, postdischarge care, remote follow-up with phone calls (day 3 and day 5).
- Clinical visits and tracking of emergency care returns of the patient (including noting down of the causes) must be meticulously done. Any requirement for readmission must be discussed by a monthly review of the robotic program committee.

Audit

Audit involves a monthly review by the robotic committee with a four-pronged approach:

1. Assessing clinical outcomes (morbidity, length of hospital stay, mortality)
2. Assessing nonclinical outcomes (cost-effectiveness, patient satisfaction)
3. Gauging compliance to ERAS/PSH/fast-tracking protocols
4. Modification of the existing multimodal concepts with inputs from new evidence

PRACTICE PRESCRIPTION (BASED ON EVIDENCE FROM PROTOCOLS/GUIDELINE REFERENCES AND LITERATURE REVIEW)

Gregg et al. compared the 90-day mortality rate in nutritionally deprived cystectomy patients with well-nourished cystectomy patients and found a 16.5% mortality in those with nutritional deficiency and 5.1% in remaining patients.[10]

Persson et al. evaluated adherence to ERAS protocol, perioperative complication rate as per the Clavien–Dindo classification, time to first stool passage, length of hospital stay, and readmission rate in 31 consecutive patients undergoing open radical cystectomy with urinary diversion with 39 comparable non-ERAS patients and found that the ERAS group had significantly shorter times to passage of feces and a lower 30-day readmission rate. [29]

Collins et al. subjected 135 patients scheduled for totally intracorporeal robot-assisted radical cystectomy to the ERAS protocol and found the postoperative length of hospital stay to be significantly reduced to 8 days compared to 9 days in the control group of 86 patients.[13] Nabhani et al. calculated expenditures accrued during the ERAS protocol for radical cystectomy at their center and noted USD 4,489 savings in 30-day costs compared to the conventional management regimen.[30]

Karl et al. prospectively applied the ERAS protocol to 62 patients undergoing radical cystectomy for carcinoma bladder and found a significant improvement in quality of life parameters (European Organization for the Research and Treatment of Cancer) compared to 39 similar patients undergoing the same surgery managed in the conventional manner.[31] A reduction in complications such as delayed wound healing, thrombosis, and pyrexia and a diminished analgesic requirement in the postoperative period were also observed in the ERAS group.

Guan et al. utilized FTS for laparoscopic radical cystectomy and ileal conduit diversion patients and found a reduced time to first flatus and shortened time to regular diet.[32] A lower total leukocyte count and C-reactive protein in these patients reflecting reduced surgical stress response was observed on the 5th and 7th postoperative days (PODs). The length and cost of hospital stay was also reduced. A multifactorial FTS system was also employed by Saar et al. for patients scheduled for robot-assisted radical cystectomy with extracorporeal urinary diversion.[33] After having a normal breakfast, the patient was admitted to the hospital a day prior to surgery. Thereafter, a liquid diet comprising soup and unrestricted clear fluids were given to the patient. Two high carbohydrate drinks were given at 6 PM followed by Fleet enema later in the evening. On the day of surgery, two high carbohydrate drinks were repeated at 5 AM, a single injectable antibiotic dose was administered intraoperatively, no abdominal drains were employed, and the nasogastric tube was removed right at the end of the procedure. Two hours after surgery, free fluids were orally allowed as tolerated; 300 mg magnesium citrate and nonopioid analgesics such as diclofenac 75 mg were administered 12 hourly and opioid was given only if required. The patients were mobilized early (after 5 hours). On the 1st POD, protein drinks, light diet, and free intake of fluids (>1500 mL) were allowed.

Diclofenac 75 mg every 12 hours and IV nonopioids and opioids for breakthrough pain were administered as required. The patients were mobilized, physiotherapy was provided, and they were allowed to remain out of bed for 8 hours, including walking in the corridor twice. In addition to above, on the 2nd POD, a rectal laxative (bisacodyl suppository) was administered. A regular diet was resumed on the 3rd POD. The 31 patients in the FTS group required remarkably lower postoperative morphine equivalents (57.3 vs. 92.4 mg) compared to the conventional group. The time to mobilization within the room was reduced from 30.2 to 17.5 hours, whereas the time to regular diet was decreased from 6.6 to 4 days.

Chang et al. utilized the post open radical retropubic prostatectomy collaborative care pathway where patients were fed a full liquid diet in the afternoon progressing to a regular diet in the evening of POD 1.[34] A full recovery of bowel function was not a prerequisite for discharge. Milk of magnesia and glycerin suppositories were prescribed on an SOS basis in the discharge instructions. This reduced the length of hospital stay from 3 to 2 days.

ERAS was introduced for 124 laparoscopic prostatectomy patients by Lin et al. who witnessed a reduction in length of hospital stay from 9.2 to 3.8 days accompanied by slashing of hospitalization costs from USD 7,200 to 6,100.[35] The time to first water intake, first ambulation, and first defecation was reduced to 2.5, 8.7, and 17 hours, respectively, in the ERAS group compared to 30.1, 73, and 81 hours in the control group.

An early and vigilant follow-up may reduce readmissions by 20% through early detection of complications and nipping them in the bud.[36] Two-way unhindered communication between the patient and his physician provides grease for smooth running of any perioperative care program, in all phases including the postoperative period. There should be early follow-up with the patient's primary care provider, in addition to early and frequent phone calls from their surgeon aided by telemedicine.[37-39]

It is nearly impossible to achieve 100% compliance to ERAS and even large multicentric trials report merely 65% adherence.

Currently, ERAS guidelines pertaining to 19 different types of surgery are available (downloaded free of cost from http://erassociety.org website). One of these guidelines pertains to bladder surgery while none exists for prostate surgery. Based on these guidelines, a review of current literature and tempered with the authors' clinical experience, we recommend the following practice prescription **(Table 1)**.

Table 1: An ERAS-compliant practice prescription for bladder and prostate oncosurgery.

ERAS item	Cystectomy	Prostatectomy
• Preoperative counseling and education[9]	Detailed oral and written discussion about surgical details, length of hospital stay, and discharge criteria Stoma education in case of ileal conduit Patient's expectations about neobladder functioning must be realistic	Detailed oral and written discussion about surgical details, length of hospital stay, and discharge criteria TURP syndrome
• Preoperative medical optimization[9]	Optimization of comorbidities such as anemia, diabetes, hypertension, and hypothyroidism Nutritional support, albumin infusion if hypoproteinemia exists Cessation of smoking, alcohol <60 mL/day Moderate physical exercises	Optimization of comorbidities Screening for glaucoma and raised intracranial pressure and offering such patients an alternative form of radical prostatectomy instead of RALP
• Oral mechanical bowel preparation[15,40]	Can omit without compromising patient safety and outcomes	Can omit without compromising patient safety and outcomes
• Preoperative carbohydrates loading[9,11,14]	All nondiabetic patients should receive maltodextrin drink	All nondiabetic patients should receive maltodextrin drink
• Preoperative fasting[41]	Oral intake of clear fluids (water, apple juice) up to 2 hours before surgery Solids allowed up to 6 hours before surgery except in diabetics with gastroparesis (8 hours)	Oral intake of clear fluids (water, apple juice) up to 2 hours before surgery Solids allowed up to 6 hours before surgery
• Preanesthesia medication	Long-acting sedatives such as diazepam avoided or switched with shorter acting ones such as midazolam, if required	Shorter acting anxiolytics preferred
• Thrombosis prophylaxis[16]	Mechanical prophylaxis: Compression stockings Pharmacological prophylaxis: LMWH as per ASRA guidelines Extended prophylaxis for 4 weeks as cystectomy patients are considered high risk	Mechanical prophylaxis and early ambulation recommended
• Epidural analgesia[9,14,42]	Pain relief with thoracic epidural catheters is superior to systemic opioids Catheter removal 72 hours postcystectomy	Lumbar epidural catheter can be used for postoperative analgesia if a combined spinal epidural has been employed
• Minimally invasive approach	Robotic/laparoscopic approach reduces surgical stress and is considered superior	Minimal-access prostate surgery in properly selected patients has good results
• Resection site drainage	Urine leak might necessitate drainage	Pelvic drain can be safely omitted
• Antimicrobial prophylaxis and skin preparation	A single prophylactic antibiotic dose 1 hour before skin incision Chlorhexidine-alcohol painting prevents/decreases surgical site infection	
• Standard anesthetic protocol	Surgical stress response and intubation response attenuation, hemodynamic stability, central and peripheral oxygenation, muscle relaxation (peripheral nerve stimulator guidance, especially in robotic surgery), adequate depth of anesthesia and analgesia	
• Perioperative fluid management[14]	Goal-directed fluid therapy with esophageal Doppler monitor, cardiac output monitoring using Vigileo/FloTrac monitor in cases where an arterial cannula is in situ or with pleth variability index measured by a noninvasive Masimo CO oximeter. Cardiac output and not CVP should be the target; clinical judgment required Vasopressors to counter hypotension in absence of hypovolemia	Goal-directed fluid therapy with esophageal Doppler monitor, cardiac output monitoring using Vigileo/FloTrac monitor in cases where an arterial cannula is in situ or with pleth variability index measured by a noninvasive Masimo CO oximeter CVP shows fallaciously high readings in ST position (RALP)
• Preventing intraoperative hypothermia	Major and prolonged surgery with fluid shifts so patients prone to hypothermia Warming convective forced air blankets to cover the patient's nonsurgical sites, hypoallergenic warming gel pad to be placed below the torso Warm IV fluids	

Contd…

Contd...

ERAS item	Cystectomy	Prostatectomy
• Nasogastric intubation[42]	Postoperative nasogastric intubation not routinely indicated Early removal of nasogastric tube (placed intraoperatively) recommended postoperatively	Early removal of nasogastric tube
• Urinary drainage	Ureteral stents and transurethral neobladder catheter are recommended. The optimal duration of ureteral stenting (at least until POD 5) and transurethral catheterization for cystectomies is unknown. (In colorectal and other surgeries, the transurethral catheter should be removed on the 1st POD)	
• Prevention of postoperative ileus[26-28]	Multimodal approach including oral magnesium and gum chewing to promote gut function Preoperative and postoperative alvimopan	Multimodal approach including oral magnesium and gum chewing to promote gut function
• Prevention of PONV[15]	Multimodal prophylaxis in patients with ≥2 PONV risk factors	Multimodal prophylaxis in patients with ≥2 PONV risk factors
• Postoperative analgesia[15,43,44]	Multimodal approach Thoracic epidural mainstay Avoid/minimize opioid use	Open prostatectomy/TURP: Subarachnoid block (bupivacaine + dexmedetomidine) RALP: Paracetamol (PCM); Ketorolac HIFU: IV PCM 1 g × 12 hourly
• Early mobilization[43,45]	Patient should be mobilized out of bed for 2 hours on POD 0 and for 6 hours on POD 1	
• Early oral diet[43]	Early oral nutrition 4 hours after surgery	
• Audit[9]	Routine audit of patient outcomes, cost-effectiveness, compliance with ERAS protocol, and deviation from protocol	Audit required

(ASRA: American Society of Regional Anesthesia; ERAS: enhanced recovery after surgery; HIFU: high-intensity focused ultrasound; IV: intravenous; POD: postoperative day; PONV: postoperative nausea vomiting; RALP: robot-assisted laparoscopic prostatectomy; ST: steep Trendelenburg; TURP: transurethral resection of prostate)

■ REFERENCES

1. Antoni S, Ferlay J, Soerjomataram I, Znaor A, Jemal A, Bray F. Bladder cancer incidence and mortality: A global overview and recent trends. Eur Urol. 2017;71(1):96-108.

2. Shah SB, Hariharan U, Bhargava AK, Rawal SK, Chaudhary AA. Robotic surgery and patient positioning: Ergonomics, clinical pearls and review of literature. Trends Anaesth Crit Care. 2017;14:21-9.

3. Shah SB, Hariharan U, Bhargava AK. High intensity focussed ultrasound therapy for prostatic tumors: Anaesthesiologists perspective. J Anest & Inten Care Med. 2016;1(2):555-9.

4. Li K, Lin T, Fan X, Xu K, Bi L, Duan Y, et al. Systematic review and meta-analysis of comparative studies reporting early outcomes after robot-assisted radical cystectomy versus open radical cystectomy. Cancer Treat Rev. 2012;39(6):551-60.

5. Shabsigh A, Korets R, Vora KC, Brooks CM, Cronin AM, Savage C, et al. Defining early morbidity of radical cystectomy for patients with bladder cancer using a standardized reporting methodology. Eur Urol. 2009;55(1):164-74.

6. Gandaglia G, Popa I, Abdollah F, Schiffmann J, Shariat SF, Briganti A, et al. The effect of neoadjuvant chemotherapy on perioperative outcomes in patients who have bladder cancer treated with radical cystectomy: A population-based study. Eur Urol. 2014;66(3):561-8.

7. Baack Kukreja JE, Kiernan M, Schempp B, Siebert A, Hontar A, Nelson B, et al. Quality improvement in cystectomy care with enhanced recovery (QUICCER) study. BJU Int. 2017;119(1):38-49.

8. Cerantola Y, Valerio M, Persson B, Jichlinski P, Ljungqvist O, Hubner M, et al. Guidelines for perioperative care after radical cystectomy for bladder cancer: Enhanced recovery after surgery (ERAS(R)) society recommendations. Clin Nutr. 2013;32(6):879-87.

9. Shah SB, Hariharan U, Chawla R. Integrating perioperative medicine with anaesthesia in India: Can the best be achieved? A review. Indian J Anaesth. 2019;63(5):338-49.

10. Gregg JR, Cookson MS, Phillips S, Salem S, Chang SS, Clark PE, et al. Effect of preoperative nutritional deficiency on mortality after radical cystectomy for bladder cancer. J Urol. 2011;185(1):90-6.

11. Nanavati AJ, Prabhakar S. Enhanced recovery after surgery: If you are not implementing it, why not? Pract Gastroenterol. 2016;151:46-56.

12. Mukhtar S, Ayres BE, Issa R, Swinn MJ, Perry MJ. Challenging boundaries: An enhanced recovery programme for radical cystectomy. Ann R Coll Surg Engl. 2013;95(3):200-6.

13. Collins JW, Adding C, Hosseini A, Nyberg T, Pini G, Dey L, et al. Introducing an enhanced recovery programme to an established totally intracorporeal robot-assisted radical cystectomy service. Scand J Urol. 2016;50(1):39-46.

14. Koupparis A, Villeda-Sandoval C, Weale N, El-Mahdy M, Gillatt D, Rowe E. Robot-assisted radical cystectomy with intracorporeal urinary diversion: Impact on an established enhanced recovery protocol. BJU Int. 2015;116(6):924-31.

15. Cerruto MA, De Marco V, D'Elia C, Bizzotto L, De Marchi D, Cavalleri S, et al. Fast track surgery to reduce short-term

complications following radical cystectomy and intestinal urinary diversion with Vescica Ileale Padovana neobladder: Proposal for a tailored enhanced recovery protocol and preliminary report from a pilot study. Urol Int. 2014;92(1):41-9.

16. Hariharan U, Shah SB. Venous thromboembolism and robotic surgery: Need for prophylaxis and review of literature. J Hematol Thrombo Dis. 2015;3:227.

17. Holzbeierlein JM, Smith JA. Radical prostatectomy and collaborative care pathways. Semin Urol Oncol. 2000;18(1):60-5.

18. Lestar M, Gunnarsson L, Lagerstrand L, Wiklund P, Odeberg-Wernerman S. Hemodynamic perturbations during robot-assisted laparoscopic radical prostatectomy in 45° Trendelenburg position. Anesth Analg. 2011;113(5):1069-75.

19. Meininger D, Byhahn C, Mierdl S, Westphal K, Zwissler B. Positive end-expiratory pressure improves arterial oxygenation during prolonged pneumoperitoneum. Acta Anaesthesiol Scand. 2005;49(6):778-83.

20. Shah SB, Bhargava AK, Chowdhury I. Noninvasive intracranial pressure monitoring via optic nerve sheath diameter for robotic surgery in steep Trendelenburg position. Saudi J Anaesth. 2015;9(3):239-46.

21. Awad H, Santilli S, Ohr M, Roth A, Yan W, Fernandez S, et al. The effects of steep Trendelenburg positioning on intraocular pressure during robotic radical prostatectomy. Anesth Analg. 2009;109(2):473-8.

22. Kim DH, Kim H, Kwak S, Baek K, Na G, Kim JH, et al. The settings, pros and cons of the new surgical robot da Vinci Xi system for transoral robotic surgery (TORS): A comparison with the popular da Vinci Si system. Surg Laparosc Endosc Percutan Tech. 2016;26(5):391-6.

23. Umemura S, Kawabata K, Sasaki K. In vivo acceleration of ultrasonic tissue heating by microbubble agent. IEEE Trans Ultrason Ferroelectr Freq Control. 2005;52(10):1690-8.

24. Yao CL, Trinh T, Wong GT, Irwin MG. Anaesthesia for high intensity focused ultrasound (HIFU) therapy. Anaesthesia. 2008;63(8):865-72.

25. Roberts T. The post-anaesthetic scoring system (PASS): A new assessment aid for the recovery room. Br J Anaesth Recovery Nursing. 2010;11(3):59-64.

26. Cui Y, Chen H, Qi L, Zu X, Li Y. Effect of alvimopan on accelerates gastrointestinal recovery after radical cystectomy: A systematic review and meta-analysis. Int J Surg. 2016;25:1-6.

27. Clyne M. Bladder cancer: Faster recovery after radical cystectomy with alvimopan. Nat Rev Urol. 2014;11(4):186.

28. Lee CT, Chang SS, Kamat AM, Amiel G, Beard TL, Fergany A, et al. Alvimopan accelerates gastrointestinal recovery after radical cystectomy: A multicenter randomized placebo-controlled trial. Eur Urol. 2014;66(2):265-72.

29. Persson B, Carringer M, Andrén O, Andersson SO, Carlsson J, Ljungqvist O. Initial experiences with the enhanced recovery after surgery (ERAS) protocol in open radical cystectomy. Scand J Urol. 2015;49(4):302-7.

30. Nabhani J, Ahmadi H, Schuckman AK, Cai J, Miranda G, Djaladat H, et al. Cost analysis of the enhanced recovery after surgery protocol in patients undergoing radical cystectomy for bladder cancer. Eur Urol Focus. 2016;2(1):92-6.

31. Karl A, Buchner A, Becker A, Staehler M, Seitz M, Khoder W, et al. A new concept for early recovery after surgery for patients undergoing radical cystectomy for bladder cancer: Results of a prospective randomized study. J Urol. 2014;191(2):335-40.

32. Guan X, Liu L, Lei X, Zu X, Li Y, Chen M, et al. A comparative study of fast-track versus conventional surgery in patients undergoing laparoscopic radical cystectomy and ileal conduit diversion: Chinese experience. Sci Rep. 2014;4:6820.

33. Saar M, Ohlmann CH, Siemer S, Lehmann J, Becker F, Stöckle M, et al. Fast-track rehabilitation after robot-assisted laparoscopic cystectomy accelerates postoperative recovery. BJU Int. 2013;112(2):E99-106.

34. Chang SS, Cole E, Smith JA Jr, Baumgartner R, Wells N, Cookson MS. Safely reducing length of stay after open radical retropubic prostatectomy under the guidance of a clinical care pathway. Cancer. 2005;104(4):747-51.

35. Lin C, Wan F, Lu Y, Li G, Yu L, Wang M. Enhanced recovery after surgery protocol for prostate cancer patients undergoing laparoscopic radical prostatectomy. J Int Med Res. 2019;47(1):114-21.

36. Kripalani S, Theobald CN, Anctil B, Vasilevskis EE. Reducing hospital readmission rates: Current strategies and future directions. Annu Rev Med. 2014;65:471-85.

37. Brooke BS, Stone DH, Cronenwett JL, Nolan B, DeMartino RR, MacKenzie TA, et al. Early primary care provider follow-up and readmission after high-risk surgery. JAMA Surg. 2014;149(8):821-8.

38. Kashiwagi DT, Burton MC, Kirkland LL, Cha S, Varkey P. Do timely outpatient follow-up visits decrease hospital readmission rates? Am J Med Qual. 2012;27(1):11-5.

39. Viers BR, Lightner DJ, Rivera ME, Tollefson MK, Boorjian SA, Karnes RJ, et al. Efficiency, satisfaction, and costs for remote video visits following radical prostatectomy: A randomized controlled trial. Eur Urol. 2015;68(4):729-35.

40. Tabibi A, Simforoosh N, Basiri A, Ezzatnejad M, Abdi H, Farrokhi F. Bowel preparation versus no preparation before ileal urinary diversion. Urology. 2007;70(4):654-8.

41. Maffezzini M, Campodonico F, Capponi G, Manuputty E, Gerbi G. Fast-track surgery and technical nuances to reduce complications after radical cystectomy and intestinal urinary diversion with the modified Indiana pouch. Surg Oncol. 2012;21(3):191-5.

42. Daneshmand S, Ahmadi H, Schuckman AK, Mitra AP, Cai J, Miranda G, et al. Enhanced recovery protocol after radical cystectomy for bladder cancer. J Urol. 2014;192(1):50-5.

43. Tyson MD, Chang SS. Enhanced recovery pathways versus standard care after cystectomy: A meta-analysis of the effect on perioperative outcomes. Eur Urol. 2016;70(6):995-1003.

44. Xu W, Daneshmand S, Bazargani ST, Cai J, Miranda G, Schuckman AK, et al. Postoperative pain management after radical cystectomy: Comparing traditional versus enhanced recovery protocol pathway. J Urol. 2015;194(5):1209-13.

45. Smith J, Meng ZW, Lockyer R, Dudderidge T, McGrath J, Hayes M, et al. Evolution of the Southampton Enhanced Recovery Programme for radical cystectomy and the aggregation of marginal gains. BJU Int. 2014;114(3):375-83.

Perioperative Management of Renal Tumor Surgeries/Nephrectomy

Jyotsna Goswami, Anshuman Sarkar, Sudipta Mukherjee

INTRODUCTION

Global incidence of carcinoma of kidney is 4.4 per 100,000.[1] American Cancer Society estimated that 73,820 new cases of kidney cancer will be diagnosed in 2019 in the US, primarily renal cell carcinoma (RCC).[2] The remainder is transitional cell carcinoma and Wilms tumor in children. Incidence is almost twice as much in men than in women, which accounts for 5% and 3% of all cancer respectively.[3,4] Incidence rate in India is lower than in Europe, North America, and Australia.[5] Incidence rate has increased since 1975, which may be due to more frequent detection by medical imaging.[2]

ETIOLOGY

Multiple environmental and genetic risk factors for RCC have been described. Smoking is the most common factor, which almost doubles the risk in dose-dependent manner. Other common etiologies are obesity and hypertension. The other established risk factors are occupational exposure to certain chemicals like trichloroethylene, benzene, benzidine, cadmium, herbicides, and vinyl chloride. Regarding long-term use of analgesics, Choueiri TK et al. in their meta-analysis, concluded that acetaminophen and nonsteroidal anti-inflammatory drugs (NSAIDs) may increase the risk.[6] Whereas Karami et al. did not find any positive association with aspirin and NSAIDs unlike acetaminophen.[7] Long-term dialysis leading to acute cystic disease of the kidney is a predisposing factor RCC. Chronic hepatitis C[8] and renal stones in males have been reported[9] to be associated with RCC. Some genetic disorders like von Hippel-Lindau syndrome,[10,11] hereditary papillary renal carcinoma, Birt-Hogg-Dube syndrome, and hereditary renal carcinoma[12] can be associated with RCC.

CLINICAL PRESENTATION

Renal cell carcinoma typically presents in the sixth and seventh decades of life.[13] As compared to the Western population, the mean age at diagnosis in Indian population is lower.[14] Symptoms associated with RCC can be due to local tumor growth, hemorrhage, paraneoplastic syndromes or metastatic disease. More than 40% of these tumors are detected incidentally by noninvasive testing for evaluation of nonspecific symptoms. The classic triad of flank pain, gross hematuria, and palpable abdominal mass is now rarely found. Patients with distant metastasis may present with cough, bone pain, cervical lymphadenopathy and constitutional symptoms such as weight loss, fever, and night sweats. 20% of the patients present with paraneoplastic syndromes of which notable are hypercalcemia, hypertension, and polycythemia and nonmetastatic hepatic dysfunction.

Angiogenic property of the tumor increases the propensity for vascular invasion and formation of venous tumor thrombus (TT). Involvement of the venous system with RCC occurs in 4–10% of patients. Tumors invading the inferior vena cava (IVC) and causing vena caval obstruction may present with bilateral lower extremity edema and nonreducing or right-sided varicocele, dilated superficial abdominal veins, pulmonary embolism or right atrial mass.

The staging of RCC has been described by the American Joint Committee on Cancer (AJCC) tumor-node-metastasis (TNM) system,[15] which is based on three parameters **(Table 1)**: (1) the size of the primary tumor (T) and its spread into adjacent areas; (2) spread to regional lymph nodes (N); and (3) metastasis to other organs (M), i.e., the bones, brain, and lungs.

Extension of TT into IVC and Atrium

Renal cell carcinoma has the tendency of invasion into the vessels or IVC (in 10% cases), which may extend up to right atrium (RA; in 2% cases).[16] Four levels of TT have been described[17] **(Table 2)**. Metastasis or extension of TT into IVC does not preclude surgery, which improves prognosis and quality of life. Five-year survival rate was reported

Table 1: Tumor-node-metastasis (TNM) classification.[17]	
T1	Tumor ≤7 cm, confined to the kidney
T1a	<4 cm
T1b	>4 cm
T2	Tumor >7 cm, confined to the kidney
T2a	≤10 cm
T2b	>10 cm
T3	Tumor extends into major veins or perinephric tissues but not into adrenal gland or beyond Gerota's fascia
T3a	Extends into renal vein or branches or perirenal sinus fat but not beyond Gerota's fascia
T3b	Extends into vena cava below the diaphragm
T3c	Extends into vena cava above the diaphragm or invades the wall of the vena cava
T4	Tumor invades beyond Gerota's fascia including into the adrenal gland
N0	No regional lymph node metastasis
N1	Metastasis in regional lymph node
M0	No distant metastasis
M1	Distant metastasis

Anatomic stage/prognostic groups			
Stage I	T1	N0	M0
Stage II	T2	N0	M0
Stage III	T1 or T2	N1	M0
	T3	N0 or N1	M0
Stage IV	T4	Any N	Any M
	Any T		M1

Table 2: Vena cava extension of tumor thrombus in renal cell carcinoma (RCC).[17]	
Levels	*Thrombus extension*
0	Thrombus limited to renal vein
I	Thrombus extending ≤2 cm above the renal vein
II	Thrombus extending >2 cm above the renal vein, but below the hepatic veins
III	Thrombus at the level of or above the hepatic veins but below the diaphragm
IV	Thrombus extending above the diaphragm

as 87%, 88%, 72%, and 46% for grade I, II, III, and IV RCC respectively.[16]

SURGICAL APPROACH AND ITS IMPLICATION

Surgery remains the mainstay for curative treatment. The surgical approach is individualized depending upon the stage of the disease, location of the tumor, preoperative baseline renal function, the presence of bilateral pathology, and surgeon preference.[16]

Open Radical Nephrectomy

It is the preferred option for patients with stage I, II, and III disease. Various incisions can be used for this surgery, i.e., flank, thoracoabdominal, and transabdominal (chevron or anterior subcostal). An extended subcostal incision using transperitoneal approach is preferred commonly. The thoracoabdominal approach is employed occasionally in case of very large and potentially invasive tumors involving the upper portion of the kidney.

Patients undergoing radical nephrectomy (RN) are left with significantly reduced renal reserve and at higher risk of developing moderately severe chronic kidney disease (CKD), especially in presence of underlying preoperative renal dysfunction. Lau et al. has reported that 22% and 11.6% of patients that underwent RN and partial nephrectomy (PN) respectively, develop chronic renal failure within 10 years following surgery.[18]

Partial Nephrectomy

Partial nephrectomy is indicated for the patients with: (a) tumor smaller than 7 cm in diameter; (b) tumor location at one pole; and (c) situations where RN will render the patient anephric; or (d) at high risk for requirement of dialysis such as those with bilateral disease or tumor involving a solitary functioning kidney. This can be performed by both open and laparoscopic or robotic techniques.

This "nephron sparing" surgical intervention targets better postoperative renal function in view of preserved glomerular filtration rate (GFR). However vascular clamping during the procedure leads to decreased blood flow, which may cause ischemic injury to healthy normal renal parenchyma. This damage depends on type (warm/cold) and duration of ischemia, age, body habitus, background, comorbidities (hypertension, diabetes and other systemic disease), and underlying CKD or previous history of renal surgery. This ischemic insult is the primary predictor of renal failure after nephron sparing surgery.[19] Studies have shown that PN for a renal tumor less than 7 cm rarely results in temporary or permanent renal failure; average loss of renal function over time was 8.8%.[20] Decreasing renal ischemia time during PN is an important intervention to preserve renal function. Usually normothermic (warm) ischemia up to 30 minutes (without specific renal protection) is recommended. In view of anticipated prolonged vascular clamping, cold ischemia has been used liberally for open PN, i.e., surface cooling of kidney to decrease medullary temperature to 15–20°C can increase safety margin to 60–70 minutes.[21] A cold ischemia time (CIT) <44 minutes significantly decreases chance of long-term renal insult,[22] even though there may be some early postsurgical estimated GFR change. This safe margin of ischemia time will be further less in solitary kidney (warm ischemia cut off <25 minutes). Intermittent renal arterial occlusion should be avoided for potential of arterial vasospasm and renal damage.

The loss of function of the operated kidney was found to depend on the maximum thickness of resected healthy parenchyma and more significantly on warm ischemia time (WIT), with worsening outcome with WIT >32 minutes.[23] Residual renal function usually stabilizes between 3 weeks and 3 months and remains at that level for a prolonged period, up to 4 years. The longer the period of decline in renal function after PN, the worse the nadir and the ultimate GFR.

Laparoscopic/Hand-Assisted/Robotic Surgery

Laparoscopic RN provides a less morbid alternative to open surgery providing equivalent oncologic outcomes. This technique is useful in tumors with low-to-moderate-volume (10 cm or smaller), localized with no local invasion, limited or no renal vein involvement, and manageable lymphadenopathy. These minimally invasive procedures require pneumoperitoneum and steep Trendelenburg position. Patients with severe ischemic or valvular heart disease and increased intracranial pressure may not tolerate these procedures.

Laparoscopic partial nephrectomy (LPN) usually needs longer ischemia time compared to open partial nephrectomy (OPN). Some modifications of surgical technique emerged to improve postoperative renal outcome, especially in LPN. These are the early unclamping technique, off-clamp PN, PN with selective clamping, laparoscopic or robotic "zero ischemia" PN, preoperative superselective embolization of feeding renal artery, etc. But while compared with traditional techniques with restricted WIT within a safe zone, these techniques provide doubtful advantage in terms of renal preservation.

▌PREANESTHESIA ASSESSMENT

Preoperative assessment for various types of nephrectomy should be directed to the impact of the surgery on the renal function in the postoperative period in addition to other concerns of the major surgery.

Important preoperative considerations for the assessing anesthesiologist are:

- These patients are usually in their sixth and seventh decades of life and may have associated cardiorespiratory comorbidities. Assessment of functional status is of paramount importance.
- Patients undergoing RN are at risk of developing postoperative renal insufficiency, which in turn is associated with morbid cardiovascular events and increased mortality rates.[24]

- Chemotherapy is not a routine preoperative therapy as expression of multidrug resistance proteins lead to the chemorefractoriness of RCC. So usual assessment of the impact of chemotherapy is not required during preanesthesia assessment.
- Surgical positions may have cardiopulmonary effects and risk of perioperative peripheral neuropathy. When deemed appropriate, the anesthesiologist must ensure that the patient can comfortably tolerate the anticipated operative position.
- Since tobacco exposure is one of the generally accepted environmental risk factors for RCC, detailed elucidation of the addiction history, proper counseling, and beneficial effects of smoking cessation program should be discussed.
- Twenty percent of the patients present with paraneoplastic syndromes. Hypercalcemia has been reported in up to 13% of patients with RCC and Stauffer syndrome or nonmetastatic hepatic dysfunction has been reported in 3–20% of cases. Other than raised liver enzymes, these patients may have an elevated prothrombin time and thrombocytopenia.

Routine preoperative tests include complete blood count, serum urea, creatinine, sodium, potassium and calcium, routine urine analysis, liver function tests, prothrombin time and international normalized ratio (INR), 12-lead electrocardiogram (ECG), and two-dimensional (2D) echocardiography.

Further investigations like cardiopulmonary exercise testing, noninvasive stress tests, pulmonary function tests, and cardiology or pulmonology referral should be guided by history and detailed physical examination. If clinical symptoms are consistent with deep venous thrombosis of the lower extremities, a Doppler ultrasound is indicated to assess the venous patency of the lower extremities.

In addition to this, a thorough review of the surgical assessment, preoperative radiological assessment and coordination with the surgical team regarding the presence of synchronous metastasis, venous TT and its cephalad extension, and the intended surgical approach is essential. Magnetic resonance imaging (MRI) is the preferred diagnostic modality for demonstrating both the presence and the cephalad extent of vena caval involvement. The preoperative imaging should be obtained as close as possible to the date of surgery because progression of the TT may mandate important changes in intraoperative management.

Preoperative pulmonary embolism does not necessitate deferral of surgical management of the venous TT. Cardiothoracic surgery backup is needed for patients with level III and IV tumor thrombi that are expected to require either venovenous bypass or cardiopulmonary bypass (CPB) with or without circulatory arrest.

PREOPERATIVE PREPARATION

- Preoperative counseling and risk explanation
- Optimization of pre-existing medical conditions
- Adequate quantities of blood products should be kept ready
- Thromboprophylaxis.

As per the European Association of Urology guidelines on thromboprophylaxis,[25] there is weak and low-quality evidence favoring mechanical prophylaxis in all patients. Although pharmacological prophylaxis has weak and low-quality evidence for use in open nephrectomies including those with thrombectomy, it has strong evidence for patients those are at risk of venous thromboembolism prophylaxis (VTE).

Inferior vena cava filters are not much into practice now in surgical candidates with venous TT as these devices increase the surgical complexity of thrombectomy and can become incorporated in the tumor but if it is needed, should be inserted within 48 hours of the surgery so that the filter cannot be infiltrated with TT.[26]

INTRAOPERATIVE

Positioning

Surgical positioning may vary as per surgical approach, but commonly both open and laparoscopic nephrectomy are performed in lateral position with varying degrees of tilt at waist. Therefore, adequate padding and support is necessary to prevent position-related complications, i.e., pressure sore, nerve damage, venous pooling, corneal abrasion, and venous congestion. Lateral positioning with Trendelenburg tilt also compromises lung function. There will be reduced functional residual volume (FRC), development of basal atelectasis leading to increased ventilation perfusion (VQ) mismatch. Pneumoperitoneum created during laparoscopic approach will further compromise this pulmonary function. It decreases venous return and cardiac output particularly if the intra-abdominal pressure is more than 20 mm Hg and/or patient has a compromised cardiac function. Pneumoperitoneum leads to decrease in renal blood flow, which is also influenced by pressure used for insufflation (>10 mm Hg), positioning (worst in the head-up position), and the fluid status of the patient. Renal physiology is also affected by carbon dioxide absorption, neuroendocrine factors and tissue damage from oxidative stress.[27]

Maintenance of Normothermia

Hypothermia should be prevented by all means: Prewarming with forced air warmer prevents redistribution hypothermia. Active warming should be initiated early and should be continued throughout the surgical procedure with a forced-air warmer, heated mattress, and fluid warmer.[28]

Analgesia

Multimodal analgesia is recommended. NSAIDs should preferably be avoided because of their nephrotoxicity. Thoracic epidural analgesia (TEA) is the most effective mode of analgesia in open approaches. Thoracic paravertebral block provides equivalent analgesia and can be considered as an alternative to TEA with favorable side effect profile.[29] In laparoscopic or robot-assisted approaches, epidural has gone out of favor because of its risk-benefit imbalance. Risks of delayed identification of compartment syndrome of the lower limbs especially in robotic surgery, side effects such as hypotension and epidural hematoma outweighs benefit of postoperative analgesia (less analgesic requirement compared to open surgery). This modality is largely replaced by newer muscle plane blocks such as transversus abdominis plane (TAP) block, quadratus lumborum (QL) block, erector spinae block, etc., which are used as part of multimodal opioid-sparing analgesia in minimal access surgery. However, adequate high-quality evidence favoring their routine use is still lacking. Wound catheter and local infiltration analgesia can also be included as part of multimodal analgesia.

Monitors

For a standard RN to treat a stage I tumor in American Society of Anesthesiologists (ASA) I patient, standard ASA monitors may suffice. More complex surgeries in patients with higher risks mandate invasive monitoring (central venous access and arterial line placement). There is major risk of bleeding, coagulopathy, and potential need of CPB. Therefore, monitoring should be directed according to the complexity of the surgery, anticipated blood loss, and comorbid status of the patients. Noninvasive cardiac output monitoring may be useful for hemodynamic monitoring and intraoperative fluid optimization.[30] Intraoperative monitoring of pulmonary artery pressure (PAP) may not be ideal as there is unknown risk of thrombus dislodgement, interference with surgery, and potential of false readings with mass in RA.[31] For level II-IV tumor thrombi, intraoperative transesophageal echocardiography (TEE) may be an useful tool to delineate the level of the thrombus prior to incision, characterization of the nature of the thrombus, assessment for thrombus embolization during IVC manipulation, as well as assessment of cardiac function.

Prevention of Ischemic Injury during PN

Duration of renal ischemia is the strongest modifiable risk factor for renal insufficiency after PN.[20] When clamping of the renal artery is required, in situ renal hypothermia by surface cooling of the kidney with ice slush for 10–15 minutes immediately after the renal artery is occluded is done to protect against ischemic renal injury. This allows up to 3 hours of safe ischemia without permanent renal injury. Prior to temporary renal artery occlusion, intravenous mannitol is administered.

Vascular Control

Anesthesiologists should be aware of the critical steps involved in achieving vascular control in patients with venous TT. After the exposure of the affected kidney and the anterior surface of the IVC and aorta, the renal artery is ligated, which reduces blood flow through venous collaterals and potentially limits blood loss.

In case of minimal extension into the IVC, the thrombus is milked back into the renal vein. Then a vascular clamp is placed around the renal vein ostium to avoid occluding the IVC completely and the thrombus can be isolated.

In case of level II tumor thrombi, IVC and the contralateral renal vein are mobilized to allow vascular control both above and below the TT. Once the IVC is circumferentially mobilized, vascular clamps are placed sequentially on the suprarenal IVC proximal to the cephalad extent of the thrombus, then on the contralateral renal vein, and lastly on the infrarenal IVC. A test clamp should be performed, as the IVC is cross-clamped initially to ensure the patient is able to remain hemodynamically stable during this procedure. In most cases when clamping below the hepatic venous confluence, bypass is not necessarily due to collateral venous return via the lumbar system and portal venous system for level II tumor thrombi. The lumen of the IVC is then inspected for residual TT, is flushed, ensuring that all thrombus and air is aspirated from the IVC lumen prior to completion of the cavorrhaphy. This is performed by placing the operative bed in the Trendelenburg position, then releasing the infrarenal clamp to allow back-bleeding prior to completing the cavorrhaphy.

Level III of TT necessitates precise characterization of the tumor level on preoperative imaging and intraoperative TEE. Although it is possible to obtain control of the suprahepatic IVC, permitting complete surgical excision of a level III TT, mobilization of the liver may be necessary, and involvement of a hepatobiliary or transplant surgeon may be helpful for this part of the procedure. IVC cross-clamp along with Pringle maneuver results in hemodynamic instability as there is insufficient venous return or substantial blood loss from venous collaterals. A test clamp is recommended prior to proceeding with cavotomy. In the case of significant hypotension, vascular bypass via either CPB with hypothermic cardiac arrest or venovenous bypass is indicated.

Level IV or supradiaphragmatic thrombi generally necessitate involvement of cardiothoracic surgery with CPB and hypothermic circulatory arrest. However, venovenous bypass may be utilized following mobilization of the liver if the thrombus is free floating and is able to be reduced below the diaphragm.

POSTOPERATIVE PERIOD

Postoperative complication rate of surgery for RCC is about 20%,[30] which could be due to pre-existing comorbidity or due to intra or postoperative complications. Immediate postoperative complications like vascular injury, splenic injury, bowel injury, etc., that need to be carefully monitored and taken for re-exploration. Subcutaneous emphysema or pneumothorax that develops after pneumoperitoneum usually treated with high flow oxygen with or without intercostal tube drainage along with intense monitoring for progression of complication. Other uncommon surgical complications like bowel obstruction or perforation, peritonitis, etc., may present in early postoperative period, which need prompt intervention.

Mortality after nephrectomy is rare (<0.5%) and mostly it is because of pulmonary embolism and myocardial infarction; so strict vigilance for these complications in postoperative phase is very important.

Postoperative acute renal failure is a serious concern, especially patients with background of CKD, bilateral malignancy requiring intervention or aorta caval involvement (prolonged cross-clamping of IVC or bypass). Renal function recovers with time in a certain subgroup of patients. Acute renal failure may progress to chronic renal failure, which is a late complication. Renal replacement therapy may be needed in the long run. High-risk patients should be counseled properly regarding the anticipated complications.

The cardiopulmonary decompensation, which may occur intraoperatively, may continue in postoperative period. Optimal supportive care is needed to resume normal physiology.[27]

Impaired hepatic venous return and hepatic ischemia can cause accumulation of toxic metabolites and hepatic failure.

Assessment of Postoperative Renal Function

Serum creatinine is most commonly used to measure postoperative renal function, but it is strongly influenced by age, sex, and muscle mass. A healthy contralateral kidney may falsely produce a normal creatinine value. Calculation of GFR as marker of renal function [24 hours urinary creatinine clearance, Cockcroft-Gault formula, the Modification of Diet in Renal Disease (MDRD), Chronic

Kidney Disease Epidemiology Collaboration (CKD-EPI) equations] is more accurate technique. Renal scintigraphy using technetium-99m-mercaptoacetylglycylglycine (99mTc-MAG3) is a more reliable method to evaluate split renal function. Role of biomarkers (e.g. neutrophil gelatinase-associated lipocalin—NGAL) in this scenario need further evaluation.[32]

NEPHROPROTECTIVE MEASURES

Strategies to prevent perioperative renal insult are of utmost importance. Patient with partial or RN will have a decrease in effective GFR in postoperative period; having add-on renal injury will make the situation worse. Underlying renal diseases, cardiac diseases, exposure to nephrotoxic agents and renal hypoperfusion are the possible predisposing risk factors[33] that cause worsening of residual renal function. Most important preventive measure is to maintain hemodynamics in the perioperative period in terms of maintaining optimum blood pressure and volume status to prevent renal hypoperfusion. Other measures are avoidance of nephrotoxic drugs, strict glycemic control and appropriate management of postoperative complications (nonrenal acute cardiac dysfunction, hemorrhage, sepsis, rhabdomyolysis and intra-abdominal hypertension). Drugs those have nephrotoxic potential include:

- Antibiotics—aminoglycosides, cephalosporins, amphotericin-B, penicillin, sulfonamides
- Calcium (hypercalcemia)
- Chemotherapeutic or immunosuppressive agents— cisplatin, cyclosporine, tacrolimus, methotrexate, nitrosourea
- Contrast agents
- Nonsteroidal anti-inflammatory drugs
- Pigments—hemoglobin myoglobin.

Ischemic and pharmacological preconditioning has been evaluated for different organs including kidney. Anesthetic agents such as volatile agents can cause ischemic preconditioning. No drug has shown to have a renoprotective effect in perioperative scenario. Different agents have been tried for this purpose such as dopamine, theophylline, fenoldopam, calcium channel blockers, sodium nitroprusside, frusemide, mannitol, natriuretic peptides, N-acetyl cysteine, statins, steroids, etc. None of them have shown any benefit over proper clinical management.

CONCLUSION

Renal cell carcinoma is the most common variety of renal cancer and usually occurs in the fifth to sixth decade of life. Smoking, obesity, and hypertension are the common etiology. Incidentally diagnosed RCC in 40% cases has a

unique feature of invading IVC and sometimes up to RA. Surgical treatment is the curative option and the choice of technique depends on the extent of the tumor and preexisting comorbidities. Surgery has significant morbidity associated with it. Preserving renal function is the main challenge as there is loss of kidney volume.

REFERENCES

1. Mahdavifar N, Mohammadian M, Ghoncheh M, Salehiniya H. Incidence, mortality and risk factors of kidney cancer in the world. World Cancer Res J. 2018;5(1):e1013.

2. American Cancer Society. (2019). Cancer Facts and Figures 2019. [online] Available from https://www.cancer.org/content/dam/cancer-org/research/cancer-facts-and-statistics/annual-cancer-facts-and-figures/2019/cancer-facts-and-figures-2019.pdf. [Last Accessed February, 2020].

3. Siegel RL, Miller KD, Jemal A. Cancer statistics, 2018. CA Cancer J Clin. 2018;68(1):7-30.

4. Capitanio U, Bensalah K, Bex A, Boorjian SA, Bray F, Coleman J, et al. Epidemiology of renal cell carcinoma. Eur Urol. 2019;75(1):74-84.

5. Ray RP, Mahapatra RS, Khullar S, Pal DK, Kundu AK. Clinical characteristics of renal cell carcinoma. Five years review from a tertiary hospital in Eastern India. Indian J Cancer. 2016;53(1):114-7.

6. Choueiri TK, Je Y, Cho E. Analgesic use and the risk of kidney cancer: a meta-analysis of epidemiologic studies. Int J Cancer. 2014;134(2):384-96.

7. Karami S, Daughtery SE, Schwartz K, Davis FG, Ruterbusch JJ, Wacholder S, et al. Analgesic use and risk of renal cell carcinoma: a case-control, cohort and meta-analytic assessment. Int J Cancer. 2016;139(3):584-92.

8. Gonzalez HC, Lamerato L, Rogers CG, Gordon SC. Chronic hepatitis C infection as a risk factor for renal cell carcinoma. Dig Dis Sci. 2015;60(6):1820-4.

9. van de Pol JAA, van den Brandt PA, Schouten LJ. Kidney stones and the risk of renal cell carcinoma and upper tract urothelial carcinoma: the Netherlands Cohort Study. Br J Cancer. 2019;120(3):368-74.

10. William G, Kaelin Jr. The von Hippel-Lindau tumor suppressor gene and kidney cancer. Clinical Cancer Research. 2004;10(18):6290s-5s.

11. Tsang SH, Sharma T. von Hippel-Lindau disease. Atlas of inherited retinal diseases. 2018;1085:201-3.

12. Maher ER. Hereditary renal cell carcinoma syndromes: diagnosis, surveillance and management. World J Urol. 2018;36(12):1891-8.

13. Joshi A, Anand A, Prabhash K, Noronha V, Shrirangwar S, Bakshi G, et al. Kidney cancer demographics and outcome data from 2013 at a tertiary cancer hospital in India. Indian J Cancer. 2017;54(4):601-4.

14. Agnihotri S, Kumar J, Jain M, Kapoor R, Mandhani A. Renal cell carcinoma in India demonstrates early age of onset and a late stage of presentation. Indian J Med Res. 2014;140(5):624-9.

15. Kim SP, Alt AL, Weight CJ, Costello BA, Cheville JC, Lohse C, et al. Independent validation of the 2010 American Joint Committee on Cancer TNM classification for renal cell carcinoma: Results from a large, single institution cohort. J Urol. 2011;185(6): 2035-9.

16. Chapman E, Pichel AC. Anaesthesia for nephrectomy. BJA Educ. 2016;16:98-101.

17. Blute M, Leibovich B, Lohse C, Cheville J, Zincke H. The Mayo Clinic experience with surgical management, complications and outcome for patients with renal cell carcinoma and venous tumour thrombus. BJU Int. 2004;94(1):33-41.

18. Lau W, Blute M, Weaver A, Torres V, Zincke H. Matched comparison of radical nephrectomy vs nephron-sparing surgery in patients with unilateral renal cell carcinoma and a normal contralateral kidney. Mayo Clin Proc. 2000;75(12):1236-42.

19. Volpe A, Blute M, Ficarra V, Gill I, Kutikov A, Porpiglia F, et al. Renal ischemia and function after partial nephrectomy: A collaborative review of the literature. Eur Urol. 2015;68(3):61-74.

20. Lane B, Babineau D, Poggio E, Weight C, Larson B, Gill I, et al. Factors predicting renal functional outcome after partial nephrectomy. J Urol. 2008;180(6):2363-9.

21. Marberger M. Renal ischemia: not a problem in laparoscopic partial nephrectomy? BJU Int. 2007;99(1):3-4.

22. Iida S, Kondo T, Amano H, Nakazawa H, Ito F, Hashimoto Y, et al. Minimal effect of cold ischemia time on progression to late-stage chronic kidney disease observed long term after partial nephrectomy. Urology. 2008;72:1083-8.

23. Porpiglia F, Renard J, Billia M, Musso F, Volpe A, Burruni R, et al. Is renal warm ischemia over 30 minutes during laparoscopic partial nephrectomy possible? One-year results of a prospective study. Eur Urol. 2007;52(4):1170-8.

24. Huang W, Levey A, Serio A, Snyder M, Vickers A, Raj G, et al. Chronic kidney disease after nephrectomy in patients with renal cortical tumors: a retrospective cohort study. Lancet Oncol. 2006;7(9):735-40.

25. Tikkinen K, Cartwrighht R, Gould M, Naspro R, Novara G, Sandset P, et al. (2018). EAU guidelines on thromboprophylaxis in urological surgery. [online] Available from https//uroweb. org/Guidelines-on-thromboprophylaxis 2018. [Last Accessed, February, 2020].

26. Woodruff DY, Van Veldhuizen P, Muehlebach G, Johnson P, Williamson T, Holzbeierlein JM. The perioperative management of an inferior vena caval tumor thrombus in patients with renal cell carcinoma. Urol Oncol Semin Orig Investig. 2013;31: 517-21.

27. Sodha S, Nazarian S, Adshead J, Vasdev N, Mohan SG. Effect of pneumoperitoneum on renal function and physiology in patients undergoing robotic renal surgery. Curr Urol. 2016;9(1):1-4.

28. Horn E, Bein B, Broch O, Iden T, Bohm R, Latz S, et al. Warming before and after epidural block before general anaesthesia for major abdominal surgery prevents perioperative hypothermia: a randomised controlled trial. EJA. 2016;33(5):334-40.

29. Baik J, Oh A, Cho C, Shin H, Han S, Ryu J. Thoracic paravertebral block for nephrectomy: a randomized, controlled, observer-blinded study. Pain Med. 2014;15(5):850-6.

30. Stapleton C, Duffy C, Duplisea J. Perioperative management of the genitourinary oncologic patient undergoing partial/radical nephrectomy. Oncol Crit Care. 2019;1-11.

31. Morita Y, Ayabe K, Nurok M, Young J. Perioperative anesthetic management for renal cell carcinoma with vena caval thrombus extending into the right atrium: case series. J Clin Anesth. 2017;36:39-46.

32. Vanmassenhove J, Vanholder R, Nagler E, Van Biesen W. Urinary and serum biomarkers for the diagnosis of acute kidney injury: an in-depth review of the literature. Nephrol Dial Transplant. 2013;28(2):254-73.

33. Bajwa S, Sharma V. Peri-operative renal protection: The strategies revisited. Indian J Urol. 2012;28(3):248-55.

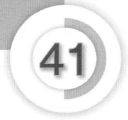
Perioperative Management of Adrenal and Extra-adrenal Pheochromocytoma

Sushil Ambesh, Amit Rastogi

INTRODUCTION

Pheochromocytomas are neuroendocrine tumors that have the potential to secrete catecholamines arising from chromaffin cells of the sympathetic adrenal medulla. Nonadrenal paragangliomas are neuroendocrine tumors arising from extra-adrenal paraganglia. The term "pheochromocytoma" is coined from the Greek words *phaios* dark, *chroma* color, *kytos* cell, and *-oma* tumor. Pheochromocytomas are derived from the adrenal gland; paragangliomas arise from parasympathetic-associated tissues, most commonly along the cranial nerves and vagus, e.g., glomus tumors, chemodectoma, and carotid body tumor, and from extra-adrenal sympathetic-associated chromaffin tissue, often designated as extra-adrenal pheochromocytomas. While paragangliomas arise mainly from chromaffin tissue adjacent to sympathetic ganglia in the abdomen and less commonly in the chest or pelvis, both adrenal and extra-adrenal tumors display similar histopathological characteristics. Extra-adrenal pheochromocytomas or paragangliomas are usually found intra-abdominally along the sympathetic chains or from the organs of Zuckerkandl. Occasionally, they may spread to other organs, known as malignant pheochromocytoma or paraganglioma.

There are probably few names that have not been used to describe the notoriousness of pheochromocytoma—from somewhat complimenting "great masquerader" to unflattering "treacherous murderer." These apparently "mixed feelings" relate to the rarity of disease. Pheochromocytoma can occur at any age, but most often it is reported in the fourth and fifth decades of life, and it occurs equally in men and women. Though the prevalence of pheochromocytoma in the general population of India is not precisely known, its reported incidence in the United States of America is about 1–2 per 100,000 adults/year.[1] The World Health Organization defines pheochromocytoma as

a tumor which is arising from catecholamine-producing chromaffin cells in the adrenal medulla—an intra-adrenal paraganglioma.[2,3] The adrenal medulla secretes two important chemical mediators, namely adrenaline and noradrenaline. Both of these mediators are responsible for blood pressure regulation, blood flow, and acute response to stress. Adrenal medulla is also a type of specialized paraganglion, specifically the sympathetic nervous system. Paraganglia are found in various locations in the body—head, neck, thorax, near the vertebral column, large blood vessels such as aorta, close to internal organs such as bladder and abdomen, and in close association with the autonomic nervous system. Intrathoracic pheochromocytomas, a rare entity, are also related to the sympathetic chain. Other extra-adrenal sites could be intrapericardial, interatrial septum, prostate, and urinary bladder. Autopsy studies have shown that significant numbers of pheochromocytomas remain undiagnosed until death and that up to 50% of these unrecognized tumors may have contributed to patient death.[4] Occasionally, occult pheochromocytoma may be associated with hyperparathyroidism and may present hypertensive crisis, a life-threatening emergency, during the perioperative period of thyroid surgery.[5]

ETIOLOGY

The majority of pheochromocytomas are found sporadically and around one-third of cases have specific gene mutations that are usually inherited as autosomal-dominant. They may also be associated with multiple endocrine neoplasia 2A and 2B, Von Hippel–Lindau disease, hereditary paraganglioma syndrome, and neurofibromatosis type 1. Historically, "Rule of 10s" was used for pheochromocytoma which explains that 10% of pheochromocytoma are "extra-adrenal," 10% are malignant, 10% are bilateral, and 10% are familial.[6] But now this statement is not absolutely true since at least 32% of pheochromocytomas and paragangliomas are familial and in familial disease, more than 80% are bilateral or multiple sites. The malignant pheochromocytoma incidence is seen to be around 10–17%.[7]

Symptoms of Pheochromocytomas

The classic symptoms of a pheochromocytoma are headache, palpitation, pallor, orthostatic hypotension, and sweating. Hypertension is seen in and around 90% of cases though it is paroxysmal in 35–50% of cases. The symptoms usually appear suddenly lasting for few minutes to several hours. However, these symptoms are nonspecific and can also occur gradually. Pheochromocytoma may also present with nonspecific symptoms such as chest pain, lethargy, anxiety, nausea, weight loss, polyuria, polydipsia tremors, and hyperglycemia. Other associated symptoms could be abdominal pain secondary to gut ischemia and visual disturbances due to malignant hypertension causing papilledema. Paragangliomas may also be diagnosed as swelling in certain parts of the body arising from the head or neck area.

DIAGNOSIS

Biochemical Investigations

Pheochromocytoma tumors produce epinephrine, norepinephrine, and rarely dopamine **(Flowchart 1)**.

Pheochromocytoma diagnosis is done by 24-hour urine estimation of catecholamines and vanillylmandelic acid (VMA) and blood estimation of the plasma level of catecholamines. A 24-hour urine sample is required for this purpose since plasma catecholamine has short half-lives. However, nowadays, metanephrine and normetanephrine levels are measured which are degradation products of epinephrine and norepinephrine, respectively. Both urine and plasma levels can be taken for estimation purpose, though the plasma levels are more sensitive and urine levels are, however, more specific. The dopamine-secreting tumors can be identified by estimating plasma or urinary dopamine levels and homovanillic acid levels. The estimation of metanephrine and normetanephrine can give false-positive results under various circumstances such as dietary factors, recent exercise, renal dysfunction, and various other drugs that can interfere with the uptake or metabolism of these catecholamines such as antidepressants, β-blockers, and sympathomimetic drugs.

Imaging

The pheochromocytoma diagnosis is first to be established biochemically followed by confirmation by imaging studies. Ultrasonography of the abdomen can easily identify a tumor or mass in the abdomen, but it is less precise in making accurate diagnosis.

Flowchart 1: Biochemical pathway for catecholamine synthesis.

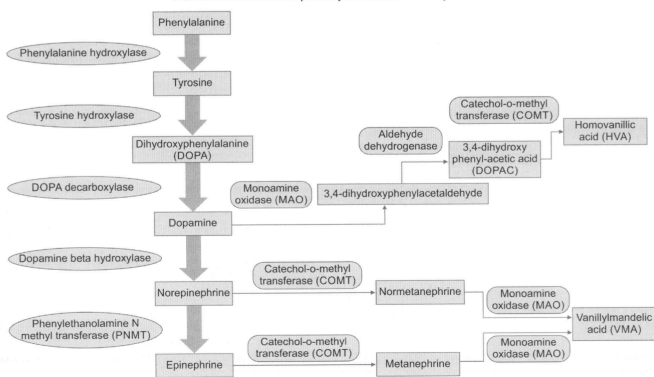

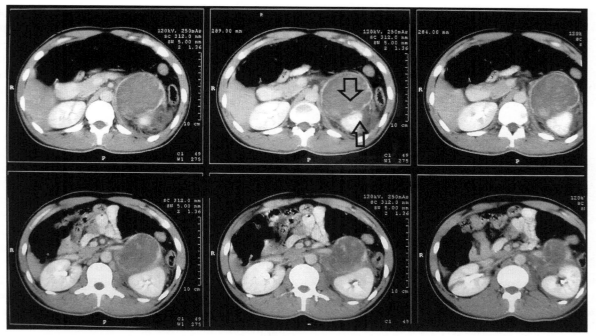

Fig. 1: Computed tomography scan of left-sided suprarenal tumor. The downward arrow in the middle slide of the top row of the CT scan slide shows left-sided pheochromocytoma and the upward arrow shows the left kidney.

Approximately 95% of extra-adrenal pheochromocytomas are found in the abdomen and pelvis.[8] Both computed tomography (CT) scan and magnetic resonance imaging (MRI) are used for localization of tumors once biochemical tests are positive. Both CT scans and MRI have got nearly equal sensitivities, but MRI is more sensitive in recognition of paragangliomas and has got higher specificity **(Fig. 1)**.

During positron emission tomography (PET) scan, a radioactive sugar is injected into the vein followed by body scan. The cancer cell takes sugar much avidly than normal tissue. In this way, the cancer area can be localized. PET is helpful in identification of adrenal tumors and metastasis as well. Functional imaging like scintigraphy is only relevant for preoperative staging in patients with extra-adrenal paragangliomas. A radioactive analogue of norepinephrine is meta-iodobenzylguanidine (MIBG)-123 and it is taken up by catecholamine-producing cells after ingestion. It can be used for diagnosing pheochromocytomas **(Figs. 2 and 3)**. MIBG is appropriate when lesions are bilateral, there is clinical suspicion of malignancy, and when pheochromocytoma cannot be found but strongly suspected.[9,10]

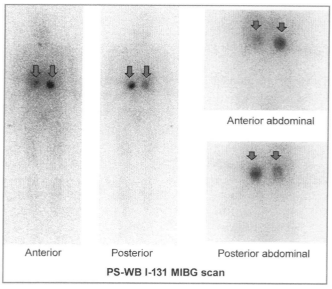

PS-WB I-131 MIBG scan

Fig. 2: MIBG scan of adrenal glands showing bilateral pheochromocytoma. See downward arrows.
(MIBG: meta-iodobenzylguanidine)

these tumors result in wide swings of blood pressure and heart rate beyond extremes.

Earlier, Roizen's criteria were used for preoperative assessment for the management of pheochromocytoma resection surgery which includes the following:

- Blood pressure of <160/90 mm Hg at least 24 hours prior to surgery

PREOPERATIVE PREPARATION

Once the diagnosis of pheochromocytoma is confirmed, appropriate medical management is a must before any operative procedure. During the surgery, manipulation of

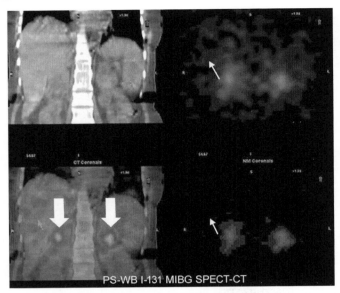

Fig. 3: MIBG SPECT-CT of patient with bilateral pheochromocytoma. See downward arrows.
(MIBG: meta-iodobenzylguanidine; SPECT-CT: single photon emission computed tomography)

- Absence of orthostatic hypotension with blood pressure < 80–45 mm Hg
- No ST-T changes in the electrocardiogram (ECG) for at least a week
- Premature ventricular complexes not more than 1 in 5 minutes

The pharmacological therapy is targeted not only to reduce blood pressure, particularly fluctuations of blood pressure that may occur during the intraoperative period, but also to prevent severe hypotension that immediately occurs following removal of the tumor.

The blood pressure can be controlled with a single antihypertensive agent or combination. Oral drugs commonly used for preoperative treatment[11-16] are:

- α-Adrenoceptor antagonists—phenoxybenzamine, prazosin, doxazosin
- Dihydropyridine calcium channel receptor blockers
- α-Methyltyrosine
- Competitive α- and β-receptor blocking drug—labetalol

The drug dosage is assessed and titrated every 2–3 days until desired therapeutic control of blood pressure is gained. The goal is to reduce blood pressure to normal values with minimal orthostatic hypotension and a heart rate of around 60–70 bpm. Treatment is usually continued for 1–2 weeks till adequate preoperative blood pressure control is achieved.[17-22]

Since this is a sympathetic overactive state, most of the patients are in relatively volume-contracted state; therefore, preoperative hydration and volume expansion are to be optimized before surgery.[23,24] Nonselective

α-adrenergic blockade may result in reflex tachycardia so addition of β-adrenergic blockade is required to prevent tachycardia. However, the β-blocker should never be started alone and always started once α-blockade is achieved, since β-blockade in absence of α-blockade can result in inhibition of β-2 adrenoceptor-mediated vasodilatation and an unopposed α-adrenergic stimulation may cause hypertensive crisis.

Phenoxybenzamine

A nonselective, noncompetitive α-blocker with a prolonged action duration is the most commonly used agent. The α-2 action causes blockade at the presynaptic receptor responsible for regulating noradrenaline secretion from sympathetic nerve terminal causing reflex tachycardia via unopposed β-1 action. The central α-2 action results in headache, somnolence, nasal stuffiness, and headache. This drug's prolonged duration of action also causes hypotension in the postoperative period.[25] In few centers, this drug is stopped and the patient is taken on short-acting agents.

Doxazosin

Doxazosin is a specific competitive inhibitor of α-1 receptor and lacks α-2 effects. There is no tachycardia or sedation with its use. The PRESCRIPT trial demonstrated equal efficacy of doxazosin and phenoxybenzamine pretreatment in intraoperative hemodynamic control during pheochromocytoma resection surgery. Patients who were pretreated with phenoxybenzamine required more β-blockers preoperatively, presumably via enhanced reflex tachycardia, but fewer vasodilating agents during surgery.[26]

β-Blockers

β-Blockers are used when there is tachyarrhythmia due to adrenaline-/dopamine-secreting tumors or as result of α-blockade after drug therapy. Most commonly, nonselective β-blockers such as propranolol are used; however, selective β1-blockers usage will not oppose β2-mediated vasodilatation. As described earlier, β-blockade is to be achieved only after α-blockade is established.

Calcium Channel Blockers

Calcium channel blockers are mainly used as an adjunctive therapy. They inhibit noradrenaline-induced calcium influx into vascular smooth muscle in patients who are already on α-blocker therapy.

α- and β-adrenoceptor Antagonists

Labetalol is a drug with both α- and β-adrenoceptor antagonist property and it is used for short-term blood pressure control and is never used as the primary choice. In few centers, calcium channel blockers are used as primary treatment in patients with pheochromocytoma who have normal blood pressure.[27]

Metyrosine

Metyrosine is a tyrosine hydroxylase inhibitor and competitively inhibits catecholamine synthesis, the rate-limiting step of catecholamine synthesis.[28] This drug is used in pheochromocytoma patients with high blood pressure having an extensive metastatic disease or preoperative patients with active tumors.[29,30] This drug is used in sync with other adrenergic blockers due to incomplete depletion of catecholamine stores regardless of the dose.[9,17,31,32]

In summary, due to lack of large, randomized, prospective, and controlled trials, retrospective data suggest that α-adrenergic blockade is the preferred choice in the preoperative management of pheochromocytoma to improve perioperative outcome. However, patients with normal blood pressure, so-called low-risk patients, sometimes show hypertensive response during induction or surgical stimulation, thereby demonstrating unpredictable response of blood pressure changes.[20,33-35] These normotensive patients must also be given α-adrenoceptor blockade or calcium channel blockers.

DRUGS THAT INTERFERE WITH CATECHOLAMINE SYNTHESIS

Various drugs are known to stimulate the catecholamine secreting tumors and may cause sudden surge of catecholamines in blood, leading to hypertensive catastrophe. Such drugs are as follows:

- Glucagon, steroids, histamine, angiotensin II, and vasopressin can cause release of catecholamines.
- Food products such as tyramine in cheese, bananas, soy sauce, wine, smoked or fermented juices can cause release of catecholamines from storage vesicles.
- Tricyclic antidepressants and other antidepressants such as amitriptyline, nortriptyline, and duloxetine also inhibit catecholamine uptake, and drugs that influence norepinephrine metabolism such as monoamine oxidase (MAO) inhibitors contribute significantly to catecholamine levels.
- Linezolid, an oxazolidinone antibiotic, has got MAO inhibitory properties so it must be used with caution in pheochromocytoma patients. Dopamine receptor antagonist drugs such as chlorpromazine, prochlorperazine, and metoclopramide used as antipsychotic and antiemetic drugs can also induce catecholamine secretion in pheochromocytoma patients.

EVALUATION OF THE PATIENT

A detailed clinical history, examination, and complete laboratory workup along with cardiac workup are imperative for considering a patient for pheochromocytoma resection surgery. Cardiac workup includes preoperative ECG and echocardiography. ECG can diagnose ventricular hypertrophy, arrhythmias, and conduction abnormalities.

Echocardiography is done to study the effects of prolonged hypertension on heart such as concentric hypertrophy, diastolic dysfunction, and cardiomyopathy. However, the value of preoperative echocardiography in the absence of any cardiac symptoms or clinical evidence of cardiac involvement is debatable.[36] Doppler echocardiography is better than conventional echocardiography to predict risk of perioperative cardiovascular collapse.[37] The optimum blood pressure control is to be achieved with the help of combination of various hypertensive drugs before considering for elective resection of tumor.

Due to underlying high catecholamine surge, all these patients are vasoconstricted and relatively volume depleted. The pharmacological control of blood pressure along with restoration of adequate fluid volume status is relevant before posting the patient for pheochromocytoma resection. The use of α-adrenergic blockade alone will result in restoration of blood volume in nearly 60% of population only.[38] Renal function must be studied to evaluate the effect of prolonged hypertension on renal tissue. A detailed renal function testing is required for such patients. Large left adrenal pheochromocytoma patients may have to undergo splenectomy also; and in such patients vaccination against Pneumococcus, Meningococcus and *Haemophilus influenzae* must be considered. Catecholamine surge can cause hyperglycemia or the patient can have preexisting diabetes; in such cases, blood glucose control is to be achieved preoperatively by shifting the patient to insulin. Serum electrolytes must be investigated and optimized if deranged. Smoking and alcohol consumption must be stopped.

Intraoperative Management

The challenge during pheochromocytoma resection mainly includes the following issues:

- Hypertensive response during manipulation of tumor
- Cardiac arrhythmias during resection process
- Hypotensive response in the postresection period

Apart from routine intraoperative monitoring of heart rate, SpO_2, $EtCO_2$, temperature and urine output these patients must also have monitoring of intra-arterial blood pressure and central venous pressure. A four-lumen central venous catheter should preferably be placed for infusion of vasoactive drugs and to guide the fluid therapy.

Pulmonary artery catheters are not used these days due to well documented risks associated with them. However, use of transesophageal ECG to guide fluid, inotropes, and vasodilators has been described.[39] Usefulness of noninvasive monitoring for cardiac output and variability of stroke volume in diagnosing fluid deficit cannot be ignored. Esophageal Dopplers can be used in pediatric patients. Underhydration or underfilling the vascular bed can cause hypotension while overfilling can cause perioperative congestive heart failure and pulmonary edema. During the intraoperative period, adequate depth of anesthesia must be ensured using bispectral indices, neuromuscular monitoring, and epidural- and opioid-based pain control. Acute hypertensive crisis and tachycardia during tumor manipulation are pharmacologically managed by intravenous (IV) agents **(Table 1)**.

Magnesium Sulfate

Magnesium sulfate acts by inhibition of release of adrenal catecholamines and also reduction of α-adrenoceptor sensitivity to catecholamines' surge. Magnesium also causes vasodilatation and reduces afterload and has got antiarrhythmic action by antagonism of L-type calcium channel blockers. James et al. have combined magnesium along with fentanyl before intubating the pheochromocytoma patients followed by infusion of IV magnesium 1–2 g/h and found stable hemodynamic during the surgery.[40]

Earlier, surgical ligation of the adrenal vein was conventionally recommended to attenuate hemodynamic instability; however, it has been seen that catecholamine levels may still rise and this approach carries a high risk of damage to the adjacent tissues, particularly when tumor is of a large size. Laparoscopic surgery is always considered superior to open surgery due to less postoperative pain, early recovery, and short hospital stay. Open surgery is preferred when the tumor is large or has got extra-adrenal location.

Steroid infusion must be supplemented when bilateral adrenalectomy is planned for such tumors, and such patients may require lifelong corticosteroid replacement. To prevent this, partial adrenalectomy is performed; however, the risk of recurrence is always there and about one-third of the gland vascularity must be preserved to retain corticotropic function.

SURGICAL TECHNIQUES

- *Anterior transabdominal approach:* This is done for unilateral tumors and is the most common approach; however, chevron incision or bucket handle incision is given for bilateral or multiple or extra-adrenal tumors.
- *Lateral flank approach:* An incision is made through bed of 11th or 12th rib, for resection of well-localized one-sided tumors.
- *Thoracoabdominal approach:* Large or malignant tumors involving adjacent visceral organs such as pancreas, kidney, spleen, or major vessels are approached by this method.
- *Laparoscopic methods:* Most abdominal pheochromocytomas measuring <6 cm can be removed laparoscopically. The procedure has significant advantages

Table 1: Intravenous agents to manage acute hypertensive crisis and tachycardia.			
Drug	*Mechanism of action*	*Doses*	*Side effects*
Phentolamine	Reversible nonselective α-adrenergic blocker	1–2 mg IV bolus followed by infusion	Hypotension, tachycardia, sedation, nasal stuffiness, dry mouth
Sodium nitroprusside	Arterial vasodilator	0.5–1.5 µg/kg/min can be increased up to 4 µg/kg/min	Hypotension, cyanide toxicity, methemoglobinemia
Nitroglycerin	Venodilator	0.5–10 µg/kg/min	Tachycardia, cyanide toxicity, tachyphylaxis
Labetalol	Blocks α1-, β1-, and β2-receptors. The ratio of α-blockade to β-blockade has been estimated to be approximately 1:7	2.5–10 mg administered intravenously over 2 minutes Slow continuous infusion at a rate of 0.5–2 mg/min	Long elimination half-life >5 hours, prolonged Infusions are not recommended
Esmolol	Short-acting selective β1-blocker	Loading dose of 0.5 mg/kg administered over 1 minute, followed by a continuous infusion of 50 µg/kg/min	Avoided in patients with sinus bradycardia, heart block greater than first degree, cardiogenic shock, or overt heart failure
Nicardipine	Calcium channel blockers arterial vasodilator action	3–5 mg/h for 15 minutes and adjusted by increments of 0.5–1 mg/h	Persistent hypotension due to elimination half-life of 40–60 minutes

(IV: intravenous)

over the open approach and the access can be achieved via the transabdominal/retroperitoneoscopic approach.

Complications During Surgery

- *Hemorrhage:* Due to injury surrounding vessels
- *Vascular:* Inadvertent ligation of renal vessels, mesenteric, or major vessels
- *Organ injury:* Injury to adjacent organs such as kidney, stomach, liver, spleen and bowel may occur. Pleural injury may cause pneumothorax and must be careful for.
- *Hypertensive crisis:* Precipitating myocardial ischemia, pulmonary edema, heart failure, and intracranial bleed
- *Embolic complication:* Carbon dioxide embolism during laparoscopic surgery

▌POSTOPERATIVE CARE

As these patients have cardiovascular and hemodynamic perturbations, they must therefore be cared in an intensive care unit (ICU) or a high dependency unit (HDU) for the next 12–48 hours. Extensive hemodynamic monitoring of the intraoperative must be continued in the postoperative period. Postoperative hypotension is very common and the incidence varies from 20 to 70% which may somewhat be dependent on the kind of preoperative preparation with α-antagonists and use of intraoperative hypotensive agents. Postoperative hypotension is most commonly present due to residual action of antihypertensive drugs and sudden withdrawal of catecholamine surge causing adrenoceptor downregulation.[41]

Brunjes et al. postulated that the physiological mechanism of low blood pressure in the postoperative period is due to a chronically volume-depleted state as a result of high catecholamine surge in the preoperative state causing long-term peripheral vasoconstriction.[42] Following tumor removal, the vascular bed expands resulting in a relatively dilated state necessitating the need of extra fluid volume. Volume replacement is the treatment of choice. Generally, following the removal of tumor, approximately 0.5–1.5 times of the patient's blood volume is required to be infused during the first 24–48 hours. Thereafter, about 125 mL/kg/h fluid infusion is required to maintain a urine output of >1 mL/kg/h. Norepinephrine is often required in the postoperative period to maintain blood pressure. Vasopressin can be considered only if hypotension is refractory to norepinephrine infusion and fluid optimization. However, sometimes even in the postoperative period, the patient may show persistent hypertension which may be secondary to postoperative pain, residual tumor, or coexistent essential hypertension. To differentiate between residual tumor and coexistent essential hypertension, biochemical testing is to be repeated after around 2 weeks of surgery. Other causes of high blood pressure in the immediate postoperative period such as autonomic instability, volume excess, and urinary retention must be ruled out. Rarely, ligation of renal artery inadvertently may cause delayed hypertension due to hyper-reninism. Approximately 25% of patients may continue to remain hypertensive, even after removal of the tumor, which can easily be controlled on antihypertensive medication.[43,44]

Hypoglycemia may occur in the postoperative period. It may be due to sudden catecholamine withdrawal after tumor removal leading to rebound hyperinsulinism and/or relative increase in sensitivity to insulin with already depleted glycogen stores. At times, presentation of hypoglycemia is masked by the concurrent use of β-blockers. Therefore, strict monitoring of blood sugar, at least for the first 24 hours, in the postoperative period is recommended to avoid severe hypoglycemia and appropriate titration of glucose infusions. Patients with bilateral adrenalectomy may require steroid replacement in the postoperative period in the form of 100 mg hydrocortisone 8 hourly for the first 72 hours, followed by switch to oral prednisolone.

Many times, patients can have excessive diuresis in the postoperative period, especially in patients who have undergone bilateral adrenalectomies. This diuresis may be due to acute mineralocorticoid deficiency or continued elevation of plasma human atrial natriuretic peptide (ANP) and brain natriuretic peptide (BNP) in response to the high blood pressure preoperatively.[45] This diuresis usually responds to hydrocortisone supplementation and fludrocortisone given sublingually.

▌SUMMARY

Pheochromocytomas are rare tumors; accurate biochemical and radiological investigation with clinical corroboration is required for proper diagnosis and treatment. Perioperative management right from the diagnosis, preoperative optimization of hemodynamic, minimizing intra-operative complications by fluid and drug therapy to intensive monitoring of vitals requires a team approach. Massive hemodynamic instability, fluid replacement, and use of antihypertensive or vasopressor medication are required in the postoperative period. Therefore, intensive hemodynamic monitoring used during the intra-operative period must be continued at least for 24–48 hours, in the ICU or HDU.

▌ACKNOWLEDGEMENT

The authors would like to acknowledge Dr Sabaretnam Mayilvaganan Associate Professor from the Department of Endocrine Surgery, for figures and scans in the chapter.

■ REFERENCES

1. Ambesh SP. Guest editorial. World J Endoc Surg. 2010;2(3):1.

2. De Lellis RA, Lloyd RV, Heitz PU, Eng C (Eds). Pathology and Genetics of Tumours of Endocrine Organs. Lyon, France: IARC Press; 2004.

3. Pacak K, Eisenhofer G, Ahlman H, Bornstein SR, Gimenez-Roqueplo AP, Grossman AB, et al. Pheochromocytoma: Recommendations for clinical practice from the First International Symposium. October 2005. Nat Clin Pract Endocrinol Metab. 2007;3(2):92-102.

4. Sutton MG, Sheps SG, Lie JT. Prevalence of clinically unsuspected pheochromocytoma. Review of a 50-year autopsy series. Mayo Clin Proc. 1981;56(6):354-60.

5. Ambesh SP. Occult pheochromocytoma in association with hyperthyroidism presenting under general anesthesia. Anesth Analg. 1993;77(5):1074-6.

6. Gimenez-Roqueplo AP, Dahia PL, Robledo M. An update on the genetics of paraganglioma, pheochromocytoma, and associated hereditary syndromes. Horm Metab Res. 2012;44(5):328-33.

7. Eisenhofer G, Bornstein SR. Surgery: Risk of hemodynamic instability in pheochromocytoma. Nat Rev Endocrinol. 2010;6(6):301-2.

8. Bravo EL. Evolving concepts in the pathophysiology, diagnosis, and treatment of pheochromocytoma. Endocr Rev. 1994;15(3):356-68.

9. Pacak K, Linehan WM, Eisenhofer G, Walther MM, Goldstein DS. Recent advances in genetics, diagnosis, localization, and treatment of pheochromocytoma. Ann Intern Med. 2001;134(4):315-29.

10. Bravo EL, Tagle R. Pheochromocytoma: State-of-the-art and future prospects. Endocr Rev. 2003;24(4):539-53.

11. Lebuffe G, Dosseh ED, Tek G, Tytgat H, Moreno S, Tavernier B, et al. The effect of calcium channel blockers on outcome following the surgical treatment of phaeochromocytomas and paragangliomas. Anaesthesia. 2005;60(5):439-44.

12. Takahashi S, Nakai T, Fujiwara R, Kutsumi Y, Tamai T, Miyabo S. Effectiveness of long-acting nifedipine in pheochromocytoma. Jpn Heart J. 1989;30(5):751-7.

13. Bravo EL. Pheochromocytoma: An approach to antihypertensive management. Ann N Y Acad Sci. 2002;970:1-10.

14. Prys-Roberts C. Phaeochromocytoma—Recent progress in its management. Br J Anaesth. 2000;85(1):44-57.

15. Steinsapir J, Carr AA, Prisant LM, Bransome ED Jr. Metyrosine and pheochromocytoma. Arch Intern Med. 1997;157(8):901-6.

16. Kanto JH. Current status of labetalol, the first alpha- and beta-blocking agent. Int J Clin Pharmacol Ther Toxicol. 1985;23(11):617-28.

17. Young WF Jr. Pheochromocytoma: Issues in diagnosis & treatment. Compr Ther. 1997;23(5):319-26.

18. Eigelberger MS, Duh QY. Pheochromocytoma. Curr Treat Options Oncol. 2001;2(4):321-9.

19. Shapiro B, Fig LM. Management of pheochromocytoma. Endocrinol Metab Clin North Am. 1989;18(2):443-81.

20. Williams DT, Dann S, Wheeler MH. Phaeochromocytoma—Views on current management. Eur J Surg Oncol. 2003;29(6):483-90.

21. Manger WM, Gifford RW Jr. Pheochromocytoma: Current diagnosis and management. Cleve Clin J Med. 1993;60(5):365-78.

22. Mannelli M. Management and treatment of pheochromocytomas and paragangliomas. Ann N Y Acad Sci. 2006;1073:405-16.

23. Kinney MAO, Narr BJ, Warner MA. Perioperative management of pheochromocytoma. J Cardiothorac Vasc Anesth. 2002;16(3):359-69.

24. Pacak K. Preoperative management of the pheochromocytoma patient. J Clin Endocrinol Metab. 2007;92(11):4069-79.

25. Connor D, Boumphrey S. Perioperative care of phaeochromocytoma. BJA Educ. 2016;16(5):153-8.

26. Prescript trial Endocrine. Abstracts 2018 56OC7.5. (2018). [online] Available from: https://www.endocrine-abstracts.org/ea/0056/ea0056oc7.5. [Last accessed March, 2020].

27. Ulchaker JC, Goldfarb DA, Bravo EL, Novick AC. Successful outcomes in pheochromocytoma surgery in the modern era. J Urol. 1999;161(3):764-7.

28. Sjoerdsma A, Engelman K, Spector S, Udenfriend S. Inhibition of catecholamine synthesis in man with alpha-methyl-tyrosine, an inhibitor of tyrosine hydroxylase. Lancet. 1965;2(7422):1092-4.

29. Kuchel O, Buu NT, Edwards DJ. Alternative catecholamine pathways after tyrosine hydroxylase inhibition in malignant pheochromocytoma. J Lab Clin Med. 1990;115(4):449-53.

30. Robinson RG, DeQuattro V, Grushkin CM, Lieberman E. Childhood pheochromocytoma: Treatment with alpha methyl tyrosine for resistant hypertension. J Pediatr. 1977;91(1):143-7.

31. Malchoff CD, MacGillivray D, Shichman S. Pheochromocytoma treatment. In: Mansoor GA (Ed). Secondary Hypertension. Totowa, NJ: Humana Press; 2004. pp. 235-49.

32. Perry RR, Keiser HR, Norton JA, Wall RT, Robertson CN, Travis W, et al. Surgical management of pheochromocytoma with the use of metyrosine. Ann Surg. 1990;212(5):621-8.

33. Kebebew E, Duh QY. Benign and malignant pheochromocytoma: Diagnosis, treatment, and follow-up. Surg Oncol Clin N Am. 1998;7(4):765-89.

34. Werbel SS, Ober KP. Pheochromocytoma. Update on diagnosis, localization, and management. Med Clin North Am. 1995;79(1):131-53.

35. Cohen DL, Fraker D, Townsend RR. Lack of symptoms in patients with histologic evidence of pheochromocytoma: A diagnostic challenge. Ann NY Acad Sci. 2006;1073:47-51.

36. Devaux B, Lentschener C, Jude N, Valensi L, Pili-Floury S, Dousset B, et al. Predictive value of preoperative transthoracic echocardiography in patients undergoing adrenalectomy for pheochromocytoma. Acta Anaesthesiol Scand. 2004;48(6):711-5.

37. Meune C, Bertherat J, Dousset B, Jude N, Bertagna X, Duboc D, et al. Reduced myocardial contractility assessed by tissue Doppler echocardiography is associated with increased risk during adrenal surgery of patients with pheochromocytoma:

Report of a preliminary study. J Am Soc Echocardiogr. 2006;19(12):1466-70.

38. Grosse H, Schröder D, Schober O, Hausen B, Dralle H. The importance of high-dose alpha-receptor blockade for blood volume and hemodynamics in pheochromocytoma. Anaesthesist. 1990;39(6):313-8

39. Matsuura T, Kashimoto S, Okuyama K, Oguchi T, Kumazawa T. Anesthesia with transesophageal echocardiography for removal of pheochromocytoma. Masui. 1995;44(10):1388-90.

40. James MF. Use of magnesium sulphate in the anaesthetic management of phaeochromocytoma: A review of 17 anaesthetics. Br J Anaesth. 1989;62(6):616-23.

41. Snavely MD, Mahan LC, O'Connor DT, Insel PA. Selective down-regulation of adrenergic receptor subtypes in tissues from rats with pheochromocytoma. Endocrinology. 1983;113(1):354-61.

42. Brunjes S, Johns VJ Jr, Crane MG. Pheochromocytoma: Postoperative shock and blood volume. N Engl J Med. 1960;262:393-6.

43. Amar L, Servais A, Gimenez-Roqueplo AP, Zinzindohoue F, Chatellier G, Plouin PF. Year of diagnosis, features at presentation, and risk of recurrence in patients with pheochromocytoma or secreting paraganglioma. J Clin Endocrinol Metab. 2005;90(4):2110-6.

44. Young JB, Landsberg L. Catecholamines and the adrenal medulla. In: Wilson JD, Foster DW (Eds). William's Textbook of Endocrinology, 9th edition. Philadelphia: WB Saunders Company; 1998. pp. 665-728.

45. Tobe M, Ito K, Umeda S, Sato A, Adaniya N, Tanaka Y, et al. Severe polyuria after the resection of adrenal pheochromocytoma. Int J Urol. 2010;17(12):1004-7.

Orthopedics

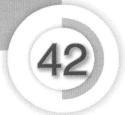
Perioperative Management of Major Orthopedic Surgeries Including Hemi-Pelvectomies

Sohan Lal Solanki, Subha Padakannaya, Atul Prabhakar Kulkarni

INTRODUCTION

Perioperative care and management of major/supramajor orthopedic surgeries like hemipelvectomy is challenging because of complex procedure with extensive tissue trauma during surgery, preoperative adjuvant chemotherapy, radiotherapy, major blood loss intraoperative, and sometimes problem of ongoing blood loss in postoperative period, ileus, and experience of severe pain because of extensive surgery.

There are three common primary bone sarcomas:[1]

1. Osteosarcoma, the most common, has an incidence of 4.6 per million people. Osteosarcoma has age preference of 10–19 years. These may also be found in patients more than 40 years of age in association with Paget's disease.
2. Ewing's sarcoma is more common during second decade of life with a peak incidence (3 per million) during 15–19 years of age.
3. Chondrosarcomas arise most commonly from the pelvis, upper femur, and shoulder girdle.

Metastatic bone tumors are more common than primary bone tumors with majority (up to 70%) of metastases from breast and prostate cancers. Other than these few more cancers such as lung, stomach, rectum, colon, uterus, kidney, and thyroid also metastasize to the bone which incidences ranging from 15 to 30% of cases.[2,3]

Major bone cancers involving knee, thigh, and pelvic bones often need megaprosthesis implantations, lower limb amputations, hip disarticulation or hemipelvectomy. These radical limb operations are mandatory due to the high risk of metastasis, especially to the lungs. External hemipelvectomy or hindquarter amputation involves amputation of the lower limb of affected side, whereas limb is spared in case of internal hemipelvectomy.[4]

Surgical goal in these cases is to reconstruct the resulting defect for optimal function and cosmesis. Prosthetic knee joints can accommodate for length of femur resected for bone cancers but for proper functioning of lower limb a residual femoral length of minimum 8 cm from greater trochanter is required.

Hemipelvectomy needs reconstruction surgery with a long posterior flap to create a proper sitting area on the prosthesis. Patients who have a diffuse/widespread cancer in pelvis, but without distant metastases, can be offered hemicorporectomy (translumbar amputation) which is often a rare procedure. This has been shown to have a good rehabilitation outcome.[5,6]

PREOPERATIVE CONSIDERATIONS

These patients who are posted for orthopedic oncologic surgeries often have received variable treatment (general treatment, radiotherapy or chemotherapy) prior to surgery. These forms of treatment, especially chemotherapy and radiotherapy can cause significant anemia, low platelets, and sometimes pancytopenia. A proper preoperative evaluation and preoperative management of anemia (if present) by intravenous iron or exogenous erythropoietin therapy and if needed platelet transfusion can be beneficial.[7]

If tumor is very vascular and there are chances of preoperative bleed or intraoperative major blood loss, preoperative embolization of the vessel to the tumor is very helpful is successful management. A large bore intravenous access is always warranted in suspicion of preoperative bleeding.[8]

A close communication between surgeon, anesthesiologist, blood bank, and intensive care specialist is mandatory prior to supramajor orthopedic oncologic surgeries like hemipelvectomy. It warrants the anesthesiologist, transfusion specialist, and surgeon appropriate planning according to the procedure, availability of blood and blood products, and monitoring arrangement.

Erythropoietin preoperatively can reduce the need for blood transfusion. It is usually started when hemoglobin (Hb) level is less than 10 mg/dL and is useful in patients receiving myelosuppressive chemotherapy. 100–150 U/kg intravenous/subcutaneous three times weekly, alternatively 40,000 U subcutaneous once weekly until completion of chemotherapy. If Hb increases >1 g/dL withhold dose and initiate at 25% below the previous dose. However, if after 4 weeks of therapy, Hb level do not rise more than 1 g/dL increase the dose by 50%. If no response after 8 weeks patient is unlikely to benefit from further doses and consider discontinuing. Erythropoietin is not indicated in patients scheduled for surgery and willing for autologous blood donation.

Autologous blood transfusion is the collection of blood from a single patient and retransfusion back to the same patient when required. There are three methods of autologous transfusion:[9]

1. *Cell salvage*: Blood is collected from surgical field, suction bottles, drains, and retransfused back to the patient after proper filtration or washing.[10,11]
2. *Preoperative autologous donation (PAD)*: Blood from surgical patient is collected well in advance of a planned surgery, kept and stored in the blood bank, and transfused back to the patient when required.[12]
3. *Acute normovolemic hemodilution (ANH)*: Immediately prior to surgery blood is collected from patient and the blood volume is replaced by adequate intravenous crystalloids and colloids. The collected blood can be retransfused when needed or after the surgery is finished in the operating room.[13]

Cell Salvage

Cell salvage is more commonly used in cardiovascular and other type of surgeries involving major blood loss. Limitations of the cell salvage technique are that it cannot be used in oncologic patients because of risk of cancer spreading systemically. Researches are being conducted on effectiveness of filtered and irradiated salvaged blood to decrease the tumor burden and prevention of spreading cancers.

Autologous transfusions do not have advantages over allogeneic or exogenous blood transfusion and long-term outcomes are similar in both. Patients who had undergone autologous donations prior to surgery had higher incidence of transfusion intraoperative or postoperatively despite the fact that blood loss was similar in both type of patients. Both autologous and allogeneic blood transfusion can be associated with transfusion-related immunomodulation and cause decreased disease free survival in cancer patients. Autologous blood transfusion is only considered when there is a high incidence of blood loss (anticipated blood loss >20%) and transfusion. There should be strict institutional protocol and guidelines for autologous blood transfusion.[14] Some of the advantages and disadvantages of autologous blood donations are discussed below.

Advantages

- Reduced risk of transmission of infection.
- Reduced risk of transfusion reaction.
- Allows safer transfusion in patients with rare blood groups and multiple autoantibodies.
- Eliminates immunosuppression.
- May be acceptable to some Jehovah's Witness patients.

Disadvantages

- Not cost effective because it require equipment and disposables are expensive and require a dedicated manpower.
- Chances of clerical error because of complex logistics for collection, storage, and transfusion of the correct unit to the correct patient.
- Unused blood is wasted and cannot be returned to the donor pool and use for other patients.
- Higher risk of bacterial and other infection/contamination.

Preoperative Autologous Deposition

The patient is required to present to the out-patient department for repeated blood donation of about 450 mL blood (up to 10.5 mL/kg). This process can be started up to 5 weeks prior to surgery and allowing the collection of up to 4 units of blood. The collected blood can be stored only up to 35 days. Erythropoiesis can be maintained after blood donation by use of oral or intravenous iron supplementation. No blood donation should be encouraged at least 2–3 days prior to surgery to allow for compensation and setting of equilibrium. It should be clearly labeled to identify it from allogeneic units. During surgery, PAD must be mentioned in surgical safety checklist and whenever required predonated blood can be asked from blood bank. The surgical team, anesthesiologist, and nursing team should be communicated about PAD and documented.

In summary the medical exclusion criteria for preoperative donation are as follows:
- Active bacterial infection
- Positive results for human immunodeficiency virus (HIV) or hepatitis C virus (HCV)
- Epilepsy
- Prolonged or frequent angina, left main stem disease, significant aortic stenosis or cyanotic heart disease
- Caution with patients on β-blockers or angiotensin-converting enzyme inhibitors: consider isovolemic replacement with crystalloids

- Uncontrolled hypertension
- Pregnancy, especially if impaired placental flow or intrauterine growth retardation, due to possible harm to the fetus
- Patients with a previous history of prolonged faint after blood donation
- Hemoglobin below 11 g/dL at the start or below 10 g/dL for subsequent donations
- In children under 8 years old or weighing less than 25 kg, PAD is technically difficult and rarely justified
- Exercise caution with patients under 50 kg may need small-volume packs (250 mL packs are available) to avoid taking more than 12% of blood volume.

Other requirements:
- The patient must have suitable venous access.
- The operation would normally require blood to be cross-matched.
- The operation date is fixed.
- There is sufficient time to donate the required number of units: the last unit should be taken 7–10 days before the planned surgery. The minimum safe interval before surgery is 72 hours, which allows the blood volume to be replenished.

Acute Normovolemic Hemodilution

Acute normovolemic hemodilution is performed after induction of anesthesia and before surgical incision is taken. A large-bore cannula (14 G) is needed to allow the collection of 15–20 mL/kg of blood prior to surgery. The collected blood volume can be replaced with intravenous crystalloid or colloid. The collected blood is carefully labeled, signed, and should be kept with the patient in the operating room at all times at room temperature. The blood is transfused back to the patient whenever required or at the end of surgery after hemostasis. ANH can be performed aggressively allowing a hematocrit of minimum 20%.

The amount of Hb spared by ANH can be calculated using the following equation:

$$(Hbi - HbANH) \times VBL$$

Where, Hbi is the initial (preinduction) Hb in g/dL, HbANH is Hb following ANH and VBL is volume of blood lost during surgery. For example, reducing the Hb from 12 to 10 g/dL will spare 20 g Hb per 1,000 mL blood loss (16%) whereas a reduction from 12 to 8 g/dL would spare 40 g per 1,000 mL (33%).

Acute normovolemic hemodilution causes an acute and significant reduction in hematocrit leading to hemodynamic instability. Cardiac patients, patients with long standing diabetes are especially vulnerable and may cause myocardial ischemia/infarction perioperatively. Other complications can also arise because of the physiological effects of acute hemodilution.

INTRAOPERATIVE CONSIDERATIONS[15,16]

Proper preoperative optimization and preparation leads to better intraoperative management. These procedures which may involve any big bone or soft tissue and need resection of large part/whole bone and major neurovascular structures, need for cementing of bones, use of local or free flap for reconstructions. Intraoperative management starts with a proper surgical safety checklist and coordination between surgeon, anesthesiologist, and nursing team. Epidural catheter can be placed if the puncture site and dressing of epidural catheter is not coming in the surgical field. These patients may experience major blood loss and prolonged surgeries, so general anesthesia can be a better choice although central neuraxial blockade like spinal anesthesia or combined spinal epidural anesthesia can be used for lower limb surgeries. For hemipelvectomies, general anesthesia is better choice than central neuraxial blockade. Adequate amount of crystalloids and colloids including albumin should be kept ready because these tumors are known for major blood loss especially in highly vascular tumor and major pelvic resections. The tumors often involve adjacent structures such as bowel and bladder needing excision of multiple organs and multidisciplinary approach. Involvement and handling of nerves can potentially lead to postoperative neuropathic pain. At least two proper large bore intravenous access should be kept in case of major blood loss and need for rapid replacement. Apart from standard American Society of Anesthesiologists (ASA) monitoring such as electrocardiogram (ECG), noninvasive blood pressure, pulse oximetry, and end-tidal CO_2; invasive arterial blood pressure can be monitored especially in cases with anticipated major blood loss like hemipelvectomies. A central venous catheter is not always required but can be placed if vasopressor or inotrope support is needed.

When placing a patient in the lateral decubitus position, special care of the neck is required to keep in a neutral/midline position, and pressure on the eyes and dependent ear should be avoided.

For position such as lateral decubitus and prone position, standard precautions have to be taken to prevent any injury to pressure points, eyes, breasts, and neck. During prone position, abdomen should not be compressed, rather it should be free, and because excessive pressure may compromise ventilation and decrease venous return from the lower extremities.[17]

Blood Loss

Major orthopedic tumors and mostly vascular and surgical procedures on or near them may lead to major bleeding throughout the intraoperative period. Monitoring blood loss is difficult as less than half of the blood loss is collected in the surgical sucker container or contained by surgical packs. The rest of blood is spilt in the drapes and the floor. Blood loss during pelvic surgery can be rapid and sometimes uncontrollable and needs rapid replacement with crystalloids, colloids, blood, and blood products.[18]

Rapid blood transfusion is although required and lifesaving in these type of procedures but it is associated with certain complications such as hypothermia (transfusion of cold blood, less time for warming blood because of ongoing loss), dilutional coagulopathy, and dilutional thrombocytopenia (because of rapid transfusion of colloids and crystalloids), metabolic acidosis, electrolyte abnormalities, citrate toxicity, transfusion-related acute lung injury (TRALI), transfusion-associated circulatory overload, and allergic reactions.

Pelvic metastases should be the ideal for preoperative embolization because these are often very vascular and hemorrhage significantly regardless of histological subtype. Myeloma may affect multiple systems from direct spread of tumor and Bence Jones proteins.[19]

Study comparing tranexamic acid with ANH to decrease intraoperative blood loss in patients undergoing total knee arthroplasty showed that fluid and vasoactive drugs requirements were significantly higher in ANH group and they attributed this to lower blood viscosity secondary to hemodilution after ANH, which leads to decreased systemic vascular resistance and requirement of vasoactive drugs.[20] There are some controversial statements about use of antifibrinolytics in oncology patients because of belief that antifibrinolytics cause in increase in thrombus formation which can lead to higher chance of deep vein thrombosis (DVT) and even pulmonary embolism, but studies failed to show any increased incidence of thrombosis.[21]

The Cochrane database meta-analysis of more than 200 studies consisting of over 20,000 patients, showed that use of aprotinin, epsilon-aminocaproic acid (EACA), or tranexamic acid in perioperative period decrease blood loss without any increase in risk of thrombus formation.[22] Aprotinin is good drug to decrease blood loss but it causes renal toxicity. EACA and tranexamic acid are better options to minimize intraoperative blood loss. Data comparing effect of EACA and tranexamic acid are very limited in orthopedic procedures, but it appears that tranexamic acid is more efficacious in other surgeries involving large blood loss. The tranexamic acid dosing regimen most commonly used is a 10 mg/kg loading dose followed by a 1 mg/kg/h infusion; it decreases intraoperative transfusion and blood loss in spine cancer patients undergoing intralesional tumor excision and instrumentation. Tranexamic acid should be avoided in cases of subarachnoid hemorrhage, acquired defective color vision, and active intravascular clotting processes, such as disseminated intravascular coagulation.

POSTOPERATIVE CONSIDERATIONS

Hematological

Anemia, coagulopathy, and thrombocytopenia are most common complications postoperatively which can be attributed to massive transfusions. It is usually managed with supportive therapy and coagulation returns to normal in 48 hours postsurgery.[23]

Hypotension

Patients may develop postoperative multiorgan dysfunction due to intraoperative massive transfusion, hypoperfusion due to hypotension following major intraoperative losses, fluid shifts, and ongoing losses postoperatively. At the postanesthesia care unit (PACU) it is important to be vigilant of drain output and local hematoma formation. Higher drains, hematoma, and drop in Hb subsequently lead to increased length of stay in intensive care unit (ICU) and hospital. Adequate fluid resuscitation before starting on vasopressors for the hypotension, pallor, cold peripheries, feeble pulse, narrow pulse pressure, and dark colored urine point towards fluid deficient status.

Hypotension may also be related to epidural boluses and a relook into opioid and epidural dosage should be considered. Also, it is important to monitor the peripheral perfusion of lower limbs watching out for local pallor or charting capillary refill time of all the limbs. A bedside Doppler can be very useful for this purpose. The perfusion could be effected not only by reconstruction or any vascular anastomoses but also hypotension.

Nerve Palsy

Tingling and numbness of one or both lower limbs could be present. These complications could be transient and recover after stopping the epidural local anesthetic if it is due to the neuraxial blockade. Neuropraxia could also be because of patient positioning, surgery or bony metastases. Brachial plexus palsy though uncommon can be present due to overhead stretching of upper limb in prone or lateral decubitus position. Severe stretch injury or disruption of femoral and sciatic nerve can be present due to tumor involvement.

Infection

Prophylactic antibiotic must be given perioperatively. Early and frequent reexplorations/interventional radiology-guided procedures may be required to prevent complications such as intra-abdomen/pelvic collection or sepsis and to minimize complications such as disturbed wound healing and fistula formation.

Pain

Phantom limb pain (PLP) is the painful sensation arising out of the amputated limb. Nonpainful sensation arising out of amputated limb is referred to as phantom limb sensation. Stump pain is defined as the pain arising out of amputated stump. Mechanism of PLP and phantom limb sensation is still debatable; however, a lot of theories had been given. Following amputation, there may be formation of neuroma showing abnormal spontaneous activity, and on mechanical and chemical stimulation, which is thought to be due to upregulation of sodium channels. Further, there is spinal plasticity, i.e., increase in the excitability of spinal neurons, more accessibility of Aδ- and c-fibers to other pathways. N-methyl-D-aspartate (NMDA) receptor systems are also believed to have a role in "wind-up" phenomenon seen in PLP. Furthermore, spinal and cerebral reorganization occurs and there is a relationship between degree of reorganization and pain.[24]

Prevalence of neuroma postsurgery around 6–8% at high risk for development of PLP and prevalence of severe postoperative pain is around 60%.[25] Preemptive analgesia which is believed to be decreasing postoperative pain by interrupting response to noxious surgical stimulus, before starting the surgical procedure, has failed to show decreased postoperative pain. In a systematic review[26] comparing nonsteroidal anti-inflammatory drugs (NSAIDs), preincisional opioids, NMDA receptor antagonists, and regional anesthesia has shown conflicting results. In this, only epidural analgesia was shown to have a beneficial effect and there were no or very little advantages of any of the preemptive analgesic strategy. One study in megaprosthesis total knee arthroplasty in bone cancers has shown epidural analgesia better in terms of postoperative pain relief as compared to intravenous opioid based patient controlled analgesia.[27]

Patients with large bone or soft tissue cancers are often on multiple analgesic regimen including opioids preoperatively. Dose and daily requirement of opioid should be noted prior to surgery so that intraoperative and postoperative pain can be managed accordingly Adjuvants like ketamine, an NMDA antagonist, can significantly decrease postoperative pain scores when given in subanesthetic doses and is of benefit in opioid tolerant patients. Memantine, another NMDA antagonist, which is used to treat Alzheimer's disease, can also be tried to postoperative pain.[28] A multimodal analgesia pattern with a multidisciplinary approach to pain management is beneficial.

Thromboprophylaxis

Venous thromboembolism (VTE) remains a serious postoperative complication especially after long and major surgery where prolonged immobilization is required. Incidence of DVT is 45–69% after hip arthroplasty without prophylaxis. There are nonpharmacological and pharmacological ways to decrease the incidence of DVT and VTE after major surgery. In nonpharmacological methods, intermittent compression devices are very efficacious in preventing the formation of DVTs, decreasing the risk to 14%. Pharmacological thromboprophylaxis agents include warfarin, low-dose heparin, low-molecular-weight-heparins (LMWH), and aspirin. Combining nonpharmacological and pharmacological thromboprophylaxis can significantly decrease incidence of DVT and VTE. Pharmacological thromboprophylaxis after orthopedic cancer surgeries for bone or soft tissue sarcomas reduced the incidence of DVT to 4% when LMWH was started on second day.

Pharmacological thromboprophylaxis for DVT is of special concerns in patients who is having epidural catheter placed for postoperative analgesia. Timing of removal of catheter and timing of dosing of LMWH or heparin should be done according to international guidelines.[29]

CONCLUSION

The perioperative management of major or supramajor orthopedic oncologic surgeries is challenging. Comorbidities optimization and preoperative anemia management can significantly improve the postoperative outcomes. These cases vary in length and complexity; the potential for massive blood loss/massive blood transfusion and hemodynamic instability and subsequent use of vasopressor must be appreciated on time and the intraoperative use of antifibrinolytics should be considered whenever required.

REFERENCES

1. Ottaviani G, Jaffe N. The epidemiology of osteosarcoma. Cancer Treat Res. 2009;152:3-13.
2. Maccauro G, Spinelli MS, Mauro S, Perisano C, Graci C, Rosa MA. Physiopathology of spine metastasis. Int J Surg Oncol. 2011;2011:107969.
3. Macedo F, Ladeira K, Pinho F, Saraiva N, Bonito N, Pinto L, et al. Bone Metastases: An Overview. Oncol Rev. 2017;11:321.
4. Merimsky O, Kollender Y, Bickels J, Inbar M, Nirkin A, Isakov J, et al. Amputation of the lower limb as palliative treatment for debilitating musculoskeletal cancer. Oncol Rep. 1997;4:1059-62.
5. Ragnarsson KT, Thomas DC. Cancer of the limbs. In: Kufe DW, Pollock RE, Weichselbaum RR (Eds). Holland-Frei Cancer Medicine, 6th edition. Hamilton (ON): BC Decker; 2003.
6. Marfori ML, Wang EH. Adductor myocutaneous flap coverage for hip and pelvic disarticulations of sarcomas with buttock contamination. Clin Orthop Relat Res. 2011;469:257-63.
7. Zhao F, Wang Y, Liu L, Bian M. Erythropoietin for cancer-associated malignant anemia: A meta-analysis. Mol Clin Oncol. 2017;6:925-30.

8. Owen RJ. Embolization of musculoskeletal bone tumors. Semin Intervent Radiol. 2010;27:111-23.

9. Walunj A, Babb A, Sharpe R. Autologous blood transfusion. Contin Educ Anaesth Crit Care Pain. 2006;6:192-6.

10. Mason L, Fitzgerald C, Powell-Tuck J, Rice R. Intraoperative cell salvage versus postoperative autologous blood transfusion in hip arthroplasty: a retrospective service evaluation. Ann R Coll Surg Engl. 2011;93(5):398-400.

11. Klein AA, Bailey CR, Charlton AJ, Evans E, Guckian-Fisher M, McCrossan R, et al. Association of Anaesthetists guidelines: cell salvage for peri-operative blood conservation 2018. Anaesthesia. 2018;73:1141-50.

12. Kassim DY, Esmat IM, Elgendy MA. Efficacy of preoperative autologous blood donation and tranexamic acid in revision total hip arthroplasty: a randomized controlled trial. Ain-Shams J Anaesthesiol. 2017;10:131-9.

13. Murray D. Acute normovolemic hemodilution. Eur Spine J. 2004;13(Suppl 1):S72-5.

14. Federici AB, Vanelli C, Arrigoni L. Transfusion issues in cancer patients. Thromb Res. 2012;129(Suppl 1):S60-5.

15. Anderson MR, Jeng CL, Wittig JC, Rosenblatt MA. Anesthesia for patients undergoing orthopedic oncologic surgeries. J Clin Anesth. 2010;22:565-72.

16. Molnar R, Emery G, Choong PF. Anaesthesia for hemipelvectomy—a series of 49 cases. Anaesth Intensive Care. 2007;35:536-43.

17. Edgcombe H, Carter K, Yarrow S. Anaesthesia in the prone position. Br J Anaesth. 2008;100:165-83.

18. Krausz MM. Initial resuscitation of hemorrhagic shock. World J Emerg Surg. 2006;1:14.

19. Patil V, Shetmahajan M. Massive transfusion and massive transfusion protocol. Indian J Anaesth. 2014;58:590-5.

20. Zohar E, Fredman B, Ellis M, Luban I, Stern A, Jedeikin R. A comparative study of the postoperative allogeneic blood-sparing effect of tranexamic acid versus acute normovolemic hemodilution after total knee replacement. Anesth Analg. 1999;89:1382-7.

21. Abdol Razak NB, Jones G, Bhandari M, Berndt MC, Metharom P. Cancer-associated thrombosis: an overview of mechanisms, risk factors, and treatment. Cancers (Basel). 2018;10(10):380.

22. Henry DA, Carless PA, Moxey AJ, O'Connell D, Stokes BJ, McClelland B, et al. Anti-fibrinolytic use for minimising perioperative allogeneic blood transfusion. Cochrane Database Syst Rev. 2007;(4):CD001886.

23. Liumbruno GM, Bennardello F, Lattanzio A, Piccoli P, Rossetti G. Recommendations for the transfusion management of patients in the peri-operative period. III. The post-operative period. Blood Transfus. 2011;9:320-35.

24. Ahmed A, Bhatnagar S, Mishra S, Khurana D, Joshi S, Ahmad SM. Prevalence of Phantom Limb Pain, Stump Pain, and Phantom Limb Sensation among the Amputated Cancer Patients in India: A Prospective, Observational Study. Indian J Palliat Care. 2017;23:24-35.

25. Hsu E, Cohen SP. Postamputation pain: epidemiology, mechanisms, and treatment. J Pain Res. 2013;6:121-36.

26. Møiniche S, Kehlet H, Dahl JB. A qualitative and quantitative systematic review of preemptive analgesia for postoperative pain relief: the role of timing of analgesia. Anesthesiology. 2002;96:725-41.

27. Solanki SL, Katwale B, Jain AA, Chatterjee A, Gehdoo RP. Comparison of continuous epidural analgesia and intravenous patient-controlled analgesia with opioids in terms of postoperative pain and their complications in mega-prosthesis total knee arthroplasty for bone cancers. Indian J Surg Oncol. 2019;10:567-9.

28. Cohen SP, Bhatia A, Buvanendran A, Schwenk ES, Wasan AD, Hurley RW, et al. Consensus Guidelines on the Use of Intravenous Ketamine Infusions for Chronic Pain From the American Society of Regional Anesthesia and Pain Medicine, the American Academy of Pain Medicine, and the American Society of Anesthesiologists. Reg Anesth Pain Med. 2018;43:521-46.

29. Cayley WE Jr. Preventing deep vein thrombosis in hospital inpatients. BMJ. 2007;335(7611):147-51.

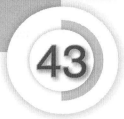

Perioperative Management of Major Orthopedic Trauma

Anila Malde, Devangi Parikh, Ruchi Jain

INTRODUCTION

Injuries to the musculoskeletal system occur in 80% of patients with polytrauma,[1] which is defined as an abbreviated injury score (AIS) ≥3 points in at least two body regions with at least one pathologic value (systolic blood pressure ≤90 mm Hg, Glasgow Coma Scale ≤8, base deficit ≥6, partial thromboplastin time ≥40 seconds, or age ≥70) with the presence of concomitant limb and pelvic fractures counting as a single body region.[2] Life-threatening musculoskeletal trauma are—major arterial hemorrhage and traumatic amputation, bilateral femoral fracture, and crush syndrome. The limb-threatening musculoskeletal injuries include open fractures and joint injuries, ischemic vascular injuries, compartment syndrome, and neurological injury secondary to fracture or dislocation. Life-threatening and limb-threatening musculoskeletal injuries should be addressed emergently, i.e., within minutes or as soon as possible. Others can be treated on an urgent basis, i.e., within 6–24 hours. Thoracic and traumatic brain (TBI) injuries are the most commonly associated injuries in polytrauma.[3] TBI and exsanguination due to hemorrhage are the leading causes of death in the polytrauma patient.[4]

GENERAL CONSIDERATIONS IN THE MANAGEMENT OF PATIENTS WITH MAJOR MUSCULOSKELETAL TRAUMA

The initial management of the patient should be as per the Advanced Trauma Life Support (ATLS)® protocol. Life-threatening extremity injuries should be identified during the primary survey and their association with severe thoracic and abdominal injuries must be recognized.[5]

Primary Survey

Primary survey consists of a quick assessment as per ABCDE (Airway, Breathing, Circulation, Disability, Exposure/ Environment). Recognition and control of hemorrhage is a component of primary survey. Bleeding may be into a closed space, not instantaneously obvious to the examiner. Major vessel injury due to deep soft tissue lacerations may lead to exsanguinating hemorrhage. Splinting of fractures can significantly reduce bleeding by decreasing motion and increasing the tamponade effect of the muscle and fascia. Direct manual pressure with a sterile dressing on the wound can control external blood loss. As there is a risk of extremity ischemia, a tourniquet should be used only when direct pressure is not effective in controlling life-threatening hemorrhage. Blindly clamping on the bleeding vessel can result in damage to nerves and veins. Appropriate replacement of intravascular volume is essential, along with definitive hemorrhage control. The patient should be covered with blankets and warm fluids should be administered to prevent hypothermia.

When fracture is suspected to be the cause of shock, fracture immobilization and X-ray examination serve as adjuncts to primary survey. Immediate application of traction, aligning the injured extremity in as close to anatomic position as possible and immobilization using a device is needed. This also controls blood loss, reduces pain, prevents neurovascular compromise and soft tissue injury. If reduction is not possible, the joint should be splinted in the position in which it was found. However, resuscitation takes precedence over application of splints.

Secondary Survey

The secondary survey includes complete history, physical examination, and reassessment of all vital signs.[5]

Fluid Resuscitation, Massive Transfusion Protocol and Damage Control Resuscitation

Hemorrhage is the most common cause of shock in trauma patients. An injured patient, who is cool to touch and is tachycardic should be considered in shock until proven otherwise.[5] Typically, two large bore (16G/18G) peripheral venous catheters are placed to administer fluid, blood, and plasma. In patients with major injury below diaphragm, venous access should be secured in drainage area of superior vena cava as there may be possible disruption of the pelvic veins or inferior vena cava. Blood samples for complete blood count, prothrombin time, and international normalized ratio are obtained, including a pregnancy test for all females of childbearing age and blood type and cross-matching. Arterial blood gases (ABG) and/or lactate level help assess the presence and degree of shock. When peripheral sites are not available, intraosseous infusion, central venous access or venesection may be used. Vigorous and continued volume resuscitation is not a replacement for definitive control of hemorrhage. Intravenous (IV) fluid therapy is initiated with warm crystalloids using fluid warming devices. A bolus of an isotonic solution (1 L in adults and 20 mL/kg in children weighing <40 kg) is administered. If a patient is unresponsive to initial crystalloid therapy, blood transfusion should be considered early as aggressive resuscitation with crystalloids before control of bleeding has been demonstrated to aggravate coagulopathy, with an increase in mortality and morbidity. Early resuscitation with blood and blood products must be considered in patients with class III and IV hemorrhage.

"Rapid responders," promptly respond to the initial fluid bolus and become hemodynamically normal. "Transient responders," respond to the initial fluid bolus. However, they begin to show worsening of perfusion indices as the initial fluids are slowed to maintenance levels suggesting continuing loss or insufficient resuscitation. Failure to respond to crystalloid and blood administration mandates immediate, definitive intervention (i.e., surgery or angioembolization) to control life-threatening hemorrhage. Patients who are transient responders or nonresponders require packed red blood cells (pRBCs), plasma, and platelets during early resuscitation. For patients who stabilize quickly, cross-matched pRBCs should be transfused when indicated. If cross-matched blood is unavailable, type O pRBCs are indicated for patients with exsanguinating hemorrhage. AB plasma is given when uncross-matched plasma is needed. To avoid sensitization and future complications, Rh-negative pRBCs are preferred for females of childbearing age. A small subgroup of patients with shock will require massive transfusion, most often defined as >10 units of pRBCs within the first 24 hours of admission or more than 4 units in 1 hour (replacement by transfusion of 50% of total blood volume in 3 hours or transfusion of 100% of total blood volume in 24 hours in pediatric patients). Eastern Society of Surgery in Trauma (EAST) recommends implementation of massive transfusion protocol (MTP) comprising of 1:1:1 ratio of plasma, platelets, and RBCs (e.g.,

6 units plasma, 1 unit apheresis platelet, and 6 units RBC) in severely injured trauma patients.[6]

Damage control resuscitation (DCR) is the standard of care which targets to minimize blood loss until definitive hemostasis is achieved.[6] This includes avoiding or reversing hypothermia, minimizing blood loss using tourniquets, hemostatic dressings, direct pressure, limiting the use of crystalloids, hypotensive resuscitation (target low normal blood pressure before definitive hemostasis), using MTPs, avoiding delays in angiographic or surgical control of hemorrhage, giving pharmacological adjuncts such as tranexamic acid to promote hemostasis and viscoelastic assays to guide ongoing transfusions, e.g., thromboelastography (TEG). First dose of tranexamic acid is usually given over 10 minutes, preferably with 3 hours of injury and the follow-up dose of 1 g is given over 8 hours. In patients who do not require massive transfusion, the use of platelets, cryoprecipitate, and fresh-frozen plasma (FFP) should be guided by coagulation studies. When necessary, calcium administration should be guided by measurement of ionized calcium.[5,7]

Management of Acute Pain

Acute pain management usually involves appropriate use of splints and pelvic binders thereby reducing pain significantly by immobilizing the fractured bones. Analgesics such as IV paracetamol and nonsteroidal anti-inflammatory drugs should be administered. Narcotics must be administered, if required, with careful monitoring of patient's consciousness, respiration, and hemodynamic parameters at the lowest dose and for the shortest time possible.[8] Low-dose ketamine (loading dose of 0.25–0.5 mg/kg followed by a continuous infusion in the range of 50–500 µg/kg/h) also can be used in select patients as an adjuvant to opioids.[9] Nerve blocks such as fascia iliaca or femoral block given as a single shot or via indwelling catheters, once the patient stabilizes, can help reduce opioid consumption.

COMMON ORTHOPEDIC INJURIES ENCOUNTERED IN TRAUMA

Pelvic Fractures

Types of Pelvic Fractures

Pelvic fractures are classified on the basis of the direction of force at the time of injury and are of the following types:[10] Anteroposterior, lateral, vertical, and combined (**Figs. 1A to D**). Fractures of the pubic symphysis and rami may result in open-book pelvic fractures which are associated with significant bleeding and often occur with severe abdominal and chest trauma. Lateral compression fractures are not associated with as much bleeding. Vertical

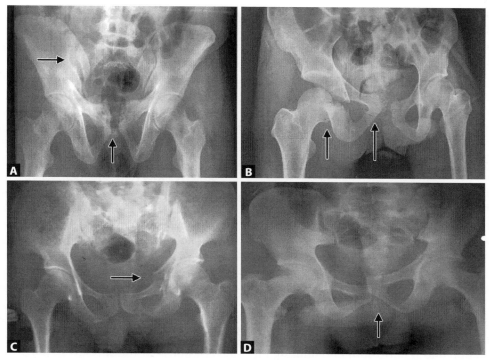

Figs. 1A to D: Types of pelvic injury. (A) Open book; (B) Vertical injury; (C) Lateral compression injury; (D) Combined injury.

shear injuries may be associated with instability of the posterior pelvic ring and stretching the lumbosacral plexus and vascular structures.

Massive hemorrhage leading to rapid exsanguination, associated injuries, and sepsis are the important causes of mortality which is 7.2–57%.[11-14] One of the important predictors of mortality is the initial hemodynamic status. Urgent resuscitation and early stabilization can minimize morbidity and mortality in these patients. Bleeding in pelvic fractures may be from fractured bony surfaces, pelvic venous plexus injury or pelvic arterial injury.[15] The amount of bleeding is related to the magnitude of displacement of the posterior pelvic ring as the extensive vasculature is closely applied to the pelvic wall. If the pelvic floor is breached, then blood leaks in large volumes into the retroperitoneal space. Bleeding from sacral venous plexus can be massive with blood loss of up to 3–10 L. The retroperitoneum of the intact pelvis can hold 4 L of blood before tamponade occurs.[16,17]

Assessment and Management

The first step in management is to identify if the patient is hemodynamically stable or not. Hemodynamically stable patients should undergo a computed tomography (CT) scan with contrast angiography followed by angiography and embolization if there is evidence of arterial bleeding. Unexplained hypotension may be the only initial indication of major pelvic disruption.[5] Mechanical instability of the

pelvic ring should be assumed if a patient with pelvic fracture is hypotensive and no other source of blood loss can be found. If the physical and radiological examination of the pelvis indicates instability of the pelvis then a pelvic binder must be applied. Distraction of the pelvis is not recommended because it may worsen or cause recurrent pelvic bleeding. The increased pelvic volume due to external rotation of the unstable pelvis holds a larger volume of blood. A pelvic binder stabilizes the pelvis and limits this expansion. The binder should be fixed over the greater trochanters instead of over the iliac crests. Pelvic stabilization helps in tamponade and reduces pain. Placement of a pelvic binder is a priority and may be lifesaving.

Focused assessment with ultrasound in trauma (FAST) is performed in patients with hemodynamic instability. If FAST is positive for significant hemoperitoneum then resuscitative endovascular balloon occlusion of aorta (REBOA) should be considered as it results in better hemorrhage control in presence of coagulopathy as compared to direct pressure with hemostatic dressing. Once the blood pressure stabilizes with REBOA, the next step involves embolization or control of hemorrhage within abdomen via laparotomy and pelvic packing with or without external pelvic fixation.[18] Embolization is 85–97% effective in controlling arterial bleeding associated with pelvic fractures;[19] however, these patients may not be stable for transfer to an angiography suite without extensive resources for ongoing resuscitation and management.

If FAST is negative for hemoperitoneum, then one can proceed directly for external fixation of pelvis. If the patient continues to remain hemodynamically unstable after pelvic packing and external fixation then one must proceed for angiography with embolization of bleeding vessel. Temporary pelvic packing via laparotomy allows time for definitive management of bleeding but has a high possibility of infection and multiorgan dysfunction.[20] In cases of major arterial injury, emergency angiography and embolization may prove to be lifesaving.

In case of suspected bladder, urethral, rectal injury, compound fracture or severe bleeding from an open wound, broad-spectrum antibiotics should be administered and the patient should be shifted to the operation room (OR) for external fixation, exploratory laparotomy to arrest bleeding or examination under anesthesia.

For patients presenting to the OR with a REBOA catheter in place, slow deflation of the balloon over several minutes once surgery or embolization has controlled most of the associated pelvic hemorrhage allows for more gradual equilibration and reperfusion. The patient may deteriorate after balloon deflation and reperfusion. Preplanning for volume loading and vasopressors may be necessary.[18]

Associated Injuries

Pelvic fractures are associated with urogenital, anorectal, sacral plexus, and sciatic nerve injuries. Urogenital injuries include rupture of bladder and urethra and injuries to external and internal genitalia. Blood at meatus is a strong indicator of urethral injury. Absence of gross hematuria does not exclude urogenital injury. To prevent worsening of the urethral injury, an intact urethra must be confirmed before urinary catheterization. A retrograde urethrogram is obligatory when the patient is unable to void, requires a pelvic binder, or has blood at the meatus, scrotal hematoma, or perineal ecchymosis. A disrupted urethra may necessitate a suprapubic cystostomy by experienced hands. Bladder rupture requires prompt diagnosis and treatment in the form of suprapubic drainage or laparotomy to avoid complications such as hyperkalemia, hypernatremia, uremia, acidosis, and peritonitis.[21] Anorectal injuries include lacerations of the rectum and perforations of small or large bowel. In case of anorectal injury, urgent laparotomy and diverting colostomy may be required as delay in obtaining fecal diversion may lead to contamination of the fracture site resulting in sepsis.

Long Bone Fractures

Multiple long bone fractures are usually associated with high-energy trauma. Average blood loss associated with long bone fractures ranges from 750 mL for humerus or tibia to 1,500 mL or more with fracture femur.

Open Fractures

Open fractures are graded by their associated soft tissue injury and contamination leading to infection. Gross contamination and particulate matter should be removed and the wound should be covered with sterile moist dressing. IV antibiotics must be administered preferably within 1 hour and definitely within 3 hours.[5] Patients with wounds less than 10 cm should be given cefazolin 1, 2 or 3 g 8 hourly for weight <50, 50–100 and >100 kg, respectively. In cases of penicillin allergy, clindamycin 600 or 900 mg is given in <80 or >80 kg, respectively. Aminoglycosides such as gentamicin (5 mg/kg) should be added, when there is severe soft tissue damage with substantial contamination and vascular injury, for gram-negative coverage. Piperacillin-tazobactam with broad-spectrum gram-positive and negative and anaerobic coverage should be administered to patients with farmyard soil or standing water contamination, irrespective of wound size.[5,22] Antibiotics should be continued up to surgery and must be continued for 24 hours postsurgery. For wound with significant contamination, antibiotic cover may be extended for 72 hours.[22] Tetanus toxoid should be administered if the last booster dose was given more than 10 years prior to evaluation or if the vaccination history is unknown or unclear. Tetanus immunoglobulin should also be given when it has been longer than 10 years since the last booster dose, or when the patient had an incomplete primary immunization.[22]

Traumatic Amputation

It is a severe form of open fracture resulting in loss of an extremity. Degloving injury with prolonged ischemia, neurologic injury, and muscle damage may require amputation. Amputation may also have to be carried out as a lifesaving measure in patients with hemodynamic instability when other measures fail.

Vascular Injury

A vascular injury should be strongly suspected in the presence of vascular insufficiency associated with a history of blunt, crushing, twisting, or penetrating injury to an extremity. Clinical signs in patients with a major arterial injury include pallor, cold limb, and decreased and/or absent pulses in an extremity. Vascular injury is suspected when there is asymmetry on palpation or Doppler. If the ankle brachial index (ABI; systolic pressure of the ankle upon systolic pressure of the arm) is <0.9, an arteriogram is indicated. Early operative revascularization is essential in vascular injuries as muscular necrosis and loss of neurological function begins within 6 hours of ischemia. Reduction and stabilization of the fracture (with either provisional or definitive methods) prior to a revascularization procedure ensures safety of the vascular repair.[1]

Timing for Operative Intervention

The ideal time for surgical intervention in orthopedic trauma is a challenging issue. There are two approaches: Early total care (ETC) and damage control orthopedics (DCO).[15] The former approach was widely used in the 1980s and it included definitive fracture fixation of all long bone fractures in one operative sitting. The advantages of early fracture fixation include decreased pain, improved mobility, lesser chances of wound infection and sepsis.[23] Even, practice management guidelines from EAST conditionally recommend early definitive fixation.[24] However, it can be used only if the patient is hemodynamically stable.

Damage control orthopedics is applied to polytrauma patients with long bone and pelvic fractures. It consists of four phases. During the acute phase, lifesaving procedures are performed. Second phase involves control of hemorrhage, temporary stabilization of major skeletal fractures, and the management of soft tissue injuries, while minimizing the degree of surgical insult to the patient. The third phase consists of a monitoring period in intensive care unit (ICU), while the fourth phase focuses on definitive fracture fixation. Rationale behind DCO is the two-hit theory in trauma patients. The initial traumatic injury is the first hit. This leads to the systemic inflammatory response syndrome (SIRS) followed by a period of recovery mediated by a counter-regulatory anti-inflammatory response (CARS). The latter can induce a prolonged immunosuppressed state. In this scenario, surgery works as a "second hit" and there is a potential risk of patient deterioration after surgery. Fat emboli and hypoxic events due to early surgery can add damage to already injured lungs in a polytrauma patient. Major lower limb orthopedic surgery increases the inflammatory, fibrinolytic and coagulation cascades.[25] DCO aims to avoid the SIRS, stabilizes the fracture, avoids compartment syndrome, and allows the patient to be mobilized for tests and improved pulmonary care. Less invasive procedures like splinting and skeletal traction and external fixators form the mainstay treatment for DCO.

Ideal Time for Definitive Surgery in DCO

The fifth to tenth days provide the "window of opportunity" for definitive osteosynthesis. The post-trauma days 2–4 have been reported to be unsuitable for performing definitive osteosynthesis.[26] However, the delay should not extend beyond 15 days in view of contamination at external fixator pin sites.

Identifying Patients for DCO Approach

The polytrauma patient can be classified into one of the four grades based on clinical parameters of shock, coagulation, temperature, and severity of injury.[27] The four grades of patients based on their clinical status are stable, borderline, unstable, and in extremis. A patient is classified into one of these four grades, if he or she meets the criteria in at least three of the four pathophysiological parameters. DCO is favored in unstable and in extremis patients. ETC is the standard of care for stable patients. The borderline patients best managed by DCO include polytrauma patient with Injury Severity Score (ISS) 20 and additional thoracic trauma, polytrauma with abdominal and pelvic trauma plus hemorrhagic shock, ISS 40 and above, bilateral lung contusion on radiography, mean pulmonary artery (PA) pressures of >24 mm Hg or an increase in PA pressure by 6 mm Hg on intramedullary nailing. Before deciding the type and timing of surgery, efforts must be focused on optimizing ventilatory and hemodynamic parameters and normalizing lactate levels, by adequate resuscitation.

Intraoperative Continuation of Resuscitation

Aggressive resuscitation and ongoing evaluation are necessary to establish effective circulating volume and oxygen transport to already hypoxic tissues. An arterial catheter provides useful information regarding hemoglobin, hematocrit, ABG, base deficit and lactate, which is an excellent marker to guide fluid resuscitation. The target base deficit should be <3 and lactate <2 mmol/L. Base deficit of 5 or more is associated with higher mortality.[28] In our institute we use normal saline as the resuscitation fluid followed by blood products. The initial transfusion strategy may be changed from MTP to laboratory parameter-based strategy to minimize wastage of blood and blood products. A disseminated intravascular coagulation (DIC) panel can be ordered in cases of massive transfusion. Thromboelastogram gives a dynamic picture of the entire clotting process, measuring the speed of clot formation, retraction, lysis and consistency, thereby guiding specific component administration. Coagulation testing may take time and visual analysis of operative field can also provide clinical evidence of microvascular bleeding, pointing toward ongoing coagulopathy.

Perioperative Concerns

Hypothermia

Resuscitation and surgical procedures, exposure to ambient temperature, immobilization, anesthesia, combined with suboptimal thermal protection renders the trauma patient hypothermic. Core temperatures between 34 and 36 °C are associated with shivering, postoperative wound infections, perioperative bleeding and transfusion requirements, adverse cardiac events, and prolonged hospital stay.[29] Hypothermic patients have higher rates of shock, organ failure, and sepsis. It is a powerful predictor of death in a severely injured trauma patient.[29] Core temperature monitoring should be instituted in the emergency room itself. Fluid warmers, convective forced-air warming systems, warming and humidification of inspired gases are methods employed to prevent hypothermia. Early control of bleeding and prevention of further heat loss are key factors to avoid the lethal triad of hypothermia, acidosis, and coagulopathy.

Crush Injury and Compartment Syndrome

Crush injury involves mechanical disruption of muscular tissue leading to edema and ischemia and subsequent reperfusion injury when treated. Edema increases compartment pressure which exceeds capillary perfusion pressure leading to hypoxia and further cell membrane damage causing a vicious cycle. Left untreated, it leads to muscle necrosis and release of intracellular components and manifestations of crush syndrome. Hypovolemic shock and hyperkalemic cardiac arrest are the major causes of complications and eventually death. Common fractures leading to compartment syndrome are tibia, forearm, and distal radius fractures. Iatrogenic causes like surgical malposition, ill-fitting casts, compression stockings, tourniquets can also lead to the same and should be observed postoperatively. The institution of epidural or peripheral nerve blocks for pain relief may mask the symptoms of acute compartment syndrome (ACS). However, this can be avoided by using lower concentrations of local anesthetic drugs which preserves motor and sensory function.[30] In this setting, continuous catheters can be advantageous as the volume and concentration can be altered.

Clinical picture is of pain out of proportion to the severity of injury. Pain in response to passive stretching of the muscle may be an early sign of ACS. Classic Ps of pallor, pulselessness and paresis develop very late and by then the limb may become unsalvageable.[30] Better objective method is direct measurement of intracompartmental pressure using a transducer connected to a catheter introduced within 5 cm of the zone of injury. Absolute value of compartment pressure >30 mm Hg or delta pressure (diastolic blood pressure—compartment pressure) <30 mm Hg in conjunction with clinical suspicion points toward ACS.[30] Near infrared spectroscopy (NIRS), is an advanced method which correlates well with tissue perfusion pressures.[31]

Blood investigations reveal hyperkalemia, hyperphosphatemia, hyperuricemia, hypocalcemia, metabolic acidosis with high anion gap, increased lactate, presence of myoglobin and creatine kinase >5,000 units/L. Electrocardiography may show tall T waves. Release of tissue factor in crush syndrome may lead to DIC and hence coagulation testing is mandatory.

Early diagnosis and treatment prevents complications of crush injury. ACS warrants immediate fasciotomies (delta pressures <20–30 mm Hg). Treatment consists of aggressive fluid resuscitation with normal saline given at the rate of 1–1.5 L/h for the first 3 hours. Precipitation of myoglobin in renal tubules can cause acute renal failure. This can be avoided by alkalization of urine with fluids and sodium bicarbonate (NaHCO$_3$ 50 mEq in 1 L of fluid) and forced diuresis with furosemide. The target urine output should be 200–300 mL/h and urine pH >6.5. Mannitol 1 g/kg can be given once urine flow is established. Mannitol is useful in therapy of crush syndrome as it is a free radical scavenger, promotes forced diuresis and can reduce intracompartmental pressure during compartment syndrome. Hyperkalemia can be treated with IV calcium, sodium bicarbonate, insulin, beta-agonist nebulization, potassium binding resins, and hemodialysis. Throughout the perioperative period, assessment of volume responsiveness, calculation of fluid requirement and serial monitoring of ABG, electrolytes, and osmolarity should be done.[32] Patients with anuria, fluid overload, potassium levels >7 mEq/L, high serum creatinine are candidates for dialysis in the setting of crush syndrome. Hyperbaric oxygen has also been used to improve tissue viability.[33]

Fat Embolism

Fat emboli into systemic circulation are a common phenomenon in long bone fractures. This can occur preoperatively due to movement of unstable bone fragments or intraoperatively while reaming the medullary canal. Fat embolism syndrome (FES) is a physiological response to fat droplets in peripheral and lung microcirculation.[34] The risk factors for the development of FES are young age, closed fractures, multiple fractures, femur fractures, and conservative therapy for long bone fractures. Factors which increase the risk of FES after intramedullary nailing are overzealous nailing and reaming of the medullary cavity, increased velocity of reaming, and increase in the gap between nail and cortical bone.[35] Femoral shaft fractures have the highest incidence of FES.[34] The presentation of FES can be gradual, developing over 12–72 hours, or fulminant leading to acute respiratory distress syndrome (ARDS) and cardiac arrest.

Fat embolism syndrome consists of a triad of neurological, pulmonary, and cutaneous symptoms. Clinical features usually include respiratory distress and hypoxemia. Pulmonary hypertension and systemic hypotension can occur in severe cases. Gurd and Wilson suggested major and minor criteria to be used for diagnosis of FES. The major features include petechial rash, mainly axillary and subconjunctival, hypoxia, pulmonary edema, and central nervous system (CNS) depression. Minor features include pyrexia, tachycardia, retinal fat emboli, jaundice, urinary fat globules, fat macroglobulinemia, anemia, thrombocytopenia, and raised erythrocyte sedimentation rate (ESR). The presence of one major and four minor findings are required for diagnosis of FES.[34] Lindeque criteria are more objective as they include ABG analysis [FES = femur fracture ± tibia fracture plus one of the following features: a sustained partial pressure of oxygen (PaO_2) <60 mm Hg, sustained partial pressure of carbon dioxide ($PaCO_2$) >55 mm Hg or pH <7.3, sustained respiratory rate >35/min even after adequate sedation, increased work of breathing judged by dyspnea, use of accessory muscles, tachycardia and anxiety].[34]

Arterial blood gases exhibit low PaO_2 due to hypoxemia and low $PaCO_2$ due to tachypnea and respiratory alkalosis. Chest X-ray includes bilateral diffuse alveolar and interstitial densities in 30-50% of the cases after 12-24 hours.[34] The most common CT features of FES are ground-glass opacity and consolidation, which correlate with disease severity.[36] Cerebral magnetic resonance imaging may show hypointense lesions on cerebral T1W images. Conventional T2W sequences typically reveal multiple diffuse foci of hyperintensity in the deep white matter, basal ganglia, corpus callosum, periventricular region, and cerebellar hemisphere.[34] Intraoperative pulmonary embolism is best diagnosed with transesophageal echocardiography with a sensitivity of 80% and a specificity of 100%.

Treatment involves early recognition of signs, oxygen administration, and reversal of aggravating factors such as hypovolemia, ventilatory and hemodynamic support, if needed. Acute right heart failure may necessitate invasive monitoring, inotropes, and other vasoactive drugs. Mechanical ventilation, if employed, mandates application of lung-protective ventilation with limited plateau pressures and increased levels of positive end-expiratory pressure (PEEP) to prevent secondary lung injury intraoperatively as well as in the postoperative period. Corticosteroids have been used in the treatment of FES, but the beneficial role of corticosteroids needs to be further studied. Continuous pulse oximetry monitoring in high-risk patients may help in detecting desaturation early, allowing early institution of oxygen. The single most important preventive measure to avoid FES is early fixation of fractures.[34]

Venous and Pulmonary Thromboembolism

Deep vein thrombosis (DVT) prophylaxis should be instituted immediately in the form of low-molecular-weight heparin or low-dose unfractionated heparin, fondaparinux, vitamin K antagonists dabigatran, rivaroxaban, apixaban, low-dose aspirin, or an intermittent pneumatic compression device.[37] If heparin is contraindicated then bilateral pneumatic compression or elastic stockings should be applied on admission to hospital and continued perioperatively. Drug prophylaxis should ideally start 12 hours before surgery. However, patients with high risk of bleeding should receive prophylaxis after the surgery. American Society of Regional Anesthesia (ASRA) guidelines should be followed for timing of spinal, epidural, peripheral nerve blocks corresponding to the last dosage of thromboprophylaxis and the same protocol should be followed at the time of removal of catheters. Detailed management is mentioned in the chapter 10.

Perioperative Concerns in Geriatric Orthopedic Trauma

Fracture femur is the most common injury in the elderly population and it is usually associated with trivial trauma. These patients have multiple comorbid conditions that may influence their perioperative care and though optimization of these comorbidities is desirable, it may not always be possible. Patients should be fully evaluated, resuscitated hemodynamically and a quick attempt should be made to correct electrolyte abnormalities, poorly controlled diabetes, congestive heart failure, anticoagulation, correctable cardiac arrhythmias, acute respiratory infection, and anemia.[38] Recent data have shown that early surgery (<24–48 hours) provides a benefit to geriatric patients with hip fractures, in comparison to delayed surgery in terms of reduced pulmonary complications and decreased length of hospital stay.[22,38-40] Surgery beyond 48 hours is associated with higher mortality risk.[39] However, recent literature which summarizes the previous available studies has concluded that it may be prudent to operate American Society of Anesthesiologists (ASA) 1 and 2 patients within 48 hours and one can wait for correctable comorbidities in ASA 3 and 4 patients, to be optimized before surgery even if it extends beyond 48 hours. This is the concept of limited delay for optimization.[41] Guidelines of preoperative testing from the American College of Cardiology and the American Heart Association do not support the use of additional cardiac investigations in most patients, as these surgeries come under emergency procedures.[42]

Recent meta-analysis in Cochrane database comparing regional vs. general anesthesia for hip fractures suggests no difference in the two techniques with regards to outcomes except for the incidence of DVT in the absence of thromboprophylaxis.[43] A large prospective UK based audit concluded that mortality was independent of type of anesthesia but was associated with fall of blood pressure perioperatively.[44] A large subset of geriatric patients is on antiplatelet or anticoagulant drugs for atrial fibrillation, stroke, ischemic heart disease, etc. ASRA guidelines for neuraxial anesthesia need to be followed in these cases.[37]

Geriatric patients do not tolerate hypovolemia or fluid overload; recent literature trends toward restricted fluid administration than had been the standard practice.[45] There is no added advantage of colloid administration in these patients.[46] Intraoperative fluid optimization using clinical methods or goal-directed fluid therapy using advanced hemodynamic monitoring has not been proven to improve outcomes in these patients.[47] In an updated meta-analysis there was no difference in outcomes such as 30-day mortality, length of hospitalization, infection rates, myocardial infarction, congestive cardiac failure when restricted transfusion practices (<8 g/dL) were followed in comparison to liberal transfusion practices (<10 g/dL).[48] Postoperative analgesia should be multimodal and care should be taken to avoid pressure sores. Air-filled mattresses should be used. Postoperative thromboprophylaxis should be instituted as early as possible. Delirium prevention or management, nutritional supplementation, detection of complications such as urinary retention, stool impaction and swallowing disorders, osteoporosis screening, early physiotherapy, and rehabilitation are important components of postoperative care following hip fracture surgery in the elderly.[40]

Postoperative Concerns

Delirium

This has been covered in the chapter 4.

Pain Management

High-quality perioperative pain management in trauma patient is of paramount importance to avoid the long-term complications of chronic pain, phantom limb and complex regional pain syndromes. Pre-emptive analgesia and multimodal analgesic regimes including dexamethasone 0.1 mg/kg, gabapentin or pregabalin, preoperative celecoxib unless contraindicated, are recommended.[8,49] Apart from the acute pain management techniques mentioned earlier in the chapter, periarticular injections, physical strategies such as cryotherapy (ice bags, gel packs, ice massage, etc.), limb elevation, transcutaneous electric nerve stimulation (TENS), and connecting patients to psychosocial interventions can be employed.[8] Both pain and sedation should be regularly assessed in patients using validated tools. Intramuscular injections and opioid-based IV patient controlled analgesia should be avoided.[49]

TACO and TRALI in Trauma Patients

Prevention of perioperative lung injury becomes especially important in trauma patients as lung injury can occur secondary to direct trauma, massive resuscitation, mobilization of fractures, aspiration or transfusion-related acute lung injury (TRALI). Aggressive resuscitation can lead to edema and inflammatory changes in alveolar spaces, elevation of inflammatory markers leading to acute lung injury (ALI) and ARDS.[50] Early transfusions of pRBCs and FFP are independent predictors of ARDS.[50] Massive transfusion can lead to respiratory complications manifesting as progressive hypoxemia, decreased lung compliance, and pulmonary edema. This could be either due to TRALI or transfusion-related circulatory overload (TACO) and it is difficult to distinguish between the two. TACO is characterized by acute pulmonary edema associated with left atrial hypertension or volume overload within 6 hours of blood transfusion. Risk factors include age >60 years, females, higher APACHE II (Acute Physiology and Chronic Health Evaluation II) score, renal failure, pre-existing cardiac dysfunction, shock, anemia, pulmonary disease, number and rate of transfusion of blood and FFP, high levels of biomarkers such as pro-B-type natriuretic peptide (proBNP) and N-terminal proBNP. Signs include acute respiratory distress, hypertension, hypoxemia, findings of congestive heart failure such as elevated venous pressures, S3 heart sound, Kerley B lines, and bilateral opacities on chest X-ray. Diagnosis of TACO can be established if there are a minimum of three signs of pulmonary edema within 6 hours of transfusion. Echocardiography will suggest findings of systolic heart failure like left ventricular dilatation and reduced ejection fraction. There may be lack of respiratory variation in inferior vena caval diameter in spontaneously breathing patient suggesting volume overload. Clinical features and echocardiography can help distinguish between the two conditions.[51]

Management of TACO follows the principles of management of cardiogenic pulmonary edema. Limiting IV fluids and blood, supplemental oxygen, elevation of head end of the bed, vasodilators, and diuretics as per hemodynamics need to be started with strict monitoring of urine output.

CONCLUSION

Musculoskeletal trauma can be life-threatening or limb-threatening and requires DCR. FES, ACS, resuscitation-induced TACO and TRALI are some of the major complications unique to musculoskeletal trauma. Vigilance to pick up early symptoms and signs and prompt measures for prevention and treatment can reduce morbidity and mortality.

REFERENCES

1. Vallier HA. Musculoskeletal trauma. In: Smith CE (Ed). Trauma Anesthesia, 2nd edition. Cambridge: Cambridge University Press; 2015.

2. Pape HC, Lefering R, Butcher N, Peitzman A, Leenen L, Marzi I, et al. The definition of polytrauma revisited: an international consensus process and proposal of the new 'Berlin definition'. J Trauma Acute Care Surg. 2014;77:780-6.

3. Banerjee M, Bouillon B, Shafizadeh S, Paffrath T, Lefering R, Wafaisade A. Epidemiology of extremity injuries in multiple trauma patients. Injury. 2013;44:1015-21.

4. Pfeifer R, Tarkin IS, Rocos B, Pape HC. Patterns of mortality and causes of death in polytrauma patients—has anything changed?. Injury. 2009;40:907-11.

5. Advanced Trauma Life Support, Student Course Manual, 10th edition. Chicago: American College of Surgeons; 2018.

6. Cannon JW, Khan MA, Raja AS, Cohen MJ, Como JJ, Cotton BA, et al. Damage control resuscitation in patients with severe traumatic hemorrhage: a practice management guideline from the Eastern Association for the Surgery of Trauma. J Trauma Acute Care Surg. 2017;82:605-17.

7. Spahn DR, Bouillon B, Cerny V, Duranteau J, Filipescu D, Hunt BJ, et al. The European guideline on management of major bleeding and coagulopathy following trauma: fifth edition. Crit Care. 2019;23:98.

8. Hsu JR, Mir H, Wally MK, Seymour RB. Clinical practice guidelines for pain management in acute musculoskeletal injury. J Orthop Trauma. 2019;33:e158-82.

9. Berti M, Baciarello M, Troglio R, Fanelli G. Clinical uses of low-dose ketamine in patients undergoing surgery. Curr Drug Targets. 2009;10:707-15.

10. Young JW, Burgess AR, Brumback RJ, Poka A. Pelvic fractures: value of plain radiography in early assessment and management. Radiology. 1986;160:445-51.

11. Yoshihara H, Yoneoka D. Demographic epidemiology of unstable pelvic fracture in the United States from 2000 to 2009: trends and in-hospital mortality. J Trauma Acute Care Surg. 2014;76:380-5.

12. Holstein JH, Culemann U, Pohlemann T. Working Group Mortality in Pelvic Fracture Patients. What are predictors of mortality in patients with pelvic fractures? Clin Orthop Relat Res. 2012;470:2090-7.

13. Eastridge BJ, Starr A, Minei JP, O'Keefe GE, Scalea TM. The importance of fracture pattern in guiding therapeutic decision-making in patients with hemorrhagic shock and pelvic ring disruptions. J Trauma. 2002;53:446-51.

14. Black EA, Lawson CM, Smith S, Daley BJ. Open pelvic fractures: the University of Tennessee Medical Center at Knoxville experience over ten years. Iowa Orthop J. 2011;31:193-8.

15. Nicola R. Early total care versus damage control: current concepts in the orthopedic care of polytrauma patients. ISRN Orthop. 2013;2013:329452.

16. Grimm MR, Vrahas MS, Thomas KA. Pressure-volume characteristics of the intact and disrupted pelvic retroperitoneum. J Trauma. 1998;44:454-9.

17. Giannoudis PV, Pape HC. Damage control orthopaedics in unstable pelvic ring injuries. Injury. 2004;35:671-7.

18. Richards JE, Conti BM, Grissom TE. Care of the severely injured orthopedic trauma patient: considerations for initial management, operative timing, and ongoing resuscitation. Adv Anesth. 2018;36:1-22.

19. Cullinane DC, Schiller HJ, Zielinski MD, Bilaniuk JW, Collier BR, Como J, et al. Eastern Association for the Surgery of Trauma practice management guidelines for hemorrhage in pelvic fracture—update and systematic review. J Trauma. 2011;71:1850-68.

20. Shim H, Jang JY, Kim JW, Ryu H, Jung PY, Kim S, et al. Effectiveness and postoperative wound infection of preperitoneal pelvic packing in patients with hemodynamic instability caused by pelvic fracture. PloS one. 2018;13:e0206991.

21. Umarji S, Bircher M. Pelvic and acetabular trauma. In: Cashman J, Grounds M (Eds). Recent Advances in Anaesthesia and Intensive Care. Cambridge: Cambridge University Press; 2007. pp. 87-108.

22. American College of Surgeons (2015). ACS TQIP best practices in the management of orthopaedic trauma. [online] Available from https://www.facs.org/-/media/files/quality-programs/trauma/tqip/ortho_guidelines.ashx?la=en. [Last accessed February, 2020].

23. Bone LB, Johnson KD, Weigelt J, Scheinberg R. Early versus delayed stabilization of femoral fractures. A prospective randomized study. J Bone Joint Surg Am. 1989;7:336-40.

24. Gandhi RR, Overton TL, Haut ER, Lau B, Vallier HA, Rohs T, et al. Optimal timing of femur fracture stabilization in polytrauma patients: a practice management guideline from the Eastern Association for the Surgery of Trauma. J Trauma Acute Care Surg. 2014;77:787-95.

25. Pape HC, Schmidt RE, Rice J, van Griensven M, das Gupta R, Krettek C, et al. Biochemical changes after trauma and skeletal surgery of the lower extremity: quantification of the operative burden. Crit Care Med. 2000;28:3441-8.

26. Stahel PF, Heyde CE, Wyrwich W, Ertel W. Current concepts of polytrauma management: from ATLS to "damage control". Der Orthopade. 2005;34:823-36.

27. Pape HC, Giannoudis PV, Krettek C, Trentz O. Timing of fixation of major fractures in blunt polytrauma: role of conventional indicators in clinical decision making. J Orthop Trauma. 2005;19:551-62.

28. Allen CF, Goslar PW, Barry M, Christiansen T. Management guidelines for hypotensive pelvic fracture patients. Am Surg. 2000;66:735-8.

29. Tsuei BJ, Kearney PA. Hypothermia in the trauma patient. Injury. 2004;35:7-15.

30. Garner MR, Taylor SA, Gausden E, Lyden JP. Compartment syndrome: diagnosis, management, and unique concerns in the twenty-first century. HSS J. 2014;10:143-52.

31. Shuler FD, Dietz MJ. Physicians' ability to manually detect isolated elevations in leg intracompartmental pressure. J Bone Joint Surg Am. 2010;2:361-7.

32. Genthon A, Wilcox SR. Crush syndrome: a case report and review of the literature. J Emerg Med. 2014;46:313-9.

33. Rajagopalan S. Crush injuries and the crush syndrome. Med J Armed Forces India. 2010;66:317-20.

34. Akhtar S. Fat embolism. Anesthesiol Clin. 2009;27:533-50.

35. Shaikh N. Emergency management of fat embolism syndrome. J Emerg Trauma Shock. 2009;2:29-33.

36. Newbigin K, Souza CA, Armstrong M, Pena E, Inacio J, Gupta A, et al. Fat embolism syndrome: Do the CT findings correlate with clinical course and severity of symptoms? A clinical-radiological study. Eur J Radiol. 2016;85:422-7.

37. Horlocker TT, Vandermeulen E, Kopp SL, Gogarten W, Leffert LR, Benzon HT. Regional anesthesia in the patient receiving antithrombotic or thrombolytic therapy: American Society of Regional Anesthesia and Pain Medicine evidence-based guidelines (fourth edition). Reg Anesth Pain Med. 2018;43: 263-309.

38. Ftouh S, Morga A, Swift C. Management of hip fracture in adults: summary of NICE guidance. BMJ. 2011;342:d3304.

39. Fu MC, Boddapati V, Gausden EB, Samuel AM, Russell LA, Lane JM. Surgery for a fracture of the hip within 24 hours of admission is independently associated with reduced short-term post-operative complications. Bone Joint J. 2017;99: 1216-22.

40. Boddaert J, Raux M, Khiami F, Riou B. Perioperative management of elderly patients with hip fracture. Anesthesiology. 2014;121:1336-41.

41. Lewis PM, Waddell JP. When is the ideal time to operate on a patient with a fracture of the hip?: a review of the available literature. Bone Joint J. 2016;98-B:1573-81.

42. Fleisher LA, Fleischmann KE, Auerbach AD, Barnason SA, Beckman JA, Bozkurt B, et al. 2014 ACC/AHA guideline on perioperative cardiovascular evaluation and management of patients undergoing noncardiac surgery: a report of the American College of Cardiology/American Heart Association Task Force on practice guidelines. J Am Coll Cardiol. 2014;64:e77-137.

43. Guay J, Parker MJ, Gajendragadkar PR, Kopp S. Anaesthesia for hip fracture surgery in adults. Cochrane Database Syst Rev. 2016;2:CD000521.

44. White SM, Moppett IK, Griffiths R, Johansen A, Wakeman R, Boulton C, et al. Secondary analysis of outcomes after 11,085 hip fracture operations from the prospective UK Anaesthesia Sprint Audit of Practice (ASAP-2). Anaesthesia. 2016;71:506-14.

45. Brandstrup B. Fluid therapy for the surgical patient. Best Pract Res Clin Anaesthesiol. 2006;20:265-83.

46. Perel P, Roberts I. Colloids versus crystalloids for fluid resuscitation in critically ill patients. Cochrane Database Syst Rev. 2012;6:CD000567.

47. Lewis SR, Butler AR, Brammar A, Nicholson A, Smith AF. Perioperative fluid volume optimization following proximal femoral fracture. Cochrane Database Syst Rev. 2016;3:CD003004.

48. Mao T, Gao F, Han J, Sun W, Guo W, Li Z, et al. Restrictive versus liberal transfusion strategies for red blood cell transfusion after hip or knee surgery: a systematic review and meta-analysis. Medicine. 2017;96:e7326.

49. Chou R, Gordon DB, de Leon-Casasola OA, Rosenberg JM, Bickler S, Brennan T, et al. Management of postoperative pain: a clinical practice guideline from the American Pain Society, the American Society of Regional Anesthesia and Pain Medicine, and the American Society of Anesthesiologists' Committee on Regional Anesthesia, Executive Committee, and Administrative Council. J Pain. 2016;17:131-57.

50. Bakowitz M, Bruns B, McCunn M. Acute lung injury and the acute respiratory distress syndrome in the injured patient. Scand J Trauma Resusc Emerg Med. 2012;20:54.

51. Roubinian NH, Murphy EL. Transfusion-associated circulatory overload (TACO): prevention, management, and patient outcomes. Int J Clin Transfus Med. 2015;3:17-28.

Head and Neck

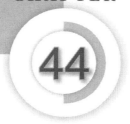

Perioperative Management of Major Head and Neck Cancers

Anuja Jain, Sohan Lal Solanki

INTRODUCTION

Head and neck malignancies form the tenth most common cancers globally and most common in India.[1] The number of patients coming for head and neck surgery is therefore the highest, implying that they remain the largest chunk of patient in postoperative care unit in an oncology set-up. Optimization and management start in preoperative period extending to postoperative critical care unit. Head and neck malignancy includes a variety of cases ranging from the base of skull cranially to larynx caudally. With all the important structures around, these surgeries are associated with various postoperative life-threatening complications. In addition to the destructive surgery, it is associated with major reconstructions a good number out of which are free flaps. Hence, it becomes imperative to have in-depth knowledge about perioperative care of head and neck cancer patients.

ETIOLOGY

Going through the literature, head and neck cancer can be attributed to smoking, tobacco chewing, alcohol, human papillomaviruses 16 and 18, and rarely due to dental trauma. All the mentioned risk factors are also blamed for comorbidities.[2] To add to the list, occupational exposure, radiation, and poor oral hygiene are other risk factors. Sometimes this can be idiopathic also.

DIAGNOSIS AND EVALUATION

Patient present with nonhealing ulcer in mouth, longstanding sore throat, change in voice, difficulty in deglutition, stuffy nose, or swelling in head and neck region. To establish cancer and ascertain the spread, imaging and supportive tissue diagnosis is mandatory. These also help in establishing the stage of disease and

formulate a management plan. Fine needle aspiration cytology (FNAC) with or without imaging done in outpatient door setting generally yields diagnosis. Imaging in form of ultrasonography, computed tomography (CT) scan, or magnetic resonance imaging (MRI) helps in establishing extent of disease and lymph nodal spread. CT scan and MRI help us to judge the airway status and formulate a plan. Flexible endoscopy gives a first-hand view of the disease status in aerodigestive tract or sinuses. Frequently FNAC does not suffice and a biopsy becomes necessary. For this direct laryngoscopy or examination under anesthesia is the option. Even for this a preanesthesia check-up is necessary.

PREOPERATIVE EVALUATION

This evaluation is the preliminary step to intraoperative and postoperative management of patient. The domain of this not only encompasses diagnosis but also includes preoperative optimization and counseling. Foremost, detail history and physical examination for comorbidities are of paramount importance. The presenting symptoms of patient give an indication toward the involvement of aerodigestive tract and are a guide for anticipating difficult airway or risk of aspiration. Airway should be examined thoroughly. One should make a habit to examine the front of neck to ensure that in emergency situation cricothyroid membrane can be located and punctured.

Cardiology and pulmonary assessment is mandatory in physical examination to rule out any comorbidities. Further evaluation is done according to American College of Cardiology/American Heart Association (ACC/AHA) guidelines for cardiac patients undergoing noncardiac surgery.[3] ACC/AHA on the basis of functional status and type of surgery predicts the risk of cardiac events in perioperative period and also guides if any further investigation or intervention is needed.

Smoking and tobacco chewing are common in these patients. Smoking leads to several cardiopulmonary changes. So, chronic obstructive pulmonary disease (COPD) is commonly encountered in these patients. A detail history of medications should be taken. Evaluation by dentist and speech therapist is also essential.

Routine screening of blood including complete blood count, liver and kidney functions, serum electrolytes, and random sugar is mandatory.[4] Depending on the age of patient, electrocardiogram is advised. Further evaluation for cardiac and COPD patients is dependent on their effort tolerance and metabolic equivalents (MET). This would include echocardiography, pulmonary function test, and cardiopulmonary exercise testing (CPET).

Emphasis should be given on Eastern Cooperative Oncology Group (ECOG) performance status and American Society of Anesthesia (ASA) classification.[5] A multidisciplinary approach and a detail discussion on management between the anesthetist, surgical oncologist, critical care physician, and medical oncologist should be done in patients with a high ASA score and ECOG score. If needed, an alternative plan of management should be suggested if the perioperative morbidity and mortality is predicted to be high for a major resection and reconstruction. On literature review many studies have concluded that with higher and uncontrolled comorbid burden the chances of recurrence are higher and disease-free survival is questionable.[6] Though other studies have shown no such correlation.[7]

Many patients with T3/T4 stage of cancer according to TNM classification might receive neoadjuvant chemotherapy (NACT) for reduction in size and make the tumor resectable or may come for salvage surgery. There are patients who have recurrence and must have received chemotherapy (CT) or radiation (RT).[8] Both these therapies have their own effect on body.

EFFECT OF MALIGNANCY AND ITS TREATMENT (CHEMOTHERAPY, RADIOTHERAPY, IMMUNOTHERAPY, SURGERY) ON BODY

not only that cancer causes various effects on body but also its treatment. Its various sequels are:
- Effects of tumor on body[9]
  - *Locally due to compression*: Commonly in mediastinal masses. This leads to compression of airway, superior vena cava, and esophagus or brachial plexus. This presents with difficulty in breathing consequently stridor, difficult deglutition, engorgement of neck veins, facial swelling, and neuropathic pain. Mechanical obstruction, tissue destruction, and ischemia can be other consequences of locally advanced malignancy.
  - *Hormonal effects*:
    Primarily due to tumor in specific organ like parathyroid tumors which causes hypocalcemia, thyroid tumors can cause deranged thyroid hormones. Paraneoplastic syndromes in form of neurological, mucocutaneous, hematological, or endocrine manifestations are also known. Although these are rarely seen in patients of head and neck cancer.
  - *Systemic effects*:[10]
    - *Renal*: Due to inadequate oral intake these patients land in to dehydration and prerenal failure.
    - *Cardiopulmonary effects*: Indirectly due to addiction of tobacco or smoking, these patients may be having cardiopulmonary comorbidities.
    - *Electrolyte derangements*: Due to poor oral intake, hyponatremia is common.
    - *Nutritional effects*: Poor oral intake due to malignancy of aerodigestive tract.
    - *Depression and anxiety*: Almost up to 70% of patients need psychological support.[11]
- Effect of treatment
  - *Chemotherapy*: Different groups of chemotherapy drugs have various effects on different systems.[12] These are described in **Table 1**.
  - *Radiotherapy*: Manifestations of this are dose dependent. Radiotherapy can be a part of multimodal therapy or individually or as palliation. It may lead to soft tissue edema in initial phases and later to fibrosis, contractures consequently restricted mouth opening and neck extension. Chondronecrosis and perichondritis of the trachea are also known which consequently lead to stenosis.[14] These can lead to difficult airway.
    Radiation also causes pulmonary and cardiac effects. Effects of radiation on lung result in reduction in compliance and radiation pneumonitis. Changes in cardiac contractility and conductivity can happen due to pericarditis and myocardial fibrosis.

Airway Assessment

These patients mostly present to the hospital at advanced stage attributed to illiteracy, lack of access to health care, and poverty especially in developing countries. As a perioperative physician challenge is to manage airway of these patients with anatomical distortions and most importantly sharing of airway with surgeon. A guaranteed airway, extending from the preoperative phase continuing to the postoperative period, to a safe discharge is responsibility of care provider. To assure this, formulation of plan is

Table 1: Various chemotherapeutic drugs and their effect on systems.[13]

System	Perioperative concerns	Chemotherapy drugs
Respiratory	Pulmonary edema	Methotrexate
	Pulmonary fibrosis	Bleomycin, ifosamide, panitumumab
Cardiovascular	Tachycardia	Procarbazine, cladribine, alemtuzumab, trastuzumab, muromonab-CD3
	Cardiac arrhythmia	Pentostatin, fludarabine, palivizumab, interferon alfa-2b, erlotinib
	Bradycardia	Docetaxel, lenalidomide
	Hypotension	Pentostatin, vincristine, alemtuzumab, daclizumab, muromonab-CD3, denileukin diftitox
	Hypertension	Pentostatin, vinblastine, vincristine, alemtuzumab, bevacizumab, trastuzumab, daclizumab, muromonab-CD3, sorafenib, sunitinib, nilotinib
	Cardiomyopathy	Doxorubicin, trastuzumab, sunitinib, dasatinib, lapatinib
Renal	Proximal tubular dysfunction	Ifosfamide
	Hypomagnesemia	Cisplatin, carboplatin
Hepatic	Coagulopathy	Asparaginase
Nervous	Peripheral neuropathy	Vinblastine, vincristine, cisplatin

indispensable starting from the preoperative visit of the patient.

Surgery for head and neck malignancies may range from a minor diagnostic procedure as direct laryngoscopy, microlaryngeal laser resection, and base of tongue biopsies to as major as tumor resection with reconstruction, total laryngectomy, tracheal resection, thyroidectomy, radical neck dissection, etc. The goal of preoperative assessment is to recognize a difficult airway. About 90% of difficult intubations can be anticipated but as high as 50% are missed which leads to major catastrophe. Most important cause of concern is the site and size of tumor, in addition to the coexistent problems such as receding jaw, restricted neck movement, etc. Central to the management of head and neck malignancies is the detection of obstructive symptoms. There might be subtle airway obstruction which gets unmasked under anesthesia when the patient is apneic. So, history of recent onset snoring, increased difficulty in breathing, noise while inspiration or expiration, change of voice, and dysphagia signify obtunding obstruction. It is substantial to differentiate these symptoms from obstructive sleep apnea and COPD.

Signs such as ankyloglossia, restricted neck movements point toward difficult intubation. History of previous easy intubation does not rule out difficulty in present setting, but prior history of difficulty definitely has a positive predictive value.

Various tests to anticipate difficult intubation has been mentioned in literature but when used alone none has a good specificity or sensitivity. When used together, they are powerful predictors of difficult airway. Before entering the operating room, one should seek answers to five questions, combining the assessment of all these are good predictors of difficult airway.

- *Mallampati class*: Worthwhile for prediction of difficult intubation. Provides information regarding the tongue size as compared to size of oral cavity.
- *Mandibular space*: Distance from submentum to hyoid bone. Space less than two fingers signify anteriorly placed larynx, greater curvature, and difficult intubation.
- *Extent of mouth opening*: For a successful laryngoscopy a minimum of 3 cm mouth opening is required less than which signifies a difficult laryngoscopy.
- *Neck movements*: Ability to assume sniffing position implies a straight axis to larynx and inability predicts a difficult position.
- *Difficult mask ventilation*: Mask ventilation assures a continuous oxygenation of the patient. Factors associated with difficult mask ventilation are beard, obese, large neck circumference, edentulous.

In addition to above, a careful palpation of the lesion helps in decision making. Other tests useful in mapping of lesion are indirect mirror or flexible nasopharyngoscopy. Mapping helps in knowing the extent of lesion involvement of tongue base and vocal cords. Ultrasonography (US) is a quick and easy technique to detect a difficult airway. US also aids in placement of endotracheal tube in awake patient, detection of esophageal intubation, calculation of appropriate size of endotracheal tube, prediction of postextubation stridor, and assessing the placement of laryngeal mask airway.[15] A CT scan or MRI of head and neck is a very good tool to have a quick look before induction of anesthesia for airway assessment and can indicate toward compromise in airway if any.

CT bronchography and virtual bronchoscopy (VB) are proven to be comparable to other assessment tools for anticipating difficult airway. Noninvasive, less time consuming, no anesthesia required, requirement of only routine CT images, and operator independent are the advantages of CT bronchography, especially useful in patients with airway strictures. However, exposure to radiation, artifacts due to secretions and blood, and nonvisualization of poorly aerated segments limits its use.[16]

PREOPERATIVE OPTIMIZATION

Enhanced Recovery after Surgery

Enhanced recovery after surgery (ERAS) in head and neck cancer patients has shown to improve outcomes. Evidence suggests that implementation of this also reduces cost of care by using resources efficiently. More so it improves efficiency of care provided in perioperative period. The components of ERAS as suggested by the society for head and neck cancer surgery are in **Table 2**.[17]

Cardiovascular System

- Control of blood pressure (BP) is important. Nonhypertensive patients with BP >180/110 in preanesthesia evaluation should be started on antihypertensive.
- Angiotensin converting enzyme inhibitors and angiotensin II antagonists should be withheld on day of surgery except when used for heart failure. Rest all the cardiac medications to be continued.
- Clopidogrel should be stopped 7 days prior and warfarin should be stopped 5 days prior and bridged with heparin.

Respiratory System

- Patients of COPD or asthma should continue with bronchodilators. While evaluating for surgery and during preanesthetic evaluation if patient is found to have infection, it should be treated with antibiotics.
- Active chest physiotherapy and incentive spirometry should be started from preoperative period.
- Preoperative nebulization with bronchodilator and steroids should be given.
- Patient should be advised to stop smoking in first visit to hospital. If needed nicotine patches or gums can be advised.[18]

Glycemic Control

- To prevent hyper- or hypoglycemia and harm associated with both, international guidelines suggest to target blood glucose levels between 79 and 144 mg/dL.[19,20]
- Guidelines suggest to continue metformin till day of surgery.[19]
- Sodium–glucose cotransporter-2 inhibitor (SGLT2i) or gliflozins, dipeptidyl peptidase 4 inhibitors (DPP4i) or gliptins and glucagon like peptide-1 receptor agonists

Table 2: Enhanced recovery after surgery recommendations for head and neck cancer patients for surgery with free flap reconstruction.[17]

Component	Evidence	Recommendation
Preoperative		
• *Preoperative education*: This should be done preadmission by qualified person	Low	Strong
• *Preoperative nutrition*: All patient should go through exhaustive nutritional assessment. With nutritional intervention for malnourished	High	Strong
• *Venous thromboembolism prophylaxis (VTE)*: Should be given pharmacologic prophylaxis in preoperative period weighing the risk of bleeding.	High	Strong
• *Nil by mouth*: Clear liquid to be allowed till 2 hours before surgery	High	Strong
Intraoperative		
• *Preoperative antibiotic*: Not to be given for clean procedures. Only for clean contaminated procedures. 1 hour prior to be continued till 24 hours.	High	Strong
• *Anesthesia protocol*: Depth enough to warrant awareness. Early awakening preferred.	Low	Strong
• *Prevent hypothermia*: Maintain normothermia.	High	Strong
• *Perioperative fluid*: Goal directed fluid. Avoid over or under hydration	Moderate	Strong
Postoperative		
• *Routine ICU admission*: Postoperative sedation and ventilation not necessary	Low	Weak
• *Pain management*: Multimodal analgesia, opioid sparing	High	Strong
• *Monitoring flap*: Hourly for first 24 hours, then taper intensity, done by experienced staff	Moderate	Strong
• *Early mobilization*: Recommended within 24 hours	Moderate	Strong
• *Urine catheter*: Remove as soon as patient can self-void in 24 hours	High	Strong
• *Tracheostomy care*		
– Decannulation and stoma closure recommended	Moderate	Strong
– Surgical closure of site recommended	Moderate	Strong
• *Wound care*		
– Vacuum assisted closure recommended for complex wound	High	Strong
– Polyurethane film or hydrocolloid film over skin donor site	High	Strong
• *Pulmonary physiotherapy*: Initiated as soon as possible	High	Strong

(GLP-1) should not be given on day of surgery and preferably should be stopped 72 hours prior.[21,22]

- Patient on insulin should be shifted to human actrapid insulin depending on blood sugar level and institutional protocol.

Nutrition

There is high prevalence of malnutrition in head and neck cancer patients due to various factors. All patients should have in depth nutritional assessment and should undergo diet modification. Various studies have proven the importance of nutritional evaluation and supplementation resulting in reduced hospital stay and early recovery. Patients with a risk of refeeding syndrome will need a nutritional plan adapted to individual patient.[23]

Presurgery Counseling

Importance of this has been stressed by many studies. Due to the psychosocial impact of a major head and neck surgery, and because of cosmetic and phonation issues, education and counseling result in better adaptation by patient.[24] The timing of counseling is still under research.

ANESTHESIA MANAGEMENT

Airway

First and foremost is the formulation of plan of airway management. Difficult airway kit should always be ready in the operation theater. All India Difficult Airway Association (AIDAA) suggests keeping these in a mobile cart or bag which can be moved easily to the place where difficult airway is encountered.[25] A great emphasis has been given to continuous supplementation of high flow oxygen by a nasal cannula or transnasal humidified rapid insufflations ventilatory exchange (THRIVE) during the time of apnea under anesthesia which significantly increases the time for apnea.[26]

Head and neck tumor patients can be encountered in following settings.

Anticipated Difficult Airway

Elective cases: Most of the cases in head and neck malignancies are anticipated as being difficult airway which is base of tongue, buccal mucosa, mandibular, supraglottic, glottic, infraglottic growths, history of prior head and neck surgery with reconstruction and radiation, and large thyroids with retrosternal extension. Post-radiation neck movements are restricted. Also due to skin changes recognition of cricothyroid membrane becomes difficult. Patients undergoing oral surgery will need nasal intubation.

Other surgeries like base of skull, salivary gland, thyroid, or neck dissections oral intubation can be done.

American Society of Anesthesia suggests first assess basic management problem and then proceeds with deciding on management choices in the form of awake intubation or under anesthesia, preservation or ablation of spontaneous ventilation, noninvasive technique or invasive technique, or using video laryngoscope as the initial method.[27] Nasal awake intubation is the choice of securing airway in these patients. For this fiberoptic bronchoscopy (FOB) is modus operandi. Where the facility is not available blind awake intubation or retrograde intubation are supplementary techniques.

When intubating, the patient under anesthesia can be induced with intravenous agents or inhalational agents. In borderline airways inducing the anesthesia and keeping patient spontaneously breathing followed by a quick check laryngoscopy with conventional laryngoscope or by video laryngoscope to ascertain the visualization of glottis is important to proceed with intubation under anesthesia. In proceeding with intubation under anesthesia, it is advisable to attach a nasal cannula with high flow oxygen till the airway is secured. Sakles et al., in their study concluded that CMAC video laryngoscope was associated with higher number of successful intubation as compared to Macintosh blade.[28] On the contrary, Levitan et al. suggest that although the visualization of glottis is good with video laryngoscope but insertion of the tube is difficult due to in congruency in vision.[29] But they also suggest after learning the technicalities and physics behind the various video laryngoscopes, intubation can be simplified. Video laryngoscopes in the form CMAC, Kings vision, and Mcgrath have steep learning curve but once learned it is the method of choice.

Head and neck cancer surgeries require nasal intubation. During nasal intubation we frequently encounter difficulty while passing the tube beyond epiglottis as the tube hits at arytenoids or inter arytenoid. Solanki et al. have described "Solanki two hand maneuver" to overcome this. They describe a novel technique, by giving a backward, upward, and rightward pressure to the larynx by an assistant anesthetist with left hand and simultaneously rotation of tube 90° counterclockwise with the right hand and pushing the tube inward either under vision of a video laryngoscope or under vision of main operating anesthetist performing direct laryngoscopy. This helps overcome the difficulty in passing nasotracheal tube through the vocal cord.[30]

Emergency Cases

Presentation of patient in such condition is principally in stridor. Advanced malignancy of base of tongue, laryngeal lesions, post radiation edema, pharyngeal and thyroid malignancy present with airway compression and stridor. Such patients when presented in emergency, after eliciting a brief history of comorbidities, past history, and fasting status, consent for tracheostomy is ensured. Patient should be wheeled in the operation theater with a high FiO_2 and propped-up position. One should ensure 100% oxygenation of the patient in operation room and a definite intravenous access. In certain conditions locating trachea becomes difficult. Such situations are when there is a mass in front of neck like thyroid, postoperative cases, postradiation. In such situations, locating the trachea with US and marking the entry point will be of help.[31]

After securing the airway by tracheostomy, end tidal CO_2 should be ascertained. Frequently it is seen that such patients have hypercarbia leading to decreased consciousness. Post-tracheostomy chest X-ray is mandatory to rule out pneumothorax.

Unanticipated Difficult Airway

Unanticipated difficult airway when encountered in both emergency and elective situation first and foremost call for help. In such situation maintaining oxygenation is of utmost importance. All guidelines have emphasized on maintaining mask ventilation if this is not possible then insertion of laryngeal mask airway but in head and neck malignancy insertion of laryngeal mask is not possible most of the times. Optimizing the patient position and changing the technique in the form of using video laryngoscope, bougie/ aid to intubate, and smaller size tubes help in successful intubation. At all steps limitation of attempts by the user is important. In an untoward situation needle or surgical cricothyrotomy is the option.

Iatrogenic Difficult Airway

Iatrogenic difficult airway occurs when ventilate can intubate becomes difficult after repeated failed attempts leading to trauma causing bleeding and difficult visualization ultimately leading to difficult mask ventilation and a cannot ventilate and cannot intubate condition. AIDAA suggests to attempt intubation only two times followed by single attempt by senior only if saturation more than 95%. Following these guidelines strictly will ensure that one does not land in iatrogenic cannot intubate cannot ventilate situation.

Monitoring

The Association of Anesthetists recommended standard monitoring in form of pulse oximeter, electrocardiogram, noninvasive blood pressure monitoring, temperature, end tidal carbon di-oxide monitor ($EtCO_2$), and urine catheter. Along with this agent gas monitoring should be used. Depending on functional status of patient invasive monitoring like arterial blood pressure monitoring or cardiac output monitoring should be used. Certain surgeries which involve manipulation of nerve such as parotidectomy or thyroidectomy will need neuromuscular monitoring. For thyroidectomies, nerve integrating monitor tube is used for locating nerve.

Positioning

A 15–20° head-up position is given for primary surgery as a technique to decrease blood loss. For neck dissection, head is tilted to opposite side. One of the complications of this positioning is air embolism. To prevent this, maintaining hemodynamic is important. Adequate padding of pressure points should be done. As the working area of surgeons is same as us, it should be ensured that the connections are tight and circuit is secured adequately.

Intravenous Fluid

Balanced salt solution should be used intravenously. Fluid should be given at a rate of 2–3 mL/Kg/h as maintenance. Maximum allowable blood loss should be calculated and blood should be replaced accordingly. Urine output should be maintained at least 0.5 mL/Kg/h. Due to tumor handling antidiuretic hormone is secreted which sometimes is the reason for reduced output which later returns to normal.

Temperature

Maintaining the temperature of patient is of vital importance. Hypothermia has been shown to increase chances of bleeding, delayed awakening from anesthesia, and arrhythmias. Along with this, it has negative influence on free flap. This might lead to total loss of flap, flap hematoma, and chances of infection.[32]

Choice of Drugs

The choice of induction agent, muscle relaxant, and maintenance agent depends upon comorbidities of patient. Multimodal analgesia should be used with opioids, paracetamol, and nonsteroidal anti-inflammatory agents. For reconstructive surgeries, morphine remains a good option as analgesic.

Intraoperative Complications

- *Injury to vessels*: There can be torrential bleeding in a major vessel injury like carotid or internal jugular vein or minimal with minor vessel. This should be managed actively by fluid and blood replacement.

- *Air embolism*: Due to head high position, risk of air embolisms increases. Anticipation helps in early recognition and intervention. The most accurate monitor for detection is transesophageal echocardiograph. As this is not routinely used among the available monitors, sudden drop in $EtCO_2$ helps in diagnosis. Management includes head low right-up position, rapid flushing of the site with saline, securing a central venous access, and aspiration of air.

- *Arrhythmias*: During neck dissection, manipulation of stellate ganglion and carotid sinus causes bradycardia, prolongation of QT interval, and sinus arrest also. Surgeon should be asked to release the stretch over these structures which temporarily improve heart rate. For persistent arrhythmias infiltration of carotid sheath with local anesthetic might help.

- In bilateral neck dissection if carotid sheath is opened, it has been shown to cause denervation of carotid bodies consequently leading to postoperative loss of hypoxic drive and autonomic dysfunction.

Extubation

During head and neck cancer surgeries, intraoral procedures are done, and it is advisable to keep the endotracheal tube in situ overnight and extubate the trachea next day in consultation with surgeons. AIDAA provides guidelines for extubation which is easy to follow.[33]

POSTOPERATIVE CARE

Postoperative ventilation: Head and neck surgery with reconstruction results in postoperative airway edema due to manipulation. With free flaps involving oral cavity intraoral space reduces dramatically because of the volume of tissue used. For all these reasons patients are kept intubated, preferably on spontaneous ventilation and eventually evaluated for extubation next day. Before extubation, should be ensured that flap is well perfused and drains are clear. There are almost 10% chances of re-exploration in free flap with variation from institute to institute. Many literatures suggest against postoperative deep sedation and mechanical ventilation as this increases the time needed to wean and chances of pulmonary complications increase. Patient should be preferably kept on spontaneous ventilation.

Monitoring of free flap in postoperative period: Every institute should have specific protocols for monitoring of free flaps. Various methods are used for same. Clinical examination to ascertain adequacy of arterial and venous flow in form of color, pin prick testing at frequent intervals, surface temperature monitoring, and capillary refill time. Other invasive techniques such as PO_2 monitors and implantable Doppler are also used.[34,35] There is no consensus as to the ideal method and timing of flap is monitoring. Various case reports and series suggest use of more than one technique as it improves the salvage rate of flap.[35] With venous congestion of flap, it appears blue, congested, and edematous, and on pin prick brisk flow of blood is present. In arterial blockade flap is pale, cold, and there is no flow on pin prick.

Analgesia: Multimodal therapy with combination of opioid and nonopioid analgesics is the choice. One can also use patient control analgesia (PCA) with opioid which has shown to be effective and has no increase in postoperative nausea and vomiting.[36]

Chyle leak (CL): Thoracic duct injury is a rare complication of head and neck surgery found in 2–8% of neck dissections and 0.5–1.4% of thyroidectomies.[37] Sudden increase in drain output which is creamy or milky in appearance after starting of feeding should indicate toward CL. If the leak continues patient develops hyponatremia, hypochloremia, hypoproteinemia, and immunocompromised status. Drain fluid should be sent for biochemical analysis which will show triglyceride level 100 mg/dL. Conservative measures in form of 30–400 head elevation, pressure dressing, and rest usually suffice in reducing drain. Dietary modification to a fat-free, low fat, or medium chain fatty acid results in reduction of chyle production. Orlistat interferes with lipid metabolism and reduces chyle production. Octreotide has been found to be more effective in reducing production. Studies have proven octreotide to be more beneficial as it significantly reduces morbidity and need for surgical intervention.[38] Surgical exploration is suggested when the drain is >500–1,000 mL/day for 4–5 days.[39]

Venous thromboembolism (VTE) prophylaxis: Postoperatively patient with free flap should be started on VTE prophylaxis in form of heparin (unfractionated or low molecular weight). More so if it is a free fibular flap as this impairs mobilization. In addition to VTE prophylaxis, this also improves microcirculation of free flap. Early mobilization reduces risk of thromboembolism.

Nutrition: Intraoral surgeries mandate enteral feed through nasogastric tube. This should be started on the first postoperative period. Diet should be modified according to the need of patient.

Refeeding syndrome: Refeeding syndrome can be defined as the potentially fatal shifts in fluids and electrolytes that may occur in malnourished patients receiving artificial refeeding (whether enterally or parenterally). These shifts can be attributed to metabolic and hormonal changes and may cause serious clinical complications. The hallmark biochemical feature of this syndrome is hypophosphatemia.[40] However, the syndrome is complex and may have abnormal sodium and fluid balance; changes in glucose, protein, and fat metabolism; thiamine deficiency; hypokalemia; and hypomagnesemia. It is recommended to follow NICE guidelines on nutritional support in adults, with particular reference to the new recommendations for best practice in refeeding syndrome.[41]

Carotid blowout or hematoma: Watchfulness on drain in head and neck surgeries is of paramount importance. Carotid blowout is a rare but dreadful complication. Any increase in volume of drain should raise suspicion. Color of drain is equally important. Surgeon should be alerted about increase in drain. This can also manifest as increased swelling in neck and difficulty in breathing. Patient might need immediate re-exploration. Blood should be reserved and coagulation profile should be checked. If patient is on VTE prophylaxis, it should be stopped immediately. Patients with impending airway compromise are candidates of awake tracheostomy but even this can be difficult due to swelling in anterior part of neck. It is advisable to open the sutures in neck first to remove hematoma and then proceed with tracheostomy. In emergency conditions this might have to be done bedside.

Nerve damage: This although happens intraoperatively manifests in postoperative period. This can be transient or permanent. After thyroidectomies there can be damage to unilateral or bilateral superficial laryngeal nerve or recurrent laryngeal nerve damage. With bilateral recurrent laryngeal nerve damage patient will need tracheostomy as the glottis space reduces dramatically. During parotidectomy, there can be damage to facial nerve either all five segments presenting as Bell's palsy or in distribution of particular segment. Patients with nerve damage steroids have definite role to play. Other nerves such as spinal accessory and marginal mandibular nerve can also be damaged.

Hypocalcemia: Damage to parathyroid glands in thyroidectomies can manifest as hypocalcemia. This can be transient <6 weeks or permanent >6 months. It usually starts in 24–48 hours after surgery. Calcium levels should be checked. In symptomatic patients with perioral tingling or Chvostek's sign intravenous calcium should be given. Nonsymptomatic cases can be managed by oral calcium and vitamin D.

Cerebrospinal fluid (CSF) leak: CSF leak can happen after base of skull surgery. Incidence is 13.2% in endoscopic cases.[42] Managed conservatively by bed rest, insertion of lumbar drain, or ventriculoperitoneal shunts for resistant cases.

Diabetes insipidus (DI): DI can manifest after pituitary surgery. This is due to reduced secretion of antidiuretic hormone (ADH) after manipulation of neurohypophysis. In these patients urine output is >3 L/24 h with hypotonic urine and osmolality <800 mOsm/Kg with increased or normal sodium level.[43] Other causes of increased urine output should be ruled out. Usually this is transient and self-limiting. Patient should have serial sodium levels. DI should be treated with desmopressin 10–40 µg intranasal three times a day in divided doses or 1–2 µg SC/IV two times a day.

TRANSORAL ROBOTIC SURGERY

Transoral robotic surgery (TORS) is relatively newer technique mostly used for oropharyngeal cancer resections and thyroid surgeries.[44] Limited access to the patient is the most important factor along with sharing of potentially difficult airway with surgeon. Logistically anesthesia providers are at the leg end of patient so long extensions for circuit and intravenous access are necessary. Complications can damage important structures. In postoperative period risk of bleeding is 3–8% occurring on 10th postoperative day.[45] Postoperative pain is very severe. PCA with opioid is effective along with other analgesics.[46] Steroid given during surgery and continued postoperatively is also effective in controlling pain.[47]

FUTURE

The future of TORS is the miniature flexible robots such as Flex systems and i-Snake system. Being miniature in size has better prospects for head and neck cancer surgery. Robotic surgery for base of skull, nasopharynx and larynx are under experiments.[48] We can expect increase in number of patients undergoing robotic surgery for head and neck cancer.

REFERENCES

1. Francis CJK. Trends in incidence of head and cancers in India. Annals Oncol. 2016;27(Suppl 9).
2. Shaw R, Beasley N. Aetiology and risk factors for head and neck cancer: United Kingdom National Multidisciplinary Guidelines. J Laryngol Otol. 2016;130:S9-S12.
3. Fleisher LA, Fleischmann K, Auerbach AD, Barnason SA, Beckman JA, Bozkurt B, et al. 2014 ACC/AHA Guideline on Perioperative Cardiovascular Evaluation and Management of Patients Undergoing Noncardiac Surgery. J Am Coll Cardiol. 2014;64:e77-e137.
4. Sahai SK. Perioperative assessment of the cancer patient. Best Pract Res Clin Anaesthesiol. 2013;27:465-80.
5. Blagden SP, Charman SC, Sharples LD, Magee LR, Gilligan D. Performance status score: Do patients and their oncologists agree? Br J Cancer. 2003;89(6):1022-7.
6. Piccirillo JF, Tierney RM, Costas I, Grove L, Spitznagel EL Jr. Prognostic importance of comorbidity in a hospital-based cancer registry. JAMA. 2004;291:2441-7.

7. Sanabria A, Carvalho AL, Vartanian JG, Magrin J, Ikeda MK, Kowalski LP. Comorbidity is a prognostic factor in elderly patients with head and neck cancer. Ann Surg Oncol. 2007;14:1449-57.

8. Allen N, Siller C, Been A. Anaesthetic implications of chemotherapy. Contin Educ Anaesth Crit Care Pain. 2012;12:52-6.

9. Heany A, Buggy DJ. Can anaesthetic techniques affect recurrence or metastasis? Br J Anesth. 2012;109:i17-i28.

10. Huettemann E, Sakka SG. Anaesthesia and anti-cancer chemotherapeutic drugs. Curr Opin Anaesthesiol. 2005;18:307-14.

11. Manzullo EF, Sahai SK, Weed GH. Preoperative evaluation and management of cancer patients. [online] Available from https://www.uptodate.com/contents/preoperative-evaluation-and-management-of-patients-with-cancer. [Last accessed March, 2020].

12. Huitink JM, Teoh WHL. Current cancer therapies: A guide for perioperative physicians. Best Pract Res Clin Anaesthesiol. 2013;27:481-92.

13. Gudaitytė J, Dvylys D, Šimeliūnaitė I. Anaesthetic challenges in cancer patients: Current therapies and pain management. Acta Med Litu. 2017;24:121-7.

14. Alraiyes AH, Alraies MC, Abbas A. Radiation-associated airway necrosis. Ochsner J. 2013;13:273-5.

15. Kundra P, Mishra SK, Ramesh A. Ultrasound of the airway. Indian J Anaesthesia. 2011;55(5):456-62.

16. Jain K, Gupta N, Yadav M, Thulkar S, Bhatnagar S. Radiological evaluation of airway: What an anaesthesiologist needs to know! Indian J Anaesth. 2019;63:257-64.

17. Dort JC, Farwell DG, Findlay M, Huber GF, Kerr P, Shea-Budgell MA, et al. Optimal perioperative care in major head and neck cancer surgery with free flap reconstruction: A consensus review and recommendations from the enhanced recovery after surgery society. 2017;143:292-303.

18. Warner DO. Preoperative smoking cessation: The role of the primary care provider. Mayo Clin Proc. 2005;80:252-8.

19. American Diabetes Association. Standards of care in diabetes 2019. Diabetes Care. 2019. Peri-operative diabetes management guidelines. [online] Available from: http://care.diabetesjournals.org/content/42/Supplement_1/S1. [Last accessed March, 2020].

20. Zwissler B. Preoperative evaluation of adult patients before elective, noncardiothoracic surgery: Joint recommendation of the German Society of Anesthesiology and Intensive Care Medicine, the German Society of Surgery; and the German Society of Internal Medicine. Anaesthesist. 2017;66: 442-58.

21. Peacock SC, Lovshin JA, Cherney DZ. Perioperative considerations for the use of sodium-glucose cotransporter-2 inhibitors in patients with type 2 diabetes. Anesth Analg. 2018;126:699-704.

22. Kuzulugi D, Papeix G, Luu J, Kerridge K. Recent advances in diabetes treatments and their perioperative implications. Curr Opin Anaesthesiol. 2019;32(3):398-404.

23. Bauer J, Capra S, Ferguson M. Use of the scored Patient-Generated Subjective Global Assessment (PG-SGA) as a nutrition assessment tool in patients with cancer. Eur J Clin Nutr. 2002;56:779-85.

24. Yarlagadda BB, Hatton E, Huettig J, Deschler D. Patient and staff perceptions of social worker counseling before surgical therapy for head and neck cancer. Health Soc Work. 2015;40:120-4.

25. Myatra SN, Shah A, Kundra P, Patwa A, Ramkumar V, Divatia JV, et al. All India Difficult Airway Association 2016 guidelines for the management of unanticipated difficult tracheal intubation in adults. Indian J Anaesth. 2016;60:885-98.

26. Patel A, Nouraei SA. Transnasal humidified rapid insufflations ventilation exchange (THRIVE): A physiological method of increasing apnea time in patients with difficult airway. Anesthesia. 2015;70:323-9.

27. Apelfbaum JL, Hagberg C, Caplan R, Blitt C, Connis R, Nickinovich D, et al. Practice guidelines for management of the difficult airway: An updated report by the American Society of Anaesthesiologists task force on management of the difficult airway. Anesthesiology. 2013:118;251-70.

28. Sakles JC, Mosier J, Chiu S, Cosentino M, Kalin L. A comparison of the C-MAC video laryngoscope to the Macintosh direct laryngoscope for intubation in the emergency department. Annals Emerg Med. 2012;60:739-48.

29. Levitan R, Heitz J, Sweeney M, Cooper R. The complexities of tracheal intubation with direct laryngoscopy and alternative intubation devices. Ann Emerg Med. 2011;57:240-7.

30. Solanki SL, Kaur J. "Two-hand-manoeuver" during nasotracheal intubation. Saudi J Anaesth. 2017;11:512.

31. Kristensen MS, Teoh WH, Graumann O, Laursen CB. Ultrasonography for clinical decision-making and intervention in airway management: From the mouth to the lungs and pleurae. Insights Imag. 2014;5:253-79.

32. Sumer BD, Myers LL, Leach J, Truelson JM. Correlation between intraoperative hypothermia and perioperative morbidity in patients with head and neck cancer. Arch Otolaryngol Head Neck Surg. 2009;135:682-6.

33. Myatra SN, Shah A, Kundra P, Patwa A, Ramkumar V, Divatia JV, et al. All India Difficult Airway Association 2016 guidelines for the management of anticipated difficult extubation. Indian J Anaesth. 2016;60:915-21.

34. Abdel-Galil K, Mitchell D. Postoperative monitoring of microsurgical free tissue transfers for head and neck reconstruction: A systematic review of current techniques—part I. Non-invasive techniques. Br J Oral Maxillofac Surg. 2009;47:351-5.

35. Chae MP, Rozen WM, Whitaker IS, Chubb D, Grinsell D, Ashton MW, et al. Current evidence for postoperative monitoring of microvascular free flaps: A systematic review. Ann Plast Surg. 2015;74:621-32.

36. Jellish WS, Leonetti JP, Sawicki K, Anderson D, Origitano TC. Morphine/ondansetron PCA for postoperative pain, nausea, and vomiting after skull base surgery. Otolaryngol Head Neck Surg. 2006;135(2):175-81.

37. Dhiwakar M, Nambi GI, Ramanikanth TV. Drain removal and aspiration to treat low output chylous fistula. Eur Arch Otorhinolaryngol. 2014;271:561-5.

38. Swanson MS, Hudson RL, Bhandari N, Sinha UK, Maceri DR, Kokot N. Use of octreotide for the management of chyle fistula following neck dissection. JAMA Otolaryngol. Head Neck Surg. 2015;141:723-7.

39. Lee YS, Kim BW, Chang HS, Park CS. Factors predisposing to chyle leakage following thyroid cancer surgery without lateral neck dissection. Head Neck. 2013;35:1149-52.

40. Crook MA, Hally V, Pantelli JV. The importance of the refeeding syndrome. Nutrition. 2001;17:632-7.

41. National Institute for Health and Clinical Excellence. (2006). Nutrition support in adults Clinical guideline CG32. [online] Available from www.nice.org.uk/page.aspx?o=cg032. [Last accessed March, 2020].

42. Naunheim MR, Sedaghat AR, Lin DT, Bleier BS, Holbrook EH, Curry WT, et al. Immediate and delayed complications following endoscopic skull base surgery. J Neurol Surg B Skull Base. 2015;76:390-6.

43. Fenske W, Allolio B. Clinical review: Current state and future perspectives in the diagnosis of diabetes insipidus: a clinical review. J Clin Endocrinol Metab. 2012;97:3426-37.

44. Grillone GA, Scharukh J. Robotic Surgery of the Head and Neck, 1st edition. New York, NY: Springer; 2015.

45. Pollei TR, Hinni ML, Moore EJ, Hayden RE, Olsen KD, Casler JD, et al. Analysis of postoperative bleeding and risk factors in transoral surgery of the oropharynx. JAMA Otolaryngol Head Neck Surg. 2013;139:1212-8.

46. Narayanasamy S, Khanna P, Bhalla A, Singh AK. Perioperative concerns in transoral robotic surgery: Initial experience of four cases. J Anaesthesiol Clin Pharmacol. 2012;28:226-9.

47. Clayburgh D, Stott W, Bolognone R, Palmer A, Achim V, Troob S, et al. A randomized controlled trial of corticosteroids for pain after transoral robotic surgery. Laryngoscope. 2017;127:2558-64.

48. Mandapathil M, Duvvuri U, Güldner C, Teymoortash A, Lawson G, Werner JA. Transoral surgery for oropharyngeal tumors using the Medrobotics(®) Flex(®) System: A case report. Int J Surg Case Rep. 2015;10:173-5.

Perioperative Management of Skull Base and Pituitary Surgeries

Nitasha Mishra, Sritam Swarup Jena

ANATOMY OF THE SKULL BASE

The skull base is a complex part of the brain that separates it from the facial structures and the suprahyoid neck. It is divided broadly into three parts, namely anterior skull base (ASB), central skull base (CSB), and posterior skull base (PSB) **(Fig. 1)**.

The ASB forms the bottom of the anterior skull, separating the anterior cranial fossa from the paranasal sinuses and the orbits. It is also the most common site of cerebrospinal fluid (CSF) leak.

The CSB forms the floor of the middle cranial fossa, the central part of which is formed by the body of the sphenoid bone. When viewed from above, the center of the sphenoid body contains the sella turcica, a saddle-shaped depression that houses the pituitary gland. It is bound anteriorly by the tuberculum sella and posteriorly by the dorsum sella. The most important anatomical contents of the CSB include cavernous sinus with branches of carotid arteries, optic nerve, superior orbital fissure with cranial nerves III, IV, V1, and VI, foramen rotundum, Vidian canal with the maxillary

artery, middle meningeal artery, and the pterygopalatine fossa. The posterior border of CSB is formed by dorsum sellae and petrous part of the temporal bone.

The PSB is formed by the clivus anteriorly, the mastoid, and petrous parts of the temporal bone. It contains foramen magnum with vital structures and jugular foramen.

This chapter will mainly focus on the critical care issues in relation to surgery of sellar and suprasellar structures. The sellar region includes the sella turcica and the pituitary gland, together with the ventral adenohypophysis and dorsal neurohypophysis. The parasellar region encompasses the cavernous sinuses, suprasellar cistern, hypothalamus, and ventral inferior third ventricle.

ANATOMY AND PHYSIOLOGY OF PITUITARY GLAND

The pituitary gland is housed within sella turcica on the surface of the sphenoid bone and consists of two parts: the anterior lobe or the adenohypophysis and posterior lobe or the neurohypophysis **(Fig. 2)**. The intermediate lobe is

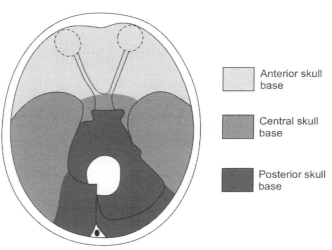

Fig. 1: Anatomy of the skull base.

Anterior skull base

Central skull base

Posterior skull base

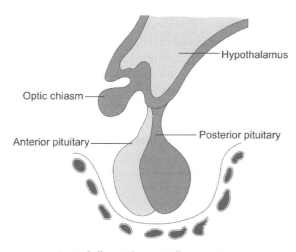

Fig. 2: Sellar and suprasellar structures.

Hypothalamus

Optic chiasm

Anterior pituitary

Posterior pituitary

a small tissue between them. The anterior pituitary plays a central role in the regulation of the endocrine system and produces seven different hormones that regulate the function of other endocrine organs. In contrast, the posterior lobe develops as a direct extension of neural ectoderm from the floor of the third ventricle. It is a projection of unmyelinated axons and specialized glial cells called pituicytes from the hypothalamus. It does not produce any hormone by itself but rather stores and releases oxytocin and vasopressin, which is produced by hypothalamic cell bodies.

Pathologies of Sellar and Suprasellar Regions

Pituitary adenomas are the most common intrasellar masses followed by others that account for nearly 10% which include the germ cell tumors, meningiomas, aneurysm, gliomas granulomatous, and metastatic and infectious diseases.[1] In children, the most common pathology is craniopharyngioma.

Preoperative Hormonal Status

Important tests that guide postoperative critical care management apart from the diagnostic test include an endocrinologic evaluation, which includes mainly the anterior pituitary function testing and hypothalamic pituitary adrenal axis testing (HPAA). Hormonal profiling includes measuring serum levels of prolactin, follicle-stimulating hormone (FSH), thyroxine, testosterone, adrenocorticotrophic hormone (ACTH), and cortisol levels at a minimum.

Assessment of the hypothalamic-pituitary-adrenal (HPA) axis, and thus defining a possible need for glucocorticoid (GC) replacement therapy, is a crucial aspect of anterior pituitary function testing. Several tests are available to help predict whether the HPA axis is able to respond normally to significant stress including basal serum cortisol, the insulin tolerance test (ITT), the glucagon stimulation test (GST), and the short Synacthen test (SST, standard- and low-dose versions). However, there is no universal agreement to which test is the best to assess pituitary reserve

- *Morning cortisol levels (MSC):* Ideally, cortisol should be measured between 8 AM and 9 AM since HPA axis activity is maximal at this time. Hagg et al. found that an MSC < 100 nmol/L clearly points to insufficiency, whereas an MSC of > 300 nmol/L almost always excludes ACTH-cortisol deficit.[2] Intermediate values of basal cortisol require dynamic testing.
- *Insulin tolerance test:* This test delivers a controlled stressful stimulus to the entire HPA axis by means of insulin-induced hypoglycemia. This test also stimulates growth hormone (GH) secretion and therefore has

the potential to test both the HPA axis and the GH reserves. However, this test is labor-intensive and is contraindicated in patients with ischemic cardiovascular disease and in spite of being a gold standard test is usually not preferred in the preoperative period.[3] A bolus dose of insulin of 0.15 U/kg is being given and cortisol response to it is noted. An increment in cortisol level of 200 nmol/L with a peak cortisol value of 550 nmol/L is considered a positive response.

- *Short Synacthen test:* Most endocrinologists prefer a standard (250 µg) or low dose (1 µg) of ACTH provocative test as preoperative evaluation in the pituitary tumors. However, since it takes 3–4 weeks to develop adrenal failure after pituitary apoplexy and surgery, it is not used for testing adrenal reserves in the postoperative period.

PERIOPERATIVE MANAGEMENT OF GLUCOCORTICOIDS

All patients with adrenal insufficiency identified preoperatively should be treated with stress-dose GC treatment both peri- and postoperatively, with GC up to a duration of 48 hours with a postoperative evaluation of HPA thyroid axis on day 3–5 with morning 8 AM cortisol levels.

In patients who have a normal preoperative cortisol level, GC supplementation is only done in cases where pituitary suppression is anticipated such as in cases of larger tumors where complete adenomectomy is done. GC supplementation can be avoided in patients with normal preoperative cortisol levels **(Flowchart 1)**.

A perioperative regimen used more commonly is dexamethasone, which is 4 mg at the induction of anesthesia, 2 mg at 8 AM on day 1, and 0.5 mg at 8 AM on day 2. Alternatively, hydrocortisone 50 mg every 8 hours on day 0, 25 mg every 8 hours on day 1, and 25 mg at 8 hours on day 2 can also be given. Dexamethasone is the preferred agent as it has a longer half-life and requires once-daily administration.

Provided there are no postoperative complications, GC supplementation should be withdrawn, after 48 hours, and measurement of 8 AM plasma cortisol levels performed daily between day 3 and day 5 postoperatively.

POSTOPERATIVE MANAGEMENT

Postoperative critical care management is a multidisciplinary approach involving neurosurgeons, neurointensivist, and endocrinologist.

Airway Management

Managing airway is of utmost importance in patients with difficult airway due to acromegaly, presence of obstructive

Flowchart 1: A structured approach to perioperative glucocorticoid (GC) replacement.

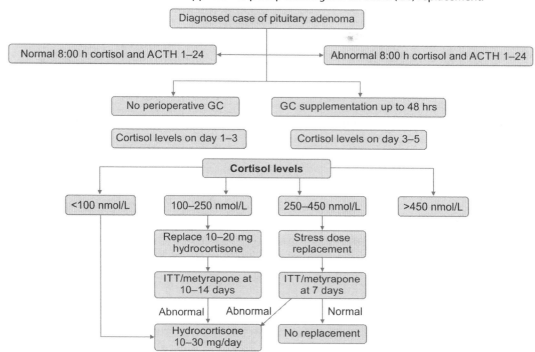

(ACTH: adrenocorticotrophic hormone; ITT: insulin tolerance test)

sleep apnea (OSA) in patients of Cushing's disease and acromegaly, nasal packing, or aspiration of blood and mucus from the nasal cavity into the airway. Meticulous suctioning of the oropharynx for secretions and residual blood is critical.

Endocrine Complications

Hypopituitarism

One of the most common complications after pituitary surgery is hypopituitarism involving either the anterior or posterior pituitary or both. As per literature evidence, the risk of postoperative hypopituitarism ranges from 5% to 25% in pituitary adenomas and peaks up to 75% in craniopharyngiomas.[4-6] Adrenal insufficiency is the most common endocrine complication seen postoperatively. The administration of the postoperative GCs depends on the preoperative status of HPA as discussed in the previous section. Postoperative adrenal responsiveness can be checked on day 1–3 if there is no preoperative GC supplementation and on day 3–5 if the patient receives perioperative GC. An algorithm to be followed for postoperative assessment of adrenal insufficiency has been shown in **Flowchart 1**.

Similarly, central hypothyroidism, hypogonadism, and GH deficiency can be diagnosed using serum thyroid-stimulating hormone (TSH), FSH and luteinizing hormone

(LH), and insulin-like growth factor-1 (IGF-1) assay, respectively and replacement provided if found to be deficient. Adrenal insufficiency should always be ruled out first before starting GH and thyroxine replacement.

Water and Electrolyte Imbalances

Surgery in the hypothalamic-pituitary area is often accompanied by disturbances of water and electrolytes due to manipulation and vascular alteration of the neurohypophysis. The incidence of water and electrolyte abnormalities is known to vary from 60% to 70% in patients undergoing surgeries for sellar and suprasellar lesions leading to considerable postoperative morbidity.[7,8] Abnormalities in blood osmolality can be life-threatening if they are not properly recognized and treated. Fluid intake and output should be recorded very accurately and reviewed every 6–8 hours. Insertion of a urinary catheter may be necessary for an accurate output record. Extra fluid losses such as stools, CSF, or drain outputs should be accounted for and replaced. Paired plasma and urine osmolality and electrolytes should be tested immediately postoperatively and every 8 hours.

The patterns of water and electrolyte disturbances after transsphenoidal surgeries can be generally categorized as periods of polyuria causing hypernatremia due to diabetes insipidus or hyponatremia, attributable to the abnormally high secretion of antidiuretic hormone [syndrome of inappropriate antidiuretic hormone secretion (SIADH)] or cerebral salt wasting syndrome (CSWS).

Central diabetes insipidus: Central diabetes insipidus (CDI) is diagnosed by the concomitant presence of inappropriate hypotonic polyuria (urine output > 3 L/24 h and urine osmolality < 300 mOsm/kg) in the presence of high or normal serum sodium. It is the most common complication after pituitary surgery. Central DI can be transient or permanent, and partial or complete, depending on the kind and extent of the damage to hypothalamic magnocellular neurons.[9]It occurs in approximately 10–30% of patients undergoing pituitary surgery, but it persists long-term only in 2–7% with approximately 50% of patients remitting in 1 week and about 80% in 3 months.[9-11] In about 1–2% of patients, it occurs in a triphasic pattern with an initial period of DI, followed by SIADH causing hyponatremia and oliguria, and then the third and final phase of permanent DI.[12] **Flowchart 2** elaborates the diagnosis and management of hypernatremia

Syndrome of inappropriate antidiuretic hormone secretion: Hyponatremia in the postoperative period is usually caused by excessive ADH release by damaged arginine vasopressin (AVP)-secreting hypothalamic neurons. SIADH may be diagnosed in a patient with hyponatremia and low plasma osmolality (osmolality < 275 mOsm/kg), highly concentrated urine in relation to plasma osmolality (>100 mOsm/kg), with elevated sodium urinary levels (>40 mmol/L), with normal sodium intake, in the presence of normal extracellular volume, and once renal failure, GC, and thyroid hormone deficiencies have been ruled out. The therapeutic intervention for SIADH is fluid restriction.[13] Sodium replacement is required only in prolonged SIADH causing total body sodium depletion. Severe symptomatic

hyponatremia with visual changes, focal neurologic deficits, encephalopathy, respiratory depression, and seizures needs to be treated with an infusion of 3% saline at 0.5–1 mmol/kg/h (1–2 mL/kg/h) for 2–3 hours, followed by conservative adjustments.[14] A rapid rate of the correction of hyponatremia can lead to a serious and permanent neurological manifestation, central pontine myelinolysis, and death and should be avoided. An algorithmic approach to hyponatremia has been presented in **Flowchart 3**.

Cerebral salt wasting syndrome: CSWS is characterized by renal loss of sodium resulting in polyuria, natriuresis, hyponatremia, and hypovolemia occurring as a result of a centrally mediated process occurring due to release of brain natriuretic peptide (BNP) from damaged neurons. It is characterized by low urine sodium, high or normal urine and serum osmolality, and raised serum hematocrit and uric acid in a dehydrated patient. However, diagnostic criteria based on accurately quantifiable factors (e.g., plasma urea, atrial natriuretic peptide, antidiuretic hormone, and other serum markers) have not been demonstrated to be accurate predictors of hyponatremia etiology in all cases, and their use in the evaluation of hyponatremia is not supported by the literature (Class III evidence).[15] Early appropriate fluid therapy and salt supplementation should be initiated to prevent further complications. Depending on the severity and clinical symptoms of hyponatremia, isotonic or hypertonic fluids are given to correct volume depletion. Sodium can be supplemented by the oral route.

Surgical Complications

Cerebrospinal fluid leak and operative site/sellar hematoma are the most common surgical complications. Due to the presence of vital structures like optic chiasm, optic nerve, and cavernous sinus, a thorough neurological assessment

Flowchart 2: Diagnosis and management of hypernatremia.

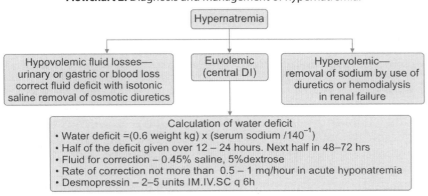

(DI: diabetes insipidus; IM: intramuscular; IV: intravenous; q6h: every 6 hours; SC: subcutaneous)

Flowchart 3: An algorithmic approach to hyponatremia in neurointensive care.

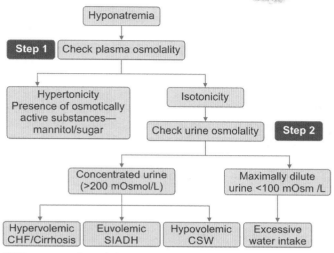

(CHF: congestive heart failure; CSW: cerebral salt wasting; SIADH: syndrome of inappropriate antidiuretic hormone)

including visual acuity should be done in the immediate postoperative period as they could be harbinger signs of sellar hematoma which needs urgent exploration. When complete resection of the tumor is not achieved, there is a possibility of residual tumor hemorrhage. This is more common after larger tumor resections. An urgent computed tomography scan is indicated in such scenario.

The incidence of CSF leak has been reported previously as 4% to as high as 40%.[4,16] Han et al. described the incidence of CSF leak to be related to tumor size, consistency, and margins with the highest incidence occurring in FSH adenomas and in those with Cushing's disease.[17] If detected intraoperatively, a fat graft may be placed and defect be repaired. Bed rest with head and torso tilt of 15–30° is usually advised in the postoperative period. A lumbar drainage catheter may be placed to drain the CSF.

Injury to the carotid artery is a known but fortunately rare complication of trans-sphenoidal surgery.[18] Following stabilization in the operating room, patients with injury of the carotid artery typically undergo postoperative angiography to evaluate for pseudoaneurysm formation. If a pseudoaneurysm is visualized, it may be treated with endovascular therapy or open surgery if endovascular therapy is not feasible. Close neurologic and hemodynamic monitoring in the intensive care unit is mandatory postoperatively to assess vasospasm and postoperative stroke.

Infections

Meningitis and bacteremia are uncommon but serious complications that can result in increased morbidity and mortality. Preoperative diabetes, intraoperative CSF leak,

revision surgery, and use of endoscopy have been identified as risk factors. Early diagnosis and appropriate use of antibiotics are vital to lower infection rates and mortality.

CONCLUSION

Pituitary tumors and other masses in the sellar and suprasellar region are commonly seen in our clinical practice. The complex pathophysiology of pituitary disease demands a multidisciplinary team involving the endocrinologist, the neurosurgeon, and the neuroanesthesiologist to optimize perioperative care. Knowledge of potential complications, their management, and strategies for avoidance are important components of postoperative care. Transsphenoidal surgery can be performed successfully and safely and critically depends on excellent postoperative care.

REFERENCES

1. Saeger W, Lüdecke DK, Buchfelder M, Fahlbusch R, Quabbe HJ, Petersenn S. Pathohistological classification of pituitary tumors: 10 years of experience with the German Pituitary Tumor Registry. Eur J Endocrinol. 2007;156(2):203-16.

2. Hagg E, Asplund K, Lithner F. Value of basal plasma cortisol assays in the assessment of the pituitary-adrenal axis. Clin Endocrinol (Oxf). 1987;44:141-6.

3. Mukherjee JJ, de Castro JJ, Kaltsas G, Afshar F, Grossman AB, Wass JA, et al. A comparison of the insulin tolerance/glucagon test with the short ACTH stimulation test in the assessment of the hypothalamo-pituitary-adrenal axis in the early post-operative period after hypophysectomy. Clin Endocrinol (Oxf). 1997;47:51-60.

4. Ciric I, Ragin A, Baumgartner C, Pierce D. Complications of transsphenoidal surgery: results of a national survey, review of the literature, and personal experience. Neurosurgery. 1997;40:225-36.

5. Roelfsema F, Biermasz NR, Pereira AM. Clinical factors involved in the recurrence of pituitary adenomas after surgical remission: a structured review and meta-analysis. Pituitary. 2012;15:71-83.

6. Lo AC, Howard AF, Nichol A, Sidhu K, Abdulsatar F, Hasan H, et al. Long-term outcomes and complications in patients with craniopharyngioma: the British Columbia Cancer Agency experience. Int J Radiat Oncol Biol Phys. 2014;88:1011-8.

7. Kristof RA, Rother M, Neuloh G, Klingmüller D. Incidence, clinical manifestations, and course of water and electrolyte metabolism disturbances following transsphenoidal pituitary adenoma surgery: a prospective observational study. J Neurosurg. 2009;111:555-62.

8. Adams JR, Blevins LS Jr., Allen GS, Verity DK, Devin JK. Disorders of water metabolism following transsphenoidal pituitary surgery: a single institution's experience. Pituitary. 2006;9:93-9.

9. Singer I, Oster JR, Fishman LM. The management of diabetes insipidus in adults. Arch Intern Med. 1997;157:1293-301.

10. Nemergut EC, Zuo Z, Jane JA, Laws ER JR. Predictors of diabetes insipidus after transsphenoidal surgery: a review of 881 patients. J Neurosurg. 2005;103:448-54.

11. Pivonello R, De Leo M, Cozzolino A, Colao A. The treatment of Cushing's disease. Endocr Rev. 2015;36:385-486.

12. Hensen J, Henig A, Fahlbusch R, Meyer M, Boehnert M, Buchfelder M. Prevalence, predictors and patterns of postoperative polyuria and hyponatraemia in the immediate course after transsphenoidal surgery for pituitary adenomas. Clin Endocrinol (Oxf). 1999;50:431-9.

13. Sherlock M, O'Sullivan E, Agha A, Behan LA, Owens D, Finucane F, et al. Incidence and pathophysiology of severe HN in neurosurgical patients. Postgrad Med J. 2009;85:171-5.

14. Verbalis JG, Goldsmith SR, Greenberg A, Korzelius C, Schrier RW, Sterns RH, et al. Diagnosis, evaluation, and treatment of hyponatremia: expert panel recommendations. Am J Med. 2013;126(10):S1-42.

15. Rahman M, Friedman WA. Hyponatremia in neurosurgical patients: clinical guidelines development. Neurosurgery. 2009;65:925-35.

16. Chowdhury T, Prabhakar H, Bithal PK, Schaller B, Dash HH. Immediate postoperative complications in transsphenoidal pituitary surgery: a prospective study. Saudi J Anaesth. 2014;8:335-41.

17. Han ZL, He DS, Mao ZG, Wang HJ. Cerebrospinal fluid rhinorrhea following trans-sphenoidal pituitary macroadenoma surgery: experience from 592 patients. Clin Neurol Neurosurg. 2008;110:570-9.

18. Solares CA, Ong YK, Carrau RL, Miranda JF, Prevedello DM, Snyderman CH, et al. Prevention and management of vascular injuries in endoscopic surgery of the sinonasal tract and skull base. Otolaryngol Clin North Am. 2010;43(4):817-25.

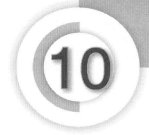
Transplantation

SECTION OUTLINE

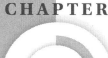
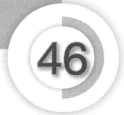

CHAPTER 46

Perioperative Management of Renal Transplantation

Divya Srivastava, Abhilash Chandra, Sohan Lal Solanki

INTRODUCTION

The true burden of end-stage renal disease (ESRD) in India remains unknown. About 120,000 patients were estimated to be on hemodialysis in 2018.[1] Kidney transplantation using organ from a deceased or living donor is considered the best form of therapy for these patients. The superiority of quality of life after transplant over patients on maintenance dialysis has been shown.[2] However, local infrastructure is of crucial importance when it comes to establishing a transplant program. It requires a good coordination between nephrologists, anesthesiologists and urologists with support of radiologists, microbiologists and pathologists. The short- and long-term graft survival is better in recipients receiving kidney from live donor as compared to those receiving from deceased donors.[3]

KIDNEY DONOR EVALUATION

In India, the transplant programs are mainly living donor based. After identification of a viable kidney donor, his willingness to donate a kidney without undue pressure or financial gains is verified. Benefits and risks associated with kidney donation are duly explained to him. His privacy and the right to withdraw from the process of donation during evaluation are given due consideration. Thereafter, a detail plan of evaluation is explained to him **(Flowchart 1)**.

Usually young donors free of comorbidities are chosen but shortage of organs has led to including extended criteria donors **(Box 1)**.[4]

Living donor renal transplants are conducted as elective procedures where we have time for proper planning. Deceased donor transplantations, on the other hand, are performed as an emergency surgery on availability of organs.

PREOPERATIVE MANAGEMENT

Initial Assessment

Patients admitted for transplantation usually have been screened properly beforehand. All their comorbidities and medications are well documented. In addition, they are on

Flowchart 1: Evaluation plan of a prospective live kidney donor.

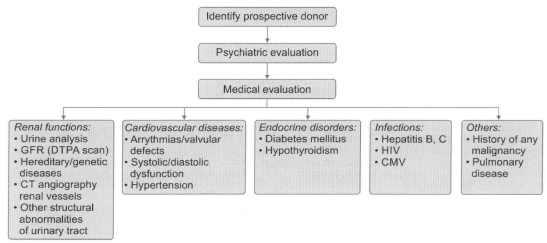

regular dialysis and follow-up. Therefore, preoperatively all they require is reassessment of previous conditions.

A detailed history is taken to know about control of comorbidities such as hypertension, diabetes, and coronary artery diseases (CAD). All ESRD patients should have undergone screening echocardiography and stress tests if required. Patients with long-standing diabetes require coronary angiography in addition to rule out any CAD.[5] The investigations routinely done[6] are shown in **Flowchart 2**. Any new symptom of angina, chest pain, dyspnea on mild exertion, and fever or symptoms suggestive of any malignancy are further evaluated **(Flowchart 3)**.

Optimization

End-stage renal disease patients are usually on multiple medications.

Antihypertensives are continued to maintain blood pressures. Beta blockers, angiotensin converting enzyme inhibitors/angiotensin receptor blockers should be continued in perioperative period. (KIDGO Recommendation 2A).[7]

Antiplatelet agents (e.g., aspirin, clopidogrel, ticagrelor): All antiplatelet agents except aspirin should be stopped 5 days prior to living donor transplant (unless cessation is contraindicated) and during the perioperative period for deceased donor transplantation.[7]

Box 1: Extended criteria for donors.

Age > 60 years or

age >50–59 years with ≥2 of the following risk factors:
- History of hypertension
- Serum creatinine ≥1.5 mg/dL
- Death due to cerebrovascular accident

Oral anticoagulants: All kidney transplant candidates (KTCs) on direct oral anticoagulants (DOACs) should be shifted to warfarin, mainly because effect of DOACs on transplant outcomes is unknown and their effect is difficult to revert. For patients receiving kidney from a living donor warfarin is stopped 5 days before and dypridimole 7 days before surgery. Unfractionated heparin is used as bridging therapy for perioperative period.[7] Warfarin can be restarted only after 4 weeks posttransplant. For patients receiving kidney from a deceased donor the effect of warfarin is reversed on admission with fresh frozen plasma and vitamin K. Despite these measures, such patients may have increased requirement of blood products intraoperatively.[7]

Oral hypoglycemic agents (OHA): All diabetic patients are converted to insulin, preferable intravenous regular insulin as per requirement in perioperative period. A good glucose control is required for early recovery. OHAs can be started after surgery when oral diet is allowed.

Other drugs: Statins, cardiac medications, erythropoietin, calcium, and vitamin D are continued.[7]

Special considerations: These patients are at particular risk of cardiac diseases and so optimization in this regard is vital. In cases of recent myocardial infarction, transplant surgery is postponed for at least a month (KIDGO recommendation 2B),[7,8] following which readiness of patient for withstanding surgery and anesthesia is reassessed. Patients with stents in coronary vessels require a gap of 1 month for bare metal and 6 months from insertion of drug eluting stent before contemplating surgery.[8,9]

Asymptomatic KTCs on dialysis for at least 2 years may have additional findings on echocardiography. If a new onset lesion or pulmonary systolic pressure greater than 45 mm Hg is found, cardiology consultation is sought.[7]

Flowchart 2: Evaluation of renal transplant recipient.

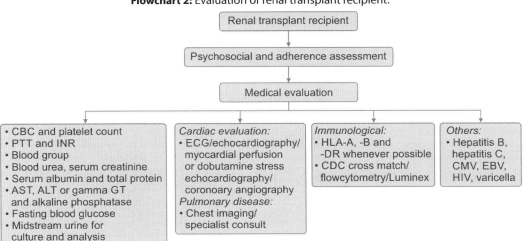

(CBC: complete blood count; PTT: partial thromboplastin time; INR: international normalized ratio; AST: aspartate aminotransferase; ALT: alanine transaminase; GT: glutamyl transpeptidase; HLA: human leukocyte antigen; CDC: Complement-dependent cytotoxicty; CMV: cytomegalovirus; EBV: Epstein-Barr virus; HIV: human immunodeficiency virus)

Flowchart 3: Evaluation of new symptoms of recipient.

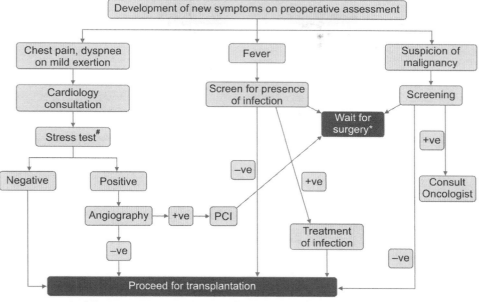

#Stress test or angiography as decided by cardiologist.
*Waiting period of 1 month required for bare metallic stent and 6 months for drug eluting stent
　Surgery is postponed till patient is free of infection. Transplant after treated malignancies depends on type of cancer and center policy.
(PCI: percutaneous coronary intervention)

Immunosuppression

An immunological risk assessment of the recipient is done and he is categorized accordingly **(Box 2)**.[10]

The immunosuppressive medication is started prior to surgery. The drugs commonly used for induction are anti-CD25 monoclonal antibody: Basiliximab, or lymphocyte-depleting antibody: antithymocyte globulin (ATG) along with intravenous methylprednisolone **(Box 3)**. The maintenance is by a combination of three agents: calcineurin inhibitor (CNI): tacrolimus + antiproliferative agent: mycophenolate + steroid: prednisolone. The blood group incompatible immunosuppression is dealt separately in **Flowchart 4**.

PREPARATION FOR SURGERY

Preparations consist of:
- *Hemodialysis* if required or peritoneal dialysis to continue. European Renal Best Practice Guideline on kidney donor and recipient evaluation and perioperative care (ERBP)[11] 2015 states hemodialysis to be repeated before transplantation only if it is clinically indicated and to avoid ultrafiltration unless there is evidence of volume overload (recommendation 1C).
- Surgical part preparation
- Notation of last mealtime (nil orally)
- Explanation of the transplant procedure to both the donor (if living donor) and recipient; signing of surgical consent form by them

Box 2: Immunological risk assessment for kidney transplantation.

Immunologic low risk:
- First-time transplant recipients who have less than 20% panel-reactive antibodies
- No donor specific antibodies.

Immunologic high risk:
- Who have rejected one or more transplants aggressively (i.e. within the first year post transplantation),
- Greater than 20% panel-reactive antibodies
- Donor specific antibodies present
- Previous pregnancies
- Previous blood transfusions
- Blood group incompatibility
- African ancestry.

- *Prophylaxis against gastric ulceration (due to stress and side effect of steroids):* Oral ranitidine 150 mg twice a day
- *Administration of prophylactic antibiotics:* At author's institute amoxycillin and clavulanic acid 1.2 g and cefoperazone 1 g are given intravenously (IV) on morning of surgery and continued TDS and BD, respectively, up to 3 days postoperatively.

INTRAOPERATIVE MANAGEMENT

Surgical Technique

Living donor nephrectomy is performed laparoscopically (ERBP Guideline[11] Recommendation 2C) or robot assisted in almost all centers. The time passed between clamping

Box 3: Induction and maintenance regimen protocol.

- *Immunological low-risk transplant candidate:*
  - Immediate release tacrolimus started 2 days prior to day of surgery (0.15–2.0 mg/kg PO/day)
  - *Basiliximab* 20 mg IV day 0 of transplant, on call to the OR. Option of no basiliximab for identical HLA match
  - *Methylprednisolone* 500 mg IV on call to OR or intraoperative
  - Two doses of mycophenolate *mofetil* (1 g each) prior to surgery
  - *Postoperative immunosuppression:*
    - *Basiliximab* 20 mg IV on day 4 of transplant. None if first dose not given
    - *Rapid steroid elimination:* Continue methylprednisolone at 40 mg IV Q12H for 24 hours postoperative. If no DGF, prednisone is not ordered. If there is DGF prednisone may be used to allow lower CNI levels. Else continue prednisone 20 mg/day until established graft function. Then taper thereafter to 5 mg/day.
    - *Tacrolimus immediate release* continued adjust for a trough level of 8–12 ng/mL (MEIA). If not able to take PO tacrolimus IV (1/4 of PO dose is given)
    - *Mycophenolate mofetil* 1 g PO bid
- *Immunological high-risk transplant candidate:*
  - *Antithymocyte globulin* 1.5 mg/kg begin on call to the OR to be continued intraoperatively
  - *Postoperative immunosuppression:*
    - *Antithymocyte globulin* for a total dose of 6.0–7.5 mg/kg over 4–10 days
    - *Not to* be considered for rapid steroid elimination
    - *Steroids: methylprednisolone until* tolerating PO fluids usually 1–2 days post-OR. Followed by prednisone 20 mg/day until establish graft function. Then taper thereafter to 5 mg/day
    - Begin *tacrolimus immediate release* 0.12–0.15 mg/kg PO/day to overlap with last dose of thymoglobulin. Adjust for a trough level of 5–10 ng/mL (MEIA). If not able to take PO tacrolimus IV (1/4 of PO dose is given)
    - *Mycophenolate mofetil* 1 g PO bid as soon as patient can take PO medications

(PO: per orally; OR: operation room; HLA: human leukocyte antigen; DGF: delayed graft function; CNI: calcineurin inhibitors; MEIA: microparticle immunoabsorption assay)

Flowchart 4: ABO incompatible renal transplant immunosuppression protocol.

(IA: immunoadsorption; TAC: Tacrolimus; MMF: mycophenolate mofetil)

of renal artery in the donor and placement of kidney in crushed ice is the *warm ischemia time* **(Fig. 1)** and is usually 5–10 minutes. The retrieved kidney is flushed with cold (2–4°C) organ retrieval solution (HTK/University of Wisconsin) till clear effluent flows out of renal vein and here begins the cold ischemia time. Eurocollins solution should not be used as preservative solution as it has been implicated in delayed graft functions (DGFs) in kidneys with prolonged ischemia time and extended criteria donors. [ERBP Guideline Recommendation[11] (1B)]. Cold Perfusion of kidney is followed by a procedure called benching. Here the surgeons remove perirenal fat and prepare the renal artery, and vein for anastomosis within the recipient.

Thereafter, the kidney is kept in cold environment till the time it is placed in recipient's body for anastomosis. The allowable cold ischemia time for kidney transplantation is 24 hours[11] (ERBP 1B)].

In the recipient a J-shaped or hockey stick incision is made in either of the iliac fossas **(Fig. 2)**. The donor kidney is placed extraperitoneally and renal vessels are anastomosed to iliac vessels of the recipient **(Fig. 3)**. The rewarm ischemia time begins when the cold organ is placed in the warm iliac fossa and is completed after anastomoses of vessel and reperfusion of the graft **(Figs. 4A and B)**. The stump of ureter of the graft is anastomosed to bladder of the recipient (ureterocystostomy). A JJ stent is placed in the

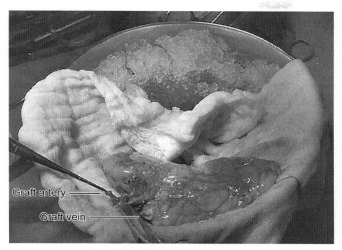

Fig. 1: Renal graft in crushed ice (Cold Ischemia) immediately after retrieval from living donor.

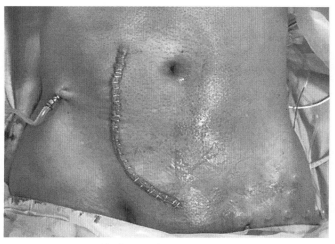

Fig. 2: Hockey stick incision in recipient.

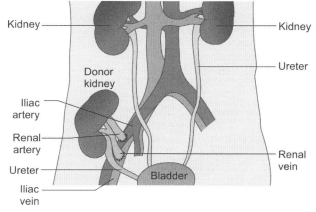

Fig. 3: Heterotopic transplantation. Renal graft placed in iliac fossa.

ureter (ERBP Guideline 2015 1B).[11] A drain is placed in the surgical field before closure which is usually removed on postoperative day (POD)2 **(Fig. 2)**.

Anesthetic Management

General anesthesia with endotracheal intubation and mechanical ventilation is generally preferred. However, regional anesthesia like combined spinal epidural with or without sedation has also been utilized.

Monitoring usually involves inserting arterial (IBP) and central venous lines (CVP) in addition to standard care. At author's institute a Flow Trac™ is used to monitor cardiac output and stroke volume variation.

Intraoperative analgesia is maintained either with epidural infusion of local anesthetics or intermittent intravenous fentanyl/sufentanyl. All nonsteroidal anti-inflammatory drugs (NSAIDs) are contraindicated. Intravenous paracetamol 1 g is usually utilized for multimodal analgesia.

Extubation in the operation room (OR) at the end of surgery is a norm unless contraindicated. The patients are shifted to a high dependency unit/kidney transplant unit for further care.

Intraoperative fluids and hemodynamics: The transplanted kidney is devoid of any nerves and autoregulation; therefore, renal allograft perfusion is solely dependent on its arterial blood flow. Maintenance of adequate intravascular volume and mean arterial pressures greater than 95 mm Hg[12] is required for this optimal graft blood flow and is vital for its early function. Historically, it was recommended to give fluids as high as 30 mL/kg/h and maintain a CVP above 15 mm Hg.[13] Gradually, however several studies have utilized goal-directed fluid therapy **(Table 1)** using either transesophageal doppler/cardiac output (CO)/ stroke volume variation to guide perioperative fluid administration.[14,15] Fernandes et al.[15] have recommended "flow directed therapy" based on "triggers" instead, for optimal organ perfusion. In this method noninvasive CO monitoring is used. If the blood pressures fall below target, the triggers, i.e., CVP and CO are seen. A cardiac output less than baseline with CVP < 12 mm Hg is managed by a bolus of crystalloid 250 mL, if it leads to rise in CO by 15% with rise of CVP by 2 mm Hg patient is considered fluid responsive.[16] In fluid nonresponsive patients vasopressor or inotrope is used for correction of hypotension.

Choice of fluid: Balanced salt crystalloids with acetate buffer are preferred fluid of choice.[17] In absence of acetate buffer a balance salt solution with lactate buffer may be used; however, there are concerns about confounding results when serum lactate values are used as a measure of end organ tissue perfusion. Colloids such as albumin may be used but they have not shown to provide any additional benefit.[18,19] The starch-based colloids are best avoided.[20] Even effect of dextran or gelatin-based colloids is questionable in renal transplant surgeries and should

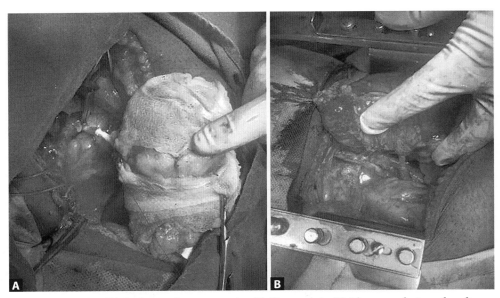

Figs. 4A and B: (A) Graft vessel anastomosis with iliac vessels; (B) After reperfusion of graft.

Table 1: Minimally invasive CO monitoring which can be used for goal-directed fluid therapy.[34]

	Device information	Advantage	Limitations
Arterial pulse wave analysis			
PiCCO	PULSION medical system, Munich, Germany	• Reliable and reproducible • Measures SVV • Can be used to measure ITBV, GEDV, EVLW	• Requires both central venous and arterial cannulation • Unpredictable during arrhythmia, rapid temperature changes, valvular insufficiencies • Affected by SVR, clot or air in circuit
Flo Trac	Edwards LifeSciences, Irvine, US	• Reliable • Requires only arterial line • Does not need calibration • Operator independent • Measures SVV	• A good arterial waveform is required • Inaccurate in arrhythmia • In severe vasoconstriction radial artery gives reduced CO readings
Pressure recording analytic method (PRAM)	Vytech, Padova, Italy	• Arterial line required • No calibration required	Not validated
EV 1000/Volume View System	Edwards Lifesciences, Irvine, CA, US	• Reliable • Measures SVV • Can be used to measure ITBV, GEDV, EVLW	Both arterial and central line required
Lithium dilution technique	Cambridge, United Kingdom	• Arterial and peripheral line required • Continuous CO measurement • Measures SV and SVV • Reliable and reproducible	• Frequent calibration required • Contraindicated in patients on Lithium therapy • Affected by valvular insufficiency intracardiac shunts, damped arterial line, arrhythmia
Esophageal doppler		Probe introduced in esophagus	• Measures flow through descending aorta: FTc • Assumptions about aortic size may not be accurate • Cannot be used in unintubated patients
Transesophageal echocardiography (TEE)		• Probe introduced in esophagus • Reliably measures volume status	• Highly operator dependent • Prolonged learning curve • Uncomfortable in unintubated patients
Noninvasive CO monitoring			
Thoracic bioimpedance	BioZ®	• Noninvasive • Electrodes placed on neck and thorax • Measure SV, VET, EPCI • Continuous CO measurement	Patient movement and arrhythmia affect accuracy

Contd...

Contd...

Partial rebreathing	NICO™	• Easy set up • Continuous CO measurement	• Tracheal intubation and fixed ventilation is required • Unsuitable in postop period
Pulsed dye densitometry	DDG-330	Noninvasive	• Intermittent assessment • Affected by position, vasoconstriction, and interstitial edema
Portable Doppler device	Ultrasonic Cardiac Output Monitors, Sydney, Australia	• Probe placed suprasternally to measure flow of aorta • Measure CO, CI SV	• Intermittent assessment • Probe positioning is important • Requires training

(CO: cardiac output; PiCCO: pulse contour cardiac output; SVV: stroke volume variation; ITBV: intrathoracic blood volume; GEDV: global end diastolic volume; EVLW: extravascular lung water; CVP: central venous pressure; SV: stroke volume; SVR: systemic vascular resistance; FTc: corrected flow time, VET: ventricular ejection time; EPCI: ejection phase contractility index; CI: cardiac index)

best be avoided until further evidence of their safety is obtained.[20] Blood products are given as per point of care coagulation studies and packed red blood cells are not given till hemoglobin of 7 g/dL.

Use of vasopressors: A mean arterial pressure of 95 mm Hg or higher is required for optimal perfusion of neograft following release of anastomosis.[12] Low dose of vasopressors like noradrenaline infusion may be used to maintain blood pressures not responding to fluid boluses. Noradrenaline infusion has not shown any greater risk of graft dysfunction when compared to patients receiving dopamine infusion.[21] Excessive use of vasopressors however either alone or in combinations has shown to have greater graft dysfunction and higher 1 year mortality.[22]

Use of drugs to enhance renal function: Many centers use *intravenous mannitol* in dose of 0.5–1 g/kg during reperfusion of graft. It is utilized for its osmotic diuresis, free radical scavenging, and decreasing tubular ischemic injury. However, there is no clear cut evidence supporting its use to improve graft function.[23]

Intravenous furosemide given during anastomosis decreases oxygen consumption of tubules and exerts diuresis by its action on ascending limb of Henle. Use of both IV furosemide or low-dose dopamine infusion has failed to show any benefit in improving renal graft function.[24]

Post-reperfusion syndrome (PRS): PRS was defined in 1988 for liver transplant surgery as drop in mean arterial blood pressure by 30% for at least 1 minute in the first 5 minutes after reperfusion of liver graft. It may be associated with persistent bradycardia and arrhythmias.[24] Though the incidence of PRS is less in renal transplantation (4%), it's presence leads to increased hospital stay and chances of graft failure.[25] The syndrome affects the cardiovascular and autonomic systems within 5 minutes of reperfusion of graft. The pathogenesis behind the manifestations remains unclear. The initial theories suggested role of transfer of

potassium, acidosis, and hypothermia from cold preserved kidney to the systemic circulation on reperfusion but further studies denied any such phenomenon.[26] Role of immunological mediators and anaphylactoid formation has also been suggested leading to decrease in systemic vascular resistance and therefore mean arterial pressure.[27] The treatment involves maintenance of hemodynamics utilizing vasopressors like noradrenaline and correction of bradycardia with atropine. Intravenous lignocaine may be used for its antiarrhythmic properties. An arterial blood gas is routinely done after reperfusion of graft to look for acidosis and dyselectrolytemia which are corrected accordingly.

Ischemic reperfusion injury (IRI) : It is local effect of reperfusion on an ischemic organ and has no systemic manifestations. The entity is more commonly seen in patients receiving kidney from deceased donors and extended criteria donors (**Box 1**). The increased duration of warm and cold ischemia also increases the risk of reperfusion syndrome. IRI leads to acute tubular necrosis (ATN) which may manifests as delayed graft function (DGF).

DGF is defined as requirement of dialysis within first week of transplantation[28] and the neo kidney regains its function later on. Optimal hemodynamic management of deceased donor prior to and during organ retrieval, adequate perfusion of harvested kidney with cold preservative solution and minimizing cold ischemia time are key to prevention of DGF. Use of pulsatile hypothermic machine perfusion instead of continuous perfusion after organ retrieval has shown to reduce the incidence of DGF,[29] although its routine use has not been recommended in ERBP Guideline 2015.[11] Several antiinflammatory strategies involving phosphodiesterase inhibitors, erythropoietin, adenosine, and antioxidant n-acetylcysteine have shown to reduce ischemic injury to the graft[30] and their use varies from center to center. Treatment of DGF is mainly supportive, both preload and blood pressures are to be maintained for adequate renal blood flow. Hemodialysis is done as and when required and immunosupressants are continued. Eventually the graft regains its function, and dialysis is no longer required.

POSTOPERATIVE MANAGEMENT

The crux of management in early postoperative period lies in maintenance of hemodynamics, continuation of immunosuppressants, infection prophylaxis, and being watchful for any deterioration in renal functions. A decline in urine output is usually the first sign of an impending problem.

Monitoring

Table 2 provides information about routine monitoring of patients postoperatively in high dependency units.[31]

Fluids and Hemodynamics

All transplant centers have a fluid replacement protocol followed postoperatively. General fluid replacement in absence of complications is shown in **Table 3**. Early oral intake of fluids is encouraged.

A close monitoring of invasive blood pressure and volume status of the patient continues in postoperative period as well. Any deficit in volume or a decrease in mean arterial pressures leads to increased risk of ATN and DGF.[32] Similarly over zealous administration of fluids may lead to pulmonary congestion specially in patients with previous cardiovascular compromise.[33] The European Best Practice Guidelines 2015 suggests utilizing central venous pressures (CVP) to guide input of fluids during this time (recommendation 2D).[11] However, several evidences have propped up questioning the reliability of CVP to predict intravascular status. Way back in 2003 Ferris et al.[34] demonstrated that there is an inevitable drop in CVP following reperfusion of graft in renal transplant recipients. This drop continues in postoperative period and is usually not responsive to fluids, neither does it determine incidence of ATN. More recently, Aref et al.[33] have suggested completely discarding the practice of using CVP for guiding fluids in renal recipients and have instead encouraged utilizing cardiac output (CO) monitoring either invasive or noninvasive in both intra and postoperative period **(Table 1)**.

Fluid of choice: Balance salt crystalloids remain fluid of choice even in postoperative period.[20] The European Best Practice Guidelines 2015[11] suggests frequent monitoring for metabolic acidosis and hyperkalemia when normal saline is used as exclusive fluid (Recommendation 1B). Colloids do not offer any additional advantage, however, if needed albumin should be preferred over other synthetic colloids.[20]

Vasopressors: Noradrenaline infusion remains vasopressor of choice if mean arterial pressure falls below 95 mm Hg despite adequate volume resuscitation.

Use of Blood Products

Low hemoglobin level is frequently observed in postoperative period and is attributed to hemodilution due to excessive intravascular fluids, surgical bleeding, or postoperative generalized oozing. These patients have chronic anemia and so have lower transfusion triggers. In the absence of cardiac issues, no transfusion is required till

Table 2: Monitoring of recipient in early postoperative period.			
Type of monitoring	*POD1*	*POD2-5*	*POD5-10*
HR, IBP, CVP	Continuously	• 2 hourly (NIBP) • Arterial line removed on POD 2 • POD2	4 Hourly (NIBP)
UO	Hourly	Hourly	Daily
Input- output charting	Hourly	Hourly	Daily
Drain output	Daily	Daily (removed in 2–5 days)	-
Body weight	Daily	Daily	Daily
Arterial blood gases	12 hourly/more if required	As per requirement	-
Serum electrolytes and lactate	Once/more if required	Daily	2–3 times
CBC, serum creatinine	Once/more if required	Daily	2–3 times/week for I month
Serum CNI levels	Once	Alternate day	2 times per week for 1 month
Blood sugars	Once	Daily	Once/week for I month
Chest X-ray	Once	As and when clinically required	
EBV, BKV screening	Once in first month		

(IBP: invasive blood pressure; UO: urine output; EBV: Ebstein-Barr virus; BKV: BK virus; POD: postoperative day).

Table 3: Suggested parenteral intake of fluids in addition to oral intake guided by thirst.

POD1	100% replacement of urine output (UO) + insensible losses
POD2	90% replacement of UO
POD3	80% replacement of UO
POD4	70% replacement of UO
POD5	60% replacement of UO
POD6	50% replacement of UO
POD7	Usually intravenous replacement is no longer required.

(POD: postoperative day).

hemoglobin of 7 g/dL. Patients with known coronary artery disease however require a higher threshold of 9 g/dL.[32] Use of any blood product increases risk of alloimunization[32] and should be given cautiously. Clinical oozing and point of care coagulation studies as thromboelastography determine platelets, plasma, and cryoprecipitate requirements.

Electrolyte Disorders

Serum electrolytes should be measured 12 hourly in early postoperative period. The main etiology behind dyselectrolytemia is excessive intravenous fluids, excessive diuresis, tubular electrolyte wasting, and side effects of immunosuppressive drugs. Common electrolyte abnormalities include hyperkalemia/hypokalemia, hypophosphatemia, hypercalcemia, hypomagnesemia, and hyponatremia.[32] Magnesium levels are maintained above 2 mg/dL to prevent lowering of seizure thresholds. Ionized calcium should be below 5.3 mg/dL. Phosphorus must be above 2.5 mg/dL to prevent weakening of respiratory muscles. Imbalances are corrected accordingly.

Use of renoprotective drugs: Low-dose dopamine has no role in renoprotection in recipients and is no longer recommended.[11,20] Fenoldopamine is a selective dopaminergic 1 agonist that causes renal and systemic vasodilatation. Though it has been shown to have some positive effect on graft function, the evidence is still not strong enough to recommend its routine use.[20]

Intravenous furosemide is used routinely to enhance urine output postoperatively in some centers. Evidence however suggests utilizing the drug only in patients with limited diuresis despite adequate intravascular volume.[20]

Some newer drugs under evaluation as renoprotective agents are oral spironolactone, N-acetylcysteine, atrial natriuretic peptide, vitamin E, and nitric oxide producers.[20] Their utility still remains doubtful.

Care of Respiratory System

In most patients, tracheal extubation is done at the end of surgery in the operation room. Respiratory exercises such as incentive spirometry and deep breathing are encouraged from day one. Early mobilization and coughing prevents atelectasis and other respiratory complications. With the advent of goal-directed fluid therapy, chances of pulmonary congestion have also deceased.

Early weaning and extubation is planned for patients who are shifted to ICU intubated. Reasons for prolonged ventilation are fluid overload, acidosis, or dyselectrolytemia mostly seen in cases of absence of immediate graft function.

Postoperative Pain Management

Adequate pain management is essential for enabling coughing, early mobilization, and recovery. Individual center protocols vary from intravenous fentanyl/morphine patient controlled analgesia (PCA)[32] or continuous epidural analgesia or patient controlled epidural analgesia. At many centers 0.2% ropivacaine with 1 ug/mL fentanyl is used for continuous epidural analgesia, rate titrated as per patient's need. 1 g intravenous paracetamol is administered thrice a day till patient starts oral diet. Thereafter, 650 mg paracetamol per orally thrice a day is continued for 3–5 days.

Care of Surgical Sites

Incision: Daily dressing and inspection of the incision is required. The ICU care provider should be watchful for any signs of infection, leaking, or dehiscence.

The drain: Drain output also requires vigilant monitoring. Any change in texture of output from serosanguinous to bloody requires prompting the urologists. If only the volume increases, creatinine values of the fluid should be checked to rule out leaking of urine from the drain. The value of creatinine in urine is far greater than that in the blood. In cases of leaking of urine a conservative management leaving the drain in situ usually suffices. The drain is usually removed in 2–5 days.[32]

Ureteral stents: Inserted at the time of anastomosing the graft ureter to native bladder, ureteral stent allows for patency of urine flow. It is usually removed in 4 weeks time by the urologist as an out patient procedure.[35]

Nutrition

Patients are allowed orally as early as POD1 if no contraindication exists. No definite guidelines on nutrition in postoperative period of renal recipient is present. Similar to every other major surgery they require high caloric diet. Total caloric requirement per day is 120–130% of basal energy expenditure (BEE). BEE is calculated by Harris–Benedict equation:[36]

Men: 66.4730 + (13.7516 × weight in kg) + (5.0033 × height in cm) − (6.7550 × age in years) Kcal/day

Women: 655.0955 + (9.5634 × weight in kg) + (1.8496 × height in cm) − (4.6756 × age in years) Kcal/day

A balanced diet with 55–65% carbohydrate, 20–30% fat should be given.[37] The protein requirement is high in initial period to tide over stress of surgery and yet keep the body in positive nitrogen balance. 1.3–2 g/kg of protein is required daily in initial period.[37] Other micronutrients such as phosphorus, magnesium, and vitamin D should also be adequately provided.

Hyperglycemia may be seen in both diabetics and nondiabetics postoperatively. It is a side effect of steroids, CNIs and surgical stress. It is managed by continuous insulin infusion[32] in early postoperative period followed by adding subcutaneous long-acting insulin supplemented with short-acting agent as and when required. Once the patient starts taking orally, an endocrinology consultation should be obtained for appropriate blood sugar management.

Deep Vein Thrombosis Prophylaxis

Sequential compressive device is used in intraoperative and early postoperative period till the patient mobilizes. As per ERBP guideline routine administration of unfractionated heparin is not required to prevent graft vascular thrombosis[11] (Recommendation 1B). However, no statement is given on use of heparin for deep vein thrombosis (DVT) prophylaxis. The incidence of venous thromboembolism (VTE) is to the extent of 1.5% in posttransplant patients which is sevenfold greater than the general population.[38] In absence of a definite guideline, practice varies from center to center. Some centers use regular 5000 units heparin subcutaneously three times a day while avoiding low molecular weight heparin (LMWH).[32] Some centers start LMWH from Day 2 till discharge.[39] Our center follows early mobilization with no pharmaceutical thromboprophylaxis.

Immunosuppression

Continued as per immunologic risk assessment of the patient and institute protocol. It has been explained in detail earlier in the chapter.

Infection Prophylaxis

These patients are highly immunosuppressed immediately after transplant. They may not have classical signs of infection like fever or leukocytosis. A deterioration in renal function or hypotension may be the first sign of sepsis, so a good infection prophylaxis and a high index of suspicion for infection is required.

Bacterial prophylaxis: No guideline on infection prophylaxis currently exists so local protocols are followed by every institute. Usually antibiotics are continued for 24–36 hours postoperatively.[40] If the donor is suffering from bacteremia or urinary tract infection, there is a risk of its transmission to the recipient and so the type and duration of antibiotic prophylaxis is changed accordingly. If the recipient during his/her previous hospital admissions had acquired a resistant or recurrent infection, he/she should be screened accordingly for presence of any occult organisms and treated before surgery.

Pneumocystis jiroveci pneumonia prophylaxis: Cotrimoxazole single strength (80 mg trimethoprim) once daily or double strength (160 mg trimethoprim) thrice weekly is given perioperatively and continued for 6 months to 1 year post discharge. Patients allergic to the drug may be given aerosolized pentamidine or oral dapsone or atovaquone.[7]

UTI: Daily dosing of cotrimoxazole provides additional prophylaxis for UTI. It is required to continue for 6 months.

Viral: Cytomegalovirus is one of most common opportunistic infection in immunosuppressed individuals. Routine prophylaxis is not required. Oral valganciclovir 900 mg daily or intravenous ganciclovir is given to recipients who were seronegative before and receiving kidney from seropositive donors and previously seropositive recipients who require antilymphocyte antibodies as part of immunosuppression therapy. The duration of prophylaxis varies from 3 months to 1 year depending on institutional practice.[41]

Fungal: Routine systemic antifungal prophylaxis is not required. Nystatin lozenges may be given to prevent oral candidiasis during hospital stay.

COMPLICATIONS IN EARLY POSTOPERATIVE PERIOD

The common complications witnessed in the postoperative period along with investigations helping in diagnosis and their treatment are mentioned in **Table 4**. If a fall in urine output is seen after initial good diuresis a urological or renovascular complication is the most likely cause.

Allograft Dysfunction

It is one of the most important complications in the postoperative period. It is manifested as decreasing urine output or a failure to decrease serum creatinine (Cr), urgent and careful evaluation of the various possible causes and their management is required **(Flowchart 5)**.

Two clinical entitities of the graft dysfunction are as follows:
1. *Delayed graft function:* It is a form of acute kidney injury where dialysis is required in the first week after transplant.[28] Utilizing deceased donor kidney especially that after cardiac death, kidney from extended criteria donor and prolonged cold ischemia time, presence of preoperative pulmonary hypertension in recipient,[45]

Table 4: Common complications seen in postoperative phase in renal transplant recipients.

	Etiology	Manifestation	Investigation	Treatment
Urological/ Surgical				
Bleeding (more common in first 48 hours)	• Difficult benching, (described in text) • Uremic thrombocytopathy • Antiplatelet drugs	• Increased drain output/pain/swelling at site of surgery • Decrease UO	• Serial fall in Hb • USG for perinephric hematoma	Resuscitation and re-exploration
Urinary obstruction	Clots in bladder, Ureterocele	Decrease in UO	–	Flushing the Foley's catheter/bladder
Urine leak/ureteric leak (in first few weeks)	–	• Localized pain and swelling at site of graft • Increase drain output	*USG*: Peritransplant collection	• *Minor leak*: Conservative • *Major leak*: Percutaneous nephrostomy • Surgical repair
Wound infection	–	Pain at incision site	–	*Depending on extent of infection*: Conservative/debridement
Wound dehiscence	–	–	–	Surgical repair
Renal vascular				
Hemorrhage	Anastomotic leak	• Increase drain output • Decrease UO • Hypotension	USG perinephric collection	Resuscitation and Re-exploration
Thrombosis (first week) (2–3%)[42]	Difficult benching, multiple vessels, prolonged cold ischemia time, vessel atherosclerosis		Doppler USG Diminished flow in vessel affected	Re-exploration
Renal artery thrombosis		Sudden decrease in UO		
Renal vein thrombosis		Pain, swelling, hematuria		
Renal artery sclerosis (rare in early period)	Donor atherosclerotic vessel is risk factor	• Hypertension • Allograft dysfunction	• *Duplex USG*: Increased velocity across anastomotic sites • A flow differential between the aorta and transplant artery	• Percutaneous transluminal angioplasty with stent placement[43] • Revision surgery
Cardiovascular				
Hypertension (60–70%)[5]	Preexisting, Iatrogenic Excess IV fluids, S/E CNI, steroid-related fluid retention	NIBP measurements		Diuretics CCB
ACS (40% within 3 months)[5]	Previous undetected disease, altered demand/supply ratio	May be absent	• ECG • Echocardio-angiography	• Cardiologist opinion • Aspirin, NTG, morphine, β blocker titrated to BP[5]
Hematological				
Anemia	• Anastomotic site leek • Generalized oozing.	• Hypotension • Drop in urine output	• Serial Hb • USG for perinephric hematoma	Resuscitation and re-exploration
	• Pretransplant anemia • Intraoperative blood loss	• No other symptoms, delayed/slow graft function		Erythropoietin 50–100 units/kg three times/week or darbepoetin 0.45 µg/kg weekly
Leukopenia	S/E of ATG, mycophenolate, cotrimoxazole, valganciclovir	Risk of infection	Absolute neutrophil count (ANC)	G-CSF 5 µg/kg/day Sc if ANC < 1,000/µL [44]
Thrombocytopenia	• S/E of Mycophenolate • TMA	–	Platelet counts investigations to rule out TMA	Transfusion if counts <50 × 10⁹/L and biopsy has to be done
Allograft dysfunction	Detailed in text			
Infection	Detailed in text			

(USG: ultrasonography; UO: urine output, CNI: calcineurin inhibitors, NIBP: noninvasive blood pressure; CCB: calcium channel blockers; ACS: acute coronary syndrome; NTG: nitroglycerine; BP: blood pressure; Hb: hemoglobin; ATG: antithymocyte globulin; TMA: thrombotic microangiopathy)

Flowchart 5: Evaluation of a patient with allograft dysfunction.

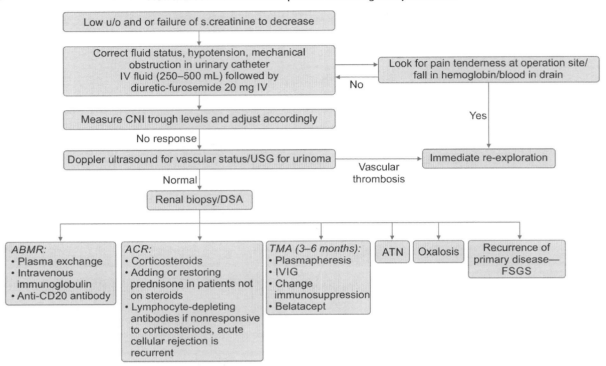

(DSA: donor specific antibodies; ABMR: antibody mediated rejection; ACR: acute cellular rejection; TMA: thrombotic microangiopathy; IVIG: intravenous immunoglobulin; ATN: acute tubular necrosis, FSGS: focal segmental glomerulosclerosis).

increases incidence of DGF. Most common pathology behind DGF is ATN and it hampers long-term graft survival.[46]

2. *Slow graft function:* It is a condition where decline in Cr in less than 30% between POD1 and 2, or the absolute value of Cr ≥3 mg/dL on POD5 or ≥ 2.5 mg/dL on POD 7.[47] It is characterized by no requirement of dialysis during this time. The risk factors and effect on outcome are similar to DGF.[47]

Whatever the clinical terminology the same scheme **(Flowchart 5)** is followed for diagnosis and management.

Infection

The renal transplant patients are highly immunosuppressed in the immediate post-transplant period and therefore are at great risk of catching nosocomial pathogens. The pathogens may also be transferred from the donor or there may be flaring up of a latent infection. Urinary tract infection (UTI) is the most common type of infection seen followed by pneumonia, surgical site infection, and septicemia.[5] Gram negative organisms are more common (*E. coli*) followed by candidiasis and gram positive enterococcus.[5] These patients do not have classic signs of sepsis, so on slightest hint of infection a complete microbiological work up of blood, urine and sputum is required. Chest and abdominal

imaging is done to rule out pathology in these regions. A broad spectrum antibiotic and an antifungal is started within an hour of presentation.

CONCLUSION

End-stage renal disease patients are known to have multisystem abnormalities and are at increased risk of morbidity and mortality. Steering these individuals through the course of a successful transplantation requires a thorough knowledge of pathophysiology of disease, expected course, and complications postoperatively. This chapter intends to provide the readers an in-depth information about a holistic perioperative management of renal transplant recipients.

REFERENCES

1. Varughese S, Abraham G. Chronic kidney disease in India. A clarion call for change. Clin J Am Soc Nephrol. 2018;13:802-4.
2. Tonelli M, Wiebe N, Knoll G, Bello A, Browne S, Jadhav D, et al. Systematic review: Kidney transplantation compared with dialysis in clinically relevant outcomes. Am J Transplant. 2011;11:2093-109.
3. Saat, TC, Van den Akker EK, IJzermans JN, Dor FJ, de Bruin RW. Improving the outcome of kidney transplantation by ameliorating renal ischemia reperfusion injury: lost in translation? J Transl Med. 2016;14:20.

4. Pascual J, Zamora J, Pirsch JD. A systematic review of kidney transplantation from expanded criteria donors. Am J Kidney Dis. 2008;52:553-86.

5. Biancofiore G, De Wolf A, Klinck JR, Niemann C, Watts A (Eds). Oxford Textbook of Transplant Anaesthesia and Critical Care, 1st edition. Oxford: Oxford University Press; 2015.

6. Dudley C, Harden P. Clinical Practice Guidelines Assessment of the Potential Kidney Transplant Recipient, 5th edition 2011. [online] Available from https://bts.org.uk/wp-content/uploads/2016/09/10_RA_KidneyRecipient-1.pdf. [Last accessed March, 2020].

7. KDIGO clinical practice guideline on the evaluation and management of candidates for kidney transplantation. 2018 draft for public review. [online] Available from https://kdigo.org/wp-content/uploads/2018/08/KDIGO-Txp-Candidate-GL-Public-Review-Draft-Oct-22.pdf on 6.10.2019. [Last accessed March, 2020].

8. Livhits M, Ko CY, Leonardi MJ, Zingmond DS, Gibbons MM, de Virgilio C, et al. Risk of surgery following recent myocardial infarction. Ann Surg. 2011;253:857-64.

9. Holcomb CN, Graham LA, Richman JS, Rhyne RR, Itani KM, Maddox TM, et al. The incremental risk of noncardiac surgery on adverse cardiac events following coronary stenting. J Am Coll Cardiol. 2014;64:2730-39.

10. Skorecki K, Chertow GM, Marsden PA, Taal MW, Yu ASL. Brenner and Rector's The Kidney, 10th edition. Philadelphia: Elsevier; 2016.

11. Abramowicz D, Cochat P, Claas FH, Heemann U, Pascual J, Dudley C, et al. European Renal Best Practice Guideline on kidney donor and recipient evaluation and perioperative care. Nephrol Dial Transplant. 2015;30:1790-7.

12. Aulakh NK, Garg K, Bose A, Aulakh BS, Chahal HS, Aulakh GS. Influence of hemodynamics and intra-operative hydration on biochemical outcome of renal transplant recipients. J Anaesthesiol Clin Pharmacol. 2015;31:174-9.

13. Marik PE, Cavallazzi R. Does the central venous pressure predict fluid responsiveness? An updated meta-analysis and a plea for some common sense. Crit Care Med. 2013;41:1774-81.

14. Srivastava D, Sahu S, Chandra A, Tiwari T, Kumar S, Singh PK. Effect of intraoperative transesophageal Doppler-guided fluid therapy versus central venous pressure-guided fluid therapy on renal allograft outcome in patients undergoing living donor renal transplant surgery: a comparative study. J Anesth. 2015;29:842-9.

15. Cavaleri M, Veroux M, Palermo F, Vasile F, Mineri M, Palumbo J, et al. Perioperative goal-directed therapy during kidney transplantation: an impact evaluation on the major postoperative complications. J Clin Med. 2019;8(1):pii: E80.

16. Calixto Fernandes MH, Schricker T, Magder S, Hatzakorzian R. Perioperative fluid management in kidney transplantation: a black box. Crit Care. 2018;22:14.

17. Castro AG, Ortiz-Lasa M, Peñasco Y, González C, Blanco C, Rodriguez-Borregan JC. Choice of fluids in the perioperative period of kidney transplantation. Nefrologia. 2017;37:572-8.

18. Abdallah E, El-Shishtawy S, Mosbah O, Zeidan M. Comparison between the effects of intraoperative human albumin and normal saline on early graft function in renal transplantation. Int Urol Nephrol. 2014;46:2221-6.

19. Shah RB, Shah VR, Butala BP, Parikh GP. Effect of intraoperative human albumin on early graft function in renal transplantation. Saudi J Kidney Dis Transpl. 2014;25:1148-53.

20. Wittebole X, Castanares-Zapatero D, Mourad M, Montiel V, Collienne C, Laterre, PF. Early postoperative ICU care of the kidney transplant recipient. In: Orlando G, Remuzzi G, Williams DF (Eds). Kidney Transplantation, Bioengineering and Regeneration. Amsterdam, Netherlands: Elsevier; 2017. pp. 199-210.

21. Feng, C, Liu, B, Piao M. Comparison of norepinephrine and dopamine in kidney transplant recipient on renal graft function. Eur J Anaesthesiol. 2011;28:139-40.

22. Choi JM, Jo JY, Baik JW, Kim S, Kim CS, Jeong SM. Risk factors and outcomes associated with a higher use of inotropes in kidney transplant recipients. Medicine (Baltimore). 2017;96: e5820.

23. Kar SK, Khurana HS, Ganguly T. Anesthesia management of renal transplantation: An update. Anaesth Pain Intens Care. 2018;22:383-91.

24. Aggarwal S, Kang Y, Freeman JA, Fortunato FL, Pinsky MR. Postreperfusion syndrome: Cardiovascular collapse following hepatic reperfusion during liver transplantation. Transplant Proc. 1987;19(4 Suppl 3):54-5.

25. Bruhl SR, Vetteth S, Rees M, Grubb BP, Khouri SJ. Post-reperfusion syndrome during renal transplantation: a retrospective study. Int J Med Sci. 2012;9:391-6.

26. Aggarwal S, Kang Y, Freeman JA, Fortunato FL Jr, Pinsky MR. Postreperfusion syndrome: Hypotension after reperfusion of the transplanted liver. J Crit Care. 1993;8:154-60.

27. Tomasdottir H, Bengtson JP, Bengtsson A. Neutrophil and macrophage activation and anaphylatoxin formation in orthotopic liver transplantation without the use of veno-venous bypass. Acta Anaesthesiol Scand. 1996;40:250-5.

28. Yarlagadda SG, Coca SG, Garg AX, Doshi M, Poggio E, Marcus RJ, et al. Marked variation in the definition and diagnosis of delayed graft function: a systematic review. Nephrol Dial Transplant. 2008;23:2995-3003.

29. Gill J, Dong J, Eng M, Landsberg D, Gill JS. Pulsatile perfusion reduces the risk of delayed graft function in deceased donor kidney transplants, irrespective of donor type and cold ischemic time. Transplantation. 2014;97:668-74.

30. Salvadori M, Rosso G, Bertoni E. Update on ischemia-reperfusion injury in kidney transplantation: Pathogenesis and treatment. World J Transplant. 2015;5:52-67.

31. KIDGO Managing Transplnat recipients. [online] Available from https://kdigo.org/wp-content/uploads/2017/02/KDIGO_TX_NephsTool-Managing-Kidney-Transplant-Recipients.pdf. [Last accessed March, 2019].

32. Naik AS, Josephson MA, Chon WJ. In: K Subramaniam, T Sakai (Eds). Postoperative Care of Renal Transplant Recipients. Anesthesia and Perioperative Care for Organ Transplantation. Berlin: Springer; 2016. pp. 297-307.

33. Aref A, Zayan T, Sharma A, Halawa A. Utility of central venous pressure measurement in renal transplantation: Is it evidence based? World J Transplant. 2018;8:61-7.

34. Ferris R, Kittur D, Wilasrusmee C, Shah G, Krause E, Ratner L. Early hemodynamic changes after renal transplantation: determinants of low central venous pressure in the recipients and correlation with acute renal dysfunction. Med Sci Monit. 2003;9:CR61-6.

35. Mehta Y, Arora D. Newer methods of cardiac output monitoring. World J Cardiol. 2014;6:1022-9.

36. Harris JA, Benedict FG. A biometric study of human basal metabolism. Proc Natl Acad Sci USA. 1918;4:370-3.

37. Fong JV, Moore LW. Nutrition trends in kidney transplant recipients: the importance of dietary monitoring and need for evidence-based recommendations. Front Med (Lausanne). 2018;5:302.

38. Lam N, Garg A, Knoll GA, Kim SJ, Lentine KL, McArthur E, et al. Venous thromboembolism and the risk of death and graft loss in kidney transplant recipients. Am J Nephrol. 2017;46:343-54.

39. Parajuli S, Lockridge JB, Langewisch ED, Norman DJ, Kujovich JL. Hypercoagulability in kidney transplant recipients. Transplantation. 2016;100:719-26.

40. Clinical Guidelines for kidney Transplantation. [online] Available from http://www.transplant.bc.ca/Documents/ Health%20Professionals/Clinical%20guidelines/Clinical%20 Guidelines%20for%20Kidney%20Transplantation.pdf. [Last accessed March, 2020].

41. Fishman JA, Alexander B. Prophylaxis of infections in solid organ transplantation. [online] Available from https://www. uptodate.com/contents/prophylaxis-of-infections-in-solid-organ-transplantation#H6. [Last accessed March, 2020].

42. Hernández D, Rufino M, Armas S, González A, Gutiérrez P, Barbero P, et al. Retrospective analysis of surgical complications following cadaveric kidney transplantation in the modern transplant era. Nephrol Dial Transplant. 2006;21:2908-15.

43. Chen W, Kayler LK, Zand MS, Muttana R Chernyak, V, DeBoccardo GO. Transplant renal artery stenosis: Clinical manifestations, diagnosis and therapy. Clin Kidney J. 2015;8:71-8.

44. Mehta HM, Malandra M, Corey SJ. G-CSF and GM-CSF in neutropenia. J Immunol. 2015;195:1341-9.

45. Goyal VK, Solanki SL, Baj B. Pulmonary hypertension and post-operative outcome in renal transplant: A retrospective analysis of 170 patients. Indian J Anaesth. 2018;62:131-5.

46. Siedlecki A, Irish W, Brennan DC. Delayed graft function in the kidney transplant. Am J Transplant. 2011;11:2279-96.

47. Wang CJ, Tuffaha A, Phadnis MA, Mahnken JD, Wetmore JB. Association of slow graft function with long-term outcomes in kidney transplant recipients. Ann Transplant. 2018;23: 224-31.

Perioperative Management of Liver Transplantation

Mozammil Shafi, Srinivas Monanga, Deepak Govil

INTRODUCTION

Liver transplantation (LT) is the mainstay of treatment for decompensated chronic liver disease (CLD) and few patients of acute liver failure (ALF). The total number of liver transplants performed worldwide has increased enormously in last few decades. Overall, perioperative outcome of these patients has improved tremendously owing to better surgical, anesthetic, and posttransplant critical care management. Nevertheless, some of them may become very sick during their pretransplant, intraoperative, and postoperative phase. In view of these challenges, an excellent teamwork between hepatologist, transplant surgeon, anesthesiologist, and intensivist is required for a successful transplant program. In this chapter, we will be focusing on perioperative issues faced by these patients and their management.

PREOPERATIVE CONSIDERATIONS

Cardiovascular Consideration

Liver failure and associated portal hypertension are characterized by hyperdynamic circulatory state. Systemic and splanchnic vasodilatation as a result of nitric oxide (NO) and other circulatory mediators mainly contribute to this hyperdynamic state. Decreased systemic vascular resistance (SVR), increased cardiac output (CO), and normal-to-low blood pressure are the hallmarks of hyperdynamic circulation.[1] Although extravascular volume is expanded, there is an effective hypovolemic state in these patients. Effective hypovolemic state leads to renin–angiotensin–aldosterone system (RAAS) activation. RAAS activation results in salt and water reabsorption inside the renal tubule and ascites formation.

Coronary Artery Disease

Contrary to the previous studies, coronary artery disease (CAD) is commonly associated with CLD patients. Incidence

varies from 5 to 26%, with 1-year posttransplant mortality as high as 50%.[2,3] Apart from common risk factors of CAD, nonalcoholic steatohepatitis (NASH) is an independent risk factor of CAD in these patients.[4] Screening for CAD should be based on the presence of risk factors. Those with two or more risk factors should be initially evaluated by computed tomography (CT) coronary angiography to look for calcium scoring. Patients with high calcium scoring must undergo noninvasive stress testing and those with positive results should be tested with coronary catheterization. Cardiologist and transplant team must decide the future course of action regarding the revascularization therapy and the type of stent. Many experienced centers have started performing combined coronary artery bypass graft (CABG) and LT with good outcome.[5]

Cardiomyopathies

Cardiomyopathies are relatively common in cirrhotics compared to general population. Many etiological factors of liver disease can also cause cardiomyopathy. Hepatitis C, hemochromatosis, and amyloidosis may result in restrictive cardiomyopathy. Chronic alcoholism can cause dilated cardiomyopathy and heart failure.[6] Cirrhotic cardiomyopathy is a distinct entity seen in patients of advance liver disease. Cardinal features of cirrhotic cardiomyopathy are impaired systolic function and diastolic relaxation, increased resting CO, repolarization abnormality, and blunted response to beta stimulation.[7] Symptoms of heart failure may not be present early or can be seen only during exercise, due to increase in baseline CO in these patients. As the disease progresses, symptoms of congestive heart failure develop, which may be difficult to differentiate from those of advance liver disease.

Portopulmonary hypertension (PPHTN) is another recognized cause of heart failure in these patients (2–16% of patients).[8] PPHTN is defined as features of portal hypertension due to advance liver disease without any

Box 1: Features of portopulmonary hypertension (PPHTN) on right heart catheterization.

- Raised resting mean pulmonary artery pressure (mPAP) of more than 20 mm Hg
- Low to normal pulmonary capillary wedge pressure (PCWP) ≤15 mm of Hg
- Increase pulmonary vascular resistance (PVR) of 240 dynes/sec/cm^{-5}

obvious extrahepatic cause. Diagnosis is established by history, physical examination, echocardiography, and lung imaging. Transthoracic echocardiography is must for estimating resting PA pressure and evaluating other cardiac abnormalities in these patients. Right heart catheterization may be required in selected cases. Diagnostic criteria for PPHTN are defined in **Box 1**.[9] In past, the presence of PPHTN was considered as absolute contraindication for LT. With availability of newer pharmacological agents such as phosphodiesterase-5 inhibitors (sildenafil and tadalafil), endothelin receptor antagonist (bosentan, ambrisentan, and macitentan), and prostacyclin agonist, many of these patients can be stabilized before LT. Pulmonary arterial hypertension (PAH)-specific therapies should only be started after consultation with experts. Diuretics are frequently prescribed for improving congestive symptoms. Calcium channel blockers are ideally avoided due to risk of hypotension and mesenteric vasodilatation. These therapies may be required to be continued in posttransplantation period. Nevertheless, PPHTN is associated with significant post-LT morbidity and risk is much higher with resting pulmonary artery (PA) pressure of >60 mm Hg.[10]

Pulmonary Consideration

Hypoxia in chronic liver failure can be caused parenchymal issues (e.g., pneumonia), extrapulmonary problems such as decreased diaphragmatic movement secondary to tense ascites, and liver specific conditions such as hepatic hydrothorax and hepatopulmonary syndrome (HPS). Pneumonia and acute respiratory distress syndrome (ARDS) are commonly seen in ALF.

Hepatopulmonary Syndrome

Hepatopulmonary syndrome is a unique syndrome seen in advance liver disease with substantial morbidity and mortality. Hallmark of this syndrome is intrapulmonary vasodilatation (IPVD) leading to ventilation perfusion mismatch and hypoxia.[11] Diagnosis is based on the demonstration of hypoxia and IPVD in patients of advance liver disease. Arterial blood analysis to look for resting partial pressure of oxygen (PaO$_2$) should be done in preoperative evaluation. HPS is graded on the basis of PaO$_2$ and alveolar arterial gradient. Severe HPS is defined as PaO$_2$ of <60

mm Hg and A-a gradient of >15 mm Hg.[12] These patients should be evaluated by bubble contrast transthoracic echocardiography for demonstrating intrapulmonary shunts. Agitated saline is pushed through a central line during echocardiography. Presence of bubbles in the left side of the heart after three to six cardiac cycles signifies IPVD and shunt. Another method to quantify shunt is radionucleotide perfusion scanning using technetium-labeled macroaggregate of albumin (MAA). MAA scan calculates shunt fraction and can discern the contribution of shunt in patients of intrinsic lung disease. Disadvantage of MAA scan is its inability to differentiate between intrapulmonary and intracardiac shunts.[13] LT is only definite therapy, especially if PaO$_2$ of <60 mm Hg.

Hepatic Hydrothorax

Hepatic hydrothorax is defined as transudative pleural effusion secondary to portal hypertension, in the absence of underlying cardiopulmonary disease.[14] It may or may not be associated with ascites and is mostly right-sided. Proposed mechanism is the migration of ascitic fluid to pleural cavity through pleuroperitoneal communication. Treatment is done with sodium restriction, diuretics, and therapeutic thoracentesis. These patients should be evaluated for liver transplantation. In selected patients, transjugular intrahepatic portosystemic shunt (TIPS) should be attempted.[15]

Renal Consideration

Acute kidney injury (AKI) is very common in both ALF and CLD. Almost 80% patients of ALF have associated AKI.[16,17] A number of etiological factors of ALF such as acetaminophen toxicity and ischemic hepatitis can result in AKI. About 30–50% of them require renal replacement therapy. AKI in CLD can be caused from prerenal, renal, and postrenal causes. Prerenal (hypoperfusion, hypovolemia, etc.) is most common form of AKI in CLD patients (about 60%). Around 30% of AKI is attributable to renal cause and <1% is caused by obstructive causes.[18]

Acute kidney injury in advance liver disease is diagnosed using RIFLE (Risk, Injury, Failure, Loss, and End-stage Kidney) or Acute Kidney Injury Network (AKIN) criteria. These two systems use serum creatinine and urine output to diagnose AKI. Creatinine level can be erroneously low in these patients due to poor muscle mass from malnutrition. Urine output may not be a good reflection of renal function, as they may have preserved glomerular filtration rate (GFR) despite of decrease urine output.

Hepatorenal syndrome (HRS) is a distinct entity seen in advance liver failure (**Box 2**).[19,20] Liver failure and associated portal hypertension leads to splanchnic vasodilation,

Table 1: Phases of liver transplant surgery.

Phases	Preanhepatic	Anhepatic	Reperfusion	Neohepatic
Timing	From initial incision to the isolation of native liver from circulation	From isolation of native liver to perfusion	Native liver is introduced to patient's circulation	From reperfusion till the completion of surgery
Characteristics	• Anesthesia induction • Lines placement • Surgical dissection • Significant fluid shift (Ascites drainage and blood loss) • Fluid management • Blood products administration • Coagulopathy correction • Avoid volume overload	• Native liver is isolated and removed • New liver is implanted • Decrease in preload depending on surgical technique • Caval cross clamping/piggyback technique/temporary portocaval bypass venovenous bypass	• New liver is introduced to circulation • Period of severe instability • Arrhythmias • Hypotension • Rise in intracranial pressure (ICP) • Cardiac arrest • Ischemia reperfusion injury leading to graft dysfunction	• Hepatic arterial and biliary anastomosis • Optimize hemodynamics • Prepare for extubation or shifting to intensive care unit (ICU)

Box 2: Diagnostics criteria of hepatorenal syndrome (HRS)

- Advance liver failure with portal hypertension
- AKI, with increase in serum creatinine 0.3 mg/dL from baseline, within 48 hours or 50% increase from baseline within 7 days
- Absence of other causes such as shock, nephrotoxic drugs, or ultrasound evidence of obstruction
- Serum creatinine not improving after 48 hours and diuretic withdrawal and volume expansion with albumin (1 g/kg to a maximum of 100 g/day)
- Urine red blood cells less 50 per high power field and urine protein less than 500 mg/day

which is the main trigger for the development of HRS. HRS can be of two types, 1 and 2, with type 1 HRS being a more serious form. Type 1 HRS is treated using a combination of vasoconstrictor (norepinephrine and terlipressin) and human albumin. TIPS can be tried in nonresponding patients. Nonresponders should be urgently evaluated for LT, as it is associated with overall very outcome.

INTRAOPERATIVE MANAGEMENT

Intraoperative management of liver transplant is challenging due to the complex nature of surgery and major hemodynamic fluctuations. Intraoperative period is divided into different phases as described in **Table 1**. Vascular access includes central line, large bore peripheral access for rapid transfusion, arterial catheter and in selected patients Swan Ganz catheter is used. Anesthesia is usually induced with propofol or etomidate or combination of both.

Anesthesia maintenance is usually done using inhalational agents. Opioid analgesics are utilized for pain control. Routine monitoring with continuous electrocardiography, oxygen saturation, capnography, temperature, etc. Invasive arterial blood pressure monitoring should be done ideally at two sites (both radial or one radial and one femoral). CO monitoring using pulmonary artery catheter (PAC) or noninvasive devices should be employed.

Routine use of PAC has fallen out of favor these days. Many centers routinely utilize transesophageal echocardiography for continuous CO monitoring. Frequent arterial blood sampling to look for acid–base and electrolytes status and lactate level is done. Although transfusion requirement has come down significantly with improvement in anesthesia and surgical technique, massive transfusion is still required at times. Good blood bank service is essential for running a successful liver transplant program. Rapid infusion devices are frequently required for massive transfusion. Transfusion is usually guided by thromboelastography and it should be available in operation theater (OT) complex itself. Additionally, heating blanket is mandatory for preventing hypothermia. Few liver transplant patients are fast tracked and can be extubated in OT itself, albeit most of them are shifted to intensive care unit (ICU) and extubated there.

POSTOPERATIVE MANAGEMENT

Once the patient is shifted to an ICU, a detail handover should be taken from anesthesia and surgical team with focus on preoperative status, intraoperative complications (bleeding and transfusion requirement, hemodynamic status, any vascular and biliary complication, etc.), warm and cold ischemia time, urine output, and blood gas and electrolyte status amongst other. Close monitoring of postoperative hemodynamic and respiratory parameters along with assessment of graft function cannot be overemphasized.

Cardiovascular Issues

Early postoperative period can be associated with significant hemodynamic perturbations. Ongoing bleeding, ischemia reperfusion injury, vasodilatation, sepsis, overt or relative hypovolemia, left ventricular (LV) dysfunction, electrolyte imbalance, acidosis, and hypothermia can complicate the situation. Intra-abdominal bleeding can be suspected from drop in hemoglobin, increase in drain output, and hemodynamic instability. Blood and blood products should be guided by thromboelastography. Overtransfusion is associated with thrombotic complications and should be avoided. Despite of coagulopathy correction, 10% of patients may require reoperation to control bleeding.[21] Fluid administration should ideally be guided by dynamic parameters (stroke volume variation, systolic pressure variation, and plethysmographic variability index) or point-of-care ultrasound examination (POCUS). Vasopressor support is required if mean arterial pressure (MAP) is not maintained by fluid boluses. Hemodynamic instability and acidosis improve with improving graft function. Antibiotic escalation may be required if sepsis is suspected and risk factors of drug-resistant infection are present.

Hypertensive response is common in postoperative period. Postoperative pain, preexisting hypertension, volume overload, and calcineurin inhibitors can contribute to this. Hypertension should be controlled by short-acting intravenous drugs such as labetalol and hydralazine.

Myocardial ischemia is relatively uncommon after liver transplant (about 5%), owing to better preoperative evaluation and management.[22] It should be managed with consultation with cardiologist and surgical team as routine treatment may be feasible in immediate postoperative period.

Acute pulmonary edema in posttransplant period can be due to ischemia reperfusion injury, Volume overload, preexisting PPHTN, cirrhotic cardiomyopathy, and myocardial ischemia. Management is supportive with fluid restriction, diuretic, and vasodilators. A small minority of patients develop stress or Takotsubo cardiomyopathy, resulting in heart failure. Treatment is entirely supportive as the condition is entirely reversible in due course.

Cardiac tamponade is a rare complication after liver transplant. Superior aspect of Mercedes Benz incision may violate pericardium resulting in pericardial effusion. Renal failure and coagulopathy are other risk factors.

Renal and Metabolic Issues

Causes of postoperative renal dysfunction include hypovolemia due to major blood loss, cardiac dysfunction, sepsis, graft dysfunction, effect of drugs, etc.[23] A good number (around 30%) of them may require short term hemodialysis.

Perioperative hyperglycemia is common and may be due to surgical stress and exogenous catecholamines, steroids, and insulin resistance secondary to liver disease. Hyperglycemia may have a bad impact on graft function.[24] Although target blood sugar range is debatable, it is prudent to maintain between 140 and 180 mg/dL in line of general critically ill patients.[25] Hypoglycemia can be detrimental and must be avoided and aggressively treated.

Infectious Complications

Infectious complications are common in post-LT period. Postsurgery immunosuppression increases the risk of infection to many folds. The risk of infection posttransplant varies with time and is based on the burden of immunosuppression and the graft function (**Table 2**).

Discussing all the infections postliver transplant is beyond this chapter. So, only perioperative infectious complications will be discussed here. System wise infections will be covered in their respective heads and generalized infections will be discussed in this head.

As immunosuppression is not fully achieved during the first month, the most common infections are nosocomial or surgery related. Overall surgical site infections posttransplant occur with a frequency of 10–37%. Risk factors for surgical site infections include diabetes, obesity, high model for end-stage liver disease (MELD score), prolonged surgical time, multiple transfusions during

Table 2: Common infections postliver transplant based on timeline.

Less than 30 days	1–6 months	6–12 months
Surgical/nosocomial	Opportunistic	Community acquired
Surgical site infections	CMV	Streptococcus
Klebsiella pneumoniae	Pneumocystis	Haemophilus influenzae
Escherichia coli	HSV (herpes simplex virus)	Mycoplasma
Acinetobacter	Aspergillosis	Herpes zoster
Enterococcus species	Mycobacterium tuberculosis	CMV
Catheter-related infections	Cryptococcus	HBV, HCV
Clostridium difficile	Nocardia	
	Toxoplasma	
Donor-derived infections		
HBV (hepatitis B virus), CMV, and HCV (hepatitis C virus)		

(CMV: cytomegalovirus)

surgery, etc. Routinely, all institutions have their own practice in choosing the prophylactic antibiotics regimen depending on local antibiogram and prevalence of resistant bugs.

Nosocomial infections generally include catheter-related infections, ventilator-associated pneumonia, etc. Mostly they are multidrug-resistant organisms such as *Klebsiella*, *Escherichia coli*, and *Acinetobacter*. Invasive fungal infections are also seen due to catheter and also in surgical site infections.

The other infections during first month are donor-derived infections such as hepatitis B virus (HBV) and hepatitis C virus (HCV). Sometimes, there will be reactivation of cytomegalovirus (CMV) that was present preoperative due to immunosuppression.[26]

Respiratory Complications

Posttransplant pulmonary complications are common ranging from 42.1 to 96.5%.[27-29] A number of perioperative risk factors are responsible for postoperative pulmonary complications. Preoperative risk factors include but not limited to are age, smoking history, presence of restrictive lung disease, prior mechanical ventilation, high MELD scores, etc. Intraoperative and postoperative factors are intraoperative bleeding volume, transfused fluid, blood volume, postoperative fluid retention, prolonged ventilation acute renal failure, etc. Perioperative respiratory complications can be infectious or noninfectious.

Pleural Effusion

Pleural effusion is the most common of all pulmonary complications with incidence ranging from 32.5 to 96.5%.[27,28] In majority of patients, it appears during the first week and involves the right lung. Multiple mechanisms have been proposed, but the exact cause is not known. Mechanisms include dissection of lymphatics during dissection, transfer of ascitic fluid through the diaphragmatic defects, hypoproteinemia, atelectasis, etc. Mostly, it is transudative in nature and does not require intervention. It resolves spontaneously in subsequent weeks as the liver function improves. Symptomatic patients with respiratory distress, inadequate cough, increased oxygen requirements, and worsening respiratory failure require drainage.

Atelectasis

Postoperative pulmonary atelectasis is extremely common after major abdominal surgery. Mostly, it is secondary to general postoperative issues such as pain during deep breathing, abdominal distension, or discomfort or related to the surgery itself. Postliver transplant diaphragmatic injury or dissection and resulting hypomobility lead to atelectasis. Other causes such as the presence of pleural effusion

lead to compression of atelectasis, decreased compliance due to increased intravascular volume, and retained secretions. Mostly, it improves by good physiotherapy, adequate analgesia, and deep breathing exercises. Drainage of effusions and fiberoptic bronchoscopy, if there is a significant lung collapse, may be required at times. Some patients may need noninvasive ventilation or high flow nasal oxygen support postextubation.

Pneumonia

Pneumonia posttransplant is mostly due to nosocomial bugs. Mostly caused by bacteria, but fungal and viral infections are not uncommon. Risk factors include prolonged ventilatory requirement due to any cause (such as presence of pleural effusion and atelectasis), multiple transfusion intra- and postoperative, severe renal impairment, surgical complications, reintubation, and need for retransplantation. Diagnosed by fever, leukocytosis, or leukopenia, new infiltrates on chest X-ray and new onset respiratory symptoms (cough, sputum, and dyspnea) are either confirmed by endotracheal aspirate or by bronchoalveolar lavage culture, which can isolate the organism. Posttransplant pneumonia is associated with high morbidity and mortality.

Bacterial pneumonia is due to both gram-positive and gram-negative organisms, but latter are more common. Gram-negative organisms include but not limited to *Klebsiella pneumoniae*, *E. coli*, *Acinetobacter*, *Haemophilus influenzae*, *Citrobacter*, and *Pseudomona* species. Gram-positive organisms include both methicillin-sensitive and resistant *Staphylococcus*; *Streptococcus* species have been reported. Antibiotics starting from beta-lactam plus beta-lactam inhibitor to carbapenems and polymyxins are used for gram-negative organisms and teicoplanin, vancomycin, and linezolid are used for gram-positive organisms.[30]

Cytomegalovirus is the most common viral infection seen in postliver transplant period. Risk factors include CMV seropositive donor with CMV seronegative recipient, previously seropositive recipient, antithymocyte globulin treatment, steroid boluses, and transfusion >10 units of packed cells. Mortality is high when there is multiorgan involvement. Treatment is done with valganciclovir or intravenous ganciclovir for a duration of 3–6 months. Foscarnet may be used in nonresponsive patients and ganciclovir resistance. Other viral etiology includes herpes simplex virus (HSV) type 1, which is seen rarely in patients receiving ganciclovir prophylaxis as it also acts on HSV 1. Adenovirus, influenza, and rhinovirus are relatively uncommon causes of pneumonia in early posttransplant period.

Fungal pneumonia in posttransplant period can be caused by *Aspergillus* species, *Cryptococcus*, *Pneumocystis jirovecii, Candida* species, and rarely *Mucorales.* Aspergillosis presents as either tracheobronchitis (which involves tracheobronchial tree) or invasive aspergillosis (which involves parenchyma). The two entities can present as phases also. The disease is diagnosed by clinical features (fever and hypoxemia), histopathological or cytopathological, radiological, and semiquantitative culture. Pneumocystis incidence is low after the starting of the prophylaxis with trimethoprim sulfamethoxazole which is given for a duration of 6–12 months postsolid organ transplant. Cryptococcal pneumonia is a rare entity and very few cases were reported. Diagnosing candida pneumonia is difficult as it is mostly recognized as a colonizer in respiratory secretions. Nevertheless, invasive candidiasis is treated aggressively. Aspergillosis is treated with voriconazole as a first-line drug followed by amphotericin B. Pneumocystis is treated by trimethoprim sulfamethoxazole. Echinocandins are the first-line agents for invasive candida infections.

Any pneumonia can worsen and can lead to ARDS. ARDS is also caused by noninfectious causes such as transfusion and drugs, managed in the same way as in an immunocompetent patient with antibiotics and lung protective ventilation. Even though it is thought that high PEEP (positive-end expiratory pressure) may lead to decreased venous return and CO affecting newly engrafted liver, the literature for the same is not adequate. Rescue therapies also can be used whenever required.[27,31]

Neurological Complications

Neurological complications are not uncommon after LT, with a frequency of 15–30%. They can be both neurological and neurocognitive and include stroke, seizures, infections, ICU-acquired weakness, decompensation of previous altered cerebral condition, etc.[32,33]

Stroke

It occurs with a frequency of 1–4% and can be both ischemic and hemorrhagic with latter being more common. Causes of hemorrhage include coagulopathy and thrombocytopenia. Risk factors are same as of general population. Diagnosis is by CT or MRI (magnetic resonance imaging) of brain.

Seizures

Seizure is one of the most common neurological complications after LT with a frequency of around 10% and can be partial or generalized. They are generally associated with hemorrhagic stroke, but can also be seen with central nervous system (CNS) infections, hyponatremia, posterior reversible encephalopathy syndrome (PRES), etc. Calcineurin inhibitors induced neurotoxicity is an important differential, especially when brain imaging is normal. Treatment is same as in nontransplant patients but potentially hepatotoxic drugs should be avoided in maintenance therapy.

Infections

Central nervous system infections occur in about 5–10% of cases and are mostly due to opportunistic infections following immunosuppressive therapy. Viral and fungal infections are common compared to bacterial infections. Viral infections are usually caused by CMV, HSV, human herpesvirus (HHV), etc. Fungal infections include *Aspergillus* and bacterial infections include *Listeria* spp., and mycobacterium tuberculosis. HSV, HHV, *Aspergillus*, and *Listeria* cause infections up to 6 months' postoperative, but tuberculosis is seen mostly after the first month (**Table 2**). Other infections that can be seen are *Nocardia*, toxoplasmosis, Japanese encephalitis virus, etc.

Posterior Reversible Encephalopathy Syndrome

It is seen in about 1% of patients and it is completely reversible as the name suggests. Clinical features include visual disturbances, headache, variable altered consciousness, and seizures. Even though CT shows changes such as multiple hypodensities in few patients, MRI is more reliable and diagnostic. Classical findings are symmetrical hyperintensities on T2- and fluid low attenuation inversion recovery (FLAIR)-weighted sequences in the white matter of the hemispheres, predominantly in the parieto-occipital regions. Frontal regions are also involved in some cases. PRES post-LT is most commonly due to endothelial dysfunction caused by calcineurin inhibitors which cause imbalance in cerebral autoregulation. The condition shows good improvement with removing the inciting agent and supportive antiepileptic treatment, if there are no hemorrhagic complications or cortical involvement.

Other complications include ICU-acquired weakness, neurocognitive complications, etc., which occur in a lesser frequency than above.

Hepatobiliary and Vascular Complications

Complications are vascular and biliary in origin with former being more common. Vascular complications include hepatic artery thrombosis (HAT), hepatic artery rupture, hepatic artery pseudoaneurysm, hepatic artery stenosis, portal venous thrombosis, portal venous stenosis, and caval anastomosis complications.[34] Biliary complications include biliary leak, obstruction, and infection.

Hepatic artery thrombosis is the most common and dreaded of all the vascular complications. It can be early (within 30 days) or late (after 30 days). It is defined as thrombotic occlusion of hepatic artery. As this artery supplies the bile duct, biliary complications such as biliary ischemia and necrosis may be associated with HAT. Possible risk factors include extended cold ischemia time, lack of ABO incompatibility, history of smoking, hypercoagulability state, transplant for primary sclerosing cholangitis, and CMV-positive donor with negative donor, and technical risk factors such as difficult anastomosis, imperfect anastomotic technique, disparity in diameters of the arteries, and small vessel size can predispose to HAT.[35] Clinically presents as raising bilirubin and serum transaminases and may lead to ischemic necrosis. Early-onset HAT is generally more severe than the late one. Decreased hepatic arterial blood supply leads to biliary injury further leading to necrosis and septic shock. Early diagnosis and management is the crux. Diagnosis is done by liver function tests, Doppler ultrasound, and CT angiography. Doppler ultrasound is very sensitive in detecting the decrease in the flow and changes in resistive index. Confirmation of finding in ultrasound is done by CT angiography. Therapeutic management includes revascularization either by surgical or endovascular intervention and by retransplantation. Late-onset HAT may not need revascularization therapy as good collateral circulation develops over time.

Portal Vein Thrombosis

Portal venous thrombosis is an uncommon complication which can occur both in early and late period post-transplantation with incidence <3%.[36] Clinically presents with features of portal hypertension such as abdominal pain, ascites, splenomegaly, etc., severe cases may present as graft dysfunction and multiorgan failure. Diagnosis is made by Doppler ultrasound, contrast-enhanced CT, portography, and MRI. Management mainly is by systemic anticoagulation. Some cases may need catheter-directed thrombolysis or stenting.[37]

Biliary Complications

Biliary complications include biliary leak, infection, and stricture. Biliary leaks occur with a frequency of approximately 4% and can be anastomotic or non-anastomotic. Anastomotic leaks are due to surgery-related issues such as difficult anastomosis, mismatch in duct size, and small ducts. Nonanastomotic leaks are due to impaired blood supply leading to necrosis and biliary leak. They present as abdominal pain, elevated bilirubin and serum transaminases, fever and septic shock (if infected), abdominal ascites, or collection (biloma or abscess). Minor leaks may not need any intervention. Major leaks need endoscopic or percutaneous drainage and sometimes biliary stenting. If fails need surgical repair with reanastomosis, biliary stricture and stenosis is late complication occurring after 1 month of transplantation.[38-40]

Immunosuppression and Graft Rejection

Immunosuppression therapy is started from the time of surgery itself. Immunosuppression protocols may vary between institutions, but a typical regimen includes steroid, calcineurin inhibitors (tacrolimus and cyclosporine), and mycophenolate. Monoclonal antibody against interleukin 2 (IL-2) that blocks T-cell proliferation (basiliximab and daciluzimab) can be tried in some patient.

Rejection can be hyperacute, acute, and chronic. Hyperacute rejection is less common than other and it is mediated by preformed antibodies in the recipient against donor's major histocompatibility complex. Acute and chronic rejections are more common. Acute responds better to treatment, compared to chronic rejection.

Acute rejection is usually seen 5–30 days' posttransplant, although it can have a late onset from 3–6 months' posttransplant. The incidence is decreased nowadays due to good immunosuppressive protocols. Risk factors include autoimmune etiology, high donor age, prolonged cold ischemia time, cytomegalovirus infection, poor compliance to immunosuppression, etc. Clinically presents as elevated serum aminotransaminases, alkaline phosphatase, and bilirubin levels, but confirmation of diagnosis needs biopsy. Histopathology shows changes such as portal, bile duct, and venous endothelial inflammation. Scores are also given to categorize the severity of rejection. Generally, acute rejection responds to steroids. Different regimens are followed. Pulse therapy of methylprednisolone 500–1,000 mg per day for 3 days followed by tapering of the dose is done. Escalation of the immunosuppression may work in some cases. Steroid-resistant rejection is managed with tacrolimus, sirolimus, antithymocyte globulin, and anti-IL-2 agents.[41,42]

▮ CONCLUSION

Perioperative care of LT patients is challenging because multisystemic nature of illness in preoperative period, complex surgery, and severe postoperative complications. With overall improvement in care of ALF and CLD patients, lots of sicker patients are being transplanted nowadays. So, transplant services now have to face more challenging and relatively unstable patients. Good coordination between specialists involve in patient management, right from beginning, is essential for improving outcome.

▮ REFERENCES

1. Iwakiri Y, Groszmann RJ. The hyperdynamic circulation of chronic liver diseases: from the patient to the molecule. Hepatology. 2006;43(2 Suppl 1):121-31.

2. Carey WD, Dumot JA, Pimentel RR, Barnes DS, Hobbs RE, Henderson JM, et al. The prevalence of coronary artery disease in liver transplant candidates over age 50. Transplantation. 1995; 59(6):859-64.

3. Plotkin JS, Scott VL, Pinna A, Dobsch BP, De Wolf AM, Kang Y. Morbidity and mortality in patients with coronary artery

disease undergoing orthotopic liver transplantation. Liver Transpl Surg. 1996;2(6):426-30.

4. Targher G, Arcaro G. Non-alcoholic fatty liver disease and increased risk of cardiovascular disease. Atherosclerosis. 2007;191(2):235-40.

5. Giakoustidis A, Cherian TP, Antoniadis N, Giakoustidis D. Combined cardiac surgery and liver transplantation: three decades of worldwide results. J Gastrointestin Liver Dis. 2011;20(4):415-21.

6. Regan TJ. Alcohol and the cardiovascular system. JAMA. 1990; 264(3):377-38.

7. Moller S, Henriksen JH. Cirrhotic cardiomyopathy. J Hepatol. 2010;53(1):179–90.

8. Hadengue A, Benhayoun MK, Lebrec D, Benhamou JP. Pulmonary hypertension complicating portal hypertension: prevalence and relation to splanchnic hemodynamics. Gastroenterology. 1991;100(2):520-8.

9. Badesch DB, Champion HC, Sanchez MA, Hoeper MM, Loyd JE, Manes A, et al. Diagnosis and assessment of pulmonary arterial hypertension. J Am Coll Cardiol. 2009; 54(1 Suppl):S55-66.

10. Huang B, Shi Y, Liu J, Schroder PM, Deng S, Chen M, et al. The early outcomes of candidates with portopulmonary liver transplantation. BMC Gastroenterol. 2018;18:79.

11. Tumgor G. Cirrhosis and hepatopulmonary syndrome. World J Gastroenterol. 2014; 20:(10)2586-94.

12. Fritz JS, Fallon MB, Kawut SM. Pulmonary vascular complications of liver disease. Am J Respir Crit Care Med. 2013;187(2):133-43.

13. Novesi MG, Tierney DF, Taplin GV, Eisenberg H. An intravenous radionuclide method to evaluate hypoxemia caused by abnormal alveolar vessels. Limitation of conventional techniques. Am Rev Respir Dis. 1976;114(1):59-65.

14. Singh C, Sager JS. Pulmonary complications of cirrhosis. Med Clin North Am. 2009;93(4):871-83. viii.

15. Rössle M, Gerbes AL. TIPS for the treatment of refractory ascites, hepatorenal syndrome and hepatic hydrothorax: a critical update. Gut. 2010;59(7):988-1000.

16. Tujios SR, Hynan LS, Vazquez MA, Larson AM, Seremba E, Sanders CM, et al. Risk factors and outcomes of acute kidney injury in patients with acute liver failure. Clin Gastroenterol Hepatol. 2015;13(2):352-9.

17. O'Riordan A, Brummell Z, Sizer E, Auzinger G, Heaton N, O'Grady JG, et al. Acute kidney injury in patients admitted to a liver intensive therapy unit with paracetamol-induced hepatotoxicity. Nephrol Dial Transplant. 2011;26(110):3501-8.

18. Garcia-Tsao G, Parikh CR, Viola A. Acute kidney injury in cirrhosis. Hepatology. 2008;48(6):2064-77.

19. Ginès P, Schrier RW. Renal failure in cirrhosis. N Engl J Med. 2009;361(13):1279-90.

20. Angeli P, Ginès P, Wong F, Bernardi M, Boyer TD, Gerbes A, et al. Diagnosis and management of acute kidney injury in patients with cirrhosis: revised consensus recommendations of the International Club of Ascites. J Hepatol. 2015; 62(5):968-74.

21. Liang TB, Bai XL, Li DL, Li JJ, Zheng SS. Early postoperative hemorrhage requiring urgent surgical reintervention after orthotopic liver transplantation. Transplant Proc. 2007;39(5):1549-53.

22. Dec GW, Kondo N, Farrell ML, Dienstag J, Cosimi AB, Semigran MJ. Cardiovascular complications following liver transplantation. Clin Transplant. 1995;9(6):463-71.

23. Cabezuelo JB, Ramirez P, Rios A, Acosta F, Torres D, Sansano T, et al. Risk factors of acute renal failure after liver transplantation. Kidney Int. 2006;69(6):1073-80.

24. Marvin M, Morton V. Glycemic control and organ transplantation. J Diabetes Sci Technol. 2009;3(6):1365-72.

25. Moghissi E, Korytkowski M, DiNardo M, Einhorn D, Hellman R, Hirsch IB, et al. American Association of Clinical Endocrinologists and American Diabetes Association consensus statement on inpatient glycemic control. Endocr Pract. 2009;15(4):353-69.

26. Lin M, Mah A, Wright AJ. Infectious complications of liver transplantation. AME Med J. 2018;3(1).

27. Feltracco P, Carollo C, Barbieri S, Pettenuzzo T, Ori C. Early respiratory complications after liver transplantation. World J Gastroenterol. 2013;19(48):9271-81.

28. Hong SK, Hwang S, Lee SG, Lee LS, Ahn CS, Kim KH, et al. Pulmonary complications following adult liver transplantation. Transplant Proc. 2006; 38(9):2979-81.

29. Levesque E, Hoti E, Azoulay D, Honore I, Guignard B, Vibert E, et al. Pulmonary complications after elective liver transplantation-incidence, risk factors, and outcome. Transplantation. 2012;94(5):532-8.

30. Xia D, Yan LN, Xu L, Li B, Zeng Y, Wen TF, et al. Postoperative severe pneumonia in adult liver transplant recipients. Transplant Proc. 2006;38(9): 2974-78.

31. Lui JK, Spaho L, Holzwanger E, Bui R, Daly JS, Bozorgzadeh A, et al. Intensive care of pulmonary complications following liver transplantation. J Intensive Care Med. 2018;33(11):595-608.

32. Živković SA. Neurologic complications after liver transplantation. World J Hepatol. 2013;5(8):409-16.

33. Weiss N, Thabut D. Neurological complications occurring after liver transplantation: role of risk factors, hepatic encephalopathy, and acute (on chronic) brain injury. Liver Transpl. 2019;25(3):469-87.

34. Cavallari A, Vivarelli M, Bellusci R, Jovine E, Mazziotti A, Rossi C. Treatment of vascular complications following liver transplantation: multidisciplinary approach. Hepatogastroenterology. 2001;48(37):179-83.

35. Bekker J, Ploem S, de Jong KP. Early hepatic artery thrombosis after liver transplantation: a systematic review of the incidence, outcome and risk factors. Am J Transplant. 2009;9(4):746-57.

36. Pérez-Saborido B, Pacheco-Sánchez D, Barrera-Rebollo A, Asensio-Díaz E, Pinto-Fuentes P, Sarmentero-Prieto JC, et al. Incidence, management, and results of vascular complications after liver transplantation. Transplant Proc. 2011;43(3):749-50.

37. Azzam AZ, Tanaka K. Management of vascular complications after living donor liver transplantation. Hepatogastroenterology. 2012;59(113):182-86.

38. Sheng R, Sammon JK, Zajko AB, Campbell WL. Bile leak after hepatic transplantation: cholangiographic features, prevalence, and clinical outcome. Radiology. 1994;192(2):413-6.

39. Wojcicki M, Milkiewicz P, Silva M. Biliary tract complications after liver transplantation: a review. Digestive Surgery. 2008;25(4):245-57.

40. Daniel K, Said A. Early biliary complications after liver transplantation. Clin Liver Dis. 2017;10:63.

41. Cohen SM. Current immunosuppression in liver transplantation. Am J Ther. 2002; 9(2):119-25.

42. Choudhary NS, Saigal S, Bansal RK, Saraf N, Gautam D, Soin AS. Acute and chronic rejection after liver transplantation: what a clinician needs to know. J Clin Exp Hepatol. 2017;7(4):358-66.

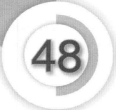
Perioperative Management of Heart Transplantation

Rahul Pandit, Amish Jasapara

INTRODUCTION

Heart transplant poises a very complex challenge to any institute that desires to develop the program. Quite often compared to final frontier in terms of complexity, clinical excellence, and epitome of success, heart transplant does carry an aura around it. Starting a program and sustaining it is an ongoing process and outcomes need to be analyzed in a dynamic fashion to keep the program sustainable. Saying this the program is based on a multidisciplinary approach which extends beyond the clinical talent pool, to laboratory, blood bank, specialized units which do tissue typing, etc. Needless to say each team has to be at par to have a successful outcome. The management of patient in intensive care unit (ICU) is perhaps as important as the surgical procedure itself, because it defines the outcome of the patient. This chapter is aimed at identifying the important aspects of care in ICU for managing these patients.

PHYSIOLOGY

Patients, who present for heart transplantation, shall have some form of systolic and diastolic heart failure. This causes increase in pulmonary artery (PA) pressures and often the left ventricular dysfunction causes a shift in the intravascular fluid thus worsening the pulmonary circulation.

The physiological changes quite often affect many other systems and they need to be understood to manage the patients.

Neurological

History of syncopal episodes, carotid stenosis, and ischemic or transient ischemic attacks needs to be taken. Many patients would be on anticoagulants or have coagulopathy and hence history of intracranial bleed/hemorrhage needs to be considered.

Respiratory

Smoking, chronic obstructive pulmonary disease (COPD), and oxygen or continuous positive airway pressure (CPAP) dependency needs to be understood. A spirometry and pulmonary diffusing capacity for carbon monoxide (DLCO) is important to know. Usually chronic heart failure decreases DLCO and the transplantation may not completely compensate for the DLCO to return normal.

Cardiovascular

The origin of cardiomyopathy: Hypertrophic, dilated, and ischemic cardiomyopathy is important to know, so that the physiological changes can be predicted especially in other organs.

Presence of other diseases responsible for cardiomyopathy like amyloidosis, sarcoidosis or autoimmune is important to know as these diseases are multisystemic and often need a different approach in management.

The most important aspect of cardiovascular physiology, which affects transplantation, is the presence of pulmonary hypertension.

Presence of pulmonary hypertension like primary pulmonary hypertension could lead to severe right heart failure. The cells lining pulmonary vasculature are inflamed and undergo mutation; the capillaries become narrow and cause obstruction in pulmonary blood flow. This leads to increase in afterload for right ventricle (RV), causing a gradual dilatation and failure. Right heart failure patients are may not benefit from heart transplant, but shall need a heart lung transplant, or optimization of medical therapy.

Contrary to that left heart failure can precipitate pulmonary hypertension and is in fact more common form of pulmonary hypertension. As the left ventricular function worsens, it leads to a passive increase in downstream pressures of left heart, this then causes incomplete/ineffective pulmonary emptying leading to inflammation of pulmonary vessel cells. A combination of increase in downstream pressures and changes in pulmonary vasculature causes pulmonary pressures to rise. The World Health Organization has classified this pulmonary hypertension as Group II.[1]

Patients who have a pulmonary vascular resistance (PVR) of >3 wood units are very high risk and may be contraindicated for transplantation.[2,3] These patients may be given a trial of reversibility by dobutamine test or by selective pulmonary vasodilators like sildenafil, as these are known to decrease the pulmonary pressures and may benefit this group of patients. Only if they respond and demonstrate reversibility then heart transplant should be considered.

Liver

Chronic heart failure patients often develop transaminitis and high bilirubin. This is due to a gradual systemic portal venous congestion. Though it does not have a bearing on decision to transplant, it does tend to change the pharmacokinetics and pharmacodynamic of the drugs which are used during transplantation.

Renal

Due to prolonged low perfusion state and coexisting disease like diabetes, many patients have chronic or acute renal dysfunction. Along with alteration in fluid and electrolyte management these patients quite often need perioperative renal replacement therapy. Also many of the immunosuppressive drugs used have a known renal toxicity and hence it is important to know the base line renal function.

Metabolic

Surgical stress and corticosteroid therapy may dramatically increase glycemic levels and which in turn may increase lactate levels during and after surgery. Hypothyroidism can worsen as the levels of triiodothyronine are often decreased for prolonged period following cardiopulmonary bypass (CPB).

▌OPERATIVE MANAGEMENT

Heart transplantation may be planed or an urgent procedure. A thorough examination focusing on the current symptoms, medications, fasting status, other organ involvement, airway difficulties, and recent blood and radiologic examination should be done. Cytomegalovirus (CMV) free and leukodepleted blood and blood products should be arranged. Timing is the most important issue in this procedure so as to minimize the period of cold ischemia

(maximum 4 hours) of the donor heart. A continuous communication between the donor retrieval team and the recipient team should be present at all times to take key decisions and to ascertain donor clamp time.

The recipient arrives into the operating room once the organ is finally accepted. Apart from standard noninvasive monitors the protocol includes cerebral oximetry, radial and femoral arterial pressure monitoring, central venous cannulation, and PA catheter insertion for central venous pressure (CVP) and pulmonary artery pressure (PAP) monitoring, respectively. These procedures should be performed under ultrasonography (USG) guidance and before induction of anesthesia. PA catheters having the ability to measure continuous mixed venous oximetry and cardiac output (CO) are preferred. Once the PA catheter is floated all measurements are recorded to ascertain PVR and transpulmonary gradient (TPG.) The PA catheter is then pulled back into superior vena cava (SVC).[4,5]

These patients are usually very apprehensive and highly dependent on intrinsic sympathetic activity. Fast induction of anesthesia can lead to a sudden cardiovascular collapse. It is always beneficial to start a small dose of inotropes and vasopressors before induction. An induction of anesthesia with etomidate (0.2–0.3 mg/kg), fentanyl (1–2 µg/kg), and rocuronium (1 mg/kg) usually maintains the hemodynamics reasonably. Maintenance of anesthesia is with volatile anesthetics particularly sevoflurane, fentanyl, and rocuronium. Regardless of the agents used, it is imperative to maintain heart rate (HR), contractility, and systemic vascular resistance (SVR) till CPB is instituted. Broad-spectrum antibiotics and immunosuppression with methylprednisolone and basiliximab 20 mg (interleukin-2 receptor antagonist) is achieved postinduction.

Transesophageal echocardiography (TEE) monitoring during this period is not of much help except for knowing the volume status, estimating pulmonary hypertension, and recognition of intracardiac thrombi and other congenital anomalies especially persistent left SVC.

Following individual vena cava and aorta cannulation CPB is initiated and the recipient diseased heart is excised leaving behind a left atrial (LA) cuff containing the opening of four pulmonary veins, both vena cava, aortic and pulmonary stumps. During this period moderate hypothermia 32–34°C and a mean arterial pressure (MAP) of around 60 mm Hg is maintained. Once the donor heart is in the operating room, the donor left atrium is anastomosed to recipient LA cuff followed by inferior vena cava (IVC) and SVC anastomosis. This method is known as the bicaval technique and is now followed in all institutions worldwide. Advantages include reduced tricuspid regurgitation (TR) and conduction disturbances in the postoperative period. The pulmonary and aortic anastomoses are then done completing the heart transplantation.

Once the anastomosis is complete, the aortic cross clamp is removed and the total ischemia time is calculated. At this time usually some electromechanical activity ensues and epicardial pacing can be initiated. Standard de-airing maneuvers are performed to achieve complete de-airing under echocardiography guidance. Rewarming is completed to 36–37°C. A rest period of around 45 minutes to 1 hour is given so as to optimize the hemodynamics. During this period RV protective ventilation and inhaled nitric oxide (iNO) 10–20 ppm is started.

Inotropic therapy is usually a combination of adrenaline (0.05–0.5 µg/kg/min) and milrinone (0.5–0.75 µg/kg/min). A bolus dose of milrinone is usually avoided as it may cause profound vasodilatation. Noradrenaline (0.05–0.5 µg/kg/min) should also be used when the measured SVR is low. The HR should be elevated to 110–120 beats/minute by epicardial pacing (AV sequential) so as to increase the RV output. The PA catheter is then floated and values measured. The heart is then loaded, CPB flow reduced gradually and changes in hemodynamics noted. Once satisfactory hemodynamics, i.e., MAP > 60 mm Hg, CVP < 10 mm Hg, mean PAP < 25 mm Hg, CO > 3 L/min, and urine output is >1 mL/kg/h, cautious separation from CPB is done followed by decannulation and complete reversal of heparinization with protamine.

The main aim in the post-CPB period is early recognition and prevention of RV dysfunction. Although the transplanted heart is preload dependent excessive preload should be avoided. RV contractility is maintained with milrinone and adrenaline and RV afterload is reduced with iNO and milrinone. Hypoxia, acidosis, hypothermia, and hypercarbia should be avoided as these can increase PVR and precipitate RV failure. TEE is invaluable to assess the RV function by eyeballing the RV contractility and RV fractional area change (RV FAC) measurement. RV FAC > 31% and < 18% suggest normal and severe RV dysfunction, respectively. Apart from this one can look for RV dilatation, worsening TR, and flattening of interventricular septum. Once the RV is examined, LV function assessment and gradients across the various anastomoses should be ascertained.

Coagulopathy is usually a concern, especially in redo cases. Performance of rotational thromboelastometry (ROTEM) analysis of coagulation system should be done to guide blood component therapy. Once satisfactory hemostasis is achieved closure of chest is completed. Chest closure can at times have tamponade effect on RV impairing its function, in that case the chest can be kept open and closed later. If all these strategies to maintain RV function fail then one may have to consider intra-aortic balloon pump (IABP), extracorporeal membrane oxygenator (ECMO) or right ventricular assist device (RVAD).

INTENSIVE CARE UNIT ADMISSION

Patient needs to be admitted to a specialty ICU, created specifically for care of heart transplant patients. An ideal setting is an isolation room, with double door, an anteroom that provides reverse isolation. The ICU should have monitors capable of continuous monitoring of several parameters, allowing three or more invasive monitoring channels, two temperature channels, end-tidal carbon dioxide along with standard electrocardiogram (ECG) and noninvasive monitoring modules. A modern ventilator, with graphic display, syringe drivers, infusion pumps, and provision for mechanical circulatory support (MCS) in form of IABP, ECMO or a cardiac (left and right ventricle) assist device (LVAD/RVAD). The room should be big to accommodate all this and should have uninterrupted power supply (UPS) of minimum of 24 points.

All personnel should practice strict hand hygiene and wear cap, mask, and clean gown. The infection control policy of the hospital and ICU should be strictly followed at all times. On arrival to ICU, a detailed hand over between anesthesiologist, nursing staff, and ICU team should be documented. Patient connected to ventilator, all invasive lines and infusions connected. A spare infusion for vasopressors/inotropes and sedation should be kept ready.

SPECIFIC MONITORING AND TREATMENT

- 12 lead ECG to document initial rhythm, if atrial fibrillation (AF) is present then along with electrolyte correction like potassium and magnesium, a loading dose of amiodarone should be given or cardioversion considered. A difficult to convert AF may be a sign of acute rejection and if needed a bolus dose of 500 mg of methylprednisolone should be administered. If bradycardia is present then usually isoprenaline or adrenaline infusion is commenced in low dose (0.01–0.04 µg/kg/min). A usual target HR is around 100 beats/minute. In severe atrioventricular (AV) block a sequential pacing should be commenced, if severe AV block persist beyond 2 weeks then a dual chamber permanent pacemaker should be inserted.
- Arterial blood gas, looking at acid base, lactates, and gas exchange. Ventilator should be adjusted accordingly and electrolytes corrected as needed.
- *Rule of 100*: Aim to keep HR around 100 beats/minute, systolic blood pressure above 100 mm Hg, urine output around 100 mL/h, temperature closer to 98.5°F, partial pressure of oxygen in arterial blood (PaO$_2$) of 100 mm Hg and, saturation of 100%.
- *Monitor pulmonary artery pressure*: A transpulmonary gradient, mean PAP, and PA capillary wedge pressure should be noted. A pressure gradient > 15 will indicate

early postoperative right ventricular dysfunction. Monitor continuous CO and a mixed venous blood sample is a good indicator of tissue oxygen utilization.

- Ventilator is adjusted with an aim to provide good oxygenation and carbon dioxide clearance. The settings are mode as per the unit policy, intending to keep fraction of inspired oxygen (FiO_2) of 0.6 and above and then adjust as per arterial blood gas values. Tidal volume of 6–8 mL/kg, ideal body weight along with a positive end-expiratory pressure (PEEP) of 5 cmH_2O or more as required.

- Request chest X-ray, full blood count, and renal, liver, and coagulation function. If drains outputs are high then thromboelastography or ROTEM should be checked along with other coagulation parameters. Thyroid and blood glucose should be noted. Check position of endotracheal tube, nasogastric tube, invasive lines, and drains on chest X-ray, along with lung fields.

- Immunosuppressive therapy should be noted and plan for immunosuppressive therapy should be clearly documented. Usually intraoperatively basiliximab is given along with methylprednisolone, calcineurin inhibitors like tacrolimus are started in a couple of days when renal function stabilizes. Usually after an initial bolus dose of steroids patients receive a decreasing dose of methylprednisolone until the steroid sparing drugs are started and levels achieved.

- Antibiotic therapy as per the hospital policy for surgical prophylaxis is initiated. If there is a suspicion of infection then as per the standard infectious disease guidelines antibiotics are initiated.

- *Support the RV*: The donor heart; particularly the RV in case of preexisting pulmonary hypertension has to deal suddenly with a high after load. Quite often coexisting hypoxia, hypercapnia, and some reperfusion injury may worsen the pulmonary hypertension.[6,7] Hence iNO in dose of 10–40 part per million is used for decreasing the pulmonary hypertension. Other drugs used and general goals of therapy are mentioned in **Table 1**. An important goal is to maintain negative fluid balance, along with good oxygenation and avoiding hypercapnia.

- A continuous and frequent monitoring of several parameters is of prime importance, HR, ECG, oxygen saturation, core body temperature, CVP, MAP, PAP, left atrial pressure (LAP), mixed venous oxygen saturation (S_VO_2), CO, cardiac index (CI), and lactate. The target values are to keep HR around 100 beats/minute, MAP > 65–70 mm Hg, LAP 8–12 mm Hg, SvO_2 > 65%, urine > 1.5 mL/kg/h (100 mL/h), and lactate < 2 mmol/L.

HEMODYNAMIC MANAGEMENT UNIQUE TO HEART TRANSPLANT

After heart transplant, hemodynamics may be compromised due to several reasons such as autonomic denervation, chronotropic and inotropic failure of ventricles, ischemia reperfusion injury, volume depletion, and at times metabolic acidosis. Drugs used for hemodynamic control are given in **Table 2**.

It is obligatory to monitor the above-mentioned parameters and to approach each problem methodologically.

Fluid Management

A goal-directed approach is the best approach to ensure optimal filling of the intravascular compartment. The above mentioned parameters, targets along with a transthoracic echocardiography (in early phase even a TEE should be used. Assessment of the vena cava along with CO, lactate,

Table 1: Pulmonary artery hypertension and right ventricular dysfunction prevention.	
Monitor by PAC	***CVP, MPAP, PCWP, CO, SvO₂***
Mechanical ventilation	PaO_2 100 mm Hg, PCO_2 30–35 mm Hg, pH 7.5. Adequate PEEP level (5–10 cmH_2O) to recruit lung and optimize PVR
Restricted fluid therapy	Monitoring filling pressure CVP 10–12 mm Hg, PCWP 12–15 mm Hg. Monitoring LVEDV and RVEDV by echocardiography
Inotropes to support RV contractility	Epinephrine 0.02–0.25 µg/kg/min
Inodilator	Milrinone 0.2–0.5 µg/kg/min
	Levosimendan 0.2 µg/kg/min ± norepinephrine (up to 0.15 µg/kg/min) to maintain right coronary perfusion pressure
iNO	5–40 ppm
Phosphodiesterase V inhibitor	Revatio 3 × 20 mg po
Systemic vasodilators	Sodium nitroprusside, prostacyclin (PGI_2) analog iloprost (2 ng/kg/min)

(CO: cardiac output; CVP: central venous pressure; iNO: inhaled nitric oxide; LVEDV: left ventricular end-diastolic volume; MPAP: mean pulmonary artery pressure; PAC: pulmonary artery catheter; PaO_2: partial pressure of oxygen in arterial blood; PCO_2: partial pressure of carbon dioxide; PCWP: pulmonary capillary wedge pressure; PEEP: positive end-expiratory pressure; PVR: pulmonary vascular resistance; RV: right ventricle; RVEDV: right ventricular end-diastolic volume; SvO_2: mixed venous oxygen saturation)

Table 2: Drugs used for hemodynamic control.

Drug	Average dosage	Advantages	Side effects
Epinephrine	0.05–0.25 µg/kg/min	Support RV overload	Tachycardia, arrhythmias, raise O_2 demand
Norepinephrine	Up to 0.15 µg/kg/min	Contrast vasodilatation	Increase PVR
Levosimendan	0.1–0.2 µg/kg/min	Support RV overload	Vasodilation
Milrinone	0.2–0.5 µg/kg/min	Support RV overload	Arrhythmias, raise O_2 demand, vasodilation
Vasopressin	2.5–5 U/h	Contrast vasodilatation	Increase SVR impair forward flow of LVAD
iNO	20–40 ppm	Reduce PVR (if not fixed)	
Inhaled milrinone	5 mg/15 minutes	Reduce PVR (if not fixed)	
Inhaled iloprost	20–30 µg/15 minutes	Reduce PVR (if not fixed)	
Methylene blue	0.5–2 mg/kg	Contrast vasodilation	

(iNO: inhaled nitric oxide; LVAD: left ventricular assist device; PVR: pulmonary vascular resistance; RV: right ventricle; SVR: systemic vascular resistance)

and monitoring of B lines on lung ultrasound often help in deciding the need for volume optimization. It is important to note that volume should only be given if there is a need to increase CO in presence of volume responsiveness as determined by either vena cava assessment or other dynamic parameters.

Passive leg raising and fluid challenge may be difficult to perform in view of brittle hemodynamics. Once decision for fluid is been made, then balanced crystalloids or 5% albumin can be administered as per the fluid responsiveness. It is important to check the volume status again at frequent intervals and guide further therapy according to need.

Pharmacological Support

The goal is to avoid excessive increase in preload and afterload at the same time maintaining an adequate CO. Sequential atrial pacing or low dose isoprenaline/adrenaline ensures an adequate chronotropy, while inotropy is maintained with low to moderate dose of adrenaline/nor adrenaline in combination of phosphodiesterase inhibitor like milrinone. A combination of vasodilators like nitroglycerine or sodium nitroprusside is helpful in conjunction with inotropes to reduce the afterload.[8]

Support for Failing Left and Right Ventricle

Despite supports and monitoring if left ventricle insufficiency is evident in form of decreasing urine output, hypoperfusion of tissues (rising lactate), dropping CO and rising LAP, then a need to increase inotropes to high dose in combination with vasopressors and very low dose of peripheral dilators (if MAP allows) may be needed. Echocardiography is a handy tool to monitor the response to therapy. An IABP can be inserted to reduce after load and help improve contraction along with improved coronary perfusion. If this fails to improve the hemodynamics then

a peripheral or central venoarterial ECMO (VA ECMO) is necessary to support the heart.

Similarly if the RV starts to dilate or the tricuspid annular peak systolic excursion (TAPSE) reduces along with dilatation of vena cava then adequate inotropic support should be started. Pulmonary vasodilators like iNO increased and if needed a mechanical circulatory device such as ECMO initiated to support RV early.

Acid-base and Kidney Support

All heart transplant recipients, come from long periods of low CO state, hence some kidney dysfunction is preexisting. Combine that with volume depletion, inflammatory reaction to extracorporeal support, and episodes of hypotension, many may have metabolic acidosis and sometimes may need renal replacement therapy. In patients who develop oliguria or anuria despite diuretic challenge with furosemide or torsemide or polyuric kidney failure with inadequate urine concentration and serum urea values > 200 mg/dL or hyperkalemia and/or increased preload as in hypervolemia, renal replacement therapy is applied without delay. Early postoperatively continuous venovenous hemodiafiltration (CVVHDF) is commenced, which is able to achieve an optimal volume balance. If the patient is on MCS, the renal replacement circuit is attached to the MCS circuit and dialysis commenced.

Weaning from Ventilatory Support

The goals of weaning from mechanical ventilation are no different from any cardiac surgery patients. The patient should be hemodynamically stable, on moderate or low dose of vasoactive supports, fully awake, and able to protect airway if extubated, adequate analgesia is ensured, drain output are minimal, stable arterial blood gases, and most importantly no evidence of RV or LV failure. It is important to remember that iNO can be given with mechanical ventilation only, once extubated, noninvasive techniques do not provide the comfort of iNO therapy and hence patient may need to be changed to oral pulmonary vasodilators like sildenafil. If extubation is not possible due to any reason then a percutaneous/surgical tracheostomy is performed as per unit policy to facilitate weaning.

Postextubation physiotherapy and early mobilization are very important. It is necessary to understand that in some cases of MCS an extubation can be tried if patient is stable to be extubated and MCS continued. This helps early mobilization.

GRAFT DYSFUNCTION

Graft dysfunction is classified as primary and secondary graft dysfunction. The primary can occur as early as 24 hours characterized by severe bi/one ventricular failure, along with poor CO and severe hypoperfusion state. A secondary graft dysfunction can occur late and is characterized by decrease contractility, pulmonary hypertension, and ultimately drop in CO and hypoperfusion. The acute management is aimed at support of heart along with therapies specifically aimed at rejection, such as steroid loading and/or plasmapheresis of intravenous immunoglobulin (IVIG).

CONCLUSION

Management of heart failure patient offers a large number of variables to be combined in to a care bundle. Quite often it is challenging, but a standard protocolized care is important to have consistent good outcomes.

REFERENCES

1. Simonneau G, Galiè N, Rubin LJ, Langleben D, Seeger W, Domenighetti G, et al. Clinical classification of pulmonary hypertension. J Am Coll Cardiol. 2004;43(12 Suppl S):5S-12S.
2. Mehra MR, Kobashigawa J, Starling R, Russell S, Uber PA, Parameshwar J, et al. Listing criteria for heart transplantation: International Society for Heart and Lung Transplantation guidelines for the care of cardiac transplant candidates—2006. J Heart Lung Transplant. 2006;25:1024-42.
3. Miller WL, Grill DE, Borlaug BA. Clinical features, hemodynamics, and outcomes of pulmonary hypertension due to chronic heart failure with reduced ejection fraction: Pulmonary hypertension and heart failure. JACC Heart Fail. 2013;1:290-9.
4. Demas K, Wyner J, Mihm FG, Samuels S. Anaesthesia for heart transplantation. A retrospective study and review. Br J Anaesth. 1986;58:1357-64.
5. Costanzo MR, Dipchand A, Starling R, Anderson A, Chan M, Desai S, et al. The International Society of Heart and Lung Transplantation Guidelines for the care of heart transplant recipients. J Heart Lung Transplant. 2010;29:914-56.
6. Fischer S, Glas KE. A review of cardiac transplantation. Anesthesiol Clin. 2013;31:383-403.
7. Kaul TK, Fields BL. Postoperative acute refractory right ventricular failure: Incidence, pathogenesis, management and prognosis. Cardiovasc Surg. 2000;8:1-9.
8. Koster A, Diehl C, Dongas A, Meyer–Jark T, Luth IU. Anesthesia for Cardiac Transplantation: A practical overview of current management strategies. Appl Cardiopulm Pathophysiol. 2011;15:213-9.

Perioperative Management of Lung Transplantation

Suresh Rao KG, Sureshkumaran K, Balakrishnan KR

INTRODUCTION

Pulmonary transplantation is the accepted treatment modality for decompensated respiratory failure and pulmonary vascular diseases. The first transplant was done in USA by James D Hardy (1918–2003) at the University of Mississippi. The patient who underwent lung transplant was John Russel, a 60-year-old male with left lung carcinoma. On June 11, 1963, the first lung transplantation surgery was done following which he had good early recovery of pulmonary function but died on 18th postoperative day secondary to renal failure.[1] In 1983, the first series of successful human lung transplantation was published which led to the beginning of a new era of pulmonary transplantation.[2] Since then, advances and success of lung transplantation made it to become a lifesaving procedure in patients with end-stage decompensated respiratory failure and pulmonary vascular diseases. However, survival rates in post lung transplant recipients in relation to other solid organ transplant recipients are sagging, because of distinct surgical technique, immunological characteristics of pulmonary parenchyma, and infectious complications post lung transplantation. In recent era, survival has increased, greatly due to advances in critical care management during the early post-transplant period.[3]

INDICATION

The indications for pulmonary transplantation have been widened to include disorders of pulmonary parenchyma, airway tract, and pulmonary vasculature. Since 1995, chronic obstructive pulmonary disorders (COPD) have been the most common indication for pulmonary transplantation. COPD was followed by interstitial lung disease (ILD), cystic fibrosis leading to bronchiectasis, pulmonary hypertension, and pulmonary fibrosis. Few uncommon indications are bronchiectasis not secondary to cystic fibrosis, sarcoidosis, and COPD due to alpha-1 antitrypsin deficiency. Nowadays, lung retransplantation has also become one of the indications accounting to 2.6% of all lung transplant recipients since many post-transplant patients develop progressive airflow limitation disorder called bronchiolitis obliterans syndrome (BOS) in the absence of other common etiologies (**Table 1**).[5]

In our Fortis Malar Hospital, Chennai, we have done 32 lung transplants of which majority were ILD (**Table 2**).

ABSOLUTE CONTRAINDICATIONS[6]

- Active viral hepatitis B, hepatitis C, human immuno-deficiency virus (HIV) infection
- Any carcinoma in the last 2 years other than cutaneous basal cell carcinoma and cutaneous squamous cell carcinoma

Table 1: Worldwide indication of patients who underwent lung transplantation.[4]

Indication	Percentage distribution
Chronic obstructive pulmonary disorders	39.3
Interstitial lung disease	23.7
Bronchiectasis associated with cystic fibrosis	16.6
Idiopathic pulmonary artery hypertension	3.1
Pulmonary fibrosis	3.7
Bronchiectasis	2.7
Retransplantation	2.6
Sarcoidosis	2.5
Connective tissue diseases	1.3
Obliterative bronchiolitis	1.1
Lymphangioleiomyomatosis	1
Congenital heart disease	0.9
Cancer	0.1
Others	1.4

Table 2: Indication of patients who underwent lung transplantation in our center.

Indication	Percentage distribution
Interstitial lung disease	13 (40.6%)
Idiopathic pulmonary arterial hypertension	8 (25%)
Bronchiectasis	4 (12.5%)
Cystic fibrosis	2 (6.25%)
Chronic obliterative bronchiolitis	1 (3.12%)
Chronic obstructive pulmonary disorders	1 (3.12%)
Retransplantation	1 (3.12%)
Fibrosing alveolitis	1 (3.12%)
Pneumoconiosis	1 (3.12%)

- Vertebral column and chest wall abnormality causing significant pulmonary restriction
- Decompensated heart failure, hepatic failure, renal failure
- Substance abuse in the last 6 months
- Noncompliance to follow drug therapy

RELATIVE CONTRAINDICATIONS

- Critically ill patient
- Very poor functional capacity
- Frail individual and age >65 years
- Individuals with colonization of highly virulent pathogens
- On mechanical ventilation
- Severe osteoporosis
- Body mass index (BMI) >30 kg/m^2

PREOPERATIVE EVALUATION AND PREPARATION

To ascertain the appropriateness of listing for lung transplantation, several studies are necessary during the preoperative evaluation process. Basic hematological and biochemical investigations to assess the functional status of the end organs such as liver function tests and renal function tests are done. Pulmonary function tests are done to assess the lung volumes and lung capacities. A 6-minute walk test is done to assess the functional capacity. Chest radiography by chest X-ray and CT scan is necessary to rule out malignancy and to ascertain the size of the chest cavity. An echocardiogram and right heart hemodynamic study are done to assess the heart function and pulmonary hypertension. In any patient >45 years of age or in patients with symptoms, electrocardiogram (ECG) and coronary angiogram are done to rule out coronary artery diseases. If single-lung transplantation is planned, lung perfusion imaging is done to determine which lung is to be transplanted depending on the perfusion

status. Few screening tests such as positron emission tomography-computed tomography (PET-CT) scan, Pap smear, endoscopy, and mammogram are done to rule out malignancy. In severe osteoporosis, bone densitometry is done to assess the fracture risk.

To assess the pathogenic colonization in lung, culture of sputum or bronchoalveolar lavage (BAL) specimen is done. Viral markers and serological status of hepatitis virus, cytomegalovirus (CMV), herpes simplex virus, varicella virus, Epstein–Barr virus, and toxoplasmosis are identified for prophylaxis and risk stratification of recipients after lung transplantation. Immunological tests such as human leukocyte antigen (HLA) typing and panel reactive antibodies are done to ensure optimal donor and recepient match to prevent acute rejection.

TYPE OF LUNG TRANSPLANT

Due to the limited donor organs, single-lung transplant may extend the organ availability but compromises on providing limited lung function. Decreased perioperative risk after single-lung transplant makes it a choice for geriatric patients undergoing lung transplant.[7] Bilateral lung transplantation is the technique of choice in suppurative lung disorders such as cystic fibrosis, since there is a risk of cross-infection to the transplanted lung from the native lung and also bilateral transplant is preferred in COPD with hyperinflated lungs due to the compression of the transplanted lung by the native lung in single-lung transplant.[8,9] Apart from few compelling indications for dual-lung transplant, it always provides long-term survival when compared to single-lung transplant.[10]

Mechanical Bridges to Transplant

Mechanical bridges refer to modalities to provide artificial support in an acutely decompensating recipient until a suitable organ is available.[11,12] An ideal bridge to transplant is that which extends the life expectancy in the pretransplant period and improves the outcome by stabilizing the clinical condition in the pretransplant period.[13] The most commonly used strategy to bridge is mechanical ventilation.[14-16] But prolonged mechanical ventilation may cause ventilator-associated pneumonia (VAP) and ventilator-associated lung injury. Many ventilated patients need to be sedated which mandates them to be bedridden and may lead to numerous secondary complications.

Nowadays, extracorporeal mechanical support by means of an extracorporeal membrane oxygenator (ECMO) is being used as a bridge to transplant, and mortality is comparable to patients without extracorporeal mechanical support.[17-20] However, extracorporeal mechanical support use is still controversial. Extracorporeal mechanical support may be venovenous (VV) ECMO or venoarterial (VA) ECMO. VV-ECMO is a low-pressure circuit, used for isolated respiratory support. VA-ECMO is a high-pressure circuit used for combined cardiorespiratory support in patients with hemodynamic instability. Extracorporeal mechanical support leads to substantial utilization of resources and is also associated with numerous vascular complications, coagulopathy, sepsis, and multiorgan failure.

DONOR ACCEPTABILITY CRITERIA[21]

- Donor age <55 years
- Compatible ABO
- Crossmatch negative
- Clear lung fields in chest X-ray
- P:F ratio >300
- Smoking <20 pack-years
- No chest wall injury or lung contusion
- No aspiration pneumonia
- Absence of sepsis
- No previous cardiothoracic surgery
- Sputum Gram stain—negative for organisms
- Bronchoscopy—no purulent secretion

Donor lungs are ventilated with lung-protective strategies, i.e., low tidal volume [6–8 mL/kg of predicted body weight (PBW),] low FiO_2, positive end-expiratory pressure (PEEP), and closed-circuit suctioning. Recruitment maneuvers after each disconnection from the ventilator will be done to prevent atelectasis. Donor hemodynamics are maintained with fluids, vasopressors, and inotropes if cardiac dysfunction is present. Donor lungs are assessed using disposable bronchoscope (Ambu® aScope™ Ambu A/S, Ballerup, Denmark) and secretions, if any, will be sent for Gram stain and culture.

LUNG PRESERVATION

Lung preservation helps to avoid primary graft dysfunction and improves graft survival. Viability of donor lungs depends on multiple factors such as type of preservation solution used, method of administration, storage temperature, lung inflation volume and pressure, mode of transportation, and ischemic time. During organ harvesting, the lungs are flushed with lung preservation solution in anterograde and retrograde manners. An ideal preservative solution is that which prevents the development of tissue edema and prevents pulmonary vasoconstriction and aerobic metabolism, thus facilitating lung preservation.[22] Perfadex solution is used in our center and is based on the low-potassium solution that was developed ideally for lung preservation.

Lung Preservation Techniques

- Ideal preservation solution containing low potassium, glucose, and dextran-40
- Anterograde and retrograde flushing at a dose of 60 mL/kg
- Flush height at 30 cm
- Preservation temperature 4–8°C
- Low FiO_2–50%
- Lung inflation up to 50% of the total lung capacity
- Prostaglandin E1, heparin, glucocorticoid additives in lung preservation solution
- Cold ischemic time, ideally <8 hours[23]
- Ex vivo lung perfusion

Ex Vivo Lung Perfusion

Ex vivo lung perfusion (EVLP) simulates the in vivo environment of the donor lung. This technique helps in further assessment and potential repair of the injured lungs. In 1970, the concept of EVLP was started. Cypel and colleagues reported 50 lung transplants where they initially used EVLP and then used those lungs for transplantation.[24] These donor lungs were borderline and hence kept on EVLP for 4–6 hours and their P:F ratio, compliance, and peak pressure were analyzed every hour. Radiography and bronchoscopy were also done every hour. Organs which showed improvement in the P:F ratio were accepted for transplantation. The Toronto technique, Vivoline system, and Organ Care System are few EVLP techniques that are currently in trials. Donor lung preservation requires a multidisciplinary team involving donor management intensivist and lung retrieval team. Newer techniques such as EVLP help in increasing the donor pool for the large number of waiting recipients.

INTRAOPERATIVE MANAGEMENT

Patients on bronchodilators, antibiotics, prostaglandins, and pulmonary vasodilators should be continued. Broad-spectrum antibiotics are given as antimicrobial prophylaxis within 1 hour of commencement of surgery, but in patients with proven infection, antibiotics are given as per the culture and sensitivity report. Donor infection is also taken into account before starting antimicrobials. The immunosuppressant regimen starts before the transplant and varies between institutions. Since these patients have poor respiratory reserve, they are vulnerable to cardiorespiratory arrest secondary to hypoxia, hypercarbia, and high pulmonary vascular resistance (PVR); hence, any premedication or sedation should be given cautiously.

THORACIC EPIDURAL ANALGESIA

Postoperative analgesia is the most important modality for early pulmonary rehabilitation required to facilitate extubation. Even though thoracic epidural analgesia may rarely cause epidural hematoma due to heparinization, it provides far better analgesia than systemic opioids. Hence, patients have to be chosen based on risk–benefit analysis. Paravertebral block and epidural catheter insertion in the postoperative period are other options to avoid risks of epidural hematoma.

Hemodynamic Monitoring Techniques

A large-bore intravenous cannula for volume resuscitation, a pulmonary artery catheter with thermistor, mixed venous oximetry for continuous cardiac output monitoring and pulmonary artery pressure monitoring, a central venous catheter for vasoactive agent infusion, and an arterial cannula for arterial gas analysis are used. Five-lead electrocardiography, pulse oximetry, invasive measurement of blood pressure and central venous pressure, urinary output measurement, temperature monitoring, capnography, and anesthetic gas analysis are also used. Near-infrared spectroscopy (NIRS), used as a cerebral oximetry analyzer, and bispectral index for depth of anesthesia monitoring are other commonly used monitors.

Transesophageal Echocardiography

Intraoperative transesophageal echocardiography (TEE) during lung transplantation can be used for assessing surgical anastomotic sites. TEE is also used for assessing preload, ventricular function, and regional wall motion abnormalities. TEE can be used to analyze the cause of unexplained refractory hypoxemia and identify intracardiac air, thrombus, shunting, and other unexpected abnormalities.

Induction

The induction of anesthesia may lead to cardiorespiratory arrest; hence, the surgeon and perfusionist need to be prepared to initiate cardiopulmonary bypass. Induction is the most critical period of anesthesia since it reduces the sympathetic drive and causes myocardial depression, vasodilation, and impairment of venous return due to positive pressure ventilation. Hence, the goals of induction are to maintain systemic vascular resistance, myocardial contractility and to prevent increase in PVR. Beta-1 and alpha-1 agonist infusions and pulmonary vasodilators before induction can be used to maintain hemodynamic goals.

Maintenance of Anesthesia

Adequate amounts of anesthetic agents have to be maintained to avoid intraoperative awareness. Propofol infusion, inhalational anesthetics, or both are used to maintain anesthesia throughout the surgery. PVR may be increased by nitrous oxide; hence, it is avoided. The intravenous anesthetics causes minimal myocardial depression and less inhibition of hypoxic pulmonary vasoconstriction. The inhalational anesthetic technique has an advantage since it can cause bronchodilatation.

One-lung ventilation (OLV) may be used during single-lung transplantation; lung with greater perfusion is better tolerated. Hypothermia should be avoided since it increases pulmonary pressure, causes coagulopathy, and increases the risk of arrhythmia. Prophylactic administration of magnesium can be done to prevent arrhythmia. Vasoactive agents can be used to maintain perfusion pressure. Optimal fluid management is done to avoid fluid overload to prevent pulmonary edema which impairs graft survival.

Cardiopulmonary Bypass

Cardiopulmonary bypass (CPB) may be electively used in patients with severe pulmonary hypertension and also in patients requiring a surgical procedure involving repair of intracardiac shunts. CPB is used in patients requiring plasmapheresis to remove donor-specific antibodies in allosensitized recipients. Emergency CPB is administered in patients having cardiorespiratory compromise, refractory hemodynamic instability, and right ventricular failure following clamping of the pulmonary artery and in patients who did not tolerate OLV.

While on CPB itself, ventilation and reperfusion of lungs is done after anastomosis to limit the ischemic time. Coagulopathy following prolonged CPB is managed with antifibrinolytic agents, protamine, platelets, fresh frozen plasma, and cryoprecipitate. Even though CPB provides hemodynamic stability and controlled reperfusion of grafts, it can cause release of inflammatory mediators that increase the risk of acute lung injury.

SURGICAL CONSIDERATION AND ANASTAMOSIS

In case of redo thoracic surgery, restrictive, suppurative lung diseases and extensive pleural adhesions make the retrieval of the diseased lung difficult. Extensive adhesions may cause increased blood loss. In bilateral sequential single-lung transplantation, if performed off pump, the lung with lower perfusion should be transplanted first to avoid instability. After bronchial anastomosis, bronchoscopic toileting of the graft is performed which is followed by venous and arterial anastomosis. Communication between the surgeon and anesthesiologists is critical since arrhythmias and hypotension can happen due to manipulation of heart during anastomosis. Deairing is done by inflating the lung before releasing the atrial clamp and before tying the final stitch. Rapid fluid shifts after clamp release may require volume replacement. Myocardial stunning may happen since the initial venous return is cold with ischemic metabolites. Inotropic support can be initiated to improve the contractility of heart. Right coronary artery air embolism may happen which is usually transient.

After clamp-release grafts are ventilated with low FiO_2, optimal PEEP and low peak inspiratory airway pressure are used to reduce lung injury. Nitric oxide (NO) can be used to decrease pulmonary pressure and to improve the lung perfusion. Minute ventilation is adjusted to remove carbon dioxide.

IMMUNOSUPPRESSANTS

Induction immunosuppression is one commonly used strategy to suppress the T-cell immune response of the recipient to the donor organ in the immediate postoperative period. All transplant programs invariably use high-dose methylprednisolone in induction immunosuppression. Apart from steroids, agents that deplete T cells and interrupt activation or proliferation are commonly used as induction agents. They can be divided into monoclonal and polyclonal agents. Use of induction agents should follow a patient-centric approach considering the comorbidities to balance the risk of infection and rejection.

The commonly used monoclonal induction agent used is basiliximab.[25] Basiliximab binds to the alpha-subunit of the interleukin-2 receptor and inhibits activation and proliferation of T cells. It is administered intraoperatively and if required repeated after 4 days. Basiliximab is well tolerated without major side effects. Another monoclonal agent used is alemtuzumab which acts on most T cells and few B cells by binding with CD52 antigen leading to direct and complement-mediated lymphocyte depletion. Antithymocyte globulin (ATG) is a polyclonal agent that is used as an induction agent as it nonspecifically binds to antigens resulting in lymphocyte depletion.

The early initiation of immunosuppressants in the postoperative period predisposes the patient to infectious complications. The tacrolimus, a calcineurin inhibitor, and cyclosporine which are most commonly used can cause renal dysfunction, by causing constriction of afferent renal arteriole. Triple-drug immunosuppressants are commonly used maintenance regimen which consist of calcineurin inhibitor, mycophenolate mofetil, and prednisone. Alternate regimens are available and are used depending on individual tolerability. Immunosuppressants such as tacrolimus, cyclosporine, sirolimus, and everolimus need to be monitored by their drug level in blood as they have a narrow therapeutic index and are also affected by many patient factors such as genetic polymorphisms of cytochrome P450 enzyme, gut absorption, and drug interaction.

POSTOPERATIVE ISSUES

Most common complications are infection, rejection, and side effects of immunosuppressants. Surgical complications include size mismatch, pulmonary venous thrombosis, bronchial anastomosis dehiscence, and pulmonary arterial stenosis. Postoperative complications can be categorized organ-wise. Respiratory complications are primary graft dysfunction, pleural effusion, pulmonary embolism, persistent air leak through chest tube, atelectasis, and native lung hyperinflation. Cardiovascular complications such as right ventricular dysfunction, arrhythmias, and myocardial infarction and neurologic complications such as calcineurin inhibitor-induced posterior leukoencephalopathy, phrenic nerve injury, critical illness, delirium, and myopathy/neuropathy are common. Other complications such as transfusion-related acute lung injury (TRALI), gastroparesis, reflux, dysphagia, ileus, colonic perforation, acute renal failure, hemolytic uremic syndrome, deep venous thrombosis causing pulmonary embolism, and autoimmune hemolysis are not uncommon.

Primary Graft Dysfunction

Primary graft dysfunction is a dreadful complication leading to acute lung injury after transplantation, leading to early morbidity and mortality. It can happen as early as lung reperfusion, with a spectrum of severity from a mild self-limiting disorder to severe fulminant respiratory failure. The primary graft dysfunction causes poor lung compliance, pulmonary edema, and high vascular resistance leading to decreased oxygenation. Severity is graded using the P:F ratio similar to acute lung injury.

Management of primary graft dysfunction is similar to the acute respiratory distress syndrome (ARDS) protocol that is lung-protective ventilation to avoid barotrauma, volutrauma, and atelectrauma. Differential ventilation can be used in a single-lung transplant. Pharmacological agents such as pulmonary vasodilators and inotropes for right ventricular support can be used. Severe primary graft dysfunction may cause severe hemodynamic instability and multiorgan dysfunction which may require extracorporeal support to maintain systemic perfusion.

Role of Nitric Oxide

Nitric oxide is the most commonly used selective inhaled pulmonary vasodilator. It is used at a dose of 10–40 ppm to treat severe hypoxia and high pulmonary pressure caused in primary graft dysfunction. NO causes increase in cyclic guanosine monophosphate (c-GMP) which relaxes the smooth muscles leading to vasodilation of capillaries adjacent to well-ventilated lung parenchyma. Hence, NO causes decrease in pulmonary pressure and maintains ventilation–perfusion matching. Pulmonary hypertension may rebound after discontinuation of NO. NO requires specialized delivery and monitoring systems to avoid toxicity.

INFECTION CONTROL

Infection is one of the most common causes for morbidity and mortality after lung transplantation. Apart from immunosuppression, the lung is as unique as compared to other solid organs since it gets continuous exposure to environmental pathogens leading to higher risk of infection. Empirical broad-spectrum antibiotic therapy is usually initiated in the operating room and continued in the postoperative period on a case-by-case basis depending on the clinical progression of the patient. Donor BAL is taken during donor assessment and it is used for Gram stain, culture, and sensitivity. Recipients with suppurative lung diseases, bronchiectasis, cystic fibrosis, cavitary lesion, and empyema antibiotics are rationalized according to the culture reports. On clinical suspicion of sepsis, focus of infection is identified depending on the clinical data of the patient and cultures are sent from blood, urine, and tracheal aspirate. In severe sepsis, antibiotics are escalated and they are de-escalated after culture report and clinical improvement.

Viral infections after lung transplantation are rare when compared to bacterial infection. CMV is the most common viral infection in post-transplant patients. It may affect all major organs in these immunosuppressed recipients. Depending on the CMV status of the donor and recipient, antiviral prophylaxis is started. Due to a large variety of opportunistic infections in the post-transplant period, clinical expertise of infectious disease specialists may help in managing these patients.

LUNG RETRANSPLANTATION

The indication for lung retransplantation is similar to the indications for initial transplantation. The risk retransplantation is more because of associated comorbidities, renal dysfunction, bleeding, and adhesion.[26] Retransplantation can be single- or dual-lung transplantation. Previous single-lung transplant may require explantation since it may be a source of infection or immunological response.[27] Retransplantation of a single lung on the same side has been found to have a higher risk than on the contralateral side.[28] Although it has numerous

confounding factors, bilateral lung retransplantation is commonly indicated nowadays.[29] Recent meta-analysis[30] found that retransplantation after bronchiolitis obliterans is found to have a better outcome than for primary graft dysfunction, and poor outcome on patients on mechanical ventilation. Even then, survival after lung retransplantation is inferior to the initial transplantation.

HEART–LUNG TRANSPLANTATION

Patients who are not amenable to only heart or lung transplantation like advanced heart failure with lung disease, uncorrectable congenital cardiac defects, severe pulmonary hypertension with right heart failure are the candidates for combined heart and lung transplantation.[31]

Severe pulmonary hypertension is defined as a systolic pulmonary artery pressure >60 mm Hg with any one of the associated factors such as elevated PVR >5 Wood units (WU), pulmonary vascular resistance index (PVRI) >6 WU, and transpulmonary pressure gradient between 16 and 20 mm Hg. These patients are given a vasodilator challenge test, if PVR reduces to <2.5 WU without a decrease in systolic blood pressure to <85 mm Hg; high-risk isolated heart transplantation is possible. But if PVR does not decrease, then these patients are at high risk of right ventricular failure and may require mechanical circulatory support to improve these indices to obviate the need for combined transplantation.

In patients with right ventricular failure secondary to severe pulmonary hypertension, isolated dual-lung transplantation has shown comparable results with.[32] The right ventricle is assessed for any infarct or fibrotic changes and cardiac size occupancy in the thoracic cavity as these can be used to determine whether isolated lung transplantation is feasible for a better outcome.

Patients with surgically correctable cardiac diseases such as coronary artery disease, valvular heart disease, and septal defects are managed along with concomitant lung transplantation.[33] Sarcoidosis and other connective tissue disorders affecting both lung and heart may require combined heart and lung transplantation.

PEDIATRIC LUNG TRANSPLANTATION

The indication and contraindication for pediatric lung transplantation are similar to adult criteria. In the pediatric age group, cystic fibrosis is the most common indication for lung transplantation.[34] Other leading causes are congenital heart disease and pulmonary hypertension.[35] Pediatric patients have a long waiting list and may require long-standing mechanical ventilation and extracorporeal support. Poor compliance is one of the reasons for graft dysfunction in pediatric and adolescent age groups. Since the waiting list is long because of limited donor availability, live lobar lung transplantation is an acceptable mode of treatment in experienced centers for long-waiting pediatric recipients.[36]

LIVE-DONOR LUNG TRANSPLANTATION

Live lobar lung donor is one of the promising alternatives for long-waiting recipients since these patients clinically deteriorate over time leading to multiorgan dysfunction making an inoperable and poor outcome even after transplant. Two donors donate each of their lobes to one recipient; each lobe becomes a right or a left lung. Live lobar lung transplantation decreases the pitfalls of a brain-dead donor such as trauma, lung contusion, aspiration, infection, neurogenic pulmonary edema, effects of prolonged ventilation on airway, and cardiac instability. Live lobar donor has decreased ischemic time and can be transplanted when the recipient is in a clinically stable condition. Hence, live lobar donor is an acceptable alternative to a brain-dead donor for the long-waiting recipients.

REFERENCES

1. Dabak G. History of lung transplantation. Eurasian J Pulmonol. 2013;15(2):82-7.

2. Christie JD, Edwards LB, Kucheryavaya AY, Benden C, Dobbels F, Kirk R, et al. The registry of the international society for heart and lung transplantation: twenty-eighth adult lung and heart-lung transplant report. J Heart Lung Transplant. 2011;30(10):1104-22.

3. Carlin BW, Lega M, Veynovich B. Management of the patient undergoing lung transplantation: an intensive care perspective. Crit Care Nurs Q. 2009;32(1):49-57.

4. Yusen RD, Edwards LB, Kucheryavaya AY, Lund LH, Benden C, Christie JD, et al. The registry of the International Society for Heart and Lung Transplantation: thirty-first adult lung and heart-lung transplant report–2014; focus theme: retransplantation. J Heart Lung Transplant. 2014;33(10):1009-24.

5. Estenne M, Maurer JR, Boehler A, Egan JJ, Frost A, Hertz M, et al. Bronchiolitis obliterans syndrome 2001: an update of the diagnostic criteria. J Heart Lung Transplant. 2002; 21:297-310.

6. David W, Benden C, Corris PA, Dark JH, Duane Davis R, Keshavjee S, et al. A consensus document for the selection of lung transplant candidates: 2014—An update from the Pulmonary Transplantation Council of the International Society for Heart and Lung Transplantation. J Heart Lung Transplant. 34(1)1-15.

7. Low DE, Trulock EP, Kaiser LR, Pasque MK, Dresler C, Ettinger N, et al. Morbidity, mortality, and early results of single versus bilateral lung transplantation for emphysema. J Thorac Cardiovasc Surg. 1992;103(6):1119-26.

8. Schulman LL, O'Hair DP, Cantu E, McGregor C, Ginsberg ME. Salvage by volume reduction of chronic allograft rejection in emphysema. J Heart Lung Transplant. 1999; 18(2):107-12.

9. Hadjiliadis D, Chaparro C, Gutierrez C, Steele MP, Singer LG, Davis RD, et al. Impact of lung transplant operation on bronchiolitis obliterans syndrome in patients with chronic obstructive pulmonary disease. Am J Transplant. 2006;6(1):183-9.

10. Thabut G, Christie JD, Ravaud P, Castier Y, Dauriat G, Jebrak G, et al. Survival after bilateral versus single-lung transplantation for idiopathic pulmonary fibrosis. Ann Intern Med. 2009;151(11):767-74.

11. Cypel M, Keshavjee S. Extracorporeal life support as a bridge to lung transplantation. Clin Chest Med. 2011;32(2):245-51.

12. de Perrot M, Granton JT, McRae K, Pierre AF, Singer LG, Waddell TK, et al. Outcome of patients with pulmonary arterial hypertension referred for lung transplantation: a 14-year single-center experience. J Thorac Cardiovasc Surg. 2012;143(4):910-8.

13. Strueber M. Bridges to lung transplantation. Curr Opin Organ Transplant. 2011;16(5):458-61.

14. Gottlieb J, Warnecke G, Hadem J, Dierich M, Wiesner O, Fuhner T, et al. Outcome of critically ill lung transplant candidates on invasive respiratory support. Intensive Care Med. 2012;38(6):968-75.

15. de Perrot M, Granton JT, McRae K, Cypel M, Pierre A, Waddell TK, et al. Impact of extracorporeal life support on outcome in patients with idiopathic pulmonary arterial hypertension awaiting lung transplantation. J Heart Lung Transplant. 2011;30(9):997-1002.

16. Vermeijden JW, Zijlstra JG, Erasmus ME, van der Bij W, Verschuuren EA. Lung transplantation for ventilator-dependent respiratory failure. J Heart Lung Transplant. 2009; 28(4):347-51.

17. Toyoda Y, Bhama JK, Shigemura N, Zaldonis D, Pilewski J, Crespo M, et al. Efficacy of extracorporeal membrane oxygenation as a bridge to lung transplantation. J Thorac Cardiovasc Surg. 2013;145(4):1065-70: [discussion 1070-1].

18. Shafii AE, Mason DP, Brown CR, et al. Growing experience with extracorporeal membrane oxygenation as a bridge to lung transplantation. ASAIO J. 2012;58:526-9.

19. Hoopes CW, Kukreja J, Golden J, Davenport DL, Diaz-Guzman E, Zwischenberger JB. Extracorporeal membrane oxygenation as a bridge to pulmonary transplantation. J Thorac Cardiovasc Surg. 2013;145(3):862-7.

20. Bittner HB, Lehmann S, Rastan A, Garbade J, Binner C, Mohr FW, et al. Outcome of extracorporeal membrane oxygenation as a bridge to lung transplantation and graft recovery. Ann Thorac Surg. 2012;94(3):942-9.

21. Bhorade SM, Vigneswaran W, McCabe MA, Garrity ER. Liberalization of donor criteria may expand the donor pool without adverse consequence in lung transplantation. J Heart Lung Transplant. 2000;19(12):1199-204.

22. Munshi L, Keshavjee S, Cypel M. Donor management and lung preservation for lung transplantation. Lancet Respir Med. 2013;1(4):318-28.

23. Thabut G, Mal H, Cerrina J, Dartevelle P, Dromer C, Velly JE, et al. Graft ischemic time and outcome of lung transplantation: a multicenter analysis. Am J Respir Crit Care Med. 2005;171(7): 786-91.

24. Cypel M, Yeung J, Machuca T, Chen M, Singer LG, Yasufuku K, et al. Experience with the first 50 ex vivo lung perfusions in clinical transplantation. J Thorac Cardiovasc Surg. 2012;144(5):1200-7.

25. Swarup R, Allenspach LL, Nemeh HW, Stagner LD, Betensley AD. Timing of basiliximab induction and development of acute rejection in lung transplant patients. J Heart Lung Transplant. 2011;30(11):1228-35.

26. Novick RJ, Stitt LW, Al-Kattan K, Klepetko W, Schafers HJ, Duchatelle JP, et al. Pulmonary retransplantation: predictors of graft function and survival in 230 patients. Pulmonary Retransplant Registry. Ann Thorac Surg. 1998;65(1):227-34.

27. Kawut SM. Lung retransplantation. Clin Chest Med. 2011;32(2):367-77.

28. Kawut SM, Lederer DJ, Keshavjee S, Wilt JS, Daly T, D'Ovidio F, et al. Outcomes after lung retransplantation in the modern era. Am J Respir Crit Care Med. 2008;177(1):114-20.

29. Brugiere O, Thabut G, Castier Y, Mal H, Dauriat G, Marceau A, et al. Lung retransplantation for bronchiolitis obliterans syndrome: long-term follow-up in a series of 15 recipients. Chest. 2003;123(6):1832-7.

30. Aigner C, Jaksch P, Taghavi S, Lang G, Reza-Hoda MA, Wisser W, et al. Pulmonary retransplantation: is it worth the effort? A long-term analysis of 46 cases. J Heart Lung Transplant. 2008;27(1):60-5.

31. Choong CK, Sweet SC, Guthrie TJ, Mendeloff EN, Haddad FJ, Schuler P, et al. Repair of congenital heart lesions combined with lung transplantation for the treatment of severe pulmonary hypertension: a 13-year experience. J Thorac Cardiovasc Surg. 2005;129(3):661-9.

32. Fadel E, Mercier O, Mussot S, Leroy-Ladurie F, Cerrina J, Chapelier A, et al. Long-term outcome of double-lung and heart-lung transplantation for pulmonary hypertension: a comparative retrospective study of 219 patients. Eur J Cardiothorac Surg. 2010;38(3):277-84.

33. Januszewska K, Malec E, Juchem G, Kaczmarek I, Sodian R, Uberfuhr P, et al. Heart-lung transplantation in patients with pulmonary atresia and ventricular septal defect. J Thorac Cardiovasc Surg. 2009;138(3):738-43.

34. Benden C. Specific aspects of children and adolescents undergoing lung transplantation. Curr Opin Organ Transplant. 2012;17(5):509-14.

35. Benden C, Edwards LB, Kucheryavaya AY, Christie JD, Dipchand AI, Dobbels F, et al. The Registry of the International Society for Heart and Lung Transplantation: sixteenth official pediatric lung and heart-lung transplantation report—2013; focus theme: age. J Heart Lung Transplant. 2013;32(10):989-97.

36. Sweet SC. Pediatric living donor lobar lung transplantation. Pediatr Transplant. 2006; 10(7):861-8.

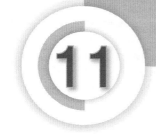
Miscellaneous

Nutrition in Perioperative Care

Subhal Bhalchandra Dixit, Khalid Ismail Khatib

INTRODUCTION

Perioperative nutrition is an important but underappreciated aspect of the overall care of the critically ill surgical patient. That, perioperative nutrition has an important impact on the surgical outcomes has been proved beyond doubt, yet it has not translated into surgical practice as much as it should have.[1-4] Use of nutrition therapy in the preoperative period and continuing into the postoperative period should be utilized to not only counteract the ill-effects of the illness, per se, but also the stress caused by surgery. The metabolic response to surgery and the corresponding hypermetabolic state in the postoperative period lead to increased nutritional strain on an already precarious nutritional state in the critically ill surgical patient. This leads to nutritional deficits. To combat these nutritional deficits, oral nutritional supplements (ONSs), enteral nutrition (EN), or parenteral nutrition (PN) is used. Also preoperative optimization of the nutritional status and use of immunonutrition are the other avenues to improve the outcome in these patients. Optimization of perioperative nutrition has become an integral part of enhanced recovery after surgery (ERAS) pathways and has also been incorporated in all International Society Guidelines of nutrition.[5-9]

ASSESSMENT OF NUTRITIONAL STATUS[5,10-12]

It is done using various tools given in **Table 1**. The aim of nutritional assessment is to identify patients at high risk and to set up interventions to modify the high risk and reduce surgical morbidity. Causes of perioperative malnutrition and types of surgical procedures, which may lead to increased risk of malnutrition, are given in **Box 1**.

Patients in the perioperative period should be screened for risk of malnutrition using the NUTRIC (Nutrition Risk in the Critically Ill) score or Perioperative Nutrition Screening, Perioperative Nutrition Score (PONS) or other screening tools [Mini Nutritional Assessment (MNA),

Table 1: Nutrition assessment tools used to determine nutrition risk in perioperative patients.

S. No.	Nutrition tools	Remarks
1.	The Malnutrition Universal Screening Tool (MUST)	Not specific for perioperative patients
2.	Nutritional Risk Index (NRI)	
3.	Nutritional Risk Screening (NRS-2002)	Validated and supported by level I evidence in perioperative patients
4.	Mini Nutritional Assessment (MNA)	
5.	Subjective Global Assessment (SGA)	Takes into account the following points—visual assessment of subcutaneous fat and muscle mass, anorexia, functional capacity, GI symptoms, and weight loss over 6 months. Has been used in surgical patients
6.	Serum albumin	Not reliable, values vary due to many other reasons
7.	Serum prealbumin	Not reliable
8.	Perioperative Nutrition Screening Perioperative Nutrition Score (PONS)[5]	Body mass index <18.5 (<20 if age > 65 years), unplanned weight loss >10% over previous 6 months, oral intake <50% of usual diet over last 7 days, serum albumin <3 mg/dL. Presence of any one should lead to referral to a dietitian for appropriate intervention

(GI: gastrointestinal)

Malnutrition Universal Screening Tool (MUST), Short Nutritional Assessment Questionnaire (SNAQ), Subjective Global Assessment (SGA), and Nutritional Risk Score-2002 (NRS-2002)]. Radiological tools include ultrasonography of quadriceps muscle (to measure muscle mass and changes during course of illness) and computed tomography (CT) scan analysis of skeletal muscle density (SMD). Patients are

Table 2: Components of a prehabilitation bundle.

S. No.	Components	Remarks
1.	Exercise tolerance	If 6 MWT < 60% of predicted value for age and sex, a program of aerobic and resistance exercise is started
2.	Weight	Identify presence of frailty using the Fried frailty score or modified frailty index
3.	Nutrition	Use ONS and/or parenteral nutrition in the preoperative period
4.	Glucose control	Should be used in patients with HbA1c values > 7. Insulin to be used to maintain mild hyperglycemia (up to 140 –220 mg/dL) and prevent hypoglycemia. Intensive glycemic control is not indicated

(HbA1c: glycosylated hemoglobin; 6MWT: 6-minute walking test; ONSs: oral nutritional supplements)

at high nutrition risk if the NUTRIC score is ≤ 5 or NRS score is > 3. MNA score value of 0–7 points denote malnourished individuals at start of the illness, while a score of 8–11 points denotes individuals at risk of malnutrition. The PONS takes into account the following factors: (1) body mass index <18.5 (<20 if age > 65 years), (2) unplanned weight loss >10% over previous 6 months, (3) oral intake < 50% of usual diet over last 7 days, and (4) serum albumin < 3 mg/dL. The presence of any one of these factors should lead to referral to a dietitian for appropriate intervention, so that nutritional status can be improved in the perioperative period.

Malignancy-related Malnutrition[8]

Malnutrition is the most common comorbidity associated with malignancy. These patients experience anorexia, food aversion, and decreased food intake leading to weight loss, muscle loss, and progressive deterioration throughout their care continuum. Malnutrition in these patients is the effect of cancer biology, cancer-induced chronic inflammatory state as well as local effects from tumor-induced changes in the digestive tracts. Patients with cancers arising in the upper digestive tract and pancreas have the highest propensity for weight loss and malnutrition. Cancer treatments including surgery, chemotherapy, and radiotherapy are well known to trigger many adverse events including loss of appetite, nausea, vomiting, altered taste, dry mouth, sore throat, diarrhea, lactose intolerance, constipation, and pain, all of which potentiates weight loss. These factors cause and sustain weight loss and malnutrition, also known as precachexia, among 30–90% of patients with cancer. If left untreated, gradually the precachexia progress to cachexia and refractory cachexia. A large number of patients with malignancy await surgery. These patients who are well nourished and even those with mild malnourishment should undergo necessary surgery when indicated. Those patients with severe malnutrition will benefit from nutritional interventions prior to surgery.

PREOPERATIVE INTERVENTIONS FOR IMPROVING NUTRITION

Optimization of the nutritional status prior to undergoing surgery (so called "prehabilitation") has an effect on the prognosis of the patient and has beneficial effect.[13] The period of time available will depend on the prior nutritional status of the patient, the underlying illness, extent and type of surgery (whether elective or emergency), response of the patient to nutritional therapy, etc. The components of a "prehabilitation bundle" have been studied and are given in **Table 2**.[11,13-15] It has been shown to be beneficial in patients undergoing colorectal surgeries for malignancy and abdominal surgeries.[15,16] In a pre- and postintervention pilot study conducted on patients undergoing surgery for colorectal malignancy, a prehabilitation intervention (lasting for a mean period of 33 days) led to an improvement in functional status and better postoperative recovery.[13] A randomized controlled trial (RCT) conducted in 77 patients with colorectal malignancy undergoing surgery randomized patients to prehabilitation (interventions prior to surgery over 1 month) or to rehabilitation (intervention after surgery). Patients in the prehabilitation group showed better postoperative functional recovery (in the form of better 6 minute walking test) with some patients having better functional capacity than baseline.[15]

Immunonutrition with arginine, omega-3-fatty acids, and glutamine may be used in patients undergoing major elective abdominal surgeries. It is to be used in patients who are malnourished and at risk for infectious complications starting 5–7 days prior to surgery.[17]

Route and Duration of Preoperative Nutrition

Enteral route is the preferred route for preoperative nutrition, and it should be used for a period of at least 7 days and even for 10–14 days. ONS (preferably containing whey protein or casein) may be started in patients at risk for nutrition to achieve a protein goal of 1.2 g/kg/d. Patients should take at least 20 grams of protein per meal and two to three such meals per day, as tolerated. If the

Box 2: Contraindications to enteral route for nutrition.

Contraindications
- Intestinal obstruction or ischemia
- Acute peritonitis
- High output fistulas
- Severe malabsorption
- Lack of bowel continuity

patient is unable to swallow or is intolerant to ONS, EN via a feeding tube may be given.[5] Some patients at high risk for malnutrition undergoing major abdominal surgeries have contraindications for enteral feeding or are unable to meet their daily requirement of calories and/or proteins via ONS or EN. These patients may be given preoperative PN for 7 days. Contraindications for enteral feeding are given in **Box 2**.[10]

Carbohydrate Loading and Avoiding Prolonged Preoperative Fasting

Patients undergoing surgery do not require overnight fasting and should be allowed to consume clear liquids up to 120 minutes prior to anesthesia. This prevents adverse events like headaches, thirst, and anxiety and stimulates gastric emptying.[18,19] Patients may be advised to consume 50 grams of carbohydrate in a clear liquid form over 5–10 minutes. This is known as carbohydrate loading and has been shown to have biochemical, metabolic, and clinical benefits.[11,20,21] The commonly used products contain maltodextrin and there may even be a case for adding amino acids to this preparation.[22]

POSTOPERATIVE INTERVENTIONS FOR IMPROVING NUTRITION

Early Oral Intake

Oral food intake in the postoperative period should be started early. It has been found to be safe, effective, and reduces postoperative complications. Even in patients undergoing gastrointestinal (GI) surgeries, feeding these patients within 24 hours of surgery did not increase mortality, morbidity, or intestinal anastomotic complications.[23,24] Patients who are not candidates for early oral intake are those with intestinal obstruction and ischemia.

Oral Nutritional Supplements, Enteral Nutrition, and Parenteral Nutrition

Nutrition in the postoperative period should consist of both adequate calories and amino acids. This will attenuate proteolysis, stimulate insulin secretion, and help in anabolism in this period. This prevents loss of muscle mass in all patients and onset of frailty in the elderly. The

amount of protein that is considered adequate for this period is 1.2–2.0 g/kg/d. Usually, this level of protein and calorie intake is not reached in a majority of these patients, without diligent nutrition support and intervention. Patients will require ONS supplementation (two to three times a day) with their meals to reach their protein targets. If patients are unable to reach >50% of their needs in this way, an enteral tube may be placed and EN may be given. Patients not reaching >50% of their nutritional targets (calorie or protein) for 7 days should receive PN. Patients receiving PN may benefit from the use of fish oil-based lipid formulations as compared to soy-based ones in the form of reduced length of stay (LOS) and infectious complications.

Patients receiving ONS, EN, or PN should do so for at least 1 month or even longer depending on the extent of malnutrition and surgical trauma. The patients who require longer supplementation up to 3–6 months (i.e., even in the posthospital discharge phase) are those with severe malnourishment and prolonged hospital or intensive care unit (ICU) stays.

Immunonutrition[17,25]

Immunonutrition (in the form of combination of arginine, glutamine, and omega-3-fatty acids) should be considered in patients undergoing high-risk GI surgery, for a period of a week postoperatively. They reduce the risk of complications (including infectious) and even anastomotic leaks. A Cochrane meta-analysis studied the effect of glutamine supplementation on patients (both critically ill and surgical). This very large meta-analysis included 53 studies and 4,671 patients.[26] It found "moderate" evidence of reduction of infections and decreased days on minute ventilation (MV). There was evidence of reduced hospital LOS in critically ill and surgical patients, though it was of "low quality." Glutamine supplementation did not reduce overall mortality or did not reduce ICU LOS. Chen et al. in 2014, conducted a meta-analysis which consisted of 18 trials with 3,383 ICU patients and found that there was no difference in either hospital mortality or mortality at 6 months in patients who received glutamine supplementation and those who did not receive glutamine supplementation.[27] Also there was no difference in hospital LOS and mortality (hospital or 6-month) among patients who received glutamine when assessed according to the route of administration (enteral or parenteral). However, when patients were classified as per the dose of glutamine administered, patients who received higher dose of glutamine had significant higher mortality rate as compared to patients who did not receive glutamine. When only surgical ICU patients were analyzed, the rate of infections was significantly lower in patients who received glutamine.

CONCLUSION

Nutritional support in the perioperative period aims to attenuate the adverse effects of surgery (surgical stress) and boost perioperative recovery with decreased morbidity, complications, frailty, loss of muscle mass, and mortality. It aims to do this by assessing the risk of nutrition in this period and then implementing interventions to combat the surgical stress. These interventions start in the preoperative period and extend into the postoperative period and beyond (into the posthospital discharge period).

REFERENCES

1. Stratton RJ, Elia M. Who benefits from nutritional support: what is the evidence? Eur J Gastroenterol Hepatol. 2007;19:353-8.
2. Benoist S, Brouquet A. Nutritional assessment and screening for malnutrition. J Visc Surg. 2015;152(Suppl 1):S3-S7.
3. Braga M, Ljungqvist O, Soeters P, Fearon K, Weimann A, Bozzetti F. ESPEN guidelines on parenteral nutrition surgery. Clin Nutr. 2009;28:378-86.
4. Williams JD, Wischmeyer PE. Assessment of perioperative nutrition practices and attitudes: A national survey of colorectal and GI surgical oncology programs. Am J Surg. 2017;213:1010-8.
5. Wischmeyer PE, Carli F, Evans DC, Guilbert S, Kozar R, Pryor A, et al. American society for enhanced recovery and perioperative quality initiative joint consensus statement on nutrition screening and therapy within a surgical enhanced recovery pathway. Anesth Analg. 2018;126:1883-95.
6. Weimann A, Braga M, Harsanyi L, Laviano A, Ljungqvist O, Soeters P, et al; DGEM (German Society for Nutritional Medicine); ESPEN (European Society for Parenteral and Enteral Nutrition). ESPEN guidelines on enteral nutrition: Surgery including organ transplantation. Clin Nutr. 2006;25:224-44.
7. McClave SA, Taylor BE, Martindale RG, Warren MM, Johnson DR, Braunschweig C, et al; Society of Critical Care Medicine; American Society for Parenteral and Enteral Nutrition. Guidelines for the provision and assessment of nutrition support therapy in the adult critically ill patient: Society of Critical Care Medicine (SCCM) and American Society for Parenteral and Enteral Nutrition (A.S.P.E.N.). J Parenter Enteral Nutr. 2016;40:159-211.
8. Arends J, Bachmann P, Baracos V, Barthelemy N, Bertz H, Bozzetti F, et al. ESPEN guidelines on nutrition in cancer patients. Clin Nutr. 2017;36:11-48.
9. Weimann A, Braga M, Carli F, Higashiguchi T, Hübner M, Klek S, et al. ESPEN guideline: clinical nutrition in surgery. Clin Nutr. 2017;36:623-50.
10. McClave SA, Kozar R, Martindale RG, Heyland DK, Braga M, Carli F, et al. Summary points and consensus recommendations from the North American Surgical Nutrition Summit. J Parenter Enteral Nutr. 2013;37(5 Suppl):99S-105S.
11. Martindale RG, McClave SA, Taylor B, Lawson CM. Perioperative nutrition: What is the current landscape? J Parenter Enteral Nutr. 2013;37(5 Suppl):5S-20S.

12. Miller KR, Wischmeyer PE, Taylor B, McClave SA. An evidence-based approach to perioperative nutrition support in the elective surgery patient. J Parenter Enteral Nutr. 2013;37(5 Suppl):39S-50S.
13. Li C, Carli F, Lee L, Charlebois P, Stein B, Liberman AS, et al. Impact of a trimodal prehabilitation program on functional recovery after colorectal cancer surgery: A pilot study. Surg Endosc. 2013;27(4):1072-82.
14. Gillis C, Carli F. Promoting perioperative metabolic and nutritional care. Anesthesiology. 2015;123:1455-72.
15. Gillis C, Li C, Lee L, Awasthi R, Augustin B, Gamsa A, et al. Prehabilitation versus rehabilitation: a randomized control trial in patients undergoing colorectal resection for cancer. Anesthesiology. 2014;121:937-47.
16. Jie B, Jiang ZM, Nolan MT, Zhu SN, Yu K, Kondrup J. Impact of preoperative nutritional support on clinical outcome in abdominal surgical patients at nutritional risk. Nutrition. 2012;28(10):1022-7.
17. Braga M, Wischmeyer PE, Drover J, Heyland DK. Clinical evidence for pharmaconutrition in major elective surgery. JPEN J Parenter Enteral Nutr. 2013;37(5 Suppl):66S-72S.
18. McLeod R, Fitzgerald W, Sarr M; Members of the Evidence Based Reviews in Surgery Group: Canadian Association of General Surgeons and American College of Surgeons evidence based reviews in surgery. 14. Preoperative fasting for adults to prevent perioperative complications. Can J Surg. 2005;48:409-11.
19. Ljungqvist O. Modulating postoperative insulin resistance by preoperative carbohydrate loading. Best Pract Res Clin Anaesthesiol. 2009;23:401-9.
20. Nygren J, Thorell A, Ljungqvist O. Preoperative oral carbohydrate therapy. Curr Opin Anaesthesiol. 2015;28:364-9.
21. Smith MD, McCall J, Plank L, Herbison GP, Soop M, Nygren J. Preoperative carbohydrate treatment for enhancing recovery after elective surgery. Cochrane Database Syst Rev. 2014;8:CD009161.
22. Perrone F, da-Silva-Filho AC, Adôrno IF, Anabuki NT, Leal FS, Colombo T, et al. Effects of preoperative feeding with a whey protein plus carbohydrate drink on the acute phase response and insulin resistance. A randomized trial. Nutr J. 2011;10:66.
23. Lewis SJ, Egger M, Sylvester PA, Thomas S. Early enteral feeding versus "nil by mouth" after gastrointestinal surgery: Systematic review and meta-analysis of controlled trials. BMJ. 2001;323:773-6.
24. Jeejeebhoy KN. Enteral feeding. Curr Opin Gastroenterol. 2005;21:187-91.
25. Evans DC, Hegazi RA. Immunonutrition in critically ill patients: Does one size fit all? JPEN J Parenter Enteral Nutr. 2015;39:500-1.
26. Tao KM, Li XQ, Yang LQ, Yu WF, Lu ZJ, Sun YM, et al. Glutamine supplementation for critically adults (review). Cochrane. 2014;9:CD010050.
27. Chen QH, Yang Y, He HL, Xie JF, Cai SX, Liu AR, et al. The effect of glutamine therapy on outcomes in critically ill patients: a meta-analysis of randomized controlled trials. Crit Care. 2014;18:R8.

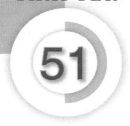
Prehabilitation and Rehabilitation

Anuradha Abhijit Daptardar, Ajeeta Mohan Kulkarni, Vincent Singh Paramanandam

INTRODUCTION

Surgical care has an important role in the treatment of various diseases.[1] Three hundred and ten million patients undergo surgery worldwide each year.[2] Research suggests that the number and severity of complications postsurgery are closely related to the preoperative functional reserve, nutritional status, habit, and psychological well-being of the patients. This has prompted a greater interest in targeting these issues preoperatively with an intervention program.[3] The history of prehabilitation dates back to 1946, for men enlisting for the second world war, who were malnourished and presented with a poor physical condition. These men were subjected to 2 months of physical and nutritional interventions, transforming these substandard recruits into standard recruits.[4] The concept of prehabilitation has evolved since then and has come a long way. Prehabilitation is a multimodal intervention program to improve the functional capacity, physical and psychological wellbeing of patients in the preoperative period to prevent or reduce postoperative consequences. The multimodal intervention includes medical optimization, exercise training, nutritional therapy, and psychological counseling to reduce anxiety.[5,6] A growing body of evidence has shown that prehabilitation has minimized length of stay, postoperative pain, and complications.[7]

COMPONENTS OF PREHABILITATION

Several weeks may elapse before the date of surgery and this period provides a window for the prehabilitation program. Many of the prehabilitation programs described in the literature are for a span of 4–12 weeks. A minimum of 4 weeks is required for prehabilitation to be effective.[8] Anything less than this is ineffective and anything more than 12 weeks may affect compliance. The multidisciplinary prehabilitation team consists of surgeons, anesthetists, physicians, physiotherapists, nutritionists, and psychologists. Prehabilitation can be a supervised hospital-based program or an unsupervised home-based program (**Flowchart 1**).

Flowchart 1: Components of prehabilitation program.

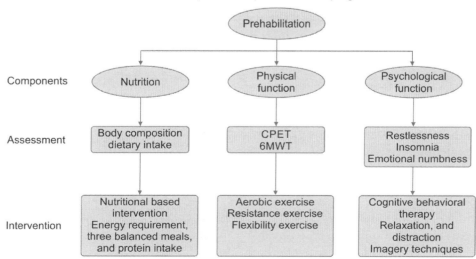

(CPET: cardiopulmonary exercise test; 6MWT: 6 minute walking test)

Assessment

A baseline assessment of the physical, functional, nutritional, and psychological status by expert clinician, physiotherapist, dietician, and psychologist is a prerequisite to understand and plan a prehabilitation regime to improve postoperative outcomes.[9] Baseline assessment includes evaluation of preoperative levels of physical activity, strength, functional capacity, nutritional status, anxiety, and depression.

Comprehensive history, medical records, demographics such as age, gender, and occupation is noted. Basic anthropometrics such as height, weight, body composition, functional capacity, dietary habits, and mood are recorded and monitored intermittently. A thorough musculoskeletal, cardiopulmonary, and neurological assessment is done to evaluate the strength, endurance, and dysfunction preoperatively.[10] There are many tests used to measure the functional capacity such as 6 minute walk test (6MWT), cardiopulmonary exercise test (CPET), Timed Up and Go test, Sit-to-Stand test, step test, and others. The two tests most frequently used are the CPET and the 6MWT. The CPET measures gas exchange and ventilation parameters to evaluate oxygen consumption during incremental exercises.[11] The 6MWT is a simple, objective inexpensive submaximal exercise test that measures functional capacity by evaluating the distance walked by a patient at a brisk pace in 6 minutes. Although it is a simple test, a standardized protocol has to be followed to get reliable results.[12] Heart rate, dyspnea, and fatigue level are recorded at the beginning and end of the test and the distance walked is measured. The 6MWT is performed again on completion of the prehabilitation regime to help quantify any change in the functional capacity.

Poor nutritional status results in poor surgical outcomes, longer stay in the hospital, higher rate of infections, and increased rate of mortality.[13] The dietician records parameters such as body mass index (BMI), sudden involuntary weight loss, dietary habits, and others to evaluate malnutrition, cachexia, and sarcopenia. The necessary nutritional support to correct the disorders and meet the energy requirement is tailor-made based on the baseline nutritional evaluation and the additional nutritional demands of the prehabilitation program. Advocacy of high protein intake balanced meal with an intake of macronutrients in adequate proportion, at regular hours and with regular intervals is a major key component of prehabilitation.[14,15]

The anxiety and fear related to surgery, anesthesia, pain, and recovery have a negative impact on postoperative recovery, wound healing, infection rate, and length of hospital stay.[16,17]

The Psychologist assesses the mood and anxiety levels and aims to reduce the preoperative anxiety symptoms and psychological distress by cognitive behavioral interventions, relaxation, and imagery techniques.[18]

Medical Optimization

It has already been established that preoperative smoking cessation reduces the risk of cardiopulmonary complications, wound infections, prolonged hospital stay, and death.[19] Alcohol misuse increases postoperative infections, bleeding, and cardiopulmonary complications. Preoperative abstinence for a minimum period of 4 weeks has known to decline postoperative morbidity.[20] Preoperative pharmacological optimization of hypertension, diabetes, heart disease, and chronic obstructive pulmonary disease (COPD) also forms an important element of prehabilitation.

Exercise Training

Diverse exercise regimes are recommended in literature; however, there are no optimal exercise regime that has been defined. A major prerequisite for prescribing exercise training is a baseline objective assessment of the cardiopulmonary system and assessment of muscle strength and endurance.[21] A generalized exercise prescription may result in an underdosing or overdosing of exercise treatment; thus, an individualized training program is recommended. Exercise training always provides a physiological stimulus that creates biological stress, which in turn challenges homeostasis, eliciting a stress response, and leading to physical adaptation. The key requirement for an effective exercise prescription is an optimization and incremental increase in the stress or load to achieve continued physiological adaptation. Appropriate rest and recovery are essential elements between training sessions to optimize physiological adaptation **(Fig. 1)**.[22]

Traditionally the prehabilitation exercise regime is tailor-made and the exercise prescription is based on the frequency, intensity, time, and type (FITT) framework. The frequency can be from two to five sessions per week.

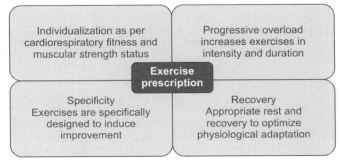

Fig. 1: Exercise prescription.

Duration of the exercises is 30–60 minutes. Type of exercise is mainly a combination of aerobic exercise and resistance exercise. The intensity of the workout is calculated based on VO_2 max, heart rate maximum (HR max) or rate of perceived exertion (RPE).

Aerobic exercises such as brisk walking, cycling, swimming, and slow dancing require minimal skills and can easily be modified to meet the individual's physical fitness levels. Aerobic training can be given with moderate to vigorous intensity of 50–75% of VO_2 max; 60–80% of HR max or RPE of 11–14. Incremental progression is achieved by increasing the duration or frequency of the session.

Resistance exercises are given to improve muscle strength or endurance. It can be customized by doing calisthenics such as push-ups, pull-ups, crunches, squats, sit-ups, rowing or can include the use of free weights or resistance bands for muscle strengthening. The intensity of resistance exercise prescription is determined by calculating the load or resistance using one repetition maximum (1RM) (the maximum amount of weight one can lift in a single repetition for a given exercise) or as per individual tolerance. The duration of resistance exercise is based on the number of repetitions and sets. 8 to 15 repetitions optimally constitute a set of exercises. The number of repetitions and load of resistance are inversely proportional to each other, i.e. greater the load, fewer repetitions required for improving muscle strength and power, whereas, lesser load and number of repetitions enhance muscular endurance. A reasonable rest period of 2 or 3 minutes, between sets may be allowed. Progression of resistance exercises can be achieved by increasing the load, increasing the repetition per set, increasing the number of set, decreasing the rest period between sets or increasing the exercise frequency. It is recommended to increase the repetition per set initially before increasing the load (5% increase) **(Table 1)**.[23]

Table 1: FITT framework.

FITT training	Aerobic	Resistance training
Frequency	Two to five times/week	Two to three times/week
Intensity	50–75% of VO_2 peak, 60–80% of HR max, or RPE of 11–14	50–70% of maximal voluntary contraction
Time	30–60 minutes	8–15 repetitions as per strength/endurance
Type	Walking, running, cycling, swimming	Free exercises such as push-ups, crunches, sit-ups, handgrips, etc.
		Resistance strength by weights/therabands

(FIIT: frequency, intensity, time, and type; HR max: heart rate maximum; RPE: rate of perceived exertion)

It is well documented that home-based prehabilitation programs are convenient and cost effective; however, compliance rates and overall improvement in functional capacity are better demonstrated with hospital-based prehabilitation program.[24]

ENHANCED RECOVERY AFTER SURGERY

Surgery being a serious invasive procedure results in some amount of complication and pain is the most common complaint. Surgical sites tend to reduce mobility due to incisional pain, resulting in a slouched and protracted posture. This result in poor breathing patterns, ineffective coughing, and retained secretions leading to more severe complications such as atelectasis and pneumonia. Other side effects of surgery are nausea, vomiting, and fatigue.[25]

The enhanced recovery after surgery (ERAS) protocol or "fast-track program" is a multidisciplinary approach to reduce patient's surgical stress, optimize their physiological function and facilitate recovery. ERAS was initiated by Professor Henrik Kehlet in the 1990s.[26]

Physiotherapy is an important element within the ERAS pathway, contributing by using evidence-based physiotherapy protocols to prevent pulmonary complications and promoting early mobilization safely and effectively for patients in the intensive care unit (ICU).[27]

POSTOPERATIVE PHYSIOTHERAPY REHABILITATION

Physiotherapists play an integral part in the multidisciplinary healthcare team in the dynamic environment of ICU, by providing postoperative respiratory care, breathing exercises, chest expansion, pain management, fatigue, postural correction, limb exercises, early mobilization, and home programs.

Postoperative Respiratory Care in Intensive Care Unit

Evidence shows that a thorough evaluation to weigh the benefits versus adverse effects, keeping in mind the patient's stability, before starting any physiotherapy intervention, makes physiotherapy treatment both safe and effective. Vital parameters such as heart rate, blood pressure, oxygen saturation, X-rays, arterial blood gas (ABG) need to be monitored when a patient is intubated.[28]

Atelectasis, pneumonitis, and pneumonia are serious problems after major surgery due to anesthesia and postoperative analgesics. Ineffective coughing and expectoration are associated with retained secretions leading to consolidation and other pulmonary complications that can be prevented by effective pulmonary evaluation and prehabilitation prior to surgery. This will enhance postoperative recovery and improve functional outcomes.[29]

Postoperatively, patients who require prolonged mechanical ventilation in the ICU may be at an increased risk for developing cardiopulmonary, neuromuscular, cognitive, and psychosocial complications, which can result in decreased quality of life and altered functional performance.

Airway management becomes predominantly important when patients require endotracheal intubation or tracheostomy during mechanical ventilation. Placement of endotracheal tube impairs mucociliary clearance and coughing mechanism. Prolonged intubation may result in further complications such as retained secretions, atelectasis, and weaning failure. Besides this, there is potential physical deconditioning, muscle weakness, and joint stiffness. Physiotherapy interventions aim at the prevention and treatment of respiratory and neuromuscular conditions. Chest physiotherapy (CPT) focuses on optimizing ventilation and clearing secretions, positioning, using various maneuvers such as percussions, vibrations, and shaking. Early mobilization, ambulation, and upright position help improve functional residual capacity and tidal volume, both in spontaneously breathing and anaesthetized patients due to the lowering of the diaphragm and alveolar expansion.[30] Pediatric patients undergoing thoracoabdominal surgery are given CPT identical to that of an adult, however, their lungs are not fully developed and this may lead to early collapse of dependent lobe of lungs. Strategies incorporated to older patients need to be modified for a child depending on their age and development **(Fig. 2)**.[31]

Breathing exercises help in increasing the transpulmonary pressure which helps to expand the lungs. Thoracic expansion exercises re-expand the lung tissue, mobilize excess bronchial secretions, and inflate the collapsed segments by exerting effective pressure that dilates the airways improves the lung volume.

Active cycle of breathing technique (ACBT) and *autogenic drainage (AD)* are interventions used for the gradual increase in inspiratory and expiratory reserve volumes, increase in the breath-holding period to improve ventilation and mobilize the secretions, decrease the atelectatic area, and prevent the collapse of the alveoli.

The ACBT starts with breathing control where the patient breathes through the nose and out through the mouth with pursed lip to create back pressure in airways. Then the chest expansion exercises with 3 seconds breath-holding are given followed by huffing or huff coughing. This helps to get more air into the smaller airways and behind the mucus if any, which can be easily brought out by huffing. The AD technique comprises of self-drainage with breathing exercises taught to the patient to assist in the removal of secretions.[32]

Incentive Spirometry

Incentive spirometry, also known as sustained maximal inspiration (SMI), is a technique used to encourage the patient to perform maximum inspiration, using a device, measuring flow or volume and providing visual feedback to increase the patient's pulmonary performance. A maximal inspiration sustained for 3 seconds may increase the transpulmonary pressure, improve inspiratory volumes, and inspiratory muscle performance, simulating the normal pattern of pulmonary hyperinflation **(Fig. 3)**. It may reverse lung atelectasis and maintain airway patency with frequent repetition. Although there is no strong evidence to support its significance in the management of surgical patients, it is still widely used in clinical setups.[33]

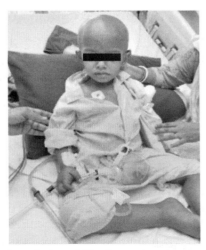

Fig. 2: Early mobilization and positioning.

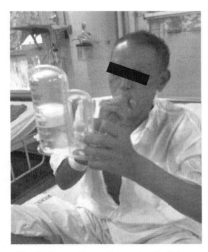

Fig. 3: Incentive spirometer training.

Pain

Postoperative pain can be debilitating for the patient. Pain prevents the patient from coughing effectively, interferes with mobilization and increases dependency. Pain medications given prior to physiotherapy intervention have known to improve the patient's functional performance. Physiotherapy interventions for postoperative pain relief include (1) transcutaneous electrical nerve stimulation (TENS), (2) cryotherapy, and (3) splinting.

Transcutaneous electrical nerve stimulation uses low voltage electrical current to stimulate nerve cells that block the transmission of pain signals. The other proposed alternative mechanism for the effect of TENS is the release of endorphins and activation of inhibitory reflex areas in the brainstem. TENS is a complementary analgesic, which helps in the reduction of pain, which in turn reduces the dose of analgesics and its side effects, improves the exercise performance, improves the lung expansion and prevents postoperative pulmonary complications.[34,35]

Cryotherapy can be given to the inflamed muscles adjacent to the incisional site. Ice application causes vasoconstriction, which reduces inflammation and swelling, decreases the sensitivity of nerve endings to pain, thereby reducing pain.[35]

Splinting: Pain during deep breathing and coughing can be reduced by proper support to the incision. The patient's hands, an abdominal binder, a thoracic binder or a pillow can achieve this. In the case of thoracotomy, physiotherapist or caregiver can support incision during exercises and coughing.[35]

Postoperative Fatigue

Postoperative fatigue sets in due to the surgery itself, prolonged anesthetic effect, analgesics, anemia, and poor coughing efforts leading to pulmonary problems. Fatigue is subjective and multidimensional. The most commonly used instrument to assess fatigue is the visual analog scale (VAS). Fatigue should be managed as per the cause and the physical activity should be gradually increased to accommodate the weariness after surgery.[36,37]

Early Mobilization

Many potential avoidable and unavoidable factors prevent the mobilization of patients in the ICU. The avoidable factors include vascular catheters, procedure timings, sedation management, and others. The unavoidable factors are predominantly respiratory instability, followed by hemodynamic instability, intracranial hypertension, and immobilization due to fractures or likewise.[38] Prolonged immobilization leads to many musculoskeletal complications such as muscle disuse atrophy, loss of muscle strength and endurance, contractures and soft tissue changes, disuse osteoporosis, and degenerative disease of the joints; and cardiovascular complications such as increased heart rate, decreased cardiac reserve, orthostatic hypotension, and venous thromboembolism.[39]

The concept of early postoperative mobilization was described, first by a surgeon, Dr Emil Ries, a gynecologist in Chicago in 1899. However, it was only in the 1940s, that surgeons accepted this concept. Until then postoperative bed rest was advised for a few weeks to reduce pain and good healing of the wound.[40]

Limb Exercises and Postural Correction

Before commencement of exercises in the ICU, the patient must be assessed for stable orthostatic pressure, core stability, and muscle strength of both upper and lower extremities. Core stability is assessed as the ability of the patient to sit erect for more than 1 minute. Stable orthostatic pressure should be assessed as the ability of the patient to stand up for more than 1 minute without developing lightheadedness, dizziness or nausea, and hemodynamic changes such as increase in heart rate by more than 30 beats/minute above baseline or decrease of systolic blood pressure by more than 20 mm Hg, should be monitored. Muscle strength grading scale is used for muscle strength charting of both upper and lower extremities. Hand dynamometer is used for the grip strength.[41]

The mobility typically begins with bed-level activities that include an active or passive activity such as side rolling, assisted and active exercises for the upper and lower extremity, and breathing exercises combined with arm movements. Ankle pumps and quadriceps exercises should be started as early as possible to minimize circulatory stasis and prevent deep vein thrombosis and pulmonary embolism. Postural correction, incorporating shoulder movements on the ipsilateral side, shoulder retraction exercises, and erect posture are encouraged for patients who have undergone thoracotomy or abdominal surgeries. The focus of mobilization then moves to transfer the patient from bed to a chair and appropriate ambulation as tolerated **(Fig. 4)**.[25]

Postoperative Ambulation

Early postoperative ambulation is initiated for patients undergoing major surgeries to improve functional capacity and to enhance recovery. Physical activities/exercises are associated with improvement in cardiopulmonary endurance, decreased fatigue symptoms, improved muscular strength, and quality of life. Despite the potential benefits of a structured postoperative rehabilitation program, there

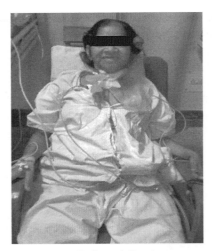

Fig. 4: Early mobilization.

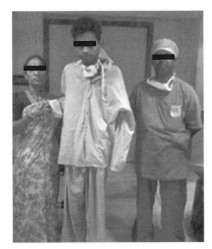

Fig. 5: Early ambulation.

is still a lack of standardized postoperative rehabilitation protocols in current guidelines of perioperative care. Early mobilization and an increased number of rehabilitation sessions beginning within the ICU has shown to reduce overall hospital length of stay **(Fig. 5)**.[42]

The exercise training based on the FITT framework, started preoperatively progresses into the postoperative period. The functional capacity measured acts as the baseline for postoperative exercise training. Safety guidelines for ambulation should be followed. Patients even with clinically stable cardiopulmonary conditions should be closely monitored during exercise/mobilization because they still may have the potential to become unstable on exertion. Short but frequent walks are recommended initially, with a gradual increase to patient's level of <13 on the RPE or 60% of HR max. A cycle ergometer or a treadmill can be used for this purpose **(Figs. 6 and 7)**. Postambulation, patient's recovery in 3/6 minutes and return of the vital parameters to baseline is subsequently monitored.[25]

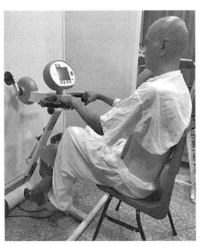

Fig. 6: Active passive trainer.

Home Exercise Program

On the day of discharge, a detailed home exercise program combined with both aerobic and resistance exercises should be chalked out on the basis of the patient's current functional capacity. Exercises should be gradually increased in intensity and duration. Walking can be gradually increased by 5 minutes duration every week. The patient can be taught to self-monitor the intensity of walking by RPE. If the patient can talk during walking without stopping for breath, then the intensity of aerobic training can be considered within moderate limits. The commonest problem with home-based programs, in spite of proper instructions, is the patient's compliance and adherence to exercises and walking. This can be resolved by emphasizing on supervised exercise training programs and regular follow-ups, whenever feasible. Studies have shown that supervised

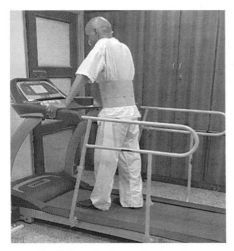

Fig. 7: Treadmill exercise training.

exercises are safe and feasible, helps regain preoperative functional capacity and improves the postoperative quality of life.[25,43]

CONCLUSION

Evidence-based perioperative care protocols include a multidisciplinary approach which helps to reduce the length of hospital stay and postoperative pulmonary complications. Prehabilitation programs have positive effects on improving health outcomes after surgery. Postoperative rehabilitation reduces postoperative pulmonary complications, prevents deconditioning, and promotes early recovery and discharge from the hospital. Home exercise programs with good compliance help patients regain their functional status and promote improved quality of life.

REFERENCES

1. Rose J, Chang DC, Weiser TG, Kassebaum NJ, Bickler SW. The role of surgery in global health: analysis of United States inpatient procedure frequency by condition using the global burden of disease 2010 framework. PLoS One. 2014;9:e89693.

2. Weiser TG, Haynes AB, Molina G, Lipsitz SR, Esquivel MM, Uribe-Leitz T, et al. Estimate of the global volume of surgery in 2012: an assessment supporting improved health outcomes. Lancet. 2015;385:S11.

3. Li C, Carli F, Lee L, Charlebois P, Stein B, Liberman AS, et al. Impact of a trimodal prehabilitation program on functional recovery after colorectal cancer surgery: a pilot study. Surg Endosc. 2013;27:1072-82.

4. Prehabilitation, rehabilitation, and revocation in the Army. Br Med J. 1946;1:192-7.

5. Carli F, Gillis C, Scheede-Bergdahl C. Promoting a culture of prehabilitation for the surgical cancer patient. Acta Oncol. 2017;56:128-33.

6. Le Roy B, Selvy M, Slim K. The concept of prehabilitation: What the surgeon needs to know? J Visc Surg. 2016;153:109-12.

7. Santa Mina D, Clarke H, Ritvo P, Leung YW, Matthew AG, Katz J. Effect of total body prehabilitation on postoperative outcomes: a systematic review and meta-analysis. Physiotherapy. 2014;100:196-207.

8. Chen BP, Awasthi R, Sweet SN, Minnella EM, Bergdahl A, Mina DS, et al. Four-week prehabilitation program is sufficient to modify exercise behaviors and improve preoperative functional walking capacity in patients with colorectal cancer. Support Care Cancer. 2017;25:33-40.

9. Minnella EM, Carli F. Prehabilitation and functional recovery for colorectal cancer patients. Eur J Surg Oncol. 2018;44:919-26.

10. Sahrmann SA. Diagnosis by the physical therapist—a prerequisite for treatment. A special communication. Phys Ther. 1988;68:1703-6.

11. Levett DZ, Grocott MP. Cardiopulmonary exercise testing, prehabilitation, and enhanced recovery after surgery (ERAS). Can J Anaesth. 2015;62:131-42.

12. ATS Committee on Proficiency Standards for Clinical Pulmonary Function Laboratories. ATS statement: guidelines for the six-minute walk test. Am J Respir Crit Care Med. 2002;166:111-7.

13. Aaldriks AA, van der Geest LG, Giltay EJ, le Cessie S, Portielje JE, Tanis BC, et al. Frailty and malnutrition predictive of mortality risk in older patients with advanced colorectal cancer receiving chemotherapy. J Geriatr Oncol. 2013;4:218-26.

14. Van Dijk DP, van de Poll MC, Moses AG, Preston T, Olde Damink SW, Rensen SS, et al. Effects of oral meal feeding on whole body protein breakdown and protein synthesis in cachectic pancreatic cancer patients. J Cachexia Sarcopenia Muscle. 2015;6:212-21.

15. Weimann A, Braga M, Carli F, Higashiguchi T, Hubner M, Klek S, et al. ESPEN guideline: clinical nutrition in surgery. Clin Nutr. 2017;36:623-50.

16. Rosenberger PH, Jokl P, Ickovics J. Psychosocial factors and surgical outcomes: an evidence-based literature review. J Am Acad Orthop Surg. 2006;14:397-405.

17. Mavros MN, Athanasiou S, Gkegkes ID, Polyzos KA, Peppas G, Falagas ME. Do psychological variables affect early surgical recovery? PLoS One. 2011;6:e20306.

18. Johnston M, Vögele C. Benefits of psychological preparation for surgery: a meta-analysis. Ann Behav Med. 1993;l5:245-56.

19. Theadom A, Cropley M. Effects of preoperative smoking cessation on the incidence and risk of intraoperative and postoperative complications in adult smokers: a systematic review. Tob Control. 2006;15:352-8.

20. Tonnesen H, Rosenberg J, Nielsen HJ, Rasmussen V, Hauge C, Pedersen IK, et al. Effect of preoperative abstinence on poor postoperative outcome in alcohol misusers: randomised controlled trial. Br Med J. 1999;318:1311-6.

21. American College of Sports Medicine. American College of Sports Medicine position stand. Progression models in resistance training for healthy adults. Med Sci Sports Exerc. 2009;41:687-708.

22. Sasso JP, Eves ND, Christensen JF, Koelwyn GJ, Scott J, Jones LW. A framework for prescription in exercise-oncology research. J Cachexia Sarcopenia Muscle. 2015;6:115-24.

23. Thompson WR, Gordon NF, Pescatello LS. ACSM's Guidelines for Exercise Testing and Prescription, 8th edition. United States: American College of Sports Medicine; 2010.

24. Carli F, Charlebois P, Stein B, Feldman L, Zavorsky G, Kim DJ, et al. Randomized clinical trial of prehabilitation in colorectal surgery. Br J Surg. 2010;97:1187-97.

25. Ahmad AM. Essentials of physiotherapy after thoracic surgery: what physiotherapists need to know. A Narrative Review. Korean J Thorac Cardiovasc Surg. 2018;51:293-307.

26. Melnyk M, Casey RG, Black P, Koupparis AJ. Enhanced recovery after surgery (ERAS) protocols: Time to change practice? Can Urol Assoc J. 2011;5:342-8.

27. Hanekom S, Louw QA, Coetzee AR. Implementations of a protocol facilitates evidence-based physiotherapy practice in intensive care units. Physiotherapy. 2013;99:139-45.

28. Qureshi SM, Pushparajah K, Taylor D, et al. Anaesthesia for paediatric diagnostic and interventional cardiological procedures. Contin Educ Anaesth Crit Care Pain. 2015;15:1-6.

29. Sugimachi K, Ueo H, Natsuda Y, Kai H, Inokuchi K, Zaitsu A. Cough dynamics in oesophageal cancer: prevention of postoperative pulmonary complications. Br J Surg. 1982;69:734-6.

30. Weeks A, Campbell C, Rajendram P, Shi W, Voigt L. A Descriptive Report of Early Mobilization for Critically Ill Ventilated Patients with Cancer. Rehabil Oncol. 2017;35:144-50.

31. Oberwaldner B. Physiotherapy for airway clearance in paediatrics. Eur Respir J. 2000;15:196-204.

32. Shingavi SS, Kazi A, Gunjal S, Lamuvel M. Effects of active cycle of breathing technique and autogenic drainage in patient with abdominal surgery. Int J Appl Res. 2017;3:373-6.

33. Wange P, Jiandani MP, Mehta A. Incentive spirometry versus active cycle of breathing technique: effect on chest expansion and flow rates in post abdominal surgery patients. Int J Res Med Sci. 2016;4:4762-6.

34. Lamuvel MW, Kazi A, Gunjal S, Jaiswal A. Effect of ACBT and TENS on Pulmonary Function and Pain Perception in Abdominal Surgeries: A Randomized Control Trial. Int J Health Sci Res. 2016;6;211-7.

35. Melzack R. Prolonged relief of pain by brief intense transcutaneous somatic stimulation. Pain. 1975;1:357-73.

36. Salmon P, Hall GM. A theory of postoperative fatigue. J R Soc Med. 1997;90:661-4.

37. Oliveira M, Oliveira G, Souza-Talarico J, Mota D. Surgical oncology: evolution of postoperative fatigue and factors related to its severity. Clin J Oncol Nurs. 2016;20:E3-8.

38. Leditschke IA, Green M, Irvine J, Bissett B, Mitchell IA. What are the barriers to mobilizing intensive care patients? Cardiopulm Phys Ther J. 2012;23:26-9.

39. Dittmer DK, Teasell R. Complications of immobilization and bed rest. Part 1: Musculoskeletal and cardiovascular complications. Can Fam Physician. 1993;39:1428-32.

40. Castelino T, Fiore JF Jr, Niculiseanu P, Landry T, Augustin B, Feldman LS. The effect of early mobilization protocols on postoperative outcomes following abdominal and thoracic surgery: A systematic review. Surgery. 2016;159:991-1003.

41. de Almeida EPM, de Almeida JP, Landoni G, Galas FRBG, Fukushima JT, Fominskiy E, et al. Early mobilization programme improves functional capacity after major abdominal cancer surgery: a randomized controlled trial. Br J Anaesth. 2017;119:900-7.

42. Needham DM, Korupolu R, Zanni JM, Pradhan P, Colantuoni E, Palmer JB, et al. Early physical medicine and rehabilitation for patients with acute respiratory failure: a quality improvement project. Arch Phys Med Rehabil. 2010;91:536-42.

43. Jones LW, Eves ND, Peterson BL, Garst J, Crawford J, West MJ, et al. Safety and feasibility of aerobic training on cardiopulmonary function and quality of life in postsurgical nonsmall cell lung cancer patients: a pilot study. Cancer. 2008;113:3430-9.

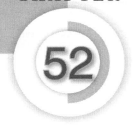
Physiotherapy and Weaning from Mechanical Ventilation

Sohan Lal Solanki, Gauri Raman Gangakhedkar, Karishma Shah

INTRODUCTION

The focus of management of critical illnesses has transformed from preventing deaths due to life-threatening illnesses to a multispecialty therapeutic intervention to not only treat the disease at hand, but also allow early resumption of normal life. A comparison of intensive care unit (ICU) outcomes among European patients over a decade revealed that in spite of admitting older patients with higher Sequential Organ Failure Assessment (SOFA) scores, recently admitted patients had a lower proportion of those requiring mechanical ventilation (53% vs. 58.8%, $P < 0.001$). ICU mortality was also reduced, particularly with those in sepsis.[1] Achieving these targets becomes particularly difficult in patients who have had required prolonged ICU stay and required prolonged ventilatory support.

Prolonged critical illnesses necessitate immobilization, which causes a myriad of adverse effects on all the organ systems. In addition to muscle wasting, reduction in muscle mass, and increased bone resorption, there is an increased incidence of cardiac deconditioning, risk of thromboembolic events, pressure ulcers, insulin resistance, development of delirium or cognitive processing impairments, and alterations in sleep patterns.[2] Furthermore, the risk of developing ICU-associated weakness (ICUAW) has been found to be anywhere between 25 and 100% in patients having an ICU stay lasting longer than 7 days.[2,3] This proves to be deleterious and contributes to delayed discharges from the ICU. The added time spent in the ICU could further complicate the patient's ICU stay with nosocomial infections and thus comprising a vicious cycle (**Fig. 1**). Moitra et al. studied 34,696 patients who were discharged from the hospital after an ICU stay. By analyzing the ICU stay and postdischarge follow-up, they correlated that every additional day of ICU stay (>7 days) increased the odds of death by 1 year of 1.04 [95% confidence interval (CI) 1.03–1.05] whether they required mechanical ventilation or not.[4]

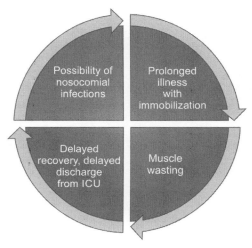

Fig. 1: Vicious cycle triggered by critical illnesses.
(ICU: intensive care unit)

As a consequence, care must be exercised at each point to ensure just as fervent a commitment to the musculoskeletal recovery as there is to the expedited recovery of the illness causing the ICU admission.

Mechanically ventilated patients comprise 15% of the total number of critically ill patients.[5] Mechanical ventilations and the use of sedation to ensure tube tolerance promote immobilization and hence form independent contributory factors for muscle wasting.[2,5] The first focus of all strategies to decrease the overall ICU stay thus remains, to rid the patient of his/her need for ventilatory support using the process of weaning. Weaning as a term comprises the whole process of liberating the patients from mechanical ventilation and endotracheal tube.[6] While various clinical and ventilatory parameters (**Table 1**) are used to identify if the patient is likely to have a successful course of weaning, the primary criterion to be fulfilled, is the successful resolution of the disease process.

Table 1: Common criteria for starting weaning process.[6]

Category	Example	
Clinical criteria	Resolution of acute phase of disease	
	Adequate cough	
	Absence of excessive secretions	
	Cardiovascular and hemodynamic stability	
Ventilatory criteria	Spontaneous breathing trial	Tolerates for 20–30 minutes
	$PaCO_2$	<50 mm Hg with normal pH
	Vital capacity	>10 mL/kg
	Spontaneous VT	>5 mL/kg
	Spontaneous f	<35/min
	f/VT	<100 breaths/min/L
	Minute ventilation	<10 L with satisfactory ABG
Oxygenation criteria	PaO_2 without PEEP	>60 mm Hg at FIO_2 up to 0.4
	PaO_2 with PEEP (<8 cm H_2O)	>100 mm Hg at FIO_2 up to 0.4
	SaO_2	>90% at FiO_2 up to 0.4
	PaO_2/FiO_2 (P/F)	≥150 mm Hg
	QS/QT	<20%
	$P(A-a) O_2$	<350 mm Hg at FiO_2 of 1.0
Pulmonary reserve	Vital capacity	>10 mL/kg
	Maximum inspiratory pressure	>–30 cm H_2O in 20 seconds
Pulmonary measurements	Static compliance	>30 mL/cm H_2O
	Airway resistance	Stable or improving
	VD/VT	<60% while intubated

(f: respiratory rate; FiO_2: inspiratory oxygen fraction; $P(A-a)O_2$: Alveolar to arterial oxygen gradient; PaO_2: arterial oxygen tension; PEEP: positive end-expiratory pressure; QS/QT: ratio of physiologic shunt to total perfusion; SaO_2: arterial oxygen saturation; VC: vital capacity; VD: dead space volume; VT: tidal volume)

It is vital that all institutes have a protocol in place to assess and assist weaning from mechanical ventilation. The presence of strong protocols enables regular screening of respiratory function and spontaneous breathing trials (SBT) and thus decreases the time to extubation, reduces the incidence of self-extubation, the incidence of tracheostomy and ICU costs, and a potentially reduced incidence of reintubation.[7]

Once these criteria are met, the next step to be applied is to subject the patient to tests to ensure a successful weaning process. This includes SBT where, using either a T-piece, continuous positive airway pressure (CPAP), or

Table 2: Factors that can potentially lead to failure of SBT.

Increased respiratory load	• Reduced compliance • Increased work of breathing • Increased airway resistance • Bronchoconstriction
Increased cardiac load	• Preexisting cardiac dysfunction • Myocardial dysfunction due to increased cardiac workload
Neuromuscular causes	• Central ventilatory command • Depressed central drive • Critical illness neuromuscular abnormalities (CINMA)
Neuropsycho-logical causes	• Anxiety • Depression • Delirium
Metabolic causes	• Role of corticosteroids • Hyperglycemia
Nutritional abnormalities	• Malnutrition • Obesity • Ventilator-induced diaphragm dysfunction
Anemia	

(SBT: spontaneous breathing trial)

automatic tube compensation (ATC), the patient is allowed to breathe spontaneously for 30 minutes. If the patient shows a normal respiratory pattern, adequate gas exchange, and hemodynamic stability during the course of SBT, either as a stand-alone measure or with the use of either oxygenation or mild pressure support supplementation, the patient can be extubated.[6] There are studies where longer durations of SBT, 60–120 minutes, have been used, but since most patients exhibit failure in the first 20–30 minutes of the test, such extended testing periods are not recommended.[8,9] If the patient fails the first attempt at SBT, supportive modes of ventilation need to be instituted while evaluating the reasons for SBT failure. The common causes for SBT failure are as mentioned in **Table 2**.[6,7]

Factors leading to failure of SBT need to be investigated and corrected before attempting the SBT again. Until such time that the patient is deemed fit to undergo another SBT trial, the patient can be put on weaning modes on the ventilator that offer partial ventilatory support. The process of weaning is described in **Figure 2**.

The modes of mechanical ventilation have been discussed in Chapter 63, so this chapter shall only briefly cover the various weaning modes with the special features of each of them:[6,7]

- *Pressure support mode (PSV):* This is one of the most popular modes for weaning with ample scientific evidence to back its use in clinical practice. PSV may be used either by itself or in conjunction with synchronized intermittent mandatory ventilation (SIMV) mode. Weaning is usually started with PSV at a level of 5–15

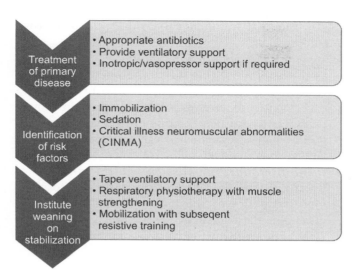

Fig. 2: Process of weaning.

cm H_2O (up to 40 cm H_2O) to augment spontaneous tidal volume until a desired volume (10–15 mL/kg) or spontaneous frequency (<25/min) is reached. The support is then gradually reduced by 3–6 cm H_2O till a level close to 5 cm H_2O is reached with the patient maintaining his/her ventilation. Extubation can be considered at this point.

- *Synchronized intermittent mandatory ventilation:* SIMV is not recommended as a stand-alone mode for weaning. The target is to shift the work of breathing from the ventilator to the patient by gradually reducing the mandatory breaths to 2–4/min, while measuring blood gases to ensure oxygenation. SIMV is sometimes used in conjunction with PSV to aid weaning.

- *Volume support (VS) and volume-assisted pressure support (VAPS):* In VS, the pressure support level adjusts automatically to achieve the target tidal volume. In VAPS, the preset tidal volume is achieved by incorporating inspiratory PSV with conventional volume-assisted cycles. VAPS can be used to deliver a stable tidal volume in patients with irregular breathing patterns.

- *Mandatory minute ventilation (MMV):* In MMV, the ventilator adjusts the frequency to achieve the target minute ventilation automatically.

- *Airway pressure-release ventilation (APRV):* This mode has two pressure levels. The tidal volume is determined by the pressure gradient between the higher airway pressure (e.g., 10 cm H_2O) and the lower release pressure (usually 0 cm H_2O). The expiration occurs during pressure release and inspiration occurs when the pressure returns to the airway pressure.

- *Automatic tube compensation:* ATC reduces the airway resistance imposed by the artificial airway (endotracheal or tracheostomy tube) and allows the patient to have a breathing pattern as if breathing spontaneously. This may facilitate breathing efficacy and reduce the work of breathing.

- *Noninvasive ventilation (NIV):* NIV is an extremely useful mode in weaning the patient off ventilatory support, since it can lead to decreased work of breathing and an increase in dynamic lung compliance, tidal volume, and inspiratory capacity with a subsequent improvement in blood gases. It has been discussed in Chapter 63.

During this rather demanding process of weaning, all efforts must be directed toward the employment of a comprehensive interdisciplinary rehabilitation program to ensure early recovery. Effective physiotherapy is paramount by assisting in both respiratory and musculoskeletal rehabilitation physiotherapy.

RESPIRATORY PHYSIOTHERAPY

The traditional role of physiotherapists in the ICU has centered around the respiratory care they provide in mechanically ventilated patients. Impaired or inhibited cough, and depressed mucociliary function due to intubation and sedation, leads to the sequestration of secretions which form a potential growth medium for bacteria and could possibly cause pneumonia.[10] Additionally, supine position leads to decreased functional residual capacity, atelectasis due to closure of dependent airways, increased airway resistance, and an increased pulmonary blood volume leading to a ventilation—perfusion (V/Q) mismatch.[10] The understanding is that optimization of ventilation, ensuring airway clearance, will prevent pulmonary complications and hasten weaning.[11,12] In keeping with this, the strategy employed is:

- *Positioning:*[11,13-15] Changing the patient from supine position aids in reducing V/Q mismatch and thus assists ventilation. In patients with unilateral lung disease, the affected lung is to be positioned at the uppermost location, thus increasing recruitment and promotes drainage from the lung segment. Rotating or kinetic frames are an innovative alternative which ensure continuous rotation with a specific rotational bed and help reduce the pulmonary complications. Delaney et al. were able to demonstrate a significant reduction in the incidence of nosocomial pneumonia, but no difference in weaning or mortality.

- *Percussion and bibration:*[10,13,16,17] While percussion uses cupped hands or the palm cup to enhance airway clearance by manually clapping the affected lung, performing postural drainage, and thus allowing shifting of secretions from the peripheral airway to the central airway, vibrations use oscillatory positive expiratory-pressure devices such as Flutter and Acapella

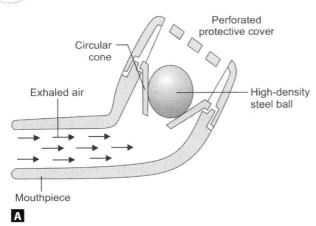

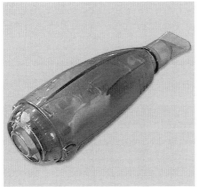

Figs. 3A and B: (A) Flutter; (B) Acapella.

(Smiths Medical, Carlsbad, CA, USA) (**Fig. 3**) to conduct chest oscillation and compression together during the expiratory phase to improve peak expiratory flow rates by >50%. These devices help reduce airway collapse and improve mucus discharge, enhancing lung function and oxygenation. They can be used three to four times a day depending on the patient's condition.

- *Hyperinflation:*[10,13,18,19] Lung hyperinflation is used to prevent pulmonary collapse and allow re-expansion of collapsed alveoli. It also improves gas exchange by promoting secretion removal and increases lung compliance. After a manometer is connected to the ventilatory circuit, expiratory flow is induced after sufficient inspiration and 2–3 seconds of inspiratory hold is maintained. The manometer helps reduce the incidence of barotrauma. The large tidal volumes and increased intrathoracic pressures are likely to reduce venous return, so hemodynamic stability must be ensured before hyperinflation is initiated. Both manual hyperinflation (MHI) and ventilator hyperinflation have been described to be equally effective but the feedback received by the physiotherapist, through the resuscitator bag, allows estimation of lung compliance. Bertie et al. conducted a randomized-controlled trial (RCT) where they were able to hasten weaning and reduce the ICU stay using MHI in combination with expiratory rib cage compression.

- *Mechanical insufflation exsufflation:*[13,18] Also known as inexsufflation, this forms a popular method of excess sputum removal in patients who are not able to expectorate by themselves because of an impaired cough reflex. The device inflates the lung to a large volume with positive pressure and then a negative pressure is rapidly applied to mimic a physiological cough.

- *Intrapulmonary percussive ventilation:*[13,18,20,21] By simultaneously providing positive pressure, high-frequency oscillations and aerosol delivery, intrapulmonary percussive ventilation can reduce the work of breathing by increasing sputum removal and lung expansion. Intrapulmonary percussive ventilation is an attractive option for patients with cystic fibrosis, bronchiectasis, chronic obstructive pulmonary disease, acute respiratory failure, and even those with tracheostomies, since it has to be given for a short duration of time (15 minutes) at a time. However, like with hyperinflation techniques, hemodynamic instability needs to be watched out for.

- *Suctioning:*[10] Once the secretions have been mobilized from the periphery to the center, they can be gently suctioned out. The recommended technique is to use a catheter no wider than half the diameter of the endotracheal/tracheostomy tube, for <15 seconds and using a pressure between 11 and 16 kPa (up to 20 kPa for thick secretions). Though either technique can be used, closed suction is recommended over open, since it minimizes interruptions during ventilation and reduces risk of both hypoxia and contamination.

MUSCULOSKELETAL PHYSIOTHERAPY

Since the culprits leading to muscle wasting are known to be immobilization, measures need to be taken to counteract the effects using techniques to retrain the muscles to endure the overload and thus mitigate the effects of immobilization.[2,22] Mobilization of patients in the critical care setup, either active or passive, provides multisystemic benefits as described in **Table 3**. Early mobilization is the key to early recovery. Even when patients are intubated, mobilization can be initiated, when hemodynamic and neurological stability is achieved. This includes use of semirecumbent (45°) positioning, 2-hourly changes in position, daily passive movement of all joints, passive bed cycling, and electrical stimulation as indicated.[14,18,23,24] In fact, Schweikert et al. published a landmark paper where they demonstrated a significantly reduced time to independent function status when exercises were started during the sedation-free time of the day, as early as day 2 of ventilation.[25] While active exercises may take longer

Table 3: Benefits of mobilization.[11]

System	Effects
Pulmonary system	Improves ventilation–perfusion rate and depth of respiration, facilitates mucociliary clearance, and improves strength and quality of cough
Cardiovascular system	Improves stroke volume and venous return, myocardial contractility, coronary perfusion, and heart rate
	Reduces peripheral vascular resistance and improves peripheral blood flow
Muscular system	Improves blood flow to exercising muscle
	Facilitates better oxygen extraction
Neurological system	Improves alertness and arousal
	Increases cerebral electrical activity
Hematological system	Reduces circulatory stasis
Lymphatic system	Improves pulmonary lymphatic flow and drainage
Endocrine system	Increases release, distribution, and degradation of catecholamines
Renal system	Improves glomerular filtration and urine output
Gastrointestinal system	Improves gut mobility
Integumentary system	Improves cutaneous circulation

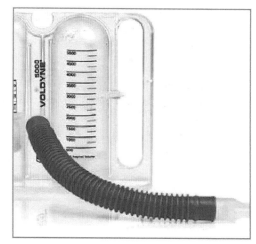

Fig. 4: Incentive spirometer.

to establish, measures such as assisted limb movements, or even use of low-voltage electrical currents to stimulate skeletal muscles, can be employed.[2,18,25,26]

The various approaches that are employed for mobilization are as follows:

- *Respiratory muscle training:*[13,18,27,28] Weakened respiratory muscles are unable to bear the load of the ventilation, which could lead to weaning failure. Additionally, the diaphragm also undergoes atrophy with prolonged ventilation. Inspiratory muscle training helps both inspiratory and expiratory muscle strengthening and can reduce the duration of ventilation and weaning. The technique used is known as threshold loading. In this, the threshold loading is set between 20% and 50% of the maximum inspiratory pressure, and five sets with 6–10 breaths per set are performed once or twice a day. The threshold is increased as the patients' respiratory strength improves.

- *Deep breathing exercises:*[10,28] Used either by itself or in conjunction with other techniques in nonintubated patients, deep breathing exercises help train the patients to breathe using their diaphragm and not accessory muscles. The goals behind instituting deep breathing are to reverse atelectasis, increase oxygenation, aid alveolar recruitment, increase functional residual capacity and tidal volumes, and potentially help removal of secretions.

- *Incentive spirometry:*[10,13,29] Incentive spirometry is a time-tested, well-established tool that helps provide a visual feedback to the patient and thus helps promote maximal inspiration, in nonintubated patients. Patients are usually asked to perform 5–10 repetitions of a sequence of performing deep breathing slowly, holding the breath for 2–3 seconds, and then exhaling slowly. Patient cooperation is essential (**Fig. 4**).

- *Intermittent positive pressure breathing:*[10,30] In spontaneously breathing patients or even tracheostomized spontaneously breathing patients, inspiratory positive pressure is applied using a mask or mouthpiece. It has the facility to also deliver aerosols. It can be used to augment inspiratory muscle training.

- *Neuromuscular electrical stimulation (NMES):*[18,31-33] NMES can be used without leading to any form of ventilatory stress, even in patients who are supine. NMES promotes muscular microcirculation, delays muscle atrophy during the immobility period, and improves muscle strength and endurance. Currently, however, there is little evidence to suggest additional clinical benefit of NMES over other techniques, but it seems to show promise in chronic obstructive pulmonary disease, congestive cardiac failure, and ICU neuromyopathy.

- *Passive range of movement (ROM) and stretching:*[13,18,26,34] Passive motion in immobilized patients prevents contracture and preserves the architecture of muscle fibers. It also helps reduce the risk of thromboembolism. A decreased length of hospital stay was found in patients who required mechanical ventilation when passive ROM using a gradual mobility protocol for both upper and lower limbs was instituted.

- *Cycle ergometer:*[13,24] Normal ROM can be maintained sedated, immobilized, and bedridden patients, using passive cycle ergometers. Active-assisted and

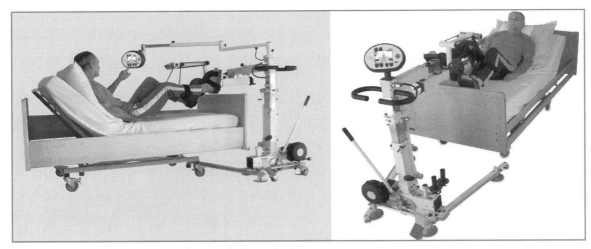

Fig. 5: Cycle ergometer.

activeresistive modes can be used once the patient recovers. Cycle ergometers help to strengthen the quadriceps force and increase exercise capacity (**Fig. 5**).

- *Tilt table:*[13,35] A tilt table provides partial weight bearing and assists in the gradual transition from bed rest to bearing the full body weight. It also helps improve lower limb strength, prevent ankle joint contracture, and enhance patient arousal.

- *Active mobilization and resistive muscle training:*[10,11,13,18,35-37] Active mobilization involves sitting at the edge of the bed, standing (with the assistance of the physiotherapist and with or without the help of standing or walking aids), transfers from bed to chair, chair-based exercises, walking in one place, and eventually walking. Active mobilization aims at optimizing oxygen transport by enhancing alveolar ventilation and V/Q matching, and it also represents a gravitational stimulus to maintain or restore normal fluid distribution in the body.

Resistive muscle training increases muscle mass and force generation. Cycle ergometers, as described above, can be used in an assistive and resistive capacity to provide the same. Exercise tools such as elastic bands and pulleys can also be used to perform exercises in bed. Tools such as the Borg Rate of Perceived Exertion are used to assess the patient's perceived fatigue before, during, and after exercise to monitor and subsequently tailor the patient's exercise intensity.

ROLE OF PHYSIOTHERAPISTS IN WEANING: CURRENT EVIDENCE AND TRENDS

Over a decade ago, the European Society of Intensive Care Medicine issued a statement suggesting that the physiotherapist should be responsible for implementing mobilization plans and exercise prescription and make recommendations for progression of these in conjunction with other team members involved in patient care.[10,14] This would be useful to setup what is now termed as therapist driven protocol (TDP).[38] There is scientific evidence to suggest that TDP is a successful gambit and indeed results in faster weaning with reduced costs and complications.[18,39] Despite the availability of evidence, recent studies show that the adoption of TDPs across the world is infrequent and not as popular as would be expected among critical care setups.

Morar et al. did a questionnaire-based study among physiotherapists working in ICU setups in South Africa, where an alarming majority (73%) reported that they were seldom or never involved in ICU decision-making, though a majority of them worked in open ICUs.[40] They responded positively, however, to performing active-assisted and active exercises for mobilization and respiratory muscle strengthening. They also reported extremely low levels of physiotherapy autonomy, with regards to weaning, and implementation of all changes was usually directly supervised by a medical colleague.

A survey conducted in Brazilian Neonatal and Pediatric Intensive Care Units had slightly better results.[41] Although 66.7% were involved in actually changing the ventilator settings, fewer number of them were a part of the decision-making process. Neonatal intensive care units (NICUs) showed better numbers with regards to their involvement in the decision and actually performing the weaning, as compared to a pediatric intensive care unit (PICU). The availability of physiotherapists in the ICU was found to be proportional to the role they were allotted. In setups where they were a part of the decision-making, therapists were available round the clock, whereas in other units they were available for around 18 hours.

Cork et al. published an interesting paper, which highlighted the role of physiotherapists in the decision-making during the weaning process.[42] Physiotherapists were asked to assess and stratify risk of extubation failure in patients just before they were extubated. Patients who were classified as high risk or with inappropriate mentation were likely to fail extubation, four and three times more than their counterparts, respectively. They also found that specialist physiotherapists were more likely to predict the feasibility extubation more accurately. What is important to note is that while the physiotherapists were consulted, the final decision for extubation rested with the ICU consultant alone. This is reflected in the cases which resulted in extubation failure. The physiotherapists classified 22% of the patients as high risk. 55.5% of these underwent reintubation. Had the physiotherapist's advice been taken into account, the numbers could potentially be much lower. This study provides additional proof that a change in ICU weaning policies is mandated.

CONCLUSION

Weaning from mechanical ventilation is an important process and usually starts with a patient's admission in an ICU. Physiotherapists play a crucial role in influencing the course of ICU stay among critically ill patients. In addition to the classical roles attributed to them for respiratory physiotherapy, by promoting early mobilization and resistive training, they are able to compound the effects of good medical care and thus enable patients to leave the ICU sooner and with fewer complications. In spite of the availability of overwhelming evidence to suggest that physiotherapy reduces the time taken for extubation, reduces in-hospital and out-of-hospital mortality, and allows earlier resumption of functional existence, there is still a sense of resistance in implementing TDP for weaning. With increasing life expectancy and easy availability of advanced medical care, increasingly sicker patients get admitted to ICUs. As a result, involving the physiotherapists as core members for decision-making in weaning from ventilatory support is likely to be a game changer with regard to critical care outcomes.

REFERENCES

1. Vincent JL, Lefrant JY, Kotfis K, Nanchal R, Martin-Loeches I, Wittebole X, et al. Comparison of European ICU patients in 2012 (ICON) versus 2002 (SOAP). Intensive Care Med. 2018;44(3): 337-44.

2. Parry SM, Puthucheary ZA. The impact of extended bed rest on the musculoskeletal system in the critical care environment. Extrem Physiol Med. 2015;4:16.

3. De Jonghe B, Sharshar T, Lefaucheur JP, Authier FJ, Durand-Zaleski I, Boussarsar M, et al. Paresis acquired in the intensive care unit: a prospective multicenter study. JAMA. 2002;288(22):2859-67.

4. Moitra VK, Guerra C, Linde-Zwirble WT, Wunsch H. Relationship between ICU length of stay and long-term mortality for elderly ICU survivors. Crit Care Med. 2016;44(4):655-62.

5. Schreiber AF, Ceriana P, Ambrosino N, Malovini A, Nava S. Physiotherapy and weaning from prolonged mechanical ventilation. Respir Care. 2019;64(1):17-25.

6. Chang DW, Hiers JH. Weaning from mechanical ventilation. In: Clinical Applications of Mechanical Ventilation, 4th edition. New York, New York: Delmar; 2014. pp. 517-44.

7. Boles JM, Bion J, Connors A, Herridge M, Marsh B, Melot C, et al. Weaning from mechanical ventilation. Eur Respir J. 2007;29(5):1033-56.

8. Yang KL, Tobin MJ. A prospective study of indexes predicting the outcome of trials of weaning from mechanical ventilation. N Engl J Med. 1991;324(21):1445-50.

9. Perren A, Domenighetti G, Mauri S, Genini F, Vizzardi N. Protocol-directed weaning from mechanical ventilation: clinical outcome in patients randomized for a 30-min or 120-min trial with pressure support ventilation. Intensive Care Med. 2002;28(8):1058-63.

10. Pathmanathan N, Beaumont N, Gratrix A. Respiratory physiotherapy in the critical care unit. Contin Educ Anaesth Crit Care Pain. 2015;15(1):20-5.

11. Bhat A, Vasanthan LT, Babu AS. Role of physiotherapy in weaning of patients from mechanical ventilation in the intensive care unit. Indian J Respir Care. 2017;6(2):813-9.

12. Strickland SL, Rubin BK, Drescher GS, Haas CF, O'Malley CA, Volsko TA, et al. AARC clinical practice guideline: effectiveness of nonpharmacologic airway clearance therapies in hospitalized patients. Respir Care. 2013;58(12):2187-93.

13. Jang MH, Shin MJ, Shin YB. Pulmonary and physical rehabilitation in critically ill patients. Acute Crit Care. 2019;34(1):1-13.

14. Gosselink R, Bott J, Johnson M, Dean E, Nava S, Norrenberg M, et al. Physiotherapy for adult patients with critical illness: recommendations of the European Respiratory Society and European Society of Intensive Care Medicine Task Force on physiotherapy for critically Ill patients. Intensive Care Med. 2008;34(7):1188-99.

15. Delaney A, Gray H, Laupland KB, Zuege DJ. Kinetic bed therapy to prevent nosocomial pneumonia in mechanically ventilated patients: a systematic review and meta-analysis. Crit Care. 2006;10(3):R70.

16. McCarren B, Alison JA, Herbert RD. Manual vibration increases expiratory flow rate via increased intrapleural pressure in healthy adults: an experimental study. Aust J Physiother. 2006;52(4):267-71.

17. Hristara-Papadopoulou A, Tsanakas J, Diomou G, Papadopoulou O. Current devices of respiratory physiotherapy. Hippokratia. 2008;12(4):211-20.

18. Ambrosino N, Venturelli E, Vagheggini G, Clini E. Rehabilitation, weaning and physical therapy strategies in chronic critically ill patients. Eur Respir J. 2012;39(2):487-92.

19. Berti JS, Tonon E, Ronchi CF, Berti HW, Stefano LM, Gut AL, et al. Manual hyperinflation combined with expiratory rib cage compression for reduction of length of ICU stay in critically ill patients on mechanical ventilation. J Bras Pneumol. 2012;38(4):477-86.

20. Paneroni M, Clini E, Simonelli C, Bianchi L, Degli Antoni F, Vitacca M. Safety and efficacy of short-term intrapulmonary percussive ventilation in patients with bronchiectasis. Respir Care. 2011;56(7):984-8.

21. Clini EM, Antoni FD, Vitacca M, Crisafulli E, Paneroni M, Chezzi-Silva S, et al. Intrapulmonary percussive ventilation in tracheostomized patients: a randomized controlled trial. Intensive Care Med. 2006;32(12):1994-2001.

22. Bruton A. Muscle plasticity: response to training and detraining. Physiotherapy. 2002;88(7):398-408.

23. Krishnagopalan S, Johnson EW, Low LL, Kaufman LJ. Body positioning of intensive care patients: clinical practice versus standards. Crit Care Med. 2002;30(11):2588-92.

24. Burtin C, Clerckx B, Robbeets C, Ferdinande P, Langer D, Troosters T, et al. Early exercise in critically ill patients enhances short-term functional recovery. Crit Care Med. 2009;37(9): 2499-505.

25. Schweickert WD, Pohlman MC, Pohlman AS, Nigos C, Pawlik AJ, Esbrook CL, et al. Early physical and occupational therapy in mechanically ventilated, critically ill patients: a randomised controlled trial. Lancet. 2009;373(9678):1874-82.

26. Griffiths RD, Palmer TE, Helliwell T, MacLennan P, MacMillan RR. Effect of passive stretching on the wasting of muscle in the critically ill. Nutrition. 1995;11(5):428-32.

27. Levine S, Nguyen T, Taylor N, Friscia ME, Budak MT, Rothenberg P, et al. Rapid disuse atrophy of diaphragm fibers in mechanically ventilated humans. N Engl J Med. 2008;358(13):1327-35.

28. Bissett B, Leditschke IA, Green M, Marzano V, Collins S, Van Haren F. Inspiratory muscle training for intensive care patients: a multidisciplinary practical guide for clinicians. Aust Crit Care. 2019;32(3):249-55.

29. Bartlett RH, Gazzaniga AB, Geraghty TR. Respiratory maneuvers to prevent postoperative pulmonary complications. A critical review. JAMA. 1973;224(7):1017-21.

30. Chen YH, Yeh MC, Hu HC, Lee CS, Li LF, Chen NH, et al. Effects of lung expansion therapy on lung function in patients with prolonged mechanical ventilation. Can Respir J. 2016;2016:5624315.

31. Ambrosino N, Strambi S. New strategies to improve exercise tolerance in chronic obstructive pulmonary disease. Eur Respir J. 2004;24(2):313-22.

32. Edwards J, McWilliams D, Thomas M, Shah S. Electrical muscle stimulation in the intensive care unit: an integrative review. J Intensive Care Soc. 2014;15(2):142-9.

33. Stiller K. Physiotherapy in intensive care: Towards an evidence-based practice. Chest. 2000;118(6):1801-13.

34. Morris PE, Goad A, Thompson C, Taylor K, Harry B, Passmore L, et al. Early intensive care unit mobility therapy in the treatment of acute respiratory failure. Crit Care Med. 2008;36(8):2238-43.

35. Stiller K, Phillips AC, Lambert P. The safety of mobilisation and its effect on haemodynamic and respiratory status of intensive care patients. Physiother Theory Pract. 2004;20:175-85.

36. Sommers J, Engelbert RH, Dettling-Ihnenfeldt D, Gosselink R, Spronk PE, Nollet F, et al. Physiotherapy in the intensive care unit: an evidence-based, expert driven, practical statement and rehabilitation recommendations. Clin Rehabil. 2015;29(11):1051-63.

37. Gosselink R, Clerckx B, Robbeets C, Vanhullebusch T, Vanpee G, Segers J. Physiotherapy in the intensive care unit. Neth J Crit Care. 2011;15(2):66-75.

38. Vitacca M. Therapist driven protocols. Monaldi Arch Chest Dis. 2003;59(4):342-4.

39. Saura P, Blanch L, Mestre L, Vallés J, Artigas A, Fernández R. Clinical consequences of the implementation of a weaning protocol. Intensive Care Med. 1996;22(10):1052-6.

40. Morar D, Van Aswegen H. Physiotherapy contributions to weaning and extubation of patients from mechanical ventilation. S Afr J Crit Care. 2016;32(1):6-10.

41. Bacci SLLDS, Pereira JM, Chagas ACDS, Carvalho LR, Azevedo VMGO. Role of physical therapists in the weaning and extubation procedures of pediatric and neonatal intensive care units: a survey. Braz J Phys Ther. 2019;23(4):317-23.

42. Cork G, Camporota L, Osman L, Shannon H. Physiotherapist prediction of extubation outcome in the adult intensive care unit. Physiother Res Int. 2019;24(4):e1793.

Perioperative Hemodynamic Monitoring

Harish MM, Sudhindra Prakash Kanavehalli, Atul Prabhakar Kulkarni

INTRODUCTION

Around 230 million surgical procedures are performed each year around the world and a significant number of patients are at risk of intra- or postoperative complications or both. Though less than 15% of in-patient procedures are performed in high-risk patients such patients account for 80% of the deaths.[1-3] The ones who survive to leave hospital, postoperative complications remain an important determinant of functional recovery and long-term survival.[4] Causes for these complications are multifactorial such as preoperative patient status and comorbidities, type of surgery performed and its duration, the degree of urgency, the skill and experience of the operating and anesthetic teams, and the postoperative management. But it is generally the tissue hypoperfusion and the imbalance between oxygen delivery (DO_2) and oxygen consumption, which plays an important role in the development of complications and poor outcomes.[5,6] Therefore, selecting the appropriate hemodynamic monitoring devices to prevent, diagnose, and treat hypo/hypervolemia and cardiac dysfunction, infusion of fluids, and prevention of fluid overload and titration of vasoactive drugs to maintain adequate DO_2 and prevent multiorgan failure is a vital first step in reducing the risk of complications.[7,8] Hemodynamic monitoring allows the "real-time" measurement of cardiovascular variables and dynamic parameters of fluid responsiveness to guide administration of intravenous fluids, and vasoactive drug therapy.[9] Therefore, selecting the most appropriate hemodynamic monitoring device may be an important first step in reducing the risk of complications. No single device exists at present that is able to provide the clinician with a complete and 100% accurate evaluation of cardiovascular status and each monitor is associated with its own benefits and limitations. In this chapter, we review the available hemodynamic monitoring systems and their use in the perioperative period.

HEMODYNAMIC MONITORING AND THE DIFFERENT VARIABLES

Previously anesthetists were using individual vital signs such as heart rate (HR), blood pressure (BP), central venous pressure (CVP), and urine output to guide their perioperative care. Even though they are ways to get at the best, these variables are neither sensitive nor specific enough to provide a definitive evaluation of the cardiovascular status as a whole.[10,11]

Mean arterial pressure (MAP) depends upon preload, cardiac output (CO), and the afterload vascular tone, so BP may remain normal in patients with hypovolemia, because of severe peripheral vasoconstriction. Similarly, under anesthesia, HR may not help in picking up hypovolemia.[12] An integrated assessment of various hemodynamic parameters helps in overall improvement of clinical status of the patient.[13] For example, the combination of arterial pressure and the partial pressure of end-tidal carbon dioxide ($ETCO_2$) can help differentiate between vasodilation and low CO as a cause of hypotension ($ETCO_2$ transiently decreases when CO decreases) and may prevent "reflex" fluid administration whenever BP decreases. Similarly, a reduction in the $ETCO_2$ value without any changes in the minute ventilation (in the absence of hypothermia) suggests decreased pulmonary blood flow (and thus CO) and may serve as an indicator for more advanced hemodynamic monitoring.

Arterial Blood Pressure

Continuous invasive measurement of arterial pressure helps identify the rapid fluctuations in arterial pressure that may occur in high-risk patients. Artifacts (overdamping or underdamping) should be carefully identified and eliminated, especially when systolic-diastolic components and the shape of waveform need to be analyzed. The arterial pressure waveform is, related to the changes between

SV and changes in vascular resistance, compliance and impedance of the system.[9] Currently available noninvasive hemodynamic monitoring for continuous measurement of BP is usually performed in peripheral arteries and may become unreliable in case of vasoconstriction or low peripheral flow.

Central Venous Pressure

Central venous pressure has previously been used to guide perioperative fluid therapy, but a CVP of between 5 mm Hg and 20 mm Hg has certainly almost no predictive value, and changes in CVP in response to a fluid bolus (fluid challenge) have not been shown to be predictive of fluid status.[14] CVP is affected by other variables, such as intrathoracic pressure, venous resistance, and pulmonary vascular resistance, and a recent study demonstrated that there is little value in using central venous oxygen saturation ($ScvO_2$) in isolation (obtained from a CVP catheter) as a marker of adequate systemic DO_2 after major surgery.[15]

▮ CARDIAC OUTPUT MONITORING

One parameter which had wide fluctuation in the perioperative period is total oxygen consumption (VO_2). The main target in the perioperative period is to maintain the adequate DO_2 to meet the fluctuating tissue oxygen requirements. This depends upon CO and the oxygen content of the arterial blood. Once you correct anemia and hypoxia, remaining parameter which determines DO_2 is CO. Although there are various methods available for monitoring CO, a survey indicated that only about 35% patients with high-risk surgical procedures underwent CO monitoring (**Table 1**).[16,17]

The various CO monitoring devices available today (**Table 2**) use methodologies based on indicator dilution, thermodilution, pulse pressure analysis, Doppler principles, and also Fick principle. Patient status dictates the type of CO monitoring required.

Pulmonary Artery Catheter

Even though lots of data criticized the utility of the pulmonary artery catheter (PAC) because of its invasiveness, some parameters like continuous monitoring of pulmonary artery pressure, right-sided and left-sided filling pressures, CO, and mixed venous oxygen saturation (SvO_2) are possible only with PAC.[18,19] Currently, many less invasive CO monitoring devices have replaced PAC, in some complex clinical situations (for example, cardiac surgery, organ transplant surgery, and surgery associated with major fluid shifts or high risk of respiratory failure or in patients with compromised RV function), the PAC still represents a valuable tool. But the clinicians should adequately trained in insertion and interpretation of the data provided by the PAC.[20] In such patients, the PAC can be inserted and used

Table 1: Hemodynamic monitoring routinely used in high-risk surgery patients.[17]

	ASA respondents (n = 237) Response percentage	ESA respondents (n = 195) Response percentage
Invasive arterial pressure	95.4%	89.7%
Central venous pressure	72.6%	83.6%
Noninvasive arterial pressure	51.9%	53.8%
Cardiac output	35.4%	34.9%
Pulmonary capillary wedge pressure	30.8%	14.4%
Transesophageal echocardiography	28.3%	19.0%
Systolic pressure variation	20.3%	23.6%
Plethysmographic waveform variation	17.3%	17.9%
Pulse pressure variation	15.2%	25.6%
Mixed venous saturation ($ScvO_2$)	14.3%	15.9%
Central venous saturation (SvO_2)	12.7%	33.3%
Oxygen delivery (DO_2)	6.3%	14.4%
Stroke volume variation	6.3%	21.5%
Near-infrared spectroscopy	4.6%	5.1%
Global end-diastolic volume	2.1%	8.2%

(ASA: American Society of Anesthesiology; ESA: European Society of Anesthesiology)

Table 2: Cardiac output monitoring devices.

Method	Monitoring system
Pulmonary thermodilution	Pulmonary artery catheter (PAC)
Transpulmonary thermodilution	PiCCO volume view
Transpulmonary indicator dilution	LiDCO
Arterial pressure waveform derived	PiCCO
	LiDCO
	FloTrac/Vigileo
	Volume clamp method (Finarpes, Nexfin)
Esophageal Doppler	CardioQ
Electrocardiography (TTE and TEE)	
Applied Fick (Partial CO_2 rebreathing)	NICO
Bioimpedance	Lifegard
	TEBCO
	HOTMAN
	BioZ
Bioreactance	NICOM

(TEE: transesophageal echocardiogram; TTE: transthoracic echocardiogram)

Tables 3: Parameters obtained with a pulmonary artery catheter.

Parameters	Calculation	Normal values
Measured Parameters		
RA pressure/CVP		2–6 mm Hg
RV systolic pressure		15–25 mm Hg
RV diastolic pressure		0–8 mm Hg
PA systolic pressure		15–25 mm Hg
PA diastolic pressure		8–15 mm Hg
Mean pulmonary artery pressure		10–20 mm Hg
PA occlusion pressure (wedge pressure)		6–12 mm Hg
Mixed venous saturation		60–80 %
Core temperature		36.5–37.2 °C
Cardiac output	$HR \times SV / 1{,}000$	4–8 L/min
Stroke volume	$CO/HR \times 1000$	60–100 mL/beat
Cardiac index	CO/BSA	2.5–4L/min/m^2
Stroke volume index (SVI)	$CI/HR \times 1{,}000$	33–47 mL/m^2/beat
Calculated Parameters		
Systemic vascular resistance (SVR)	$80 \times (MAP - RAP)/CO$	800–1,200 dynes sec/cm^{-5}
Systemic vascular resistance index (SVRI)	$80 \times (MAP - RAP)/CI$	1970–2390 dynes sec/cm^{-5}/m^2
Pulmonary vascular resistance (PVR)	$80 \times (MPAP - PAOP)/CO$	<250 dynes–sec/cm^{-5}
Pulmonary vascular resistance index (PVRI)	$80 \times (MPAP - PAOP)/CI$	255–285 dynes – sec/cm^{-5}/m^2
Left ventricular stroke work (LVSW)	$SI \times MAP \times 0.0144$	8–10 g/m/m^2
Left ventricular stroke work index (LVWI)	$SVI \times (MAP - PAOP) \times 0.0136$	50–62 g/m^2/beat
Right ventricular stroke work (RVSW)	$SI \times MAP \times 0.0144$	51–61 g/m/m^2
Right ventricular stroke work index (RVSWI)	$SVI \times (MPAP - CVP) \times 0.0136$	5–10 g/m^2/beat
Oxygen delivery (DO$_2$)	$CaO_2 \times CO \times 10$	950–1150 mL/min
Oxygen consumption (VO$_2$)	$C(a - v)O_2 \times CO \times 10$	200–250 mL/min
Oxygen extraction ratio (O$_2$ER)	$(CaO_2 - CvO_2)/CaO_2 \times 100$	22–30%
Oxygen extraction index (O$_2$EI)	$(SaO_2 - SvO_2)/SaO_2 \times 100$	20–25 %
Coronary artery perfusion pressure (CCP)	Diastolic BP – PAOP	60–80 mm Hg

(CVP: central venous pressure; CO: cardiac output; HR: heart rate; MAP: mean arterial pressure; MPAP: mean pulmonary artery pressure; PA: pulmonary artery; RA: right Atrial; RAP: right atrial pressure; RV: right ventricular)

for a limited period of time and removed when no longer necessary. **Table 3** describes parameters obtained from using a PAC.

PiCCO and Volume View (Transpulmonary Thermodilution)

The PiCCO (Pulsion Medical Systems, Munich, Germany) and VolumeView (Edwards Life Sciences, USA) devices allow CO to be measured by minimal invasive method. They use central venous and a femoral arterial catheter, rather than a catheter in the pulmonary artery. These devices use a thermistor placed at the arterial site to measure the changes in temperature after running a thermodilution calibration.

Calibration—this can be done by injecting about 20 mL of normal saline (with temperature < 8°C or at least room temperature < 24°C) through the central line which have temperature sensor. At the arterial end the changes in temperature of the cold saline will be measured by the thermistor and finally the CO will be calculated by area under the curve of thermodilution curve by using modified Stewart–Hamilton algorithm.

PiCCO and VolumeView will provide information on extravascular lung water (EVLW), which gives an idea about pulmonary edema.

Single measurement of CO: Ice cold fluid is injected into the central line and the change in temperature measured downstream to calculate CO. Thus they are referred to as "transpulmonary." It is advised to calibrate the device at least once in 8 hours or when some unexpected changes happened in hemodynamic or when there is requirement for adjustment of vasoactive agent infusion dosage.

Continuous CO (CCO): This is derived by analyzing the systolic portion of the arterial pressure waveform using an algorithm to calculate the CO.[21]

The accuracy of PiCCO may be affected by the vascular compliance, aortic impedance, air bubbles in the system, clotting of the catheter, valvular regurgitation, aortic aneurysm, significant arrhythmias, and rapidly changing temperature.[22]

Validation studies have found a good correlation with PAC in cardiac surgery with the exception of off-pump coronary artery bypass surgery (OPCAB).[23]

In addition to CO measurements, transpulmonary thermodilution also provides advance volumetric parameters such as global end-diastolic volume (GEDV) and EVLW. Other parameters obtained are global ejection fraction, intrathoracic blood volume, and pulmonary vascular permeability index.[24-26]

Global End-diastolic Volume

Global end-diastolic volume is a hypothetical volume that assumes the situation that the four heart chambers are simultaneously in the diastolic phase. GEDV is the combined EDVs of all the four cardiac chambers. In addition, it also includes volume of central vein and aorta from point of injection of injectate to site of measurement. It is calculated as the difference between the intrathoracic thermal volume (ITTV) and pulmonary thermal volume (PTV).[27-29] It has been found to be a reliable indicator of cardiac preload in critically ill patients.[28] GEDV indexed to the body surface area is GEDV index. Normal GEDVI—680–800 mL/m^2.

Extravascular Lung Water

Extravascular lung water is the amount of water that is contained in the lungs outside the pulmonary vasculature. It corresponds to the sum of interstitial, intracellular, alveolar, and lymphatic fluid, not including pleural effusions.[30] An increase in EVLW is the pathophysiological hallmark of hydrostatic pulmonary edema and acute respiratory distress syndrome (ARDS).[31] EVLW is also high in many septic shock[32] and critically ill[33] patients. EVLWI is the ratio of EVLW with the patient's actual or predicted body weight (PBW) to nullify the variation due to patient's anthropometric measures. Normal value of EVLWI less than 10 mL/kg (**Figs. 1A to C**).

LiDCO (Transpulmonary Indicator Dilution)

The LiDCO (lithium diluted cardiac output) (LiDCO, London, UK), this devise uses an indicator (lithium chloride) instead of changes in temperature.

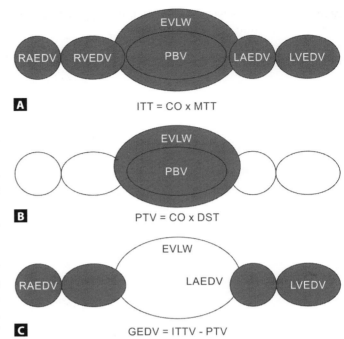

Figs. 1A to C: Extravascular lung water (EVLW) and global end diastolic volume (GEDV).

(ITTV: intrathoracic thermal volume; LAEDV: left atrial EDV; LVEDV: left ventricular EDV; PBV: pulmonary blood volume; PTV: pulmonary thermal volume; RAEDV: right atrial EDV; RVEDV: right ventricular EDV)

- *Single CO measurement:* For the purpose of calibration, a small volume of lithium chloride can be injected through either central or peripheral line and measured downstream using a lithium-selective electrode attached to the patient's arterial line. This single measurement is used to calibrate the device and is recommended on set-up, every 8 hours and in periods of hemodynamic instability or after adjustment of vasopressor infusion rates.
- *Continuous CO:* This is derived by analyzing the arterial pressure waveform with what is called the pulse power analysis and uses an algorithm to calculate CO.

The *LiDCOplus* using pulse power analysis[9] converts the arterial waveform into a volume-time waveform to calculate CO.[34] The *LiDCOrapid* system uses a nomogram to calculate the patient's specific aortic compliance, and therefore prior calibration with lithium dilution is not required.[35]

The use of both LiDCO systems in perioperative goal-directed therapy (GDT) has been extensively studied and evidence has demonstrated both reduced length of stay and postoperative outcomes.[36]

This technique has also been validated against PAC.[37] Its accuracy is also affected by aortic regurgitation, postaortic reconstruction, intra-aortic balloon pump (IABP), damped arterial line, severe peripheral arterial vasoconstriction, arrhythmia, and intra- or extracardiac shunts. It requires regular calibrations as well.[22] Thus, it is not considered a favorable technique in cardiac surgery.

FloTrac/Vigileo (Arterial Pressure-based Cardiac Output—APCO)

FloTrac and Vigileo is the monitor introduced by Edwards Life science for monitoring CO continuously. It is not a calibrated device as it does not require thermodilution or dye dilution, but it requires arterial wave form and pre-entered demographic data to calculate CO. It is easy to use, operator independent, and requires an existing arterial line. The parameters measured include:

- Stroke volume (SV)
- Stroke volume variation (SVV)
- Mean arterial pressure
- Systemic vascular resistance (SVR)
- Continuous CO (CCO)

Its accuracy is affected in patients with altered vascular tone and problems with the arterial waveform.

Studies thus far indicate that it is robust and accurate over a wide range of CO and clinical conditions.[38-40]

FloTrac/Vigileo analyses the waveform 100 times/second over 20 seconds, capturing 2,000 data points for analysis. This is then incorporated into a proprietary formula to calculate CO. The FloTrac, since its introduction in 2005, has been continuously updated, and now integrates "third-generation" software; studies have shown reasonable agreement with pulmonary artery thermodilution.[41] The third-generation algorithm in FloTrac is considered to be useful in sepsis and other critical illnesses as well.[42]

Although it has not been extensively studied in GDT, there are limited data showing beneficial effects in reducing postoperative complications.[43]

Use of FloTrac in cardiopulmonary bypass, coronary artery bypass grafting in a multicentric trial,[44] was found to be advantageous in terms of shorter duration of mechanical ventilation and intensive care unit and hospital length of stay as compared to the control group.

Volume Clamp Method (Finapres/Nexfin)

This newer noninvasive technique uses an inflatable finger cuff (consisting of bladder with an infrared plethysmograph) and stand-alone monitor. *Calibration: An inflatable cuff is attached to the middle phalanx* of the finger; the whole system is "zeroed" at the level of the right atrium.

By repeated inflation and deflation of the cuff beat-to-beat continuous BP is measured. On the basis of Windkessel model, CO and SV are calculated and the same principle has been used to get SVV and pulse pressure variation (PPV)

is also measured. Data to date on the usefulness of this technique in the critically ill is limited.

Esophageal Doppler

The esophageal Doppler monitor (EDM) is another most commonly used minimally invasive method of hemodynamic monitoring. This uses pulse wave Doppler to get CO, many studies have showed improved clinical outcome by using esophageal Doppler to optimize fluid therapy.[45] Doppler probe has been inserted into the esophagus up to the midthoracic level, CO is measured by using the blood flow velocity which transverses in the descending aorta and by calculating the aortic root diameter. The British National Institute for Health and Care Excellence recommended the use of EDM as the data suggest that it helps in reducing the length of hospital stay in patients undergoing major high-risk surgeries.[46]

Bioreactance

It is one of the newer methods of CO using noninvasive method. In this device, high-frequency transthoracic current has been applied and the changes in the voltage with each heart beat are measured. This device consists of four pads placed across the anterior chest wall and connected to a monitor. The main advantage is that it can be used in both ventilated and spontaneously breathing patient even with nonsinus rhythm.[10]

A recent study using bioreactance technology in GDT demonstrated similar performance compared with the EDM, and some studies have shown encouraging results regarding its precision compared with pulmonary artery thermodilution in terms of CO monitoring.[47] The use of electrocautery, however, interferes with the thoracic bioimpedance signal which is a major disadvantage of this device for intraoperative use.

PITFALLS IN THE INTERPRETATION OF CARDIAC OUTPUT

Even though we are able to measure CO using above devices with good accuracy, it is very difficult to tell what is the optimal CO for a particular patient during critical illness. A "normal" or even high CO does not preclude the presence of inadequate regional and microcirculatory flow, and a low CO may be adequate in a context of low metabolic demand, especially during surgery under general anesthesia. Moreover, simple identification of a low CO does not tell us what to do about it. To correctly interpret the data acquired by any of the described devices, we need to combine/integrate several variables to help decide whether the CO/SV is adequate and how it can be optimized in the most effective manner.

How to select the best system for CO monitoring in the perioperative period?

All monitoring systems have unique characteristics in terms of accuracy, precision, validity, stability, and reliability.[16] Not all monitoring devices have been evaluated against the same set of criteria, and uncertainty remains regarding acceptance thresholds for the performance of CO monitors and the used reference techniques.[48]

Several questions can be raised when considering choice of CO monitoring in the perioperative period:

- Are we ready to accept a less accurate measurement in order to limit invasiveness? A less accurate measurement may be acceptable, if the trend analysis is reliable. Cost may also be an important issue.
- Do we need continuous, semicontinuous, or intermittent measurements? Most complications after surgery do not have a sudden onset (except sudden cardiac failure, for example due to myocardial infarction or pulmonary embolism) or an obvious cause (for example, massive bleeding during surgery) but develop slowly; therefore, semicontinuous or intermittent measurements may be acceptable. However, it should be noted that only beat-by-beat measurement of SV allows assessment of the response to preload-modifying maneuvers, such as a fluid challenge or passive leg raising (PLR) test.
- Are calibrated or uncalibrated systems preferable? Non-calibrated systems are acceptable for the operating room (OR) or the postanesthesia care unit (PACU) but may not be suitable for more complex cases, especially in the ICU. In unstable patients, there is a necessity to "recalibrate" more often because of frequent changes in vascular tone and also because derived variables (for example, EVLW and GEDV) need to be recalculated. A practical option may be to use an uncalibrated system in the OR/PACU and replace it with a calibrated system in the ICU.
- What alarms do we need? A major problem for patient surveillance by telemetric monitoring is artifact robustness. Any system with too many false alarms is prone to failure as personnel become desensitized.
- What kind of monitoring for what kind of patient? This is not a "one size fits all" decision; rather, the optimal monitoring technique for each patient will vary depending on the degree of risk and the extent of the surgical procedure.

METHODS TO ASSESS FLUID RESPONSIVENESS: FUNCTIONAL HEMODYNAMIC PARAMETERS

A simple preload or fluid status assessment is not useful at the bedside. Under-resuscitation carries the hazard of possible organ failure in the future, while enthusiastic fluid infusion can lead to positive fluid balance. There is enough evidence now to suggest that higher the cumulative positive fluid balance, higher is the chance of poor outcome.[49,50] What we need to know, is if patient is given fluid bolus, will he respond by increasing his CO. Fluid responsiveness can be defined as an increase in SV or CO by 10–15% in response to a fluid challenge, although the rate and volume of fluid is variable.[14] Fluid infusion is titrated in such a manner that the CO does not increase any further in response to fluid administration, which in physiological terms is the plateau of the Frank–Starling curve, various methods of assessing fluid responsiveness are discussed in **Table 4**.[51]

In patients who are paralyzed and mechanically ventilated, the cyclical variations in the intrathoracic pressure lead to changes in SV of both right and left heart, which are reflected in the SV. These changes in the SV (and therefore pulse pressure and systolic pressure) can be used to predict fluid responsiveness before giving fluids.

Intrathoracic pressure changes and effect on the hemodynamic parameters—during inspiration on mechanical ventilation, there will be increase in intrathoracic pressure which leads to decrease in right-sided venous return and hence right ventricular SV. After couple of beats, the overall impact is reduced left ventricular output because of pulmonary blood transit time. On the other hand, in the left side there will be squeezing of pulmonary veins result in increased left atrial filling, which leads to increase in left ventricular output. Due to the decrease in the transmural aortic pressure that is equivalent to an effective decrease in LV afterload.[52,53]

A mechanical breath will lead to changes in LV CO in relation to respiration, these changes are going to be get exaggerated in severe hypovolemia and represents probability of fluid responsiveness. At the patient's bedside changes in arterial waveform tells about the measurable parameter of fluid responsiveness (**Figs. 2 and 3**).

Systolic Pressure Variation

Systolic pressure variation (SPV) is the difference between the maximal and minimal values of systolic arterial pressure during one mechanical breath (**Fig. 2**). The SPV is composed of an early augmentation of systolic BP during inspiration, termed delta up (dUp), which reflects the inspiratory augmentation of the CO, and a later decrease in systolic BP, termed delta down, which reflects the decreased CO due to the decrease in venous return (**Fig. 2**).[54]

The SPV has been validated and used to guide fluid therapy in surgical patients, including those undergoing major abdominal,[55] neurosurgery,[56] vascular surgery,[57] cardiac,[58] and scoliosis surgery.[59] Although the SPV has been found to be somewhat less accurate than PPV,[58] its accuracy in predicting fluid responsiveness is similar to that of SVV.[60] When PPV and SVV are not measured automatically, SPV has a distinct practical advantage over

Table 4: Preload and preload responsiveness assessment.

Parameter	Type	Advantage	Disadvantages
CVP	Static	Commonly used, gives a number	*Invasive, saline manometry:* Not very good, too many assumptions, does not reflect preload responsiveness
PAOP	Static	Gives a number	Invasive, skill required, too many assumptions, does not reflect preload responsiveness
RVEDA	Static	Gives a number	Noninvasive, skill required, does not reflect preload responsiveness
LVEDA	Static	Gives a number	Noninvasive, skill required, does not reflect preload responsiveness
IVC diameter	Static	Gives a number	Noninvasive, skill required, does not reflect preload responsiveness
Pulse pressure variation (PPV)	Dynamic	Predict fluid responsiveness	Only works when patient is sedated and paralyzed (all DP and TV > 8 mL/kg), needs arterial line and software in the monitor + Needs CO monitoring
Systolic pressure variation (SPV)	Dynamic		
Stroke volume variation (SVV)	Dynamic	Predict fluid responsiveness	
Plethysmography variability index (PVI)	Dynamic	Noninvasive, predict fluid responsiveness	Not reliable in vasoconstricted state (cold peripheries, hypotension)
End-expiratory occlusion test (EEOT)	Dynamic	Negates effect of increased intrathoracic pressure during inspiration	Requires continuous CO monitoring device
Tidal volume challenge (TVC)	Dynamic	Improves reliability of PPV, can be used in low TV settings(transiently)	Needs further validation, may not be fully reliable in ARDS settings
Passive leg raise (PLR)	Dynamic	Noninvasive, predict fluid responsiveness even in patients with spontaneous breathing, arrhythmias, low tidal volume ventilation, low lung compliance situations	Can't be used intraoperative and when patient positioning is contraindicated

(CVP: central venous pressure; IVC: inferior vena cava; LVEDA: left ventricular end-diastolic area; PAOP: pulmonary wedge pressure; RVEDA: right ventricular end-diastolic area)

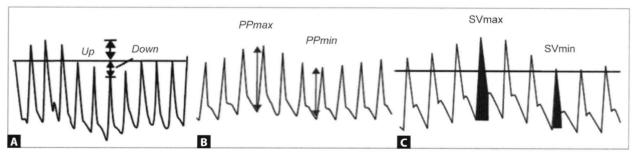

Figs. 2A to C: (A) SPV; (B) PPV; (C) SVV.
(PPV: pulse pressure variation; SPV: systolic pressure variation; SVV: stroke volume variation)

the other two parameters in that it can easily and accurately be estimated from visual examination.[61,62]

Pulse Pressure Variation

Pulse pressure variation reflects the changes in pulse pressure in relation to inspiration and expiration within each cycle of respiration, and is calculated as the difference between the maximum and minimum pulse pressure values during one mechanical breath divided by the mean pulse pressure.[63] PPV is more accurate than SPV since, under constant conditions, the SV is proportional to the pulse pressure, and since the changes in the systolic BP may be influenced by some degree of transmission of airway

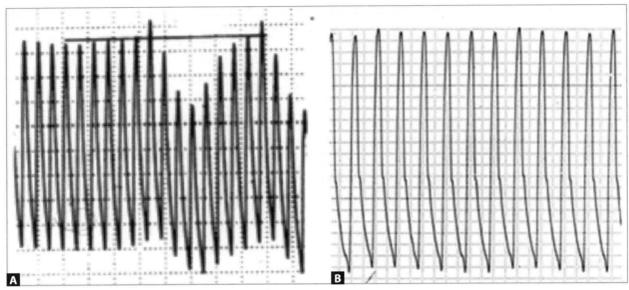

Figs. 3A and B: (A) Responders; (B) Nonresponders.

pressure.[60] In patients with severe hypovolemia filling of the aorta is greatly decreased, the changing relation of the SV to the pulse pressure causes the associated increase in PPV to be much greater than the simultaneous increase in SPV and SVV.[64] Numerous studies have repeatedly shown that PPV is an accurate predictor of fluid responsiveness with threshold values of 11–13%.[65] PPV has been validated and used to guide fluid therapy in a variety of surgical patients, which include those undergoing major abdominal procedures,[66] liver transplantation,[67] cardiac surgery,[68] and scoliosis surgery.[69] Also a high PPV value was associated with higher inflammatory response and lower organ yield in brain-dead organ donors.[70] Automatic measurement of PPV is available in most monitors that use pulse contour analysis for the measurement of CCO, and also in some standard high end monitors.

Stroke Volume Variation

Stroke volume variation is the difference between the maximum and minimum SV during one mechanical breath divided by the mean SV (**Fig. 2**). SVV values around 10–13% accurately predict fluid responsiveness, with reported predictive values of more than 0.85[71] in patients who are in sinus rhythm without arrhythmias. This is in stark contrast to the 50% accuracy rate of a clinician to predict whether a patient is fluid responsive based on clinical criteria alone.[72]

Continuous measurement of this parameter has become possible with the introduction of pulse contour methods for the continuous measurement of CO. SVV has been validated and used to guide fluid therapy in a variety of surgical patients, including patients undergoing cardiac,[73] major abdominal,[74] and liver transplant surgery.[75] In addition, because of different nonstandardized proprietary algorithms, SVV values measured by one monitor cannot be used interchangeably with those measured by another monitor without great caution.[76]

Plethysmographic Variability Index (PVi® Masimo, Japan)

Since pulse oximetry is a standard noninvasive intraoperative monitor, respiratory plethysmographic (Pleth Variability Index PVi® Masimo, Japan) is another dynamic parameter available in mechanically ventilated anesthetized patients.[77] PVi can be calculated as the difference between the maximal and minimal plethysmographic signal amplitudes divided by the amplitude of the signal during apnea or by the mean of the two values.[78]

In the absence of an automated measurement,[79] the variations in the plethysmographic signal should be simply eyeballed, although there are no data regarding the sensitivity and accuracy of such observation. PVi has been shown to accurately reflect changes in circulating blood volume intraoperatively and in fluid responsiveness in patients undergoing major abdominal and cardiac surgery.[78,80,81]

The major problem with the clinical use of PVi is the significant impact of vasoconstriction on the plethysmographic waveform (for example, during hypotension or hypothermia). An increase in PVi may be the first sign for development of a still-occult hypovolemia and should prompt the anesthesiologist to consider the immediate administration of fluids.

End-expiratory Occlusion Test

In patients with mechanical ventilation during inspiration, there will be increased intrathoracic pressure and in turn decrease in CO. EEO prevents any variation in intrathoracic pressure induced by mechanical ventilation. This leads to an increase in venous return, cardiac preload, and SV in preload-responsive patients. Thus, an increase in cardiac index during an EEO could predict fluid responsiveness. In order to identify the rapid and transient increase in cardiac index during the EEO, a real time continuous and instantaneous CO and index monitoring is necessary (pulse contour analysis/TTE). SVV/PVV can be recorded 30 seconds after an end-expiratory occlusion test (EEOT) and after volume expansion (250 mL saline 0.9% given over 10 minutes). Patients with an increase in SV ≥ 10% after volume expansion are defined as fluid responsive patients.[82]

Tidal Volume Challenge Test

Several studies have shown that PPV does not reliably predict fluid responsiveness during lung protective low tidal volume ventilation.[83] De Backer et al.[84] showed that PPV was a good predictor of fluid responsiveness only when the tidal volume was at least 8 mL/kg PBW. During low tidal volume ventilation, PPV value may be low and may indicate a nonresponsive status even in responders as the tidal volume might be insufficient to produce a significant change in the intrathoracic pressure.[85]

The "tidal volume challenge (TVC)" is a novel test proposed to improve the reliability of PPV during low tidal volume ventilation. The test involves transiently increasing tidal volume from 6 mL/kg PBW to 8 mL/kg PBW, in a paralyzed patient, for 1 minute and observing the change in PPV/SVV ($\Delta PPV_{6-8}/\Delta SVV_{6-8}$) from baseline ($PPV_6/SVV_6$) to that at 8 mL/kg PBW (PPV_8/SVV_8). ΔPPV_{6-8} of ≥ 3.5% and ΔSVV_{6-8} of ≥ 2.5% reliably predicts fluid responsiveness.[86]

Passive Leg Raising Test

In acute circulatory failure, PLR is a test that predicts whether CO will increase with volume expansion.[87] By transferring a volume of around 300 mL of venous blood[88] from the lower body toward the right heart, PLR mimics a fluid challenge. However, no fluid is infused and the hemodynamic effects are rapidly reversible[87,89] thereby avoiding the risks of fluid overload.

This test has the advantage of remaining reliable in conditions in which indices of fluid responsiveness that are based on the respiratory variations of SV cannot be used,[87] like spontaneous breathing, arrhythmias, low tidal volume ventilation, and low lung compliance. The steps of doing a PLR test are depicted in **Figure 4**. It may not be feasible to this intraoperatively but can be done pre- or postoperatively if no contraindications exist for patient positioning. CO must be measured in real time not only before and during PLR but also after PLR when the patient has been moved back to the semirecumbent position, in order to check that it returns to its baseline. Pain, cough, discomfort, and awakening could provoke adrenergic stimulation, resulting in mistaken interpretation of CO changes.

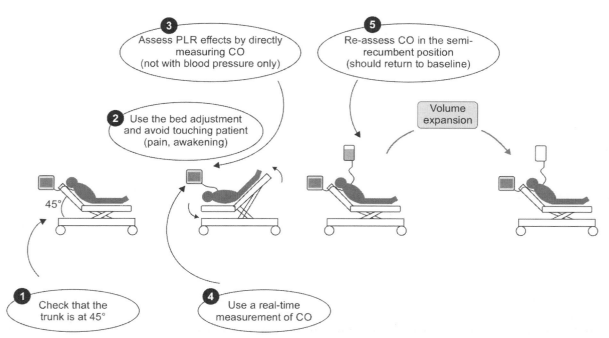

Fig. 4: Steps of a passive leg raise (PLR) test.

LIMITATIONS OF FUNCTIONAL HEMODYNAMIC PARAMETERS

There are many limitations of functional hemodynamic monitoring (FHM) in relation to its measurement and interpretation, in fact that any dynamic parameter is composed of a stimulus and a response[90] makes the process vulnerable to many confounding factors, because of this we cannot use these parameters in many anesthetized patients.[77]

Spontaneous Breathing

The hemodynamic effects of a spontaneous breath are physiologically different from those of a mechanical one and are greatly affected by the inspiratory effort of any particular patient. Dynamic parameters, especially when automatically measured, can therefore be very misleading in the presence of spontaneous or assisted ventilation. This is a major limitation of functional hemodynamic parameter (FHP) and is responsible for the large number of anesthetized patients (for example, those under regional anesthesia) in whom these parameters cannot be used and in patients who are recovering from anesthesia in the postoperative period.[77]

Nonstandardized Tidal Volume

Tidal volume more than 8 mL may exaggerate the size of dynamic parameters at similar preload conditions.[91] On the other hand, low tidal volume may produce an inadequate change in CO and considerably reduce the reliability of dynamic parameters like PPV, SPV, and SVV. It is accepted that such reliability can be achieved only with tidal volume $\geq$ 8 mL/kg[92] or $\geq$ 7 mL/kg.[93]

Nonstandardized Airway Pressure/ Respiratory Rate

A very high respiratory rate was shown to reduce the respiratory variations in SV and its derivatives, whereas respiratory variations in the superior vena cava diameter were unaltered.[94] Decreased chest wall compliance will have an exaggerated response of dynamic parameters

Prone positioning has been shown to significantly increase PPV and SVV, although it did not alter their ability to predict fluid responsiveness.[69] Another clinical condition which may also increase dynamic variables significantly even in the absence of fluid responsiveness is increased intra-abdominal pressure.[95] Air-trapping and positive end-expiratory pressure may result in high values of dynamic parameters denoting a real compromise of venous return and CO.

Decreased lung compliance is usually not a limitation of FHPs as long as the tidal volume remains adequate. But recent evidence also suggests that low compliance of the respiratory system reduces the accuracy of PPV.[96]

Open-chest conditions may affect the ability of respiratory variations in the arterial pressure to predict fluid responsiveness and have been the subject of some debate.[97] Since during open-chest conditions, there is no inspiratory impediment to venous return, we believe that these variations are entirely due to augmentation of CO (dUp) following inspiratory squeezing of the pulmonary blood volume, that they reflect LV fluid responsiveness, and that their absence should be a cause for concern.[54]

Nonsinus (Abnormal) Rhythm

Since the dynamic parameters measurement and interpretation depend upon arterial trace, arrhythmia can alter the contour of arterial wave form and can lead to inaccuracies. Since the respiratory-induced dynamic parameters rely on the individually measured maximal and minimal SV (or its surrogates); any arrhythmias may cause significant inaccuracies. Nodal rhythm leads to loss of atrial kick, which causes inappropriate increase the size of respiratory-induced dynamic parameters by effectively decreasing preload.

Right Heart Failure

If any elevated RV afterload is there, it leads to erroneous increase in SPV, PPV, or SVV in the presence of right ventricular failure, which should be suspected when patients have large variations in dynamic parameters, but they do not respond to fluids.

A Neglected Termed Delta Up

In patients with hypervolemia and congestive heart failure, early augmentation of LV ejection, which may become the dominant.[98] This has a very little volume sensitivity.[99] Since this augmentation reflects the maximal SV and hence impacts the calculation of SPV, SVV, and PPV, it may reduce their accuracy in predicting fluid responsiveness, especially when their values are in midrange. The presence of a significant dUp may explain, in part at least, the recently reported inability of PPV values between 9 and 13% to accurately predict fluid responsiveness (gray zone).[100] If it is possible to identify a dominant dUp, it reflects that the patient is not fluid responsive, but mechanical ventilation is helping in good LV output.

CONCLUSION

A vast array of devices is available to monitor preload, CO, and afterload. CO monitoring devices and the FHPs offer unique information about delivery of oxygen to the tissues and fluid responsiveness, which may help detect fluid needs and avoid unnecessary fluid loading. Despite their limitations and confounding factors, these parameters should be used to guide fluid therapy in all surgical patients in whom their use is appropriate, as part of, or independently of, GDT strategies.

REFERENCES

1. Weiser TG, Regenbogen SE, Thompson KD, Haynes AB, Lipsitz SR, Berry WR, et al. An estimation of the global volume of surgery: a modelling strategy based on available data. Lancet. 2008;372:139-44.

2. Jhanji S, Thomas B, Ely A, Watson D, Hinds CJ, Pearse RM. Mortality and utilisation of critical care resources amongst high-risk surgical patients in a large NHS trust. Anaesthesia. 2008;63:695-700.

3. Pearse RM, Harrison DA, James P, Watson D, Hinds C, Rhodes A, et al. Identification and characterisation of the high-risk surgical population in the UK. Crit Care. 2006;10:R81.

4. Khuri SF, Henderson WG, DePalma RG, Mosca C, Healey NA, Kumbhani DJ. Determinants of long-term survival after major surgery and the adverse effect of postoperative complications. Ann Surg. 2005;242:326-41.

5. Bennett-Guerrero E, Welsby I, Dunn TJ, Young LR, Wahl TA, Diers TL, et al. The use of a postoperative morbidity survey to evaluate patients with prolonged hospitalization after routine, moderate-risk, elective surgery. Anesth Analg. 1999;89:514-9.

6. Lugo G, Arizpe D, Dominguez G, Ramírez M, Tamariz O. Relationship between oxygen consumption and oxygen delivery during anaesthesia in high-risk surgical patients. Crit Care Med. 1993;21:64-9.

7. Marjanovic G, Villain C, Juettner E, zur Hausen A, Hoeppner J, Hopt UT, et al. Impact of different crystalloid volume regimes on intestinal anastomotic stability. Ann Surg. 2009;249:181-5.

8. Kulemann B, Timme S, Seifert G, Holzner PA, Glatz T, Sick O, et al. Intraoperative crystalloid overload leads to substantial inflammatory infiltration of intestinal anastomoses—a histomorphological analysis. Surgery. 2013;154:596-603.

9. Cove ME, Pinsky MR. Perioperative Haemodynamic Monitoring. Best Prac Res Clin Anesthesiol. 2012;26:453-62.

10. Suehiro K, Joosten A, Alexander B, Cannesson M. Guiding goal directed therapy. Curr Anesthesiol Rep. 2014;4:360-5.

11. Bundgaard-Nielsen M, Holte K, Secher NH, Kehlet H. Monitoring of peroperative fluid administration by individualized goal-directed therapy. Acta Anaesthesiologica Scandinavica. 2007;51:331-40.

12. Pizov R, Eden A, Bystritski D, Kalina E, Tamir A, Gelman S. Hypotension during gradual blood loss: waveform variables response and absence of tachycardia. Br J Anaesth. 2012;109:911-8.

13. Vincent JL, Rhodes A, Perel A, Martin GS, Della Rocca G, Vallet B, et al. Clinical review: update on hemodynamic monitoring - a consensus of 16. Crit Care. 2011;15:229.

14. Marik PE, Cavallazzi R. Does the central venous pressure predict fluid responsiveness? An updated meta-analysis and a plea for some common sense. Crit Care Med. 2013;41:1774-81.

15. Litton E, Silbert B, Ho KM. Clinical predictors of a low central venous oxygen saturation after major surgery: a prospective prevalence study. Anaesth Intensive Care. 2015;43:59-65.

16. Thiele RH, Bartels K, Gan TJ. Cardiac output monitoring: a contemporary assessment and review. Crit Care Med. 2015;43:177-85.

17. Cannesson M, Pestel G, Ricks C, Hoeft A, Perel A. Hemodynamic monitoring and management in patients undergoing high risk surgery: a survey among North American and European anesthesiologists. Crit Care. 2011;15:R197.

18. Rhodes A, Cusack RJ, Newman PJ, Grounds RM, Bennett ED. A randomised, controlled trial of the pulmonary artery catheter in critically ill patients. Intensive Care Med. 2002;28:256-64.

19. Harvey S, Harrison DA, Singer M, Ashcroft J, Jones CM, Elbourne D, et al. Assessment of the clinical effectiveness of pulmonary artery catheters in management of patients in intensive care (PAC-Man): a randomised controlled trial. Lancet. 2005;366: 472-7.

20. Vincent JL. The pulmonary artery catheter. J Clin Monit Comput. 2012;26:341-5.

21. Jansen JR. The thermodilution method for the clinical assessment of cardiac output. Intensive Care Med. 1995;21(8):691-7.

22. Mehta Y, Arora D. Newer methods of cardiac output monitoring. World J Cardiol. 2014;6:1022-9.

23. Buhre W, Weyland A, Kazmaier S, Hanekop GG, Baryalei MM, Sydow M, et al. Comparison of cardiac output assessed by pulsecontour analysis and thermodilution in patients undergoing minimally invasive direct coronary artery bypass grafting. J Cardiothorac Vasc Anesth. 1999;13:437-40.

24. Godje O, Peyerl M, Seebauer T, Dewald O, Reichart B. Reproducibility of double indicator dilution measurements of intrathoracic blood volume compartments, extravascular lung water, and liver function. Chest. 1998;113:1070-7.

25. Costa MG, Pompei L, Rocca GD. Transpulmonary thermodilution technique for cardiac output measurements: Single versus double indicator. Crit Care. 2003;7(Suppl 2):192.

26. Sakka SG, Rühl CC, Pfeiffer UJ, Beale R, McLuckie A, Reinhart K, et al. Assessment of cardiac preload and extravascular lung water by single transpulmonary thermodilution. Intensive Care Med. 2000;26:180-7.

27. Reuter DA, Huang C, Edrich T, Shernan SK, Eltzschig HK. Cardiac output monitoring using indicator-dilution techniques: Basics, limits, and perspectives. Anesth Analg. 2010;110:799-811.

28. Michard F, Alaya S, Zarka V, Bahloul M, Richard C, Teboul JL. Global end-diastolic volume as an indicator of cardiac preload in patients with septic shock. Chest. 2003;124:1900-8.

29. Newman EV, Merrell M, Genecin A, Monge C, Milnor WR, McKeever WP. The dye dilution method for describing the central circulation. An analysis of factors shaping the time-concentration curves. Circulation. 1951;4:735-46.

30. Perel A, Monnet X. Extravascular lung water. In: Vincent J, Hall J (Eds). Encyclopedia of Intensive Care Medicine. Berlin Heidelberg: Springer-Verlag; 2011.

31. Kushimoto S, Taira Y, Kitazawa Y, Okuchi K, Sakamoto T, Ishikura H, et al. The clinical usefulness of extravascular lung water and pulmonary vascular permeability index to diagnose and characterize pulmonary edema: a prospective multicenter study on the quantitative differential diagnostic definition for acute lung injury/acute respiratory distress syndrome. Crit Care. 2012;16:R232.

32. Martin GS, Eaton S, Mealer M, Moss M. Extravascular lung water in patients with severe sepsis: a prospective cohort study. Crit Care. 2005;9:R74-82.

33. Sakka SG, Klein M, Reinhart K, Meier-Hellmann A. Prognostic value of extravascular lung water in critically ill patients. Chest. 2002;122:2080-6.

34. Donati A, Loggi S, Preiser JC, Orsetti G, Münch C, Gabbanelli V, et al. Goal-directed intraoperative therapy reduces morbidity and length of hospital stay in high-risk surgical patients. Chest. 2007;132:1817-24.

35. Broch O, Renner J, Gruenewald M, Meybohm P, Schöttler J, Steinfath M, et al. A comparison of third-generation semi-invasive arterial waveform analysis with thermodilution in patients undergoing coronary surgery. Scientific World J. 202312;2012:451081.

36. Miller T, Thacker J, White W, Mantyh C, Migaly J, Jin J, et al. Reduced length of hospital stay in colorectal surgery after implementation of an enhanced recovery protocol. Anesth Analg. 2014;118:1052-61.

37. Linton RA, Band DM, Haire KM. A new method of measuring cardiac output in man using lithium dilution. Br J Anaesth. 1993;71:262-6.

38. Breukers RM, Sepehrkhouy S, Spiegelenberg SR, Groeneveld AB. Cardiac output measured by a new arterial pressure waveform analysis method without calibration compared with thermodilution after cardiac surgery. J Cardiothorac Vasc Anesth. 2007;21(5):632-5.

39. Zimmermann A, Kufner C, Hofbauer S, Steinwendner J, Hitzl W, Fritsch G, et al. The Accuracy of the Vigileo/FloTrac Continuous Cardiac Output Monitor. J Cardiothorac Vasc Anesth. 2008;22(3):388-93.

40. Lorsomradee S, Lorsomradee S, Cromheecke S, De Hert SG. Uncalibrated arterial pulse contour analysis versus continuous thermodilution technique: Effects of alterations in arterial waveform. J Cardiothorac Vasc Anesth. 2007;21(5):636-43.

41. De Backer D, Marx G, Tan A, Junker C, Van Nuffelen M, Hüter L, et al. Arterial pressure-based cardiac output monitoring: a multicenter validation of the third-generation software in septic patients. Intensive Care Med. 2011;37:233-40.

42. Staylor A. Recent trends in haemodynamic monitoring. USA: Medtech Insight; 2010.

43. Benes J, Chytra I, Altmann P, Hluchy M, Kasal E, Svitak R, et al. Intraoperative fluid optimization using stroke volume variation in high risk surgical patients: results of prospective randomized study. Crit Care. 2010;14:R118.

44. Kapoor PM, Bhardwaj V, Sharma A, Kiran U. Have we reached our goal? Global end diastolic volume (GEDV) An emerging preload marker, vis a vis other markers. Ann Card Anaesth. 2016;19:3.

45. Mowatt G, Houston G, Hernandez R, de Verteuil R, Fraser C, Cuthbertson B, et al. Systematic review of the clinical effectiveness and cost-effectiveness of oesophageal Doppler monitoring in critically ill and high-risk surgical patients. Health Technol Assess. 2009;13:1-95.

46. National Institute for Health and Clinical Excellence. (2011). CardioQ-ODM oesophageal Doppler monitor: Medical technologies guidance [MTG3]. [online] Available from http://www.nice.org.uk/MTG3 [Lasst accessed March, 2020]

47. Waldron NH, Miller TE, Thacker JK, Manchester AK, White WD, Nardiello J, et al. A prospective comparison of a non-invasive cardiac output monitor versus oesophageal Doppler monitor for goal-directed fluid therapy in colorectal surgery patients. Anesth Analg. 2014;118:966-75.

48. Critchley LA, Lee A, Ho AM. A critical review of the ability of continuous cardiac output monitors to measure trends in cardiac output. Anesth Analg. 2010;111:1180-92.

49. Koonrangsesomboon W, Khwannimit B. Impact of positive fluid balance on mortality and length of stay in septic shock patients. Indian J Crit Care Med. 2015;19:708-13.

50. Lee J, de Louw E, Niemi M, Nelson R, Mark RG, Celi LA, et al. Association between fluid balance and survival in critically ill patients. J Intern Med. 2015;277(4):468-77.

51. Ramsingh D, Alexander B, Cannesson M. Clinical review: does it matter which haemodynamic monitoring system is used? Crit Care. 2013;17:208

52. Perel A. The physiological basis of arterial pressure variation during positive-pressure ventilation. Réanimation. 2005;14: 162-71.

53. Magder S. Further cautions for the use of ventilatory-induced changes in arterial pressures to predict volume responsiveness. Crit Care. 2010;14:197.

54. Perel A. Assessing fluid responsiveness by the systolic pressure variation in mechanically ventilated patients. Anesthesiology. 1998;89:1309-10.

55. Mallat J, Pironkov A, Destandau MS, Tavernier B. Systolic pressure variation (Deltadown) can guide fluid therapy during pheochromocytoma surgery. Can J Anaesth. 2003;50:998-1003.

56. Deflandre E, Bonhomme V, Hans P. Delta down compared with delta pulse pressure as an indicator of volaemia during intracranial surgery. Br J Anaesth. 2007;100:245-50.

57. Coriat P, Vrillon M, Perel A, Baron JF, Le Bret F, Saada M, et al. A comparison of systolic blood pressure variations and echocardiographic estimates of end-diastolic left ventricular size in patients after aortic surgery. Anesth Analg. 1994;78: 46-53.

58. Preisman S, Kogan S, Berkenstadt H, Perel A. Predicting fluid responsiveness in patients undergoing cardiac surgery: functional haemodynamic parameters including the Respiratory Systolic Variation Test and static preload indicators. Br J Anaesth. 2005;95:746-55.

59. Pizov R, Segal E, Kaplan L, Floman Y, Perel A. The use of systolic pressure variation in hemodynamic monitoring during deliberate hypotension in spine surgery. J Clin Anesth. 1990;2:96-100.

60. Marik PE, Cavallazzi R, Vasu T, Hirani A. Dynamic changes in arterial waveform derived variables and fluid responsiveness in mechanically ventilated patients: a systematic review of the literature. Crit Care Med. 2009;37:2642-7.

61. Thiele RH, Colquhoun DA, Blum FE, Durieux ME. The ability of anesthesia providers to visually estimate systolic pressure variability using the 'eyeball' technique. Anesth Analg. 2012;115:176-81.

62. Rinehart J, Islam T, Boud R, Nguyen A, Alexander B, Canales C, et al. Visual estimation of pulse pressure variation is not reliable: a randomized simulation study. J Clin Monit Comput. 2012;26:191-6.

63. Michard F, Boussat S, Chemla D, Anguel N, Mercat A, Lecarpentier Y, et al. Relation between respiratory changes in arterial pulse pressure and fluid responsiveness in septic patients with acute circulatory failure. Am J Respir Crit Care Med. 2000;162:134-8.

64. Berkenstadt H, Friedman Z, Preisman S, Keidan I, Livingstone D, Perel A. Pulse pressure and stroke volume variations during severe haemorrhage in ventilated dogs. Br J Anaesth. 2005;94:721-6.

65. Michard F, Lopes MR, Auler JOC. Pulse pressure variation: beyond the fluid management of patients with shock. Crit Care. 2007;11:131.

66. Lopes MR, Oliveira MA, Pereira VOS, Lemos IPB, Auler JOC, Michard F. Goal-directed fluid management based on pulse pressure variation monitoring during high-risk surgery: a pilot randomized controlled trial. Crit Care. 2007;11:R100.

67. Gouvea G, Diaz R, Auler L, Toledo R, Martinho JM. Evaluation of the pulse pressure variation index as a predictor of fluid responsiveness during orthotopic liver transplantation. Br J Anaesth. 2009;103:238-43.

68. Kramer A, Zygun D, Hawes H, Easton P, Ferland A. Pulse pressure variation predicts fluid responsiveness following coronary artery bypass surgery. Chest. 2004;126:1563-8.

69. Biais M, Bernard O, Ha JC, Degryse C, Sztark F. Abilities of pulse pressure variations and stroke volume variations to predict fluid responsiveness in prone position during scoliosis surgery. Br J Anaesth. 2010;104:407-13.

70. Murugan R, Venkataraman R, Wahed AS, Elder M, Carter M, Madden NJ, et al. Preload responsiveness is associated with increased interleukin-6 and lower organ yield from brain-dead donors. Crit Care Med. 2009;37:2387-93.

71. Zhang Z, Lu B, Sheng X, Jin N. Accuracy of stroke volume variation in predicting fluid responsiveness: a systematic review and meta-analysis. J Anesthesiol. 2011;25:904-16.

72. McGuiness S, Parker R. Using cardiac output monitoring to guide perioperative haemodynamic therapy. Curr Opin Crit Care. 2015;21:364-8.

73. Reuter DA, Felbinger TW, Schmidt C, Kilger E, Goedje O, Lamm P, et al. Stroke volume variations for assessment of cardiac responsiveness to volume loading in mechanically ventilated patients after cardiac surgery. Intensive Care Med. 200228:392-8.

74. Kobayashi M, Koh M, Irinoda T, Meguro E, Hayakawa Y, Takagane A. Stroke volume variation as a predictor of intravascular volume depression and possible hypotension during the early postoperative period after esophagectomy. Ann Surg Oncol. 2009;16(5):1371-7.

75. Biais M, Nouette-Gaulain K, Cottenceau V, Revel P, Sztark F. Uncalibrated pulse contour-derived stroke volume variation predicts fluid responsiveness in mechanically ventilated patients undergoing liver transplantation. Br J Anaesth. 2008;101:761-8.

76. Perel A. Automated assessment of fluid responsiveness in mechanically ventilated patients. Anesth Analg. 2008;106:1031-3.

77. Maguire S, Rinehart J, Vakharia S, Cannesson M. Respiratory variation in pulse pressure and plethysmographic waveforms. Anesth Analg. 2011;112:94-6.

78. Pizov R, Eden A, Bystritski D, Kalina E, Tamir A, Gelman S. Arterial and plethysmographic waveform analysis in anesthetized patients with hypovolemia. Anesthesiology. 2010;113:83-91.

79. Cannesson M, Desebbe O, Rosamel P, Delannoy B, Robin J, Bastien O, et al. Pleth variability index to monitor the respiratory variations in the pulse oximeter plethysmographic waveform amplitude and predict fluid responsiveness in the operating theatre. Br J Anaesth. 2008;101:200-6.

80. Solus-Biguenet H, Fleyfel M, Tavernier B, Kipnis E, Onimus J, Robin E, et al. Non-invasive prediction of fluid responsiveness during major hepatic surgery. Br J Anaesth. 2006;97(6):808-16.

81. Wyffels PAH, Durnez PJ, Helderweirt J, Stockman WM, De Kegel D. Ventilation-induced plethysmographic variations predict fluid responsiveness in ventilated postoperative cardiac surgery patients. Anesth Analg. 2007;105:448-52.

82. Matthieu B, Larghi M, Henriot J, Courson H, Sesay M, Nouette-Gaulain K. End-expiratory occlusion test predicts fluid responsiveness in patients with protective ventilation in the operating room. Anesth Analg. 2017;125:1889-95.

83. Lakhal K, Ehrmann S, Benzekri-Lefèvre D, Runge I, Legras A, Dequin PF, et al. Respiratory pulse pressure variation fails to predict fluid responsiveness in acute respiratory distress syndrome. Crit Care. 2011;15:R85.

84. De Backer D, Heenen S, Piagnerelli M, Koch M, Vincent J. Pulse pressure variations to predict fluid responsiveness: influence of tidal volume. Intensive Care Med. 2005;31:517-23.

85. Teboul JL, Monnet X. Pulse pressure variation and ARDS. Minerva Anestesiol. 2013;79:398-407.

86. Myatra SN, Prabu NR, Divatia JV, Monnet X, Kulkarni AP, Teboul JL. The changes in pulse pressure variation or stroke volume variation after a "tidal volume challenge" reliably predict fluid responsiveness during low tidal volume ventilation. Crit Care Med. 2017;45:415-21.

87. Monnet X, Rienzo M, Osman D, Anguel N, Richard C, Pinsky MR, et al. Passive leg raising predicts fluid responsiveness in the critically ill. Crit Care Med. 2006;34:1402-7.

88. Jabot J, Teboul JL, Richard C, Monnet X. Passive leg raising for predicting fluid responsiveness: importance of the postural change. Intensive Care Med. 2009;35:85-90.

89. Boulain T, Achard JM, Teboul JL, Richard C, Perrotin D, Ginies G. Changes in BP induced by passive leg raising predict response to fluid loading in critically ill patients. Chest. 2002;121:1245-52.

90. Perel A. The value of functional hemodynamic parameters in hemodynamic monitoring of ventilated patients. Anaesthesist. 2003;52:1003-4.

91. Reuter DA, Bayerlein J, Goepfert MS, Weis FC, Kilger E, Lamm P, et al. Influence of tidal volume on left ventricular stroke volume variation measured by pulse contour analysis in mechanically ventilated patients. Intensive Care Med. 2003;29:476-80.

92. Backer D, Heenen S, Piagnerelli M, Koch M, Vincent JL. Pulse pressure variations to predict fluid responsiveness: influence of tidal volume. Intensive Care Med. 2005;31:517-23.

93. Lansdorp B, Lemson J, van Putten MJ, de Keijzer A, van der Hoeven JG, Pickkers P. Dynamic indices do not predict volume responsiveness in routine clinical practice. Br J Anaesth. 2012;108:395-401.

94. De Backer D, Taccone FS, Holsten R, Ibrahimi F, Vincent JL. Influence of respiratory rate on stroke volume variation in mechanically ventilated patients. Anesthesiology. 2009;110:1092-7.

95. Malbrain ML, de Laet I. Functional hemodynamics and increased intra- abdominal pressure: same thresholds for different conditions? Crit Care Med. 2009;37:781-3.

96. Monnet X, Bleibtreu A, Ferré A, Dres M, Gharbi R, Richard C, et al. Passive leg-raising and end-expiratory occlusion tests perform better than pulse pressure variation in patients with low respiratory system compliance. Crit Care Med. 2012;40:152-7.

97. Wyffels PA, Sergeant P, Wouters PF. The value of pulse pressure and stroke volume variation as predictors of fluid responsiveness during open chest surgery. Anaesthesia. 2010;65:704-9.

98. Tavernier B, Makhotine O, Lebuffe G, Dupont J, Scherpereel P. Systolic pressure variation as a guide to fluid therapy in patients with sepsis-induced hypotension. Anesthesiol. 1998;89: 1313-21.

99. Cannesson M, Aboy M, Hofer CK, Rehman M. Pulse pressure variation: where are we today? J Clin Monit Comput. 2010;25: 45-56.

100. Cannesson M, Le Manach Y, Hofer CK, Goarin JP, Lehot JJ, Vallet B, et al. Assessing the diagnostic accuracy of pulse pressure variations for the prediction of fluid responsiveness: a 'gray zone' approach. Anesthesiology. 2011;115:231-41.

Vasoactive Agents

Suhail Sarwar Siddiqui, Abdullah Zoheb Azhar, Atul Prabhakar Kulkarni

INTRODUCTION

Hypotension in perioperative period may occur due to multiple reasons, which include but not limited to patient's comorbid conditions, anesthesia technique, mechanical ventilation, drugs, surgical procedure itself, and intraoperative surgical complications such as blood loss or preexisting sepsis. Maintenance of optimal mean arterial pressure (MAP) during the perioperative period is important to achieve good surgical outcomes. In this chapter, we will review the blood pressure (BP) targets, whether they differ from perfusion targets, the perfusion targets, and the appropriate choice of vasopressors in the perioperative management of patients undergoing major surgical procedures.

CAUSES OF PERIOPERATIVE HEMODYNAMIC INSTABILITY

The causes of perioperative hemodynamic instability can be any or all of the following.

Preoperative State and Type of Surgery

Contrary to the perception, preoperative fasting does not reduce intravascular volume significantly.[1] However, dehydration preoperatively should be avoided by limiting "excess fasting". Gastrointestinal surgeries, for example, make patients more susceptible to large volume shifts and may make the hemodynamics unstable in patients.

Factors Related to Anesthesia

Most anesthetic drugs cause a dose-dependent vasodilation and/or myocardial depression that may contribute to hypotension.[2] Deep plane of anesthesia may be another contributor.

Sympathetic blockade, as widely known, leads to vasodilation, which causes further hypotension.

Mechanical ventilation with high positive end-expiratory pressure (PEEP) causes decreased venous return leading to a reduction in cardiac output (CO). Anesthetic drugs or perioperative antibiotic therapy may cause anaphylaxis.

Factors Related to Surgery

Intraoperative bleeding/volume loss should be corrected as soon as possible as it is a direct cause of volume loss and hypotension. The lethal triad of trauma (hypothermia, coagulation abnormality, and acidosis) can lead to uncontrolled hemorrhage.[3] In patients undergoing laparoscopic surgeries, CO_2 embolism or raised intra-abdominal pressure due to iatrogenic pneumoperitoneum may impede venous return, thereby compromising CO. Surgeries of long bone may cause fat embolism, thus causing hypotension and shock. Any surgical procedure of base of neck, thorax, or upper abdomen may cause pneumothorax.

Insensible loss can be a significant contributor during prolonged open abdominal surgeries and should be judiciously accounted for.[4] An obvious question is why should we consider vasopressor use and avoid hypervolemia in such patients. The answer lies in studies that have found increased morbidity, length of intensive care unit (ICU) stays, and mortality in patients with significant fluid retention (weight gain >10% over preoperative state).[5] Increased fluid leading to tissue edema has effect on practically all organ systems contributing to pathologies such as postoperative respiratory failure, pulmonary edema, ileus, anastomotic dehiscence, abdominal compartment syndrome, coagulation abnormality, and impaired wound healing.[6]

PERIOPERATIVE HEMODYNAMIC INSTABILITY AND OUTCOMES

Blood pressure is an important vital sign monitored intraoperatively. It is also clinically and physiologically relevant for patients, in context of surgery, under anesthesia, and for those patients who are critically ill, as hemodynamic perturbations, especially intraoperative hypotension (IOH), have important clinical impact on different vital organs function and thus influence postoperative outcomes.[7,8] As different organs have their own autoregulatory threshold, the organ blood flow is preserved during BP fluctuation within the range of autoregulation and on the extremes of that range, perfusion becomes pressure dependent. Episodes of IOH cause decreased perfusion of vital organs and consequently have potential to cause ischemia reperfusion injury and thus negatively impact the surgical outcome. However, the flaw is that the incidence of IOH cannot be exactly calculated as there does not exist a formal definition of IOH.[9] IOH has been variously defined based on absolute or relative BP threshold and use of different cut-offs such as systolic blood pressure (SBP) or MAP.[7] A recent systematic review analyzing 42 studies on association between IOH and organ injury risk has suggested that organ injury risk increases when MAP decreases below 80 mm Hg for a duration exceeding 10 minutes.[10]

A study by Walsh et al.,[11] in which they retrospectively analyzed data from 33,330 noncardiac surgeries, observed an association between IOH and postoperative acute kidney and myocardial injury. The study is unique in the sense that the analysis included various MAPs (<55, 55–59, 60–64, 65–69, and 70–74 mm Hg) with periods varying from 1 to 20 minutes for each threshold analyzed. The study concluded that intraoperative MAP <55 mm Hg even for 1–5 minutes was associated with acute kidney and myocardial injury, and the odds for these organ injuries increased as the time spent below this MAP threshold increased.[11]

Salmasi et al.[7] retrospectively studied data of 57,315 noncardiac surgery patients and observed the effect of IOH, defined on the basis of absolute or relative MAP threshold, on acute kidney and myocardial injury. They reported that both MAP values below 65 mm Hg and MAP values 20% below preoperative baseline MAP were progressively associated with postoperative organ injury. Increase in the duration of exposure to IOH was associated with increased odds for postoperative acute kidney and myocardial injury. It is notable in this study the baseline MAP was described as the average of all MAP readings taken within 6 months prior to surgery, excluding measurements during a hospital stay, which makes the study more pragmatic.[7]

Monk et al.[8] in a retrospective cohort study analyzed the data of 18,756 noncardiac major surgery patients to study the association between intraoperative BP deviation (both hypotension and hypertension) and 30-day mortality. They concluded that there was an independent association between IOH (SBP <70 mm Hg for ≥5 minutes, MAP <49 mm Hg for ≥5 minutes, and diastolic BP <30 mm Hg for ≥5 minutes, MAP decreases to >50% from baseline for ≥5 minutes) and 30-day mortality; however, intraoperative hypertension was not associated with poor outcome.[8]

In summary, IOH leads to deleterious consequences and every attempt should be made to avoid it, and in case it occurs, it should be immediately addressed and BP should be restored to levels normal for that patient.

Not only degree of IOH but also the duration of IOH is an important predictor of postoperative organ injury and mortality. Recently, detection of hypotension is now being superseded by prediction of hypotension by devices and indices based on machine learning tools to preemptively detect the possibility of hypotension.[12]

Despite all these things, there are certain positive things about BP. First, it can easily be monitored invasively or noninvasively and continuously or intermittently depending on the need. Second, it is a modifiable factor, which can be addressed to improve postoperative outcomes unlike patient's baseline demographic characteristics. Lastly, there are various measures available which can be instituted for the management of hemodynamic perturbations. However, the question arises "What BP is to be targeted?" A multicenter randomized controlled trial (RCT) [INPRESS (Intraoperative Noradrenaline to Control Arterial Pressure) trial][13] addressing the issue has evaluated individualized (achieving a SBP within 10% of resting SBP) versus standard (treating SBP <80 mm Hg or <40% from the reference value) BP management strategy in 292 adult patients undergoing major surgery under general anesthesia. The study[13] concluded that BP management strategy targeting an individualized SBP is associated with reduced risk of postoperative organ dysfunction as opposed to standard management. Additionally, one more consideration while we decide target BP is perfusion pressure which is the difference between inflow (MAP) and outflow pressure (interstitial pressure of the organ viz. intra-abdominal or intracranial pressure).[14] Another important concern is the perioperative management of patients with chronic systemic hypertension. Asfar et al.[15] in a multicenter RCT of 776 septic shock patients observed that a target MAP of 65–70 mm Hg for patients without prior chronic hypertension and MAP of 80–85 mm Hg for patients with history of systemic hypertension significantly decreased the incidence of acute kidney injury (AKI) and need for renal replacement therapy. In the same line but in perioperative context, Wu et al.[16] conducted an RCT, including 646 elderly patients with chronic systemic hypertension as a comorbidity, undergoing major gastrointestinal surgery. The primary outcome was incidence of postoperative AKI. The patients were randomized to one of the groups based on MAP target: I (65–79 mm Hg), II (80–95 mm Hg), and

III (96–110 mm Hg). In this trial, they observed that the incidence of AKI was significantly lower (6.3%) in patients allocated to the 80–95 mm Hg target group, as compared to those allocated to 65–79 mm Hg (13.5%) and 96–110 mm Hg (12.9%) groups.[16] This forms the basis of the concept that a higher MAP may be needed in patients with chronic systemic hypertension; however, a larger study is needed. BP depends on the CO, preload, and afterload. A decrease in either of these determinants will cause IOH.

PREOPERATIVE OPTIMIZATION OF THE PATIENTS FOR SURGERY

Patients for emergency surgeries can be found to be in shock state and need quick assessment and simultaneous resuscitation to maintain required MAP preoperatively or they may soon be taken for surgery while the hemodynamic optimization is ongoing in order to control the source of sepsis or bleeding. Shock could be of any etiology in operative patients and not necessarily hypovolemic but may include cardiogenic, distributive, and obstructive pathology. There can be a combination of multiple underlying etiologies, which needs assessment and may require point-of-care ultrasound or pulmonary artery catheter values. For example, multiple etiologies may have interplay in attributing to hypotension, for example, a trauma patient who is having overt or concealed bleeding (hypovolemic shock) may have pericardial effusion or tension pneumothorax (obstructive shock) and/or may have spinal cord injury (distributive shock). Comprehensive yet simultaneous assessment and resuscitation should be instituted based on individual situation.

The basic preoperative management could be guided by the principles given below.

General Assessment of Patient

Vital Signs

Shock could be inferred with basic assessment of patient's peripheries, mentation, urine output, and biomarkers such as lactates. It should be supplemented with patient's baseline history (e.g., current BP may be misleading in hypertensive patient). Based on the patient's premorbid BP, target should be defined. A target of MAP >65 mm Hg seems decent for a nonhypertensive adult patient. However, a higher MAP may be required in patients with systemic hypertension. Patients with raised organ pressure like those with intracranial or abdominal hypertension may need higher MAP in order to achieve adequate organ perfusion. Inference on the type of shock could be made based on history and clinical and laboratory variables. Pulse pressure has been a useful adjunct as it provides an indirect inference of dynamics between CO and systemic vascular resistance (SVR). Reduced pulse pressure is seen in most types of shocks with elevated diastolic BP due to increased vasoconstriction. Increased pulse pressure is seen in distributive shock with reduced diastolic BP such as in anaphylactic, spinal, and septic shocks.

Preoperative Tests

Assessment of patient's condition can be done with tests such as hemoglobin, complete blood counts, prothrombin time, renal and liver function tests, electrocardiography, echocardiogram, arterial blood gas, mixed venous oxygen saturation, chest/abdominal X-ray, and computed tomography (CT) scan; however, they should not be an impediment in initial resuscitation of the patient.

Point-of-care Ultrasound

Rapid ultrasound in shock (RUSH) is increasingly being used both in preoperative and intraoperative state to guide further management. Assessment of pump (heart), tank [inferior vena cava (IVC), internal jugular (IJ) vein, lungs, and pleural and peritoneal cavity], and pipes (aorta and distal veins such as femoral and popliteal veins) can be a part of cursory examination.

Monitoring

Standard anesthesia monitors should be placed. Invasive monitoring should be done with intra-arterial catheter, it helps in continuous monitoring of arterial BP as well as monitoring of respirophasic variation in arterial pressure with positive pressure ventilation. Patients may be assumed to be enough fluid-filled when systolic pressure variation (SPV) is <15% with different phases of respiration. Central venous catheter (CVC) placement should be done especially when large blood loss/fluid shifts or vasopressors usage is anticipated, although CVP measurement by itself is a poor predictor of volume status. Pulmonary artery catheter is routinely not placed as it has not shown to improve outcomes.[17] However, it may be used in specific situations such as in severe pulmonary arterial hypertension, right ventricular (RV) failure, and acute valvular disease. Transesophageal echocardiography may be employed for monitoring of volume status, regional and global left and right ventricular function. Additionally, other CO monitoring devices may be instituted, which may help in deciding amongst various vasoactive agents based on CO and SVR. Various invasive and noninvasive options are available including arterial pulse wave waveform, electrical thoracic bioimpedance, pulmonary/transpulmonary thermodilution, and carbon dioxide rebreathing, the details of which are described in other chapter of the book.

INTRAOPERATIVE MANAGEMENT OF HYPOTENSION

Vasopressors

Vasopressors should be instituted in patients to treat hypotension that is unresponsive to fluid administration or change in the depth of anesthesia. Vasopressors increase SVR whereas inotropes typically raise CO through effects on heart rate (HR) and cardiac force of contraction (contractility). Specific agents may alter venous return differently by changes in splanchnic circulation and preload reduction. Such changes may be detrimental in patients such as those with ischemic heart disease and left ventricular outflow tract (LVOT) obstruction. Hence, knowledge about individual vasopressors is required. Commonly used vasoactive agents are given below.

Ephedrine

It stimulates α, β-1, and β-2 receptors. It is particularly useful in patients with bradycardia because of its effect on HR. It is used in 5–10 mg bolus doses. It causes presynaptic release of norepinephrine and also has an additional effect on postsynaptic release and uptake of norepinephrine.[18] It increases BP, CO, and HR; therefore, it is particularly useful in patients with bradycardia, especially if its origin is within or above the atrioventricular node (e.g., secondary to beta-blocker use).[19]

It can be beneficial in patients with bronchospasm due to its effect via the β-2 receptors.[20]

It has better cerebral oxygenation and preservation of cerebral blood flow than phenylephrine.[21]

Disadvantages: Inability to use it as continuous infusion, tachyphylaxis is common, particularly with repeated doses. Drugs such as cocaine and reserpine that impair synaptic uptake can alter its action. Fetal acidosis is common when used in obstetric patients.

Phenylephrine

Among the most common used vasopressors, especially when HR is normal or elevated. It acts via stimulation of α-1 adrenergic receptors causing vasoconstriction and hence baroreceptor-mediated reflex decreases in HR. It is used in doses of 50–100 μg as bolus or in an infusion at 10–100 μg/min. Ischemic heart disease patients benefit from decrease in HR.[21] Phenylephrine is beneficial for patients with LVOT obstruction, aortic stenosis (AS), and tetralogy of Fallot (TOF). Phenylephrine can be used a bolus. There is a concern regarding reduced CO with phenylephrine due to its effect on α-1 receptor. As it causes bradycardia, it is not ideal for regurgitant valvular diseases.

Vasopressin

This is a naturally acting nonapeptide released from posterior pituitary gland in response to decreased intravascular volume, increased plasma osmolarity, pain, and nausea. It acts via V_1 receptor and causes vasoconstriction, thereby increasing BP. Exogenous administration as a continuous infusion at 0.01–0.04 units/min is recommended. It is often used in patients when shock is refractory to conventional vasopressors as a second-line therapy. It also augments the vasoconstrictive effect of norepinephrine. Direct coronary and cerebral vasoconstriction are comparatively lesser than catecholamines; however, this effect may be offset by dose-dependent increase in SVR and increased vagal tone.[22]

Vasopressin as compared to norepinephrine has less severe vasoconstrictive effect on pulmonary vasculature, thus it can be used safely in cardiogenic shock with RV failure and in patients with pulmonary hypertension,[23] and also its role can be utilized perioperatively in cardiac surgeries.[24]

The VASST (Vasopressin and Septic Shock Trial) study,[25] a multicenter RCT, tested hypothesis that low-dose vasopressin as compared with norepinephrine would decrease mortality among patients with septic shock in 778 patients. It concluded that there was no difference in 28-day mortality between the two groups. However, analysis of apriori subgroup demonstrated survival advantage among patients receiving low-dose (5–14 μg/min) norepinephrine with the addition of vasopressin.[25]

The VANISH (Vasopressin vs. Norepinephrine as Initial Therapy in Septic Shock) trial,[26] a 2 × 2 factorial RCT, evaluated 409 septic shock patients with early use of vasopressin with placebo or hydrocortisone versus norepinephrine with placebo or hydrocortisone for kidney failure-free days as outcome. The conclusion stated that early use of vasopressin compared with norepinephrine did not improve the number of kidney failure-free days.[26]

Current recommendation for sepsis and septic shock guidelines consider vasopressin as a second-line vasopressor agent in patients where MAP cannot be maintained with norepinephrine.[27]

Dopamine

Dopamine is a precursor of norepinephrine. It has a differential dose-dependent action on cardiac contractility and vascular smooth muscles. Low-dose dopamine <2 μg/kg/min was said to improve renal output. However, this notion was challenged and a randomized control study by Bellomo et al.[28] showed that in patients low-dose dopamine does not improve serum peak creatinine level, need of renal replacement therapy, duration of ICU, or hospital stay. In a moderate dose, 5–10 μg/kg/min acts on β-1 receptors increasing cardiac contractility and in doses >10 µg/kg/min shows predominantly α-1 receptor-mediated predominantly vasoconstrictor effect.[22] Historically, it has been used as a first-line vasopressor for various shock states. However, it has gone into disrepute when it was observed that it increases mortality.[29] Later, it was studied in an RCT head-to-head with norepinephrine and concluded that it does not increase 28-day mortality but increases arrhythmic events.[30] With this concern and observed increased mortality in cardiogenic shock, cohort has decreased its usage restricted to special situations and dopamine is no more a first-line vasopressor for septic shock.[27] Additionally, dopamine use has potential for negative endocrine and immune effects.[31,32]

Norepinephrine

Norepinephrine is an endogenous catecholamine (epinephrine is derived from norepinephrine by phenylethanolamine N-methyl transferase) in adrenal medulla. Norepinephrine has predominantly α-receptor agonist action, thereby causing vasoconstriction and consequently increasing BP. It also has β-agonist action and results increase in stroke volume which is less marked than α-receptor action. A recent RCT comparing dopamine versus noradrenaline in 1,679 patients of various shock states has observed no difference in 28-day mortality; however, it was found that patients who received dopamine as first-line vasopressors had higher incidence of arrhythmias.[30] In the same study,[30] subgroup analysis of cardiogenic shock patients revealed higher 28-day mortality in patients who received dopamine as first-line vasopressor.

Vasu et al.[33] in a systematic review evaluated six studies comparing noradrenaline versus dopamine as first-line vasopressor in 2,043 septic shock patients. In their analysis, they concluded that norepinephrine was superior to dopamine in terms of in-hospital mortality or 28-day mortality.[33] Current guideline for septic shock[27] and expert recommendations for cardiogenic shock[34] recommend using norepinephrine as first-line vasopressor in septic and cardiogenic shocks.

Norepinephrine has both inotropic and vasopressor action.[35] It is used as the first-line agent for most types of shocks. Recent data suggests safety of norepinephrine in obstetric anesthesia.[36]

Like other vasopressor agents, its peripheral extravasation can cause tissue necrosis. CVC is needed for prolonged administration due to fear of tissue damage.[37]

Epinephrine

Epinephrine exerts its effects by direct stimulation of both α and β receptors, though unlike norepinephrine, the β effects are much more pronounced. At low doses (0.01–0.02 µg/kg/min), it has a predominant β-2 action which may cause vasodilation. Intermediate doses (0.02–0.1 µg/kg/min) cause β-1 and β-2 action, causing both increase in BP and HR and vasodilation. There is predominance of α stimulation at high doses and bolus doses. β-2 stimulation can cause adverse metabolic effects such as hyperglycemia, lipolysis, and metabolic acidosis.[38] Epinephrine use as a first-line agent during intraoperative phase is usually restricted to anaphylactic shock or cardiac arrest. It may be used intramuscularly or via endotracheal tube, if intravenous access is not available. It may also be used as a bolus or as continuous infusion. However, reduction of splanchnic blood circulation is an important concern, especially in septic shock scenarios.[39,40]

In a prospective, double-blind RCT, Myburgh et al.[41] compared epinephrine with norepinephrine in 280 critically ill patients with shock and found essentially no difference in time to achieve BP targets, 28-day mortality, or 90-day mortality; however, 18 out of 139 patients in the epinephrine group were withdrawn from the study because of side effects (lactic acidosis or tachycardia). In another RCT, Annane et al.[42] studied 330 patients of septic shock who were allocated to receive either epinephrine or norepinephrine with dobutamine titrated to maintain an MAP of ≥70 mm Hg. In both groups, time to hemodynamic success, mortality rates at discharge from ICU, at hospital discharge, 28-day mortality, and 90-day mortality were similar. As it is known that epinephrine administration causes lactate production, hence this lactate production confounds with using lactate clearance as a marker of response to resuscitation. Currently, epinephrine is recommended as a second-line agent for septic shock in surviving sepsis campaign guidelines.[27]

Angiotensin II

Angiotensin II is an endogenous vasopressor, which is an integral part of renin–angiotensin–aldosterone system (RAAS). Renin is a proteolytic enzyme which is secreted by juxtaglomerular apparatus in response decrease BP and/or hypovolemia. Angiotensinogen is produced by the liver and released into circulation where it is converted by renin to angiotensin I, and then cleaved by angiotensin-converting enzyme (ACE) into angiotensin II. This occurs mostly by endothelial-bound ACE in the lungs. Exogenous administration of angiotensin II has catecholamine-sparing effect and effectively improves the MAP in a patient on high-dose norepinephrine with high output shock.[43] US Food and Drug Administration has approved use of angiotensin II as a vasopressor agent in high CO shock; however, it has given warning with its use to continue thromboprophylaxis as it may create a prothrombotic state with arterial/venous thrombosis events.[44]

Inotropes

Inotropic support is needed to improve cardiac contractility. Various inotropes used in clinical practice are discussed below.

Dobutamine

It acts predominantly by stimulating β-1 and β-2 receptors. It increases CO by β-1 receptor activity by increasing cardiac contractility and also HR; however, it may have a variable effect on BP. Dobutamine should be used to treat low CO in cardiogenic shock[34] and in cases where hypoperfusion persists despite adequate fluid loading and vasopressor institution.

Dobutamine can be added to norepinephrine for better tolerance and avoidance of negative effects of epinephrine use. The combination gives advantage of less arrhythmia, less myocardial oxygen consumption, and a lower increase in lactate concentration as compared to epinephrine.[45]

Phosphodiesterase 3 Inhibitors

Phosphodiesterase 3 (PDE3) enzyme causes hydrolysis of cyclic adenosine monophosphate (cAMP) to AMP. PDE3 inhibitors are the competitive inhibitors of phosphodiesterase enzymes and thus lead to increased levels of cAMP intracellularly in myocardium and vascular smooth muscle. This causes the release of calcium from sarcoplasmic reticulum, thereby increasing cardiac contractility. It has inotropic, vasodilatory, and lusitropic (through phospholamban) effects. However, its prolonged administration may lead to sudden cardiac death.[46] This group of drugs include amrinone, milrinone, and enoximone. Amrinone use has declined because it causes dose-related thrombocytopenia.[22]

Levosimendan

Levosimendan is a calcium sensitizer that exerts its effect without any increased metabolic demand of the heart. It increases myocardial cell sensitivity to Ca without increasing intracellular free Ca and additionally it causes vasodilation. It has a dual mechanism of action—one that increases inotropy and other that causes decrease in SVR—thus decreasing afterload by opening the adenosine triphosphate (ATP)-dependent potassium channel. Its therapeutic efficacy is marred by increased risk of arrhythmias and hypotension. Two of its active metabolites have half-lives of 70–80 hours, causing the duration of hemodynamic effect to last as long as 7 days.[47]

Gordon et al. in an RCT investigated the role of levosimendan added to standard care of sepsis patients for prevention of organ dysfunction in 516 adult patients. The study concluded that addition of levosimendan to standard treatment in adults with sepsis was not associated with less severe organ dysfunction or decreased mortality, on the other hand, they found that there was lower likelihood of successful weaning from mechanical ventilation and a higher risk of supraventricular tachyarrhythmia in patients allocated to levosimendan group as compared to placebo.[48] Levosimendan can be used as an alternative to dobutamine in second-line treatment of cardiogenic shock after cardiac surgery.[34] However, its use should be considered under close monitoring for hypotension and arrhythmia.

The properties of the vasoactive agents are summarized in **Table 1**.

Adrenal insufficiency should always be high on the list of differential diagnosis intraoperative period with hypotension unresponsive to standard therapy. Management is done with a "stress dose" of 100 mg of hydrocortisone.

POSTOPERATIVE CRITICAL CARE MANAGEMENT IN ICU OR RECOVERY ROOM

Patients with intraoperative shock should ideally not be extubated unless the vasopressor requirements are minimal. They should be transported to ICU for continual monitoring.

Even during the transport, patients should be continuously monitored. During transport, ECG (electrocardiogram), pulse oximeter, and continuous invasive BP should be monitored. These are as per transport guidelines of Society for Critical Care Medicine (SCCM).[49] Upon arrival to ICU, patient information should be provided ideally through a written checklist from operative team to the ICU team by a formal process of "handover."[50]

PERIOPERATIVE GOAL-DIRECTED THERAPY

Another important usage of vasoactive agents during perioperative period is guiding the hemodynamic and oxygen-derived variables to predefined goals in order to mitigate tissue hypoxia, cardiac dysfunction, and hypoperfusion. Perioperative goal-directed therapy (PGDT) has been variably used in major surgeries in high-risk surgical patients (individual or undergoing procedure having >5% mortality risk).[51] The concept of liberal and restrictive fluid strategies may lead to fluid overload and occult hypoperfusion respectively and their attendant side effects and increased mortality.[52-54]

Tissue trauma during moderate-to-high risk surgical procedures causes release of inflammatory mediators with consequent vasodilatation, capillary leakage, and cardiac dysfunctions.[55] Optimization of oxygen delivery (DO_2) by optimizing its determinants is considered to be the way forward. DO_2 predominantly depends on CO, hemoglobin (Hb) concentration, and arterial blood hemoglobin oxygen

Table 1: Vasoactive drugs.

Vasoactive drugs	Clinical indication	Dose range	Receptor binding/ mechanism of action Alpha-1, Beta-1, Beta-2, and dopamine	Side effect
Dopamine	Shock (cardiogenic, vasodilatory) HF Symptomatic bradycardia unresponsive to atropine or pacing	2.0–20 µg/kg/min (maximum 50 µg/kg/min)	+++ ++++ ++ +++++	Severe hypertension (especially in patients taking nonselective beta-blockers) Ventricular arrhythmias Cardiac ischemia Tissue ischemia/gangrene (high doses or due to tissue extravasation)
Dobutamine	Low CO (decompensated HF, cardiogenic shock, sepsis-induced myocardial dysfunction) Symptomatic bradycardia unresponsive to atropine or pacing	2.0–20 µg/kg/min (maximum 40 µg/kg/min)	+ +++++ +++ N/A	Tachycardia Increased ventricular response rate in patients with atrial fibrillation Ventricular arrhythmias Cardiac ischemia Hypertension (especially nonselective beta-blocker patients) Hypotension
Norepinephrine	Shock (vasodilatory and cardiogenic)	0.01–3 µg/kg/min	+++++ +++ ++ N/A	Arrhythmias Bradycardia Peripheral (digital) ischemia Hypertension (especially nonselective beta-blocker patients)
Epinephrine	Shock (cardiogenic and vasodilatory) and cardiac arrest Bronchospasm/anaphylaxis, symptomatic bradycardia, or heart block unresponsive to atropine or pacing	Infusion: 0.01–0.10 µg/kg/ min Bolus: 1 mg IV every 3–5 minutes (maximum 0.2 mg/kg) IM: (1:1000): 0.1–0.5 mg (maximum 1 mg)	+++++ ++++ +++ N/A	Ventricular arrhythmias Severe hypertension resulting in cerebrovascular hemorrhage Cardiac ischemia Sudden cardiac death
Isoproterenol	Bradyarrhythmias (especially torsade de pointes)	2–10 µg/min	0 +++++ +++++ N/A	Ventricular arrhythmias Cardiac ischemia Hypertension Hypotension
Phenylephrine	Hypotension (vagally mediated and medication-induced) Increase MAP with AS and hypotension Decrease LVOT gradient in HCM	Bolus: 0.1–0.5 mg IV every 10–15 minutes Infusion: 0.4–9.1 µg/kg/ min	+++++ 0 0 N/A	Reflex bradycardia Hypertension (especially with nonselective beta-blockers) Severe peripheral and visceral vasoconstriction Tissue necrosis with extravasation
Milrinone	Low CO (decompensated HF, after cardiotomy)	Bolus: 50 µg/kg bolus over 10–30 minutes Infusion: 0.375–0.75 µg/ kg/min (dose adjustment necessary for renal impairment)	N/A N/A N/A N/A Acts by increasing cellular level of cyclic AMP	Ventricular arrhythmias Hypotension Cardiac ischemia Torsade des pointes
Amrinone	Low CO (refractory HF)	Bolus: 0.75 mg/kg over 2–3 minutes Infusion: 5–10 µg/kg/min	N/A N/A N/A N/A Acts by increasing cellular level of cyclic AMP	Arrhythmias, enhanced AV conduction (increased ventricular response rate in atrial fibrillation) Hypotension Thrombocytopenia Hepatotoxicity
Vasopressin	Shock (vasodilatory and cardiogenic) Cardiac arrest	Infusion: 0.01–0.1 U/min (common fixed dose 0.04 U/min) Bolus: 40 U IV bolus	V1 receptors (vascular smooth muscle) V2 receptors (renal collecting duct system)	Arrhythmias Hypertension Decreased CO (at doses >0.4 U/min) Cardiac ischemia Severe peripheral vasoconstriction causing ischemia (especially skin) Splanchnic vasoconstriction
Levosimendan	Decompensated HF	Loading dose: 12–24 µg/kg over 10 minutes Infusion: 0.05–0.2 µg/kg/min	N/A N/A N/A N/A Sensitizes troponin C to calcium	Tachycardia, enhanced AV conduction Hypotension

(AMP: adenosine monophosphate; AS: aortic stenosis; AV: atrioventricular; CO: cardiac output; HCM: hypertrophic cardiomyopathy; HF: heart failure; IM: intramuscular; IV: intravenous; LVOT: left ventricular outflow tract; MAP: mean arterial pressure; NA: not applicable)

saturation (SaO_2). CO optimization with fluids and use of vasoactive agents play a major role in optimizing DO_2. CO optimization concept is based on qualitative figures rather than quantity or value. Thus, an adequate CO is said to be when there is normal range of downstream markers of tissue perfusion. Giving fluids in a fluid responsive patient based on dynamic parameters of fluid responsiveness is advocated. With advent of technology, minimally invasive techniques are now available to measure beat-to-beat CO along with provision of measuring dynamic parameters of fluid responsiveness. Giving fluids to increase CO in fluid responsiveness and adding vasopressors or inotropes to increase CO when patient is no more fluid responsive have been guiding principles in avoiding pumping unnecessary fluid. PGDT has considerable variations in choice of CO monitors, fluid responsiveness parameters, and use of vasopressors or inotropes. However, it has been found to have a positive impact on the outcome of patients.[56]

Early observation of Shoemaker et al. that nonsurvivors had low DO_2 led to the foundation of optimization of DO_2 by attempts to improve the components which determine the DO_2.[57] Rationale of targeting supraphysiological DO_2 led to improved outcomes in moderate-to-high risk surgical patients which defined the PGDT utility.[58-60] Improvement of technology [pulse pressure variation (PPV), stroke volume variation (SVV), and minimally invasive CO monitoring] further helped in individualizing the therapy and fine-tuning it to specific requirement of each patient.

CONCLUSION

Blood pressure monitoring is of vital importance as a part of perioperative monitoring protocol. IOH has been found to be an important modifiable factor causing various postoperative complications ranging from AKI, acute myocardial injury, and thus negatively affects postoperative outcome. However, the downside of IOH is that its exact incidence cannot be known as there is no formal definition of IOH. To improve postoperative outcomes, IOH should be avoided and in case it occurs, it should be immediately be reversed. IOH is an interplay between CO, preload, and afterload. Management should be done based on the cause of IOH. Fluids, vasoactive agents, and control of bleeding are commonly employed measures. Decision of BP target should be based on the patient's comorbid conditions and perfusion pressure. After appropriate fluid resuscitation, appropriate vasoactive drug(s) should be used to match the therapeutic goal. Choice of vasopressor agent is based on the pathobiology of shock. Vasopressors are also drugs with side effects, so the shock condition should be appropriately managed to avoid prolonged exposure of vasoactive drugs. By and large, noradrenaline is the first-line vasopressor

agent for a variety of shock. Vasopressin and adrenaline can be used as second-line vasopressors and dopamine can be used in special circumstances. Dobutamine is usually the first-line inotrope with PDE3 inhibitors and levosimendan as second line wherever appropriate.

REFERENCES

1. Danielsson EJD, Lejbman I, Åkeson J. Fluid deficits during prolonged overnight fasting in young healthy adults. Acta Anaesthesiol Scand. 2019;63(2):195-9.
2. Connolly CM, Kramer GC, Hahn RG, Chaisson NF, Svensen CH, Kirschner RA, et al. Isoflurane but not mechanical ventilation promotes extravascular fluid accumulation during crystalloid volume loading. Anesthesiology. 2003;98(3):670-81.
3. Ferrara A, MacArthur JD, Wright HK, Hastings IM, Mcmillen MA. Hypothermia and acidosis worsen coagulopathy in the patient requiring massive transfusion. Am J Surg. 1990;160(5):515-8.
4. Lamke LO, Nilsson GE, Reithner HL. Water loss by evaporation from the abdominal cavity during surgery. Acta Chir Scand. 1977;143(5):279-84.
5. Thacker JK, Mountford WK, Ernst FR, Krukas MR, Mythen MM. Perioperative fluid utilization variability and association with outcomes: considerations for enhanced recovery efforts in sample US surgical populations. Ann Surg. 2016;263(3):502-10.
6. Holte K, Sharrock NE, Kehlet H. Pathophysiology and clinical implications of perioperative fluid excess. Br J Anaesth. 2002;89(4):622-32.
7. Salmasi V, Maheshwari K, Yang D, Mascha EJ, Singh A, Sessler DI, et al. Relationship between intraoperative hypotension, defined by either reduction from baseline or absolute thresholds, and acute kidney and myocardial injury after noncardiac surgery: a retrospective cohort analysis. Anesthesiology. 2017;126(1):47-65.
8. Monk TG, Bronsert MR, Henderson WG, Mangione MP, Sum-Ping ST, Bentt DR, et al. Association between intraoperative hypotension and hypertension and 30-day postoperative mortality in noncardiac surgery. Anesthesiology. 2015;123(2):307-19.
9. Bijker JB, van Klei WA, Kappen TH, van Wolfswinkel L, Moons KG, Kalkman CJ. Incidence of intraoperative hypotension as a function of the chosen definition: literature definitions applied to a retrospective cohort using automated data collection. Anesthesiology. 2007;107(2):213-20.
10. Wesselink EM, Kappen TH, Torn HM, Slooter AJC, van Klei WA. Intraoperative hypotension and the risk of postoperative adverse outcomes: a systematic review. Br J Anaesth. 2018;121(4):706-21.
11. Walsh M, Devereaux PJ, Garg AX, Kurz A, Turan A, Rodseth RN, et al. Relationship between intraoperative mean arterial pressure and clinical outcomes after noncardiac surgery: toward an empirical definition of hypotension. Anesthesiology. 2013;119(3):507-15.
12. Vos JJ, Scheeren TW. Intraoperative hypotension and its prediction. Indian J Anaesth. 2019;63(11):877-85.

13. Futier E, Lefrant JY, Guinot PG, Godet T, Lorne E, Cuvillon P, et al. Effect of individualized vs standard blood pressure management strategies on postoperative organ dysfunction among high-risk patients undergoing major surgery: a randomized clinical trial. JAMA. 2017;318(14):1346-57.

14. Saugel B, Reuter DA, Reese PC. Intraoperative mean arterial pressure targets: can databases give us a universally valid "magic number" or does physiology still apply for the individual patient? Anesthesiology. 2017;127(4):725-6.

15. Asfar P, Meziani F, Hamel JF, Grelon F, Megarbane B, Anguel N, et al. High versus low blood-pressure target in patients with septic shock. N Engl J Med. 2014;370(17):1583-93.

16. Wu X, Jiang Z, Ying J, Han Y, Chen Z. Optimal blood pressure decreases acute kidney injury after gastrointestinal surgery in elderly hypertensive patients: a randomized study: Optimal blood pressure reduces acute kidney injury. J Clin Anesth. 2017;43:77-83.

17. Rajaram SS, Desai NK, Kalra A, Gajera M, Cavanaugh SK, Brampton W, et al. Pulmonary artery catheters for adult patients in intensive care. Cochrane Database Syst Rev. 2013;(2):CD003408.

18. Kobayashi S, Endou M, Sakuraya F, Matsuda N, Zhang XH, Azuma M, et al. The sympathomimetic actions of l-ephedrine and d-pseudoephedrine: direct receptor activation or norepinephrine release? Anesth Analg. 2003;97(5):1239-45.

19. Goertz AW, Hübner C, Seefelder C, Seeling W, Lindner KH, Rockemann MG, et al. The effect of ephedrine bolus administration on left ventricular loading and systolic performance during high thoracic epidural anesthesia combined with general anesthesia. Anesth Analg. 1994;78(1):101-5.

20. Westfall TC, Westfall DP. Adrenergic agonists and antagonists. In: Brunton LL, Chabner BA, Knollman CB (Eds). Goodman and Gilman's The Pharmacological Basis of Therapeutics, 12th edition. New York: McGraw Hill; 2011. p. 300.

21. Schwinn DA, Reves JG. Time course and hemodynamic effects of alpha-1-adrenergic bolus administration in anesthetized patients with myocardial disease. Anesth Analg. 1989;68(5):571-8.

22. Overgaard CB, Dzavík V. Inotropes and vasopressors: review of physiology and clinical use in cardiovascular disease. Circulation. 2008;118(10):1047-56.

23. Gordon AC, Wang N, Walley KR, Ashby D, Russell JA. The cardiopulmonary effects of vasopressin compared with norepinephrine in septic shock. Chest. 2012;142(3):593-605.

24. Morozowich ST, Ramakrishna H. Pharmacologic agents for acute hemodynamic instability: recent advances in the management of perioperative shock-A systematic review. Ann Card Anaesth. 2015;18(4):543-54.

25. Russell JA, Walley KR, Singer J, Gordon AC, Hébert PC, Cooper DJ, et al. Vasopressin versus norepinephrine infusion in patients with septic shock. N Engl J Med. 2008;358(9):877-87.

26. Gordon AC, Mason AJ, Thirunavukkarasu N, Perkins GD, Cecconi M, Cepkova M, et al. Effect of early vasopressin vs norepinephrine on kidney failure in patients with septic shock: the VANISH randomized clinical trial. JAMA. 2016;316(5):509-18.

27. Rhodes A, Evans LE, Alhazzani W, Levy MM, Antonelli M, Ferrer R, et al. Surviving sepsis campaign: international guidelines for management of sepsis and septic shock: 2016. Intensive Care Med. 2017;43(3):304-77.

28. Bellomo R, Chapman M, Finfer S, Hickling K, Myburgh J. Low-dose dopamine in patients with early renal dysfunction: a placebo-controlled randomised trial. Australian and New Zealand Intensive Care Society (ANZICS) Clinical Trials Group. Lancet. 2000;356(9248):2139-43.

29. Sakr Y, Reinhart K, Vincent JL, Sprung CL, Moreno R, Ranieri VM, et al. Does dopamine administration in shock influence outcome? Results of the Sepsis Occurrence in Acutely Ill Patients (SOAP) Study. Crit Care Med. 2006;34(3):589-97.

30. De Backer D, Biston P, Devriendt J, Madl C, Chochrad D, Aldecoa C, et al. Comparison of dopamine and norepinephrine in the treatment of shock. N Engl J Med. 2010;362(9):779-89.

31. Oberbeck R, Schmitz D, Wilsenack K, Schüler M, Husain B, Schedlowski M, et al. Dopamine affects cellular immune functions during polymicrobial sepsis. Intensive Care Med. 2006;32(5):731-9.

32. Beck GCh, Brinkkoetter P, Hanusch C, Schulte J, van Ackern K, van der Woude FJ, et al. Clinical review: immunomodulatory effects of dopamine in general inflammation. Crit Care. 2004;8(6):485-91.

33. Vasu TS, Cavallazzi R, Hirani A, Kaplan G, Leiby B, Marik PE. Norepinephrine or dopamine for septic shock: systematic review of randomized clinical trials. J Intensive Care Med. 2012;27(3):172-8.

34. Levy B, Bastien O, Karim B, Cariou A, Chouihed T, Combes A, et al. Experts' recommendations for the management of adult patients with cardiogenic shock. Ann Intensive Care. 2015;5(1):52.

35. Mets B. Should norepinephrine, rather than phenylephrine, be considered the primary vasopressor in anesthetic practice? Anesth Analg. 2016;122(5):1707-14.

36. Hasanin AM, Amin SM, Agiza NA, Elsayed MK, Refaat S, Hussein HA, et al. Norepinephrine infusion for preventing postspinal anesthesia hypotension during cesarean delivery: a randomized dose-finding trial. Anesthesiology. 2019;130(1):55-62.

37. Loubani OM, Green RS. A systematic review of extravasation and local tissue injury from administration of vasopressors through peripheral intravenous catheters and central venous catheters. J Crit Care. 2015;30(3):653.e9-17.

38. Totaro RJ, Raper RF. Epinephrine-induced lactic acidosis following cardiopulmonary bypass. Crit Care Med. 1997;25(10):1693-99.

39. Levy B, Bollaert PE, Charpentier C, Nace L, Audibert G, Bauer P, et al. Comparison of norepinephrine and dobutamine to epinephrine for hemodynamics, lactate metabolism, and gastric tonometric variables in septic shock: a prospective, randomized study. Intensive Care Med. 1997;23(3):282-7.

40. Zhou SX, Qiu HB, Huang YZ, Yang Y, Zheng RQ. Effects of norepinephrine, epinephrine, and norepinephrine-dobutamine on systemic and gastric mucosal oxygenation in septic shock. Acta Pharmacol Sin. 2002;23(7):654-8.

41. Myburgh JA, Higgins A, Jovanovska A, Lipman J, Ramakrishnan N, Santamaria J. A comparison of epinephrine and norepinephrine in critically ill patients. Intensive Care Med. 2008;34(12):2226-34.

42. Annane D, Vignon P, Renault A, Bollaert PE, Charpentier C, Martin C, et al. Norepinephrine plus dobutamine versus epinephrine alone for management of septic shock: a randomised trial. Lancet. 2007;370(9588):676-84.

43. Khanna A, English SW, Wang XS, Ham K, Tumlin J, Szerlip H, et al. Angiotensin II for the treatment of vasodilatory shock. N Engl J Med. 2017;377(5):419-30.

44. Jadhav AP, Sadaka FG. Angiotensin II in septic shock. Am J Emerg Med. 2019;37(6):1169-74.

45. Levy B, Perez P, Perny J, Thivilier C, Gerard A. Comparison of norepinephrine-dobutamine to epinephrine for hemodynamics, lactate metabolism, and organ function variables in cardiogenic shock. A prospective, randomized pilot study. Crit Care Med. 2011;39(3):450-5.

46. Movsesian M. New pharmacologic interventions to increase cardiac contractility: challenges and opportunities. Curr Opin Cardiol. 2015;30(3):285-91.

47. Annane D, Ouanes-Besbes L, de Backer D, DU B, Gordon AC, Hernández G, et al. A global perspective on vasoactive agents in shock. Intensive Care Med. 2018;44(6):833-46.

48. Gordon AC, Perkins GD, Singer M, McAuley DF, Orme RM, Santhakumaran S, et al. Levosimendan for the prevention of acute organ dysfunction in sepsis. N Engl J Med. 2016;375(17):1638-48.

49. Warren J, Fromm RE Jr, Orr RA, Rotello LC, Horst HM; American College of Critical Care Medicine. Guidelines for the inter- and intrahospital transport of critically ill patients. Crit Care Med. 2004;32(1):256-62.

50. Starmer AJ, Spector ND, Srivastava R, West DC, Rosenbluth G, Allen AD, et al. Changes in medical errors after implementation of a handoff program. N Engl J Med. 2014;371(19):1803-12.

51. Boyd O, Jackson N. Clinical review: how is risk defined in high-risk surgical patient management? Crit Care. 2005;9:390-6.

52. Brandstrup B, Tønnesen H, Beier-Holgersen R, Hjortsø E, Ørding H, Lindorff-Larsen K, et al. Effects of intravenous fluid restriction on postoperative complications: comparison of two perioperative fluid regimens: a randomized assessor-blinded multicenter trial. Ann Surg. 2003;238(5):641-8.

53. Mythen MG, Swart M, Acheson N, Crawford R, Jones K, Kuper M, et al. Perioperative fluid management: consensus statement from the enhanced recovery partnership. Perioper Med. 2012;1:2.

54. Varadhan KK, Lobo DN. A meta-analysis of randomised controlled trials of intravenous fluid therapy in major elective open abdominal surgery: getting the balance right. Proc Nutr Soc. 2010;69(4):488-98.

55. Lin E, Lowry S. Inflammatory cytokines in major surgery: a functional perspective. Intensive Care Med.1999;25(3):255-7.

56. Hamilton MA, Cecconi M, Rhodes A. A systematic review and metaanalysis on the use of preemptive hemodynamic intervention to improve postoperative outcomes in moderate and highrisk surgical patients. Anesth Analg. 2011;112(6): 1392-402.

57. Shoemaker WC, Appel PL, Kram HB, Waxman K, Lee TS. Prospective trial of supranormal values of survivors as therapeutic goals in high-risk surgical patients. Chest. 1988;94(6):1176-86.

58. Gan TJ, Soppitt A, Maroof M, el-Moalem H, Robertson KM, Moretti E, et al. Goal-directed intraoperative fluid administration reduces length of hospital stay after major surgery. Anesthesiology. 2002;97(4):820-6.

59. Cecconi M, Fasano N, Langiano N, Divella M, Costa MG, Rhodes A, et al. Goal-directed haemodynamic therapy during elective total hip arthroplasty under regional anaesthesia. Crit Care. 2011;15(3):R132.

60. Lobo SM, Ronchi LS, Oliveira NE, Brandão PG, Froes A, Cunrath GS, et al. Restrictive strategy of intraoperative fluid maintenance during optimization of oxygen delivery decreases major complications after high-risk surgery. Crit Care. 2011;15(5):R226.

Blood Transfusion in the Perioperative Period

Ruchira Wasudeo Khasne, Atul Prabhakar Kulkarni, Pradnya Atul Kulkarni

INTRODUCTION

Blood transfusion (BT) is one of the most common procedures performed in hospitals all over the world with considerable geographic variations in practices.[1] BT may be lifesaving in few situations, but many studies have shown an increased morbidity and mortality patients who were transfused.[2] It is an independent predictor of organ dysfunction, nosocomial infection, and acute respiratory distress syndrome, and it should be undertaken only if it improves patient outcome.[3] Thus, patient-centered, multimodality, and multidisciplinary approach focusing on better clinical outcomes should be implemented. This review is restricted to perioperative BT with preoperative assessment and optimization, transfusion trigger, blood component therapy, transfusion reactions, restrictive transfusion strategy, impact on patient outcome, massive transfusion protocol (MTP), storage lesions, adjuncts to prevent and/or treat bleeding, current place of leukodepleted, and artificial blood.

PATIENT EVALUATION AND PREOPERATIVE PREPARATION

Preoperatively every patient should be evaluated in detail **(Tables 1 and 2)** with review of medical records including previous history of BT and reactions to transfusions if any. Additional test should be advised based on clinical conditions such as anemia and coagulopathy, etc. The anesthetist and the intensivist (if needed) should discuss with the patient and family preoperatively regarding the possible need for BT and associated risk during perioperative course, if blood loss is anticipated.

IDENTIFICATION OF IDEAL HEMOGLOBIN TRANSFUSION TRIGGERS

Transfusion trigger is defined as that value of hemoglobin (Hb) below which RBC transfusion is indicated.

Traditionally, the rule of "10/30" (Hb level 10 g/dL or a hematocrit 30%) has been followed for RBC transfusion. Due to variable transfusion practices, the exact transfusion trigger has not been defined. Although decisions to transfuse should be individualized on case-to-case basis, but overall "restrictive transfusion strategy" is widely accepted. Clinical factors such as patient's age, severity scores, comorbidities such as IHD with reduced cardiopulmonary reserve, ongoing bleeding or potential for bleeding, hemodynamic instability, volume status with ongoing ischemia, patients consent, etc., should be considered. Blood should be administered unit-by-unit, with frequent re-evaluation. But broad guidelines should not surpass the clinical judgment in making the decisions regarding transfusion.

A recent audit of transfusion practices[1] found that the transfusion trigger is slightly lower in patients admitted to the intensive care units (ICUs) in Western Europe (8.1 g/dL) or North America (7.9 g/dL) than those reported in the older studies such as ABC (Anemia and Blood Transfusion in the Critically Ill) (8.4 g/dL) and CRIT (Anemia and blood transfusion in the critically ill – Current clinical practice in the United States) (8.6 g/dL).

Clinical Practice Guideline 2016 from the American Association of Blood Banks (AABB)[7] recommends a "restrictive transfusion strategy" with two different Hb levels for RBC transfusion. First group comprises of hemodynamically stable ICU patients with Hb of 7 g/dL and is recommended as a restrictive RBC transfusion threshold whereas in the second group, patients undergoing orthopedic or cardiac surgery, and those with pre-existing cardiovascular disease, Hb level of 8 g/dL is recommended as a restrictive RBC transfusion threshold with strong recommendation based on moderate-quality evidence. However, guideline suggests that these recommendations are not applicable to patients with acute coronary syndrome (ACS), severe thrombocytopenia (patients treated for hematological or oncological reasons

Table 1: Preoperative preparation and preadmission evaluation.[4]

Preoperative preparation	Evaluate risk factors for organ ischemia such as ischemic heart disease (IHD), respiratory disease, surgical risk of bleeding, e.g., cardiac, hepatic, orthopedic surgery	Transfuse as per transfusion protocol. Reserve blood products in anticipation
	Evaluate cause and diagnosis of anemia and optimize Hb to reduce unnecessary red blood cell (RBC) transfusion	Preoperative—oral or intravenous iron (the route will depend on when the surgery is planned), vitamin B_{12}, folic acid, and erythropoietin (EPO), which reduces subsequent RBC transfusion
	Detailed drug history of oral anticoagulants, antiplatelets agents, and herbal medicines should be obtained Depending on the drug intake history and the clinical condition, a bridging therapy (with intravenous unfractionated heparin) may be planned	Consider the risk of thrombosis vs. bleeding while altering anticoagulation status Perioperative management of these medications should follow the latest guidelines with cautious withholding of dual antiplatelet therapy, especially in case of recent percutaneous coronary interventions (PCIs) (will depend on when the stent was placed, the type of stent, etc.) Aspirin may be continued on case-to-case basis. Reversal of anticoagulant effect of vitamin K antagonists (warfarin) by administration of fresh-frozen plasma (FFP) or four-factor prothrombin complex concentrate (PCC) (if urgent) or intravenous vitamin K (when nonurgent) Change over to short-acting anticoagulants such as intravenous unfractionated heparin in selected patients. The NOACs should be reversed with nonspecific pharmacologic strategies by coagulation factor concentrates, such as inactive PCCs (Octaplex, Beriplex/KCentra), activated PCCs (FEIBA), and recombinant activated factor VII (rFVIIa, Novoseven®) or drug-specific antidotes idarucizumab for dabigatran or class-specific antidote, andexanet alfa for anti-Xa direct-acting oral anticoagulant as needed and universal antidote, ciraparantag[5]
	Management of thrombocytopenia coagulopathy or any thrombotic history	Causes should be identified and corrected prior to surgery
Preparation of large expected blood loss	Elective surgery	Assure availability of blood components, e.g., cardiac surgery, hepatic resection
	Emergency surgery	Assure availability of blood components, e.g., polytrauma, aortic aneurysm, obstetric surgeries
	Blood conservation techniques for high-risk planed surgeries	Preoperative autologous blood donation (PAD), intraoperative acute normovolemic hemodilution (ANH), and/or intraoperative blood salvage therapy Though use is declining, these techniques minimize the need for allogeneic transfusions
Consents and advance directives	Acceptance or declining various blood components and conservation modalities should be discussed preoperatively and related consents and advanced directives should be obtained and documented	Patient wishes (Jehovah's witness)

(FEIBA: factor eight inhibitor bypassing activity; NOAC: novel oral anticoagulant)

who are at risk of bleeding), and chronic transfusion–dependent anemia.

Following recommendations are made by an American Society of Anesthesiologist's Task Force:[8]

- Hb level is above 10 g/dL: Transfusion is rarely indicated.
- Hb level is below 6 g/dL: Transfusion is almost always indicated.
- Hb level is 6–10 g/dL: Transfusion should be based on any ongoing sign of organ ischemia or bleeding, the rate and magnitude of any potential or actual bleeding, and the patient's intravascular volume status.

RECOMMENDATIONS FOR USE OF COMPONENT THERAPY

Significant advances have been made in transfusion medicine and we are now in the era of blood component therapy as per **Table 3**. Evidence suggests that whole BT does not have any benefit rather it may prove harmful.

TRANSFUSION REACTIONS

It is recommended that all patients undergoing BT are monitored for adverse reactions, although they are rare **(Table 4)**.

Table 2: Intraoperative and postoperative strategies.

Intraoperative strategies	Surgical techniques to minimize bleeding	Electrocautery Hemostatic agents Antifibrinolytics Tissue adhesives ANH
Intraoperative and postoperative strategies	Fluid management and monitoring of blood loss	Appropriate fluids preferably crystalloids, for initial resuscitation and maintain euvolemia until threshold for transfusion is met Monitor blood loss by periodic evaluation and quantitative measurement including checking suction canisters, surgical sponges, and surgical drains Monitor organ perfusion
	Temperature management and coagulopathy management	Avoid hypothermia as it impairs platelets aggregation and coagulation cascade Even mild hypothermia (<1°C) is associated with an increase in blood loss by approximately 16% (4–26%) and increases the relative risk for transfusion by approximately 22% (3–37%)[6] Tests such as INR, activated partial thromboplastin time (APTT)], fibrinogen concentration, and platelet count may need to be done in some patients
	Blood products and adverse effect of BT	Prefer component therapy as per trigger. Do not treat abnormal labs in absence of obvious bleeding Monitor for adverse effects and treat
	Treatment of excessive bleeding and blood salvage	Surgical re-evaluation to rule out bleeder along with supportive transfusion therapy

(ANH: acute normovolemic hemodilution; BT: blood transfusion; INR: international normalized ratio)

Table 3: Recommendations for transfusion of blood components.

Blood component	Indications	Evidence
Red blood cells (RBCs)[4]	Threshold of Hb < 8 g/dL (hematocrit ≤ 25%)	Restrictive transfusion strategy reduces RBC transfusion with equivocal outcome
Platelets[9,10]	Active bleeding in the presence of platelet defects Platelet count of < 50,000/mm³ in patients with active bleeding. In hematology, patients having active bleeding associated with dengue, malaria, kala azar, and autoimmune platelet disorders *In oncology patients:* Patients with platelet counts < 20,000/mm³, in the presence of risk factors Patients with platelet counts < 10,000/mm³ with no risk factors *In patients needing surgical or any other interventions:* Platelet count < 50,000/mm³, if there is minimal risk of bleeding Platelet < 100,000/mm³, for any ophthalmic or central nervous system surgeries Part of MTP as specific blood component therapy In severe uncontrolled bleeding, post-cardiopulmonary by pass	One RDP contains 24,000 platelets and one SDP contains at least 55,000 platelets Avoid prophylactic platelet transfusions in patients with counts below thresholds, unless they are excessively low and/or bleeding Equivocal evidence regarding obtaining a test of platelet function, if available, in patients with suspected or drug-induced (e.g., clopidogrel) platelet dysfunction[4]
Fresh-frozen plasma (FFP)[4]	Prophylaxis in patients with coagulopathy undergoing surgery or with invasive procedures when intravenous vitamin K therapy is deemed inadequate to reverse the warfarin effect Patients with proven coagulopathy with severe bleeding with PT > 1.5, international normalized ratio (INR) > 2, aPTT > twice normal limit *Component of MTP:* • During plasma exchange • Congenital or acquired factor deficiency with no alternative therapy • Reversal of warfarin, when need of urgent surgery or active bleeding if a prothrombin complex concentrate (PCC) is not available • Replacement of factor deficiency (factor V and XI) • Dilutional coagulopathy needing procedure or active bleeding • Liver diseases with coagulopathy in presence of active bleeding or needing intervention	FFP contains all clotting factors, fibrinogen, albumin, protein C, protein S, antithrombin, tissue factor pathway inhibitor Dose: 10–15 mL/kg FFP is not indicated, if PT or INR and aPTT are normal, solely for augmentation of plasma volume or albumin concentration

Contd…

Contd...

Blood component	Indications	Evidence
Cryoprecipitate	Life-threatening intraoperative bleeding in patients with DIC Fibrinogen levels < 100 mg/dL in patients with bleeding Massive transfusion Factor XIII deficiency Liver disease in the presence of active bleeding	A single unit of cryoprecipitate contains fibrinogen (factor I), factor VIII, factor XIII, von Willebrand's factor (VWF), and fibronectin In patients with excessive bleeding, assess fibrinogen levels before administrating cryoprecipitate, if possible[4] Transfusion of cryoprecipitate is rarely indicated, if fibrinogen concentration is >150 mg/dL in nonpregnant patients[4]
Prothrombin complex concentrate (PCC)	Recommended for urgent reversal of vitamin K-dependent oral anticoagulants[11] Consider in life-threatening post-traumatic bleeding patients treated with novel oral anticoagulants and in bleeding patients based on evidence of delayed coagulation initiation using viscoelastic monitoring[11] In congenital or acquired deficiency of vitamin K-dependent clotting factors and hemophilia B or for bleeding episodes or prior to surgical procedures if individual components or factors are not available They are also recommended in the presence of inhibitors to native coagulation factors	Three-factor (i.e., factors II, IX, and X) or four-factor (i.e., factors II, VII, IX, and X) concentrates with a concentration approximately 25 times higher than in normal plasma and associated with reduction in blood loss and normalization of INR values. Four-factor PCC is now available in India (Octaplex® one vial contains 500 units of 4F PCC) Care should be taken to avoid hypercoagulation Dose of PCC is 1–2 mL/kg, which is much lower than FFP and it does not cause transfusion-associated acute lung injury (TRALI)

(DIC: disseminated intravascular coagulation; MTP: massive transfusion protocol; PT: prothrombin time; RDP: random donor platelet; SDP: single donor *platelet*)

RESTRICTIVE BLOOD TRANSFUSION STRATEGY

Hemoglobin criteria for transfusion < 8 g/dL and hematocrit values < 25% are typically reported as restrictive as per current literature.[4] However, there are equivocal results about restrictive strategy as regards to mortality, cardiac, neurologic, or pulmonary complications, and length of hospital stay.[4]

The TRICC (Transfusion Requirements in Critical Care) trial from Canada was the first trial in critical care to suggest that restritctive transfusion strategy may be as safe as liberal strategy of blood transfusion. Results of this study influenced the BT practice in ICUs by raising concerns related to BT and encouraged intensivists to limit the use of BT. In this study, liberal strategy (Hb 10–12 g/dL) and restrictive strategy (Hb 7–9 g/dL) of transfusion, except in patients with acute myocardial infarction and unstable angina was compared. They reported a nonsignificant trend toward lower 30-day mortality for the restrictive group (18.7% vs. 23.3 L%, $P = 0.11$). However, the mortality rate during hospitalization was significantly lower in the restrictive strategy group (22.2% vs. 28.1%, $P = 0.05$). Thus, they recommended that Hb concentrations should be maintained between 7.0 g/dL and 9.0 g/dL.[12]

The results of the TRICC study have been validated by two recent studies, the Transfusion Requirements After Cardiac Surgery (TRACS) study[13] and "FOCUS" (Functional Outcomes in Cardiovascular Patients Undergoing Surgical Hip Fracture Repair).[14] TRACS trial (502 postcardiac surgical patients) compared liberal strategy (hematocrit ≥ 30%) to a restrictive strategy (hematocrit ≥ 24%). The 30-day mortality was similar between the two groups (10% liberal vs. 11% restrictive; between-group difference, 1%; 95% CI, – 6–4%; $P = 0.85$). However, the study also suggested that irrespective of transfusion strategy, the number of transfused RBC units was an independent risk factor for clinical complications or death at 30 days [hazard ratio (HR) for each additional unit transfused 1.2; 95% CI, 1.1–1.4; $P = 0.002$]. FOCUS trial showed that even in elderly patients, it is acceptable to limit the RBC transfusion except for those with either symptoms of anemia or an Hb of 8 g/dL. Average Hb level in liberal strategy was 1.3 g/dL higher as compared to restrictive-strategy ($P < 0.001$). They observed that the mortality rate or an inability to walk without human assistance at 60-day follow-up were similar in liberal strategy and restrictive-strategy groups (35.2% vs. 34.7%, $P = 0.90$).

The AABB guidelines on RBC transfusion strongly recommend adherence to restrictive transfusion strategy (7–8 g/dL) in hospitalized, stable patients.[15] The committee

Table 4: Transfusion reactions.

	Reaction	Mechanism
Acute reactions	Acute hemolytic transfusion reaction	Incompatible transfused red cells
		Patient's own anti-A or anti-B antibodies or other alloantibodies anti-rhesus (Rh) D to red cell antigens
	Nonhemolytic febrile reactions to transfusion of platelets and red cell	Due to patient antibodies to transfused white cells
	Transfusion-associated dyspnea (TAD), transfusion-related acute lung injury (TRALI)	Due to donor plasma containing antibodies against the patient's leukocyte
	Mild-to-severe allergic reaction or anaphylaxis	Patient's antibodies that react with proteins in transfused blood components
	Transfusion-associated circulatory overload (TACO)	Rapid administration of blood products leading to pulmonary edema and acute respiratory failure
	Citrate toxicity	An anticoagulant present in significant amounts, which readily binds calcium and magnesium resulting in hypocalcemia- and hypomagnesemia-associated cardiac manifestations
Delayed reactions	Delayed hemolysis of transfused cells	5–10 days post-transfusion, a rapid, secondary immune response raises the antibody level drastically, leading to the rapid destruction of transfused cells
	Alloimmunization	Development of anti-RhD in RhD-negative patients who have received RhD-positive cells, which is fatal
	Development of antibodies that react with antigens of white cells or platelets	Development of leukocyte and/or platelet antibodies causing nonhemolytic febrile transfusion reactions in the future
	Post-transfusion purpura	Platelet-specific alloantibodies
	Graft vs. host reactions	Caused by T-lymphocytes, result in immunologic reaction against immunodeficient host. It is devastating and fatal
	Iron overload	Each unit of blood contains 250 mg of iron and those receiving red cells over a long period may develop iron accumulation in cardiac and liver tissues
	Infection	Though rare but risk of HIV, hepatitis B, or hepatitis C from transfusion is present
		Nonendemic infection such as human T-cell leukemia virus type 1 (HTLV-1) and type 2 (HTLV-2), West Nile virus, malaria, and *Trypanosoma cruzi* (causing Chagas' disease) and variant Creutzfeldt-Jakob disease (vCJD) are also transmitted by BT
	Transfusion-related immunomodulation (TRIM)	Leukocytes are responsible for immunomodulatory effect

reported that 11 out of 19 trials showed lower mortality with restrictive transfusion strategy [risk ratio (RR), 0.85; 95% CI, 0.7–1.03].

Restrictive transfusion strategy is also supported by a Cochrane Review, which included 19 trials (6,264 patients) in the settings of surgery (including cardiac surgery), critical care, trauma, and acute hemorrhage. This strategy was associated with a reduction in RBC transfusion by 39% (RR 0.61; 95% CI 0.52–0.72) and the average units of RBCs transfused were reduced by 1.19 units (95% CI 0.53–1.85 units). However, heterogeneity between trials was statistically significant ($P < 0.00001$; I^2 93%) for these outcomes. They added that restrictive transfusion strategies did not impact the rate of adverse events compared to liberal transfusion strategies, in terms of mortality, cardiac events, myocardial infarction, stroke, pneumonia, and thromboembolism. In fact, restrictive transfusion strategy is associated with a statistically significant reduction in hospital mortality (RR 0.77, 95% CI 0.62–0.95) but not 30-day mortality (RR 0.85, 95% CI 0.70–1.03). However, this review

did not comment on transfusion strategies in patients with ACS.[16]

Another Cochrane review (31 trials, n = 12,587)[17] compared restrictive transfusion strategy (Hb trigger for transfusion = 7 g/dL or 8 g/dL) to liberal transfusion threshold (higher Hb trigger for transfusion = 9–10 g/dL). Restrictive transfusion strategy reduced the proportion of participants exposed to RBC transfusion by 43% across a broad range of clinical specialties (RR for transfusion 0.57, 95% CI 0.49–0.65). However, there was a large amount of heterogeneity between trials (I 2 = 97%). Besides that, restrictive transfusion strategies had no impact on 30-day mortality and morbidity (such as cardiac events, myocardial infarction, stroke, pneumonia, thromboembolism, infection) with RR 0.97, 95% CI 0.81–1.16. However, there was insufficient data to inform the safety of transfusion policies in certain clinical subgroups, including acute coronary syndrome, myocardial infarction, neurological injury/traumatic brain injury (TBI), acute neurological disorders, stroke, thrombocytopenia, cancer, hematological malignancies, and bone marrow failure. Currently, the results of an ongoing large-scale RCT (ClinicalTrials.gov Identifier: NCT02981407) on liberal transfusion strategy in patients with acute coronary syndrome are awaited.[18]

A meta-analysis of three trials (2,364 participants) showed that a restrictive transfusion strategy using a Hb transfusion trigger of < 7 g/dL results in a significant reduction in ACS (RR, 0.44; CI, 0.22–0.89), pulmonary edema (RR, 0.48; CI, 0.33–0.72), rebleeding (RR, 0.64; CI, 0.45–0.90), bacterial infections (RR, 0.86; CI, 0.73–1.00), in-hospital mortality (RR, 0.74; CI, 0.60–0.92), and total mortality (RR, 0.80; CI, 0.65–0.98), compared with a more liberal strategy. Also, there was a reduction in number of units transfused by 40%, with an average of 2 units less per person.[19]

Another study reported no significant differences in 90-day mortality, number of ischemic events, adverse reactions, and use of life support in patients with lower Hb threshold transfusion strategy versus higher Hb threshold. The patients with lower-threshold group received 50% less units of blood compared to higher-threshold group.[20]

A systematic review of 31 randomized trials (9,813 patients) found that with restrictive transfusion the incidence of myocardial infarction remained unaltered (RR, 1.28; 95% CI, 0.66–2.49; $P = 0.46$). Thus, restrictive transfusion strategies were found to be safer, and liberal transfusion strategy did not offer any benefit.[21] This was also supported by Cochrane review of six trials (2,722 participants) of RBC transfusion for patients undergoing hip fracture surgery.[22]

IMPACT OF BLOOD TRANSFUSION ON PATIENT OUTCOMES

Association of Blood Transfusion with Mortality in Cardiac Patients

Benefit of BT in patients with myocardial infarction is debatable. In a meta-analysis, liberal BT strategy was associated with higher risk for mortality independent of baseline Hb level, nadir Hb level, and change in Hb level during the hospital stay in a multivariate analysis. It showed an increase in all-cause mortality with a strategy of BT versus no BT (18.2% vs. 10.2%) (RR, 2.91; 95% CI, 2.46–3.44; P <0.001), with a weighted absolute risk increase of 12%. Besides that BT was significantly associated with a higher risk for subsequent myocardial infarction (RR, 2.04; 95% CI, 1.06–3.93; $P = 0.03$).[23] Practice of routine or liberal BT in cardiac patients should be discouraged.

As per AABB guidelines, the transfusion should be considered for patients associated with symptoms or Hb level ≤ 8 g/dL as there is no mortality benefit. Further it reduces transfusion cost and risks for adverse effects.[10] However, there is some uncertainty about the risk for perioperative myocardial infarction associated with a restrictive transfusion strategy as evidence supporting this is not large enough. The British Committee for Standards in Haematology (BCSH) guidelines, in patients with ACS, suggests transfusion to keep Hb at > 8 g/dL, maintain Hb >7 g/dL if the patient is anemic, and has stable angina.[24]

Blood Transfusion in Sepsis

The Surviving Sepsis Campaign Guidelines 2016 have strongly recommended that RBC transfusion should occur only when Hb concentration decreases to < 7.0 g/dL in adults in the absence of myocardial ischemia, severe hypoxemia, or acute hemorrhage.[25] The Transfusion Requirements in Septic Shock (TRISS) trial, a prospective randomized multicenter trial, which included patients with septic shock, compared a transfusion thresholds of 7 versus 9 g/dL.[20] The lower-threshold group received less number of transfusions (median of 1 unit of blood vs. median of 4 units). They found a similar 90-day mortality (43.0% vs. 45.0% in lower vs. higher threshold group, with RR, 0.94; 95% CI, 0.78–1.09; $P = 0.44$). The number of patients with ischemic events [0.90 (0.58–1.39)] and use of life support were similar in both groups.

Blood Transfusion in Trauma

Trauma is one of the leading causes of mortality worldwide and massive bleeding leading to hypovolemia remains the primary cause of death in initial 24 hours after injury. Traditionally any hypotensive bleeding trauma patient, resuscitation should be initiated with isotonic crystalloid solutions. Administration of larger crystalloid volume is independently associated with increase risk of bleeding and decreased survival rate in trauma. Hypotonic solutions such as Ringer's lactate should be avoided in patients with severe head trauma and use of colloids might be restricted. Damage control resuscitation strategy, i.e., rapid control of bleeding along with early supplementation of blood components has been recommended. Patients with severe hemorrhage should undergo the MTP to restore the blood volume and clotting factors.[27] Treatment should aim to achieve a target Hb of 7–9 g/dL. Initial management of patients with expected massive hemorrhage should include either plasma (FFP or pathogen-inactivated plasma) in a plasma-RBC ratio of at least 1:2 as needed or fibrinogen concentrate and RBC according to Hb level.[11] Besides that measures to reduce heat loss and warm the hypothermic patient should be employed to achieve and maintain normothermia.

Following are the strategies for transfusion in actively bleeding patient:[26]

Fixed ratio approach: It involves transfusion of RBCs, fresh-frozen plasma (FFP), and platelets in a fixed ratio, i.e., 1:1:1 in order to provide a composition similar to whole blood. The PROPPR (Pragmatic, Randomized Optimal Platelet and Plasma Ratios) trial in 2015, randomized control trial (n = 680) compared transfusion of FFP, platelets, and RBC in a 1:1:1 versus 1:1:2 ratio in severely bleeding trauma patients. No significant differences in mortality at 24 hours or at 30 days were observed. There was more deaths due to exsanguination in low-ratio group. The treatment group was not associated with increase in transfusion-related complications suggestive of safety of high-fixed transfusion ratios.[28] PROMMTT (the PRospective Observational Multicenter Major Trauma Transfusion) study in 2013,[29] a prospective observational study (n = 905), compared plasma to RBC ratios of 1:1 versus 1:2. They observed that higher ratio of plasma to RBC was associated with reduced 6 hours mortality, although there was no difference in 24 hours mortality in those who required more than three blood products.

Thromboelastometry-guided approach: It is based on the current understanding of the pathophysiology of trauma, coagulopathy, and selective replacement of blood products. Currently available blood tests for coagulation such as prothrombin time (PT), international normalized ratio (INR), activated partial thromboplastin time (APPT), fibrinogen level/activity, and platelet count are not designed for diagnosis of coagulopathy or to guide hemostatic therapy. These tests also require prolonged turnaround time. Thus, goal-directed therapy for the replacement of coagulation factors is specifically required. The use of viscoelastic testing, i.e., rotational thromboelastometry (ROTEM) or thromboelastography (TEG) has become accepted standard of care in such settings. TEG provides a more appropriate approach to monitor hemostasis, as it quickly provides information about the polymerization of fibrin in the presence of platelet activity, fibrinogen deficiency assessment, and factor XIII deficiency.[26] Tapia et al. have shown that MT guided by TEG is superior in resuscitating patients with penetrating trauma when compared to standard MT practice.[30] Meyer et al. demonstrated that ROTEM clot firmness at 10 minutes is helpful in predicting who would require MT in a trauma population.[31]

Strategy of transfusion in trauma patients (STATA): A randomized trial, included patient with severe trauma and high-injury severity score and compared fixed ratio protocol (1:1:1) versus TEG-guided approach. The primary outcome is organ dysfunction at day 1, 5, 7, and 28 days, and secondary outcomes are number of transfusions within 48 hours, LOS in hospital, duration of ventilator-free days, and cost of treatment.[26] This trial has finished recruitment in 2016, but the results are yet to be published. An interim analysis after recruitment of 50% participants showed no difference in two groups. A meta-analysis has shown that the use of point-of-care assay (TEG or ROTEM) in patients receiving massive blood transfusion (MBT) does not decrease the mortality, morbidity, or the use of platelets and FFP.[32] Controversy remains at present regarding the utility of viscoelastic methods for the detection of post-traumatic coagulopathy.[11,33]

Other strategies to reduce transfusion requirements in trauma patients: Several other strategies to reduce the BTs in ICU can be implemented because of concerns of safety, storage lesions, limited availability, and costs associated with blood products.[8,11,24]

- Measures should be undertaken to stop ongoing bleeding
- Damage control surgery
- Pelvic ring stabilization and in case of ongoing hemodynamic instability despite pelvic ring stabilization, patient should undergo early preperitoneal packing, angiographic embolization, and/or surgical bleeding control
- Correct the lethal triad of hypothermia, acidosis, and coagulopathy
- Consider stopping unnecessary anticoagulation and antiplatelet agents
- Consider reversal of anticoagulation with vitamin K antagonists for nonurgent reversal and PCC or FFP in urgent reversal
- Use of antifibrinolytic agents [tranexamic acid or epsilon-aminocaproic acid (EACA)] especially in early in trauma [CRASH II (Clinical Randomization of an Antifibrinolytic in Significant Hemorrhage II) trial]
- Techniques of cell salvage during surgery
- Use blood conservation devices while sampling.

Massive Transfusion Protocol

Massive transfusion protocol must be initiated in life-threatening situation in a massively bleeding patient after trauma and/or during a procedure to optimize the delivery of blood product with an intention to minimize the adverse effects of hypovolemia and dilutional coagulopathy.[18] The standard pRBC:FFP:platelet ratio suggested by MTPs is 1:1:1. With unknown patient blood type, group O pRBCs and group AB for FFP and platelets are recommended to be transfused. Group O RhD-negative pRBC is recommended, but RhD-positive pRBC may be used if RhD-negative pRBC is not available. It results in a higher transfusion of FFP:pRBC ratio and a decrease in the use of crystalloids, with maintenance of normothermia to bring Hb to optimum level. It has been observed to lead to a significant decrease in mortality with improvement in compliance with timely activation and type of product given as per MTP protocol[34] and should be initiated early in emergency room itself. However, this protocol has raised the concern that use of blood products in such a large amount may cause subsequent shortage of products and about complications associated with massive BT such as TRALI, ARDS, TACO, TRIM, infections, hypokalemia, hyperkalemia, hypocalcemia, citrate toxicity, hypothermia, dilutional coagulopathy, hemolytic transfusion reactions, post-transfusion *graft-versus-host disease* (GVHD), etc.

Blood transfusion in neurocritical care: Although anemia is consistently associated with worse outcomes among patients with TBI, there is insufficient evidence regarding the relative benefit of a liberal over a restrictive transfusion strategy. In patients with TBI, the target Hb can be kept between 7 and 9 g/dL. In those with TBI associated with evidence of cerebral ischemia, consider target Hb > 9 g/dL, and in those with subarachnoid hemorrhage (SAH), the target Hb should be between 8 and 10 g/dL. If patients are presenting with an acute ischemic stroke, the Hb should be maintained above 9 g/dL.[24] There is clear agreement in literature that critically ill patients with TBI and Hb < 7 g/dL should be transfused. However, the exact threshold between 7 and 10 g/dL remains a debatable issue.

Although the overall quality of the evidence is low, but recent data from a review article found no difference in neurological outcomes between the restrictive and liberal transfusion strategies.[35] In a recent international survey conducted on RBC transfusion practices for patients with acute brain injury in five critical care medicine societies, 54% intensivists reported an Hb threshold of < 8 g/dL for transfusing pRBCs. However, >50% of these physicians transfused blood at higher Hb values.[36] Randomized trials evaluating the optimal transfusion threshold for TBI patients are currently ongoing, which may answer this question in near future.

Role of Recombinant Factor VIIa in Patients with Uncontrolled Bleeding

Recombinant factor VIIa (rFVIIa) binds to the surface of activated platelets and promotes factor X activation, which facilitates thrombin generation localized at the site of injury (without widespread thrombosis) which is independent of tissue factor. It has an amino acid sequence identical to that of plasma-derived factor VII and is produced by transfection of the human factor VII gene into baby hamster kidney cells cultured in bovine albumin. It is recommended to consider administration of rFVIIa, when traditional options for treating excessive bleeding due to coagulopathy have been exhausted.[4] It should be given in dose of 90–120 μg/kg and should be repeated every 2–3 hours till effective hemostasis is achieved.

Following are US Food and Drug Administration (FDA) approved uses of rFVIIa:
- To treat bleeding episodes or to prevent bleeding in surgical interventions or invasive procedures in hemophilia A or B patients (with inhibitors to factor VIII)
- To treat or to prevent bleeding episodes in patients with congenital FVII deficiency

Besides that there are some off-label indications. rFVIIa may be considered only if major bleeding and traumatic coagulopathy persist despite standard attempts to control bleeding such as traumatic bleeding.[11] Other off-label indications are perioperative blood loss, postpartum hemorrhage, spontaneous intracerebral hemorrhage, bleeding in liver diseases, and anticoagulant-associated bleeding.

Evidence: A systematic review and meta-analysis of 12 studies (1,244 patients) with acquired hemophilia found that rFVIIa is effective in control of bleeding with good safety profile.[37]

Its efficacy and safety for treatment of bleeding in major abdominal, urological, and vascular surgery has been evaluated in a meta-analysis. The authors concluded that use of rFVIIa was associated with reduction of bleeding with increased probability of survival in patients responding to rFVIIa, and that its use was not associated with an increased risk of thromboembolism compared with placebo.[38] Its use in intracerebral hemorrhage in one randomized control trial (n = 841 patients) showed reduced expansion of the hematoma but without survival benefit or improved functional outcome.[39]

Hsia et al.[40] included 22 randomized controlled trials of rFVIIa (n = 3,184 patients) of trauma and found that there was less need for additional transfusions and its use was not associated with increased risk of thrombosis, but also that there was no mortality benefit.

Another meta-analysis by Yank et al.[41] including 16 randomized controlled trials and 26 comparative observational studies and 22 noncomparative observational studies found that there was no overall survival benefit of rFVIIa in surgeries such as cardiac, intracranial hemorrhage, body trauma, liver transplantation, and prostatectomy. Besides this, there is an increased risk of thromboembolism mainly in cardiac surgery and intracranial hemorrhage. In addition to that, it is expensive without any proven benefit in off-label indications. Thus, rFVIIa should be used cautiously in nonapproved situations.

Table 5: Association of RBC storage duration with mortality and morbidity.

Study	Population	Type of study	Sample size	Outcome
ABLE (Age of Blood Evaluation) trial[43] Lacroix et al. 2015	Critically ill adults with a high risk of death with 15% trauma	Double-blind, multicenter RCT Fresh blood (<8 days) vs. older blood	2,430	No significant difference in 90-day mortality
INFORM (Informing Fresh versus Old Red Cell Management) trial[44] Eikelboom JW et al. 2016	Hospitalized patient who required BT > 18 years 13% trauma	Unblinded, randomized fresh blood vs. old blood	20,858	No significant difference in 90-day mortality
TRANSFUSE (STandaRd Issue TrANsfusion versuS Fresher red blood cell Use in intenSive carE) trial[42] Cooper et al. 2017	Critically ill adult patient 10% trauma	Multicenter, RCT Fresh available RBC vs. standard issue	4,919	No significant difference in 90-day mortality
RECESS (Red Cell Storage Duration Study) trial[45] Steiner et al. 2015	12 years or more, undergoing complex cardiac surgery	Multicenter, RCT <10 days vs. >21 days	1,098	No difference in MODS

(BT: blood transfusion; RBC: red blood cell; MODS: multiple organ dysfunction syndrome; RCT: randomized controlled trial)

STORAGE LESIONS

The "storage lesions" refer to the multiple complex biochemical and biomechanical alterations that occur during ex vivo storage of RBCs. Prolonged storage has been associated with changes that may render red cells ineffective as oxygen carriers by metabolic changes such as decrease in 2-3 DPG (*2,3-diphosphoglycerate)*, oxidative stress, and altering the shape. Also, they are associated with decrease in pH, increased K^+ concentrations, and accumulation of pro-inflammatory cytokines causing untoward biologic effects.[42] Current regulations permit the storage of red cells for up to 42 days depending on manufacturing process, additive solution, and local policies.

However, there is no strong evidence for an increased risk of adverse events and 30-day mortality with transfusion of RBC within recommended storage time as mentioned in **Table 5**. There is no impact of fresh versus old RBCs on the in-hospital and 30-day post-hospitalization mortality, infectious complications, and ICU or hospital length of stay.[18] AABB has recommended to use pRBC units within the recommended storage time rather than limiting the use to fresh units within 10 days after collection.[7] Various studies have shown that there is no evidence that fresh RBCs transfusion reduces mortality.[7]

MEASURES TO REDUCE BLEEDING WITH USE OF ADJUNCT MEDICATIONS

Pharmacologic treatments for excessive bleeding include **(Table 6)**:
- Aprotinin
- Antifibrinolytics (i.e., ε-aminocaproic acid, tranexamic acid)
- Desmopressin
- Ethamsylate
- Tissue sealants.

ROLE OF IRON THERAPY (IV OR ORAL) AND ERYTHROPOIETIN IN PREOPERATIVE OPTIMIZATION

Till date evidence on perioperative EPO with or without iron therapy are based on studies with significant heterogeneity related to dosing, timing of administration, severity of preoperative anemia, its cause, and type of surgery. There is no strong recommendation but EPO can be administered possibly to reduce the need for allogeneic blood in selected group of patients, e.g., renal insufficiency, anemia of chronic disease, refusal of transfusion, and iron can be administered to patients with iron deficiency anemia if time permits.[7]

A systematic review and meta-analysis (32 RCT n = 4,750) evaluated the effect of preoperative EPO or placebo on perioperative BT in orthopedic and cardiac cases. There was a decrease in the use of allogeneic BT in all patients (n = 28 studies; RR, 0.59; 95% CI, 0.47–0.73; $P < 0.001$) as well as patients undergoing cardiac (n = 9 studies; RR, 0.55; 95% CI, 0.37–0.81; $P = 0.003$) and elective orthopedic (n = 5 studies; RR, 0.36; 95% CI, 0.28–0.46; $P < 0.001$) surgery compared to placebo, respectively. Beside that the rate of thrombotic complications was not different between the groups although the P value was not significant (n = 28 studies; RR, 1.02; 95% CI, 0.78–1.33; $P = 0.68$). But heterogeneity of study populations, variation in EPO dosing, etc. were the limitations.[48]

One prospective RCT evaluated the efficacy of EPO, intravenous iron, vitamin B12, and oral folic acid in patients with preoperative anemia or isolated iron deficiency anemia in cardiac surgical patients compared with placebo. They observed reduced RBC and total allogeneic blood product transfusions in treatment group compared to placebo [odds ratio (OR), 0.70; 95% CI, 0.50–0.98). However, it is still not clear whether IV iron therapy without EPO

Table 6: Adjunct medications to reduce bleeding.

Drug	Mechanism	Indication	Recent recommendation
Aprotinin	Broad-spectrum protease inhibitors, bovine in origin, reduces fibrinolysis, stabilizes platelet function, potential anti-inflammatory effect	Reduces blood loss and transfusion requirements in patients undergoing cardiothoracic, liver transplant, orthopedic surgeries	Withdrawn from the market in 2007 due to its adverse effect on renal function and the high incidence of anaphylactic reactions Increased risk of myocardial infarction, heart failure, stroke, encephalopathy, and mortality
Tranexamic acid	Synthetic lysine derivative and inhibits fibrinolysis by reducing conversion of plasmin to plasminogen Cardiac surgery: 10 mg/kg (IV) immediately preoperatively followed by IV infusion of 1 mg/kg/h Traumatic hemorrhage in adults (CRASH-2): 1 g IV within 3 hours of the event followed by 1 g infused over 8 hours Women with postpartum hemorrhage (WOMAN trial): 1 g IV followed by a further 1 g if bleeding continues or recurs CRASH-3 trial: In intracranial bleed, patients were given TA (loading dose 1 g over 10 minutes then infusion of 1 g over 8 hours, within 3 hours of injury) or placebo	Its use is strongly recommended and should be included in major traumatic hemorrhage protocols Effective in reducing risk of receiving BT by 30% and need of further surgeries due to rebleed, e.g., cardiopulmonary bypass, primary orthotopic liver transplantation, knee arthroplasty, hip replacement[18]	CRASH 2 trial[46] (n = 20,000) demonstrated improvement in all-cause mortality when used in traumatic hemorrhage patients within 3 hours from the time of injury without increase in thromboembolic events A major international trial of tranexamic acid in WOMAN trial (n = 15,000) showed significant reduction in hemorrhage and need for surgery, with no differences for stroke, myocardial infarction, renal failure, re-exploration, or mortality[4] In the CRASH-3 trial, the risk of head injury-related death reduced with tranexamic acid in patients with mild-to-moderate head injury (RR, 0.78; 95% CI, 0.64–0.95) but not in patients with severe head injury (RR, 0.99; 95% CI, 0.91–1.07). The incidence of seizures was similar in TA and placebo group[48]
Epsilon-aminocaproic acid (EACA)	Competitive inhibitor of plasminogen activation and inhibits plasmin	Prophylaxis of bleeding episodes in hemophiliacs, control of menorrhagia, gastrointestinal bleeding, obstetrical bleeding, and in bleeding following cardiac and thoracic surgery and orthotopic liver transplantation	EACA is as effective as tranexamic acid in reducing estimated blood loss and transfusion and decreased intraoperative blood loss and showed a trend toward improved graft and patient survival Effective in reducing total perioperative blood loss and the number of patients transfused in major cardiac, orthopedic, or liver surgery and equivocal findings are reported for the volume of blood transfused[4] EACA can cause renal dysfunction; therefore, its use should be restricted to patients with high risk of bleeding
Vasopressin analogue desmopressin	Release of endothelial factor VIII and von Willebrand's factor into the plasma which forms a complex with platelets and enhance their aggregation The standard dose is 0.3 µg/kg subcutaneously or intravenously	Hemophilia A Von Willebrand's disease Uremic thrombocytopathy Bleeding due to platelet dysfunction	Should not consider its use routinely in the bleeding trauma patient[11]
Ethamsylate	Reduces thromboxane A2 and prostacyclin biosynthesis and improving platelet homo- and heterotypic adhesiveness	Dysfunctional uterine bleeding, periventricular hemorrhage in very low-birth weight babies, perioperative scenarios	
Tissue sealants	Derived from human or animal clotting factors such as fibrinogen or synthetic hydrogel polymers Collagen-based, gelatin-based, absorbable cellulose-based, fibrin synthetic glues, and polysaccharide based	Sprayed on surgical fields or raw surfaces to promote hemostasis and reduce blood loss	They can reduce surgical bleeding and exposure to donor blood, the effect being most significant in orthopedic surgery Although the evidence is mainly observational, these agents have become widely used[11]

(BT: blood transfusion; CRASH: Clinical Randomization of an Antifibrinolytic in Significant Hemorrhage II; IV: intravenous; TA: tranexamic acid; WOMAN: World Maternal Antifibrinolytic Trial)

is equally effective as in patients with iron deficiency and/or additional supplement of vitamin B_{12} and folate offer any additional benefit.[49] Additionally, the efficacy of perioperative intravenous iron therapy (IVIT) on transfusion and recovery profiles in orthopedic surgery has been evaluated in 12 clinical trials including four RCTs (n = 616 patients) and eight case control studies n = 1,253 patients). IVIT significantly showed a good recovery profile with reduction in proportion of patients transfused by 31% (RR, 0.69; $P = 0.0002$), and in the units of RBCs transfused by 0.34 units/person (MD, –0.34; P= 0.0007), with shorter LOS and decreased infection rate, without change in mortality rate. Due to inadequacy of satisfactory statistical analysis with low to high risk of bias, larger, prospective, well-designed RCTs are needed to confirm its efficacy in perioperative patients.[50]

BLOOD SALVAGE THERAPY

Blood salvage comprises preoperative autologous donation (PAD) and acute normovolemic hemodilution (ANH) where patient's blood is collected prior to occurrence of surgical blood loss. Intraoperative blood salvage/blood recovery is retrieval and salvaging blood that has already been shed and which is collected, washed, or filtered and returned to the patient, whenever transfusion is needed. PAD may be considered if there is sufficient time for RBC regeneration prior to surgery, patients are not anemic, and expected to lose significant amount of blood during the surgical procedure. Nowadays, PAD practice has been declining because of expense, inconvenience, being cumbersome, need for planning beforehand, wastage of PAD units, and creation of anemia by serial donation preoperatively.

Acute normovolemic hemodilution may be considered in selected patients with normal initial hemoglobin levels and are expected to lose two or more units of blood ($\geq$ 1,000 mL) intraoperatively such as cardiac, thoracic, major orthopedic, and hepatic surgeries. It involves removal of blood from a patient shortly after induction of anesthesia, with maintenance of normovolemia using crystalloid and/or colloid as replacement fluids. It is a safer technique when used in healthy, young adults with high risk for excessive bleeding and is a good option for Jehovah's witnesses (if they accept the procedure). Meta-analyses of RCTs indicate that ANH is effective in reducing the volume of allogeneic BT for major cardiac, orthopedic, thoracic, or liver surgery.[51]

Blood salvage is generally safe and is recommended in procedures with high blood loss ($\geq$ 1,000 mL) or $\geq$ 20% of the expected blood loss, low hemoglobin levels and high risk of bleeding, rare blood group or multiple unexpected antibodies, and patient's refusal to receive allogeneic BT.[18] It is associated with a very low incidence of adverse events and is beneficial. Intraoperative and postoperative

blood recovery and reinfusion with recovered RBCs using leukoreduction filters may be considered as a blood sparing intervention and it reduces the frequency of allogeneic BTs particularly in major surgeries.[4] Leukoreduction filters efficiently reduce the risk of contamination through amniotic fluid and fetal RBCs in obstetric surgeries or in cancer surgeries; however, bowel contamination is considered as contraindication for intraoperative blood salvage.

ROLE OF LEUKODEPLETED BLOOD

Leukoreduced (LR) RBCs are prepared by prestorage filtration of donor leukocytes from packed RBC units. LR is effective in reducing the rate of febrile nonhemolytic transfusion reaction (FNHTR) by reducing leukocyte count.[52] Also, it reduces the risk of transfusion transmitted-CMV (TT-CMV)[53] and HLA alloimmunization,[54] and graft rejection in cases of multiple transfusions related to solid organ transplants.[55] It also plays a key role in the prevention of transfusion-transmitted Epstein-Barr virus (EBV), HTLV infections. With prion reduction filters, it provides promising results for the prevention of transmission of Creutzfeldt-Jakob disease. Leukoreduced RBCs are recommended when repeated BTs are required such as in patients with leukemia, aplastic anemia, myelodysplastic syndrome, bone marrow failure, bone marrow transplant recipients, patients scheduled for allogeneic or autologous stem cell transplantation, immunocompromised patients with hematologic malignancy, congenital or acquired immune deficiency, and patients receiving chemotherapy.[18] It has shown advantages by reducing ischemia-reperfusion injury in patients with cardiopulmonary bypass, and reduced postoperative morbidity and mortality.[56] However, it has its own drawbacks too. Up to 10% of RBCs may be inadvertently removed and also hemolyzed during the filtering process affecting its oxygen-delivering capacity.[57] Thus, clinical benefits of LR are not large as per the current evidence and RCTs are equivocal regards to LR versus non-LR blood products transfusion in postoperative infections and infectious complications.[4] Further studies are required to elucidate the benefits of LR for the purpose of reducing the complications associated with BT with an additional concern about the cost effectiveness.

CURRENT EVIDENCE ON USE OF ARTIFICIAL BLOOD

Blood transfusion carries various risks, is expensive, and often its supply is scarce. Development of artificial RBC substitutes or synthetic oxygen transporters products are under intensive focus due to increasing demand for blood products. The products studied are of mainly two types:

(1) perfluorocarbon (PFC) and (2) Hb-based oxygen carriers (HBOCs) (polymerized HBOCs, cross-linked HBOCs, conjugated HBOCs).[58] The risk of spreading an infectious disease is eliminated with use of these products. However, these products have limitations of having a short half-life (most of the Hb-based products last not >20–30 hours in the body). They do not perform other functions of blood such as coagulation. Thus, the current status of artificial blood products is limited to only short-term blood replacement applications. In the future, it is anticipated that new materials to carry oxygen in the body will be found having longer half-life and less side effects.

CONCLUSION

A comprehensive perioperative BT treatment algorithm should be implemented for the management of bleeding in surgical patients in perioperative period. Blood products improve O_2 carrying capacity; their use is associated with better outcome provided need of transfusion is individualized based on clinical scenario. An assessment of the risk-to-benefit ratio considering comorbidities of the patient and surgical risk are the key considerations to optimize patient outcomes. Restrictive strategy (7–9 g/dL) has almost replaced liberal strategy which would have a large effect on RBC use and related risks of complications. General attempts to minimize the use of blood products and nontransfusion-based strategies (e.g., antifibrinolytic drugs such as tranexamic acid) and other measures to control bleeding, and use of blood conservation devices should be pursued. RBC transfusion should be undertaken when Hb drops to < 7.0 g/dL in hemodynamically stable critical patients (in absence of myocardial ischemia, severe hypoxemia, or acute hemorrhage). In later conditions, higher Hb threshold of 9 g/dL should be aimed at. Prospective randomized studies are required to determine the thresholds of BT in ACS. The transfusion threshold in patients undergoing neurosurgery and those with head injury is unknown, with current evidence suggesting a need for higher threshold for transfusion. Development of artificial RBC substitutes will open a new horizon in the field of transfusion.

REFERENCES

1. Vincent JL, Jaschinski U, Wittebole X, Lefrant JY, Jakob SM, Almekhlafi GA, et al. Worldwide audit of blood transfusion practice in critically ill patients. Crit Care. 2018;22:102.

2. Lelubre C, Vincent JL. Red blood cell transfusion in the critically ill patient. Ann Intensive Care. 2011;1:43.

3. Marik PE, Corwin HL. Efficacy of red blood cell transfusion in the critically ill: a systematic review of the literature. Crit Care Med. 2008;36:2667-74.

4. Apfelbaum JL, Nuttall GA, Connis RT, Harrison CR, Miller RD, Nickinovich DG, et al. Practice Guidelines for Perioperative Blood Management An Updated Report by the American Society of Anesthesiologists Task. Am Soc Anesthesiol. 2015;122:241-75.

5. Burnett A, Siegal D. Specific antidotes for bleeding associated with direct oral anticoagulants. BMJ. 2017;357:j2216.

6. Rajagopalan S, Mascha E, Na J, Daniel IS. The effects of mild perioperative hypothermia on blood loss and transfusion requirement. Am Soc Anesthesiol. 2008;108:71-7.

7. Carson JL, Guyatt G, Heddle NM, Grossman BJ, Cohn CS, Fung MK, et al. Clinical practice guidelines from the AABB red blood cell transfusion thresholds and storage. JAMA. 2016;316(19):2025-35.

8. Practice Guidelines for Perioperative Blood Transfusion and Adjuvant Therapies An Updated Report by the American Society of Anesthesiologists Task Force on Perioperative Blood Transfusion and Adjuvant Therapies. Anesthesiology. 2006;105:198-208.

9. Kaufman RM, Benjamin D, Gernsheimer T, Kleinman ST, Tinmouth AT, Kelley EC, et al. Platelet transfusion: a clinical practice guideline from AAB. Ann Intern Med. 2015;162:205-13.

10. Slichter SJ, Kaufman RM, Assmann SF, McCullough J, Triulzi DJ, Strauss RG, et al. Dose of prophylactic platelet transfusions and prevention of hemorrhage. N Engl J Med. 2010;362:600-13.

11. Rossaint R, Bouillon B, Cerny V, Coats TJ, Duranteau J, Fernández-mondéjar E, et al. The European guideline on management of major bleeding and coagulopathy following trauma: 4th edition. Crit Care. 2016;20:100.

12. Hébert PC, Wells G, Blajchman MA, Marshall J, Martin C, Pagliarello G, et al. A multicenter, randomized, controlled clinical trial of transfusion requirements in critical care. Transfusion Requirements in Critical Care Investigators, Canadian Critical Care Trials Group. N Engl J Med 1999;340(6):409-17.

13. Silva CM, Filho RK, Sundin MR, Lea WC. Transfusion requirements after cardiac surgery. JAMA. 2015;304:1559-67.

14. Carson JL, Terrin M. Liberal or restrictive transfusion in high-risk patients after hip surgery. N Engl J Med. 2011;365:2453-62.

15. Carson JL, Grossman BJ, Kleinman S, Tinmouth AT, Marques MB, Fung MK, et al. Annals of Internal Medicine Clinical Guideline Red Blood Cell Transfusion : A clinical practice guideline from the AABB. Ann Intern Med. 2012;1:49-58.

16. Carson JL, Stanworth SJ, Roubinian N, Fergusson DA, Triulzi D, Doree C, et al. Transfusion thresholds and other strategies for guiding allogeneic red blood cell transfusion. Cochrane Database Syst Rev. 2016;2016:1-69.

17. Carson JL, Stanworth SJ, Roubinian N, Fergusson DA, Triulzi D, Doree C, et al. Transfusion thresholds and other strategies for guiding allogeneic red blood cell transfusion (Review). Cochrane Database Syst Rev. 2016;10:CD002042.

18. Koo B, Kwon MA, Kim S, Kim JY, Moon Y, Park SY, et al. Korean clinical practice guideline for perioperative red blood cell transfusion from Korean Society of Anesthesiologists. Korean J Anesthesiol. 2019;72:91-118.

19. Salpeter SR, Buckley JS, Chatterjee S. Impact of more restrictive blood transfusion strategies on clinical outcomes: a meta-analysis and systematic review. Am J Med. 2014;127:124-131.e3.

20. Holst LB, Haase N, Wetterslev J, Wernerman J, Guttormsen AB, Karlsson S, et al. Lower versus higher hemoglobin threshold for transfusion in septic shock. N Engl J Med. 2014;371:1381-91.

21. Holst LB, Petersen MW, Haase N, Perner A, Wetterslev J. Restrictive versus liberal transfusion strategy for red blood cell transfusion: systematic review of randomised trials with meta-analysis and trial sequential analysis. BMJ. 2015;350:h1354.

22. Brunskill SJ, Millette SL, Shokoohi A, Pulford EC, Doree C, Murphy MF, et al. Red blood cell transfusion for people undergoing hip fracture surgery. Cochrane Database Syst Rev. 2015;(4):CD009699.

23. Chatterjee S, Wetterslev J, Sharma A, Lichstein E, Mukherjee D. Association of blood transfusion with increased mortality in myocardial infarction: a meta-analysis and diversity-adjusted study sequential analysis. JAMA Intern Med. 2013;173:132-9.

24. Retter A, Wyncoll D, Pearse R, Carson D, Mckechnie S, Stanworth S, et al. Guidelines on the management of anaemia and red cell transfusion in adult critically ill patients. Br J Haematol. 2013;160:445-64.

25. Rhodes A, Evans LE, Alhazzani W, Levy MM, Antonelli M, Ferrer R, et al. Surviving sepsis campaign: International Guidelines for Management of Sepsis and Septic Shock: 2016. Intensive Care Med. 2016;43:304-77.

26. Rodrigues R, Oliveira R, Lucena L, Paiva H, Cordeiro V, Carmona MJ, et al. STATA- strategy of transfusion in trauma patients: a randomized trial. J Clin Trials. 2016;6:CD007871.

27. Sihler KC, Napolitano LM. Massive transfusion: new insights. Chest. 2009;136:1654-67.

28. Holcomb JB, Tilley BC, Baraniuk S, Fox EE, Wade CE, Podbielski JM, et al. Transfusion of plasma, platelets, and red blood cells in a 1:1:1 vs a 1:1:2 ratio and mortality in patients with severe trauma: the PROPPR randomized clinical trial. JAMA. 2015;313:471-82.

29. Holcomb JB, del Junco DJ, Fox EE, Wade CE, Cohen MJ, Schreiber MA, et al. The Prospective, Observational, Multicenter, Major Trauma Transfusion (PROMMTT) study: comparative effectiveness of a time-varying treatment with competing risks. JAMA Surg. 2013;148:127-36.

30. Haas T, Fries D, Tanaka KA, Asmis L, Curry NS, Schöchl H. Usefulness of standard plasma coagulation tests in the management of perioperative coagulopathic bleeding: is there any evidence? Br J Anaesth. 2015;114:217-24.

31. Laursen TH, Meyer MA, Meyer AS, Gaarder T, Naess PA, Stensballe J, et al. Thrombelastography early amplitudes in bleeding and coagulopathic trauma patients: results from a multicenter study. J Trauma Acute Care Surg. 2018;84:334-41.

32. Afshari A, Wikkelsø A, Brok J, Møller AM, WJ. Thrombelastography (TEG) or thromboelastometry (ROTEM) to monitor haemotherapy versus usual care in patients with massive transfusion. Cochrane Database Syst Rev. 2015;CD007871.

33. Hunt H, Stanworth S, Curry N, Woolley T, Cooper C, Ukoumunne O, et al. Thromboelastography (TEG) and rotational thromboelastometry (ROTEM) for trauma induced coagulopathy in adult trauma patients with bleeding. Cochrane Database Syst Rev. 2016;2:CD010438.

34. Bawazeer M, Ahmed N, Izadi H, Mcfarlan A, Nathens A, Pavenski K. Compliance with a massive transfusion protocol (MTP) impacts patient outcome. Injury. 2015;46:21-8.

35. East JM, Viau-Lapointe J, McCredie VA. Transfusion practices in traumatic brain injury. Curr Opin Anaesthesiol. 2018;31(2):219-26.

36. Badenes R, Oddo M, Suarez JI, Antonelli M, Lipman J, Citerio G, et al. Hemoglobin concentrations and RBC transfusion thresholds in patients with acute brain injury: an international survey. Crit Care. 2017;21:1-10.

37. Tiede A, Worster A. Lessons from a systematic literature review of the effectiveness of recombinant factor VIIa in acquired haemophilia. Ann Hematol. 2018;97:1889-901.

38. von Heymann C, Jonas S, Spies C, Wernecke KD, Ziemer S, Janssen D, et al. Recombinant activated factor VIIa for the treatment of bleeding in major abdominal surgery including vascular and urological surgery: a review and meta-analysis of published data. Crit Care. 2008;12:R14.

39. Mayer SA, Brun NC, Begtrup K, Broderick J, Davis S, Diringer MN, et al. Efficacy and safety of recombinant activated factor VII for acute intracerebral hemorrhage. N Engl J Med. 2008;358:2127-37.

40. Hsia CC, Chin-Yee IH, McAlister VC. Use of recombinant activated factor VII in patients without hemophilia: a meta-analysis of randomized control trials. Ann Surg. 2008;248:61-8.

41. Yank V, Tuohy CV, Logan AC, Bravata DM, Staudenmayer K, Eisenhut R, et al. Systematic review: benefits and harms of in-hospital use of recombinant factor VIIa for off-label indications. Ann Intern Med. 2011;154:529-40.

42. Cooper DJ, McQuilten ZK, Nichol A, Ady B, Aubron C, Bailey M, et al. Age of red cells for transfusion and outcomes in critically ill adults. N Engl J Med. 2017;377(19):1858-67.

43. Lacroix J, Hébert PC, Fergusson DA, Tinmouth A, Cook DJ, Marshall JC, et al. Age of transfused blood in critically ill adults. N Engl J Med. 2015;372:1410-8.

44. Eikelboom JW, Cook RJ, Barty R, Liu Y, Arnold DM, Crowther MA, et al. Rationale and design of the Informing Fresh versus Old Red Cell Management (INFORM) Trial: an International pragmatic randomized trial. Transfus Med Rev. 2016;30:25-9.

45. Steiner ME, Ness PM, Assmann SF, Triulzi DJ, Sloan SR, Delaney M, et al. Effects of red-cell storage duration on patients undergoing cardiac surgery. N Engl J Med. 2015;372:1419-29.

46. Roberts I, Shakur H, Coats T, Hunt B, Balogun E, Barnetson L et al. The CRASH-2 trial: a randomised controlled trial and economic evaluation of the effects of tranexamic acid on death, vascular occlusive events and transfusion requirement in bleeding trauma patients. Health Technol Assess (Rockv). 2013;17:1-79.

47. CRASH-3 trial collaborators. Articles effects of tranexamic acid on death, disability, vascular occlusive events and other morbidities in patients with acute traumatic brain injury (CRASH-3): a randomised, placebo- controlled trial. Lancet. 2019;394:1713-23.

48. Cho BC, Serini J, Zorrilla-vaca A, Scott MJ, Gehrie EA, Frank SM, et al. Impact of preoperative erythropoietin on allogeneic blood transfusions in surgical patients: results from a systematic review and meta-analysis. Anesth Analg. 2019;128:981-92.

49. Spahn DR, Schoenrath F, Spahn GH, Seifert B, Stein P, Theusinger OM, et al. Articles Effect of ultra-short-term treatment of patients with iron deficiency or anaemia undergoing cardiac surgery: a prospective randomised trial. Lancet. 2019;6736: 1-12.

50. Shin HW, Park JJ, Kim HJ, You HS, Choi SU, Lee M. Efficacy of perioperative intravenous iron therapy for transfusion in orthopedic surgery : a systematic review and meta-analysis. PLoS One. 2019;14:e0215427.

51. Zhou X, Zhang C, Wang Y, Yu L, Yan M. Preoperative acute normovolemic hemodilution for minimizing allogeneic blood transfusion: a meta-analysis. Anesth Analg. 2015;121:1443-55.

52. Bianchi M, Vaglio S, Pupella S, Marano G, Facco G, Liumbruno GM, et al. Leucoreduction of blood components: an effective way to increase blood safety? Review Blood Transfus. 2016;14:214-27.

53. Hall S, Danby R, Osman H, Peniket A, Rocha V, Craddock C, et al. Transfusion in CMV seronegative T-depleted allogeneic stem cell transplant recipients with CMV-unselected blood components results in zero CMV transmissions in the era of universal leukocyte reduction: a UK dual centre experience. Transfus Med. 2015;25:418-23.

54. Seftel MD, Growe GH, Petraszko T, Benny WB, Le A, Lee CY, et al. Universal prestorage leukoreduction in Canada decreases platelet alloimmunization and refractoriness. Blood. 2004;103:333-9.

55. Sarkar RS, Philip J, Yadav P. Transfusion medicine and solid organ transplant - Update and review of some current issues. Med J Armed Forces India. 2013;69:162-7.

56. Bilgin YM, van de Watering LM, Eijsman L, Versteegh MI, Brand R, van Oers MH, et al. Double-blind, randomized controlled trial on the effect of leukocyte-depleted erythrocyte transfusions in cardiac valve surgery. Circulation. 2004;109:2755-60.

57. Kim Y, Xia BT, Chang AL, Pritts TA. Role of leukoreduction of packed red blood cell units in trauma patients: a review young. Int J Hematol Res. 2017;2:124-9.

58. Moradi S, Jahanian-Najafabadi A, Roudkenar MH. Artificial blood substitutes: first steps on the long route to clinical utility. Clin Med Insights Blood Disord. 2016;9:33-41.

Role of Point-of-care Ultrasound in the Perioperative Period

Sachin Gupta, Deeksha Singh Tomar

INTRODUCTION

Point-of-care ultrasound (POCUS) plays a very important role in the modern daily practice of anesthesiologists. To understand the various applications of POCUS, we need to be well versed with the definition of POCUS which is defined as rapid bedside ultrasound examination by the physician to answer specific but limited diagnostic questions, form a diagnosis, and impart treatment on the basis of these findings.[1] It is also called as "modern day stethoscope" for the anesthesiologist.

Anesthesiologists have been masters in the use of ultrasound technology in transesophageal echocardiography (TEE),[2] establishing central venous access[3] and regional anesthesia.[4] The utility of POCUS in critical care and emergency medicine is an established fact[5] now but the same extrapolation in perioperative care is still lacking.

The scope of POCUS in various perioperative issues such as airway management, determination of prandial status and gastric volume, assessment of pulmonary status, detection of free gas or free fluid in abdomen, and assessment of cardiovascular system is growing rapidly.[6,7]

POCUS utilizes the three basic transducers on the machine: Cardiac or phased array transducer, curvilinear or famously known abdominal transducer, and linear or vascular transducer. We will see the utility of each one in various indications **(Figs. 1A to C)**.

AIRWAY ULTRASOUND

The airway management is one of the most important task that an anesthetist carries out in the operative room.

Placement of Endotracheal Tube

The correct placement of endotracheal tube is the most important step in airway control. Unrecognized malpositioning of the endotracheal tube can lead to serious

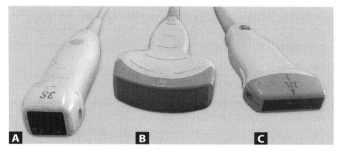

Figs. 1A to C: The three transducers used in POCUS. (A) Cardiac or phased array transducer; (B) Curvilinear or abdominal transducer; (C) Linear or vascular transducer.

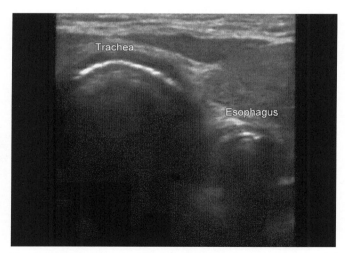

Fig. 2: Esophageal intubation. The esophagus appears as a mini trachea if the endotracheal tube is inserted in the esophagus.

complications in the perioperative period and may also terminate into death of the patient.[8] POCUS can be used to detect correct placement of endotracheal tube real time dynamically and can also prevent esophageal intubation. The sensitivity and specificity to predict esophageal intubation is very high (0.93 and 0.97, respectively)[9] **(Fig. 2)**.

The correct placement of endotracheal tube can be viewed real time by placing the linear transducer in a transverse manner at the suprasternal notch. The movement of tube in the trachea and not in the esophagus is a conformational of endotracheal intubation.[10] The indirect way of confirmation of endotracheal intubation is to look for bilateral lung sliding postintubation by placing the linear transducer in a longitudinal manner at the mid-axillary line,[11] but this may not be very confirmatory as endobronchial intubation may cause lung sliding to cease on the side which is not ventilating.

Prediction of Difficult Airway

Difficult airway is the biggest nightmare for an anesthetist and any modality which can correctly predict it will be of greatest help. The studies carried out by Adhikari et al.[12] concluded that difficult laryngoscopy can be predicted on the basis of the measurements of anterior neck soft tissue thickness measured at the level of the hyoid bone, although further validation studies are missing.

Extubation Assessment

Role of POCUS in identifying the patients who can develop stridor postextubation is now increasing. Ding et al.[13] in their pilot study demonstrated that if the air column width during cuff deflation was less, then it was a good predictor of postextubation stridor as it represented laryngeal edema. Another reason for postextubation stridor or breathing difficulty could be vocal cord palsy. The classical way of detecting is by doing direct laryngoscopy but patients may not tolerate laryngoscopy without sedation and so POCUS can be utilized here. By keeping the linear transducer in a transverse manner at the level of thyroid cartilage and

visualizing the movement of vocal cords, one can easily identify vocal cord palsy.[14]

LUNG ULTRASOUND

Ultrasound of the pleura and thorax is a simple but an essential tool for the perioperative physician. The wide subset of patients with various pulmonary issues are landing into operation theater and their management in the perioperative period by the anesthesiologist has an impact in the overall outcome of the patients. Ultrasound findings have been shown to be more sensitive and specific as compared to the chest radiograph for diagnosing conditions such as pleural effusion, pneumothorax, consolidation, and alveolar interstitial syndrome.[15] The learning curve required for this examination is not high and even a novice learner with a handheld device can generate the same images as done by a trained person with a fully equipped ultrasound machine.[16]

For the perioperative physician, the most important pathologies to deal with are pneumothorax, pulmonary edema, atelectasis, pleural effusion, and consolidation. These all can be assessed and monitored with the help of POCUS. The Bedside Lung Ultrasound in Emergency (BLUE) protocol[17] was investigated to reach to a diagnosis for patients in acute respiratory distress and it was found to have a sensitivity over 90% for all of the above conditions. Lung ultrasound is an analysis of various artifacts which are produced due to reflection of ultrasound beam coming in contact with the air either in lung parenchyma or outside the parenchyma. For lung ultrasound, each hemithorax is divided into six zones by a horizontal line at the level of nipple and two vertical lines, one is anterior axillary and the other is posterior axillary **(Figs. 3A and B)**.

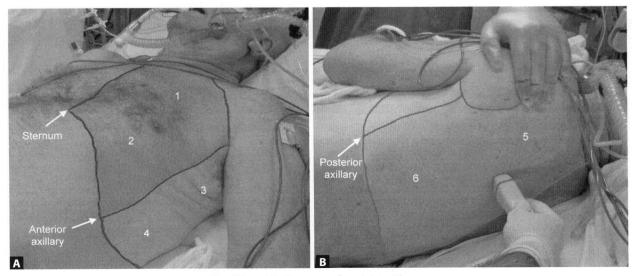

Figs. 3A and B: Six zones of each hemithorax.

Lung Sliding

Lung ultrasound examination is done by using both the linear and the curvilinear transducers. The first examination should be to ascertain whether the lung is aerated and contributing in ventilation. For this, the linear transducer is kept on various zones of the lung on both sides and the "to-and-fro" movement of sliding of visceral and parietal pleura over each other is appreciated. This is called as "lung sliding"[18] and is indicative that the lung zone where the transducer is placed is ventilating and there is no sign of pneumothorax (**Fig. 4**). When an M-mode is put on this lung sliding, a granular appearance is seen on the screen which is called as "sea-shore" sign[19] as it looks similar to sand on a beach pattern (**Fig. 5**).

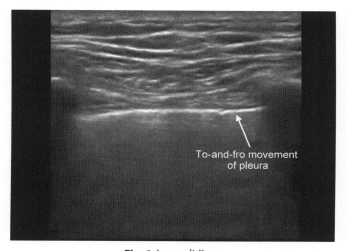

Fig. 4: Lung sliding.

A-Lines

The presence of "A-lines" represents that the lung is aerated and does not have pneumothorax, pleural effusion, or consolidation. They are seen as horizontal line under the pleural line at a distant equal to the skin and the pleural line (**Fig. 6**). They do not just represent healthy lung but may be present in bronchial asthma, chronic obstructive pulmonary disease (COPD), and pulmonary embolism.

B-Lines

The presence of "B-lines" is always associated with pathology and is produced due to increase in the fluid component of the lung leading to a change in the air:water ratio of lung parenchyma. In very simple words, B-lines represent wet lungs. These "comet tail artifact"[20] appears as hyperechoic lines from pleura, moves with lung sliding, reaches the base of the frame, and obliterates the A-lines (**Figs. 7A to C**). They are present classically in pulmonary edema in bilateral lung zones, consolidation only in the area affected, and lung contusion due to trauma. In acute respiratory distress syndrome (ARDS), the B-lines appear in different forms as the pathology is nonhomogenous. The finding of B-lines is important for a perioperative physician in managing a patient with previous normal findings.

Lung Pulse

The "lung pulse" is a sign which is seen in immobile lung. On B-mode ultrasound, it appears as small movement of lung which is synchronous with the heartbeat of the patient. On M-mode, it is seen as vertical lines (representing cardiac oscillations) overlying the horizontal lines of absent

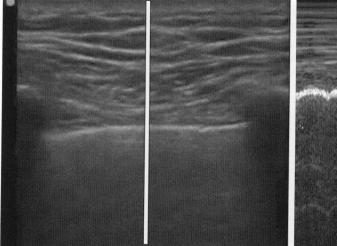
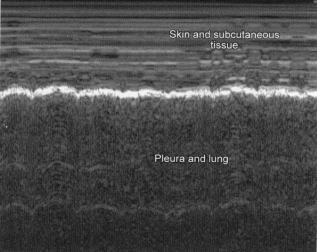

Fig. 5: Sea-shore sign.

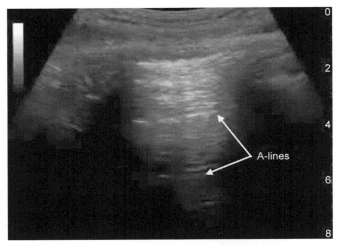

Fig. 6: A-lines.

ventilation **(Figs. 8A and B)**. This is very commonly seen in one-lung ventilation, mucus plugging one of the mainstem bronchus, atelectasis, or even in situations where the lung is surrounded by massive pleural effusion. This sign can be easily used to determine to rule out endobronchial intubation as we should have bilateral lung sliding after intubation. The sensitivity and specificity of lung pulse for diagnosing atelectasis ranges from 70 to 99% and 92 to 100%, respectively.[21]

Air Bronchograms

Consolidation represents the loss of aeration of the lung and it appears like a hard tissue, just like liver and so has been staged as red or gray hepatization. On ultrasound, consolidation has many pathognomonic signs, but the most

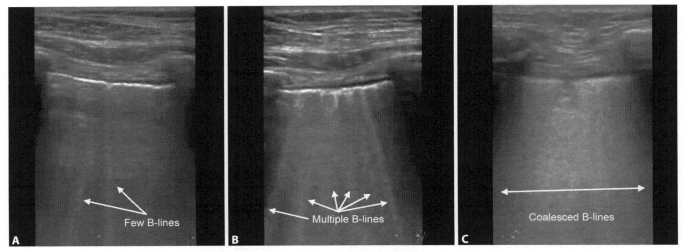

Figs. 7A to C: Phases of B-lines. (A) Occasional or very few B-lines; (B) The lines increase in number due to increase in disease process as in pulmonary edema; (C) Coalesced B-lines as happens in ARDS and consolidation.

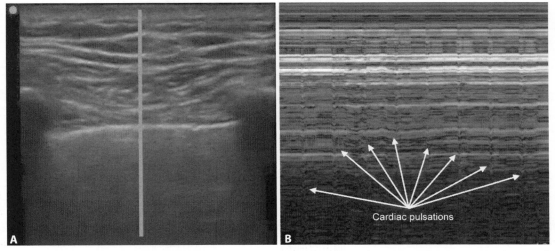

Figs. 8A and B: M-mode image of lung pulse showing transmission of cardiac pulsations on the nonmoving lung and pleura.

characteristic sign is "dynamic air bronchogram."[22] This is seen as to-and-fro movement of air in the alveoli with the phases of respiration and is seen as white color. This is differentiated from atelectasis as in this the air is trapped inside the alveoli and do not move in and out with phases of respiration, so on ultrasound, it appears like white dots during both phases of respiration. This is called as "static air bronchogram" **(Figs. 9A and B)**.

Lung Point

Risk of pneumothorax is always present during central venous cannulation and more so during subclavian vein (SV) cannulation. Chest X-rays are not very sensitive in detecting small pneumothoraces as compared to ultrasound. The ultrasound finding of "lung point"[23] in

B-mode and "stratosphere sign" in M-mode is nearly 100% sensitive and specific for pneumothorax. Lung point denotes the point where there is breach in the pleura and is seen as a junction where on one side pleural sliding is present and on the other side, static A-lines are seen. If M-mode is put on this static area, it appears like horizontal lines with no transmission of cardiac pulsation and this is called as stratosphere sign **(Figs. 10A and B)**.

Pleural Effusion

Identification of pleural effusion is difficult on chest X-ray as blunting of costophrenic (CP) angles happens only when a moderate amount of fluid has accumulated. On ultrasonography, presence of anechoic or hypoechoic fluid between the lung and the diaphragm in B-mode

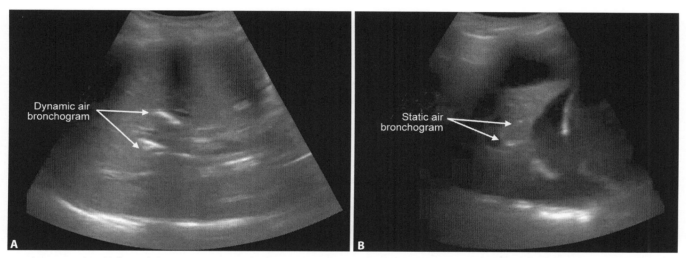

Figs. 9A and B: Air bronchograms. (A) Dynamic air bronchogram as seen in consolidation where air is seen going in and out with respiration; (B) Static air bronchogram as seen in atelectasis where air is seen trapped in both phases of respiration.

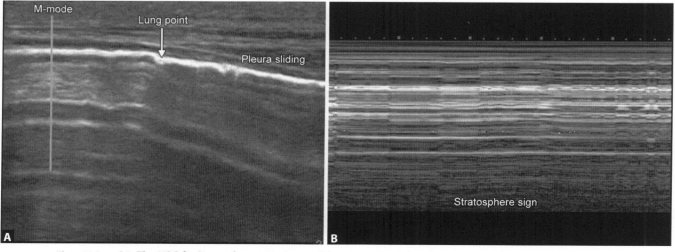

Figs. 10A and B: The USG findings of pneumothorax. (A) Lung point, defined as junction point where the pleura is still attached to the lung; (B) Stratosphere sign, an M-mode finding of pneumothorax.

is confirmatory of pleural effusion. The evaluation of pleural effusion is done by the curvilinear probe with the marker pointed cephalad with the lung and the diaphragm being visualized. If the pleural effusion is in significant amounts, then the underlying lung appears collapsed and consolidated[24] **(Figs. 11A and B)**.

CARDIAC ULTRASOUND

The word echocardiogram is very specific for a cardiologist. The assessment of cardiac function and the necessity of rapid decision-making required in emergency and intensive care have included cardiac evaluation in POCUS. The main objective of cardiac assessment is to diagnose and manage undifferentiated shock. An anesthesiologist may utilize this knowledge in managing the variety of etiologies. To evaluate the cause of hemodynamic instability intraoperatively or postoperatively, there is a structured algorithm to rule out or rule in most of the causes **(Fig. 12)**.

Fluid Responsiveness

This information is frequently required by anesthesiologist during intraoperative hypotension. Static parameters such as central venous pressure (CVP) do not correlate with the actual fluid status and has been advised not to use.[25] Measuring the inferior vena cava (IVC) diameter just distal to the insertion of hepatic vein is a reliable tool in diagnosing fluid responsiveness. End-expiratory diameter of <1 cm correlates with the need for fluid administration in the event of hypotension. This is measured by keeping the cardiac-phased array probe at the subxiphoid position and pointing the marker at 90° cephalad. The IVC variability with respiration without even measuring the diameter is also a reliable estimate of fluid responsiveness. This is called as "eye balling" **(Fig. 13)**.

Another technique of measuring fluid responsiveness is by measuring the velocity time integral (VTI). It is a Doppler measurement of flow across a valve. It is measured by putting a pulse wave Doppler at the center of the jet of the aortic valve in apical five chamber view. A trace is obtained on the screen. In most modern machines, there is an option of measuring the VTI by marking the trace. This becomes the baseline value for the patient. Now after a fluid bolus, if there is an incremental change in VTI, it indicates that the patient is fluid responsive.[26] Even while performing passive leg raising test, if there is an increase in VTI, it also has the same inference. This is one of the fastest noninvasive techniques when assessing the fluid responsiveness of the patient **(Fig. 14)**.

Assessment of Left Ventricular Function

Perioperative assessment of left ventricular (LV) function can be of value to anesthesiologist while managing patients with LV systolic dysfunction. The knowledge becomes all the more important when the evaluation is done for patients planned for an emergency surgery where the availability of an echocardiographer may be absent. There is evidence that the validity of such assessments is almost at par with the trained echocardiographers.[27]

Cardiac Arrest

The most important information that can be achieved during cardiac arrest is the presence of cardiac contractility during pulseless electrical activity (PEA) as these patients have a higher chance of survival. This condition is known as "pseudo-PEA." Focus-assessed transthoracic echocardiography (FATE)[28] protocol has been studied in the event of cardiac arrest to rule out conditions such as pulmonary embolism, pericardial tamponade, tension

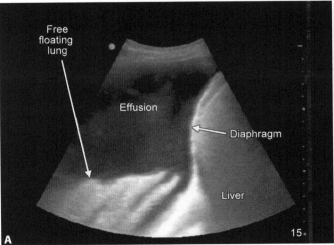
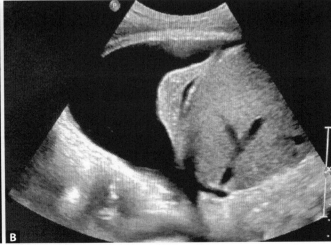

Figs. 11A and B: Large pleural effusion. (A) Freely floating lung in massive pleural effusion; (B) Consolidated appearance of lung due to weight of large pleural effusion.

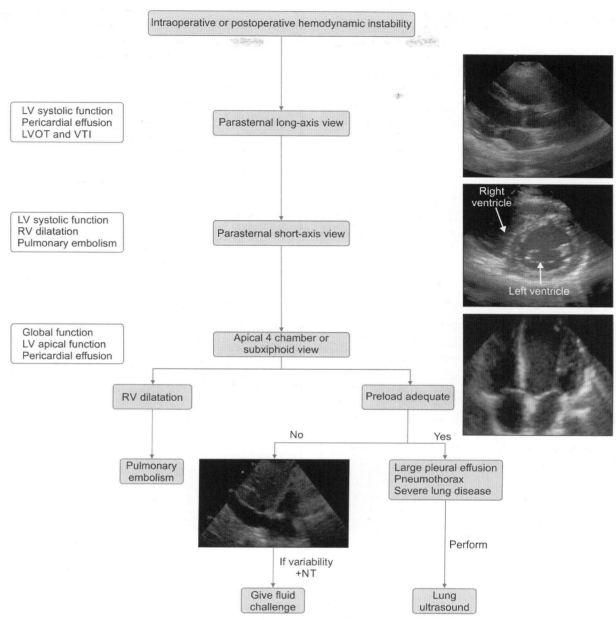

Fig. 12: Algorithm for intraoperative hemodynamic instability.

pneumothorax, and myocardial ischemia as the cause of arrest. This evaluation is done by placing the probe in the subxiphoid area and scanning the heart during the 10-second pulse check in cardiopulmonary resuscitation (CPR). The ongoing CPR is not halted for the ultrasound examination **(Figs. 15 and 16)**.

ABDOMINAL ULTRASOUND

The role of abdominal ultrasound has been used maximally during the Focused Assessment by Sonography in Trauma (FAST) scan in emergency and intensive care unit (ICU) settings. The utility of abdominal ultrasound for a

perioperative physician is to evaluate the volume of gastric content, correct placement of orogastric or nasogastric tube, and assessment of urinary bladder fullness status in the postoperative period.

Gastric Content Volume

The risk of aspiration of gastric contents is always on the priority list of the anesthesiologist during intubation. The various techniques such as Sellick maneuver or rapid sequence intubation have been in practice for long to prevent this but none of this technique can ascertain the content and the volume of the content in the stomach. POCUS can

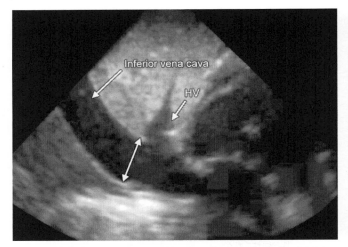

Fig. 13: Inferior vena cava and its site of measurement which is just next to the insertion of hepatic vein (HV).

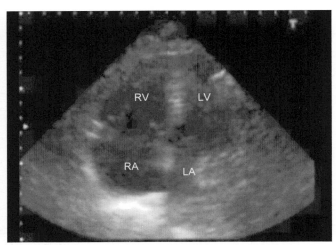

Fig. 15: Massive pulmonary embolism with RA, RV dilated and the interventricular septum is convex towards left ventricle.

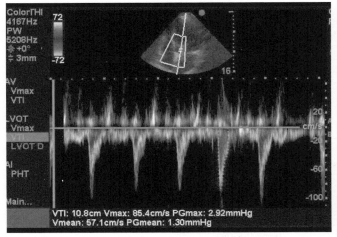

Fig. 14: Velocity time integral (VTI). The pulsed wave Doppler is kept at the center of the jet of the aortic valve and the trace is obtained. Marking the trace gives the VTJ.

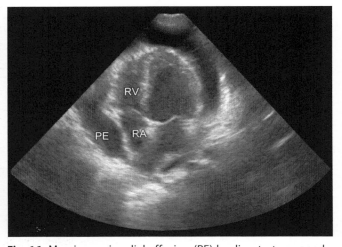

Fig. 16: Massive pericardial effusion (PE) leading to tamponade. The RA is collapsed during late diastole and RV is collapsed during early diastole.

ascertain the gastric content volume with good precision by visualizing the gastric antrum in the right lateral position.[29] This is done by keeping the curvilinear abdominal transducer just beneath the left rib cage to visualize the gastric antrum. The content would appear anechoic if it is just liquid in nature but if there are ring down artifacts present, then it indicates the presence of particulate matter which can cause chemical pneumonitis, if aspirated. Similarly, if the walls of the stomach are opposed to each other with a white line visible, it is suggestive of an empty stomach and this white line stands for air in the stomach **(Fig. 17)**.

Placement of Orogastric/Nasogastric Tube

The correct placement of orogastric or nasogastric tube is confirmed by listening to the bubbling sound in

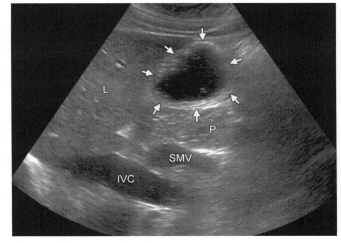

Fig. 17: Stomach filled with fluid.

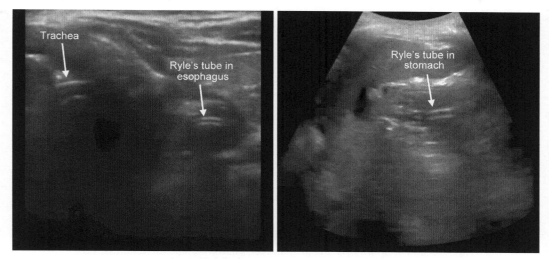

Fig. 18: Ryle' tube insertion and visualization.

epigastrium by stethoscope or by getting a chest X-ray done. The use of ultrasound can confirm the correct placement by observing it real time.[30] The linear transducer is placed on the left side of trachea so that the collapsed esophagus is visible. Now the tube is made to pass and one can appreciate that the collapsed esophagus starts showing two hemispherical artifacts which are the walls of the orogastric tube. This is the first confirmation that the tube is in the esophagus and not in trachea. Second, after the requisite length has passed, one can attempt visualizing the tube in the stomach as a double lumen structure **(Fig. 18)**.

This is very vital in patients who are not fully alert or whose airway reflexes are obtunded as they may not cough if the tube goes in the trachea.

Urinary Bladder Assessment

Postoperatively, the patients may have decreased urine output and this can be a matter of concern. The use of pelvic view of the FAST scan can be done to look for retention of urine, especially in elderly patients or decreased urine output in general.

OPTIC ULTRASOUND

Optic Nerve Sheath Diameter

Managing a patient with raised intracranial pressure (ICP) is a challenging task. Optic nerve sheath diameter (ONSD) is a useful surrogate of ICP and has excellent sensitivity and specificity (85% and 92% respectively).[31] ONSD is measured at the retrobulbar part 3 mm below the retina by keeping the linear transducer over the closed eyelid with adequate amount of jelly. The diameter of >5.6 mm is taken as a cut-

off for ICP >20 mm Hg. This examination is more useful in managing liver transplant for an acute liver failure patient or managing an eclampsia patient intraoperatively as they are at very high risk for developing cerebral edema and raised ICP **(Figs. 19A and B)**.

Other Optic Findings

Patients coming with facial trauma may not give the opportunity to examine the pupils and other injuries in the eye. Optic ultrasound can detect the pupillary size and reaction to light. One can also appreciate retinal detachment, lens dislocation, and even vitreous hemorrhage in such patients.[32] The entire examination is done by keeping the linear transducer over the closed eyelid with the help of adequate jelly as interface.

VASCULAR ACCESS

This is the only skill-based part in the entire POCUS and requires certain training. Classically, central and arterial cannulation has been done in a blind manner by following the anatomical landmarks. But this practice is associated with various observed and various concealed complications. The most common complications seen with the traditional technique are arterial puncture, hematoma, pneumothorax, failed cannulation, and multiple attempts.

The recent systematic reviews[33] have highlighted the safety of ultrasound in performing central venous cannulation and the practice recommendations[34] have come into place to use ultrasound for cannulation. The dynamic technique of central venous cannulation is superior to the static technique wherein the anatomy is visualized with the help of ultrasound, but the cannulation is still done blindly without using ultrasound.

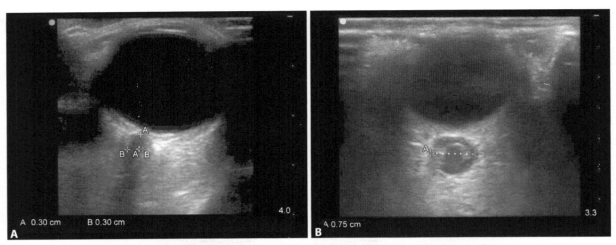

Figs. 19A and B: Optic nerve sheath diameter. (A) Normal size; (B) Abnormal size.

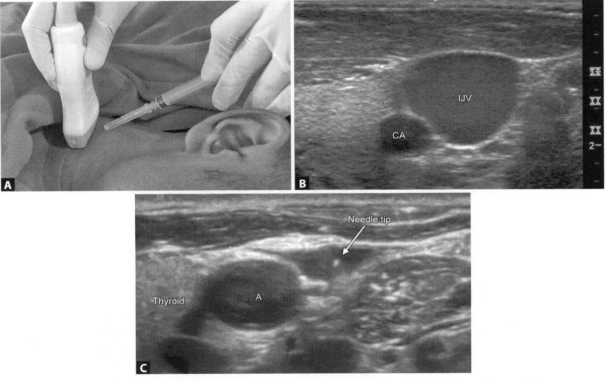

Figs. 20A to C: Short-axis view of IJV. (A) Orientation of the transducer; (B) Ultrasound view of IJV; (C) Ultrasound view of needle tip in IJV.

Internal Jugular Vein

The various orientations of internal jugular vein (IJV) cannulation are short or transverse-axis (SAX), long or longitudinal-axis (LAX), and the oblique-axis.

Short-axis

Visualizing the structures surrounding the vein is the main advantage of this view. The artery is usually present in close proximity to the vein and to avoid inadvertent cannulation of the artery is the prime objective while cannulation. In this view, the performer directs the needle at 45° toward the vein by following the Pythagorean Theorem, and hence enters the vein **(Figs. 20A to C)**.

Long Axis

The advantage of this axis is the better visualization of the entire path of the needle entering the vein. In this technique, the transducer is kept in longitudinal direction over the IJV, so that only the vein is visualized and then the needle is

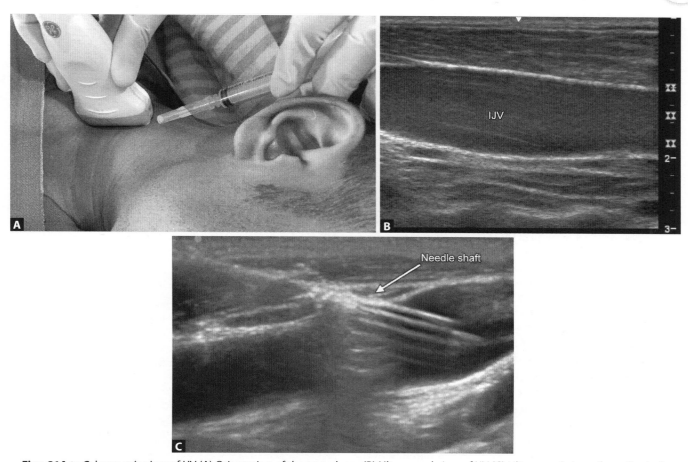

Figs. 21A to C: Long axis view of IJV (A) Orientation of the transducer (B) Ultrasound view of IJV (C) Ultrasound view of needle shaft.

entered just under the transducer so that it is always under the footprint of the transducer. This way the entire shaft of the needle is visualized.

A prospective randomized observation study comparing the ease of insertion with SAX versus LAX concluded that SAX was more easier for beginners as it gave the visualization of both the vascular structures and also the hand-eye coordination required for LAX was difficult[35] **(Figs. 21A to C)**.

Oblique View

This view exploits the advantages of both the above mentioned views. The transducer is kept in an oblique manner over the IJV so that both the vascular structures are visualized in an oval shape. The needle is then inserted under the transducer as in LAX and so the entire path of the needle is seen. This is more useful in short neck patients where there is vertical length available to place the transducer for LAX technique **(Figs. 22A to C)**.

Subclavian Vein

The most dreaded complication during SV cannulation is pneumothorax due to its very close proximity to pleura. In the traditional anatomical approach, the needle is inserted

infraclavicularly at the junction of medial one-third and lateral two-thirds of the clavicle and is directed toward the suprasternal notch. In ultrasound technique, the transducer is kept in transverse orientation over the vein, so that the vein appears tubular in shape and then the needle is inserted as in LAX technique of IJV, visualizing the entire path of the needle. The angle of the needle is kept as parallel to the skin as increasing the angulation increases the risk of puncturing the pleura.

In a trial comparing the utility of ultrasound for SV cannulation versus the traditional technique, it was found that ultrasound-guided procedures had a higher success rate (92% vs. 44%), less attempts (1.1% vs. 2.5%), and less minor complications (1 vs. 11). They concluded that ultrasound should be used to cannulate SV.[36]

The recommendation[37] for using ultrasound for SV cannulation is weak and can be used only for high-risk cases to locate the site and ascertain the patency of the vein.

Femoral Vein

This is generally the choice for cardiac catheterization and also for securing a venous access in emergency scenarios. The femoral artery (FA) and the femoral vein (FV) lie in

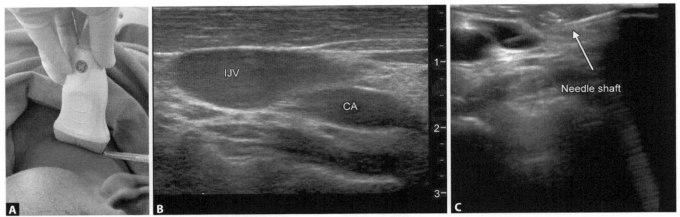

Figs. 22A to C: Oblique view of IJV. (A) Orientation of the transducer; (B) Ultrasound view of IJV; (C) Ultrasound view of needle shaft.

the femoral triangle with vein lying medially to artery. The ease of puncturing and a large size of the vessel make it less prone to complications, thus achieving higher success rate with the traditional technique. Ultrasound has been used for securing FV access and FA access as the anatomy is better defined. It has been shown that the use of ultrasound reduces the number of complications such as inadvertent arterial puncture during FV cannulation.[38]

The recommendation[37] is still weak for using ultrasound for FV cannulation as the complication rate is low with traditional technique. The ultrasound use should be for detailing of the anatomy and ascertain the patency of the vein.

Arterial Cannulation

Hypotension, shock, repeated arterial puncture, arterial vasospasm, edema at the site of puncture, nonpalpable arterial pulse, and morbid obesity are some of the indications for the use of ultrasound for arterial cannulation.[39] Radial artery is generally the first choice due to superficial nature, predictable anatomy, ease in palpation, and low complication rate. The first attempt successful cannulation rate of radial artery with the help of ultrasound is between 62 and 87% as compared to 34–50% with palpation technique[40] **(Fig. 23)**.

Similarly, the FA can be accessed with much ease with the help of ultrasound as compared to palpation technique.

The recommendation[37] is to use ultrasound for radial artery cannulation to improve first attempt cannulation.

Peripheral Inserted Central Catheters

Peripheral inserted central catheters (PICC) lines are inserted in superficial veins but may be difficult in patients with arm edema, obesity, chronic drug abusers, or even in elderly with thin fragile veins. Ultrasound has shown

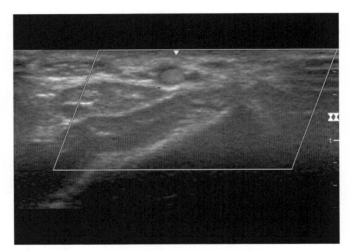

Fig. 23: Radial artery with Doppler.

to improve the success rate of PICC line insertion in such population. Both SAX and LAX orientations can be used depending on the expertise of the performer.

The recommendation[37] is to use ultrasound to look for patency and anatomy of the superficial vein but does not strongly recommend for using it during the procedure.

CONCLUSION

Incorporating POCUS in daily anesthesia practice improves the outcome of the patients as it helps in managing life-threatening situations in a more protocolized manner. The improved diagnostic accuracy of various pulmonary and cardiac etiologies by the perioperative physician helps to plan the technique of anesthesia and be ready for the expected complications. The inclusion of FATE in advanced cardiac life support (ACLS) announces the importance of this modality. The procedural guidance has changed the way central venous cannulation is being done and is now an important quality indicator. The neuromonitoring with the help of ONSD estimation has lot of literature support and should be made a part of the anesthesia routine while managing patients prone to raised ICP. An anesthesiologist should undergo a formal training of various aspects of POCUS to increase the safety and precision in managing such cases intraoperatively.

REFERENCES

1. Moore CL, Copel JA. Point-of-care ultrasonography. N Engl J Med. 2011;364(8):749-57.

2. Shore-Lesserson L, Moskowitz D, Hametz C, Andrews D, Yamada T, Vela-Cantos F, et al. Use of intraoperative transesophageal echocardiography to predict atrial fibrillation after coronary artery bypass grafting. Anesthesiology. 2001;95(3):652-8

3. Wu SY, Ling Q, Cao LH, Wang J, Xu MX, Zeng WA. Real-time two-dimensional ultrasound guidance for central venous cannulation: a meta-analysis. Anesthesiology. 2013;118(2): 361-75.

4. Gray AT. Ultrasound-guided regional anesthesia: current state of the art. Anesthesiology. 2006;104(2):368-73.

5. AHRQ issues critical analysis of patient safety practices. Qual Lett Healthc Lead. 2001;13(8):8-12.

6. Canty DJ, Royse CF, Kilpatrick D, Bowman L, Royse AG. The impact of focused transthoracic echocardiography in the preoperative clinic. Anaesthesia. 2012;67(6):618-25.

7. Perlas A, Chan VW, Lupu CM, Mitsakakis N, Hanbidge A. Ultrasound assessment of gastric content and volume. Anesthesiology. 2009;111(1):82-9.

8. Keenan RL, Boyan CP. Cardiac arrest due to anesthesia. A study of incidence and causes. JAMA. 1985;253(16):2373-7.

9. Chou EH, Dickman E, Tsou PY, Tessaro M, Tsai YM, Ma MH, et al. Ultrasonography for confirmation of endotracheal tube placement: a systematic review and meta-analysis. Resuscitation. 2015;90:97-103.

10. Kristensen MS. Ultrasonography in the management of the airway. Acta Anaesthesiologica Scandinavica. 2011;55(10): 1155-73.

11. Rudraraju P, Eisen LA. Confirmation of endotracheal tube position: a narrative review. J Intensive Care Med. 2009;24(5):283-92.

12. Adhikari S, Zeger W, Schmier C, Crum T, Craven A, Frrokaj I, et al. Pilot study to determine the utility of point-of-care ultrasound in the assessment of difficult laryngoscopy. Acad Emerg Med. 2011;18(7):754-8.

13. Ding LW, Wang HC, Wu HD, Chang CJ, Yang PC. Laryngeal ultrasound: a useful method in predicting postextubation stridor: a pilot study. Eur Respir J. 2006;27(2):384-9.

14. Vats A, Worley GA, de Bruyn R, Porter H, Albert DM, Bailey CM. Laryngeal ultrasound to assess vocal fold paralysis in children. J Laryngol Otol. 2004;118(6):429-31.

15. Lichtenstein D, Goldstein I, Mourgeon E, Cluzel P, Grenier P, Rouby JJ. Comparative diagnostic performances of auscultation, chest radiography, and lung ultrasonography in acute respiratory distress syndrome. Anesthesiology. 2004;100(1):9-15.

16. Andersen GN, Haugen BO, Graven T, Salvesen Ø, Mjølstad OC, Dalen H. Feasibility and reliability of point-of-care pocket-sized echocardiography. Eur J Echocardiogr. 2011;12(9):665-70.

17. Lichtenstein DA, Mezière GA. Relevance of lung ultrasound in the diagnosis of acute respiratory failure. Chest. 2008;134(1):117-25.

18. Volpicelli G, Elbarbary M, Blaivas M, Lichtenstein DA, Mathis G, Kirkpatrick AW, et al. International evidence-based recommendations for point-of-care lung ultrasound. Intensive Care Med. 2012;38(4):577-91.

19. Stefanidis K, Dimopoulos S, Nanas S. Basic principles and current applications of lung ultrasonography in the intensive care unit. Respirology. 2011;16(2):249-56.

20. Lichtenstein D, Mezičre G, Biderman P, Gepner A, Barré O. The comet-tail artifact. An ultrasound sign of alveolar-interstitial syndrome. Am J Respir Crit Care Med. 1997;156(5):1640-6.

21. Lichtenstein DA, Lascols N, Prin S, Mezičre G. The "lung pulse": an early ultrasound sign of complete atelectasis. Intensive Care Med. 2003;29(12):2187-92.

22. Lichtenstein D, Mezière G, Seitz J. The dynamic air bronchogram. A lung ultrasound sign of alveolar consolidation ruling out atelectasis. Chest. 2009;135(6):1421-5.

23. Lichtenstein DA, Menu Y. A bedside ultrasound sign ruling out pneumothorax in the critically ill. Lung sliding. Chest. 1995;108(5):1345-8.

24. Soni NJ, Franco R, Velez MI, Schnobrich D, Dancel R, Restrepo MI, et al. Ultrasound in the diagnosis and management of pleural effusions. J Hosp Med. 2015;10(12):811-6.

25. Marik PE, Cavallazzi R. Does the central venous pressure predict fluid responsiveness? An updated meta-analysis and a plea for some common sense. Crit Care Med. 2013;41(7):1774-81.

26. Lamia B, Ochagavia A, Monnet X, Chemla D, Richard C, Teboul JL. Echocardiographic prediction of volume responsiveness in critically ill patients with spontaneously breathing activity. Intensive Care Med. 2007;33(7):1125-32.

27. Cowie BS. Focused transthoracic echocardiography in the perioperative period. Anaesth Intensive Care. 2010;38(5):823-36.

28. Neskovic AN, Hagendorff A, Lancellotti P, Guarracino F, Varga A, Cosyns B, et al. Emergency echocardiography: the European Association of Cardiovascular Imaging recommendations. Eur Heart J Cardiovasc Imaging. 2013;14(1):1-11.

29. Van de Putte P, Perlas A. Ultrasound assessment of gastric content and volume. Br J Anaesth. 2014;113(1):12-22.

30. Vigneau C, Baudel JL, Guidet B, Offenstadt G, Maury E. Sonography as an alternative to radiography for nasogastric feeding tube location. Intensive Care Med. 2005;31(11):1570-2.

31. Liu D, Li Z, Zhang X, Zhao L, Jia J, Sun F, et al. Assessment of intracranial pressure with ultrasonographic retrobulbar optic nerve sheath diameter measurement. BMC Neurol. 2017; 17(1):188.

32. Mahmood F, Matyal R, Skubas N, Montealegre-Gallegos M, Swaminathan M, Denault A, et al. Perioperative ultrasound training in anesthesiology: a call to action. Anesth Analg. 2016;122(6):1794-804.

33. Lalu MM, Fayad A, Ahmed O, Bryson GL, Fergusson DA, Barron CC, et al. Ultrasound-guided subclavian vein catheterization: a systematic review and meta-analysis. Crit Care Med. 2015;43(7):1498-507.

34. NICE Guidelines. Guidance on the use of ultrasound locating devices for placing central venous catheters. ASA Task Force on Central Venous Access. Practice guidelines for central venous access. A report by the American Society of Anesthesiologists Task Force on Central Venous Access. Anesthesiology. 2012;116:539-73.

35. Blaivas M, Brannam L, Fernandez E. Short-axis versus long-axis approaches for teaching ultrasound-guided vascular access on a new inanimate model. Acad Emerg Med. 2003;10(12):1307-11.

36. Gualtieri E, Deppe SA, Sipperly ME, Thompson DR. Subclavian venous catheterization: greater success for less experienced operators using ultrasound guidance. Crit Care Med 1995;23(4):692-7.

37. Troianos CA, Hartman GS, Glas KE, Skubas NJ, Eberhardt RT, Walker JD, et al. Guidelines for Performing Ultrasound Guided Vascular Cannulation: Recommendations of the American Society of Echocardiography and the Society of Cardiovascular Anesthesiologists. J Am Soc Echocardiogr. 2011;24(12): 1291-318.

38. Seto AH, Abu-Fadel MS, Sparling JM, Zacharias SJ, Daly TS, Harrison AT, et al. Real-time ultrasound guidance facilitates femoral arterial access and reduces vascular complications: FAUST (Femoral Arterial Access with Ultrasound Trial). JACC Cardiovasc Interv. 2010;3(7):751-8.

39. Sandhu NS, Patel B. Use of ultrasonography as a rescue technique for failed radial artery cannulation. J Clin Anesth 2006;18(2):138-41.

40. Shiver S, Blaivas M, Lyon M. A prospective comparison of ultrasound-guided and blindly placed radial arterial catheters. Acad Emerg Med. 2006;13(12):1257-79.

Perioperative Management of Hypertension

Vijay Chakkaravarthy KR, Nagarajan Ramakrishnan

INTRODUCTION

The overall prevalence of hypertension is 25.3% in India, with greater prevalence in men (27.4%) than women (20.0%). This translates to 207 million persons with hypertension.[1] Hypertension was also found to be the second most common risk factor for surgical morbidity.[2]

High blood pressure (BP) can be associated with life-threatening complications such as ischemic heart disease, heart failure, renal impairment, and cerebrovascular accidents. While these complications can be reduced by effective BP management, setting a target for systolic and diastolic BP or mean arterial pressure and achieving it still remains a challenge.

Perioperative hypertension management includes effective control during the preoperative, intraoperative, and postoperative periods.

PREOPERATIVE HYPERTENSION

Preoperative evaluation involves:
- Blood pressure control
- Review of antihypertensive drugs patient is receiving
- Continuation of certain antihypertensive drugs till surgery
- Evaluating for evidence of end-organ damage.

There is no sufficient recommendations for systolic BP above which the therapy should be initiated,[3] but any hypertension in which the systolic BP is ≥180 mm Hg or diastolic BP ≥110 mm Hg, constitutes a risk factor for perioperative ischemic events.[4,5] Although BP is regularly monitored in preoperative care, it is difficult to assign a specific BP target for all patients as studies have defined goals based on patient population and type of surgery.

We quote here the Perioperative Quality Initiative consensus statement on preoperative BP management:
- Whenever available, ambulatory (as opposed to single office or clinic reading) arterial pressure should be used to establish the relevant preoperative arterial pressure to avoid white coat hypertension and inaccurate readings.[6]
- Elevated diastolic, but not systolic, pressure is noted to be associated with increased postoperative mortality with the association beginning at diastolic BPs of >90 mm Hg.[7]

While treating the BP in surgical patients, the threshold for initiation of antihypertensive therapy depends on the patient's preoperative BP. For any increase in systolic or diastolic hypertension 20% increase over the baseline often defines a treatment threshold. Chronic hypertensive patients are generally able to tolerate a higher BP level but they do not tolerate hypotension compared with normotensive individuals.[8] Generally, a systolic cutoff of 180 mm Hg and/or a diastolic pressure is used to take decision on canceling or postponing a surgery.[9]

Deferring Elective Surgeries

Any patient with a stage 3 hypertension, surgery should be deferred especially if it is associated with any other cardiovascular risk factors or end-organ damage, which further increases the perioperative risk. For any patient with stage 4 hypertension, it is recommended to defer anesthesia and surgery whenever possible and the BP should be treated.[10] There is little evidence regarding lowering the BP in preoperative period for reducing the perioperative risk. Perioperative use of extended-release metoprolol may reduce the risk of myocardial infarction, new clinically significant atrial fibrillation (AF) but significantly increased risk of death, stroke and clinically significant bradycardia and hypotension.[11] So, routine initiation of β-blocker perioperatively should be avoided.

There are various classes of antihypertensives available to control the BP before surgery. Most common groups include angiotensin-converting enzyme inhibitor/angiotensin receptor blocker (ACE inhibitor/ARB), β-blocker, calcium channel blockers and diuretics. The Perioperative Quality Initiative consensus statement on use of these medications is summarized here[12]:

- Withhold ACE inhibitors/ARB 24 hours before surgery as it may reduce the risk of mortality, stroke, and myocardial injury by avoiding intraoperative hemodynamic instability.
- Restart ACE inhibitors/ARBs as soon as possible within 48 hours in the immediate postoperative period.
- Do not initiate β-blockers in the immediate perioperative period which have been associated with higher risk of stroke.
- For patients already on chronic β-blocker therapy (such as congestive heart failure or acute coronary syndrome within the past 2 years, β-blockers should be continued.
- Initiation or withholding of loop diuretics should be considered on an individualized basis. Since it may be associated with volume depletion and electrolyte imbalance, it is ideal to hold these medications on the morning of surgery in most cases.
- Discontinuation of α-2 agonists before surgery has the risk of clonidine withdrawal syndrome. So, it is suggested to continue clonidine (patch if available) in those patients who have been on clonidine already.

INTRAOPERATIVE HYPERTENSION

Increased sympathetic activity is the main reason for intraoperative hypertension, which may be associated with arrhythmias. Inadequate analgesia or anesthesia, surgical stimulation, or airway handling during laryngoscopy causes intraoperative hypertension. Other causes include hypoxemia, hypercapnia, or increased use of vasopressors and inotropes for any reason. However, any unexpected intraoperative hypertension must prompt exclusion of malignant hyperthermia as its cause.[13]

The response to sympathetic activation during anesthesia can be exaggerated in patients with uncontrolled hypertension, as the systolic BP can increase by up to 90 mm Hg and the heart rate by up to 40 bpm in contrast to the response in normotensive individuals where the BP generally increases by 20–30 mm Hg and the heart rate to increase by 15–20 bpm.[14] Any patient with renal or cerebrovascular complication of hypertension has higher intraoperative systolic pressure. Common causes of intraoperative hypertension are outlined in **Box 1**.

Intraoperative Management[15]

- Limit duration of direct laryngoscopy
- Balanced anesthesia to blunt hypertensive responses
- Invasive hemodynamic monitoring
  - Recheck and rule out technical errors before treating

Box 1: List of causes of intraoperative hypertension.[15,16]

- *Measurement errors*
  - Calibration drift of invasive device
  - Sphygmomanometer cuff herniation
  - Calibration error of noninvasive device
- *Ventilation/equipment errors*
  - Stuck valve
  - Hypoventilation
  - Soda lime exhaustion
  - Endobronchial intubation
  - Failure to deliver volatile agents/nitrous oxide
- *Patient related factors*
  - Undiagnosed or poorly controlled HTN
  - Pregnancy-induced hypertension
  - Withdrawal of antihypertensive treatment
  - Anxiety or pain
- *Increased sympathetic tone*
  - Sympathetic tone leading to vasoconstriction
  - Inadequate analgesia
  - Inadequate anesthesia
  - Hypoxemia
  - Hypercapnia
  - Hypothermia
  - Airway manipulation
  - Surgical stimulation
- *Vasoconstrictor use (intentional or unintentional)*
  - Vasopressors
  - Adrenaline with local anesthetic
- *Other causes*
  - Aortic cross-clamping
  - Raised intracranial pressure
  - Pheochromocytoma
  - Malignant hyperthermia
  - Thyroid storm
  - Fluid overload

(HTN: hypertension)

- Monitor intraoperative awareness (bispectral index) and deepen anesthesia, if inadequate
- Titrate down or stop the vasopressors if on flow
- Airway manipulation to be done only under deep anesthesia
- Interrogate with the surgeon and cease the stimulation, if possible
- Review drugs and the delivery of anesthesia
- End tidal CO_2 and SpO_2 monitoring and maintain adequate ventilation.

POSTOPERATIVE HYPERTENSION

Acute postoperative hypertension (APH) is one of the most common complications after surgery. Any extremes of BP warrant intervention because postoperative hypertension may predispose to bleeding, while hypotension may compromise organ perfusion and carry a risk of stroke.[17] It is defined by values of systolic hypertension >190 mm Hg with or without a diastolic BP ≥100 mm Hg in, at least, two consecutive measurements during the postoperative

Box 2: Causes of postoperative hypertension.

- *Patient related factors*
  - Withdrawal of antihypertensive medications
  - Anxiety
  - White coat syndrome
- *Increased sympathetic tone*
  - Pain
  - Inadequate analgesia
  - Inadequate anesthesia
  - Hypoxemia
  - Hypercapnia
  - Hypothermia
  - Airway manipulation
  - Surgical stimulation
- *Overuse of drugs*
  - Vasoconstrictors
  - Inotropes
  - Intravenous fluids

period. The APH that occurs is manifested in the first 20 minutes after surgery and lasts approximately 3 hours[18,19] (**Box 2**).

PATHOPHYSIOLOGY

- *Neuroendocrine response:* The stress response to surgery results in significantly upregulated neuroendocrine activity including the sympathetic nervous system.[20] The hypovolemia caused by cytokine mediated capillary fluid sequestration leads to salt and water retention to maintain circulating volume and cardiovascular homeostasis.
- *Sympathetic response:* The plasma catecholamine levels increase immediately after injury and peak between 24 and 48 hours due to stimulation of autonomic receptors. Arginine vasopressin secreted from the posterior pituitary gland promotes water retention and the production of concentrated urine by direct action on the kidney. The release of vasopressin may continue up to 5 days also. As a result of sympathetic efferent stimulation, renin is released from the juxtaglomerular cells which in turn result in the production of angiotensin II. This, in addition to adrenocorticotropic hormone (ACTH), leads to sodium and water reabsorption from the distal tubules of the kidney.

Complications of Untreated Hypertension

Untreated postoperative hypertension may lead to decreased left ventricular ejection fraction, increased myocardial oxygen demand thereby precipitating ischemia, cerebrovascular accidents, arrhythmias, and bleeding.

MANAGEMENT

The patient should first be assessed for other treatable causes of hypertension such as pain and anxiety, as well as ensuring

that the urinary catheter is appropriately positioned and draining urine. The patient's current medications should also be reviewed to ensure that the patient is not having an adverse reaction to a medication that has been acutely stopped such as β-blockers. The perioperative strategy suggested is targeting a BP within 20% of preoperative values to prevent end-organ hypoperfusion.[21] Hypertension should be individualized and defined by the patient's preoperative BP. A 20% increase over the baseline BP, either systolic or diastolic BP should be the treatment threshold. Compared with a normotensive individual, a chronic hypertensive patient often tolerates higher BP than a significant drop in BP due to shift in autoregulatory system.[8]

Pharmacotherapy in Perioperative Hypertensive Emergencies

In general, the BP target should be based on the patient's preoperative BP. Conservatively targeting a BP of around 10% above that baseline would be appropriate but a more aggressive approach to lower BP may be targeted for patients who have bleeding risk or patients with risk of heart failure. Major concern should be about balancing the risks associated with hypertension versus the risk of end-organ hypoperfusion with the earlier described drugs. Choice of agent should be individualized depending on the clinical situation, patient's characteristics, the hospital settings, and the experience of individual (**Table 1**).

Apart from individualizing the BP, the perfusion pressure should be targeted during perioperative period and not the mean arterial pressure alone. A generalized mean arterial pressure target cannot be set for everyone because the perfusion pressure for an organ is the difference between "inflow pressure" and "outflow pressure". Mean arterial BP should be individualized for every patient and adjusted according to the individual patient's outflow pressures such as central venous pressure, intrathoracic pressure, intra-abdominal pressure.

- For example, in case of reduced abdominal perfusion pressure (APP) in patients with abdominal compartment syndrome, the target mean arterial pressure should be kept above 65 mm Hg after measuring the intra-abdominal pressure. APP = Mean arterial pressure – Intra-abdominal pressure.

CONCLUSION

Hypertension is prevalent and needs to be appropriately managed preoperatively, intraoperatively, and postoperatively to avoid complications. Understanding the pathophysiology, setting appropriate goals and responding appropriately with clinical changes that could reduce the sympathetic response or using titratable medications is the key to successful management.

Table 1: Pharmacotherapy in perioperative hypertensive emergencies.[22,23]

Drug	Class	Dose	Onset, duration of action and side effects
Clevidipine	It is a dihydropyridine 3rd generation calcium channel blocker (CCB)	Infusion to be started at 0.4 µg/kg/min, titrated by doubling increments every 90 seconds up to 3.2 µg/kg/min (maximum of 2.5 g/kg/24 hours)	• Half-life of 1-minute, duration of action 5–15 minutes • Infusion set up should be changed every 4 hours • Avoid in patients with egg or soy allergy
Nicardipine	It is a second generation dihydropyridine CCB	Infusion to be started at 5 mg/h, titrated by 2.5 mg/h every 5 minutes up to a maximum of 15 mg/h	• Onset of action is 5–15 minutes, duration of action is 4–6 hours • Increased half-life may result in prolonged action within 24 hours of use
Nitroglycerin	It is a direct arterial and venous dilator	• Starting dose is 5 µg/kg/min, to be titrated at 5 µg/kg/min every 3–5 minutes • Once dose exceeds 20 µg/kg/min, further titrations may be at 20 µg/kg/min	• Onset of action is 2–5 minutes, duration of action is 3–5 minutes • Hypotension and reflex tachycardia may occur. Tachyphylaxis may occur within 4 hours • Methemoglobinemia may occur with prolonged infusion
Nitroprusside	It is a direct arterial and venous dilator with rapid action	0.25–0.5 mg/kg/min titrated every 1–2 minutes	• Onset of action in seconds, the duration of action is 1–2 minutes, and plasma half-life is 3–4 minutes • Decreases renal blood flow and function and may also cause coronary steal phenomenon. Decreases cerebral blood flow but increases intracranial pressure • Coronary steal • Prolonged infusion may result in cyanide toxicity
Hydralazine	It is a directly acting arteriolar dilator	IV bolus of 10–20 mg may be given and repeated every 1–4 hours as needed. IV, if infusion required suggested loading dose is 0.1 mg/kg, followed by a continuous infusion of 1.5–5 µg/kg/min	• Onset of action is 5–25 minutes, drop in BP can last up to 12 hours. Circulating half-life is 3 hours • Reflex tachycardia in ischemic heart disease may result in iatrogenic acute coronary syndrome • Avoid in patients with dissecting aneurysms • It may increase intracranial pressure
Labetalol	Combined alpha- and beta-blocker	Suggested loading dose is 20 mg followed by 20–80 mg every 10 minutes. After initial dose, a 1–2 mg/min infusion titrated until desired effect has been achieved	• Onset of action is 2–5 minutes, it reaches a peak at 5–15 minutes and lasts up to 4 hours, its elimination half-life is 5.5 hours • Should not be used in patients with acute heart failure, bradycardia, second- or third-degree heart block, bronchospasm
Esmolol	It is a beta-blocker	500–1,000 µg/kg loading dose in 1 minute, followed by infusion starting at 50 µg/kg/min and may be titrated up to 300 µg/kg/min	• Onset of action in 60 seconds and a short duration of action of 10–20 minutes • Anemia can prolong its half-life. Avoid use in patients with acute heart failure, bradycardia, second- or third-degree heart block, bronchospasm
Enalaprilat	It is an ACE inhibitor	Recommended dose is 1.25 mg (over 5 minutes) every 6 hours titrated by increments of 1.25 mg at 12–24 hours to a maximum of 5 mg every 6 hours	• Onset of action is 15 minutes with peak effect in an hour. Duration of action is 6 hours • Limitations include variable response, slow onset of action, difficult to titrate to effect

(ACE: angiotensin-converting enzyme)

REFERENCES

1. Gupta R, Gaur K, S Ram CV. Emerging trends in hypertension epidemiology in India. J Hum Hypertens. 2019;33(8):575-87.
2. Howell SJ, Sear JW, Foëx P. Hypertension, hypertensive heart disease and perioperative cardiac risk. Br J Anaesth. 2004;92(4):570-83.
3. Sessler DI, Bloomstone JA, Aronson S, Berry C, Gan TJ, Kellum JA, et al. Perioperative quality initiative consensus statement on intraoperative blood pressure, risk and outcomes for elective surgery. Br J Anaesth. 2019;122(5):563-74.
4. Chobanian AV, Bakris GL, Black HR, Cushman WC, Green LA, Izzo JL Jr, et al. The seventh report of the Joint National Committee on prevention, detection, evaluation, and treatment of high blood pressure: The JNC 7 report. JAMA. 2003;289(19):2560-72.
5. Eagle KA, Berger PB, Calkins H, Chaitman BR, Ewy GA, Fleischmann KE, et al. ACC/AHA guideline update for perioperative cardiovascular evaluation for noncardiac surgery—executive summary a report of the American College of Cardiology/American Heart Association Task Force on Practice Guidelines (Committee to Update the 1996 Guidelines

on Perioperative Cardiovascular Evaluation for Noncardiac Surgery). Circulation. 2002;105(10):1257-67.

6. Ackland GL, Brudney CS, Cecconi M, Ince C, Irwin MG, Lacey J, et al. Perioperative quality initiative consensus statement on the physiology of arterial blood pressure control in perioperative medicine. Br J Anaesth. 2019;122(5):542-51.

7. Venkatesan S, Myles PR, Manning HJ, Mozid AM, Andersson C, Jørgensen ME, et al. Cohort study of preoperative blood pressure and risk of 30-day mortality after elective non-cardiac surgery. Br J Anaesth. 2017;119(1):65-77.

8. Goldberg ME, Larijani GE, Pharm D. Perioperative hypertension. Semin Anesth. 1998;17(2):87-92.

9. Prys-Roberts C, Meloche R, Foëx P. Studies of anaesthesia in relation to hypertension. I. Cardiovascular responses of treated and untreated patients. Br J Anaesth. 1971;43(2):122-37.

10. Dix P, Howell S. Survey of cancellation rate of hypertensive patients undergoing anaesthesia and elective surgery. Br J Anaesth. 2001;86(6):789-93.

11. Devereaux PJ, Yang H, Yusuf S, Guyatt G, Leslie K, Villar JC, et al. Effects of extended-release metoprolol succinate in patients undergoing non-cardiac surgery (POISE trial): a randomised controlled trial. Lancet. 2008;371(9627):1839-47.

12. Sanders RD, Hughes F, Shaw A, Thompson A, Bader A, Hoeft A, et al. Perioperative quality initiative consensus statement on preoperative blood pressure, risk and outcomes for elective surgery. Br J Anaesth. 2019;122(5):552-62.

13. Graham SG, Aitkenhead AR, Alan R. Complications during anaesthesia. In: Smith G, Aitkenhead AR, Moppett IK, Thompson JP (Eds). Smith and Aitkenhead's Textbook of Anaesthesia. New York: Churchill Livingstone/Elsevier; 2013. pp. 853-86.

14. Wolfsthal SD. Is blood pressure control necessary before surgery? Med Clin North Am. 1993;77(2):349-63.

15. Paix AD, Runciman WB, Horan BF, Chapman MJ, Currie M. Crisis management during anaesthesia: hypertension. Qual Saf Health Care. 2005;14(3):e12.

16. Hazzi R, Mayock R. Perioperative management of hypertension. J Xiangya Med. 2018;3(6):25.

17. Erstad BL, Barletta JF. Treatment of hypertension in the perioperative patient. Ann Pharmacother. 2000;34(1):66-79.

18. Halpern NA, Goldberg M, Neely C, Sladen RN, Goldberg JS, Floyd J, et al. Postoperative hypertension: a multicenter, prospective, randomized comparison between intravenous nicardipine and sodium nitroprusside. Crit Care Med. 1992;20(12):1637-43.

19. Gal TJ, Cooperman LH. Hypertension in the immediate postoperative period. Br J Anaesth. 1975;47(1):70-4.

20. Desborough JP, Hall GM. Endocrine response to surgery. In: Kaufman L (Ed). Anesthesia Review, Vol 10. Edinburgh: Churchill Livingstone; 1993. pp. 131-48.

21. Dodson GM, Bentley WE 4th, Awad A, Muntazar M, Goldberg ME. Isolated perioperative hypertension: clinical implications & contemporary treatment strategies. Curr Hypertens Rev. 2014;10(1):31-6.

22. Marik PE, Varon J. Perioperative hypertension: a review of current and emerging therapeutic agents. J Clin Anesth. 2009;21(3):220-9.

23. Gerber JG, Nies AS. Antihypertensive agents and the drug therapy of hypertension. In: Goodman-Gilman A, Rall TW, Nies AS, Taylor P (Eds). Goodman and Gilman's the Pharmacological Basis of Therapeutics, 8th edition. New York: Pergamon Press; 1990. pp. 784-813.

Antibiotic Strategies in Postoperative Period

Ashit Hegde

INTRODUCTION

Antibiotics may be considered in the postoperative period in three situations.
1. As prophylaxis
2. For treatment of an infection as an adjuvant to surgical source control
3. For the treatment of a nosocomial infection acquired after surgery.

ANTIBIOTICS AS PROPHYLAXIS

Most guidelines including the ones issued by the Indian Council of Medical Research (ICMR) recommend against continuing prophylactic antibiotics postoperative. Some guidelines recommend a maximum duration of 24 hours of antibiotic prophylaxis.

The only exception to this recommendation is cardiac surgery, where 48 hours of antibiotics as prophylaxis are allowed.

ANTIBIOTIC PROPHYLAXIS GUIDELINES ISSUED BY ICMR[1]

The antibiotic prophylaxis guidelines issued by ICMR is given in **Box 1**.

ANTIBIOTICS AS AN ADJUNCT TO SURGICAL SOURCE CONTROL

Complicated intra-abdominal infections, complicated urinary tract infections (UTIs), and severe skin and soft tissue infections (SSTI) are situations where urgent surgery is often needed for source control. Antibiotics are complementary to surgery.

Antibiotic Strategies for Complicated Intra-abdominal Infections[2]

The choice of empirical antibiotics for complicated intra-abdominal infection (IAI) should be based on local epidemiology, severity of infection, the source of infection, and the patient's risk factors for resistant pathogens.[3]

In India, gut carriage of extended spectrum beta-lactamase (ESBL)-producing organisms is quite high even in otherwise healthy patients who have not had recent exposure to antibiotics.[4]

Drugs effective against ESBL are therefore recommended in the empiric treatment of patients with complicated IAI. Carbapenems are usually recommended for such patients who are sick enough to be in the intensive care unit (ICU).

Beta-lactam/beta-lactamase inhibitor (BL/BLI) combinations might be an alternative in patients who are not very sick, who have not been exposed to antibiotics recently and have undergone early source control.

Tigecycline is an option for patients who have an allergy to the beta-lactam antibiotics.

Additional cover for anaerobes is needed if the source of the infection is the distal gastrointestinal (GI) tract and if the patient is not receiving a carbapenem or piperacillin/tazobactam. Metronidazole is preferred over clindamycin in this situation.

If the source of infection is the proximal GI tract and if source control is performed early and if the patient is stable, ceftriaxone alone is a reasonable option.

Antibiotics for Emphysematous Pyelonephritis[5]

Emphysematous pyelonephritis (EP) is a severe form of renal parenchymal infection associated with collection of gas in the renal tissues. Diabetes is the most important risk factor for the development of EP. A nephrectomy (partial or complete) might be necessary for the treatment of severe EP. *Escherichia coli* and *Klebsiella* are implicated in the majority of cases of EP. Carbapenems are therefore the antibiotics of choice for the empiric treatment of severe EP.

Box 1: Antibiotic prophylaxis guidelines issued by ICMR

R. Surgical Antimicrobial Prophylaxis

- To be administered within 1 hour before the surgical incision
- Single dose is recommended. Consider for second intraoperative dose in prolong surgery based on the choice of antibiotic used for prophylaxis
- Prophylaxis should not be given beyond surgery duration (except for cardiothoracic surgery, up to 48 hours permissible)
- Choice of the prophylaxis should be based on the local antibiogram

Surgery	Medication
Breast	Inj. cefazolin 2 g or inj. cefuroxime 1.5 g IV stat
Gastroduodenal and biliary	Inj. cefoperazone—sulbactam 2 g IV stat and BD for 24 h (maximum)
ERCP	Inj. piperacillin-tazobactum 4.5 g or Inj. cefoperazone—sulbactam 2 g
Cardiothoracic	Inj. cefuroxime 1.5 g IV stat and BD for 48 h
Colonic surgery	Inj. cefoperazone—sulbactam 2 g IV stat and BD for 24 h (maximum)
Abdominal surgery (hernia)	Inj. cefazolin 2 g or Inj. cefuroxime 1.5 g IV stat
Head and neck/ENT	Inj. cefazolin 2 g IV stat
Neurosurgery	Inj. cefazolin 2 g or Inj. cefuroxime 1.5 g IV stat
Obstetrics and gynecology	Inj. cefuroxime 1.5 g IV stat
Orthopedic	Inj. cefuroxime 1.5 g and BD for 24 h (maximum) or Inj. cefazolin 2 g IV stat Open reduction of closed fracture with internal fixation—Inj. cefuroxime 1.5 g IV stat and q 12 h or Inj. cefazolin 2 g IV stat and q 12 h (for 24 hrs)
Trauma	Inj. cfuroxime 1.5 g IV stat and q 12 h (for 24 hrs) or Inj. ceftriaxone 2 g IV OD
Urologic procedures	Antibiotics only to patients with documented bacteriuria
Transrectal prostatic surgery	Inj. cefoperazone—sulbactam 2 g IV stat

Antibiotics for Severe Skin and Soft Tissue Infections[6]

Along with complete surgical debridement, appropriate antibiotics are an important component in the management of severe SSTI.

Severe SSTIs involving the extremities are usually caused by gram-positive organisms (*Staphylococcus* or *Streptococcus*). Ceftriaxone or cefazolin are the recommended antibiotics in this situation. A protein synthesis inhibitor such as clindamycin is usually combined with the beta lactam in order to suppress toxin production by the bugs. Linezolid may be an alternative to clindamycin especially if the patient has risk factors for CA-MRSA (community-acquired methicillin-resistant *Staphylococcus aureus*).

For severe SSTIs closer to the perineum, additional cover for gram-negative bacteria is necessary. A carbapenem is the recommended additional antibiotic for the severely ill patients. Tigecycline is an alternative in carbapenem allergic patients.

ANTIBIOTICS FOR THE MANAGEMENT OF POSTOPERATIVE NOSOCOMIAL INFECTIONS

Nosocomial Intra-abdominal Infections[2,7]

The choice of empiric antibiotics for severe nosocomial IAI depends upon the local epidemiology and upon the antibiotic that the patient has already received.

Carbapenems are a reasonable option in patients who have not been exposed to carbapenems or BL/BLIs recently. Fluconazole as prophylaxis may be prescribed for patients who i) have an anastamotic leak ii) have undergone repeat surgery.

Patients who have already received carbapenems or BL/BLIs are at risk of developing infections caused by a host of resistant organisms—CRO (carbapenem-resistant organisms), enterococci, MRSA, *Candida*.

Empiric treatment for nosocomial IAIs in such patients will have to include a polymyxin along with either tigecycline or fosfomycin. Both these drugs might have some action against CREs and also cover MRSA and enterococci. Empiric antifungal therapy might also need to be administered to patients with risk factors [proximal GI or pancreato-biliary surgery, candida colonization, receipt of broad-spectrum antibiotics, anastomotic leak, multiple instrumentation, and total parenteral nutrition (TPN)] for invasive candidiasis.[8]

Tertiary peritonitis:[9] It is defined as IAI that persists or recur ≥48 hours following successful and adequate surgical source control. In this condition also the microbiology shifts toward the more resistant gram-negative bugs (CRO), MRSA, enterococci, and *Candida*. Antibiotics to cover these organisms will need to be administered.

Other Nosocomial Infections Acquired by the Postsurgical Patient

Hospital-acquired pneumonia (HAP):[10,11] Patients may be transferred back to the ICU postoperatively if they have developed an HAP. In patients who were not being mechanically ventilated before development of a pneumonia, the most likely causative organisms are gram-negative organisms. Carbapenems are the drugs of choice for patients admitted/transferred to the ICU with a severe postoperative HAP. The incidence of HAP caused by *S. aureus* is very low in our country, empiric cover for *Staphylococcus* may be safely omitted if a Gram stain of the sputum does not reveal any gram-positive organisms. If, however, the Gram stain does reveal gram-positive organisms either linezolid or a glycopeptide (in adequate doses) must be added pending cultures.

Postoperative Ventilator-associated Pneumonia

Some patients might need prolonged mechanical ventilation post major surgery and might go on to develop a ventilator-associated pneumonia (VAP). The empiric treatment of the VAP depends on (1) the antibiotics that the patient has been exposed to and (2) (*probably more important*) the epidemiology of the ICU. In India CROs— *Klebsiella, Acinetobacter*, and *Pseudomonas* seem to be the bugs predominantly responsible for VAP. A polymyxin in combination with another drug (which is also sensitive or the least resistant) will be the treatment of choice for severely ill patients. In ICUs where the predominant bugs responsible for VAP are not CROs, patients can be treated with a carbapenem. Also patients who are not seriously ill and who have not been exposed to carbapenems or BL/BLIs may be treated with a carbapenem to begin with.

Catheter-associated Urinary Tract Infections[12]

Catheter-associated urinary tract infection (CAUTI) is probably overdiagnosed. Pyuria and bacteriuria are almost inevitable after Foley's catheterization. Most patients have catheter-associated bacteriuria (CAB) which does not require antibiotic treatment.

Catheter-associated urinary tract infection should be diagnosed only if the patient has fever, dysuria and no other focus of infection or if he develops fever after a urologic procedure.

Quite often patients develop a significant postvoid residue after removal of the Foley's catheter and this may be a cause of UTI. Postvoid residue should therefore be routinely checked in immobile or elderly patients after removal of the Foley's catheter.

Carbapenems are again the drugs of first choice for empiric treatment of CAUTI because ESBL-producing organisms are usually the offending bacteria. If the patient has had previous episode of UTI or has received broad-spectrum antibiotics in the recent past and is severely ill empiric cover for CROs will have to be considered. Of the polymyxins, only colistin should be prescribed for the treatment of UTI because polymyxin B does not achieve adequate levels in urine.

Central Line-associated Bloodstream Infections

As in the case of VAP, empiric antibiotic choices for central line-associated bloodstream infection (CLABSI) depend on the epidemiology of the ICU and on the previous antibiotic exposure of the patients. A carbapenem with a glycopeptide may be a reasonable option in patients who have not had prior exposure to broad-spectrum antibiotics.

Patients who have been previously exposed to broad-spectrum agents will merit treatment with a polymyxin and another companion drug (fosfomycin, tigecycline, high dose carbapenem) depending on the local epidemiology. Cover for MRSA might also be necessary especially if there is evidence of exit site inflammation. Empiric antifungal therapy might be added for severely ill patients with risk factors for invasive candidiasis (upper abdominal surgery, TPN, steroid therapy, fungal colonization, etc.).[13]

GENERAL PRINCIPLES OF GOOD ANTIBIOTIC PRESCRIBING PRACTICE[14-16]

In critically ill patients, the antibiotics should be administered as soon as possible.

Appropriate cultures (*only from suspected foci*) should be sent before antibiotics are administered.

Drain cultures are notoriously unreliable and prescribing antibiotics on the basis of drain cultures should be avoided.

The antibiotics should be adequately and appropriately dosed, keeping pharmacokinetic-pharmacodynamic (pK/pD) principles in mind.

A loading dose of the antibiotic should be administered to all seriously ill patients irrespective of their renal or hepatic function. Subsequent doses may be modified depending on the clearance of the drug and organ dysfunction. For time-dependent antibiotics the antibiotic should be administered as a prolonged infusion. If the patient has renal dysfunction, the dose may be decreased but the duration of dosing should remain unchanged. For concentration-dependent antibiotics the antibiotic should preferably be administered as a single high dose. If there is renal dysfunction, the dosing intervals should be increased but the administered dose should remain unchanged.

Antibiotics should be de-escalated if possible once the results of culture are available.

In most situations antibiotics can be safely stopped once the patient is afebrile and well.[17] This would usually mean that approximately 5–7 days of antibiotics is sufficient for most patients and probably even fewer for CAUTI. The exceptions to this rule are *S. aureus* bacteremia and candidemia. Measuring procalcitonin (PCT) levels may give the clinician the confidence to discontinue antibiotics in certain situations (*infections caused by nonlactose fermenters, CRO*).

If a patient remains unwell in spite of 5 days of appropriate antibiotics, merely prolonging the antibiotic will not be of much use. The clinician needs to analyze the probable reasons for the nonresponse and quite often this is because of inadequate source control.

SUMMARY

Antibiotics are not needed in most postoperative patients even if they have undergone major surgery and are in the ICU. In the few situations when antibiotics are indicated, principles of antimicrobial stewardship should be adhered to, viz., "the right antibiotic only for the right patient at the right time at the right dose causing the least harm to the patient and future patients."

REFERENCES

1. Ministry of Health and Family Welfare. National Treatment Guidelines for Antimicrobial Use in Infectious Diseases: Version 1.0 (2016) NATIONAL CENTRE FOR DISEASE CONTROL Directorate General of Health Services. New Delhi: Ministry of Health and Family Welfare, Government of India; 2016.
2. Sartelli M. A focus on intra-abdominal infections. World J Emerg Surg. 2010;5:9.
3. Kurup A, Liau KH, Ren J, Lu MC, Navarro NS, Farooka MW, et al. Antibiotic management of complicated intra-abdominal infections in adults: the Asian perspective. Ann Med Surg (Lond). 2014;3:85-91
4. Antony S, Ravichandran K, Kanungo R. Multidrug-resistant *Enterobacteriaceae* colonising the gut of adult rural population in South India. 2018;36:488-93.
5. Eswarappa M, Suryadevara S, John MM, Kumar M, Reddy SB, Suhail M. Emphysematous pyelonephritis case series from south India. Kidney Int Rep. 2018;3:950-55.
6. Laxminarayan R, Chaudhury RR. Antibiotic resistance in India: drivers and opportunities for action. PLoS Med. 2016;13:e1001974.
7. Augustin P, Kermarrec N, Muller-Serieys C, Lasocki S, Chosidow D, Marmuse JP, et al. Risk factors for multidrug resistant bacteria and optimization of empirical antibiotic therapy in postoperative peritonitis. Crit Care. 2010;14:R20.
8. Dupont H, Paugam-Burtz C, Muller-Serieys C, Fierobe L, Chosidow D, Marmuse JP, et al. Predictive factors of mortality due to polymicrobial peritonitis with Candida isolation in peritoneal fluid in critically ill patients. Arch Surg. 2002;137:1341-6; discussion 1347.
9. Mishra SP, Tiwary SK, Mishra M, Gupta SK. An introduction of tertiary peritonitis. J Emerg Trauma Shock. 2014;7:121-3.
10. Kalil AC, Metersky ML, Klompas M, Muscedere J, Sweeney DA, Palmer LB, et al. Management of adults with hospital-acquired and ventilator-associated pneumonia: 2016 Clinical Practice Guidelines by the Infectious Diseases Society of America and the American Thoracic Society. Clin Infect Dis. 2016;63:e61-e111.
11. Khilnani GC, Zirpe K, Hadda V, Mehta Y, Madan K, Kulkarni A, et al. Guidelines for antibiotic prescription in intensive care unit. Indian J Crit Care Med. 2019;23:S1-S63.
12. Sangamithra V, Sneka, Praveen S, Manonmoney. Incidence of catheter associated urinary tract infection in medical ICU in a tertiary care hospital. Int J Curr Microbiol App Sci. 2017;6:662-9.
13. Pappas PG, Kauffman CA, Andes DR, Clancy CJ, Marr KA, Ostrosky-Zeichner L, et al. Clinical practice guideline for the management of candidiasis: 2016 update by the Infectious Diseases Society of America. Clin Infect Dis. 2016;62:e1-e50.
14. Shani V, Muchtar E, Kariv G, Robenshtok E, Leibovici L. Systematic review and meta-analysis of the efficacy of appropriate empiric antibiotic therapy for sepsis. Antimicrob Agents Chemother. 2010;54:4851-63.
15. Pea F, Viale P. Bench-to-bedside review: appropriate antibiotic therapy in severe sepsis and septic shock—does the dose matter? Crit Care. 2009;13:214.
16. Johnson I, Banks V, Antibiotic stewardship in critical care. BJA Education. 2017;17(4):111-6.
17. Sartelli M, Catena F, Ansaloni L, Coccolini F, Di Saverio S, Griffiths EA. Duration of antimicrobial therapy in treating complicated intra-abdominal infections: a comprehensive review. Surg Infect (Larchmt). 2016;17:9-12.

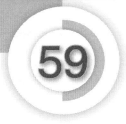

Transthoracic Echocardiography

Amol Kothekar, Anuja Bidkar

INTRODUCTION

Echocardiography (ECHO) is routinely used in the perioperative period for various indications. This chapter covers intraoperative and postoperative transthoracic echocardiography (TTE) by point-of-care ultrasound (POCUS) which is done by the perioperative physician (anesthesiologists and intensivists). Detailed preoperative ECHO for risk assessment for an elective procedure is beyond the scope of this chapter.

Transthoracic echocardiography POCUS provides information about the cardiorespiratory status of the patient and also provides assessment of hemodynamic parameters critical for patient management.[1] The "point-of-care echocardiography" done by the trained critical care or emergency physician provides rapid assessment of the cardiorespiratory status in the setting of resuscitation and helps in planning further management.

Comprehensive POCUS assessment of the cardiorespiratory status requires integration of cardiac assessment by TTE, lung ultrasound, deep vein thrombosis (DVT), and focused assessment with sonography in trauma (FAST). Rapid Ultrasound in SHock (RUSH) is one of the protocols which integrates ultrasound information from heart, chest, abdomen, and major arteries and veins to assess "the pump, the tank, and the pipes".[2] This chapter deals with the indications, techniques, and interpretation of TTE with respect to emergent clinical scenarios commonly seen in the emergency department, critical care units, and intraoperative scenario. Other components of ultrasound (DVT, FAST, and lung) assessment are discussed elsewhere in the textbook.

INDICATIONS

Common indications of TTE-POCUS during the perioperative period are as follows:[3]

- Shock or hemodynamic instability*: To differentiate etiology of shock, namely, hypovolemic, cardiogenic, or obstructive
- Assessment of volume status
- Identification of patients who are likely to be fluid responsive
- New-onset chest pain or ECG changes suggestive of coronary artery disease. TTE provides quick assessment of regional wall motion abnormality (RWMA)
- Hypoxia (desaturation), decreased lung compliance (tight bag or increased airway pressure), respiratory distress (in awake patients)
- Identification of weaning failure of cardiac origin
- For perioperative cardiac arrest for differentiating pulseless electrical activity (PEA) arrest from pseudo-PEA and also for identification of cause of arrest. [Good-quality *cardiopulmonary resuscitation (*CPR) is the primary treatment of cardiac arrest and TTE-POCUS should not interfere with chest compressions.]

PHYSICS AND TECHNICAL ASPECTS OF ECHOCARDIOGRAPHY

Basics of physics of ultrasound is discussed elsewhere in the textbook. In this chapter, we will discuss physics specific to ECHO. In conventional two-dimensional (2D) ECHO, brightness at a given pixel is determined by the amplitude of the returned echo signal at that particular depth. Hence, it is known as B (brightness) mode. ECHO also uses M or

---

*For shock or hemodynamic instability in postcardiac surgery settings, POCUS should also include transesophageal echocardiography (TEE) along with TTE as these patients can have small loculated collections compressing left atrium (LA) or ventricle in absence of abnormalities of the right heart.[4]

motion mode for measurement of fast-moving structures such as ventricular walls valve leaflets and Doppler mode for measurement of blood flow velocities. M-mode and Doppler are discussed later in the chapter.

Acoustic Windows

The heart is covered by a bony rib cage and aerated lungs; both are considered the biggest enemies of the echocardiographer due to poor ultrasound penetration. Imaging of the heart is possible through the small areas devoid of air and bone known as acoustic window. Acoustic windows relevant to TTE are shown in **Figure 1**. The image acquisition of TTE is considered to be one of the most difficult skills to acquire for the sonographer.

Patient Positioning

Majority of postoperative TTE-POCUS are done in supine position. If the patient's condition allows, left lateral decubitus position (LDP) with the left arm extended behind the head can be used as it offers a better acoustic window for TTE.[5] The position of intraoperative TTE is dictated by the position for surgery unless the patient is made supine for the crisis situation. If the patient is already in left LDP, TTE can be done in the same position as it may provide better ECHO. If the patient is in right LDP for surgery and TTE window is poor, the patient can be turned supine if possible, provided it is critical to do TTE as this will halt the surgery. We did not come across any TTE in prone position but an apical four-chamber (A4C) view may be tried in prone position if the need arises.

Probe and Scanner Settings

The cardiac phased array probe is commonly used for TTE. The probe is made of many small transducers, which emit ultrasound waves at different times independent of each other (in a pulsed manner). The data obtained from the multiple transducers are combined together to get the complete picture. A phased array transducer probe typically has frequency of 2–5 MHz which allows deeper penetration (**Fig. 2**). Pediatric echo probe has higher frequency and lesser depth. The probe has the following features, which help in better visualization of cardiac structures during TTE:

- It has a triangular beam originating from a small footprint (**Fig. 2**) allowing visualization of cardiac structures through the small acoustic windows.
- It offers a higher frame rate (images/second) which helps in imaging of fast-moving structures (cardiac tissues and valves).
- It has a capacity of continuous transmission and reception of ultrasound waves which is used in continuous-wave Doppler for accurate measurement of higher velocities typically seen in regurgitations.

Alternative Probe

A curvilinear probe has frequency similar to a phased array probe and can be used as an alternative if the latter is not available. However, there are few limitations:

- It has bigger footprint and it is difficult to obtain a complete cardiac image through the ribs.
- It has a lower frame rate and is not designed to image fast-moving structures; hence, the quality of images will be inferior.
- Cardiac calculations, e.g., ejection fraction (EF) and velocity time integral (VTI), are not possible.
- Continuous-wave Doppler is not available.
- The sonographer may find it difficult to keep steady probe position with fine manipulations due to a larger size of the probe.

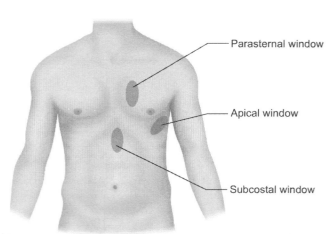

Fig. 1: Acoustic windows of transthoracic echocardiography.

Parasternal window

Apical window

Subcostal window

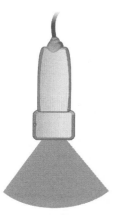

Fig. 2: Schematic image of a cardiac phased array probe with a triangular beam originating from a small footprint with an indicator (red dot) on one side.

Holding the Probe

Holding the probe close to the patient helps the echo cardiographer to obtain a steady image and allows the probe manipulation if necessary. Resting fingers or palmer surface on the patient provides stability. Holding the probe at the cable or away from the patient should be discouraged as it is difficult to obtain a steady image with this grip.

Probe Manipulation

Manipulation of the transducer is essential for optimum visualization of the organ of interest (heart for TTE) and can be split into five basic movements known as sweeping and sliding, rocking, tilting/fan, rotating, and compression. A fine blend of these movements allows optimum anatomy visualization.

Sweep and Slide

The transducer is moved over the patient's chest in the direction of ultrasound plane (slide) or perpendicular to it (sweep) to find the best window (**Figs. 3A and B**).

Rocking

Rocking is also known as in-plane motion as the transducer is moved in the visualized plane either toward or away from

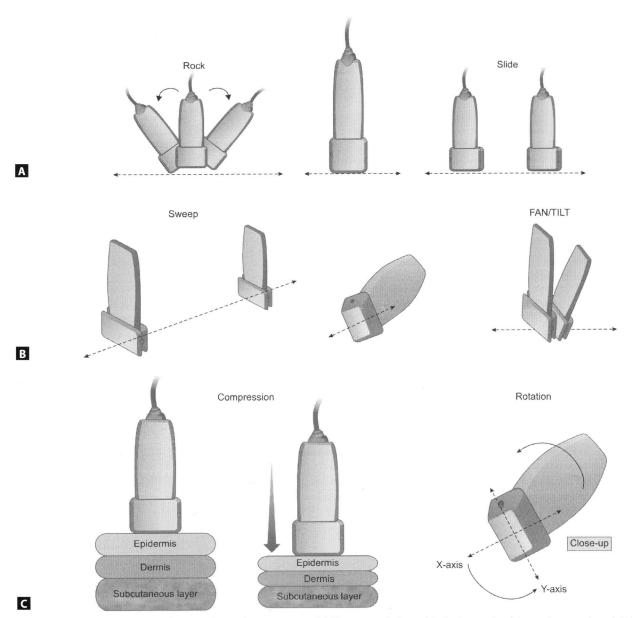

Figs. 3A to C: Schematic image showing the probe maneuvers. (A) Maneuvers in line with the long axis of the probe—rock and slide; (B) Probe maneuvers along an axis that is perpendicular to the long axis—sweep and tilt/fan; (C) Probe maneuvers—compression and rotation.

the indicator and the image plane is moved parallel to the visualized plane. This allows extension of the field of view in one or another direction allowing focusing to the area of interest (**Fig. 3A**).

Tilting/Fan

This is known as cross-plane motion as the image plane is moved perpendicular to the visualized plane. Tilting allows visualization of other planes in the same axis without sliding the transducer around the body. For example, in a parasternal short-axis (PSAX) view, tilting the probe allows complete visualization of the heart from the base to the apex (**Fig. 3B**).

Rotating

Rotation of the transducer allows scanning in the same window in different planes. For example, in the apical window, a four-chamber view allows visualization of septal and lateral walls of the left ventricle (LV). Rotating the probe 60° in a counterclockwise direction gives a two-chamber view in which the anterior and inferior walls of LV are seen (**Fig. 3C**).

Compression

Transducer compression is mainly used for compression ultrasound for detection of deep venous thrombosis. In a subcostal view, transducer compression may help in pushing the bowel gas out of the field of view. The compression should be kept gentle and minimal as higher degrees of compression can be uncomfortable to the patient (**Fig. 3C**).

Concept of Long and Short Axes

Ultrasound is a 2D modality. Based on the orientation of ultrasound beam, the heart can be scanned in either short-axis plane or two long-axis planes perpendicular to each other (**Figs. 4A to C**). It is impossible to scan all

parts of the heart in a single image, and multiple views are recommended for interpretation.

Common Transthoracic Echocardiography Windows and Views

Commonly used windows and views for emergency TTE are mentioned below.

Parasternal Window

Parasternal window is an acoustic window seen at intercostal spaces that directly overlies the long axis of the heart. It is usually identified as an area next to the left sternal border in the 3rd, 4th, and 5th intercostal space.

Parasternal long-axis (PLAX) view: This view can be obtained in supine position. If the patient's condition allows, a better view can be obtained in left LDP. The method of obtaining this view is described in **Table 1**. In an ideal PLAX view, the cardiac axis [interventricular septum (IVS)] is horizontal and LV apex is not seen. PLAX view allows visualization of LV inflow and outflow tracts, IVS, right ventricle (RV), and descending thoracic aorta (**Figs. 5A to D**). Descending thoracic aorta can help differentiating pericardial effusion from pleural as the former is above the descending thoracic aorta.

Troubleshooting: If poor or no acoustic window is observed, move the probe as medially as possible. Once view is achieved, note the position of IVS. If IVS is not horizontal, try to get the view at higher intercostal space with tilting if necessary. Avoid interpretation and measurements in suboptimal view, which can be inaccurate and nonreproducible. Adjust depth to see all structures including descending aorta. Use maneuvers such as rock, tilt, fan, sweep, or slide to get a view with an ideal image. If image quality is still poor, change the patient's position to left LDP if feasible.

Table 1: Views in the parasternal window with appropriate probe placement and maneuvers.

View	Probe position	Marker	Tilt	Direction of probe (ultrasound beam)
Long-axis view	3rd, 4th, or 5th intercostal space just left to sternum	Right shoulder	Fine-tune to see aortic valve opening and closing	Vertically down
Short-axis view		Left shoulder	Tilt from cranial to caudal to get view at various levels • Aortic valve and right ventricle inflow and outflow tract • Mitral valve • Chordae • Papillary muscle • Apex	Vertically down

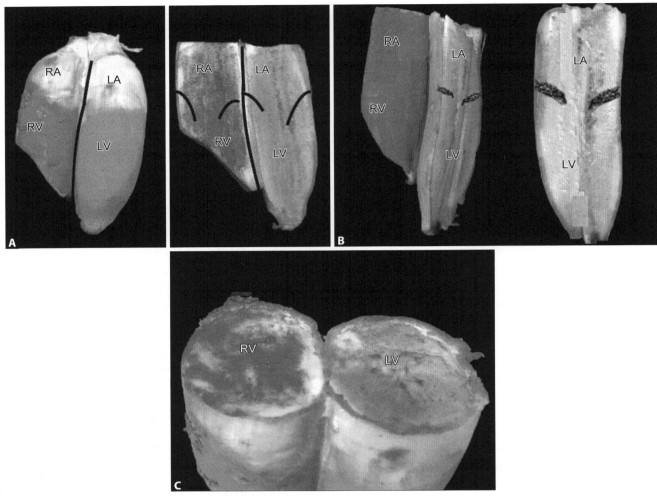

Figs. 4A to C: Schematic image showing the planes. (A) Depicting the long axis or coronal plane; (B) Depicting the long axis in the sagittal plane; (C) Depicting the short axis or transverse plane. (*Courtesy:* Dr Amol Kothekar.)

(LA: left atrium; LV: left ventricle; RA: right atrium; RV: right ventricle)

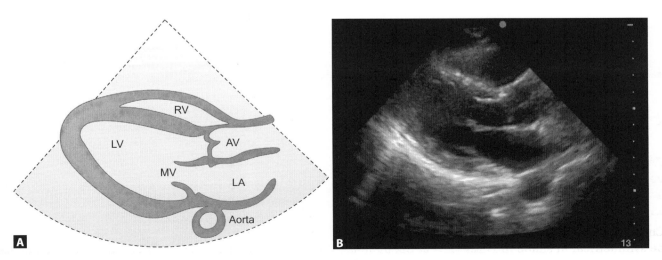

Figs. 5A and B

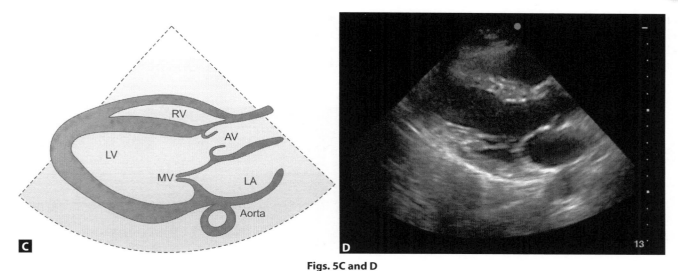

Figs. 5C and D

Figs. 5A to D: Parasternal long-axis view. (A) Schematic image and (B) echo image in ventricular diastole with open mitral valve and closed aortic valve; (C) Schematic image and (D) echo image in ventricular systole with closed mitral valve and open aortic valve. Also, note the papillary muscles attached to mitral valve.

(AV: aortic valve; MV: mitral valve; LA: left atrium; LV: left ventricle; RV: right ventricle)

Principal applications:
- Visual assessment of LV systolic function
- Diameter of left ventricular outflow tract (LVOT) for calculation of stroke volume (SV)
- Differentiating pericardial effusion from pleural effusion
- Calculation of EF using M-mode
- RWMA of the anterior and inferior walls of LV.

Parasternal short-axis view: Once an optimum PLAX view is obtained as described previously, the probe is rotated 60–90° clockwise to obtain PSAX view. Similar to PLAX view, this view can be obtained both in supine and in left lateral positions using methods described in **Table 1**.

The structures seen in PSAX view depend on the level of section as described below:
- At the level of aortic valve—RV inflow and outflow tract views (**Figs. 6A and B**)
- At the level of mitral valve (MV)—for RV, IVS, anterior and posterior mitral leaflets, LV (**Figs. 6C and D**)
- Papillary muscles—visualize RV, IVS, posteromedial and anterolateral papillary muscles, LV. Both papillary muscles should be symmetrical in shape (**Figs. 6E and F**).
- Left ventricular apex – to visualize LV apex (**Figs. 6G and H**)

Troubleshooting: Adjust depth of assessment (10–16 cm); use maneuvers such as rock, tilt, fan, sweep, or slide to get a view with an ideal image. Changing patient position to left LDP may help.

Characteristics of ideal view: Both papillary muscles should be symmetrical in shape in PSAX view at the papillary muscles.

Principal applications:
- Visual assessment of LV systolic function
- RWMA of all walls of LV
- RV pressure overload based on the shape of LV.

Apical Window

Apical window is the acoustic window seen at intercostal space that directly overlies the apex of the heart. Usually identified as the point of maximal impulse (PMI), it is typically found at the 5th or 6th intercostal space in the mid-clavicular line or nipple line. Similar to PLAX view, views in this window can be obtained both in supine and in left lateral positions using methods described in **Table 2**.

Apical four-chamber view

Structures seen: The right and left atria and the RV and LV, the IVS, interatrial septum (IAS), and the atrioventricular valves (**Figs. 7A to D**).

Characteristics of ideal view: The following structures should be demonstrable for optimal examination—LA, MV, LV, IAS, right atrium (RA), tricuspid valve (TV), RV, and IVS. The septum should be vertical. Both the MV and TV opening and closing should be seen in the single view.

Foreshortening: Ultrasound beam should obtain an image of the heart through the true apex. True apex can be identified by bullet shape and pinching during each contraction. In case of foreshortening, the ultrasound beam should obtain an image of the heart through the LV wall rather than true apex. This can be identified by more rounded "apex" which moves with the contraction rather than pinching. A foreshortened image may cause inaccurate interpretation as the image is off-axis causing shortened left ventricular long axis.

Principal applications:
- Visual assessment of LV systolic function
- To assess left ventricular ejection fraction (LVEF) using Simpson's method
- RV dilatation, tricuspid regurgitation (TR), McConnell's sign in pulmonary embolism (PE)
- Tricuspid annular plane systolic excursion (TAPSE)
- Mitral regurgitation

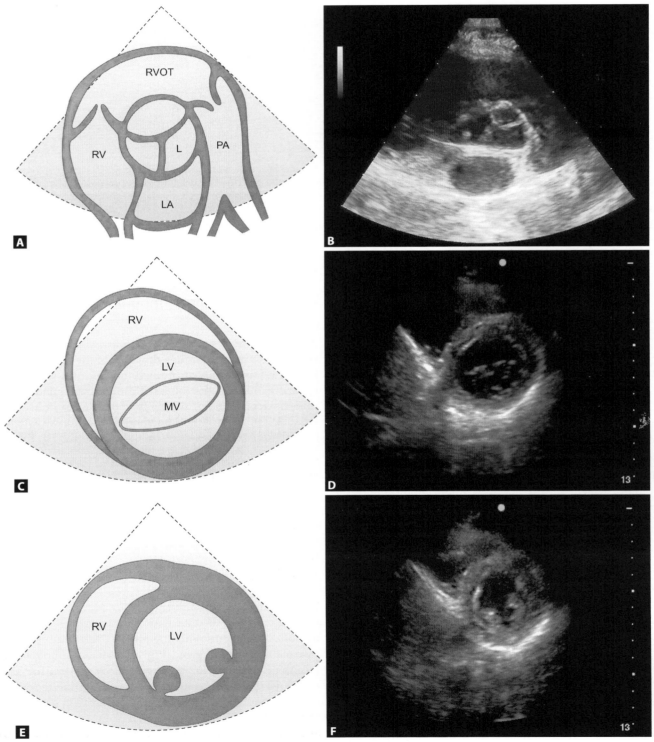

Figs. 6A to F

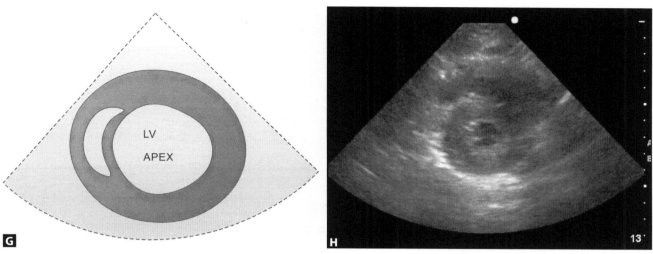

Figs. 6G and H

Figs. 6A to H: Parasternal short-axis view. (A) Schematic image and (B) echo image at the level of aortic root with right ventricular inflow and outflow tract; (C) Schematic image and (D) echo image in ventricular diastole with open anterior and posterior mitral valve leaflets; (E) Schematic image and (F) echo image at the level of posteromedial and anterolateral papillary muscles; (G) Schematic image and (H) echo image of the left ventricular apex.

(L: left coronary cusp; LA: left atrium; LV: left ventricle; MV: mitral valve; N: noncoronary cusp; PA: pulmonary artery; R: right coronary cusp; RV: right ventricle)

Table 2: Views in apical window with appropriate probe placement and maneuvers.

View	Probe position	Marker	Tilt	Direction of probe (ultrasound beam)
Four-chamber	Point of maximal impulse (PMI) typically at 5th or 6th intercostal space in midclavicular line or nipple line	Left side below the shoulder	Fine-tune to see opening and closing of both mitral and tricuspid valves	Pointing toward right shoulder
Five-chamber			Tilt ventrally	
Two-chamber		60° in counterclockwise rotation. Between suprasternal notch and right shoulder	Fine-tune to keep LV and LA in the center of the screen	
Three-chamber, also known as long-axis view	Rotating the transducer even further in counterclockwise direction from the two-chamber view (approximately a further 60°)	Further 60° in counterclockwise Close to right shoulder		

(LA: left atrium; LV: left ventricle)

- Diastolic dysfunction
- RWMA of septum or lateral wall.

Apical five-chamber (A5C) view: Start with a four-chamber view and tilt the probe.

Principal applications: To assess LVOT and aortic valve pathology.

Troubleshooting: Use maneuvers such as rock, tilt, fan, sweep, or slide to get a view with an ideal image. Change patient position to left semilateral decubitus.

Probe manipulation gives A2C (LA and LV), A3C (LA, LV, LVOT, and aortic valve), and A5C (LA, LV, RA, RV + RVOT, and aortic valve) views as well.

Apical two-chamber (A2C) view: Obtain by rotating the transducer approximately 60° in a counterclockwise direction from A4C view. The IVS should not be seen.

Principal applications: To assess LV global function and regional wall motion abnormalities.

Apical three-chamber (A3C) view or apical long-axis view: Ideal view to study LVOT flow, e.g., aortic regurgitation due to angle of insonation.

Subcostal Window

Subcostal window is the acoustic window seen just below the xiphisternum. It is an especially useful window where

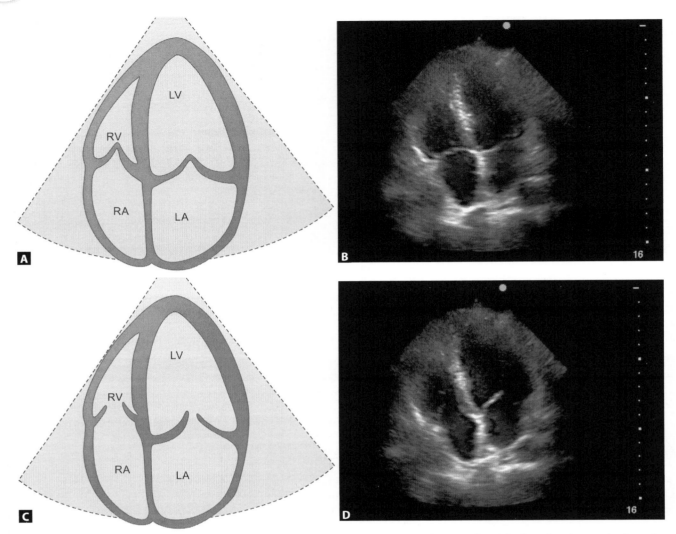

Figs. 7A to D: Apical view. (A) Schematic image and (B) echo image in ventricular systole with closed atrioventricular valves; (C) Schematic image and (D) echo image in ventricular diastole with open atrioventricular valves.

(LA: left atrium; LV: left ventricle; RA: right atrium; RV: right ventricle)

the liver provides a good medium for transmission of ultrasound. The subcostal window takes the advantage of liver window avoiding bone or lung tissue, thereby allowing imaging patients in supine position. Turning the patient to left lateral position may not help to improve image. The methods for obtaining various views are described in **Table 3**.

Subcostal four-chamber view

Structures seen in subcostal view:
- *Subcostal four-chamber view:* RV, RA, LV, LA (**Figs. 8A and B**).
- *Subcostal short-axis view:* Short-axis views can be obtained at different levels by moving the transducer more to the left to view the ventricular segments and to

the right to view the basal segments. It is useful to assess pericardial effusion.
- *Subcostal caval view to visualize inferior vena cava (IVC):* To obtain this view, start with a four-chamber view with RA in the center of the image, then rotate the transducer counterclockwise, and direct it to the right. The IVC will be visualized in the long axis. In an ideal view, the IVC is seen as it enters the RA, along with the hepatic veins, which drain into the IVC below the diaphragm (**Figs. 8C and D**). The hepatic veins are important to help differentiate the IVC from the abdominal aorta (**Figs. 8E and F**).

Troubleshooting: Adjust depth of assessment (15–20 cm); use maneuvers such as rock, tilt, fan, sweep, or slide to

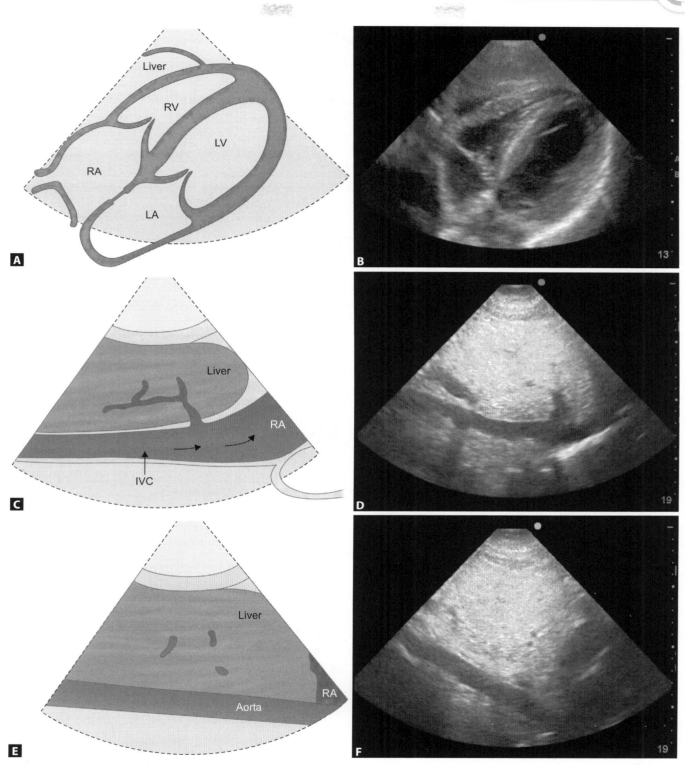

Figs. 8A to F: Subcostal view. (A) Schematic image and (B) echo image of all four chambers of heart; (C) Schematic image and (D) echo image of the inferior vena cava at the cavoatrial junction; (E) Schematic image and (F) echo image of the abdominal aorta which is pulsatile and has no branches. Note the liver provides good acoustic window.

(L: left coronary cusp; LA: left atrium; LV: left ventricle; MV: mitral valve; N: noncoronary cusp; PA: pulmonary artery; R: right coronary cusp; RV: right ventricle)

Table 3: Views in the subcostal/subxiphoid window with appropriate probe placement and maneuvers.

View	Probe position	Marker	Tilt	Direction of probe (ultrasound beam)
Four-chamber view	Subcostal or subxiphoid space	Left shoulder		Toward left shoulder
Two-chamber short-axis view		Suprasternal notch counterclockwise rotation from four-chamber view	Tilt from cranial to caudal to get view at various levels: Aortic valve and RV inflow and outflow tracts Mitral valve Chordae Papillary muscle Apex	
IVC long-axis view		Pointing toward suprasternal notch		Vertically down, slight cranial angulation and very little angulation toward right side

(IVC: inferior vena cava; RV: right ventricle)

get a view with an ideal image. Ask the patient to relax the abdomen by flexing knees.

Principal applications:
- Frequently, it is the only view available in patients on ventilator, especially in chronic obstructive pulmonary disease (COPD) patients
- Pericardial effusion (most dependent part of pericardium)
- To assess LV contractility by eyeballing
- RV strain/dilatation TR
- RWMA of septum or lateral wall
- Volume status with IVC view
- RWMA of any wall with short-axis view.

Right lateral transhepatic caval view: In patients with no access to the subcostal window due to surgical incision or due to bowel gas, the right lateral transabdominal coronal long axis (also known as rescue view or transhepatic view) may be helpful.

Principal applications: To assess IVC dimensions and variability with respiration.

Key points for optimum image acquisition and interpretation:
- Adjust the depth to optimum, aiming for maximum screen utilization so that all relevant structures are seen.
- Adjust the gain to optimum so that the endocardial border is seen. This is particularly important for eyeballing of contractility.
- For 2D or B-mode, ultrasound beam should be perpendicular to the surface of the structure of interest.
- For Doppler, ultrasound beam should be parallel to the flow.
- Know your ultrasound machine; many modern machines are equipped with the enhancement software such as

tissue harmonic imaging (THI) which helps in better image quality.
- Integrate images from different views. Integrate ECHO findings with ultrasound of lung, DVT, etc.

APPLICATIONS OF TRANSTHORACIC ECHOCARDIOGRAPHY

Transthoracic echocardiography can be used for assessment of preload and contractility and can also be used for diagnosis of etiology of shock.

Specific Diagnostic Targets of Transthoracic Echocardiography Point-of-care Ultrasound[1]

- Presence of pericardial effusion and evidence of cardiac tamponade
- Right ventricular enlargement or dysfunction suggestive of PE
- Preload assessment by volume status and fluid responsiveness
- Left ventricular systolic dysfunction including hypokinesia or RWMA of the LV
- Left ventricular diastolic dysfunction (LVDD) (for weaning failure)
- Gross chronic heart disease
- Gross valvular disease or gross intracardiac masses.

Pericardial Effusion and Tamponade

Pericardial effusion is a pathologic accumulation of excessive fluid in the pericardial cavity (**Fig. 9**). Cardiac tamponade is a life-threatening condition caused by accumulation of fluid in the pericardial space that compresses the cardiac

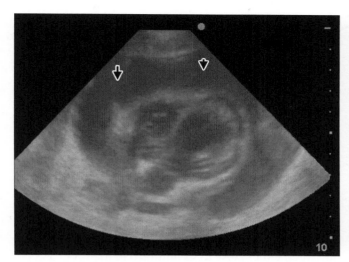

Fig. 9: An echo image in the subcostal four-chamber view showing a massive pericardial effusion (identified by the arrows).

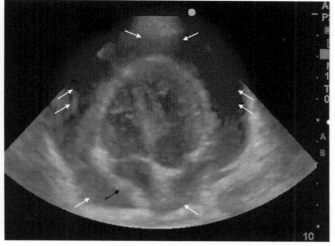

Fig. 10: An echo image in the subcostal four-chamber view showing a large amount of pericardial effusion (identified by the white arrows). Also note the right atrium collapse during ventricular systole (black arrow).

chambers and restricts them from normal filling.[6] Diastolic collapse is seen with RA (**Fig. 10**) in early cases and both RA and RV in severe cases.

Echocardiographic assessment for pericardial effusion should include:

- Identification and quantification of effusion
- Differentiation between global and localized effusion
- Ruling in or out associated tamponade

The presence of tamponade and hemodynamic instability is not dependent on the amount of fluid around the heart, but on the speed of accumulation of the pericardial fluid. Very large effusions that appear over a long period of time may permit the pericardium to stretch and accommodate that much fluid with minimal to mild hemodynamic consequences. Acute effusions may cause hemodynamic compromise despite having a lower volume of pericardial fluid.

As the pressure in the RA is the lowest during systole, the first sign will be a collapse of the RA during systole, which can be seen as an inversion of the free wall on the RA during systole.[7] The duration of atrial collapse (collapse longer than one-third of the cardiac cycle) has been described as an almost 100% sensitive and specific sign of clinical cardiac tamponade.[8]

Pulmonary Embolism

Pulmonary embolism is one of the most important differential diagnoses to be considered in a critically ill patient with unexplained hemodynamic instability or cardiac arrest. Pulmonary angiography is considered as the gold standard for diagnosis of PE; however, in an acute

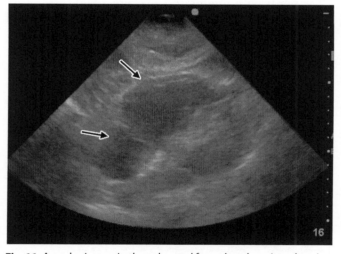

Fig. 11: An echo image in the subcostal four-chamber view showing RA and RV dilatation suggestive of pulmonary embolism (identified by the arrows).

(RA: right atrium; RV: right ventricle)

care setting, there may be practical difficulties in transport of a critically ill patient.

Acute RV dilatation (**Fig. 11**) with hemodynamic instability suggests PE. Identification of DVT in a shocked patient in an appropriate scenario is highly suggestive of PE (RUSH protocol). ECHO cannot be used for diagnosis of PE, except for the rare case of direct visualization of the thrombus in RV or pulmonary artery (PA). TTE probably is more useful in prognostication rather than diagnosis of PE. Few echocardiographic signs suggestive of PE are listed below.

Echocardiographic Signs Suggestive of Pulmonary Embolism

- Dilated RV (RV to LV ratio in A4C view > 1 or RV area equal to or more than LV area)
- D-shaped LV with displacement of septum toward LV in PSAX view at papillary muscles level
- Presence of TR
- McConnell's sign: It is the akinesia of the mid-RV free wall with relatively preserved apical contractility; it is not very sensitive (25–77%);[9] hence, the absence of McConnell's sign does not rule out a PE. However, presence of McConnell's sign in an appropriate clinical context is very specific (94–100%) for PE in the absence of other causes of RV strain.

Other Differential Diagnoses of Right Ventricle Enlargement

Patients with preexisting pulmonary hypertension or COPD can have chronic RV enlargement and hypertrophy.

Patients with moderate-to-severe acute respiratory distress syndrome (ARDS) especially on high positive end expiratory pressure (PEEP), can have acute RV dilatation.

Acute cor pulmonale can be easily diagnosed in TTE by RV dilation. A right ventricular end diastolic area (RVEDA)/ left ventricular end diastolic area (LVEDA) ratio > 0.60 in A4C view and septal dyskinesia in the short axis are considered surrogates for diagnosis of PE.[10] However, these signs are neither sensitive nor specific and does not confirm or exclude a diagnosis of PE. Other conditions causing RV dilatation and septal dyskinesia include long-standing COPD, pulmonary hypertension, and right ventricular infarction.

Preload Assessment

Preload is defined as the ventricular wall stress at the end of diastole which is determined by ventricular end-diastolic volume, wall thickness, and end-diastolic pressure. With TTE, ventricular end-diastolic pressure can be estimated by calculating and IVC diameter. LVEDA can be used as a surrogate for ventricular end-diastolic volume (LVEDV) as discussed below.

Inferior Vena Cava Size and Respiratory Variation

Inferior vena cava measures can provide quick assessment of volume status and preload. IVC is visualized in the subcostal window. Measurements are done commonly in the longitudinal or long-axis view. IVC diameter is measured either close to its entrance to the RA or 1–2 cm caudal to the hepatic vein opening. IVC diameter and its respiratory variation can be measured with either M-mode or B-mode. If M-mode is used, care should be taken to put the cursor of M-mode perpendicular to the long axis of IVC (**Figs. 12A and B**). If IVC is difficult to visualize in the subcostal window due to surgical incision or bowel gas, the right lateral transabdominal coronal long axis (transhepatic view) can be used.

During spontaneous respiration, there is collapse in IVC diameter due to negative intrathoracic pressure which can be quantified as IVC collapsibility index by the following formula:

IVC collapsibility index (IVCc) = $D_{max} - D_{min}/D_{max}$

During controlled mechanical ventilation, intrathoracic pressure causes inspiratory distension of IVC which can be measured by either IVC$_{distensibility}$ index (dIVC) or delta IVC (ΔIVC) as follows:

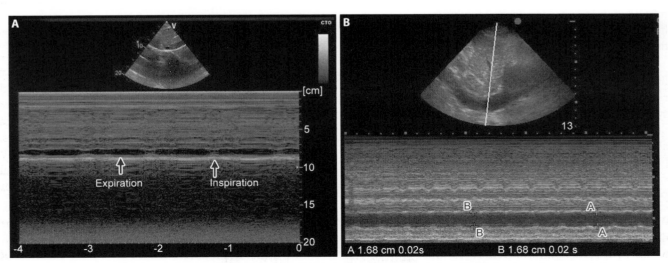

Figs. 12A and B: Subcostal view of IVC in M-mode. (A) Marked respiratory variation; (B) Minimal respiratory variation.

(IVC: inferior vena cava)

Distensibility index $(dIVC) = D_{max} - D_{min}/D_{min}$
(threshold value of 18%)

Delta IVC $(\Delta IVC) = D_{max} - D_{min}/D_{mean}$
(threshold value of 12%)

In the absence of raised intra-abdominal pressure, IVC size and its variability correlates well with central venous pressure and preload as given in **Table 4**. The dynamic indices of IVC respiratory variation are not very sensitive for prediction of fluid responsiveness. A patient can be fluid responsive even in the absence of IVC respiratory variation. The algorithm for fluid therapy in shock using IVC size and respiratory variations is described in **Table 5**.

Left Ventricular End-diastolic Area and Index

Left ventricular end-diastolic area measured at the mid-papillary level in PSAX view is used as a surrogate of LV ventricular end-diastolic volume, one of the indicators of LV preload. Reported normal range of PSAX left ventricular

end-diastolic area and index (LVEDAI) [LVEDA/body surface area (BSA)] is between 8 and 12 cm/m². In patients with gross hypovolemia, "kissing papillary muscle sign" can be observed. LVEDA of <10 cm² or LVEDA index of <5.5 cm/m² indicates significant hypovolemia. LVEDA measurement is not possible in many patients as it requires presence of good acoustic window. Presence of severe concentric left ventricular hypertrophy makes interpretation of LVEDA inaccurate, and these patients are known to have low LVEDA in the absence of hypovolemia. Barring these limitations, LVEDA is a good indicator of preload; however, it is not a reliable indicator of volume responsiveness.[13]

ASSESSMENT OF LEFT VENTRICULAR CONTRACTILITY OR SYSTOLIC FUNCTION

It can be done with either gross assessment (visual estimation or eyeballing) or measurement of EF. Eyeballing to differentiate good, moderate, or poor LV function is usually sufficient for management during resuscitation. Accurate measurement of LVEF is time-consuming and may not change patient management. For LVEF estimation, care should be taken to adjust the view and gain so that movement of endocardial border is clearly seen; thickening of the myocardium, movement of the tricuspid annulus, and change in geometry of the ventricle should be noted for visual estimation of LVEF.[14] Integration of two or more views can increase the accuracy of estimation (**Figs. 13A and B**).

The absolute value or estimation of LVEF should be interpreted in the context of LV afterload.[15]

A borderline or failing LV can have a normal value of LVEF in the presence of severe mitral regurgitation (MR) or profound vasoplegia in septic shock. Correction of vasodilation of septic shock with norepinephrine can unmask global left ventricular hypokinesia with EF of <45%.[16]

PREDICTION OF FLUID RESPONSIVENESS

As discussed previously IVC diameter, respiratory variation, or LVEDA are not accurate indicators of fluid responsiveness. *Respiratory variations of VTI or V_{max} are surrogates of SV variations.* These dynamic indices utilize heart–lung interactions for predicting fluid responsiveness. LVOT or aortic VTI or V_{max} may be used as surrogates of SV in the patients getting mechanically ventilated with tidal volumes of at least 8 mL/kg and without arrhythmias or raised abdominal pressure (**Figs. 14A and B**).[17]

Respiratory variations in VTI > 20% or peak aortic flow (V_{max}) > 12% predict fluid responsiveness.[18]

These indices can be calculated rapidly and do not require invasive line insertion or setup. Hence, they are an attractive choice for prediction of fluid responsiveness.

Table 4: Correlation of IVC diameter and respiratory variation in spontaneously breathing patients with central venous pressure.[11,12]

CVP	IVC diameter	IVC collapsibility index in spontaneously breathing patients
<10	<2 cm	≥50%
>10	≥2 cm	<50%

(CVP: central venous pressure; IVC: inferior vena cava)

Table 5: Algorithm for fluid therapy in shock using IVC size and respiratory variations.

	Small (<2 cm) or variable IVC present	Large (≥2 cm) IVC or minimal respiratory variation
Shock* present	Fluid boluses are indicated	Fluid boluses may be needed
		Dynamic indices, such as PPV, SVV, LVOT or VTI, should be used for identifying patients who would be fluid responsive
		Patients are at higher risk for developing pulmonary edema
Shock* absent	Fluid boluses are not indicated as the patient is not in shock	Fluid restriction and diuretics can be considered if weaning from ventilator is planned or the patient is at high risk of pulmonary edema

(IVC: inferior vena cava; LVOT: left ventricle outflow tract; PPV: pulse pressure variation; SVV: stroke volume variation)

*Shock is defined as base of clinical or biochemical criteria

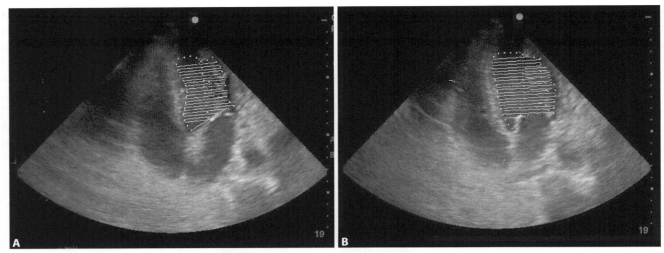

Figs. 13A and B: Measurement of left ventricular ejection fraction (LVEF) in apical four-chamber view. (A) Left ventricular area in systole; (B) Left ventricular area in diastole.

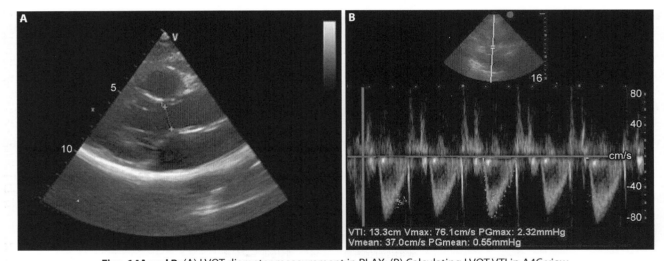

Figs. 14A and B: (A) LVOT diameter measurement in PLAX; (B) Calculating LVOT VTI in A4C view.

(A4Cs: area of left ventricle in systole in apical four-chamber view; LVOT: left ventricular outflow tract; PG_{max}: peak gradient; PLAX: parasternal long axis; VTI: velocity time integral; V_{max}: maximum velocity; V_{mean}: mean velocity); PG_{mean}: mean peak gradient

However, they require a good acoustic window and skilled hand.

ECHOCARDIOGRAPHY IN PERIOPERATIVE CARDIAC ARREST

Echocardiography can be used for identification of reversible causes of cardiac arrest such as hypovolemia, cardiac tamponade, or myocardial infarction, and PE. It can be integrated with the fast vascular and lung USG for identification of pneumothorax, DVT or hemoperitoneum or hemothorax. Care should be taken not to interfere with components of CPR, mainly chest compression.

During a resuscitation, ECHO should not interrupt chest compressions for more than 10 seconds and should be done by dedicated operator using subcostal window.

PHYSICS AND TECHNICAL ASPECTS OF M-MODE AND DOPPLER

M-Mode Ultrasound Imaging

As discussed previously, M-mode is primarily used for quantification or measurement of magnitude of movement of structures such as walls of chambers and also valve leaflets. In PLAX, M-mode can be used to measure fractional

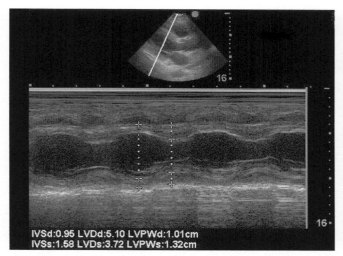

Fig. 15: Measurement of left ventricular ejection fraction in parasternal long-axis view using fractional shortening.

(IVSd: interventricular septum in diastole; IVSs: interventricular septum in systole; LVDd: left ventricular internal diameter in diastole; LVDs: left ventricular internal diameter in systole; LVPWd: left ventricular posterior wall in diastole; LVPWs: left ventricular posterior wall in systole)

shortening (FS) of LV which can be used to calculate EF (**Fig. 15**). In A4C view, TAPSE can be measured for estimation of RV function (**Figs. 16A and B**). Respiratory variation of IVC can be quantified using M-mode (*see* **Fig. 12**).

Doppler Phenomenon and its Application in Transthoracic Echocardiography

Many of us have observed that the pitch of siren of ambulance reaching us is different from the ambulance leaving. Christian Doppler, in 1842 has described the phenomenon of change in frequency of a moving sound source proportional to its speed. TTE uses this principle for calculation of blood flow velocities.

Change in frequency with Doppler is proportional to the blood flow velocity and cosine of the angle between ultrasound beam and blood flow (cos θ). The echocardiographer should align the axis of Doppler interrogation as close as possible with direction of blood flow (θ = 0–30, cos θ = 1–0.86).

The most commonly used Doppler modalities in TTE are pulsed-wave Doppler (PWD), continuous wave Doppler (CWD), and tissue Doppler imaging (TDI). Color flow Doppler (CFD) is representation of the Doppler flow superimposed on the 2D image. CFD conventionally uses blue color for flow going away from the probe and red color for the flow toward the probe [BART (blue away red toward) pneumonic].

Color flow Doppler is used for screening of flow and for identifying regurgitant flow and the area with maximal

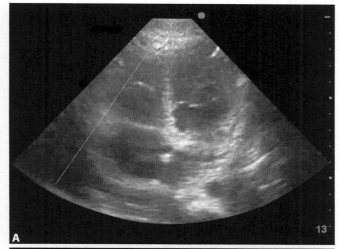

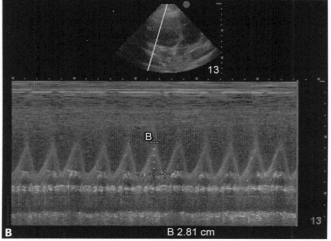

Figs. 16A and B: Tricuspid annular plane systolic excursion (TAPSE) using apical four-chamber view. (A) Location of cursor for M-mode; (B) Measurement of TAPSE with M-mode.

flow. For calculation of blood flow velocity at a particular point, PWD should be measured as it provides accurate flow measurement at a particular point (spatial resolution). PWD is used for calculation of flow across MV for diastole dysfunction, LVOT, and aortic valve for calculation of volumes.

Continuous wave Doppler can measure higher flow rates which are common in vulvar regurgitations. These higher flows are beyond the measuring capacity of PWD. CWD should not be used for measurements of other flow given above due to lack of spatial resolution. Common application of CWD is measurement of TR jet. Further, using simplified Bernoulli equation, pressure gradient across a valve can be calculated as given below:

$$\text{Pressure gradient} = 4 \times (V_{peak})^2$$

V_{peak} is maximal flow velocity.

Adding CVP to this value provides right ventricular systolic pressure (RVSP).

Measurement of Stroke Volume and Cardiac Output

Transthoracic echocardiography can be used for noninvasive measurement of SV and cardiac output.

Stroke volume can be calculated by the following formula:

$$SV = LVOT \text{ area} \times LVOT \text{ VTI}$$

where LVOT is left ventricular outflow tract and VTI is velocity time integral.

Left ventricular outflow tract diameter is measured in the PLAX view (*see* **Fig. 13A**) to calculate LVOT area by drawing a line perpendicular to the walls of the LVOT in mid-systole, with maximal separation of leaflets.

Left ventricular outflow tract VTI is calculated by placing the pulsed Doppler sample volume in the LVOT in A4C view. Care should be taken to put the sample volume exactly in LVOT and not in the aorta. Placement of sample volume in aorta will provide an inaccurately higher measurement. Second, pulse-wave Doppler should be used for measurement as CWD would be inaccurate due to the absence of spatial orientation.

As LVOT diameter remains constant in a given patient, serial measurements of LVOT VTI can be used as a surrogate of changes in cardiac output. For LVOT VTI measurement, the operator must manually trace the ejection graph (*see* **Fig. 13B**). Newer machines can automatically trace this graph eliminating human error. Peak aortic flow (V_{max}) at LVOT is easy to calculate and can be used instead of VTI for monitoring changes in cardiac output.

Normal range of LVOT VTI is between 18 and 22 cm. In RUSH protocol, interventions are targeted to maintain LVOT VTI > 18 cm. LVOT VTI in the range of 9.5 cm is seen in cardiogenic shock and higher values up to 30 cm are reported in septic shock.

Measurement of cardiac output by ECHO is not accurate compared with the gold standard (PA catheter) and errors in the calculation due to angulation between the ultrasound beam and blood flow at LVOT should be kept in mind.

Precise measurement of cardiac output using ECHO is time-consuming.

LEFT VENTRICULAR DIASTOLIC DYSFUNCTION

Left ventricular diastolic dysfunction refers to a preclinical state involving abnormalities in cardiac filling, which results from a combination of slowed LV relaxation and increased stiffness. Evidence of abnormal LV relaxation, filling, diastolic distensibility, and diastolic stiffness can be acquired noninvasively by cardiac ECHO. Mitral inflow velocities are commonly used to determine patterns of diastolic dysfunction.

Left ventricular diastolic dysfunction can be assessed using one of the two techniques:

1. Pulsed-wave Doppler (PWD) **(Figs. 17A to C)**
2. Tissue Doppler imaging (TDI) **(Fig. 17D)**

Techniques of measurement of LVDD are beyond the scope of this chapter.

INTEGRATED AND PROTOCOLIZED USE OF TRANSESOPHAGEAL ECHOCARDIOGRAPHY

As discussed previously, finding of TTE should not be used in isolation but should be used in the clinical context along with ultrasound of lungs abdomen and veins (DVT). RUSH can be used for etiological diagnosis in a patient with shock.[2] The bedside lung ultrasound in emergency (BLUE)-protocol provides bedside identification of cause of acute respiratory failure.[19] FALLS (Fluid Administration Limited by Lung Sonography) protocol, an extension of BLUE protocol, can be extremely helpful for fluid management in patients with shock.[20]

Rapid Ultrasound for Shock Protocol

Rapid Ultrasound for SHock (RUSH) is a protocol describing the use of TTE, usually performed by noncardiologists. The original RUSH ultrasound protocol was devised by Dr Weingart in 2006 and late modified by Perera et al. in 2010.[2] The scanning sequence is easy to remember with pneumonic—HI-MAP. Based on the scanning, cardiovascular system is divided into Pump Tank and Pipes.[2]

HI-MAP scanning sequence:

- **H**eart—apical four-chamber and parasternal long- and short-axis views using cardiac probe
- **I**nferior vena cava—using the same probe. Change probe to abdominal
- **M**orrison's pouch and bladder
- **A**orta and other veins at depth
- **P**leura, **P**ericardium—using same probe to look for any collection.

Pump tank and pipes:

- The pump—LV contractility, RV strain, and pericardium
- The tank—IVC, other pleural, pericardial or abdominal leaks
- The pipes—Aortic aneurysm, dissection, DVT.

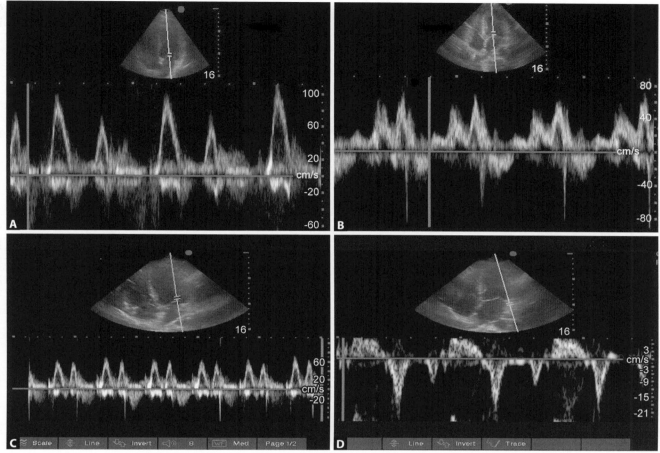

Figs. 17A to D: Echocardiographic assessment of Diastolic functions in apical four-chamber view with pulse Doppler (A, B and C) and tissue Doppler (D) imaging at the mitral annulus. (A) Normal diastolic function; (B) and (C) Diastolic dysfunction; (D) Tissue Doppler at lateral mitral annulus showing normal diastolic function.

FALLS Protocol[20]

FALLS protocol was originally described as extension of BLUE protocol of lung ultrasound.

- As soon as the heart is scanned with echo, one should look for presence of pericardial effusion with diastolic collapse of RA and RV suggestive of pericardial tamponade or right heart enlargement suggestive of PE. This examination can be combined with lung ultrasound to identify pneumothorax. Absence of pericardial tamponade, PE, and pneumothorax make the diagnosis of obstructive shock less likely.
- In the next step, contractility of LV is assessed with visual method (eyeballing). Hypocontractile LV along with B-profile in lung suggestive of pulmonary edema, indicates cardiogenic shock.
- Once both obstructive shock and left cardiogenic shock are systematically ruled out, hypovolemic or distributive shock becomes the likely diagnosis. Such patients should be treated with fluid therapy along with monitoring of lung ultrasound for B lines.

ADVANTAGES AND LIMITATIONS OF TRANSTHORACIC ECHOCARDIOGRAPHY

Advantages and limitations of echocardiographic indices are described in **Table 6**. There are no absolute contraindications of perioperative TTE. However, limitations of TTE in the following areas should be kept in mind:

- Limited access to precordium in perioperative period due to patient positioning, drapes and preparation and dressings
- Poor acoustic window due to ventilation, surgical emphysema, etc.
- Unavailability of equipment. A curvilinear ultrasound probe may be used if echo probe is not available and if echocardiographer is familiar with the probe.
- Inability to perform continuous monitoring similar to lesser invasive cardiac output monitors.
- Intraobserver and interobserver variation in measurements
- Limitations as an upstream parameter: TTE findings should be correlated with the clinical and biochemical parameters to identify shock or adequacy of perfusion.

Table 6: Advantages and limitations of echocardiographic indices.

TTE parameter	Cutoff	Advantages	Limitations
All parameters with TTE	–	Quick (except stroke volume using LVOT diameter and VTI), noninvasive, and can be repeated multiple times	Most of the TTE parameters are operator dependent and are known to have both intra- and interobserver variations. TTE parameters require good acoustic window. In ventilated patients and patients with COPD, apical and parasternal windows may be poor
IVC size and variability	Size < 2 cm respiratory variation • ≥50% in spontaneously breathing patient • Distensibility index >18% • Delta IVC (ΔIVC) = >12%	Provides estimation of CVP and volume status **(Table 4)** Serial measurement provides information about change in volume status Can be visualized in majority of ventilated and COPD patients with apical and parasternal windows	There is no agreement on the ideal method of IVC measurement with respect to the exact location of measurement and technique of measurement (M-mode vs B-mode) and scanning axis (long vs short-axis) Pseudo-variability or "pseudocollapse" may occur due to relative movement between the transducer probe and IVC due to respiratory mechanics as well as operator drift. With raised intra-abdominal pressure, IVC diameter can be falsely low even in presence of euvolemia or hypervolemia. IVC size and variability do not accurately predict fluid responsiveness
Left ventricular end-diastolic area (LVEDA)	Significant hypovolemia • Kissing papillary muscle sign (eyeballing) • LVEDA < 10 cm^2 • VEDA index < 5.5 cm/m^2	Unlike CVP and IVC, LVEDA is not influenced by intrathoracic pressure or intra-abdominal pressure	Measurement is operator dependent A good acoustic window is required for its assessment Patients with severe concentric left ventricular hypertrophy can have low LVEDA in the absence of hypovolemia
Respiratory variation of LVOT VTI/V max	VTI > 20% V_{max} >12%	Noninvasive dynamic index of fluid responsive-ness	VTI calculation can be inaccurate due angulation between the ultrasound beam and blood flow at LVOT Time-consuming Not reliable in conditions like aortic regurgitation or presence of pathologic LVOT gradient
Stroke volume using LVOT diameter and VTI		Noninvasive cardiac output measurement Serial measurements provide idea about changes in cardiac output with respect to change in patient's hemodynamic status	All limitations of LVOT VTI/ V_{max} Stroke volume calculation needs expertise and can be tedious Change in cardiac output with hemodynamic optimization may have more value than the single value of cardiac output

(COPD: chronic obstructive pulmonary disease; CVP: central venous pressure; IVC: inferior vena cava; LVEDA: left ventricular end-diastolic area; LVOT: left ventricle outflow tract; TTE: transthoracic echocardiography; V$_{max}$: maximum velocity; VTI: velocity time integral)

REFERENCES

1. Via G, Hussain A, Wells M, Reardon R, ElBarbary M, Noble VE, et al. International evidence-based recommendations for focused cardiac ultrasound. J Am Soc Echocardiogr. 2014;27(7):683. e1-683.e33.

2. Perera P, Mailhot T, Riley D, Mandavia D. The RUSH exam: Rapid Ultrasound in SHock in the evaluation of the critically ill. Emerg Med Clin North Am. 2010;28(1):29-56,vii.

3. Neskovic AN, Hagendorff A, Lancellotti P, Guarracino F, Varga A, Cosyns B, et al. Emergency echocardiography: the European Association of Cardiovascular Imaging recommendations. Eur Heart J Cardiovasc Imaging. 2013;14(1):1-11.

4. Carmona P, Mateo E, Casanovas I, Peña JJ, Llagunes J, Aguar F, et al. Management of cardiac tamponade after cardiac surgery. J Cardiothorac Vasc Anesth. 2012;26(2):302-11.

5. Jensen MB, Sloth E, Larsen KM, Schmidt MB. Transthoracic echocardiography for cardiopulmonary monitoring in intensive care. Eur J Anaesthesiol. 2004;21(9):700-7.

6. Roy CL, Minor MA, Brookhart MA, Choudhry NK. Does this patient with a pericardial effusion have cardiac tamponade? JAMA. 2007;297:1810-8.

7. Gillam LD, Guyer DE, Gibson TC, King ME, Marshall JE, Weyman AE. Hydrodynamic compression of the right atrium: a new echocardiographic sign of cardiac tamponade. Circulation. 1983;68(2):294-301.

8. Weitzman LB, Tinker WP, Kronzon I, Cohen ML, Glassman E, Spencer FC. The incidence and natural history of pericardial effusion after cardiac surgery—an echocardiographic study. Circulation. 1984;69(3):506-11.

9. McConnell MV, Solomon SD, Rayan ME, Come PC, Goldhaber SZ, Lee RT. Regional right ventricular dysfunction detected by

echocardiography in acute pulmonary embolism. Am J Cardiol. 1996;78(4):469-73.

10. Vieillard-Baron A, Page B, Augarde R, Prin S, Qanadli S, Beauchet A, et al. Acute cor pulmonale in massive pulmonary embolism: incidence, echocardiographic pattern, clinical implications and recovery rate. Intensive Care Med. 2001;27(9):1481-6.

11. Kircher BJ, Himelman RB, Schiller NB. Noninvasive estimation of right atrial pressure from the inspiratory collapse of the inferior vena cava. Am J Cardiol. 1990;66(4):493-6.

12. Prekker ME, Scott NL, Hart D, Sprenkle MD, Leatherman JW. Point-of care ultrasound to estimate central venous pressure: a comparison of three techniques. Crit Care Med. 2013;41(3): 833-41

13. Marik PE, Cavallazzi R, Vasu T, Hirani A. Dynamic changes in arterial waveform derived variables and fluid responsiveness in mechanically ventilated patients: a systematic review of the literature. Crit Care Med. 2009;37(9):2642-7.

14. 123sonography. (2019). 3.2.3 Left ventricular function. [online] Available from: https://www.123sonography.com/ebook/left-ventricular-function. [Last accessed March, 2020].

15. Vieillard-Baron A. Septic cardiomyopathy. Ann Intensive Care. 2011;1(1):6.

16. Vieillard-Baron A, Caille V, Charron C, Belliard G, Page B, Jardin F. Actual incidence of global left ventricular hypokinesia in adult septic shock. Crit Care Med. 2008;36(6):1701-6.

17. Charron C, Fessenmeyer C, Cosson C, Mazoit JX, Hebert JL, Benhamou D, et al. The influence of tidal volume on the dynamic variables of fluid responsiveness in critically ill patients. Anesth Analg. 2006;102(5):1511-7.

18. Feissel M, Michard F, Mangin I, Ruyer O, Faller JP, Teboul JL. Respiratory changes in aortic blood velocity as an indicator of fluid responsiveness in ventilated patients with septic shock. Chest. 2001;119(3):867-73.

19. Lichtenstein DA, Mezière GA. Relevance of lung ultrasound in the diagnosis of acute respiratory failure: the BLUE protocol. Chest. 2008;134(1):117-25.

20. Lichtenstein D. Fluid administration limited by lung sonography: the place of lung ultrasound in assessment of acute circulatory failure (the FALLS-protocol). Expert Rev Respir Med. 2012;6(2):155-62.

Transesophageal Echocardiography

Ajay Kumar, Poojitha Reddy Gunnam, Sohan Lal Solanki

INTRODUCTION

Readily available ultrasound and echocardiography in an intensive care unit (ICU) has positive impact on critical care practice. It provides crucial help not only in diagnosis but also in monitoring when the hemodynamic profile is changing. It has been found to have prognostic importance in patients with sepsis and septic shock. Hospitals where echocardiography was used had declining rates of hospital mortality.[1]

As we know "seeing is believing," the transthoracic echocardiography (TTE) is helpful to diagnose the cause of hemodynamic instability around 70% of the time. But when TTE is not diagnostic or images are suboptimal, transesophageal echocardiography (TEE) becomes helpful to make appropriate diagnosis and proper intervention. TEE provides unique window to heart such as posterior structures and great vessels which are not visualized with TTE. The therapeutic impact of TEE can be gauged from the fact that it was able to solve 97% (95/98) of the clinical problems in comparison to 38% (60/158) in TTE and had therapeutic impact on 36% (35/96) of the cases in comparison to 16% (20/128) in TTE.[2] Early diagnosis facilitates early intervention, reducing mortality. TEE can be used as a sole diagnostic intervention but at several times it is complementary to TTE.

PERIOPERATIVE TRANSESOPHAGEAL ECHOCARDIOGRAPHY IN NONCARDIAC SURGERY

Perioperative echocardiography is recommended in known or suspected cardiovascular pathology that might result in hemodynamic, pulmonary, and neurologic compromise. It is also recommended in persistent and unexplained hypotension and hypoxemia. It helps in strategic management triage of patients according to need and decides on use of enhanced monitoring tools.[3]

TRANSESOPHAGEAL ECHOCARDIOGRAPHY IN CARDIAC SURGICAL INTENSIVE CARE UNIT

In cardiac surgical patients, echocardiography by a cardiac anesthesiologist starts from the preoperative phase. He/she not only reconfirms the diagnostic findings but also prognosticates a patient's perioperative outcome and plans management accordingly. In critically ill cardiac patients, TEE is helpful for diagnosing infective endocarditis, presence of left atrial (LA) thrombus in patients who are candidates for balloon mitral valvotomy (BMV), to rule out LA clot during cardioversion, smoke, or thrombus in stroke patients (**Fig. 1**). During the early postoperative period, TTE imaging is difficult due to drains, collection of blood, surgical dressings, and difficulty in patient positioning for optimum image acquisition. An intensivist must rely on TEE to evaluate regional tamponade (**Figs. 2A to D**), hemodynamic

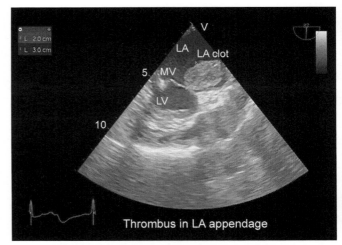

Fig. 1: Clot observed in ME left atrial appendage view in a case of mitral stenosis.

(LA: left atrial; LV: left ventricular; ME: mid-esophageal; MV: mitral valve)

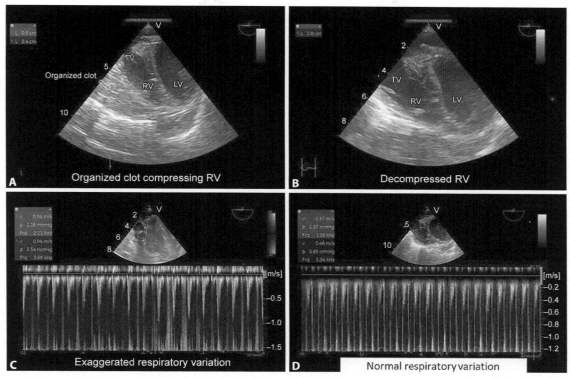

Figs. 2A to D: (A) Organized clot seen in ME four-chamber view compressing the RV (Hollow arrow) and tricuspid valve annulus (0.8 cm); (B) Respiratory variation of tricuspid inflow is >25%; (C) Tricuspid annulus 2.0 cm after removal of clot. (D) Respiratory variation of tricuspid inflow is <25%

(RV: right ventricular; ME: mid-esophageal; TV: tricuspid valve; LV: left ventricular)

instability, low cardiac output (CO) state, right ventricular (RV) dysfunction, prosthetic heart valve dysfunction, and unexplained hypoxemia. There is exaggerated respiratory variation (>25%) in RV inflow in presence of tamponade.

APPLICATIONS OF TRANSESOPHAGEAL ECHOCARDIOGRAPHY IN CRITICAL CARE

In a critical care setup, TEE is mostly used in categorization of shock, diagnosis of life-threatening disease, intermittent monitoring of hemodynamic profiles, and interventions such as extracorporeal membrane oxygenation (ECMO) and intra-aortic balloon pump (IABP). It was indicated in 45% of cases to assess hemodynamic instability, in 22% to assess infective endocarditis, in 20% due to poor TTE window, and in another 20% to ascertain the cause of cardiac arrest.[4] It impacted decision-making regarding fluid administration in 25%, change of inotropic drug in 23%, confirm/rule out diagnosis in 19%, and surgical intervention in 19%. It helped in knowing the reasons of cardiac arrest of ambiguous origin.[4] It ruled out the cardiac cause of arrest in 43% cases and ascertained etiology in 14%, left ventricular (LV) dysfunction in 8%, and shock in 5%. It helped therapeutic decision in 67% of the cases in terms of cardiopulmonary resuscitation (CPR)

management, prognostication, volume/blood transfusion, inotropes, and vasopressor infusion.[5]

Left Ventricular Structure and Function

Contractility: Though qualitative in nature, "eyeballing" the left ventricle in transgastric mid-papillary short-axis (TG SAX) view gives an overall idea of the systolic function (contractility) of myocardium. It is helpful in assessment of LV size, volume status, and regional and global function. It is widely used in "rescue" TEE for rapid assessment of myocardial function. Myocardial segments supplied by all three coronaries are assessed simultaneously in this view. Regional wall motion abnormality (RWMA) is estimated quickly in 17 segments—six at the base of heart at the mitral valve (MV) level, six at the mid-papillary level, four at the apical level, and one at the apical cap. RWMA is classified as follows:

- Normal or hyperkinetic
- Hypokinetic (reduced thickening)
- Akinetic (absent thickening)
- Dyskinetic (systolic thinning or aneurysmal changes)

Quantitative estimation of systolic function is done by Simpsons biplane method of ejection fraction which is gold standard, and by fractional area change (FAC) in TG mid-SAX view. The fractional area change is measured in the TG mid-SAX view of the LV cavity; the resultant area change depicts the systolic function.[6] Normal values are men 56–62% and women 59–65%.

$$FAC (\%) = [(LVAd - LVAs)/LVAd] \times 100$$

where LVAd is left ventricle area in diastole and LVAs is left ventricle area in systole.

Sometimes, it is difficult to get an accurate TG mid-SAX view, perpendicular to the long axis due to the prolate ellipse shape of the left ventricle. TG LV two-chamber view which lies orthogonal to TG mid-SAX view (**Fig. 3**)[7] can be used with diameter measurements perpendicular to TG LV two-chamber view to obtain ventricular volume using linear measurements with M mode or calliper.[7] Measurements are obtained 1 cm distal to MV leaflets. Reference ranges for LV internal diastolic diameter (LVIDd) are from 3.9 to 5.2 cm for women and 4.2 to 5.9 cm for men.[8] These measurements are used to measure EF and differentiate etiology of hypotension during hemodynamic assessment (**Table 1**).[9]

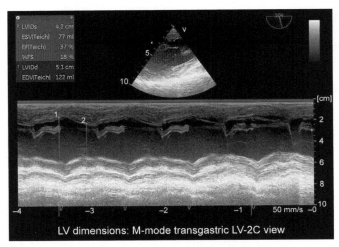

LV dimensions: M-mode transgastric LV-2C view

Fig. 3: Application of M-mode echocardiography or calliper orthogonal to transgastric two-chamber view helps in calculation of ventricular dimensions and ejection fraction.
(EDV: end-diastolic volume; EF: ejection fraction; ESV: end-systolic volume; LV: left ventricular; LVIDd: left ventricular internal diastolic diameter; LVIDs: left ventricular internal systolic diameter)

There are various causes of LV hypokinesia in perioperative and critically ill patients such as myocardial ischemia or infarction, sepsis, and inflammation, or it may be stress induced. These causes must be differentiated, as acute myocardial infarction (MI) has to be managed with immediate revascularization whereas other causes are transient and can be managed with supportive treatment.

Diastolic Function

Diastole is no longer considered a simple passive phase of ventricular filling; rather it is a complex interaction between ventricular relaxation, compliance, systolic function, and atrial contraction in late diastole. Filling pressures measurement in the left side of cardiac chambers requires direct invasive tools whereas echocardiography provides a safe and noninvasive means to evaluate diastolic function. It is assessed perioperatively in patients having shortness of breath despite normal systolic function. It should also be investigated in patients who are difficult to wean or patients with repeated weaning failures from a ventilator. Diastolic dysfunction leads to increased left atrial pressure (LAP > 15 mm Hg). In mid-esophageal (ME) four-chamber view, the mitral inflow pattern is assessed first with pulse wave Doppler at the tip of MV. From the four-chamber view, the lateral MV annular velocity is measured by placing the tissue Doppler imaging (TDI) sample volume on the lateral MV annulus where e′, a′, and s′ measure early relaxation, late atrial contractility, and ventricular systole, respectively.[6] If the ratio of early to late filling (E/A) is ≤1 (impaired relaxation) or >2 (restrictive filling pattern), then further data are not required (**Figs. 4A to D**). If the value of E/A lies between the two extremes, then three factors such as average E/e′ ratio > 14, LA maximum volume index > 34 mL/m³, and peak tricuspid regurgitation (TR) 2.8 m/s velocity are assessed. If any two of the three factors are raised, then LAP is >15 mm Hg.[10]

Right Ventricular Function

Assessment of RV function encompasses RV size, shape, interatrial septum, interventricular septum (IVS), and

HD state	TEE findings					Hemodynamic findings		
	Contractility	LVIDd	LVIDs	VTI	EF	RAP	MAP	CI
Hypovolemia	Vigorous	↓	↓	↓	↔	↓	↓	↓
Reduced LV compliance	Vigorous	↓	↓	↓	↔	↔	↓	↓
Low SVR	Vigorous	↔	↓	↑	↑	↑	↓	↑
Systolic dysfunction	Poor	↑	↑	↓	↓	↑	↓	↓

Table 1: TEE findings in some common hemodynamic conditions.[9]

(CI: cardiac index; EF: ejection fraction; LV: left ventricle; LVIDd: left ventricular internal diastolic diameter; LVIDs: left ventricular internal systolic diameter; MAP: mean arterial pressure; RAP: right atrial pressure; SVR: systemic vascular resistance; TEE: transesophageal echocardiography; VTI: velocity time integral)

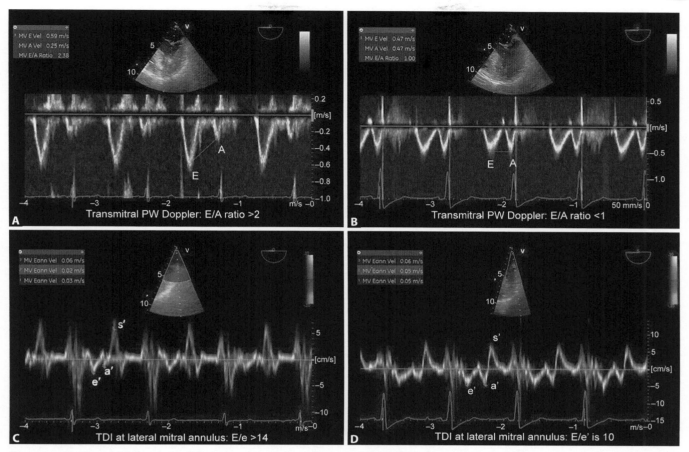

Figs. 4A to D: (A) and (C) Restrictive filling pattern seen by pulse wave (PW) Doppler across transmitral flow in a case of coronary artery disease. (B) and (D) Impaired relaxation seen in a case of severe aortic stenosis with LV hypertrophy. (TDI: tissue Doppler imaging)

tricuspid annular plane systolic excursion (TAPSE). The RV size is estimated in ME four-chamber view. The RV area is measured in systole and diastole by the planimetry method and RV FAC < 35% is considered abnormal.[11] A normal RV/LV area ratio is 0.6 and is seen when pulmonary artery pressures are normal. The ratio changes when there is RV enlargement (**Figs. 5A and B**). If the apex of the heart is made by RV, then it is called severely enlarged RV. The echocardiographic signs of RV failure are bowing of interatrial septum toward right atrium (RA), hypokinesia of RV free wall (seen best in ME four-chamber view), loss of crescentic shape, D-shaped RV due to flattening of IVS, or loss of convexity of IVS (observed best in TG mid-SAX view) (**Figs. 6A and B**).[12] In TEE examination, TAPSE is measured in TG RV inflow-outflow view from 0 to 20° or 110° where M-mode beam can be aligned with tricuspid annular excursion.[7] RV contractility is considered significantly decreased if TAPSE is <17 mm, where the normal value is around 20–25 mm (**Figs. 7A and B**). Pulmonary thromboembolism with thrombus is occasionally seen; however, associated features such as severe RV dysfunction,

hypokinesia of LV free wall, flattening of IVS, and decreased TAPSE are commonly observed (**Figs. 8A and B**).

A mid-esophageal modified bicaval tricuspid view (at 90–110°) is considered most appropriate to measure TR by color and spectral Doppler as a regurgitant jet is aligned parallel to the insonation beam. A visible TR jet is interrogated with continuous wave Doppler to measure its peak velocity. Simplified Bernoulli's equation ($\Delta P = 4V^2$; P = pressure gradient across tricuspid valve; V = peak TR jet velocity) is then used to estimate the transvalvular pressure gradient, which is then further added to right atrial pressure (RAP) to estimate RV peak systolic pressure. This right ventricular systolic pressure (RVSP) is a good estimate of pulmonary artery systolic pressure (PASP) (**Figs. 7A and B**).[13]

Pulmonary artery systolic pressure: RVSP or PASP = $4(V^2)$ + RAP

Preload

The assessment of preload status of a patient can be estimated quickly by "eyeballing" at LV cavity in transgastric

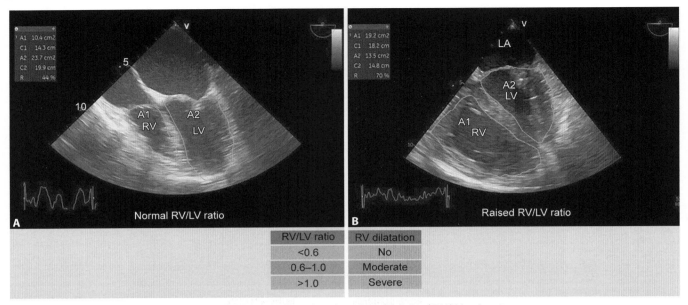

Figs. 5A and B: (A) Normal RV/LV ratio <0.6 seen in ME four-chamber view; (B) Raised RV/LV ratio >1.
(LV: left ventricular; ME: mid-esophageal; RV: right ventricular; IVS: interventricular septum)

RV/LV ratio	RV dilatation
<0.6	No
0.6–1.0	Moderate
>1.0	Severe

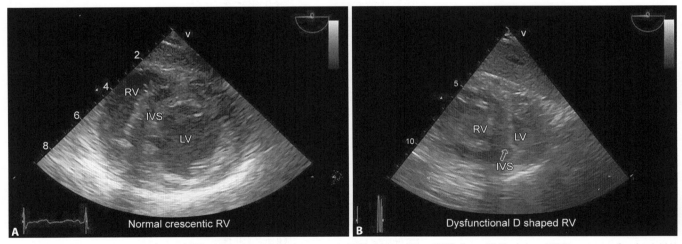

Figs. 6A and B: (A) Crescent-shaped RV with normal function seen in TG mid-papillary SAX view; (B) D-shaped RV in a case of pulmonary thromboembolism.
(LV: left ventricular; RV: right ventricular; SAX: short-axis view; TG: transgastric; IVS: interventricular septum)

mid papillary (TG mid SAX or TG SAX) view. "Kissing papillary muscles" indicate hypovolemia and need for fluid administration (**Figs. 9A to D**). Quantitative measurements of LV dimensions can be taken in systole and diastole as mentioned earlier and they reflect the amount of fluid in the left ventricle (**Fig. 3**).[8] LVIDd and LVIDs change in different clinical scenarios as shown in **Table 1**.

Filling pressure can be raised in case of diastolic dysfunction as mentioned earlier. Although LAP measurement may not reflect the intravascular volume status, a large increase in LAP during fluid administration warns of impending pulmonary edema that may be hastened by further volume.

Filling pressures on the right side of heart can be measured by the TEE 2D method or M-mode. Low filling pressure is high likely if absolute inferior vena cava (IVC) diameter < 1 cm and abnormally high filling pressure increasing likely if IVC diameter is > 2 cm. However, changes in collapsibility or distensibility index with respect to positive pressure ventilation are helpful in classifying filling pressures [(al venous pressure (CVP)] in patients who have IVC diameter between 1 and 2 cm. In mechanically ventilated patients, the increase in intrathoracic pressure during inspiration collapses superior vena cava (SVC) and distends IVC. The extent of these variations with respiration increases when there is volume deficit. The change in

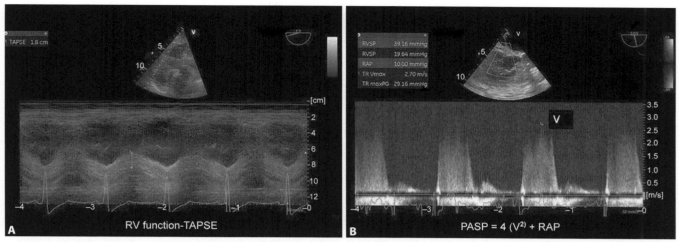

Figs. 7A and B: (A) Tricuspid annular plane systolic excursion (TAPSE) in TG inflow–outflow view at 20°; (B) Continuous wave (CW) Doppler image of tricuspid regurgitation. A sample calculation of pulmonary artery systolic pressure in modified bicaval view: ΔP = 4(2.7)²; systolic pulmonary artery pressure or RVSP = 29 + right atrial pressure; PASP is approximately 39 mm Hg.
(RVSP: right ventricular systolic pressure; PASP: pulmonary artery systolic pressure)

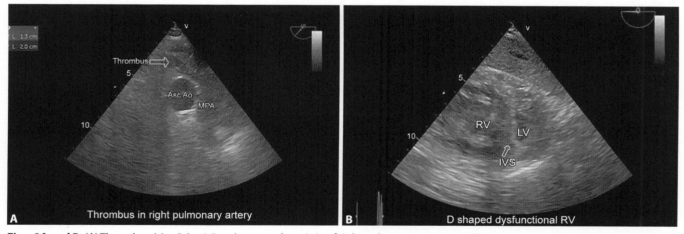

Figs. 8A and B: (A) Thrombus (size 2.0 × 1.3 cm) seen at the origin of right pulmonary artery in ME ascending aorta SAX view; (B) D-shaped dysfunctional RV due to severe pulmonary hypertension seen in TG mid-papillary SAX view.
(IVS: interventricular septum; LV: left ventricular; ME: mid-esophageal; RV: right ventricular; SAX: short axis view; TG: transgastric)

diameter that is ΔSVC and ΔIVC of >36% and >18% indicates volume responsiveness (**Fig. 10**). ΔSVC is found to be more specific in various studies, the limitation being that these parameters become less reliable with low tidal volumes, arrhythmias, acute respiratory distress syndrome (ARDS), and pulmonary hypertension.

Dynamic Parameters of Stroke Volume and Cardiac Output

Stroke volume (SV) and CO can be calculated by biplane Simpson's method as explained earlier in ME four-chamber and ME two-chamber views. As both the above measurements are static parameters, dynamic methods are increasingly being used to assess whether change in preload or afterload or contractility has led to change in SV. Principles of continuity equation are used here to measure SV. The velocity time integral (VTI) of the LV outflow tract or aortic valve is measured in deep transgastric (deep TG) view (**Figs. 11A and B**). The diameter of left ventricular outflow tract (LVOT) and aortic valve can be measured in ME long-axis view. The product of LVOT area [cross-sectional area (CSA) = πr^2] and LVOT VTI gives SV.[13]

$$\text{LVOT CSA} \times \text{LVOT VTI} = \text{SV}$$

$$\text{Stroke volume} \times \text{Heart rate} = \text{CO}$$

As the LVOT diameter is a static parameter, only VTI will change if fluid challenge or passive leg raising (PLR) is done. Therefore, prediction of fluid responsiveness with bolus fluid administration or PLR has been advocated. Because of

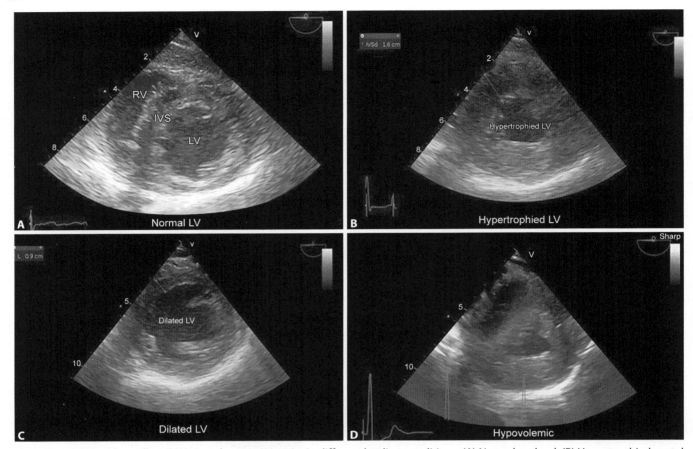

Figs. 9A to D: TG mid-papillary SAX view showing LV cavity in different loading conditions. (A) Normal preload; (B) Hypertrophied septal thickness of 1.6 cm; (C) Dilated LV with RWMA; (D) Hypovolemic LV.
(IVS: interventricular septum; LV: left ventricular; RV: right ventricular; RWMA: regional wall motion abnormality; SAX: short axis view; TG: transgastric)

Fig. 10: Respiratory variation seen in ME bicaval view in superior vena cava.
(LA: left atrial; ME: mid-esophageal; RA: right atrium)

being an internal preload challenge, PLR has been indicated in surviving sepsis campaign. The increase in ΔVTI > 12% or greater indicates volume responsiveness as indicated by a simultaneous increase in SV with 77% sensitivity and 100% specificity.[14] This is more accurate than change in LV dimensions to fluid challenge.

Though a patient is predicted to be fluid responsive, the decision to administer fluids should always be made by assessment of risk of organ damage and benefit of giving fluids, especially in high-risk patients.

Systemic vascular resistance (SVR): Once SV and CO are calculated, SVR can be calculated by a simple formula where RAP is estimated by IVC collapsibility and arm blood pressure measurement to measure mean arterial pressure (MAP). The unit of SVR is dyne. sec. cm^{-5}.

Systemic vascular resistance: SVR = [MAP – RAP (mm Hg)/ CO(L/min)] × 80

Echocardiographic Assessment in Different Clinical Situations

Hemodynamic instability seen in patients with normal EF may be attributed to hypovolemia, diastolic dysfunction,

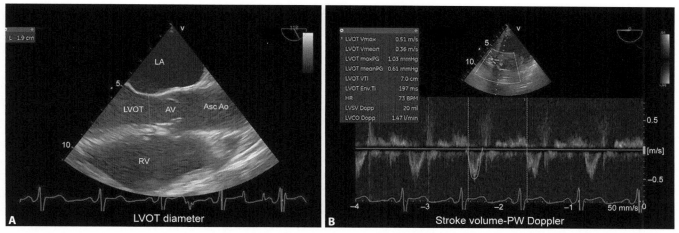

Figs. 11A and B: (A) Measurement of the LVOT diameter (1.9 cm) from the mid-esophageal long-axis view; (B) Pulse wave (PW) Doppler measurement of blood flow velocities across the LVOT (LVOT VTI) from the deep transgastric LVOT view. The VTI is 7 cm. The cross-sectional area of the LVOT (CSA_{LVOT}) is calculated from the measured diameter using the equation $\pi(D/2)^2$. The calculated area of the LVOT (2.8 cm²) multiplied by VTI (7.0 cm) yields a stroke volume of 20 mL/beat. When multiplied by heart rate (HR), the cardiac output is obtained. (HR: heart rate; LVOT: left ventricular outflow tract; VTI: velocity time integral)

decreased SVR, obstructive pathologies such as pulmonary artery hypertension (PAH), and regional tamponade. More commonly reduced afterload or preload is the cause of hemodynamic instability. Assessment of volume and afterload begins with LV dimensions in systole and diastole in TG mid-papillary SAX view and TG LV two-chamber view and Doppler quantification of SV.[7] In hypovolemia, both LVIDd and LVIDs as well as cardiac index parameter VTI also decrease, whereas EF remains the same.[9] In case of hypotension due to decreased SVR, LVIDd is normal and LVIDs is decreased, and EF and VTI are increased. Hypotension is rarely due to diastolic dysfunction; it has parameters similar to hypovolemia. However, there is elevated LAP which can easily be confirmed by using pulse wave and TDI of annulus. It warns against excess fluid infusion. When there is systolic dysfunction [heart failure with reduced ejection fraction (HFrEF)], LVIDd and LVIDs increase whereas EF and VTI decrease. Fluid administration is done within these limits and treatment is monitored with increase in VTI (**Table 1**).

A vasodilator in a normal patient manifests as a hypovolemic patient with increased venous capacitance, more stressed volume turning to nonstressed volume in the circulatory system resulting in decreased preload, and SV manifesting as decreased VTI (**Table 1**). The opposite happens when vasopressors are used in a normal patient. In contrast, in patients of congestive heart failure, when vasopressors are used, they cause increased preload and increased MAP due to increase in SVR, but contractility remains the same or deteriorates. There is insignificant or no increase in SV despite increase in preload making infusion of vasopressors futile or deleterious for patients.

So, VTI should be preferred in place of indirect indicators, i.e., vena cava diameter or indices that are inconsistent or misleading such as pulse pressure variation (PPV). Inter- and intraobserver variability is <10% making it a reliable tool to monitor a patient during his/her course of ICU stay.[15]

Septic cardiomyopathy may be masked due to low SVR and normal EF with normal LVIDd and decreased LVIDs. When these patients are challenged with norepinephrine, EF decreases; however, their filling pressures or LAPs are normal. It is one of the reasons that septic cardiomyopathy is diagnosed very late or not diagnosed at all.[16]

Positive pressure ventilation increases transpulmonary pressure, which reduces RV preload and increases RV afterload. It reduces RV SV, which manifests as a decrease in VTI instantaneously in right ventricular outflow tract (RVOT) or after —three to four beats in LVOT. Change in VTI is exaggerated if the patient is on a steeper portion of the Frank–Starling curve. If there is increased afterload such as in ARDS, and PAH or patient is euvolemic, then respiratory variability in VTI will not be significant.

Thirty percent patients of ARDS present with acute cor pulmonale. It requires ventilation strategy protective to RV function, which is less driving pressure and avoids overt hypercapnia.[17] TEE is the only modality of hemodynamic monitoring which makes accurate diagnosis of acute cor pulmonale.

Rescue Transesophageal Echocardiography

Limited TEE examination with 11 views has been suggested as "rescue TEE" to know the reasons of persistent hypotension or hypoxemia when cause is not understood. The reported incidence of identifying the cause of cardiac arrest is

64–86%.[18] ME four-chamber view is assessed for biventricular function, hypovolemia, and acute chordal rupture. ME long-axis (LAX) view is assessed for aortic dissection and pleural effusion and TG SAX view for cardiac contractility and tamponade. Pericardial effusion can be quantified as small (<1 cm), moderate (1–2 cm), and large (>2 cm).

Transesophageal echocardiography is reliable in ruling out any aortic dissection as a cause of hemodynamic instability in patients of traumatic incident and has no time for workup. Early diagnosis and management improve prognosis. True lumen has a smaller size, shape systolic expansion, and laminar flow with color flow Doppler. False lumen has large size and irregular or crescent slope with spontaneous echo contrast (**Figs. 12A to D**).

Left Ventricular Outflow Tract Obstruction

Left ventricular outflow tract obstruction (LVOTO) is seen with hypovolemia and low afterload as seen in sepsis. There is dynamic obstruction of LVOT in mid- and late systole. The systolic anterior motion of MV results in mild-to-moderate mitral regurgitation (MR). This results in hypotension which is worsened with administration of inotropes.

Takotsubo Cardiomyopathy/Stress Myocardial Infarction

It is similar in presentation as acute MI with ST elevation patterns in ECG and raised serum level of cardiac markers. It is differentiated from acute MI by hypokinesia and ballooning of apex and normal or hyperkinetic basal segments on TEE. However, coronary angiography is confirmatory which is normal.

Extracorporeal Membrane Oxygenation

It helps in making a choice whether the patient needs venovenous or venoarterial ECMO depending on RV dysfunction. Thermodilution methods of CO are inaccurate in patients of ECMO where pulmonary circulation is bypassed. The bicaval view helps in correct placement of a dual lumen cannula in orifices of SVC and IVC in venovenous ECMO and outflow port across the tricuspid

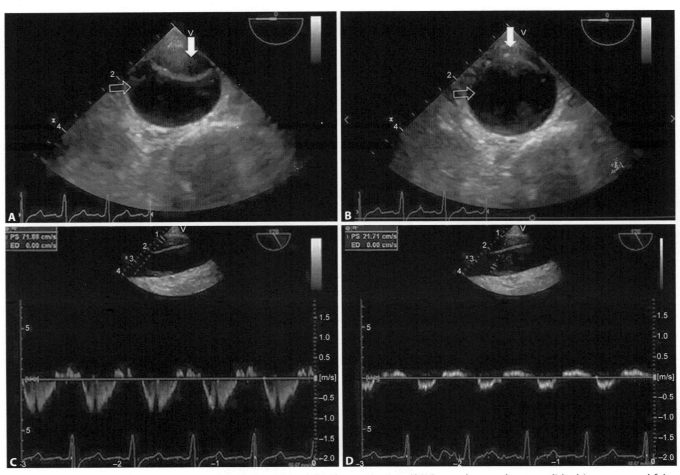

Figs. 12A to D: Dissection seen in descending aorta. (A) and (B) Short-axis view (SAX); see the true lumen solid white arrow and false lumen hollow arrow. (C) and (D) Descending aorta long-axis view (LAX) true lumen has high forward flow and false lumen has low flow.

valve in venoarterial ECMO. Regular TEE helps in decision-making about cardiac performance and weaning from ECMO.[15]

Intra-aortic Balloon Pump

Transesophageal echocardiography helps in placement of aortic balloon in the descending aorta (DA) distal to origin of the left subclavian artery to avoid ischemia to the left upper limb. Guidewire is visualized in DA LAX and SAX views. Then, the TEE probe is withdrawn slowly where the left subclavian artery originates. Guidewire is secured distal to the origin of the left subclavian artery.[15]

Intensive Care Unit Performance

It helps in early decision-making in severely ill patients and establishes beneficial cooperation among intensivists, cardiac anesthesiologists, cardiac surgeons, and cardiologists. It helps in understanding circulatory failure pathophysiology and thus improves decision-making.[15]

Suggested Transesophageal Echocardiography Views

Knowledge of echocardiography machine, its knobology, selection of appropriate probe, and familiarity with various echocardiographic modalities such as 2D, color flow Doppler, tissue Doppler, and spectral Doppler is required by an intensivist.[13] Mayo et al. have suggested a 21-set of TEE views for comprehensive echocardiographic measurements in critical care practice.[6]

Training and Credentialing

About 30 studies are considered enough to achieve the level of competence for TEE.[19] Simulation (Symbionix™) based training modules are available which split the entire course into various modules of image acquisition and image interpretation.[20] The fellows are expected to perform 10–12 examinations on these platforms before starting on patients. Unlike TTE where there are two different training modules—basic and advanced TTE, there is a single module in critical care TEE practice,[6] which comprises qualitative as well as quantitative measurements. An association with cardiac anesthesiologists is of great help where TEE is conducted routinely.

Safety Profile

Transesophageal echocardiography is a safe procedure with a reported mortality rate of 0.0098%. The complication rate would be reduced when placed in sedated and paralyzed patients. The TEE probe is usually placed blindly with slight neck extension and jaw thrust. In case of difficulty with

Box 1: List of contraindications to transesophageal echocardiography.[22]

- *Absolute contraindication*
  - Perforated viscus
  - Esophageal stricture
  - Esophageal tumor
  - Esophageal perforation
  - Active upper GI bleed
- *Relative contraindications*
  - History of radiation to neck and mediastinum
  - History of GI surgery
  - Recent upper GI bleed
  - Barrett's esophagus
  - History of dysphagia
  - Restriction of neck mobility
  - Symptomatic hiatal hernia
  - Esophageal varices
  - Coagulopathy
  - Thrombocytopenia
  - Active esophagitis
  - Active peptic ulcer disease

(GI: gastrointestinal)

jaw thrust maneuver, direct laryngoscopy should be done. TEE probe placement by neck and jaw thrust maneuver is known to have a lower complication rate with respect to laryngoscopy. Continuous hemodynamic monitoring using a single-use TEE probe for 72 hours has been seen without any complication.[21] Contraindications to TEE probe insertion are given in **Box 1**. Before probe placement, relevant history about any associated contraindications, risk benefits, and informed consent should be taken from close relatives.

Future Direction

There is no randomized trial to evaluate the impact of TEE in critical care. An ideal trial may show beneficial effect of TEE -directed diagnosis and intermittent monitoring. It can be compared with other invasive monitors based on arterial waveform analysis and pulmonary artery catheters. Newer modalities of TEE which can be used continuously for at least 72 hours can be further evaluated. An analysis should be made about its cost-effectiveness in critical care.

CONCLUSION

Transesophageal echocardiography provides diagnostic, prognostic, and intermittent monitoring in ICU. It is very helpful in diagnosis and management of shock where TTE imaging is inadequate. It efficiently differentiates RV dysfunction from LV dysfunction which is not possible with other modalities. It has been able to find false-positive cases of fluid responsiveness with the use of dynamic indices such as VTI. It performs a critical role in rescue echocardiography in cases of sudden hemodynamic collapse and cardiac arrest making early diagnosis and management. It plays a significant role in placement of IABP and ECMO. It has improved ICU performance by expediting clinical decision-making among different clinicians.

■ REFERENCES

1. Papolos A, Narula J, Bavishi C, Chaudhry FA, Sengupta PP. U.S. hospital use of echocardiography: Insights from the Nationwide inpatient sample. J Am Coll Cardiol. 2016;67(5):502-11.

2. Vignon P, Mentec H, Terré S, Gastinne H, Guéret P, Lemaire F. Diagnostic accuracy and therapeutic impact of transthoracic and transesophageal echocardiography in mechanically ventilated patients in the ICU. Chest. 1994;106(6):1829-34.

3. American Society of Anesthesiologists and Society of Cardiovascular Anesthesiologists Task Force on Transesophageal Echocardiography. Practice guidelines for perioperative transesophageal echocardiography. An updated report by the American Society of Anesthesiologists and the Society of Cardiovascular Anesthesiologists Task Force on Transesophageal Echocardiography. Anesthesiology. 2010;112(5):1084-96.

4. Arntfield R, Lau V, Landry Y, Priestap F, Ball I. Impact of critical care transesophageal echocardiography in medical-surgical ICU patients: Characteristics and results from 274 consecutive examinations. J Intensive Care Med. 2018;885066618797271.

5. Arntfield R, Pace J, Hewak M, Thompson D. Focused transesophageal echocardiography by emergency physicians is feasible and clinically influential: Observational results from a novel ultrasound program. J Emerg Med. 2016;50(2):286-94.

6. Mayo PH, Narasimhan M, Koenig S. Critical care transesophageal echocardiography. Chest. 2015;148(5):1323-32.

7. Hahn RT, Abraham T, Adams MS, Bruce CJ, Glas KE, Lang RM, et al. Guidelines for performing a comprehensive transesophageal echocardiographic examination: Recommendations from the American Society of Echocardiography and the Society of Cardiovascular Anesthesiologists. J Am Soc Echocardiogr. 2013;26(9):921-64.

8. Lang RM, Bierig M, Devereux RB, Flachskampf FA, Foster E, Pellikka PA, et al. Recommendations for chamber quantification. Eur J Echocardiogr. 2006;7(2):79-108.

9. Choudhury M. Transoesophageal echocardiography: What a neuroanaesthesiologist should know? J Neuroanaesth Crit Care. 2015;2:3-14.

10. Nagueh SF. Non-invasive assessment of left ventricular filling pressure. Eur J Heart Fail. 2018;20(1):38-48.

11. Porter TR, Shillcutt SK, Adams MS, Desjardins G, Glas KE, Olson JJ, et al. Guidelines for the use of echocardiography as a monitor for therapeutic intervention in adults: A report from the American Society of Echocardiography. J Am Soc Echocardiogr. 2015;28(1):40-56.

12. Rudski LG, Lai WW, Afilalo J, Hua L, Handschumacher MD, Chandrasekaran K, et al. Guidelines for the echocardiographic assessment of the right heart in adults: A report from the American Society of Echocardiography endorsed by the European Association of Echocardiography, a registered branch of the European Society of Cardiology, and the Canadian Society of Echocardiography. J Am Soc Echocardiogr. 2010;23(7):685-713.

13. Perrino AC, Reeves ST. A Practical Approach to Transesophageal Echocardiography, 4th edition. Philadelphia: Lippincott Williams and Wilkins, a Wolter Kluwer Business; 2019.

14. Lamia B, Ochagavia A, Monnet X, Chemla D, Richard C, Teboul JL. Echocardiographic prediction of volume responsiveness in critically ill patients with spontaneously breathing activity. Intensive Care Med. 2007;33(7):1125-32.

15. Vignon P, Merz TM, Vieillard-Baron A. Ten reasons for performing hemodynamic monitoring using transesophageal echocardiography. Intensive Care Med. 2017;43(7):1048-51.

16. Chauvet JL, El-Dash S, Delastre O, Bouffandeau B, Jusserand D, Michot JB, et al. Early dynamic left intraventricular obstruction is associated with hypovolemia and high mortality in septic shock patients. Crit Care. 2015;19:262.

17. Vieillard-Baron A, Price LC, Matthay MA. Acute cor pulmonale in ARDS. Intensive Care Med. 2013;39(10):1836-8.

18. Memtsoudis SG, Rosenberger P, Loffler M, Eltzschig HK, Mizuguchi A, Shernan SK, et al. The usefulness of transesophageal echocardiography during intraoperative cardiac arrest in noncardiac surgery. Anesth Analg. 2006;102(6):1653-7.

19. Charron C, Prat G, Caille V, Belliard G, Lefèvre M, Aegerter P, et al. Validation of a skills assessment scoring system for transesophageal echocardiographic monitoring of hemodynamics. Intensive Care Med. 2007;33(10):1712-8.

20. TEE module. [online] Available from https://simbionix.com/simulators/us-mentor/us-library-of-modules/us-tee/. [Last accessed March, 2020].

21. Cioccari L, Zante B, Bloch A, Berger D, Limacher A, Jakob SM, et al. Effects of hemodynamic monitoring using a single-use transesophageal echocardiography probe in critically ill patients - study protocol for a randomized controlled trial. Trials. 2018;19(1):362.

22. Vieillard-Baron A, Caille V, Charron C, Belliard G, Page B, Jardin F. Actual incidence of global left ventricular hypokinesia in adult septic shock. Critical Care Med. 2008;36(6):1701-6.

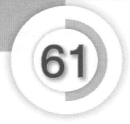

61

Perioperative Renal Replacement Therapy

Natesh Prabu R, Atul Prabhakar Kulkarni

INTRODUCTION

Acute kidney injury (AKI) is a common problem in the intensive care unit (ICU) and the perioperative period. The incidence varies between 5 and 20% and usually occurs as part of multiorgan failure[1] with approximately 5% requiring renal replacement therapy (RRT).[2] In the AKI-EPI (Acute Kidney Injury-Epidemiologic Prospective Investigation) study, the incidence of AKI within the 1st week of ICU admission was 52% after scheduled surgery and 56% after emergency surgery.[3] Patients with AKI, requiring mechanical ventilation and having other organ dysfunction have higher mortality (>50%).[4,5] RRT is needed in patients with an advanced stage of AKI and who have complications due to AKI. As a general saying, earlier the better, early RRT may prevent the acute life-threatening complications of renal failure such as refractory hyperkalemia, severe metabolic acidosis, pulmonary edema, and uremic complications. There exists a controversy in the literature regarding RRT for acute renal failure in the ICU. There are no clear guidelines about when to start, what mode to use, which anticoagulants to use, when to stop, and what is the optimum dose of dialysis. Therefore, there are differences in practice in the management of RRT for AKI in different ICUs. Moreover, in the perioperative setting, RRT need may be different, especially when it is done for nonrenal causes, e.g., rhabdomyolysis or when surgery is performed in patients with end-stage renal disease (ESRD). Also, perioperative RRT may be done even before, during, and after surgery depending on patient needs.

ACUTE KIDNEY INJURY AND RENAL REPLACEMENT THERAPY IN THE PERIOPERATIVE PERIOD: RISK FACTORS AND PATHOPHYSIOLOGY

Perioperative complications are more common in high-risk patients, especially those undergoing major surgeries (either the individual risk is >5% compared to population undergoing surgery or surgery itself has >5% mortality).[6] Sepsis and major surgeries are common causes of perioperative AKI, i.e., AKI associated with surgery.[2]

Sepsis-associated AKI (SA-AKI) is associated with adverse outcomes. There is a stepwise increase in adverse outcomes with increased severity of AKI.[3] The effect may be due to the affection of distant organs probably due to the systemic effects of renal failure predominantly mediated by inflammation.[7] In a recent follow-up study on patients with AKI treated with RRT, a large proportion of survivors had evidence of chronic kidney disease. Also, the 5-year mortality of patients who survived 90 days was 30%.[8] Patients with baseline deranged renal functions and undergoing major surgeries, especially cardiac surgery, are potential risk factors influencing the need for perioperative RRT.[9] Though thoracic and abdominal surgeries increase the risk of perioperative AKI and need of RRT, the majority of studies has been done in cardiac surgical patients, probably due to its unique nature, i.e., involving high-risk patients, need for cardiopulmonary bypass, and increased postoperative complications. Preoperative risk factors for postoperative RRT after cardiac surgery are female gender, diabetes, hypertension, heart failure, and pre-existing renal dysfunction.[10] The predominant factor that influences the need for perioperative RRT is preexisting renal dysfunction, i.e., increased baseline creatinine.

Pathophysiology

The kidney is at risk for many insults during the perioperative period. The common modes of injury are hemodynamic disturbances, inflammation, nephrotoxic drug usage, and urinary tract obstruction. More commonly, it is a combination of patient risk factors, surgery-related risk, and perioperative circumstances, which influences perioperative AKI and need of RRT. Major surgeries cause significant tissue trauma and an exaggerated inflammatory response mediated by tumor necrosis factor-α, interleukin- (IL-) 6,

IL-10, and other cytokines secreted by inflammatory cells. This is well described in surgery, trauma, and sepsis.[11] The inflammation due to surgical insult leads to vasodilatation, capillary leakage, and intravascular volume deficit, causing hypovolemia and reduced cardiac output. Moreover, major surgeries are associated with increased oxygen demand requiring higher global oxygen delivery (DO_2), which may lead to hypoperfusion and further multiorgan failure, as a result of massive inflammation but the exact mechanism is not known.[12] The kidney is sensitive to many drugs used in the perioperative period, e.g., fluids, analgesics, antibiotics, etc. Excess fluid loading leads to more organ dysfunction and adverse events.[13] Recent studies have shown that resuscitation with normal saline may cause AKI in both critically and noncritically ill patients.[14,15] A recent meta-analysis (over 4,500 patients) showed that hydroxyethyl starch (HES) use leads to an increased need for RRT in surgical patients.[16] In addition to the above factors, inadvertent urinary tract obstruction either due to complications of colorectal or genitourinary surgeries may also contribute to perioperative AKI.

RENAL REPLACEMENT THERAPY IN THE PERIOPERATIVE PERIOD

Renal Replacement Therapy: Acute Kidney Injury in Surgery-associated Critically Ill Patients

Renal replacement therapy is chosen to treat or prevent acute life-threatening complications of renal failure. Though a lot of studies are done on the timing and mode of RRT, controversies still exist.[17,18] Moreover, the patient populations may differ, i.e., we may have patients who develop perioperative AKI, AKI on chronic kidney disease, and also patients with ESRD on maintenance dialysis. The preference of modality of RRT, its timings, and conduct of RRT may differ in each group of patients. As a matter of discussion, we can divide the patients in to those who are on maintenance dialysis (chronic renal failure patients) and those who develop AKI during perioperative setting.

Indications and Timing of Renal Replacement Therapy in AKI Associated with Surgery

Renal replacement therapy was believed to improve outcomes when used early, i.e., before complications set in, to prevent adverse outcomes. But, there is no clear definition of what is early versus late initiation. Clinical studies that have shown better outcomes with early initiation used urine output, uremic toxin levels, and biomarkers to initiate RRT. A meta-analysis that included both medical and surgical patients (cardiac surgical) showed better outcomes with

early RRT.[19] The majority of studies included in this meta-analysis are observational studies with only two randomized controlled trials (RCTs), and the studies are of low quality. Recently conducted RCTs tried to answer this question of appropriate timing of RRT with more objective inclusion criteria, using AKIN (The Artificial Kidney Initiation in Kidney Injury) or KDIGO (The Kidney Disease Improving Global Outcomes) criteria to define early dialysis. In AKIKI (The Artificial Kidney Initiation in Kidney Injury) trial, patients received RRT within 6 hours of diagnosis of KDIGO stage 3 in early RRT group.[20] It was a multicenter trial that included predominantly medical septic shock patients and demonstrated comparable mortality at 60 days between the groups (48.5% vs. 49.7%; early vs. late, respectively). Many patients in delayed RRT group (nearly half the patients) averted RRT compared to early group. In another well-conducted single center, RCT, the ELAIN (Early vs. Late Initiation of Renal Replacement Therapy in Critically Ill Patients With Acute Kidney Injury) trial from Germany, the patients were initiated on RRT within 8 hours of diagnosis of KDIGO stage 2 in early group and within 12 hours of KDIGO stage 3 in late RRT group.[21] The study included predominantly postoperative patients, especially after cardiac surgery, and used only continuous modes of RRT, as compared to AKIKI trial. The authors also included a biomarker of kidney injury, neutrophil gelatinase-associated lipocalin (NGAL), to ensure that the injury was significant enough so that the patients were likely to require dialysis, rather than improving spontaneously. The study showed a significant reduction in mortality at 90 days (39.3% vs. 54.7%, P = 0.03) with early RRT initiation. Also, the median duration of RRT need was less in early RRT group. Both these trials were well-conducted, but had contrasting results. Later the researchers of the AKIKI trial conducted a post hoc subgroup analysis in patients with sepsis and acute respiratory distress syndrome (ARDS) and also divided patients based on disease severity [simplified acute physiology score (SAPS score].[22] Interestingly, none of the groups showed benefit of early RRT, but nearly 50% of patients in sepsis and ARDS group did not required RRT in the late group.[22] So, delaying RRT may help to avoid complications related to dialysis. A recent meta-analysis which only included RCTs (including these two recent RCTs) showed no mortality benefit with early RRT with risk ratio of 0.98 (95% CI 0.78–1.23, P = 0.84).[18] Also, there were no differences in other outcomes such as ICU length of stay (LOS) or hospital LOS, renal function recovery, RRT dependence, and requirement of mechanical ventilation. In recent IDEAL-ICU (the Initiation of Dialysis Early Versus Delayed in the Intensive Care Unit) trial in septic shock patients with AKI, the patients were initiated on RRT within 12 hours of failure stage of RIFLE (Risk, Injury, and Failure; and Loss; and End-stage kidney disease) criteria before the onset of life-threatening signs of AKI, as compared to delayed initiation, i.e., within 48 hours of failure stage (RIFLE criteria). This study did not show any difference in mortality at 90 days in severe AKI patients.[23] Another meta-analysis by Cochrane group included five RCTs (over 1,050 patients), and showed better outcomes but with increased harm with early RRT, due to wide confidence interval (CI).[17] They concluded that further good-quality studies are needed in the field. Contrastingly, another meta-analysis that was done only in cardiac surgical patients, where dialysis was done for AKI postoperatively showed beneficial outcomes with early RRT.[24] The meta-analysis included both RCTs and observational trials. Doing RRT early, i.e. within 24 hours had shown to reduce 28-day mortality [odds ratio (OR) 0.36; 95% CI 0.23–0.57; I^2 60%] and reduction of RRT duration especially when initiated within 12 hours of AKI after cardiac surgery, These studies and meta-analysis added uncertainty about early RRT and there is no definite answer to the question, whether early RRT is beneficial in improving mortality in critically ill patients and in perioperative setting. Interestingly, if you see the studies that had shown benefits with early RRT are done predominantly in surgical patients, so whether early RRT should be used preferentially in surgical critically ill patients is not explored and requires further studies focusing on this population.

Modes of Renal Replacement Therapy

Many modes of RRT are practiced globally with certain preferences for a particular modality in every ICU. The choice may differ based on advantages, limitations of mode, ease of use, safety, availability, and familiarity with modes of RRT. The modes are classified based on the principles on these work; diffusion, convection, or based on the duration of dialysis; and intermittent techniques [intermittent hemodialysis (IHD), sustained low-efficiency daily dialysis (SLEDD), and continuous techniques (continuous RRT—CRRT)]. The common-modes used in continuous techniques are continuous venovenous hemofiltration (CVVHF), continuous venovenous hemodiafiltration (CVVHDF), continuous venovenous hemodialysis (CVVHD), and slow continuous ultrafiltration (SCUF). In general, IHD is done in chronic renal failure patients and in hemodynamically stable patients with AKI in ICU. Rapid fluid shifts, hypotension, and electrolyte disturbances are more common with IHD, so there is global preference for CRRT in hemodynamically unstable patients and also in critically ill patients with multiorgan involvement. Studies done to compare different modes of RRT are not conclusive and had varied results.[25] Knowing advantages and limitations of IHD (easy to do, no anticoagulation needed, less time required, rapid clearance of metabolic products, easy nursing, less costly)

and CRRT (titrated ultrafiltration, more hemodynamically tolerated, easy to manage medications, removal of higher molecular weight compounds, can be combined with other extracorporeal therapies), hybrid therapies such as sustained low-efficiency dialysis (SLED), prolonged intermittent RRT (PIRRT), and extended daily dialysis (EDD) emerged to balance the advantages of both IHD and CRRT.[26] Though hybrid techniques were believed to have good solute removal with hemodynamic stability, it was not proven in clinical studies, rather it had more hemodynamic instability.[27] A meta-analysis that compared intermittent techniques with continuous techniques did not show any difference between two modalities.[25]

How to decide which mode of RRT to choose? It is a challenging question at the bedside. The logical answer may be to choose a particular mode for particular needs at that point in time, considering patient and logistic factors in mind. So in perioperative setting, it may be more reasonable to choose modalities based on individual patient needs rather than preferring a particular mode. CRRT is better in guardedly removing fluids when it is done only for fluid overload, especially in patients with complex hemodynamics (e.g., heart failure with renal failure). In patients who have high-solute load and hyperkalemia, IHD may be preferred when dealing with hemodynamically stable patients. When hemodynamic instability is anticipated or dealing with other organ failures such as liver failure, heart failure, comatose patients with cerebral edema, CRRT may be preferred where controlled ultrafiltration, minimal electrolyte disturbances, and osmotic shifts are warranted. KDIGO Clinical Practice Guideline 2012 recommends CRRT for hemodynamically unstable patients and patients with raised intracranial pressure and cerebral edema.[28] The modes are complementary to each other; the choice of mode may change in same patient from time to time-based on needs. The physician may choose any mode, considering the patient's needs, staff experience, cost, and potential adverse effects.

Dosing and Conduct of Renal Replacement Therapy

Adequate dialysis dose is important for the effective clearance of solutes. In IHD, solute clearance is calculated by Kt/V_{urea}. It is a dimensionless index of dialysis dose in which K is the urea clearance of the dialyzer, t is the duration of dialysis, and V is the volume of distribution of urea. It is commonly used for chronic renal failure patients on maintenance dialysis with an accepted target of 1.2. The solute clearance in continuous techniques depends on the effluent rate: in CVVHF, its ultrafiltration rate; in CVVHD, its consumed dialysate; and in CVVHDF, its sum of ultrafiltration rate and consumed dialysate. The volumes are represented usually as volume/kg/h. There are many studies that have compared low- and high-volume filtration involving various dialysis modalities. Though initial studies showed better hemodynamic stability, outcome with high-intensity therapy, later RCTs challenged the practice. In the ATN (The Acute Renal Failure Trial Network) study, high-intensity therapy was compared with standard-intensity therapy (IHD/SLED, six times/week in hemodynamically stable patients, Kt/V_{uera} = 1.2 or CVVHDF at effluent flow rate of 35 mL/kg/h in hemodynamically unstable patients versus IHD three times/week, Kt/V_{urea} = 1.4 or CVVHDF 20 mL/kg/h respectively representing the concerned groups).[29] The authors did not find any difference in mortality or renal recovery. But there were increased episodes of hypotension and requirement of vasopressor support in the high-intensity group. Another large RCT, the RENAL (The Randomized Evaluation of Normal versus Augmented Level) trial, compared high-intensity versus low-intensity treatment (40 mL vs. 20 mL/kg/h), where both groups received only CVVHDF.[30] No difference in mortality at 90 days or renal recovery was found between two groups but the incidence of hypophosphatemia was more in high-intensity groups. Later, IVOIRE study, an RCT done in septic shock patients (70 mL vs. 35 mL/kg/h) also did not show any benefit of high-intensity treatment. To note, in both groups in both the trials, the intensity of treatment was high compared to previous studies.[31] Recent Cochrane review also showed no mortality benefit with high-intensity therapy in patients with AKI and septic shock.[32] Another RCT that compared three dose ranges, <20 mL/kg/h versus 21–34 mL/kg/h versus ≥35 mL/kg/h (least, less, and high-intense RRT, respectively) also did not show any difference in mortality and renal recovery.[33]

Though the results of various RCTs and meta-analysis do not favor high-volume filtration, there is no clarity on the optimal dose range. The observation in previous RCTs is that the actual dose delivery was lower than the prescribed dose. As less intense therapy is equally effective, it may be reasonable to prescribe little more to achieve the desired dose. KDIGO also suggests aiming at around 35 mL/kg/h to achieve around 20–25 mL/kg/h.[28] This practice may seem logical as there may be problems with filter efficiency, blood flows, and frequent discontinuation of dialysis in ICU patients due to the need for imaging, surgery, etc. For patients on IHD, a reasonable target of Kt/V_{urea} =1.2–1.4 can be tried on thrice-weekly dialysis and the frequency may be increased if the targets are not met.

Anticoagulation

Anticoagulation is commonly used to prevent clotting and to increase the life span of the dialysis filter. Commonly used methods in current practice are systemic anticoagulation, regional anticoagulation, and no anticoagulation (i.e., using saline). Systemic anticoagulation may be more effective but there is an increased bleeding risk compared to regional anticoagulation (citrate-calcium, heparin-protamine). Regional heparin anticoagulation (RHA) and regional citrate anticoagulation (RCA) are two common regional anticoagulation techniques used in clinical practice. A study that compared both practices showed more adverse effects with RHA, due to protamine component and increased bleeding risk.[34] Recent literature is favoring RCA due to its efficacy and minimal adverse events.[35] Though the trials have not shown any mortality benefit or increased filter life span with either RCA versus systemic anticoagulation, the trend toward preferring RCA does exist. Among systemic anticoagulation, heparin may be preferred due to its easy reversibility rather low molecular weight heparin (LMWH). KDIGO guidelines recommend RCA over systemic anticoagulation, though there is no robust evidence.[28] It is more accepted as well as a common practice to do anticoagulation-free dialysis in patients with coagulopathy, thrombocytopenia, and who have the potential to bleed. In such conditions, the filter survival can be prolonged by minimizing hemoconcentration either by predilution with saline or intermittent saline flushes.[36] In the perioperative setting, the anticoagulation preference may be influenced by bleeding risk, planned invasive procedures, mode of dialysis, and presence of catheters such as epidural catheters. As of now, there is no clear consensus which anticoagulation to use, but it should be tailored to patient needs, and if available RCA can be considered a preferred choice, while heparin could be a reasonable alternative.

Other Special Situations: Requiring Intraoperative Renal Replacement Therapy

Certain surgeries and certain patient profile pose a real challenge to perform RRT in such situations. Patients undergoing liver transplantation are at high risk of fluid and electrolyte disturbances and reperfusion injury. Many studies have used intraoperative dialysis to manage fluid balance with successful outcomes.[37] Many studies were done with continuous modes of RRT considering the risk of massive fluid shifts and cerebral dysfunction in such patients. Also in patients where handling potassium is difficult, intraoperative dialysis was performed especially in cardiac surgeries with cardioplegia.[38] Patients with compromised baseline renal functions may require intraoperative dialysis to maintain fluids and electrolyte balance; this is commonly practiced in heart surgeries in ESRD patients.[39]

End-stage Renal Disease Patients

Patients with chronic kidney disease (and also ESRD) are increasing and number of these patients who require major surgeries is also increasing. It is a real challenge when we face dialysis-dependent chronic renal failure patients undergoing complex surgeries. When to schedule dialysis before surgery, its timing, and how to prevent conditions that may require emergency dialysis such as fluid overload, acidosis, hyperkalemia is a matter of debate and is more often based on clinical judgment. Moreover, the situation becomes more complex when such patients undergo cardiac surgeries since the heart is also very sensitive to fluid overload, acidosis, and electrolyte disturbances. Many studies have addressed this issue with different approaches to obtain a favorable outcome.[40] The common approach was to do intraoperative dialysis with ultrafiltration during cardiac surgeries (especially during coronary artery bypass surgeries). Both hemodialysis and continuous RRT were tried with each having its own advantages and limitations.

End-stage renal disease patients may have fluid overload, hypertension, electrolyte disturbances, high urea, and other metabolic derangements that may affect the outcome of the surgery. Also, surgery and medicines used during surgery including anesthesia may cause hemodynamic disturbances, fluid shifts further adding to complications. In general, to optimize the ESRD patient before surgery, perioperative dialysis is required to correct fluid status, electrolyte, and metabolic abnormalities to remove uremic toxins. As common practice, ESRD patients undergo dialysis 24 hours prior to surgery to achieve euvolemia, i.e., closer to their dry weight and to correct metabolic abnormalities.[41] The appropriate timings of preoperative dialysis are not clear due to scarcity of clinical data. The decision may depend on several factors including patient-related and also anticipated increased bleeding risk due to anticoagulation given during dialysis. Heparin may be preferred over other long-acting agents to reduce perioperative bleeding risk. As heparin is short-acting, elective surgeries can be scheduled after 6 hours. In patients at higher risk, anticoagulant free or saline dialysis can be done knowing the high risk of filter clotting. Postoperatively, the patients may require dialysis for fluid and electrolyte balance and to facilitate extubation, especially when there is influence of sedative drugs and metabolic abnormalities. In general, hemodialysis is preferred due to ease of use, less time need, and nursing ease in hemodynamically stable patients. CRRT/SLEDD may be considered over HD in hemodynamically unstable patients or patients with multiorgan dysfunction.

Renal Replacement Therapy in Perioperative Setting—A Rational and Reasonable Approach

Perioperative patients have high metabolic demands, nutritional needs, and are at risk of organ dysfunction. Choosing timing, mode, and conduct of RRT cannot be predetermined to specific groups of patients based on set criteria (AKIN, KDIGO). Patients even at advanced stages of these grading, AKIN-III, KDIGO-3, may recover their kidney function without the need of dialysis. RRT should be chosen based on the kidney capacity to meet the demand (solute, fluids, etc.), dynamics of demand (requirement of more volume, hypercatabolic state, (increased metabolic demand—common after major surgeries), electrolyte imbalances e.g. hyperkalemia, etc.), and patient organ tolerance to meet the demand (e.g., cardiac function to meet excessive fluids, acidosis).[42] Patients may pose various dynamic challenges during perioperative period with changing metabolic demand and increased risk of compromising different organ functions. So, facing patients with compromised baseline kidney function (chronic kidney disease) with normal demands may also pose a threat compared to facing high demand in patients with good renal function. So, it is reasonable to judge the demand and renal capacity and balance out the decision on initiating RRT. Also, attention to intraoperative details (bleeding risk, presence of epidural catheter, risks of renal injury during surgery, hypotension, aortic clamping, myocardial injury, rhabdomyolysis, etc.) is important to anticipate postoperative deterioration of renal function and to plan preemptive RRT.

The selection of a particular mode in the perioperative period may depend on patient characteristics, availability, and experience of staff. CRRT is preferred in patients who cannot tolerate fluid and osmotic shifts, hemodynamically unstable patients such as those undergoing cardiac surgeries with compromised heart function, liver transplant surgeries, and comatose patients with cerebral edema.[42] When the need is to rapidly remove the toxins and electrolyte, then IHD may be preferred for quick benefits. Hybrid therapies can be chosen as alternative to the other two approaches, tailoring to individual patients pending more evidence.

Personalizing and tailoring the RRT to suit the patient is of prime importance in perioperative setting, knowing the dynamics of metabolic demand and renal capacity. Also, choice of modality may change from time to time. RRT dosing and indications should be individualized for demand. More evidence is required to answer some of these unresolved questions.

▌CONCLUSION

Acute kidney injury requiring RRT is common in the perioperative period. There are no clear guides on when to initiate and how to conduct of RRT; the existing evidence is inconclusive and controversial. warranting an individualized approach. Due attention should be paid and focused on all events occurring during the perioperative period that may help to tailor the RRT for the patient. Balancing the metabolic demand and renal capacity to handle the demand is crucial to decide on RRT, and this may be a reasonable approach to manage patients with renal failure.

REFERENCES

1. Liaño F, Junco E, Pascual J, Madero R, Verde E. The spectrum of acute renal failure in the intensive care unit compared with that seen in other settings. Kidney Int Suppl. 1998;66:S16-24.

2. Uchino S, Kellum JA, Bellomo R, Doig GS, Morimatsu H, Morgera S, et al. Acute renal failure in critically ill patients: a multinational, multicenter study. JAMA. 2005;294:813-8.

3. Hoste EA, Bagshaw SM, Bellomo R, Cely CM, Colman R, Cruz DN, et al. Epidemiology of acute kidney injury in critically ill patients: The multinational AKI-EPI study. Intensive Care Med. 2015;41:1411-23.

4. Metnitz PG, Krenn CG, Steltzer H, Lang T, Ploder J, Lenz K, et al. Effect of acute renal failure requiring renal replacement therapy on outcome in critically ill patients. Crit Care Med. 2002;30:2051-8.

5. Cole L, Bellomo R, Silvester W, Reeves JH. A prospective, multicenter study of the epidemiology, management, and outcome of severe acute renal failure in a "closed" ICU system. Am J Respir Crit Care Med. 2000;162:191-6.

6. Boyd O, Jackson N. Clinical review: How is risk defined in high-risk surgical patient management? Crit Care. 2005;9:390-6.

7. Scheel PJ, Liu M, Rabb H. Uremic lung: New insights into a forgotten condition. Kidney Int. 2008;74:849-51.

8. Gallagher M, Cass A, Bellomo R, Finfer S, Gattas D, Lee J, et al.; POST-RENAL Study Investigators and the ANZICS Clinical Trials Group. Long-term survival and dialysis dependency following acute kidney injury in intensive care: extended follow-up of a randomized controlled trial. PLoS Med. 2014;11:e1001601.

9. Ichai C, Vinsonneau C, Souweine B, Armando F, Canet E, Clec'h C, et al. Acute kidney injury in the perioperative period and in intensive care units (excluding renal replacement therapies). Ann Intensive Care. 2016;1:48.

10. Sato Y, Kato TS, Oishi A, Yamamoto T, Kuwaki K, Inaba H, et al. Preoperative factors associated with postoperative requirements of renal replacement therapy following cardiac surgery. Am J Cardiol. 2015;116:294-300.

11. Lin E, Lowry SF. Inflammatory cytokines in major surgery: A functional perspective. Intensive Care Med. 1999;25:255-7.

12. Shoemaker WC, Appel PL, Kram HB, Waxman K, Lee TS. Prospective trial of supranormal values of survivors as therapeutic goals in high-risk surgical patients. Chest 1988;94:1176-86.

13. Malbrain ML, Marik PE, Witters I, Cordemans C, Kirkpatrick AW, Roberts DJ, et al. Fluid overload, de-resuscitation, and outcomes in critically ill or injured patients: a systematic review with suggestions for clinical practice. Anestezjol Intens Ter. 2014;46:361-80.

14. Semler MW, Self WH, Wanderer JP, Ehrenfeld JM, Wang L, Byrne DW, et al. Balanced crystalloids versus saline in Critically Ill adults. N Engl J Med. 2018;378:829-39.

15. Self WH, Semler MW, Wanderer JP, Wang L, Byrne DW, Collins SP, et al. Balanced crystalloid versus saline in noncritically ill adults. N Engl J Med. 2018;378:819-28.

16. Wilkens MM, Navickis RJ. Postoperative renal replacement therapy after hydroxyethyl starch infusion: A meta-analysis of randomised trials. Netherlands J Crit Care. 2014;18:4-9.

17. Fayad AI, Buamscha DG. Timing of renal replacement therapy initiation for acute kidney injury. Cochrane Database Syst Rev. 2018;12:CD010612.

18. Yang XM, Tu GW, Zheng JL, Shen B, Ma GG, Hao GW, et al. A comparison of early versus late initiation of renal replacement therapy for acute kidney injury in critically ill patients: An updated systematic review and meta-analysis of randomized controlled trials. BMC Nephrol. 2017;18:264.

19. Karvellas CJ, Farhat MR, Sajjad I, Mogensen SS, Leung AA, Wald R. A comparison of early versus late initiation of renal replacement therapy in critically ill patients with acute kidney injury: a systematic review and meta-analysis. Crit Care. 2011;15:R72.

20. Gaudry S, Hajage D, Schortgen F, Martin-Lefevre L, Pons B, Boulet E, et al. Initiation strategies for renal-replacement therapy in the intensive care unit. New Engl J Med. 2016;375:122-33.

21. Zarbock A, Kellum JA, Schmidt C, Van Aken H, Wempe C, Pavenstädt H, et al. Effect of early vs delayed initiation of renal replacement therapy on mortality in critically ill patients with acute kidney injury: the ELAIN randomized clinical trial. JAMA. 2016;315:21909.

22. Gaudry S, Hajage D, Schortgen F, Martin-Lefevre L, Verney C, Pons B, et al. Timing of renal support and outcome of septic shock and acute respiratory distress syndrome. A post hoc analysis of the AKIKI randomized clinical trial. Am J Respir Crit Care Med. 2018;198:58-66.

23. Barbar SD, Clere-Jehl R, Bourredjem A, Hernu R, Montini F, Bruyère R, et al. Timing of renal-replacement therapy in patients with acute kidney injury and sepsis. New Engl J Med. 2018;397:1431-42.

24. Zou H, Hong Q, Xu G. Early versus late initiation of renal replacement therapy impacts mortality in patients with acute kidney injury post cardiac surgery: a meta-analysis. Crit Care. 2017;21:150.

25. Truche AS, Darmon M, Bailly S, Clec'h C, Dupuis C, Misset B, et al. OSG. Continuous renal replacement therapy versus intermittent hemodialysis in intensive care patients: Impact on mortality and renal recovery. Intensive Care Med. 2016;42:1408-17.

26. Birne R, Branco P, Marcelino P, Marum S, Fernandes AP, Viana H, et al. A comparative study of cardiovascular rability with slow extended dialysis versus continuous haemodiafiltration in the ical patient. Port J Nephrol Hypertens. 2009;23:323-30.

27. Zhang L, Yang J, Eastwood GM, Zhu G, Tanaka A, Bellomo R, et al. Extended daily dialysis versus continuous renal replacement therapy for acute kidney injury: A meta-analysis. Am J Kidney Dis. 2015;66:322-30.

28. Khwaja A. KDIGO clinical practice guidelines for acute kidney injury. Nephron Clin Pract. 2012;120:c179-84.

29. VA/NIH Acute Renal Failure Trial Network, Palevsky PM, Zhang JH, O'Connor TZ, Chertow GM, Crowley ST, et al. Intensity of renal support in critically ill patients with acute kidney injury. N Engl J Med 2008;359(1):7-20.

30. RENAL Replacement Therapy Study Investigators, Bellomo R, Cass A, Cole L, Finfer S, Gallagher M, et al. Intensity of continuous renal-replacement therapy in critically ill patients. N Engl J Med 2009;361(17):1627-38.

31. Joannes-Boyau O, Honoré PM, Perez P, Bagshaw SM, Grand H, Canivet JL, et al. High-volume versus standard-volume haemofiltration for septic shock patients with acute kidney injury (IVOIRE study): A multicentre randomized controlled trial. Intensive Care Med. 2013;39:1535-46.

32. Borthwick EM, Hill CJ, Rabindranath KS, Maxwell AP, McAuley DF, Blackwood B. High-volume haemofiltration for sepsis in adults. Cochrane Database Syst Rev 2017;1:CD008075.

33. Vesconi S, Cruz DN, Fumagalli R, Kindgen-Milles D, Monti G, Marinho A, et al. Delivered dose of renal replacement therapy and mortality in critically ill patients with acute kidney injury. Crit Care. 2009;13:R57.

34. Gattas DJ, Rajbhandari D, Bradford C, Buhr H, Lo S, Bellomo R. A randomized controlled trial of regional citrate versus regional heparin anticoagulation for continuous renal replacement therapy in critically ill adults. Crit Care Med. 2015;43:1622-9.

35. Hetzel GR, Schmitz M, Wissing H, Ries W, Schott G, Heering PJ, et al. Regional citrate versus systemic heparin for anticoagulation in critically ill patients on continuous venovenous haemofiltration: A prospective randomized multicentre trial. Nephrol Dial Transpl. 2011;26:232-9.

36. Joannidis M, Oudemans-van Straaten HM. Clinical review: Patency of the circuit in continuous renal replacement therapy. Crit Care. 2007;11:218.

37. Dinorcia J, Meouchy J, Genyk YS, Nadim MK. Perioperative renal replacement therapy in liver transplantation. Int Anesthesiol Clin. 2017;55:81-91.

38. Khoo MS, Braden GL, Deaton D, Owen S, Germain M, O'Shea M, et al. Outcome and complications of intraoperative hemodialysis during cardiopulmonary bypass with potassium-rich cardioplegia. Am J Kidney Dis. 2003;41:1247-56.

39. Ilson BE, Bland PS, Jorkasky DK, Shusterman N, Allison NL, Dubb JW, et al. Intraoperative versus routine hemodialysis in end-stage renal disease patients undergoing open-heart surgery. Nephron. 1992;61:170-5.

40. Kamohara K, Yoshikai M, Yunoki J, Fumoto H, Murayama J, Hamada M, et al. Safety of perioperative hemodialysis and continuous hemodiafiltration for dialysis patients with cardiac surgery. Gen Thorac Cardiovasc Surg. 2007;55:43-9.

41. Renew JR, Pai SL. A simple protocol to improve safety and reduce cost in hemodialysis patients undergoing elective surgery. Middle East J Anaesthesiol. 2014;22:487-92.

42. Ostermann M, Joannidis M, Pani A, Floris M, De Rosa S, Kellum JA, et al. Patient selection and timing of continuous renal replacement therapy. Blood Purif. 2016;42:224-37.

62

Postoperative Pulmonary Complications

Suresh Ramasubban

INTRODUCTION

More than 230 million patients undergo surgery every year with a mortality figure ranging from 1 to 4%. Patients who survive, also suffer significant morbidity. Postoperative pulmonary complications (PPCs) are a major cause of the postoperative mortality and morbidity around the world. Until recently, PPC has been loosely defined under various individual complications; however, it is only recently that an all-encompassing definition of PPC has been made. Due to the vagaries of definition and the varying patient population and type of surgery, the incidence of PPC ranges from 20 to 80%. In this chapter, we aim to understand the impact of PPC, why it occurs, i.e., its pathophysiology, how to identify at-risk patients, prediction tools for PPC, prevention of PPC, and the clinical manifestations and management of PPC.

DEFINITION

Postoperative pulmonary complications were a medley of various conditions such as pneumonia, respiratory failure, atelectasis, etc., and the literature abounds with definitions of these individual entities. It is only after 2015, when a European Joint Task Force published guidelines defining European Perioperative Clinical Outcomes (EPCO), which we have an all-inclusive, composite definition of PPC.[1] The EPCO guidelines defined outcome measures into four categories: (1) individual adverse events definitions, (2) composite outcome measures, (3) healthcare resource use, and (4) quality of life measures. According to the EPCO guidelines, PPC includes respiratory infections, respiratory failure, pleural effusion, atelectasis, pneumothorax, bronchospasm, and aspiration pneumonitis (**Table 1**), while pneumonia, acute respiratory distress syndrome (ARDS), and pulmonary embolism are defined as individual adverse events. The definitions are evidence-based and self-explanatory and are enumerated in the **Table 1**.

Table 1: Definitions of postoperative pulmonary complications (PPC): Based of the European Perioperative Clinical Outcome (EPCO) definitions.

Outcome measures	Definition
Respiratory infection	*Initiation of antibiotics for suspected infection with one or more of the following:* new or changed sputum, new or changed lung opacities, fever, leukocytosis
Respiratory failure	Postoperative PaO_2 <60 mm Hg on room air, PaO_2/FiO_2 ratio <300 mm Hg, or oxyhemoglobin saturation <90%
Pleural effusion	Chest X-ray with blunting of costophrenic angle, loss of sharp silhouette of the hemidiaphragm in upright position, or hazy opacity in supine films in one hemithorax with preserved vascular shadows
Atelectasis	Lung opacification with shift of mediastinum, hilum, or hemidiaphragm toward the affected side with hyperinflation of nonatelectatic lungs
Pneumothorax	Presence of air in the pleural space with no vascular bed surrounding the visceral pleura
Bronchospasm	Presence of a newly detected expiratory wheeze treated with bronchodilators
Aspiration pneumonitis	Acute lung injury following aspiration of gastric contents
Pneumonia	Chest X-ray with at least one of the following: infiltrate, consolidation, cavitation *plus* any one of the following: fever, leukopenia, or leukocytosis, elderly with altered mental status and no other cause *plus* at least two of the following: new purulent sputum, increased secretions/suctioning requirement, new/worsening cough/dyspnea/tachypnea/worsening gas exchange
ARDS	Standard Berlin definition is acceptable
Tracheobronchitis	No specific definition as per EPCO guidelines
Pulmonary edema	No definition
Exacerbation of pre-existing lung disease	No definition
Pulmonary embolism	Standard definition
Death	

(ARDS: acute respiratory distress syndrome; FiO_2: fraction of inspired oxygen; PaO_2: partial pressure of oxygen)

EPIDEMIOLOGY

With >230 million surgeries being performed annually across the world, the impact of PPC is obvious. The incidence of PPC in major surgeries ranges from <1% to 23%. In fact several studies have shown a higher incidence of PPC as compared to cardiac complications. Among the PPC, postoperative respiratory failure is the most common cause of PPC. The mortality without a proper composite definition of PPC, i.e., before 2010 varies from 0.2 to 19%. In the era following composite definition of PPC, the major studies such as Assess Respiratory Risk In Surgical patients in Catalonia (ARISCAT)[2] and Prospective Evaluation of a Risk Score for Postoperative Pulmonary Complications in Europe (PERISCOPE)[3] have demonstrated a mortality of 8.3–19.5%. The impact of PPC is such that one in five patients who have a PPC will die within 30 days of major surgery in contrast to 0.2–3% in those without PPC undergoing major surgery. The impact of PPC on long-term mortality is also significant, 45.9% versus 8.7% at 1 year. PPC also influences morbidity, and the length of stay is increased by 13–17 days. An obvious corollary to the increased mortality and morbidity is an increased health care cost, which has been quantified in some studies to be as high as $25,000. There are no studies regarding cost increase in a developing country such as India.

PATHOPHYSIOLOGY

Postoperative pulmonary complication being an assortment of various disease processes ranging from atelectasis to pleural effusion to pulmonary embolism, the pathophysiology leading to PPC are better understood in terms of the changes to the respiratory system during the intraoperative period, immediate postoperative period, and postoperative period.[4]

Intraoperative Changes

There are multiple, universal changes in the respiratory system after induction of anesthesia; some of the important ones are described here:

- Depression of central respiratory drive following general anesthesia (GA) resulting in prolonged apnea and a decrease in minute ventilation.
- Decrease in ventilatory responses to hypercapnia and hypoxemia is noted after GA.
- *Decrease in functional residual capacity (FRC):* Increased curvature of the spine, cephalad displacement of the diaphragm, airway obstruction, and decrease in expiratory muscle tone, all lead to a 15–20% decrease in FRC on induction of anesthesia.
- Abnormal regional distribution of ventilation and perfusion ($\dot{V}/\dot{Q}$). Ventilation is affected due to a decrease

in FRC and perfusion is affected due to a decrease in cardiac output. This, along with regional maldistribution of ventilation can lead to areas of both high and low ($\dot{V}/\dot{Q}$) ratios, i.e., dead space fraction and shunt fraction leading to an increased partial pressure of carbon dioxide ($PaCO_2$) and decreased partial pressure of oxygen (PaO_2).

- *Development of atelectasis:* Atelectasis develops due to direct compression of lung tissue by cephalad displacement of diaphragm. Closure of airways when FRC decreases below closing volume and rapid resorption of gases from the airways beyond these closed airways also results in atelectasis. The resorption of gases is exacerbated by using 100% O_2, due to the absence of nitrogen in the narrow airways and absorption of oxygen into the alveolar capillaries.

Immediate Postoperative Changes

The change seen in the respiratory system in the immediate postoperative period, whilst the patient is in the postoperative recovery room, predominantly is hypoxia. This is due to a decreased respiratory drive from continued effects of sedation and narcotics. The ventilatory response to hypoxia and hypercapnia continues to be decreased for a few hours after GA. Neuromuscular blocking drugs (NMBD) have a residual effect on the tone of the muscles of the pharynx and airway even after conventional tests demonstrate recovery from paralysis. This residual effect of NMDB can persist up to 6 hours and lead to airway obstruction and hypoxia. The decrease in FRC seen after GA also persists in this period especially after major surgery. After minor surgery, FRC returns to normal within a few hours. Atelectasis can also persist in the immediate postoperative period. A consequence of all these effects on the respiratory system is hypoxia.

Postoperative Changes

In the postoperative period beyond the recovery room, changes in the respiratory system persist. These include a persistent low FRC, especially after upper abdominal surgeries, which reaches its lowest value 1–2 days after surgery and returns to normal after 5–7 days. Atelectasis too can persist after major surgery, so also the abnormal respiratory response to hypoxia and hypercapnia. The effort-dependent pulmonary function tests such as forced expiratory volume in the first second (FEV1) and forced vital capacity (FVC) remain low for a few days.

All these abovementioned pathophysiologic changes especially reduced FRC, residual atelectasis, and abnormal respiratory response in the intraoperative, immediate postoperative, and postoperative period lead to the development of PPC.

RISK FACTORS FOR DEVELOPING POSTOPERATIVE PULMONARY COMPLICATION

Factors that contribute to the development of PPC are numerous and they are classified by the American College of Physicians (ACP) as patient-related, procedure-related, or laboratory-testing–related risk factors.[5] All the factors are as described in **Table 2**; only a few relevant factors are described in the text that follows. The relevant nonmodifiable factors are:

- *Age*: It is a nonmodifiable risk factor and advancing age is an important risk factor for predicting PPC. Age >60–65 is considered as risk factor in multiple studies. The factor that is not represented by age is frailty. Frailty even when adjusted for age is a risk factor for PPC.
- *Surgery*: The type of surgery is one of the most important nonmodifiable risk factors that affects the incidence of PPC. The surgery with the highest risk of PPC is repair of abdominal aortic aneurysm. This is followed by with thoracic surgery, upper abdominal surgery, neck surgery, neurosurgery, and major vascular surgery. Among the abdominal surgeries, laparotomy with an upper abdominal incision has a 15-fold higher risk for PPC as compared to a lower abdominal incision.
- *Preoperative investigations*: Traditionally, spirometry, arterial blood gases (ABG), and chest X-ray (CXR) have been deemed as a predictors of PPC. However, statistical analysis has not shown any superiority of these factors; and clinical assessment alone is good enough in most cases. To this extent, the National Institute for Health and Care Excellence (NICE) guidelines[6] recommend spirometry and ABG to be performed only on the request of a senior anesthetist in patients with American Society of Anaesthesiology (ASA) class III and IV, and there is no role of routine CXR. What has shown to be predictive of PPC seems to be a simple bedside supine saturation on room air [peripheral capillary oxygen saturation (SpO_2)]. Patients with SpO_2 in supine position < 90% were 10 times as likely to get a PPC as patients with SpO_2 >96%.

Modifiable Risk Factors

The modifiable risk factors for PPC are also numerous and the relevant factors are discussed here:

- *Comorbidity*: Comorbidities such as presence of chronic obstructive pulmonary disease (COPD), congestive heart failure (CHF), chronic liver disease (CLD), and obstructive sleep apnea (OSA) are independent risk factors for PPC. Comorbidities are modifiable only to a certain extent, such that preoperative optimization is possible. COPD should be treated with bronchodilators and oral or inhaled steroids. In the event of a respiratory infection in the last 30-days prior to surgery, elective surgery should be postponed until symptoms and lung function return to baseline. However, if the surgery is urgent, an individual patient decision must be made. CHF should be optimized to ensure minimal symptoms and maximal functionality. OSA patients should be initiated on continuous positive airway pressure (CPAP) therapy and their compliance assessed prior to surgery. Similarly, CLD patients should be optimized by the hepatologists prior to surgery.

Table 2: Risk factors for developing postoperative pulmonary complications (PPC) categorized as per the American College of Physicians Guidelines (ACP).

Patient-related factors	Procedure-related factors	Laboratory testing

Nonmodifiable:
• Age
• Male sex
• ASA > II
• Frailty
• Acute respiratory infection
• Impaired cognition
• Impaired sensorium
• Cerebrovascular accident
• Malignancy
• Weight loss > 10% within last 6 months
• Long-term steroid use
• Prolonged hospitalization
	Nonmodifiable
	• Type of surgery
	  – Upper abdominal
	  – AAA
	  – Thoracic
	  – Neurosurgery
	  – Head and Neck
	  – Vascular
	• Emergency surgery
	• Duration of surgery
	• Reoperation
	• Multiple GA
		• Urea >21 mg/dL
		• Increased creatinine
		• Abnormal LFT
		• Positive cough test*
		• Abnormal preoperative chest x-ray
		• Preoperative anemia (<10 g/dL)
		• Low albumin
		• FEV_1/FVC <0.7 and FEV_1 <80% of predicted

Modifiable: • Smoking • COPD • Asthma • CHF • OSA • BMI >40 kg/m² or <18.5 kg/m² • Hypertension • Chronic liver failure • Renal failure • Diabetes • Preoperative sepsis • Alcohol	Modifiable: • Mechanical ventilation strategy • GA versus regional • Long-acting NMBD and TOF ratio <0.7 • Perioperative nasogastric tube • Neostigmine • Open abdominal surgery versus laparoscopic • Blood transfusion	

*Positive cough test, patient takes a deep breath and coughs once, and a positive test is ongoing coughing after the cough

(AAA: Abdominal aortic aneurysm; ASA: American Society of Anesthesiology; BMI: body mass index; CHF: congestive heart failure; COPD: chronic obstructive pulmonary disease; FEV_1: forced expiratory volume in one second; FVC: forced vital capacity; GA: general anesthesia; LFT: liver function test; NMDB: neuromuscular blocking drugs; OSA: obstructive sleep apnea; TOF: train of four)

- *Smoking*: Active smoking is a risk factor for PPC. Ex-smokers, i.e., those who have not smoked for >4 weeks have a reduced incidence of PPC as compared to current smokers. Comparing never smokers to ex-smokers (>1 year) and current smokers, the risk of PPC decreases from smokers to ex-smokers to never smokers. Smoking cessation before major surgery and achieving a 30-day abstinence decreases rates of PPC. Actual rates of PPC decline much more as cessation time increases, thus farther the time of cessation from time of surgery, less is the likelihood of PPC. A 4-week cessation reduces PPC by 23% and by 8 weeks reduces PPC by 47%.

- *Anemia*: Preoperative hemoglobin values <10 g/dL increase risk of PPC almost three times. Since transfusion also increases risk of PPC, methods to improve hemoglobin should target nontransfusion methods. Treatment options thus include folate, vitamin B12, and iron supplements.

- *General anesthesia*: GA as compared to regional anesthesia for the same surgery has a higher incidence of PPC. However, it is not possible to use local/regional anesthesia in all surgeries. Anesthesia and operating time >2 hours are also risk factor for increased PPC, thus having an experienced surgeon perform surgeries to decrease operating and anesthesia time is a way of decreasing PPC.

- *Ventilatory strategies in operating theater (OT)*: Lung protective ventilation (LPV) in ARDS is well studied and is shown to improve outcomes. Now good evidence exists for the benefit of LPV in the OT to prevent PPC. LPV consists of low tidal volume (TV) ventilation, optimal positive end-expiratory pressure (PEEP), and recruitment maneuvers (RM). Low TV (<8 mL/kg) has been shown to decrease PPC as compared to high TV (>8 mL/kg) irrespective of PEEP values. Moderate PEEP (10 cmH$_2$O) along with RM also have shown to decrease PPC; however, there are studies which have not shown any benefit of moderate-to-high PEEP and in fact these studies have pointed to harm. Hemodynamic compromise is significant in the higher PEEP group.

- *Neuromuscular blockers*: The association between NMBD and PPC has long been known since the era of curare. Recent studies with long-acting NMBD such as pancuronium, with a train of four (TOF) ratio <0.7 are also associated with increased incidence of PPI. As described in the pathophysiology section, NMBD causes airway obstruction even after traditional tests for reversal are positive. Even reversal agents such as neostigmine have effects on the genioglossus and upper airway musculature leading to airway obstruction and hypoxia. Newer reversal agents such as Sugammadex also have effects like laryngospasm and negative pressure

pulmonary edema. The use of even short-acting and intermediate-acting NMBD is paradoxically associated with PPC. The best preventive strategy would thus be avoidance of NMBD as much as possible.

CLINICAL MANIFESTATION AND MANAGEMENT OF POSTOPERATIVE PULMONARY COMPLICATIONS

Since the term PPC describes a heterogeneous group of clinical disorders, it is not possible to describe the management of all the complications. There are chapters which deal with certain conditions such as OSA, infection/sepsis, and respiratory failure. So this chapter will focus on the clinical manifestation and management of certain important conditions such as atelectasis, respiratory infections, pneumonia, chemical pneumonitis, and pulmonary edema.

Atelectasis

Atelectasis is one of the most common PPCs; the highest incidence is seen after upper abdominal and thoracic surgeries. The pathophysiology has already been discussed and this section will focus on clinical presentation and management.

Clinical Presentation

Majority of the patients with atelectasis are asymptomatic, whilst others may present with tachypnea and hypoxemia. The onset of hypoxia due to atelectasis is usually not seen in the immediate postoperative period; the severity of atelectasis is maximum during the 2nd postoperative day (POD) and continues through to the 4th or 5th POD. Hypoxia occurring in the immediate postoperative period, i.e., in the recovery room, should be investigated for other causes such as hypoventilation due to residual effects of NMBD and upper airway obstruction due to airway edema.

Management

Management of atelectasis depends on the respiratory secretions. Patients can be categorized into two groups, one with profuse secretions and the other without. Presence of profuse secretions is defined as frequent expectorations, expectoration of large quantities of sputum, and/or significant rhonchi on auscultation of the chest.

Management of atelectasis without profuse secretions: CPAP may be beneficial in patients with hypoxemia or in patients with increased work of breathing. The benefit of CPAP in patients with hypoxemia due to postoperative (major abdominal surgeries) atelectasis has been compared with oxygen alone, and CPAP decreases the incidence of endotracheal intubation, pneumonia, infection, and sepsis as compared to oxygen alone. Despite the limitations of such studies, CPAP use is intuitive in atelectasis and hypoxemia.

Management of atelectasis with profuse secretions: All patients with profuse secretions and atelectasis should undergo frequent suctioning and vigorous chest physiotherapy. Chest physiotherapy refers to postural drainage and percussion; this is especially helpful if there is a unilateral collapse/lobar collapse. Ideally, chest physiotherapy should be performed every 4 hours and consists of 5 minutes of chest percussion, 5 minutes of postural drainage, deep breathing to total lung capacity for 3 minutes using an incentive spirometer, and coughing or tracheal suctioning if cough is ineffective. On mechanically ventilated patients, deep breathing can be performed using an anesthesia bag to provide multiple 1–2 L inflations. The role of therapeutic suctioning using a flexible fiberoptic bronchoscope (FOB) is uncertain. FOB and therapeutic aspiration of secretion is indicated only on failure of suctioning and chest physiotherapy. Role of mucolytics such as N-acetylcysteine is also uncertain and evidence for their benefit is lacking. In patients with profuse secretions, CPAP becomes a relative contraindication and should be avoided.

Bronchospasm

In the postoperative period, bronchospasm is a common complication, presenting as either dyspnea, chest tightness, or wheezing and manifesting with small tidal volumes, prolonged expiratory time, and hypercapnic respiratory failure. Bronchospasm can be precipitated by aspiration, histamine release due to drugs (e.g., atracurium, opiates etc.), allergic reaction to drugs, and exacerbation of underlying chronic diseases such as asthma/COPD. Bronchospasm is also a result of smooth muscle constriction due to stimulation due to suctioning, intubation, and other surgical stimulation. Treatment is mainly directed at the underlying cause, removing the inciting medication/ agent, and bronchodilators. Bronchodilation is achieved preferably with short acting β-2-agonists and systemic glucocorticoids are reserved for patients unresponsive to β-2-agonists. For patients with exacerbations of their asthma/COPD, management is as it would remain in any other case.

Pneumonia

Pneumonia in the postoperative period has clinical manifestations and management similar to those of any other type of hospital-acquired (HAP) and ventilator-associated pneumonia (VAP). However, pneumonia as a PPC has certain characteristic risk factors and treatment considerations. Postoperative pneumonia tends to occur in the first 5 PODs. Clinical recognition is based on the presence of an infiltrate, consolidation, cavitation plus one of the following:

- Fever >38°C, with no other cause
- White blood cell count <4 or >12 × 10^3 mm^3
- More than 70 years of age with altered mental status with no other cause
- *Plus at least two of the following:*
  - New purulent secretions
  - Increased secretions/suctioning requirement
  - New cough/dyspnea/rales/bronchial breath sounds/ worsening gas exchange.

The diagnosis is however difficult, as there are many other causes of postoperative fever and abnormal X-ray; most important is atelectasis and pulmonary embolism. The other unique feature of pneumonia as a PPC is in the pathogen causing pneumonia. Pathogens are usually resistant organisms and are predominantly gram-negative organisms, especially *Pseudomonas* and *Acinetobacter* species. Certain surgeries have a predilection for certain pathogen, for instance, *Staphylococcus* with neurosurgery, *Streptococcus pneumoniae* with trauma. Management involves collecting respiratory specimen before initiation of empiric treatment. Empiric treatment should follow the guidelines for antibiotics as outlined for HAP/VAP by the Indian Society of Critical Care Medicine (ISCCM). However, antibiotic selection for a pneumonia following an operation should consider gram-negative pathogens as the predominant pathogen, especially *Pseudomonas* and *Acinetobacter*. Routine anaerobic coverage is probably not necessary but may be considered following thoracoabdominal surgeries.

Aspiration Pneumonitis

Postoperative patients are at risk of aspirating the acidic gastric contents resulting in aspiration pneumonitis, which is a chemical pneumonitis. The incidence of aspiration is less common in adults and is much more commonly seen in infants and children. In adults aspiration is rare, with a reported incidence of 1 in 3,200 procedures. It is classically reported as Mendelson's syndrome, i.e., aspiration pneumonitis in pregnant patients on a full stomach following ether anesthesia. Pneumonitis manifests as abrupt onset of dyspnea and tachycardia. They may also present with fever, bronchospasm, hypoxemia, cyanosis, and/or pink frothy sputum. The clinical course of the acute lung injury after aspiration of gastric contents varies. Patients can develop secondary bacterial pneumonia, may progress to ARDS, but most of the patients do make a full recovery, especially those who do not develop a cough, wheeze, >10% oxyhemoglobin desaturation, or radiological abnormalities within 2 hours of aspiration. Management of a witnessed aspiration involves immediate turning of the head to the side (lateral position) and suctioning of the patient's oropharynx. Management of chemical pneumonitis is careful monitoring and supplemental oxygen, intubation, and ventilation as required. There is no evidence of any benefit by administering corticosteroids or antibiotics. Antibiotics should be considered if symptoms of pneumonitis are not showing signs of resolution in 48 hours.

Pleural Effusion

It is not uncommon to find small pleural effusions in the postoperative period, within first 48–72 hours. In fact, almost 50% of patients after major thoracoabdominal surgeries will have small effusions, exudate by nature, and will resolve spontaneously. Most of the effusions are picked up radiologically, with blunting of costophrenic angle on CXR. A diagnostic testing is not warranted in most of the cases; it is required only if there are atypical clinical characteristics or atypical characteristics of the effusion. Diagnostic work up follows the same pattern as in a nonoperative patient and management principles also remain the same. Effusions associated with subphrenic abscess are slightly different in that they develop after >10 days after surgery rather than within the first three postoperative days.

Pulmonary Edema

Pulmonary edema that develops in the postoperative period can be cardiogenic, noncardiogenic, or a combination of both. ARDS is a form of noncardiogenic pulmonary edema; however, EPCO defines it as a separate entity. Since management of ARDS would fundamentally be the same as in a nonoperative patient, ARDS will not be discussed in this section.

Cardiogenic Pulmonary Edema

Postoperative cardiogenic pulmonary edema would typically develop within the first 36 hours of the surgery and is positively correlated with fluid retention. The diagnosis and management of cardiogenic pulmonary edema would also be dealt in the chapter on postoperative cardiac complications.

Negative Pressure Pulmonary Edema

It is one of the most important causes of noncardiogenic pulmonary edema in the postoperative period, especially following extubation. Extubation can result in laryngospasm and upper airway obstruction which leads to a generation of negative pressure in the thorax consequent to the patient trying to inhale against a fully or partially closed glottis (Mueller maneuver). Patients usually develop dyspnea

with pink frothy sputum and radiological features of pulmonary edema immediately following relief of upper airway obstruction. Occasionally, the pulmonary edema can develop a few hours after the relief of obstruction. The incidence of negative pressure pulmonary edema is estimated at 0.05–0.1% of all procedures requiring intubation and GA. Risk factors for developing negative pressure pulmonary edema are the same as that of developing upper airway obstruction, i.e., obesity, short neck, OSA, or acromegaly. However, laryngospasm-related negative pressure pulmonary edema has no such risk factor, but it has been noted that young, healthy, athletic adults tend to develop more edema than others. Treatment of patients with negative pressure pulmonary edema is mainly supportive with supplemental oxygen. Diuretics may be useful in patients who are hypervolemic. CPAP may be helpful, provided there is no upper airway obstruction. A few patients will require to be reintubated, otherwise in most of the patients it resolves on its own.

CONCLUSION

Postoperative pulmonary complications are a major cause of morbidity and mortality worldwide. PPC encompasses a wide range of different conditions, which have now been merged under the umbrella term of PPC by the EPCO study group. The impact of PPC using these definitions gives us a clear picture of the incidence, which is about 5–7.9% for a multispecialty elective and emergency surgery. The pathogenesis of PPC relates to the change in respiratory physiology starting intraoperatively and continuing in the immediate and late postoperative phase. The decrease in respiratory drive, the ventilatory response to hypoxia and hypercapnia, the decrease in FVC, all start intraoperatively and continue to be a major pathophysiologic feature in the postoperative period. The main consequence is atelectasis and hypoxia, which is the main manifestation of the PPC. The PPC can be abrogated to a great extent by identifying at-risk patients and taking preventive measures. Clinical manifestation is varied as the diseases which are lumped under the term PPC is myriad. However, the focus of this chapter has been on identifying and treating atelectasis, pneumonia, chemical pneumonitis, and negative pressure pulmonary edema.

REFERENCES

1. Jammer I, Wickboldt N, Sander M, Smith A, Schultz MJ, Pelosi P, et al. Standards for definition and use of outcome measure for clinical effectiveness research in perioperative medicine. European perioperative clinical outcome (EPCO) definitions: A statement from the ESA-ESICM joint taskforce on perioperative outcome measures. Eur J Anaesthesiol. 2015;32:88-105.

2. Canet J, Gallart L, Gomar C, Paluzie G, Vallès J, Castillo J, et al. Prediction of postoperative pulmonary complications in a population based surgical cohort. Anesthesiology. 2010;113:1338-50.

3. Mazo V, Sabate S, Canet J, Gallart L, de Abreu MG, Belda J, et al. Prospective external validation of a predictive score for postoperative pulmonary complications. Anesthesiology. 2014;121:219-31.

4. Miskovic A, Lumb AB. Postoperative pulmonary complications. Br J Anaesth. 2017;118 (3):317-34.

5. Smetana GW, Lawrence VA, Cornell JE. Preoperative pulmonary risk stratification for non-cardiothoracic surgery: systematic review for the American college of Physicians. Ann Intern Med. 2006;144:581-95.

6. Routine preoperative tests for elective surgery. (2016) NICE guidelines (NG45). [online] Available from https://www.nice.org.uk/guidance/ng45 [Last accessed March, 2020].

Perioperative Mechanical Ventilation

Rajesh Chawla, Prashant Nasa, Aakanksha Chawla Jain

INTRODUCTION

The mechanical ventilation (MV) is an integral part of general anesthesia (GA). Conventionally MV during perioperative period was targeted to attain physiological normal partial pressure of oxygen (PO_2) and carbon dioxide (PCO_2). The negative effect of GA and perioperative ventilation on oxygenation even in patients with normal lungs is known since decades. The understanding of the direct effect of MV on perioperative outcomes in particular, the postoperative pulmonary complications (PPCs) is relatively new. PPCs are currently the second most common perioperative complication after wound infections and contributes to significant morbidity and mortality.[1-3] There is enough good quality evidence of benefit of lung protective ventilation (LPV) to reduce perioperative lung injury (PLI) and PPCs. The understanding of LPV during perioperative period is important because its knowledge has been directly linked to its use in GA.[4] The anesthesiologists should have in depth knowledge of respiratory physiology, understanding of impact of GA and MV on respiratory mechanics and must tailor MV settings to reduce PLI.

PERIOPERATIVE LUNG INJURY

The term PLI is coined for pathophysiological process which includes spectrum of pulmonary inflammation, impaired gas exchange, radiographic abnormalities, and respiratory failure and it is seen after receiving GA in patients with previously noninjured lung.[5-7]

There has been increased understanding of PLI and its contribution to PPCs in last few years. Patients undergoing thoracic and abdominal surgeries have higher risk of PLI. The average incidence of PLI and respiratory failure in thoracic and abdominal surgery is 1.3–4% and 1.2–2.3%, respectively which may increase to 25–28% in high-risk cardiac and aortic surgeries.[8-10] The other preoperative risk predictors for PLI are emergency surgery, advanced age, renal failure, chronic obstructive pulmonary disease

(COPD), pneumonia, alcohol consumption, and low serum albumin.[11] The PLI can have wide presentations from common atelectasis, ventilator-induced lung injury (VILI) to acute respiratory distress syndrome (ARDS).[12,13]

Atelectasis

Atelectasis is common and can occur in up to 90% of the patients after GA.[12,14]

The mechanism of perioperative atelectasis includes:
- *Absorption atelectasis*: Higher fraction of oxygen (FiO_2 more than 80%) concentration during induction and/or maintenance of anesthesia.
- Loss of muscle tone with the use of neuromuscular blockers and anesthetics.
- Reduction of functional residual capacity (FRC) seen during GA and supine positioning.
- *Compression atelectasis:* Compression of lungs and either deficient or abnormal surfactant during anesthesia.

The risk factors of atelectasis are preexisting obstructive airway disease, obesity, smoking, and pregnancy.[14] Preoxygenation with high fraction of oxygen concentration (FiO_2) is a major risk factor for absorption atelectasis and higher the FiO_2, bigger is the risk which may involve typically 10% or more of the lung tissue and in some cases, it may exceed 25% to 40%.[14,16] The atelectasis is common in specific situations like thoracic and abdominal surgery, CO_2 pneumoperitoneum and one-lung ventilation.[14-16] The impact of atelectasis is not only impaired gas exchange, but it also increases the risk of infection or pneumonia postoperatively by impaired clearance of bronchial secretions and lymphatic flow.[15] Atelectasis once developed could persist or even worsen for several days postoperatively.[17]

Ventilator-induced Lung Injuries

The VILI is believed to be result of volutrauma, barotrauma and finally biotrauma due to positive pressure ventilation causing local and systemic inflammatory response and worsening of oxygenation. The pathophysiology of VILI involves a local inflammatory reaction, production of free oxygen radicals, that cause disruption of the alveolar-capillary barrier and alveolar flooding.[6,18] There is accumulation of protein-rich fluid in the interstitial space and alveoli causing gas-exchange abnormalities.[18] VILI initially was described in patients with preexisting lung injury and ARDS undergoing ventilation. Whether intraoperative MV can cause VILI is a matter of debate for some time now. The positive pressure used in MV can cause lung hyperinflation and cyclic stretching of the lungs, which along with higher FiO_2 can causes VILI even in patients with no previous lung injury.[19] Traditional higher TV [10–12 mL/kg of predicted body weight (PBW)] is been recognized as main risk factors for VILI in patients with ARDS undergoing MV. Subsequently, the possibility of it developing in patients undergoing routine GA was studied. Choi et al. found conventional TV of 12 mL/kg without positive end expiratory pressure (PEEP) in major abdominal surgery was associated with systemic inflammation and lung injury in patients with no previous lung disease.[20] The same group then studied the effect of TV of 12 mL/kg PBW versus 6 mL/kg with PEEP of 10 cm H_2O in elective surgeries lasting more than 5 hours and found higher inflammatory markers such as interleukin (IL)-8, myeloperoxidase, and elastase with higher TV.[21] There are other factors which contribute to VILI besides high TV like lateral position and defective or reduced surfactant production. The role of PEEP in VILI is controversial with both nil and high level of PEEP worsening lung injury.[21,22]

Perioperative lung injury is associated with poor perioperative outcomes. The hospital mortality rate of patients with PLI is 22–24% which is 5–10 times of perioperative mortality.[11,23,24] PLI is also associated with more frequent ICU admissions, need of postoperative MV, increased hospital length of stay (LOS), and increased healthcare costs.[25]

Intraoperative Lung Protective Ventilation

Traditionally anesthesiologists were trained to ventilate with tidal volume (TV) intraoperatively of 10–15 mL/kg PBW. The landmark trials of lower TV and moderate PEEP also called LPV in patients with ARDS which changed practice in intensive care units (ICU) in last two decades did not change MV intraoperatively.[26-28]

The practice of intraoperative MV continued with higher TV and little or no PEEP because of lack of enough evidence of LPV in noninjured lung for short duration of anesthesia.[29,30] The research in last decade has been focused to understand the effect of intraoperative lung protective ventilation (ILPV) in and its impact on perioperative outcomes including reduction of PPCs. The ILPV is a combination of TV <8 mL/kg PBW and ≥5 cm H_2O of PEEP, with or without a recruitment maneuver (RM) with aim to reduce VILI and PPCs.

Evidence on ILPV

The PROtective Ventilation group (PROVE) is a group of researchers which have done extensive work on ILPV. In a large scale RCT (IMPROVE trial, 2013), in abdominal surgery ILPV reduces incidence of PILI to 0.5% as compared to 3% in patients who received conventional ventilation.[31]

In thoracic, laparoscopic, and neurosurgeries similar results were found with use of ILPV during GA.[32,33] Recently, trials have found ILPV can also decrease driving pressures (DP) in patients who underwent abdominal surgery.[34,35]

In a Cochrane meta-analysis in 2018 on ILPV during surgery the available evidence showed significant effect of LPV in reducing postoperative pneumonia and other PPCs, the need for ventilatory support (invasive or noninvasive) and hospital LOS. The effects on mortality, barotrauma, and ICU-LOS however are uncertain.[36]

VENTILATOR SETTINGS FOR PERIOPERATIVE VENTILATION

Tidal Volume

The low TV is the most effective component of ILPV strategy. The intraoperative ventilation continues to be with TV > 6 mL/kg despite ARDSnet group trials because of failure of anesthesiologists to calculate PBW, traditional belief that lower TV is harmful and can cause atelectasis or simple lack of knowledge about effect of LPV on PPCs.[4,28] There is however no evidence that low TV is associated with atelectasis.[37] In a RCT on patients undergoing cardiac surgery, a TV of 12 mL/kg PBW versus 6 mL/kg was found to be associated with poorer postoperative lung compliance (14.9 vs. 5.5 mL/cm H_2O; p = 0.002), a higher risk of barotrauma (mean peak airway pressure 7.1 vs. 2.4 cm H_2O; p < 0.001), and increased intrapulmonary shunt (15.5% vs. 21.4%; p = 0.021).[38] In another RCT of around 150 patients in cardiac surgery TV of 6 mL/kg PBW compared to 10 mL/kg was associated with reduced proportion of patients needing ventilator support postoperatively at 6 hours (37.3% vs. 20.3%; p = 0.02) and the incidence of reintubation (1.3% vs. 9.5%; p = 0.03).[39] In 2015, a meta-analysis of 15 studies, found TV of 7 mL/kg PBW versus 10 mL/kg was associated with a significantly reduced risk of PPCs.[40] Yang et al. in another meta-analysis found TV of 6 mL/kg was associated with reduced PPCs reduced hospital LOS in patients undergoing general surgery.[41] Finally a Cochrane meta-analysis in 2018 found that TVs (6–8 mL/kg PBW) was associated with decrease incidence pneumonia and the need for postoperative ventilatory support as compared to TV of 10 mL/kg PBW.[36]

The PBW for TV calculation is important, as studies have shown female sex and extremes of weight and female sex where erroneous calculation of PBW is possible, are risk factors for inadvertent higher TV calculation.[42] The international expert panel on LPV in surgical patients recommends based on the above evidence use of a low-tidal-volume ILPV strategy at 6–8 mL/kg PBW.[43]

Positive End Expiratory Pressure

Tidal ventilation without PEEP causes cyclical opening and closing of the collapsed alveoli with each breath cycle producing VILI. The ventilation with zero end expiratory pressure (ZEEP) causes loss of lung volume at end expiration (EELV) and atelectasis.[44-46] The atelectasis will favor loss of lung compliance in some areas and overinflation in others. There are lot of studies which showed the negative effects of MV with low PEEP or ZEEP intraoperatively.[44-48] Anesthesiologists generally avoid using PEEP intraoperatively because of fear of hemodynamic instability due to its effect on cardiac output mandating volume expansion or optimization and perhaps even requirement of vasopressors to maintain blood pressure.[49] The trials of ILPV with low TV (6–8 mL/kg PBW) and moderate PEEP (6–10 cm H_2O) showed reduction of PPCs, cyclical opening of alveoli and atelectasis, and improved respiratory mechanics, compliance, EELV, and oxygenation.[50-53]

The PROVHILO trial, however, comparing high versus low PEEP found no difference in PPCs with either high or low levels of PEEP (≤ 2 cm H_2O vs. 12 cm H_2O) when added to low TV.[49] In another recent RCT higher PEEP was not found useful to reduce PPCs in obese patient undergoing surgery.[54]

The ZEEP is harmful and ILPV (low TV with moderate PEEP) reduces PPCs, there is however debate on optimal level of PEEP perioperatively.[45]

Instead of selecting a fixed PEEP, individualization has been found to be useful.[51] The individualized PEEP could also decrease DP and increase PO_2/FiO_2 ratio, EELV, and lung compliance.[51] Recently in another study in patients undergoing abdominal surgery, the individualized PEEP could reduce postoperative atelectasis and DP and improved oxygenation.[55] In a meta-analysis similar beneficial effect of individualized PEEP was seen.[56] The international expert panel on ILPV recommends an initial PEEP of 5 cm H_2O intraoperatively and thereafter titration or individualized PEEP to target DP and oxygenation.[43]

Fraction of Inspired Oxygen

There is conflicting evidence that MV with high FiO_2 and/or high arterial oxygen levels (hyperoxia) is harmful and is associated with increased PPCs and mortality in critically ill patients.[57-60]

There is moderate evidence of benefit of high oxygen concentration in reducing surgical site infections (SSI) as per recent World Health Organization (WHO) guidelines on prevention of SSI.[61] This recommendation was however criticized due to wide heterogeneity and doubtful reliability of the studies used in the meta-analysis. In another meta-analysis in 2018 with more reliable studies, supplemental oxygen was not associated with reduction of wound infection risk.[62,63] The pathophysiology of complications due to hyperoxia is because of free oxygen radicals induced oxidative stress, coronary and even peripheral vasoconstriction, direct cardiotoxicity, and resorption atelectasis.[64-66]

SpO_2 using pulse oximetry is commonly used to monitor oxygenation and hypoxia intraoperatively but SpO_2 does not detect hyperoxia. FiO_2 should be set to achieve normoxia ($SpO_2 \geq 94\%$) and target FiO_2 as low as possible to achieve desired SpO_2.[43]

Modes of Ventilation

The use of NMBs during GA is quite common in operation room (OR). The loss of respiratory drive thus mandates use one of controlled modes, namely volume-controlled ventilation (VCV), pressure-controlled ventilation (PCV), and dual-controlled modes.

In VCV mode, TV is independent variable while pressure is a dependent variable which rises initially to overcome the respiratory resistance, until the peak is reached and then exhalation starts with the opening of expiratory valve. The anesthesiologist can set VT, respiratory rate (RR), inspiratory to expiratory (I:E) ratio and PEEP. In PCV mode, pressure (Pi) is the independent variable and TV dependent, with a flow-time curve which has a decelerating waveform with initial vertical increment to reach the desired pressure and then a decremental trend. The anesthesiologist can set Pi, RR, I:E ratio, and PEEP. The dual modes are mostly assuring TV and pressure regulated. They have different names depending on the ventilator manufacturer. There is target VT and primarily mode is PCV ventilation with decelerating inspiratory flow, P_i is adjusted to deliver within the set limits to achieve the desired target VT as per the compliance of the lung.[67]

There is no evidence of superiority of one mode over another. In an observational study, VCV was associated with lower incidence of PPCs as compared to PCV.[67] Similarly, VCV is found to beneficial over PCV in obese patients.[68] In other studies PCV was found to be better than VCV because of lower peak inspiratory pressures.[69-71] Currently due to the heterogeneity of the available data, no particular mode can be recommended over other.[43]

Recruitment Maneuvers

Recruitment maneuvers are usually used during GA for reopening of the collapsed alveoli and thus to improve lung mechanics and oxygenation.[72,73] The RM are mostly used after intubation or any other episode of desaturation due to release of positive pressure from breathing circuit disconnection. RMs are not completely safe and complications like hypoxemia and hemodynamic instability are commonly reported so risk-benefit ratio should be assessed before performing RM.[33,49,51,72]

In a recent meta-analysis on use of RM along with LPV intraoperatively in nonobese patients, authors concluded that RM can improve oxygenation and reduce incidence PPCs but caution was advised in view of heterogeneity of studies analyzed.[74]

Recruitment maneuver can be done manually or by using the ventilator. The manual RM is actually sustained lung inflation with higher than usual VT using a reservoir. It is usually difficult to control and may lead to derecruitment of alveoli when patient is switched to ventilator circuit and is thus generally not advocated.

Ventilator-driven RM are of three types: (1) vital capacity, (2) pressure-controlled, or (3) volume-controlled cycling manoeuvres.[34,43]

Vital capacity RM is similar to manual RM with ventilator is used to deliver sustained lung inflation using inspiratory hold.

Pressure controlled RM: Higher PIP is kept for few breaths using PCV for ten consecutive breaths and PIP is decided on the basis of BMI.

Volume controlled RM: There is progressive increase the *VT* by usually 4 mL/kg is done every 3–6 breaths until target P_{plat} of 30–40 cm H_2O is achieved.

The RM should be done with close monitoring of SpO_2 and BP, and RM should be aborted as soon as any desaturation or hypotension is noted. In view of safety reasons the lowest effective PIP, shortest possible time and fewest number of breaths must be used to achieve desired targets while performing RM. There is always a risk of desaturation even if RM is successful, because of resorption atelectasis especially, if higher FiO_2 is used with RM, so lowest possible FiO_2 must be used.[43]

Emergence from Anesthesia

The emergence from anesthesia is critical phase because of loss of inspiratory efforts on the part of the patient to prevent atelectasis and alveolar derecruitment with residual effect of general anesthesia on lungs and body.

There are various steps which can be taken to prevent alveolar decruitment during emergence from anesthesia and desaturation:
- Avoid ZEEP and patient positioning to head elevation at least 30° to combat the effect of reduced FRC.
- Avoid coughing and bucking on the endotracheal tube.
- Assess and treat any cause of upper airway obstruction after extubation.
- Monitor residual effects of anesthesia avoid and treat apnea and hypopnea.

The routine use of continuous positive airway pressure in all patients and ARM to prevent atelectasis before extubation was not found to be useful.[75] Higher FiO_2 (>0.8) is found to be associated with resorption atelectasis especially during emergence of anesthesia. FiO_2 during emergence may be reduced to prevent atelectasis. Lower FiO_2 (≤0.4) should be used during emergence and SpO_2 target should be >94% in most patients.[76-78]

Postoperative noninvasive ventilation (NIV) is another strategy to reduce atelectasis, desaturation, and to prevent reintubation. In obese patients, postoperative CPAP was found to be useful in reducing risk of PPCs and improve oxygenation and pulmonary function.[79] In patients with abdominal surgery, NIV using CPAP also reduced the incidence of PPCs but optimum CPAP settings is unknown and authors recommended CPAP use should be individualized in such patients.[80]

Intraoperative Monitoring of Lung Mechanics

The plateau pressure (P_{plat}) is the pressure in the alveoli at the end of inspiration and is directly linked to VILI and PPCs.[81] The P_{plat} should be monitored intraoperatively and must be kept less than 30 cm H_2O as advocated in various LPV trials.

The DP (i.e., Plateau pressure [P_{plat}]–PEEP) has recently been recognized as a better marker than P_{plat} as determinant of lung injury and is also linked to PPCs. The target is to achieve a DP as low as possible to reduce the MV-associated complications.[56,82] The P_{plat} is dependent on the respiratory system compliance and hence DP is better tool to predict alveolar distention than P_{plat}. However DP can reflect changes in lung compliance only as long as PEEP is not causing alveolar overinflation. If PEEP causes EEV to increase above FRC then DP may not reflect change in compliance.[83]

Further studies are required to recommend use of DP as intraoperative tool for monitoring.[84] Besides the DP and P_{plat}, dynamic compliance (Crs) should also be measured intraoperatively.[43]

High Flow Nasal Cannula

High flow nasal cannula (HFNC) consists of humidified oxygen at high flow (up to 60 L/min) with a maximum FiO_2 of 1.0 and is increasingly being used in ICU and postoperatively to prevent and treat respiratory failure. RCTs on use of HFNC in postoperative period for prevention of PRF found HFNC is better tolerated and equally efficacious as NIV.[85,86] In another major trial in abdominal surgery patients, HFNC failed to produce any significant reduction of postoperative respiratory failure and PPCs.[87]

Further evidence is thus required to recommend its routine role in either the treatment or prevention of postoperative RF.

POSTOPERATIVE VENTILATION

The ventilation if required postoperatively, it should be also based on similar principles as used intraoperatively. Limited evidence that bundle of prophylactic ILPV and the continuation of LPV postoperatively can reduce the incidence of PPCs.[87]

The indications of postoperative mechanical ventilation can be based on surgical and/or anesthesia related factors.
- Apnea:
  - Residual neuromuscular blockade effect.
  - Altered pulmonary mechanics during surgery (corrected spine surgery, cervical spine or thoracic surgery).
  - Iatrogenic hypothermia
- Pre-existing reduced cardiopulmonary reserve.
- Transplant patients and cardiothoracic surgery: minimize postoperative cardiopulmonary stress
- Surgical factors
  - Unplanned or excessive resection, bleeding and/or fluid shifts during surgery
  - Intraoperative cardiac arrest

The mechanical ventilation in postoperative period as intraoperatively should be aim to prevent any further harm to the patient and to prevent any VILI. The ventilation if required postoperatively, it should be also based on similar principles as used intraoperatively. LPV using low TV of 4–6 mL/kg/PBW with period monitoring of P_{plat} and DP is the core strategy of postoperative ventilation. The FiO_2 should be adjusted to achieve SpO_2 90–94% and adequate PEEP to prevent atelectasis. Limited evidence that bundle of prophylactic ILPV and the continuation of LPV postoperatively can reduce the incidence of PPCs.[87,88]

Sedation for postoperative MV is matter of debate for some time now. Conventionally sedation assessment and weaning of these patients was based on the primary indication for postoperative ventilation. However continuous sedation without assessment may cause oversedation which

is directly linked to increase duration of MV.[89] The sedation assessment should be periodical and the general principles of target-based sedation using objective measures of pain (visual/objective pain assessment scale-VAS/OPAS), agitation (Richmond Agitation-Sedation Scale-RASS), and delirium [Confusion Assessment Method -CAM-ICU] can decreases ventilator days, ICU and hospital LOS.[90,91] The use of shorter acting sedatives like newer alpha-2 agnoists (dexmedetomidine) instead of conventional sedatives like propofol and benzodiazepines are associated with a shorter time to extubation, shorter ICU- LOS, and shorter hospital LOS in postoperative cardiac surgery patients.[92]

Early weaning using spontaneous breathing trials have been found to reduce the number of ventilation days and ICU stay. For most of the surgical cases rapid weaning is effective and well tolerated instead of gradual weaning.[93,94] The factors like preoperative medical conditions of a patient, especially cardiopulmonary status using PaO_2/FiO_2 ratio, ASA class, and surgery whether done in emergency, have to be considered to wean the postoperative mechanical ventilator support and to extubate.[95]

The conventional mode of ventilation like volume-controlled ventilation [VCV], pressure-controlled ventilation [PCV] were shown to have higher ventilator dysynchrony as compared to spontaneous ventilation modes in routine postoperative cardiac surgery patients.[96] Similarly weaning using newer automated modes may reduce the workload on healthcare staff and equally safe.[97] However other advantages like reduced duration of weaning, ventilation, and ICU-LOS is not seen with surgical patients as seen in Medical ICU patients.[98] Weaning using tools rapid shallow breathing index (RSBI) increases the rate of successful extubation than Vital capacity (VC) and Pimax.[95]

CONCLUSION

Intraoperative lung protective ventilation is safe, effective and evidence proof strategy to be used perioperatively in all patients undergoing anesthesia and perioperative ventilation to prevent VILI and PPCs. The TV of less 8 mL/kg PBW and $\geq$5 cm H_2O of PEEP, with or without a RM, FiO_2 to keep SpO_2 >94% are recommended settings for perioperative ventilation.

REFERENCES

1. Shander A, Fleisher LA, Barie PS, Bigatello LM, Sladen RN, Watson CB. Clinical and economic burden of postoperative pulmonary complications: patient safety summit on definition, risk-reducing interventions, and preventive strategies. Crit Care Med. 2011;39(9):2163-72.

2. Miskovic A, Lumb AB. Postoperative pulmonary complications. Br J Anaesth. 2017;118(3):317-34.

3. Rao VK, Khanna AK. Postoperative respiratory impairment is a real risk for our patients: the intensivist's perspective. Anesthesiol Res Pract. 2018;2018:3215923.

4. Kim SH, Na S, Lee WK, Choi H, Kim J. Application of intraoperative lung-protective ventilation varies in accordance with the knowledge of anaesthesiologists: a single-center questionnaire study and a retrospective observational study. BMC Anesthesiol. 2018;18:33.

5. Jabaudon M, Futier E, Roszyk L, Sapin V, Pereira B, Constantin JM. Association between intraoperative ventilator settings and plasma levels of soluble receptor for advanced glycation end-products in patients without pre-existing lung injury. Respirology. 2015;20:1131-8.

6. Zupancich E, Paparella D, Turani F, Munch C, Rossi A, Massaccesi S, et al. Mechanical ventilation affects inflammatory mediators in patients undergoing cardiopulmonary bypass for cardiac surgery: a randomized clinical trial. J Thorac Cardiovasc Surg. 2005;130:378-83.

7. O'Gara B, Talmor D. Perioperative lung protective ventilation. BMJ. 2018;362:k3030.

8. Serpa Neto A, Hemmes SN, Barbas CS, Beiderlinden M, Fernandez-Bustamante A, Futier E, et al. Incidence of mortality and morbidity related to postoperative lung injury in patients who have undergone abdominal or thoracic surgery: a systematic review and meta-analysis. Lancet Respir Med. 2014;2(12):1007-15.

9. Winkler EA, Yue JK, Birk H, Robinson CK, Manley GT, Dhall SS, et al. Perioperative morbidity and mortality after lumbar trauma in the elderly. Neurosurg Focus. 2015;39(4): E2.

10. Kor DJ, Lingineni RK, Gajic O, Park PK, Blum JM, Hou PC, et al. Predicting risk of postoperative lung injury in high-risk surgical patients: a multicenter cohort study. Anesthesiology. 2014;120(5):1168-81.

11. Jin Z, Chun Suen K, Ma D. Perioperative "remote" acute lung injury: recent update. J Biomed Res. 2017;31(3):197-212.

12. Duggan M, Kavanagh BP. Pulmonary atelectasis: a pathogenic perioperative entity. Anesthesiology. 2005;102:838-54.

13. Kogan A, Preisman S, Levin S, Raanani E, Sternik L. Adult respiratory distress syndrome following cardiac surgery. J Card Surg. 2014;29:41-6.

14. Hedenstierna G, Rothen HU. Atelectasis formation during anesthesia: causes and measures to prevent it. J Clin Monit Comput. 2000;16:329-35.

15. Hedenstierna G, Rothen HU. Respiratory function during anesthesia: effects on gas exchange. Compr Physiol. 2012;2(1):69-96.

16. Hedenstierna G, Edmark L. Mechanisms of atelectasis in the perioperative period. Best Pract Res Clin Anaesthesiol. 2010;24(2):157-69.

17. Hedenstierna G, Edmark L. The effects of anesthesia and muscle paralysis on the respiratory system. Intensive Care Med. 2005;31(10):1327-35.

18. Chu EK, Whitehead T, Slutsky AS. Effects of cyclic opening and closing at low-and high-volume ventilation on bronchoalveolar lavage cytokines. Crit Care Med. 2004;32(1):168-74.

19. Meier T, Lange A, Papenberg H, Ziemann M, Fentrop C, Uhlig U, et al. Pulmonary cytokine responses during mechanical ventilation of noninjured lungs with and without end-expiratory pressure. Anesth Analg. 2008;107(4):1265-75.

20. Choi G, Wolthuis EK, Bresser P, Levi M, van der Poll T, Dzoljic M, et al. Mechanical ventilation with lower tidal volumes and positive end-expiratory pressure prevents alveolar coagulation in patients without lung injury. Anesthesiology. 2006;105:689-95.

21. Wolthuis EK, Choi G, Dessing MC, Bresser P, Lutter R, Dzoljic M, et al. Mechanical ventilation with lower tidal volumes and positive end-expiratory pressure prevents pulmonary inflammation in patients without preexisting lung injury. Anesthesiology. 2008;108(1):46-54.

22. Hong CM, Xu DZ, Lu Q, Cheng Y, Pisarenko V, Doucet D, et al. Low tidal volume and high positive end-expiratory pressure mechanical ventilation results in increased inflammation and ventilator-associated lung injury in normal lungs. Anesth Analg. 2010;110(6):1652-60.

23. Zielinski MD, Jenkins D, Cotton BA, Inaba K, Vercruysse G, Coimbra R, et al. Adult respiratory distress syndrome risk factors for injured patients undergoing damage-control laparotomy: AAST multicenter post hoc analysis. J Trauma Acute Care Surg. 2014;77(6):886-91.

24. Canet J, Gallart L, Gomar C, Paluzie G, Vallès J, Castillo J, et al. Prediction of postoperative pulmonary complications in a population-based surgical cohort. Anesthesiology. 2010;113(6):1338-50.

25. Ruhl AP, Lord RK, Panek JA, Colantuoni E, Sepulveda KA, Chong A, et al. Health care resource use and costs of two-year survivors of acute lung injury. An observational cohort study. Ann Am Thorac Soc. 2015;12(3):392-401.

26. Hickling KG, Walsh J, Henderson S, Jackson R. Low mortality rate in adult respiratory distress syndrome using low-volume, pressure-limited ventilation with permissive hypercapnia: a prospective study. Crit Care Med. 1994;22:1568-78.

27. Hess DR, Kondili D, Burns E, Bittner EA, Schmidt UH. A 5-year observational study of lung-protective ventilation in the operating room: a single-center experience. J Crit Care. 2013;28:533.e9-15.

28. Blum JM, Maile M, Park PK, Morris M, Jewell E, Dechert R, et al. A description of intraoperative ventilator management in patients with acute lung injury and the use of lung protective ventilation strategies. Anesthesiology. 2011;115:75-82.

29. Amato MB, Barbas CS, Medeiros DM, Magaldi RB, Schettino GP, Lorenzi-Filho G, et al. Effect of a protective-ventilation strategy on mortality in the acute respiratory distress syndrome. N Engl J Med. 1998;338:347-54.

30. Brower RG, Matthay MA, Morris A, Schoenfeld D, Thompson BT, Wheeler A. Acute Respiratory Distress Syndrome Network ventilation with lower tidal volumes as compared with traditional tidal volumes for acute lung injury and the acute respiratory distress syndrome. N Engl J Med. 2000;342:1301-8.

31. Futier E, Constantin JM, Paugam-Burtz C, Pascal J, Eurin M, Neuschwander A, et al. A trial of intraoperative low-tidal-

volume ventilation in abdominal surgery. N Engl J Med. 2013;369(5):428-37.

32. Sutherasan Y, Vargas M, Pelosi P. Protective mechanical ventilation in the non-injured lung: review and meta-analysis. Crit Care. 2014;18(2):211.

33. Park SJ, Kim BG, Oh AH, Han SH, Han HS, Ryu JH. Effects of intraoperative protective lung ventilation on postoperative pulmonary complications in patients with laparoscopic surgery: prospective, randomized and controlled trial. Surg Endosc. 2016;30(10):4598-606.

34. Ferrando C, Suarez-Sipmann F, Tusman G, León I, Romero E, Gracia E, et al. Open lung approach versus standard protective strategies: effects on driving pressure and ventilatory efficiency during anesthesia: a pilot, randomized controlled trial. PLoS One. 2017;12:e0177399.

35. Ferrando C, Soro M, Unzueta C, Suarez-Sipmann F, Canet J, Librero J, et al. Individualized PeRioperative Open-lung VEntilation (iPROVE) Network Individualised perioperative open-lung approach versus standard protective ventilation in abdominal surgery (iPROVE): a randomised controlled trial. Lancet Respir Med. 2018;6:193-203.

36. Guay J, Ochroch EA, Kopp S. Intraoperative use of low volume ventilation to decrease postoperative mortality, mechanical ventilation, lengths of stay and lung injury in adults without acute lung injury. Cochrane Database Syst Rev. 2018;7:CD011151.

37. Cai H, Gong H, Zhang L, Wang Y, Tian Y. Effect of low tidal volume ventilation on atelectasis in patients during general anesthesia: a computed tomographic scan. J Clin Anesth. 2007;19:125-9.

38. Chaney MA, Nikolov MP, Blakeman BP, Bakhos M. Protective ventilation attenuates postoperative pulmonary dysfunction in patients undergoing cardiopulmonary bypass. J Cardiothorac Vasc Anesth. 2000;14:514-8.

39. Sundar S, Novack V, Jervis K, Bender SP, Lerner A, Panzica P, et al. Influence of low tidal volume ventilation on time to extubation in cardiac surgical patients. Anesthesiology. 2011;114:1102-10.

40. Serpa Neto A, Hemmes SN, Barbas CS, Beiderlinden M, Biehl M, Binnekade JM, et al. Protective versus conventional ventilation for surgery: a systematic review and individual patient data meta-analysis. Anesthesiology. 2015;123:66-78.

41. Yang D, Grant MC, Stone A, Wu CL, Wick EC. A meta-analysis of intraoperative ventilation strategies to prevent pulmonary complications: is low tidal volume alone sufficient to protect healthy lungs? Ann Surg. 2016;263(5):881-7.

42. Jaber S, Coisel Y, Chanques G, Futier E, Constantin JM, Michelet P, et al. A multicentre observational study of intra-operative ventilatory management during general anaesthesia: tidal volumes and relation to body weight. Anaesthesia. 2012;67(9):999-1008.

43. Young CC, Harris EM, Vacchiano C, Bodnar S, Bukowy B, Elliott RRD, et al. Lung-protective ventilation for the surgical patient: international expert panel-based consensus recommendations. Br J Anaesth. 2019;123(6):898-913.

44. Futier E, Constantin JM, Petit A, Jung B, Kwiatkowski F, Duclos M, et al. Positive end-expiratory pressure improves end-

expiratory lung volume but not oxygenation after induction of anaesthesia. Eur J Anaesthesiol. 2010;27(6):508-13.

45. Güldner A, Kiss T, Serpa Neto A, Hemmes SN, Canet J, Spieth PM, et al. Intraoperative protective mechanical ventilation for prevention of postoperative pulmonary complications: a comprehensive review of the role of tidal volume, positive end-expiratory pressure, and lung recruitment maneuvers. Anesthesiology. 2015;123(3):692-713.

46. Östberg E, Thorisson A, Enlund M, Zetterström H, Hedenstierna G, Edmark L. Positive end-expiratory pressure alone minimizes atelectasis formation in nonabdominal surgery: a randomized controlled trial. Anesthesiology. 2018;128(6):1117-24.

47. Wirth S, Kreysing M, Spaeth J, Schumann S. Intraoperative compliance profiles and regional lung ventilation improve with increasing positive end-expiratory pressure. Acta Anaesthesiol Scand. 2016;60(9):1241-50.

48. Sato H, Nakamura K, Baba Y, Terada S, Goto T, Kurahashi K. Low tidal volume ventilation with low PEEP during surgery may induce lung inflammation. BMC Anesthesiol. 2016;16(1):47.

49. Hemmes SN, Gama de Abreu M, Pelosi P, Schultz MJ. High versus low positive end-expiratory pressure during general anaesthesia for open abdominal surgery (PROVHILO trial): a multicentre randomised controlled trial. Lancet. 2014;384(9942):495-503.

50. Severgnini P, Selmo G, Lanza C, Chiesa A, Frigerio A, Bacuzzi A, et al. Protective mechanical ventilation during general anesthesia for open abdominal surgery improves postoperative pulmonary function. Anesthesiology. 2013;118(6):1307-21.

51. Nestler C, Simon P, Petroff D, Hammermüller S, Kamrath D, Wolf S, et al. Individualized positive end-expiratory pressure in obese patients during general anaesthesia: a randomized controlled clinical trial using electrical impedance tomography. Br J Anaesth. 2017;119(6):1194-205.

52. Satoh D, Kurosawa S, Kirino W, Wagatsuma T, Ejima Y, Yoshida A, et al. Impact of changes of positive end-expiratory pressure on functional residual capacity at low tidal volume ventilation during general anesthesia. J Anesth. 2012;26(5):664-9.

53. Cinnella G, Grasso S, Spadaro S, Rauseo M, Mirabella L, Salatto P, et al. Effects of recruitment maneuver and positive end-expiratory pressure on respiratory mechanics and transpulmonary pressure during laparoscopic surgery. Anesthesiology. 2013;118(1):114-22.

54. Bluth T, Bobek I, Canet JC, Cinnella G, de Baerdemaeker L, Gama de Abreu M, et al. Effect of intraoperative high positive end-expiratory pressure (PEEP) with recruitment maneuvers vs low PEEP on postoperative pulmonary complications in obese patients: a randomized clinical trial. JAMA. 2019;321(23): 2292-305.

55. Pereira SM, Tucci MR, Morais CCA, Simões CM, Tonelotto BFF, Pompeo MS, et al. Individual positive end-expiratory pressure settings optimize intraoperative mechanical ventilation and reduce postoperative atelectasis. Anesthesiology. 2018;129(6):1070-81.

56. Neto AS, Hemmes SN, Barbas CS, Beiderlinden M, Fernandez-Bustamante A, Futier E, et al. Association between driving

pressure and development of postoperative pulmonary complications in patients undergoing mechanical ventilation for general anaesthesia: a meta-analysis of individual patient data. Lancet Respir Med. 2016;4(4):272-80.

57. Staehr AK, Meyhoff CS, Henneberg SW, Christensen PL, Rasmussen LS. Influence of perioperative oxygen fraction on pulmonary function after abdominal surgery: a randomized controlled trial. BMC Res Notes. 2012;5:383.

58. Staehr-Rye AK, Meyhoff CS, Scheffenbichler FT, Vidal Melo MF, Gätke MR, Walsh JL, et al. Intraoperative inspiratory oxygen fraction and risk of major respiratory complications. Br J Anaesth. 2017;119(1):140-9.

59. Girardis M, Busani S, Damiani E, Donati A, Rinaldi L, Marudi A, et al. Effect of conservative vs conventional oxygen therapy on mortality among patients in an intensive care unit: the oxygen-ICU randomized clinical trial. JAMA. 2016;316(15):1583-9.

60. Meyhoff CS, Jorgensen LN, Wetterslev J, Christensen KB, Rasmussen LS. Increased long-term mortality after a high perioperative inspiratory oxygen fraction during abdominal surgery: follow-up of a randomized clinical trial. Anesth Analg. 2012;115(4):849-54.

61. Allegranzi B, Zayed B, Bischoff P, Kubilay NZ, de Jonge S, de Vries F, et al. New WHO recommendations on preoperative measures for surgical site infection prevention: an evidence based global perspective. Lancet Infect Dis. 2016;12:e288-303.

62. Cohen B, Schacham YN, Ruetzler K, Ahuja S, Yang D, Mascha EJ, et al. Effect of intraoperative hyperoxia on the incidence of surgical site infections: a meta-analysis. Br J Anaesth. 2018;120(6):1176-86.

63. Zhang HY, Zhao CL, Ye YW, Zhao HC, Sun N. A meta-analysis of perioperative hyperoxia for the surgical site infections in patients with general surgery. Zhonghua Yi Xue Za Zhi. 2016;96(20):1607-12.

64. Harten JM, Anderson KJ, Angerson WJ, Booth MG, Kinsella J. The effect of normobaric hyperoxia on cardiac index in healthy awake volunteers. Anaesthesia. 2003;58(9):885-8.

65. Austin MA, Wills KE, Blizzard L, Walters EH, Wood-Baker R. Effect of high flow oxygen on mortality in chronic obstructive pulmonary disease patients in prehospital setting: randomised controlled trial. BMJ. 2010;341:c5462.

66. Kilgannon JH, Jones AE, Shapiro NI, Angelos MG, Milcarek B, Hunter K, et al. Association between arterial hyperoxia following resuscitation from cardiac arrest and in-hospital mortality. JAMA. 2010;303(21):2165-71.

67. Bagchi A, Rudolph MI, Ng PY, Timm FP, Long DR, Shaefi S, et al. The association of postoperative pulmonary complications in 109,360 patients with pressure-controlled or volume-controlled ventilation. Anaesthesia. 2017;72:1334-43.

68. Wang C, Zhao N, Wang W, Guo L, Guo L, Chi C, et al. Intraoperative mechanical ventilation strategies for obese patients: a systematic review and network meta-analysis. Obes Rev. 2015;16(6):508-17.

69. Choi EM, Na S, Choi SH, An J, Rha KH, Oh YJ. Comparison of volume-controlled and pressure-controlled ventilation in steep Trendelenburg position for robot-assisted laparoscopic radical prostatectomy. J Clin Anesth. 2011;23(3):183-8.

70. Dion JM, McKee C, Tobias JD, Sohner P, Herz D, Teich S, et al. Ventilation during laparoscopic-assisted bariatric surgery: volume-controlled, pressure-controlled or volume-guaranteed pressure-regulated modes. Int J Clin Exp Med. 2014;7(8): 2242-7.

71. Gupta SD, Kundu SB, Ghose T, Maji S, Mitra K, Mukherjee M, et al. A comparison between volume-controlled ventilation and pressure-controlled ventilation in providing better oxygenation in obese patients undergoing laparoscopic cholecystectomy. Indian J Anaesth. 2012;56(3):276-82.

72. Whalen FX, Gajic O, Thompson GB, Kendrick ML, Que FL, Williams BA, et al. The effects of the alveolar recruitment maneuver and positive end-expiratory pressure on arterial oxygenation during laparoscopic bariatric surgery. Anesth Analg. 2006;102(1):298-305.

73. Pang CK, Yap J, Chen PP. The effect of an alveolar recruitment strategy on oxygenation during laparoscopic cholecystectomy. Anaesth Intensive Care. 2003;31(2):176-80.

74. Cui Y, Cao R, Li G, Gong T, Ou Y, Huang J. The effect of lung recruitment maneuvers on post-operative pulmonary complications for patients undergoing general anesthesia: a meta-analysis. PLoS One. 2019;14(5):e0217405.

75. Lumb AB, Greenhill SJ, Simpson MP, Stewart J. Lung recruitment and positive airway pressure before extubation does not improve oxygenation in the post-anaesthesia care unit: a randomized clinical trial. Br J Anaesth. 2010;104(5): 643-7.

76. Edmark L, Auner U, Lindbäck J, Enlund M, Hedenstierna G. Post-operative atelectasis: a randomised trial investigating a ventilatory strategy and low oxygen fraction during recovery. Acta Anaesthesiol Scand. 2014;58(6):681-8.

77. Kleinsasser AT, Pircher I, Truebsbach S, Knotzer H, Loeckinger A, Treml B. Pulmonary function after emergence on 100% oxygen in patients with chronic obstructive pulmonary disease: a randomized, controlled trial. Anesthesiology. 2014;120(5): 1146-51.

78. Edmark L, Auner U, Enlund M, Ostberg E, Hedenstierna G. Oxygen concentration and characteristics of progressive atelectasis formation during anaesthesia. Acta Anaesthesiol Scand. 2011;55(1):75-81.

79. Neligan PJ, Malhotra G, Fraser M, Williams N, Greenblatt EP, Cereda M, et al. Continuous positive airway pressure via the Boussignac system immediately after extubation improves lung function in morbidly obese patients with obstructive sleep apnea undergoing laparoscopic bariatric surgery. Anesthesiology. 2009;110(4):878-84.

80. Singh PM, Borle A, Shah D, Sinha A, Makkar JK, Trikha A, et al. Optimizing prophylactic CPAP in patients without obstructive sleep apnoea for high-risk abdominal surgeries: a meta-regression analysis. Lung. 2016;194(2):201-17.

81. Ladha K, Vidal Melo MF, McLean DJ, Wanderer JP, Grabitz SD, Kurth T, et al. Intraoperative protective mechanical ventilation and risk of postoperative respiratory complications: hospital based registry study. BMJ. 2015;351:h3646.

82. Amato MB, Meade MO, Slutsky AS, Brochard L, Costa EL, Schoenfeld DA, et al. Driving pressure and survival in the acute respiratory distress syndrome. N Engl J Med. 2015;372(8): 747-55.

83. Grieco DL, Russo A, Romanò B, Anzellotti GM, Ciocchetti P, Torrini F, et al. Lung volumes, respiratory mechanics and dynamic strain during general anaesthesia. Br J Anaesth. 2018;121:1156-65.

84. Chamala V, Nileshwar A. Ventilation during anesthesia: from automatic human hand to intelligent machine! Indian J Respir Care. 2019;8:1-3

85. Hernández G, Vaquero C, Colinas L, Cuena R, González P, Canabal A, et al. Effect of postextubation high-flow nasal cannula vs noninvasive ventilation on reintubation and postextubation respiratory failure in high-risk patients: a randomized clinical trial. JAMA. 2016;316:1565-74.

86. Stéphan F, Barrucand B, Petit P, Rézaiguia-Delclaux S, Médard A, Delannoy B, et al. BiPOP study group: high-flow nasal oxygen vs noninvasive positive airway pressure in hypoxemic patients after cardiothoracic surgery: a randomized clinical trial. JAMA. 2015;313:2331-9.

87. Futier E, Paugam-Burtz C, Godet T, Khoy-Ear L, Rozencwajg S, Delay JM, et al. Effect of early postextubation high-flow nasal cannula vs conventional oxygen therapy on hypoxaemia in patients after major abdominal surgery: a French multicentre randomised controlled trial (OPERA). Intensive Care Med. 2016;42:1888-98.

88. Park SH. Perioperative lung-protective ventilation strategy reducespostoperative pulmonary complications in patients undergoing thoracic and major abdominal surgery. Korean J Anesthesiol. 2016;69:3-7.

89. Simpson JR, Katz SG, Laan TV. Oversedation in postoperative patients requiring ventilator support greater than 48 hours: a 4-year National Surgical Quality Improvement Program-driven project. Am Surg. 2013;79:1106-10.

90. Robinson BR, Mueller EW, Henson K, Branson RD, Barsoum S, Tsuei BJ. An analgesia-delirium-sedation protocol for critically ill trauma patients reduces ventilator days and hospital length of stay. J Trauma. 2008;65:517-26.

91. Dale CR, Kannas DA, Fan VS, Daniel SL, Deem S, Yanez ND 3rd, et al. Improved analgesia, sedation, and delirium protocol associated with decreased duration of delirium and mechanical ventilation. Ann Am Thorac Soc. 2014;11:367-74.

92. Nguyen J, Nacpil N. Effectiveness of dexmedetomidine versus propofol on extubation times, length of stay and mortality rates in adult cardiac surgery patients: a systematic review and meta-analysis. JBI Database System Rev Implement Rep. 2018; 16: 1220-39.

93. Jacob B, Chatila W, Manthous CA. The unassisted respiratory rate/tidal volume ratio accurately predicts weaning outcome in postoperative patients. Crit Care Med 1997; 25: 253-7.

94. Savi A, Teixeira C, Silva JM, Borges LG, Pereira PA, Pinto KB, Gehm F, Moreira FC, Wickert R, Trevisan CB, Maccari JG, Oliveira RP, Vieira SR; Gaúcho Weaning Study Group. Weaning predictors do not predict extubation failure in simple-to-wean patients. J Crit Care. 2012;27:221.e1-8.

95. CH Chang, YW Hong, SK Koh. Weaning approach with weaning index for postoperative patients with mechanical ventilator support in the ICU. Korean Journal of Anesthesiology. 2007; 53:47-51.

96. Souza Leite W, Novaes A, Bandeira M, Olympia Ribeiro E, Dos Santos AM, de Moura PH, et al. Patient-ventilator asynchrony in conventional ventilation modes during short-term mechanical ventilation after cardiac surgery: randomized clinical trial. Multidiscip Respir Med. 2020;15:650.

97. Fot EV, Izotova NN, Yudina AS, Smetkin AA, Kuzkov VV, Kirov MY. Automated Weaning from Mechanical Ventilation after Off-Pump Coronary Artery Bypass Grafting. Front Med (Lausanne). 2017;4:31.

98. Rose L, Schultz MJ, Cardwell CR, Jouvet P, McAuley DF, Blackwood B. Automated versus non-automated weaning for reducing the duration of mechanical ventilation for critically ill adults and children. Cochrane Database Syst Rev. 2013;(6):CD009235.

Sepsis and Infection Control in Perioperative Care

Debashree P Lahiri, Vijaya Patil

INTRODUCTION

Healthcare-associated infections (HCAI) lead to considerable morbidity, mortality, increased number of hospital days, increased antimicrobial resistance, and hence increasing the overall healthcare costs. The incidence of HCAI reported in developed countries is 7 per 100 hospitalized patients while in low- and middle-income countries it is two to three times more.[1]

PREOPERATIVE FACTORS

Various endogenous (patient-related) and exogenous (procedure-related) factors **(Box 1)** increase the risk of surgical site infection.[2]

Preoperative bathing: The World Health Organization (WHO) global guidelines for the prevention of surgical site infection, recommend preoperative bathing with either plain soap or antimicrobial soap (moderate quality of evidence). It does not recommend the use of chlorhexidine gluconate (CHG) impregnated cloths for the purpose of reducing surgical site infection due to the very low quality of evidence.[3] Perioperative intranasal applications of mupirocin 2% ointment with or without a combination of CHG body wash is recommended in nasal carriers of *Staphylococcus aureus* undergoing cardiothoracic and orthopedic surgery.[4]

Box 1: Endogenous risk factors for surgical site infection.

- Diabetes
- Chronic renal failure
- Advanced age
- Hypoalbuminemia
- Chemotherapy
- Radiotherapy
- Immunotherapy
- Evidence of active infection at a remote site
- Smoking
- Poor physical conditions

Timing of preoperative surgical antibiotic prophylaxis: The indiscriminate use of higher antibiotics has led to the emergence of multidrug-resistant organisms. Hence, clinicians need to be careful while using antibiotics. The time of administration of preoperative antibiotic prophylaxis is highly debatable because of paucity of strong evidence. It is, however, evident that administration of antibiotic after incision increase the risk of surgical site infection. The WHO panel for the prevention of surgical site infection strongly recommends administration of surgical antibiotic prophylaxis 120 minutes before incision taking into account the half-life of the antibiotic.[3] Antibiotics such as Cefazolin, Cefoxitin, and Penicillins which have short half-life, should be administered closer to the incision time (<60 min). While, drugs such as fluoroquinolones and vancomycin which are given as prolonged infusion should be administered 120 minutes before surgical incision. Redosing during prolonged surgery should be considered for single half-life antibiotics. The same recommendations are extrapolated to the pediatric patients in the absence of any data in this group of patients.[3]

Mechanical bowel preparation and use of oral antibiotics: In the early 20th century, the high incidence of infectious complications in abdominal surgeries compelled the surgeons to evacuate the gastrointestinal tracts prior to surgery with laxatives.[5] According to Cochrane collaboration, bowel preparation is not required in right-sided colectomy but is recommended for left hemicolectomy and distal resections. The WHO global guidelines panel recommends that in adult patients undergoing elective colorectal surgery, mechanical bowel preparation alone (without oral antibiotics) should not be used.[3] There are no major randomized controlled trials (RCTs) available regarding mechanical bowel preparation in the pediatric patients. Polyethylene glycol or sodium phosphate are mainly used for mechanical bowel preparation. The choice of antibiotic should depend on availability and local antimicrobial resistance prevalence. The bowel preparation can lead to patient discomfort, electrolyte disturbances, and dehydration in the preoperative period.

Hair removal: Presence of body hair can interfere with surgical incision, suturing, and wound dressing. Also it was believed that hair removal would reduce the incidence of surgical site infection. Thus, hair removal became an important component of preoperative preparation. The WHO panel strongly recommends that in patients undergoing surgical procedure hair should either not be removed or if it is needed, a clipper should be used. Shaving is strongly discouraged under all situations.[3] This recommendation can be applied to pediatric patients also. Razor with a sharp blade is directly used on the skin causing microscopic trauma while clippers remove hair without touching it.

Enhanced nutritional support: Hypoalbuminemia is considered to be an independent risk factor for surgical site infection leading to increased hospital stay.[6] Stress conditions, e.g. surgery produce a negative nitrogen balance. Perioperative nutritional support by increasing protein and caloric intake helps in the recovery from inflammation. Though the quality of evidence is poor, administration of oral or enteral nutritional formulas is suggested especially in underweight patients undergoing major surgeries.[3] However, surgery should not be delayed to improve the nutritional status. It is considered inappropriate to give parenteral nutrition for preventing surgical site infection because of the infectious complications of intravenous access. No evidence of enhanced nutritional support in preventing perioperative infection is available in the pediatric population. Various commercially available nutritional formulas usually contain a combination of arginine, glutamine, omega-3 fatty acids, and nucleotides.

Glycemic control: In the perioperative period, the combined effect of relative hypoinsulinemia, insulin resistance and excessive catabolism due to counter-regulatory hormones increase the chance of hyperglycemia, even in nondiabetic individuals. Perioperative hyperglycemia increases the risk of surgical site infections in the postoperative period. The WHO global guidelines panel recommends intensive perioperative blood glucose control in both diabetic and nondiabetic adult patients undergoing surgery.[3] However, hypoglycemia should be avoided at all times. The benefit of perioperative glycemic control is not yet proven in pediatric population.

INTRAOPERATIVE FACTORS

It is now established beyond any doubts that contaminated operating environments increase the incidence of HCAI.[7]

Each hospital should have their own protocols for cleaning and disinfecting surgical instruments and operation theaters. The details of the same are beyond the scope of this chapter.

Ventilation of operation theaters: Positive-pressure ventilation should be maintained in the operating rooms (OR), the corridors and adjacent areas with a minimum of 15 air changes per hour in the OR, of which minimum 3 should be fresh air. Both recirculated and fresh air should be appropriately filtered. Air ought to be introduced at the ceiling and exhausted close to the floor. UV radiation is not needed in the OR to prevent surgical site infections. OR doors should be kept closed except when needed for passage of equipment, personnel, and the patient. High-efficiency particulate air (HEPA) filters remove airborne particles of 0.3 μm and above. HEPA filters can either be ceiling mounted (vertical flow) or wall mounted (horizontal flow).[8] Laminar airflow systems are frequently used when particulate contamination is undesirable, like in orthopedic surgeries. Because of low quality evidence, the WHO global guidelines panel suggests against the use of laminar airflow ventilation in total arthroplasty surgeries.[3]

Cleaning: A disinfectant approved by an Environmental Protection Agency (high-level disinfectants, e.g., glutaraldehyde, peracetic acid, and hydrogen peroxide; intermediate-level disinfectants, e.g., sodium hypochlorite; and low-level disinfectant, e.g., quaternary ammonium compounds, some phenols)[9] should be used to clean areas and surfaces where visible soiling or contamination with blood or other body fluids occurs during the surgery. There is no need to perform special cleaning or closing of ORs after contaminated surgeries. Blood pressure cuffs, pulse oximeter probes, ECG leads, and cables that come in direct contact with patients should be thoroughly cleaned. High-touch surfaces on an anesthesia work station should be disinfected with an EPA-approved disinfectant between cases that is compatible with the equipment.

Surgical site preparation: It refers to preparing the broader area of the intact skin around the intended incision site in the operation theater. The WHO global discussion group strongly recommends the use of alcohol based antiseptic solutions preferably based on CHG for surgical site skin preparation.[3] No recommendation on the concentration of the antiseptic solution is made. The effectiveness of alcohol-based antiseptic solution in pediatric patient is yet to be proven. The purpose of using an alcohol-based solution is to decrease the microbial load of the skin as much as possible before incising the skin. One should be careful to not use alcohol-based antiseptic solutions on neonates and in direct contact of mucosa, eyes, ear, and meninges. These solutions can cause allergies and skin irritation. They must be allowed to dry by evaporation before draping or else alcohol being highly flammable can ignite when a diathermy is used.

Surgical hand preparation: It is also known as "hand scrubbing." The skin flora, mainly coagulase-negative *Staphylococci*, *Propionibacterium* spp. and *Corynebacteria* spp., rarely cause surgical site infections, but the presence of a foreign body or necrotic tissue, can trigger such infections.[10] The main aim of surgical hand preparation is to eliminate transient flora, reduce the resident flora and inhibit the growth of bacteria under the gloved hand. On the other hand, routine hand hygiene removes dirt, organic material, and reduces transient flora. Surgical hand preparation thus decreases the release of skin bacteria from the hands of the surgeons to the open wound during the surgery, particularly in case of an unnoticed puncture of the surgical glove. The WHO panel on prevention of surgical site infections strongly recommends that hands and forearm should either be (but not combined) scrubbed with a suitable antimicrobial soap and water or with a suitable alcohol-based handrub before donning sterile gloves.[3] No recommendations on the duration of hand scrubbing has been laid down and depends on manufacturer's recommendation for the product, which is usually 2–5 minutes. The WHO guidelines on hand hygiene in health care, 2009[11] recommends to keep nails short and remove all jewelry, artificial nails, or nail polish before scrubbing. The surgical scrub rooms should have no-touch or elbow-operated dispensers for alcohol-based handrubs. Alternatively, there should be antimicrobial soap, clean running water, and disposable clean towels for each healthcare worker. According to the European Committee for Standardization[12,13] and the American Society for Testing and Materials,[14] antiseptic preparations used for surgical hand preparations should be able to reduce both transient and resident flora from the hands.

Drapes and gowns: Sterile drapes are used to prevent contact with unclean surfaces and thus maintain the sterility of the patients surroundings. Similarly, sterile surgical gowns also help to maintain the sterility of the surgical field.[15] The chances of transmission of pathogens increase when drapes and gowns become wet. The panel suggests the use of either sterile, disposable, nonwoven drapes or sterile, reusable woven drapes, and gowns during surgical procedures to prevent surgical site infections.[3] The panel suggests not to use plastic adhesive incise drapes. Ideally the entire body of the patient should be draped for all kind of surgeries with four sterile towels placed around the line of incision and finally a laparotomy sheet with fenestration for the incision.

Maintaining normothermia: Cold operating theaters, anesthesia-induced impairment of central thermo-regulatory control and cold intravenous and irrigation fluids make the patients hypothermic. The WHO global guidelines panel recommends using warming devices in the operating theaters to warm patients to prevent surgical site infections.[3] However, no consensus could be reached for the lower limit or optimal timing for normothermia. Usually a core body temperature of more than 36°C is maintained. In pediatric patients also it is recommended to avoid hypothermia. Many studies have evaluated the effect of forced air warmers on operation theater laminar airflow pattern. Some authors suggest that the exhausted heat from forced air warmer blankets increase the temperature of the surgical site by >5°C. This leads to warm air rising up to produce thermal convection currents transferring the floor level contaminants to the surgical site.[16,17] However, the association of disrupted laminar flow, increased contaminant count, and surgical site infection needs to be further investigated. In view of paucity of evidence, it is recommended that clinicians weigh the risks and benefits of various kinds of warmers before using one.[18]

Anesthesia practices: Risky practices such as reuse of single use vials, reuse of multidose vials, reuse of syringes after changing needle, multiple patients, preparing intravenous injections using the same bag and administration channels for patients receiving the same therapy in 1 day can lead to transmission of microorganisms. In a recent systematic review of the risk of infections with the use of Propofol, it was found that all HCAIs associated with Propofol have been reported in developed countries.[19] Amongst all anesthetic drugs, Propofol most often leads to infections due to presence of lipid emulsion which promotes bacterial growth and also due to its frequent wrongful handling such as reusing syringes or vials in multiple patients, poor external disinfection of the vial facilitating its contamination. Propofol available as single use prefilled syringes should be used within 6 hours of opening the syringe while vials should be used for single patient within 12 hours of opening or puncturing the vial.[20] It is therefore necessary to emphasize safe injection practices among the trainee and consultant anesthesiologists. Some recommendations of safe injection practices are as follows:[21-23]

- Prevent contamination of sterile injection equipment.
- Use alcohol to clean outer surface (plug, rubber) of vials or ampoules before use.
- Syringes, needles, cannulas should not be reused (in the same or different patients).
- Medications from the same syringe should not be administered to different patients even if the needle or cannula is changed.
- Single use vials should not be used in multiple patients.
- As far as possible, multidose vials should be used in one single patient.

- Multidose vials should be stored as per manufacturer's recommendations.
- Intravenous solution bags or bottles should not be used in more than one patient.
- Syringes, needles or cannulas should be considered contaminated upon contact with patient or after they are being used to connect the infusion equipment.
- When not in use syringes should be capped.
- Used single or multidose ampoules/vials, needles, syringes must be immediately discarded or latest by the end of patient's anesthesia.
- Unused syringes, needles should be stored in a clean area to avoid cross contamination from used items.
- The injection ports should be accessed only after disinfection.
- A needleless connector should be used to access intravenous administration sets. A split septum valve is preferred over mechanical valves due to increased risk of infection with the later.
- In patients, receiving continuous intravenous fluids (except blood, blood products or fat emulsions) administration sets including secondary sets and add-on devices, should be replaced no more frequently than every 96 hours but at least every week.
- No recommendations regarding the replacement of intermittently used administration sets are available.
- Sets used to administer blood, blood products, or fat emulsions should be replaced within 24 hours of infusion.
- No recommendations are available regarding replacing peripherally inserted intravenous catheters in adults unless clinically indicated. The catheter site should be directly examined at least once in a day.
- Central venous catheters should not be routinely replaced to prevent catheter-related infections, however, the catheter should be removed promptly, when it is no longer essential.
- Arterial catheters should be removed as soon as they are no longer needed. It is not advised to routinely replace arterial catheters to prevent blood stream infection. They should be replaced only when indicated.
- Disposable or reusable transducers along with the tubing, continuous-flush device, and flush solution should be replaced every 96 hours.

Microbes such as coagulase-negative staphylococci, *Bacillus* spp, and methicillin-resistant *Staphylococcus aureus* (MRSA) are found on the anesthesia station, computer touchscreens and keyboards.[24] Hand hygiene should ideally be performed before aseptic tasks (e.g., inserting central venous catheters, inserting arterial catheters, drawing medications, spiking IV bags), after removing gloves; when hands are soiled with oropharyngeal secretions, blood or other body fluids before touching anything in the surrounding; when entering and exiting the operation theaters.[21]. In the presence of visible contamination with blood or body fluids hand washing with soap (antimicrobial or nonantimicrobial) should be performed and alcohol-based handrubs can be used when there is no visible contamination. Anesthetist are vulnerable to acquire pathogens from direct contact with secretions, saliva, blood, or urine of hospitalized patients, and become vectors to transmit these organisms to others by direct touch. The ASA Recommendations for Infection Control for the Practice of Anesthesiology (3rd edition) recommends use of gloves during contact with blood, body fluids, mucous membranes, or nonintact skin, and that gloves should not be reused as removal of microorganisms and integrity cannot be ensured.[21] When gloves are contaminated they should be removed and hand hygiene should be performed. Same pair of gloves should not be used in more than one patient **(Fig. 1)**.

During airway management and endotracheal intubation, anesthetist's hands may get contaminated with airway secretions. It may not be possible to perform hand hygiene immediately leading to cross contamination of anesthesia work area. It is thus recommended to wear double gloves during airway management and remove the outer gloves soon after airway manipulation. Inner gloves should be removed as soon as possible and hand hygiene should be performed.

The laryngoscope blades and handles often get contaminated with blood and lymphoid tissue. The standard direct laryngoscope and the reusable video-laryngoscope handles and blades should undergo high-level disinfection.[22] It is advisable to replace reusable laryngoscopes with single-use standard direct laryngoscopes or video-laryngoscopes.

Hospitals should conduct regular audits to assess the adequacy of environmental disinfection, adherence to

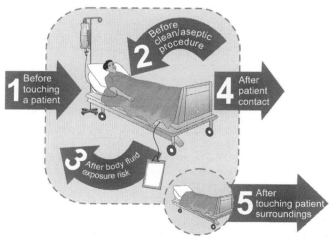

Fig. 1: WHO recommended "my five moments of hand hygiene".

disinfection protocols by the hospital staff, and invest in research to develop better modules to reduce the risk of infection.

Role of teaching in infection control: It has been found that while entering intraoperative data in computers, many times anesthetists do not remove soiled gloves, contaminating the keyboard.[23] Interactive educational sessions which include a comprehensive infection prevention and control curriculum improves knowledge, implementation of knowledge in practice. CDC guidelines give level 1 recommendation for regular education of healthcare personnel and periodic assessment of their knowledge.[24] Educational intervention targeting healthcare providers significantly improves infection prevention practices leading to effective patient care.[25]

REFERENCES

1. Arora A, Bharadwaj P, Chaturvedi H, Chowbey P, Gupta S, Leaper D, et al. A review of prevention of surgical site infections in Indian hospitals based on global guidelines for the prevention of surgical site infection, 2016. J Patient Saf Infect Control. 2018;6:1-12.

2. Buggy D. Can anaesthetic management influence surgical wound healing? Lancet. 2000;356(9227):355-7.

3. WHO. Global Guidelines for the Prevention of Surgical Site Infection, 2nd edition. Geneva: World Health Organization; 2018.

4. WHO. Global Guidelines for the Prevention of Surgical Site Infection, 2nd edition (Web Appendix 3). Geneva: World Health Organization; 2018.

5. Duncan JE, Quietmeyer CM. Bowel preparation: current status. Clin Colon Rectal Surg. 2009;22(1):14-20.

6. Hennessey DB, Burke JP, Ni-Dhonochu T, Shields C, Winter DC, Mealy K. Preoperative hypoalbuminemia is an independent risk factor for the development of surgical site infection following gastrointestinal surgery: a multi-institutional study. Ann Surg. 2010;252:325.

7. Dancer SJ. Controlling hospital-acquired infection: focus on the role of the environment and new technologies for decontamination. Clin Microbiol Rev. 2014;27(4):665-90.

8. Spagnolo AM, Ottria G, Amicizia D, Perdelli F, Cristina ML. Operating theatre quality and prevention of surgical site infections. J Prev Med Hyg. 2013;54:131-7.

9. CDC. (2003). Guidelines for Environmental Infection Control in Health-Care Facilities. [online] Available from https://www.cdc.gov/infectioncontrol/guidelines/environmental/background/services.html [Last accessed February, 2020].

10. Elek SD, Conen PE. The virulence of *Staphylococcus pyogenes* for man; a study of the problems of wound infection. Br J Exper Pathol. 1957;38(6):573-86.

11. WHO. WHO Guidelines on Hand Hygiene in Health Care. Geneva: World Health Organization; 2009.

12. European standard EN 1499. Chemical Disinfectants and Antiseptics. Hygienic Handwash. Test Method and Requirements. Brussels: European Committee for Standardization; 1997.

13. European standard EN 1500. Chemical Disinfectants and Antiseptics. Hygienic Handrub. Test Method and Requirements. Brussels: European Committee for Standardization; 1997.

14. ASTM. Standard test method for evaluation of the effectiveness of health care personnel or consumer handwash formulations. (Designation: E 1174). American Society for Testing and Materials (ASTM International); 1999.

15. Rutala WA, Weber DJ. A review of single-use and reusable gowns and drapes in health care. Infect Control Hosp Epidemiol. 2001;22(4):248-57.

16. Reed M, Kimberger O, McGovern PD, Albrecht MC. Forced-air warming design: Evaluation of intake filtration, internal microbial buildup, and airborne-contamination emissions. AANA J. 2013;81:275-80.

17. Albrecht M, Gauthier RL, Belani K, Litchy M, Leaper D. Forced-air warming blowers: an evaluation of filtration adequacy and airborne contamination emissions in the operating room. Am J Infect Control. 2011;39:321-8.

18. Ackermann W, Fan Q, Parekh AJ, Stoicea N, Ryan J, Bergese SD. Forced-air warming and resistive heating. Updated perspectives on safety and surgical site infections. Front Surg. 2018;5:64.

19. Zorrilla-Vaca A, Arevalo J, Escandón-Vargas K, Soltanifar D, Mirski M. Infectious diseases risk and propofol anesthesia, 1989–2015. Emerg Infect Dis. 2015;22:981-92.

20. Zorrilla-Vaca A, Escandón-Vargas K. La importancia del control y prevención de enfermedades infecciosas en anestesiología. Rev Colomb Anestesiol. 2017;45:69-77.

21. Stackhouse R, Beers R, Brown D, Brown M, Greene E, McCann ME, et al. Recommendations for Infection Control for the Practice of Anesthesiology, 3rd edition. Illinois: ASA; 2003.

22. Munoz-Price LS, Bowdle A, Johnston BL, Bearman G, Bernard CC, Dellinger EP, et al. Infection prevention in the operating room anesthesia work area. Infect Control Hospital Epidemiol. 2019;40:1-17.

23. Fukada T, Iwakiri H, Ozaki M. Anaesthetists' role in computer keyboard contamination in an operating room. J Hosp Infect. 2008;70:148-53.

24. CDC (2011). Guidelines for the Prevention of Intravascular Catheter-Related Infections. [online] Available from https://www.cdc.gov/infectioncontrol/guidelines/bsi/recommendations.html#rec17 [Last accessed February, 2020].

25. Koo E, McNamara S, Lansing B, Olmsted RN, Rye RA, Fitzgerald T, et al. Making infection prevention education interactive can enhance knowledge and improve outcomes: results from the targeted infection prevention (TIP). Am J Infect Control. 2016;44(11):1241-6.

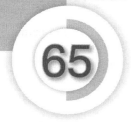

65

Perioperative Nursing

Amrit Kaur

PERIOPERATIVE NURSING CARE

The perioperative period is a term used to describe the three distinct phases of any surgical procedure, which includes the preoperative phase, the intraoperative phase, and the postoperative phase.

Perioperative nursing care (POC) is defined as the practice of patient-centered, multidisciplinary, and integrated medical and nursing care of patients from the moment of contemplation of surgery until full recovery.

The objective is to offer healthier surroundings for patients before, during, and after the surgery.

Principles of Critical Care Nursing[1]

Anticipation: It is to recognize the high-risk patients and anticipate the requirements, complications and be prepared to meet any emergency.

Early detection and prompt action: The prognosis of the patient depends on the early detection of variation, prompt and appropriate action to combat complications with monitoring of cardiorespiratory function as primary factor of assessment.

Collaborative practice: Collaborative practice between physicians and nurses working in critical care unit is indispensable to ensure quality patient care and better outcome. Collaborative practice is more and more warranted in critical care area than in any other field.

Communication: Intraprofessional, interdepartmental and interpersonal communication has a significant importance in the smooth treatment of the patient and a nurse is the key person in interpersonal communication regarding patient care.

Prevention of infection: Critically ill patients requiring intensive care are at a greater risk than other patients due to their already immunocompromised state with the antibiotic usage and stress, invasive lines, mechanical ventilators, prolonged stay, severity of illness, and environment of critical care unit.

Quality nursing care combined with a vigilant surveillance program can minimize the incident of nosocomial infection.[2]

Crisis intervention and stress reduction: As patient advocates, nurses assist the patient to express fear and identify their grieving pattern and provide avenues for positive coping. Listening is a skill to be developed by every critical care nurse (CCN), to handle the extreme complex feeling of patients who are in crisis situation. Empathy is the attitude to be developed by the CCN to make herself a good counselor to the patients.

Surgical Critical Care

Critical nursing care is one of the indispensable components of surgical critical care (SCC). It includes pediatric patients as well as adult and geriatric patients who are undergoing a major surgical procedure. Pediatric SCC is a very challenging area. A child is not a mini adult and as such comprehensive care of critically ill child requires provision of intensive care tailored to the needs of the individual child. Illness or injury becomes critical when one or more organ system fail or begin to fail.

Surgical critical care requires the ability to shift rapidly between the demands of the various age groups. The response of a neonate, toddler or a geriatric patient to surgery is definitely different from that of healthy adult. A major chunk of pediatric SCC is the care of neonates with congenital anomalies. Unless these are managed in the best possible manner, the child and the parents are saddled with a host of problems for the foreseeable future.

Comprehensive care is incomplete without medical, surgical, and critical meticulous nursing care. The standard of nursing care provided is directly proportion to quality of care provided by the intensive care unit.

Nurses are crucial component of the team that is involved in the evaluation, decision making, and execution of virtually all life-saving interventions in a critically ill surgical patient. By virtue of their presence at bedside, they complement the physician's observations and help identify subtle changes in patient's overall condition. More importantly nurses are the biggest emotional support to the parents in the pediatric as well as adult ICU's hostile environment.

Monitoring and Surveillance in Surgical Intensive Care

In the care of postoperative surgical critical patients (both adult and pediatric), the use of basic and advanced monitoring technology should always be evidence-based and patient-centered and individualized. There are continuous research activities going on around the globe for frequency and types of monitoring that can affect the best patient outcomes in surgical patients. Newer bedside technologies are growing rapidly and ensuring good outcomes.[3]

These basic and advanced monitoring allow calculation of patients' physiological reserve and effectiveness of interventions but practitioners must be familiar with the pitfalls associated with these interventions in areas of acute and critical care.[4] Despite the expansiveness of monitoring, we are seeing paucity of evidence of its effectiveness mainly in the arena of fluid management and hemodynamic monitoring where studies have been equivocal regarding the effectiveness of monitoring data to influence patient outcomes.

Surveillance

Surveillance is "a process to identify threats to patients' health and safety through purposeful and ongoing acquisition, interpretation, and synthesis of patient data for clinical decision making in the acute care setting."[5] Surveillance is a core role of critical care; while not unique to nursing, surveillance is applied continuously in critical care units worldwide. It was identified importance of surveillance in critical care nursing for patient safety was identified by use of checklist, interdisciplinary rounds, clinical decisional support and other monitoring systems which are important to surveillance and prevention of errors.[4] Practices that do not improve patient outcomes should be eliminated. The chances and margin of error is very narrow in today's complex hospital systems and the critical care unit is the hub of such concentrated complexity, making surveillance essential for safe patient care. Clear consideration for technology advancement and the effects on both nursing practice and patient outcomes is needed.

Nursing Certification and Competency in Critical Care Units

Consistent patient care and safe patient outcome need training and certification in critical care practice for physicians as well as nurses. All critical care nurses should have proper curriculum and certified teaching program to attain national or institutional certification. The American Association of Critical Care Nurses has developed a series of practice alerts for teaching care providers.[6]

Role of Nurse in Critical Care[7]

Nurses in critical care setting are highly committed, responsible, and accountable. The role of nurse extends from handling critical situations like cardiopulmonary arrest or death or life-threatening emergencies to health teaching and support of families.

Intensive nursing: It involves round the clock responsibility of a nurse for comprehensive and individualized patient care. Allocating a primary nurse for an individual critically ill patient throughout the ICU stay can promote better nurse patient interaction, better assessment, identification, and meeting all needs of patient and hence better holistic care. It is just like taking care of your own child and having that sense of parental instincts.

Therapeutic relationship: Therapeutic nurse-patient/family relationship is very essential in providing quality nursing care. It enhances family centered care and fulfil the concept of holistic care.

Support and counseling: Intensive care unit is a critical area and is very stressful for patients, families as well as healthcare personnel. Nurse should utilize good communication and counseling skills to handle these issues.

Health teaching: Health education is an inseparable part of critical care nursing. Key messages regarding health care can be communicated to the families. It is very essential as family ultimately takes care, once the patient recovers from the acute illness.

Ethical decision making: Ethical dilemmas arise in all critical care settings. The nurse should keep in mind ethical principles during decision making and performing interventions.

Why Supportive Care for Critically Ill Surgical Patients?

Early recognition of critical illness is crucial to institution of life-saving measures. This is especially true for geriatric patients, children, and patients with severe comorbidities because they have very little physiological reserve and provide a very small-time frame for intervention, before lapsing into irreversible organ damage. So, the nursing care forms a very important component of the stabilization of these patients.[8]

Components of Supportive Care of a Critically Ill Patient[7]

- General supportive care
- Care of eyes

- Bowel care
- Care of bladder
- Pressure ulcers and skin care
- Thrombophlebitis
- Mouth care
- Positioning and physiotherapy

Critical Nursing Care of the Ventilated Patient

- *Care of advanced airway:*
  - Humidification and heating
  - Suctioning and pulmonary toileting.
- Care of ventilator circuit
- *Other supportive care of ventilated patient:*
  - Repositioning
  - Provision of adequate calories
  - Adequate sedation and analgesia.
- Intravenous fluids
- Nasogastric tube
- Physiotherapy.

General Nursing Consideration in the Operating Room

Although standards of nursing practice are followed in the operating room, it is necessary to have a tailored approach for caring surgical patients. Issues that can affect patient status in the operating room and postoperatively include, but are not limited to, temperature regulation, fluid and electrolyte balance, positioning and skin integrity.[9]

Patient sfety is underlying theme for all nursing interventions.

Checklist

World Health Organization (WHO) safety checklist is mandatory for any surgical patient in adult as well as pediatric patients and it can be modified according to the institute's requirement. Nursing personals (scrub nurse as well as circulating nurse) are an important part of WHO safety checklist and must be actively participating in first, second, and third part of WHO safety checklist.[10]

Surgical Preparation and Positioning

While the patient is being prepared for the surgical procedure, maintenance of the patient's temperature is crucial.[11] Infants and children are sensitive to their environment, and changes in core body temperature can occur rapidly. Temperature regulation is more difficult because a child has a higher body surface/weight ratio than an adult. A thermoneutral environment should be provided. Nursing intervention includes adjustment of temperature of the operating room (a minimum of 10 minutes before the patient is expected to enter), warming lights, warming

pads, plastic covering, and loosely wrapping areas that will not be in the surgical field.

The nursing intervention in avoiding convective heat loss is by using careful technique with surgical preparation and by using gauze sponges and suction devices to absorb excess drainage. The result of hypothermia causes the patient's metabolism to increase, which leads to an increase in oxygen consumption and potential hypoxemia. Young infants and children are more flexible than their older counterparts. Hyperextension and/or hyperflexion should be avoided when positioning the patient.

During the Surgery

During the operation, placement of heavy instruments on the patient should be avoided. Prolonged accidental pressure caused by instruments placed on the sterile field or scrubbed personnel leaning on the patient can cause an alteration in skin integrity.

Transfer to Postanesthesia Care Unit (PACU)[12]

Once the child has been transported to the PACU, the OR nurse gives a verbal or documented report (as per institutional protocol) to the PACU nurse which includes:

- Current status of the child (vital signs, assesment of pain)
- Surgical procedure planned and surgical procedure done (if any change in plan intraoperatively)
- Assessment of surgical wounds and drains.

Main priorities of PACU nurse:

- Continuous monitoring of cardiopulmonary status
- Maintaining a patent airway
- Maintaining oxygenation
- Maintenance of fluid balance
- Electrolyte balance
- Maintaining adequate perfusion
- Promoting comfort
- Minimizing anxiety
- Counseling of relatives
- Controlling postoperative pain.

Record Keeping

Record keeping is an important aspect of patient care and everything has to be documented in electronic as well as in patient's file. Communication of documentation and documentation of communication with the family and ICU staff should be mentioned on daily basis for each patient.

Immediate Postoperative Care of Surgical Patients

Hypothermia

Hypothermia is more common in intraoperative and postoperative period after major surgery. Neonates undergoing major operative procedures are at increased risk of thermal instability. Hypothermia can cause more respiratory and cardiac instability, requiring interventions.[13]

Nursing interventions include:

- Applying warm temperature regulating blankets,
- Decreasing skin exposure, and
- Warming operative/PACU rooms.

Hypoxemia

Immediate postoperatively patient may become hypoxemic because of combined effect of opioids, anesthetic agents, and residual effect of neuromuscular blockers. Ensuring adequate oxygenation by giving oxygen and monitoring for oxygen saturation of blood is mandatory in postoperative period. If the patient is shifted with endotracheal tube in situ and placed on mechanical ventilation, frequent arterial blood gas monitoring along with oxygen saturation monitoring helps to ensure adequate oxygenation. A chest X-ray is routinely advised in a ventilated patient immediate postoperatively and on regular basis on subsequent days.

Hypovolemia and Anemia

During prolonged surgery and major fluid and blood loss, patients may end up having hypovolemia and low hemoglobin in postoperative period if adequate fluid and blood is not replaced. These patients may need more fluids in postoperative period than the other patients. Blood products should be replaced as per recent investigation reports.

After abdominal surgeries, the nursing intervention is to look for abdominal compartment syndrome in the context of abdominal closures with decreased perfusion and the potential for decreased urine output.

Glycemic Control

Prolonged surgery and major surgery can cause hyperglycemia secondary to stress and increased fluid administration. Pediatric patients are more prone for hypoglycemia during surgery and in postoperative period. Diabetic patients need special attention for glycemic control perioperatively. Pediatric patients should be given glucose-based crystalloids to avoid hypoglycemia. Patients on preoperative insulin therapy should be started on intravenous regular insulin or SC insulin based on sliding scale to keep blood sugar below 180 mg/dL.

Hemodynamic Stability

Hypotension secondary to hypovolemia may be treated with fluid boluses according to volume status of patient and type of surgery. Use of vasopressors and inotropes should be considered in patients not responding to fluids or in patients where excessive fluid intake can deterriorate the patient's condition. If anemic, packed red blood cells may be used.

Drain Output

Replacement of any gastric output should be considered with 0.45 normal saline with 10 mEq of KCL/liter. If output is large, consider replacing more frequently (i.e., every 4 hours to run over 4 hours versus once a shift over 1 hour if lower output). Replacement of gastric fluid is important to maintain fluid balance and must be balanced with urine output and overall body edema.

Infection Control

One of the most important aspects in nursing care of critically ill patients is infection control. A proper infection control helps in reducing cost of intensive care because of less use of antibiotics. All the invasive lines, tubes, drains, and any wound dressing changes should be handled in a strict aseptic fashion. A proper hand washing before and after touching the patient and their equipment is very crucial and have shown good results in preventing cross infection in patients.

Wound Care

The nurse along with surgical team must provide careful wound care in an attempt to prevent infection. Even though wound healing follows a pattern and is consistent for humans of any age, but neonates have this unique ability to heal rapidly. There is less scar hypertrophy occurring from birth to age 1.[14] However, wound healing can be compromised for number of reasons. Infections, poor nutrition, impaired circulation, hematomas, and seromas can all contribute to wound dehiscence which can further be managed with wet-to-dry dressing to allow the wound to granulate and contract.

THE SURGICAL NEONATE

The surgical neonate is a unique individual requiring specialized care and a distinct approach to his/her medical management during the preoperative, intraoperative, and postoperative period. Neonates with congenital birth defects needing surgery require very specialized care.[13,14] Understanding the unique needs of these babies is imperative throughout the perioperative period. Care of surgical neonate requires careful consideration of many aspects including the impact of anesthesia and surgery on multiple organ systems. Neonatal care should include, close attention to achieving homeostasis and stability in the perioperative period. Surgical neonates who require a lengthy hospital stay should get their schedule series of immunization once stable.

Management of surgical neonate involves stabilization and ongoing assessment of cardiopulmonary status, thermoregulation, fluid and electrolyte balance, drug therapy, wound care, and nutritional support.

Neonates have different IV fluid requirements because of their excess total body water in comparison with muscle mass and fat. The more the neonate is preterm, the more increase in ECF. After birth, there is a shift of fluid from the extracellular compartment, that results in salt and water diuresis in 48–72 hours and physiological weight loss in the first week of life. Neonates are more sensitive to hypovolemia due to relatively low cardiac contractility. Maintenance fluid replacement should allow for the initial loss of ECF diuresis over the first week of life while maintaining normal intravascular volume and tonicity reflected by heart rate, urine output, electrolytes, and acid/base status.

NUTRITION MANAGEMENT

The surgical patient carries the challenge of satisfying the increased nutritional and metabolic demands of surgical stress and along with this pediatric surgical patients have to bear high energy requirement for growth.[15] As a perioperative CCN, nutritional assessment should be performed perioperatively. This is necessary to identify patients in need of nutritional therapy and those at risk of malnutrition who may benefit from nutrition support in pre- and postoperative period. Estimation of dietary energy, protein, and micronutrient intake helps explain possible causes for failure to thrive, establish the nutritional risk of surgical patient, and determine needs in the postoperative setting. Nutrition can be given by oral, enteral, or parenteral route.

Oral intake is mostly suitable for small surgical procedure where bowel handling is not done or minimally done. In major surgery involving gastrointestinal (GI) tract, oral route is not suitable for at least first one or two days.

Enteral route (EN) is the preferred method for meeting nutritional requirements in most of the major surgical patients including GI surgeries who have a functioning or partially functioning GI tract but are unable to achieve oral intake. Enteral nutrition is used in conjunction with an oral diet if intake is suboptimal. Enhanced recovery after surgery (ERAS) protocol recommend early start of nutrition and it showed to have better outcomes after major surgical procedures.[16]

Nutrient administration is primarily achieved by means of gastric or duodenal/jejunal feedings and it can be continuous feeding or intermittent feeding. Formula of feeding should be selected based on multiple factors such as:

- Identify patient specific nutrient requirement which includes energy, protein, and fluid

- Clinical status
- Disease status
- GI function
- Length of nutrition support
- Age
- Disease specific [e.g., cystic fibrosis, necrotizing enterocolitis (NEC), short bowel syndrome, immune deficiency, burn or head trauma].

Parenteral Nutrition Support

Parenteral nutrition support (PN) should be considered for postoperative patients or medical patients in whom enteral nutrition is either contraindicated or poorly tolerated.

Indication for PN

- Congenital GI malformations
- NEC
- Hypermetabolic states
- Severe organ failure
- Total colectomy
- Inadequate nutrition with enteral feed
- Bowel obstruction

Parenteral nutrition can be given mainly by 2 access:
- Peripheral-vein parenteral nutrition (PPN)
- Central venous catheters access parenteral nutrition. Central venous access catheter needs special care including strict aseptic precautions while handling, connecting for nutrition, fluids, medications, vasopressor/inotropes and also during sampling of blood for culture and investigations.

Nursing care and maintenance of CVC needs:[17]
- Use of antiseptic agents—2% chlorhexidine
- Dressing materials preferably use of transparent semipermeable dressing.

Cleaning of catheter junction/caps needs:
- *Antiseptic agents:* 70% alcohol and/or povidone-iodine (according to institute's protocol)
- Change the cap at least every 7 days and immediately if residual blood is observed or if the integrity of the cap may have been compromised.

Twiddle's Syndrome

Patient with the nervous habit of "twiddling" their implanted ports could actually displace, curl, or kink the catheters or tubes. The nurse should observe for itching, scrubbing or excess touching of the port and the need to obtain a history, when the port appears to be tender, to have changed location, or has signs of infections present.

Cannula dislodgment and extravasation: Displacement of intravenous cannula and extravasation of fluid or vasopressors can cause serious problem in ICU and common causes are:

- Port placed in excessive adipose tissue, near breast tissue, pectoral muscles near axilla
- Movements of arms and shoulders
- Conditions that change intrathoracic pressure (coughing, sneezing, heavy lifting or forceful flushing).

Sedation and Analgesia

Sedation and analgesia are important requirement in ICU specially if the patient is on mechanical ventilation and even in nonventilated postsurgical patients.

There are various sedation agents like opioids, alpha-2 agonist, propofol, midazolam, etc. and there are certain scales used in ICU to assess sedation score like *The Richmond agitation sedation scale (RASS), Ramsay sedation score,* etc. and these can be used to assess adequate level of sedation. Analgesia should be assessed and adequate pain relief is required in postoperative period for faster healing and effortless respiration specially in abdominal and thoracic surgeries. Postoperative analgesia is given by epidural (thoracic or lumbar) analgesia, opioid- or nonopioid-based patient-controlled analgesia, clinician-based boluses of opioids or nonopioids, intravenous paracetamol and/or nonsteroidal anti-inflammatory drugs (NSAIDS) or other agents. Regular pain assessment on rest and on movement should be done in postoperative period and analgesic drugs should be scheduled according to that pain assesment is done most commonly by visual analog scale (VAS) or numeric rating scale (NRS) in adult but pain assesment in pediatric patients is tricky and difficult to comprehend.

Infection and Sepsis

Sepsis remains a frequent cause of morbidity and mortality in ICU, despite significant advances in diagnosis and management of infections. It is one of the most common admission diagnoses in the ICUs. Early recognition and treatment remain the mainstay of care, whether caring for neonates, young children or adults. Sepsis encompasses a clinical continuum of established infection with physiologic evidence of systemic inflammatory response syndrome (SIRS), which may progress to severe sepsis, and ultimately septic shock. The goal of early therapy with broad spectrum antibiotics is to interrupt this progression, minimise organ dysfunction, and provide supportive care, while treating the source of infection. It should be stressed that suspicion of infection alone is sufficient to establish the diagnosis of sepsis and initiate timely therapy.

COMMON COMPLICATIONS IN SURGICAL INTENSIVE CARE UNIT[18]

Surgical and trauma intensive care units provide the facilities, resources, and personnel needed to care for patients who have been severely injured, present with acute surgical emergencies, require prolonged and complex elective surgical procedures or have severe underlying medical conditions. Correcting the immediately evident physiologic derangement is only the first step in care of these patients. The final outcome of critically ill patients depends, to a larger extent, on events that take place after the original injury, surgical emergency, or elective procedure. Today, the concept of patient safety has grown to the point of being considered a "new healthcare discipline." Caring for surgical and trauma patients only raises the bar in terms of patient safety, because we have to take into account secondary injuries, missed injuries, and procedural complications; all of these in patients, for the most part, were fully ambulatory and with good functional status before their accident or elective procedure. Although complications occur at a relatively consistent rate, any adverse drug event, new infection, or other complication is generally perceived as unfair and unexpected.

Health Care-associated Infections

Health care-associated infection (HAI) or nosocomial infection is defined as a localized or systemic condition, resulting from an adverse reaction to the presence of an infectious agents or its toxins.[19] There must be no evidence that the infection was present at the time of admission to the acute care setting. HAIs can lead to functional disability, emotional distress, increased ICU and hospital stay, and possible other long-term sequel with reduced quality of life.

Hospital-acquired Pneumonia (HAP) and Ventilator-associated Pneumonia (VAP)

Hospital-acquired pneumonia is defined as an inflammatory condition of the lung parenchyma caused by infectious agents not presenting or incubating at the time of admission. VAP is a subset of HAP and refers to pneumonia that arises >48–72 hours after endotracheal intubation. VAP occurs almost exclusively in the ICU and represents >85% of ICU HAP. HAP is the second most common HAI and has been clearly associated with elevated morbidity and mortality. VAP is associated with increase in the length of ICU stay, hospital stay, and ventilator days.

Catheter-related Bloodstream Infections

Bloodstream infections (BSIs) are most common infections which occur in ICU patients who have central venous catheters in place and are reported as central line catheter associated BSI (CLABSI).

The surveillance definition of BSI requires positive blood cultures, with or without signs of inflammatory response and no evidence of other sources of infection. In some circumstances, a strong clinical suspicion with subsequent treatment for sepsis will be enough to configure the diagnosis of BSI even without positive cultures, particularly in pediatric population. In a patient with systemic evidence of sepsis and no other source, an infection would be considered CLABSI if a central catheter was used during the 48-hour period before its development even with negative blood cultures.

Venous Thromboembolism

Deep vein thrombosis (DVT) and pulmonary embolism (PE) are the two clinical manifestations of venous thromboembolism (VTE). Most thrombi are asymptomatic and confined to the deep veins in the calf, but when left untreated, 20–30% will extend to the thigh where they pose a 40–50% risk of embolization to the pulmonary circulation. VTE remains the most common preventable cause of hospital death. The ICU population is particularly susceptible; many of the patients already have thrombi before being transferred to the unit, with a prevalence on admission of 2–10%, and during the ICU stay, the incidence of new onset DVT is 9–40%.

◼ REFERENCES

1. Udwadia FE. Principles of Critical Care. New Delhi: Oxford University Press; 2008.
2. Henneman EA, Gawlinski A, Giuliano KK. Surveillance: a strategy for improving patient safety in acute and critical care units. Crit Care Nurse. 2012;32:e9-e18.
3. Funk M. As health care technology advances: benefits and risks. Am J Crit Care. 2011;20:285-91.
4. Andrews FJ, Nolan JP. Critical care in the emergency department: Monitoring the critically ill patient. Emerg Med J. 2006;23:561-4.
5. Bérubé M. Evidence-based strategies for the prevention of chronic post-intensive care and acute care-related pain. AACN Adv Crit Care. 2019;30:320-34.
6. American Association of Critical-Care Nurses (AACN). (2013a). Clinical Practice Alerts and Evidence Based Practice. [online] Available from http://www.aacn.org/wd/practice/content/practice alerts.pcms? menu=practice. [Last accessed February, 2020].
7. Kuruvilla J. General aspects of care. In: Essentials of Critical Care Nursing. Jaypee Brothers Medical Publishers (Pvt) Ltd.; 2008.
8. Saharan S, Lodha R, Kabra SK. Supportive care of a critically ill child. Indian J Pediatr. 2011;78:585-92.
9. Leack KM. Perioperative management of the child. In: Wise BV, McKenna C, Garvin G, Harmon BJ (Eds.). Nursing Care of General Pediatric Surgical Patient. Maryland: ASPEN Publication; 2000.
10. WHO. Surgical Safety Checklist. [online] Available from https://www.who.int/patientsafety/safesurgery/checklist/en/. [Last accessed February, 2020].
11. Haug S, Farooqi S, Banerji A, Hopper A. Perioperative care of the neonate. In: Baerg J (Ed.). Pediatric and Neonatal Surgery. London: IntechOpen Limited; 2017.
12. Liddle C. Postoperative care 1: Principles of monitoring postoperative patients. Nurs Times. 2013;109:22, 24-26.
13. Advanced Cardiac Life Support. H's and T's of ACLS. [online] Available at https://acls-algorithms.com/hsandts/. [Last accessed on February, 2020].
14. Keener KE, Knoerlein KD, McKenney WM, McNamara LM, Mullaney DM, Quinn SM. The Surgical Neonate: Nursing Care of General Pediatric Surgical Patient. Maryland: ASPEN Publication; 2000.
15. Weimann A, Braga M, Carli F, Higashiguchi T, Hübner M, Klek S, et al. ESPEN guideline: clinical nutrition in surgery. Clin Nutr. 2017;36:623-50.
16. Wang WK, Tu CY, Shao CX, Chen W, Zhou QY, Zhu JD, et al. Impact of enhanced recovery after surgery on postoperative rehabilitation, inflammation, and immunity in gastric carcinoma patients: a randomized clinical trial. Braz J Med Biol Res. 2019;52:e8265.
17. Kenney MA. Vascular access. In: Nursing Care of General Pediatric Surgical Patient. Maryland: ASPEN Publication; 2000.
18. To KB, Napolitano LM. Common complications in the critically ill patient. Surg Clin North Am. 2012;92:1519-57.
19. Wise BV, McKenna C, Garvin G, Harmon BJ. Nursing Care of the General Paediatric Surgical Patient. Maryland: ASPEN Publications; 2000.

CHAPTER

66

Audit and Quality Improvement

Subhash Todi, Chandan Biswas

INTRODUCTION

Historically, anesthesia and perioperative care have been in the forefront of quality and safety movement in health care industry. With increasing consumer demand and medicolegal pressures, accountability is increasing in all disciplines of medicine and more so in perioperative field. Quality movement started with the seminal report by Institute of Medicine "To err is human: building a safer health system" which described that 98,000 people die in any given year from medical errors that occur in hospitals.[1] That is more than that die from motor vehicle accidents, breast cancer, or AIDS—three causes that receive far more public attention. This declaration broke the mythical perception of medical practice as being safe. Though it is accepted that to err is human but not to learn from these mistakes is inhuman. Quality and Safety are two terms, which are used interchangeably and are like two sides of the same coin. Quality implying acts of omission, i.e., things are not done which should have been done, e.g., omission of perioperative deep vein thrombosis (DVT) prophylaxis, which can also be a patient safety issue, as it can lead to fatal pulmonary embolism. Safety on the other hand implies act of commission, i.e., things are done which should not have been done, e.g., administration of heparin in a bleeding patient. The term "error" should be avoided as it may be mistaken as negligence in the part of healthcare worker. In most of the circumstances the deficiency in quality care is due to system failure rather than an individual mistake and all measures should be taken to correct the underlying root cause by fact-finding exercise and not by fault finding and penalizing individuals. It is only by correcting systematic errors one can prevent mistakes from happening in future.[2]

THREE PILLARS OF QUALITY

Many principles of quality control in medicine has been borrowed from other industries and are managerial principles applicable to any service organization. Donabedian[3,4] described three pillars on which quality indicators may be constructed, i.e., structure, process, and outcome. Structural domain (what we have) relates to the human resource availability, design aspects, model of health care delivery and is dependent on financial resources and is predominantly controlled by hospital administrators with minimal input from clinicians. Process measures (what we do) is related to the proper implementation and compliance with policies and protocols. Outcome indicators (what we get) reflect mortality and morbidity parameters. These pillars of quality measures provide quantitative aspects of estimating quality and reflects on variability of clinical practices and outcome. Though some variability in patient outcome could be due to patient risk factors but others could be due to variable structure and processes of care. This chapter will review the application of principles of quality control as applicable to perioperative care.

In a recent systematic review of the literature on the subject of quality indicators in perioperative care, structure (**Box 1**) and process (**Box 2**) indicators were summarized.[5]

Box 1: Structural indicators or perioperative quality of care.

- A designated area suitable for private communication with patients should be available. Patients are given adequate information to make decision about informed consent
- Multidisciplinary team meetings to discuss patients preoperatively
- *Locally agreed policies for preoperative preparation:* Preoperative fasting, preoperative investigations, blood cross-match, thromboprophylaxis, diabetes management, allergies
- Standardized preoperative assessment protocols

Contd...

Contd...

- Up-to-date, clear, and complete information about operating lists should be immediately available. Any changes are agreed by all relevant parties
- *Additional support for patients with special needs including children:* Patients and/or advocates have access to an interpreter
- Unscheduled surgical care should be managed in a surgical ward or critical care environment
- If the patient is to go directly to theater after imaging, and decisions need to be made on the report, a provisional report is available within 30 minutes and a definitive report within 1 hour
- Availability of cardiopulmonary exercise testing for all patients undergoing major surgery
- A consultant anesthetist should lead the anesthetic preoperative assessment service, and this is factored into their job plan
- Locally agreed specialty risk scoring mechanisms in place and these are applied to all patients admitted as an emergency
- Before surgery, except in the case of acute, life-threatening situations, in the absence of patient records, information from family/surrogate specially for unconscious/elderly/confused patients
- Special precaution for elderly in preoperative period for assessments of patients admitted as emergency general surgical patients
- A written policy document to address the airway management of patients in the emergency department
- Availability of a protocol on performing prospective risk analysis preoperatively
- *Availability of anesthetic equipment in the operating room:* Measurement of inspired gas concentrations, saturations, tidal volumes, temperature, noninvasive blood pressure equipment available
- The recovery room staff are appropriately trained in all relevant aspects of postoperative care and are present in appropriate numbers
- Fully resourced, dedicated daytime emergency and trauma lists are available
- Devices for maintaining or raising the temperature of the patient are available including control of theater temperature
- Access to blood and blood conservation techniques (cell salvage or acute normovolemic hemodilution) are available
- There is a planned maintenance and replacement program for all anesthetic equipment as required
- All patients should have a named and documented supervisory anesthetist who has overall responsibility for the care of the patient intraoperatively
- After general or regional anesthesia, or sedation, all patients recover in an especially designated area which meets AAGBI and Department of Health guidelines (UK)
- There are agreed criteria for discharge from recovery
- Equipment to provide a full range of local and regional blocks is available in the operating suite
- In every site where anesthesia is given, emergency drugs including intralipid, sugammadex, and dantrolene are available and an in-date supply is maintained
- After agreed criteria for discharge have been met, an appropriately trained member of staff accompanies patients during transfer
- In a usual week, how many dedicated and planned consultant anesthetic sessions (i.e., outside of on-call and other duties) support those operating theaters available for adult general surgical emergency cases?
- All records for anesthesia and sedation contain the relevant portion of the recommended anesthetic data set and are kept as a permanent document in the patient's record
- Where sedation is provided by an anesthetist, there is a policy for the provision of this service in all subspecialty areas and the specifications of the facilities provided
- An emergency call system is in place and understood by all relevant staff; verbal confirmation of the system and how it is used should be given by any member of staff when asked
- People having surgery for inflammatory bowel disease have it undertaken by a colorectal surgeon who is a core member of the inflammatory bowel disease multidisciplinary team
- Clinicians performing endoscopy supported by dedicated endoscopy staff as opposed to other nursing staff (e.g., theater staff)
- Drugs intended for regional anesthesia are stored separately from those intended for intravenous (IV) use
- There is a written policy for the management of complications of neuraxial blockade
- Blood storage facilities are in close proximity to emergency theaters and contain O rhesus negative blood
- Equipment for fluid and blood warming and rapid infusion is available
- Equipment is available to administer oxygen to all patients undergoing procedures under sedation by an anesthetist
- There is specialized equipment for the management of difficult airways available in every area where anesthesia is given. The equipment on it should be checked. All members of staff should be able to confirm its location.
- Facilities for external cardiac pacing are available. Defibrillators should be checked to ensure they include pacing mode
- Clinicians wishing to perform ultrasound-guided regional anesthesia should be experienced in the administration of regional nerve blocks and trained in ultrasound guidance techniques
- There is regular (at least bimonthly) review of all deaths following emergency general surgery
- Postanesthesia care unit (PACU) bed area, capacity, and equipment are all maintained to national standards
- Regular education and training of PACU staff to national standards
- Transfer from operating room to PACU is with a formal handover process
- *There is a policy for the postprocedural review of all patients:* Surgical and anesthetic
- Availability of postoperative elderly medicine review for postoperative patients
- Presence of postoperative multidisciplinary consultation for facilitated discharge of patients
- Patients and supporters are given clear information on discharge from the service and are able to make contact with a healthcare professional for advice and support
- Availability of inpatient and postdischarge rehabilitation
- There is specialized equipment for the management of postoperative pain. An adequate number of PCAs epidural pumps and the arrangements for their use should be available for the services being provided

Contd...

Contd...

- Presence of a surveillance system for postoperative wound infections
- Availability of surgical follow-up within 30 days following hospital discharge
- Each PACU should have suitable recovery and discharge criteria
- Audit and critical incident systems should be in place in PACU
- Hospital annual case volume
- *Protocols exist for the perioperative management of*—venous thromboembolism prophylaxis, avoidance of hypothermia, management of diabetes mellitus, handover, anesthetic emergencies, morbidly obese patients, handling of complaints, elderly patients, remote site anesthesia, end of life care, and critical care referral
- Surgical monthly/annual case volume by surgical specialty
- *Availability of specialist services:* Burn care, transplant, trauma, endoscopic retrograde cholangiopancreatography (ERCP), prosthetics, brachytherapy, radiotherapy, sexual function, specialist continence, psychological counselling, diabetes nurse specialist, physiotherapy, and acute medical admissions
- 24 hours availability of X-ray, computed tomography, ultrasound, isotope bone scan, multiparametric magnetic resonance imaging, teleradiology, reporting by radiologist, reporting by specialized radiologist
- *Availability of:* Malignant hyperthermia kit, difficult intubation kit, and cardiac arrest cart in the theater complex
- *24 hours availability of:* Biochemistry, hematology, microbiology, and blood bank laboratories
- Surgical on-call rota is in compliance with national guidance
- *Formal staff training in:* Use of equipment, clinical practice guidelines, technical and nontechnical skills of perioperative care
- All perioperative services are consultant led
- Availability of appropriate facilities for rest and refreshment. Availability of consultant within 30 minutes of base site
- How many operating theaters in the hospital? (Excluding radiology suites, dedicated obstetric, minor ops but including day case theaters)
- *Number of general surgical beds:* The number of funded level 2 and 3 beds available for adult (>18) general surgical patients
- Availability of elderly medicines on site. Routine daily assessment of surgical patients?
- Rotas should be provided and include the allocation of formal handover time and place as well as which staff should be present at this handover
- Does the hospital accept emergency surgical admissions?
- 24 hours availability of diagnostic and interventional radiology
- The service submits data to prescribed national audits. Regular audit of critical incidents
- The department has a funded and staffed acute pain service
- *Bed size of hospital:* How many adult inpatient/overnight/23 hours stay available within the hospital
- Perioperative team size and composition
- The service has mechanisms to receive feedback from patients and supporters. Printed patient information and alternative language leaflets available
- Availability of dedicated office space, swipe card access, admin staff, and skilled assistance for surgical staff
- There are formal protocol/pathways for emergency general surgical patients
- University affiliation of the general surgery subsection
- Pharmacists are readily available to consult with nurses and medics on noncritical care units; pharmacy formularies are accessible
- Day surgery patients should have access to a 24 hours staffed telephone line for advice and help
- Theater suite conforms to Department of Health building standards
- Presence of a formal handover process for consultants and nonconsultant clinicians
- There is a trained resuscitation team for adults
- Accreditation of the surgical unit by the joint commission or cancer commission
- Dedicated operating rooms are available for each surgical specialty
- There is adequate protection provided for staff in hazardous situations
- Are admitted patients retained by the on-call consultant or are they handed over? Is there a formal handover policy?
- All research is R and D reviewed and Research Ethics Committee (REC) reviewed. Opportunities to engage in research are prioritized by the unit/network
- The emergency surgical service has an identified medical and nurse lead (separate to the leads of elective surgery)
- There is a resuscitation officer responsible for coordinating and training of staff
- Adequate surgeon training and experience for each specialty in compliance with national training guidance
- Anesthetists offering perioperative analgesia services should provide, in collaboration with other healthcare professionals as appropriate, ongoing education in analgesia
- The presence of centralization of hospital specialties
- Anesthetists and other healthcare providers should use standardized, validated instruments to facilitate the regular evaluation and documentation of pain intensity, the effects of pain therapy, and side effects caused by the therapy
- Presence of appropriate operating room equipment in compliance with national standards
- Does the hospital participate in clinical trials?
- Does the hospital disseminate reports to its community on quality and costs of healthcare services?
- Number of accredited surgeons professionals
- Number of accredited anesthesia professionals
- Dedicated surgical scrub nurses for each surgical specialty are present
- Modified early warning scores are used on surgical wards
- There is a defined governance structure to assure the quality of the service and allow for continuous improvement

Contd...

Contd...

- Senior clinicians are involved in the discussion of end-of-life pathways. Written policy should be provided as well as a verbal account of discussions of end of life pathways
- Presence of agreed protocols to defer elective activity in order to give adequate priority to unscheduled admissions
- Suitable administrative and secretarial support is available at all times for the emergency surgical team
- A representative range of resuscitation equipment, matching that in use and including mannequins, is available for training purposes by the resuscitation training officer
- There is a local resuscitation policy in compliance with national guidelines
- Surgical specialty under which amputation was performed (vascular, general, foot, and ankle surgeons)
- Availability of a perioperative antibiotic protocol
- Availability of a perioperative anticoagulant protocol

(AAGBI: Association of Anaesthetists of Great Britain and Ireland)

Box 2: Process indicators for perioperative quality indicators.

- Percentage of patients who have received an anesthetic assessment before the day of surgery
- Each patient should have his or her expected risk of death estimated and documented prior to intervention and due adjustments made in urgency of care and seniority of staff involved
- The following medical history should be documented in the medical record prior to the operation—past medical history, past surgical history, drug history, allergies
- Elapsed time between admission and entry into operating theater is measured
- Each patient should have appropriate preoperative tests—hemoglobin or hematocrit, platelets, sodium, potassium, chloride, glucose, urea, creatinine, chest X-ray, height, and weight
- Patients and their advocates understand the risks and outcomes associated with their procedure
- For alcohol abusers 1 month abstinence before surgery. For daily smokers, 1 month abstinence before surgery. Offer smoking cessation advice
- *Adequate preoperative fasting:* Clear fluids up to 2 hours prior to surgery, solids up to 6 hours prior to surgery
- Consultant surgeon review before surgery
- What proportion of patients had a CT scan before surgery?
- Time from diagnosis/referral to operation should be <2 months
- The following review of systems should be documented in the medical prior to the operation—skin (lesions/rash), cardiovascular (peripheral vascular disease, thromboembolic disease), respiratory (upper respiratory tract infection), urology (urinary tract infection, urinary retention), musculoskeletal (arthralgia, inflammatory arthritis), endocrine (diabetes mellitus)
- All patients, on admission, receive an assessment of venous thromboembolism and bleeding risk using risk assessment criteria
- Patient nutritional status assessed within 48 hours of admission to hospital by a dietician
- What proportion of patients was reviewed by a consultant surgeon within 12 hours of emergency presentation at hospital
- No routine administration of preoperative anesthetic medication or sedation
- Mechanical bowel preparation not used routinely for colonic surgery
- What proportion of patients had preoperative prophylactic venothromboembolism therapy?
- Performance of risk assessment for pressure ulcers using a standardized scale upon admission
- The proportion of cancer patients discussed by a multidisciplinary team preoperatively
- Was a discharge or rehabilitation plan discussed and recorded at the pre-assessment clinic?
- Preoperative oral carbohydrate treatment used routinely for all nondiabetic patients
- Proportion of patients with hip fracture operated on within 48 hours of hospital admission
- *Cancer care plan intent documented in the medical notes:* Curative, palliative, or no active treatment (supportive)
- Presence of an up-to-date medication list is documented in the medical record
- Percentage of surgery patients who do not see an anesthesia provider before day of operation
- Percentage of patients having a preoperative specialist falls assessment
- Patients and/or their advocates are given information about the possible side effects of pain relief drugs
- Preoperative methicillin-resistant *Staphylococcus aureus* patient screening is undertaken and documented
- Elderly patients should have a preoperative mobility and cognitive assessment
- If a patient is to undergo intestinal surgery, then the plan for surgery should be communicated to the referring physician and the patient's primary care physician
- Preoperative glucose monitoring for patients with diabetes mellitus is undertaken
- Days from fracture injury to admission to hospital measured and documented
- Proportion of patients who have a chlorhexidine shower preoperatively
- Percentage of patients with malignancy who undergo adjuvant chemotherapy preoperatively
- Written instructions for specific medicines are handed out to patients preoperatively. This includes information on—anticoagulants, diabetic medications, cardiovascular medications, and hormonal medications
- Percentage of patients/carers who are offered verbal and written information on venous thromboembolism prevention as part of their hospital admission process
- Patients provided with antiembolism stockings have them fitted and monitored in accordance with National Institute for Health and Care Excellence guidance
- Elapsed time between admission/referral to when first seen by consultant surgeon is measured and documented

Contd...

Contd...

- The maternity team is notified when a pregnant woman is admitted with a nonobstetric surgical problem
- Hip fracture patients are admitted under the joint care of a consultant geriatrician and a consultant orthopedic surgeon
- People having surgery are advised not to remove hair from the surgical site and to have a shower/bath the day on or before surgery
- Percentage of patients who had preoperative physiotherapy
- If the patient was admitted with ischemia or diabetic foot sepsis, did a consultant vascular surgeon review them within 24 hours of admission?
- Was the patient seen by an amputation/discharge coordinator preoperatively?
- Patient seen by inpatient acute pain team preoperatively
- Stoma care—patients with colorectal cancer who require a stoma are assessed and have their stoma site marked preoperatively by a nurse with expertise in stoma care
- Any changes to surgical lists are agreed by all relevant parties
- Prophylactic antibiotics are administered within 60 minutes before start of surgery
- Adults having surgery under general or regional anesthesia have normothermia (temperature >36°C) maintained before, during, and after surgery
- Proportion of patients who have had appropriate prophylactic antibiotic selection for surgical patients
- An appropriately trained and experienced anesthetist is present throughout the conduct of all general and regional anesthesia for operative procedures
- If hair removal is required, it should not be performed with a razor but with clippers
- A multimodal approach for postoperative nausea and vomiting prophylaxis should be adopted in all patients with ≥2 risk factors
- The World Health Organization surgical safety checklist (or a local variant thereof) is used for all surgical procedures in theater
- Number of cancelled planned operations
- Percentage of patients receiving a blood transfusion in accordance with National Health and Medical Research Council guidelines during the surgical procedure
- Duration of surgery measured and documented
- Surgical procedures with a predicted mortality >10% should be conducted under direct supervision of consultant surgeon and anesthetist
- Recommended standards of monitoring are met for each patient. This should be visible on the anesthetic chart
- Appropriate surgical approach for current operative procedure used
- *Optimized perioperative fluid management:* Targeting cardiac output, avoiding over-hydration, and judicious use of vasopressors. Targeted fluid therapy using the Doppler is recommended
- Patients for whom a central venous catheter was inserted with all elements of sterile barrier technique followed Documentation of daily examination of line site for signs of infection and continued need for central line
- Mechanical thromboprophylaxis used intraoperatively
- Percentage of 1st cases starting on time measured and recorded
- Operating room turnover time (minute) measured
- Epidural analgesia used intraoperatively
- Intraoperative blood loss is measured and recorded
- Critically ill patients in the recovery area are cared for by appropriately trained staff and have appropriate monitoring and support
- *Postanesthetic transfer of care:* Use of a checklist or protocol for direct transfer of care from procedure room to intensive care
- Surgical field preparation with chlorhexidine-alcohol
- What proportion of patients received goal directed fluid therapy during surgery?
- *Maintenance of euglycemia perioperatively:* Use of standardized protocol to maintain serum glucose <200 mg/day
- Measures to ensure proper positioning on table documented to prevent peripheral nerve damage and maintain skin integrity
- Number of patients receiving light or moderate sedation
- Adequate perioperative management of patient's current medications
- Induction time (minute) and emergence time (minute) are recorded
- Measurement and documentation of pain intensity scores after major surgery
- Elapsed time between admission and first dose of antibiotics in theater
- Intraoperative use of forced air warming
- *Surgical pathology specimens are correctly labeled:* Labeled, filled container, correct laterality, correct tissue type, patient name, correct patient name
- Wound catheters or transversus abdominis plane block used for intraoperative analgesia
- Multimodal approach to optimizing postoperative gut function is used
- Surgeons use explicit procedure specific intraoperative checklists
- Intravenous analgesia (patient controlled analgesia or IV lidocaine)
- Perioperative urine output monitored carefully in patients with renal failure
- All anesthetic equipment is checked before use according to AAGBI published guidelines and the checks are documented
- Type of anesthesia administered documented
- Physician Quality Reporting System/Surgical Care Improvement Project documentation available and completed
- People with hip fracture have their schedule on a planned trauma list, with consultant or senior staff supervision
- No systemic morphine used intraoperatively
- Proportion of surgical patients who had an order for venous thromboembolism prophylaxis to be given within 24 hours before incision/after surgery end
- Proportion of patients whose prophylactic antibiotics were discontinued within 24 hours after surgery end time
- Patients should be encouraged to sit out of bed and begin mobilizing the day after surgery, within 24 hours or as determined by the surgeon
- Discharge needs assessment, venous thromboembolism prophylaxis, rehabilitation, and follow-up are organized postoperatively for patients

Contd...

Contd...

- Urinary catheter removed on postoperative day 1 or postoperative day 2 with day of surgery being day 0, or reason for continuing use documented
- Postoperative treatment of diabetes mellitus (or documentation of attempt) to keep BM <10 mmol/L on day of surgery and the first 2 postoperative days
- Postoperative nasogastric tubes should not be used routinely
- Pain should be controlled with oral or nonparenteral medications on the day of surgery and before discharge, and be adequate enough to allow acute rehabilitation
- Postoperative pain assessments should be performed with each set of vital signs
- Enteral route for postoperative fluid used as soon as possible, IV fluids discontinued as soon as is practicable
- Postoperative delirium screening for all patients
- Postoperative normothermia maintained at—36–38°C
- People having surgery and their carers receive information and advice on wound and dressing care
- Cognitive and functional assessment performed daily postoperatively and at discharge
- Official postanesthesia care unit (PACU) to ward handover undertaken for all patients
- Patient's condition and vital signs evaluated continuously in the PACU
- PACU length of stay measured
- Documentation of a systematic, multidisciplinary team approach to supported discharge of suitable patients
- Stimulation of bowel movements using an even fluid balance, laxatives and chewing gum
- Percentage of recovery nurses following acute pain protocols
- Early warning system used on postoperative wards
- Patients with a risk of death >10% should be admitted to a critical care location postoperatively
- Immediately postsurgery a member of the medical/nursing team updates the patient's supporter(s) of the outcome of surgery
- Postanesthesia documentation is documented to the agreed national standard
- Visual phlebitis scores are measured daily postoperatively
- The head of the bed is elevated postoperatively
- Hydration, pressure care, assessment and treatment of pain, and attention to nutrition and continence are begun in the emergency room and are continued in the orthopedic ward postoperatively
- Patients having a postoperative physician review (not critical care)
- Waiting time from time appointed for surgical procedure until discharge
- Days from surgery until discharge from hospital
- Patients receiving prescribed antiemetic treatment when nausea and vomiting are present during acute pain management
- Time from operation until adjuvant chemotherapy
- All patients given supplemental oxygen as required
- At the end of surgery, was the decision made to place the patient on an end of life pathway; was this documented
- Review by a specialist from Elderly Medicine in the postoperative period
- What proportion of patients were admitted directly to a high dependency unit or intensive therapy unit following surgery
- After fracture surgery there is communication with the physicians responsible for postsurgical care
- Patients undergoing a procedure with an anesthetist who have a documented evidence of a postanesthesia review
- Structured assessment of patient mortality and morbidity risk, carried out at the end of surgery
- Daily anesthetist review following epidural analgesia
- Chronic beta blocker use is continued in perioperative period (24 hours before incision to first 2 postoperative days)
- Percentage of surgery patients who received appropriate venous thromboembolism prophylaxis within 24 hours prior to surgery to 24 hours after surgery
- Surgery takes place during standard daytime working hours (including weekends) except in exceptional circumstances
- Documentation of oral intake during the hospitalization
- Cooperation between orthopedic, physicians, and anesthetists in preoperative, operative, and postoperative medical management, and in the rehabilitation of hip fracture patients
- Perioperative continued use of aspirin for patients with drug-eluting coronary stents
- Information is provided to patients and supporters at each stage of the care pathway. Communication with patients and supporters is consultant-led
- Clinical audit of all emergency surgical procedures whether undertaken in an operating theater or another area (e.g., emergency resus room) is regularly undertaken
- Named supervisory consultants are available to all nonconsultant anesthetists. Those they are supervising know their identity, location, and how to contact them. In situations where a trainee is remotely supervised, the trainee must contact their supervising consultant immediately who should attend as soon as is possible
- The perioperative anesthetic care of all patients is, at all times, led by a consultant anesthetist. Clinical care may be delegated to a supervised, clinically competent trainee of sufficient seniority
- Perioperative care following GIFTASUP fluid guidelines
- Patient transfer is carried out to standards described by the AAGBI
- A consultant in intensive care medicine reviews all emergency surgical admissions to the ICU within 12 hours
- A geriatrician assesses hip fracture patients within 72 hours of admission

Contd...

Contd...

- *National policy for patient identification is followed:* Evidence that patients are labelled, that labels are replaced and that patient name and number are both used at every stage of the World Health Organization process should be seen
- Enhanced recovery used perioperatively
- Anesthetists offering perioperative analgesia services should provide, in collaboration with others as appropriate, patient and family education regarding their important roles in achieving comfort, reporting pain, and in proper use of recommended analgesic methods
- Percentage of patients whose anesthesia provider is the same during preoperative, intraoperative, and postoperative care

(AAGBI: The Association of Anaesthetists of Great Britain and Ireland; GIFTASUP: British Consensus Guidelines on Intravenous Fluid Therapy for Adult Surgical Patients)

Outcome Indicators[6-8]

As part of the International Standardised Endpoints in Perioperative Medicine (StEP) initiative, a study was conducted to derive a set of standardized and valid clinical outcome indicators for use in perioperative clinical trials, which may be useful in clinical practice as well. A final list of eight outcome indicators was generated: Surgical site infection at 30 days, stroke within 30 days of surgery, death within 30 days of coronary artery bypass grafting, death within 30 days of surgery, admission to the intensive care unit within 14 days of surgery, readmission to hospital within 30 days of surgery, and length of hospital stay (with or without in-hospital mortality). They were rated by the majority of experts as valid, reliable, easy to use, and clearly defined.

Electronic Medical Records

These are the digital equivalent of paper records, or charts. Electronic medical records (EMRs) typically contain general information such as treatment and medical history about a patient as it is collected by the individuals involved in the patient care. By implementing EMR, patient data can be tracked over an extended period of time by multiple healthcare providers. EMRs are designed to help organizations provide efficient and precise care and can impact the quality of perioperative care. EMR records are universal, meaning that instead of having different charts at different healthcare facilities, a patient will have one electronic chart that can be accessed from any healthcare facility using EMR software. EMR also ensures improvisation of quality and safety of perioperative care. It ensures easy access of all patient information such as allergies, comorbidities, any adverse complications of any medication. Thus a safer, more efficacious care is ensured towards the patients end.

Anesthesia information management systems (AIMS) is a type of electronic medical record system that collects, stores and makes available all the necessary information about the patient in the perioperative period. It is an important tool to record and present database that can reveal subtle but vital information that indicates quality of perioperative care. It also prevents suppression of any information and details of the patient care that ensures proper vigilance of the healthcare providers.

Logistics and infrastructure to ensure good quality perioperative care: There are various logistics issues involved in improvising the quality. Placement of the operating rooms and intensive care units (ICU) in the same floor will allow for easier transit and safety of the patients. Correct positioning of the entry, exit and holding areas in the perioperative period not only provide the ease of transport but also the easy monitoring the patients and thus allaying mishaps. Especially in transit of patients from and to the ICU are complicated by the various invasive lines and monitors, which are inevitable. Proper transport mechanism for the patients also are a key in the safety and quality of the perioperative care. Patients with trauma, patients on neuromuscular blockers, morbidly obese patients need special attention during the transit and shifting to the ICU beds. Specialized trolleys, sliders or rollers along with proper knowledge and training of the healthcare staff are required for the same.

Audit and training in perioperative care: Special training on a regular basis for upgradation of knowledge and skills involved in perioperative care should be provided to all stakeholders. This should include the doctors, nursing staff, health assistants, technicians, and paramedics involved in the care. Audit about the quality of the care is a key in the improvement of the quality. A monthly or at most a quarterly audit of the quality and indicators should be performed to ensure an early recognition of flaws and measures.

CONCLUSION[9,10]

Based on the above-mentioned parameters, each healthcare facility, small or large should create its own dashboard for indicators of quality. Quality control data can be used for research, accreditation and foremost patient care. Quality control through regular audit should be followed religiously in all aspects of health care delivery and specifically for perioperative care. It has been wisely quoted in our scriptures that one needs to do their processes correctly and good outcome will eventually follow.

REFERENCES

1. Kohn LT, Corrigan JM, Donaldson MS. To err is human: building a safer health system. Institute of Medicine (US) Committee on Quality of Health Care in America. Washington (DC): National Academies Press; 2000.

2. Pronovost PJ, Nolan T, Zeger S, Miller M, Rubin H. How can clinicians measure safety and quality in acute care? Lancet. 2004;363:1061-7.

3. Donabedian A. Special article: the quality of care: how can it be assessed? JAMA. 1988;260:1743-8.

4. Donabedian A. Evaluating the quality of medical care. Milbank Mem Fund Q. 1966;83:691-729.

5. Chazapis M, Gilhooly D, Smith AF, Myles PS, Haller G, Grocott MPW, et al. Perioperative structure and process quality and safety indicators: A systematic review. Br J Anaesth. 2018;120(1):51-66.

6. Bampoe S, Cook T, Fleisher L, Grocott MPW, Neuman M, Story D, et al. Clinical indicators for reporting the effectiveness of patient quality and safety-related interventions: a protocol of a systematic review and Delphi consensus process as part of the International Standardised Endpointsfor Perioperative Medicineinitiative (StEP). BMJ Open. 2018;8:e023427.

7. Boney O, Moonesinghe SR, Myles PS, Grocott MP. Standardizing endpoints in perioperative research. Can J Anaesth. 2016; 63(2):159-68.

8. Myles PS, Grocott MPW, Boney O, Moonesinghe SR. Standardizing end points in perioperative trials: towards a core and extended outcome set. Br J Anaesth. 2016;116:586-9.

9. Haller G, Stoelwinder J, Myles PS, McNeil J. Quality and safety indicators in anesthesia: a systematic review. Anesthesiology. 2009;110:1158-75.

10. Mainz J. Defining and classifying clinical indicators for quality improvement. Int J Qual Health Care. 2003;15:523-30.

Communication in the Perioperative Period

Shivakumar Iyer, Nishant Agrawal

"The most important thing in communication is hearing what isn't said."

—Peter Drucker

INTRODUCTION

Communication in the perioperative period is a different entity in itself encompassing four main areas of delivery of information to the patient and his/her relatives. First, the initial communication of information regarding the need for surgery and the preanesthetic evaluation of the patient. Second, the re-emphasis on the benefits of the surgery and risks involved during the surgical process and administration of anesthesia and obtaining a written informed consent. Third, the immediate postoperative period where the relatives are briefed about the conduct of surgery and joint counseling performed by critical care team, anesthesia, and surgical team. Fourth, before discharge from the ICU, a joint counseling by the critical care team and the surgeon to plan the goals of care, pain management and other ancillary care such as nutrition.

Various experts also participate for the safe conduct of surgery and management of patient in the perioperative period. The team of surgeons, anesthetists, nursing, blood bank staff, and last but not the least the staff involved in transport of patient to and from the theater all contribute to the safe conduct of the surgery and postoperative care. Poor interprofessional communication in the perioperative setting may contribute to an unsafe operative room culture, decision making, and productivity. Hence improving communication between professionals will provide competent and efficient care to the patient and promote a sense of harmonious teamwork and facilitate better cost containment.[1]

PRINCIPLES OF COMMUNICATION

The root of the word communication from latin is "communicare" which means to share or receive.

Communication can be defined as "a process by which information is exchanged between individuals through a common system of symbols, signs, or behavior".[2] Good communication, therefore, requires a shared verbal language and an understanding of the components of nonverbal behavior. Both these components are also culturally and geographically determined and will therefore vary from place to place. Nonetheless, there are certain common principles of good communication.

The four principles elucidated by the Institute of Medicine Committee on Quality of Health Care in America are:
1. Obtaining and grasping the patient's viewpoint.
2. Taking into account the patient's psychological state and social reality.
3. Arriving at a joint understanding of the patient's clinical problem and looking at solutions in the context of the patient's preferences and values.
4. Respecting patient's autonomy and empowering the patient through shared decision making.[3]

The Kalamazoo consensus statement describes seven tasks that need to be done during the medical encounter.[4]
1. Building the doctor patient relationship
2. Opening the discussion
3. Gathering information
4. Understanding the patient's perspective
5. Sharing information
6. Reaching agreement on problems and plans
7. Providing closure.

SPIKES Model

The SPIKES (Setting, Perception, Invitation, Knowledge, Emotion, and Summary) model was first described by Baile et al. in 2000 for breaking bad news to cancer patients and has since been used extensively in several settings including critical care **(Table 1)**.[5]

TOOLS AND MODELS FOR GOOD COMMUNICATION

The Cardiff six-point toolkit is a useful aid for ensuring good communication in end of life and palliative care communication **(Box 1)**.[6]

Comfort

Putting the patient at ease before starting the interview is extremely important. It includes ensuring a quiet room, comfortable seating, a pleasant atmosphere, making water and tissues available, putting the phones off, and minimizing interruptions. An appropriate beginning would be to make introductions and ask a question like *"How are you today?"*

Question Style

One generally starts by asking an *open-ended question* that allows the patient or family to set the content and pace of the conversation. It gives no idea of the expected answer. A typical example would be "How have things been?" If the patient or family chooses to answer such a question by enquiring about future difficult topics such as disease progression or prognosis it helps us to take the discussion forward by asking further focused questions.

Focused questions generally narrow down on a particular area or symptom. A special type of focused question is a hypothetical question which involves a possibility for the future, for example, "Have you wondered what might happen if we do not operate on the lump you have in your tummy?"

Table 1: SPIKES Model.

Principle	Explanation
Setting	Ensuring a comfortable physical and psychological setting
Perception	Exploring the patient/family understanding
Invitation	Judging the patient/family's readiness for receiving bad news
Knowledge	Delivering knowledge in a form that the patient/family can understand
Emotion	Watching/listening to verbal and nonverbal cues and acknowledging emotions
Summary	Summarize the meeting and draw up further plans

Box 1: Cardiff six-point toolkit.

1. Comfort
2. Question style
3. Language
4. Listening/use of silence
5. Reflection/acknowledgment
6. Summarizing

Closed-ended or direct questions are usually used to clarify matters and generally have yes or no type of responses.

It is better to avoid asking leading questions or multiple questions at the same time.

Language

It is important to try and speak in a language that the patient understands and is familiar with. Culture and ethnicity are reflected in language and may give important clues about the patient or family's emotions and state of mind. People often communicate through their gestures, facial expressions, and tone of voice. In fact the spoken word is only 7% of communication, 33% is the tone, and 60% is nonverbal. While giving medical information it is paramount to avoid using medical jargon and keeping it as simple as possible.

Listening/Use of Silence

In a good family meeting or interview, listening should occur 80% of the time and talking only 20%. Listening requires one to be calm, mindful, and to use silence effectively. Attentive silence tells the patient/family that they are being listened to and facilitates the expression of their concerns. It allows them to assimilate information and ask appropriate questions. It may also encourage them for broaching difficult or uncomfortable issues.

Reflection/Acknowledge Emotions or Distress

Reflection is a technique in which the healthcare provider reflects back a significant word or cue, encouraging the patient or family to elaborate on that word or the feeling behind that word. Sometimes a question like *"Am I really gonna get better?"* will need to be met by a question like *"That is a really difficult question to ask, what makes you ask it now?"* This acknowledges the distress without giving a banal answer and if followed by silence, may help the patient to voice their concerns underlying this question.

Summarizing/Recapping

It is important to give information in small understandable chunks and summarize and recap as we go along in order to check understanding.

FIVE FUNDAMENTAL PRINCIPLES IN COMMUNICATION SKILLS

Robert Arnold et al. describe five fundamental principles in communication skills that are complementary to the Cardiff toolkit and the SPIKES model.[7] These are:

1. "Ask-Tell-Ask"
2. "Tell Me More"

3. "Using Reflections"
4. "Responding to Emotion"
5. "Assessing the Informational, Coping, Decision-making Style"

"Ask-Tell-Ask"

Ask the patient/family to describe their current understanding of the situation by asking open-ended questions. This allows us to explore their understanding and gives the family a chance to voice their concerns. Asking permission also helps to establish mutual trust. This helps us negotiate the agenda for the meeting and also gives us an idea about the informational and decision-making style of the family.

Tell the family in clear simple language about the situation, being mindful about avoiding the use of medical jargon.

Ask what they understand now and clarify further, if necessary.

"Tell Me More"

Conversations about serious issues are generally occurring at three levels. At a superficial level, the family is trying to understand the information being provided. At a deeper level, the information elicits emotional responses that the patient/family may or may not be aware of. At a third level, the conversation may be about what the new information means to the patient or family member in terms of their own self. "Tell Me More" is a technique that allows us to explore these levels by asking questions like *"What more information do you need? How does this make you feel? How will this affect you in your day-to-day life?"*

"Using Reflections"

Restating or paraphrasing a patient/family statement can be a powerful method for eliciting further information or exploring understanding.

Simple reflections may just repeat what the family member said.

Mother—I can see what you mean but how can I give up hope?

Doctor—Give up hope? —— (Reflection)

Mother—What will I do if he gets sicker or does not make it?

Complex reflections interpret what the family member is saying and include the clinician's ideas, values or beliefs. This may be riskier but may also help change the perspective of the family member.

Patient's brother-in-law—I get what you are saying doctor, but please—do not tell my sister, she will be

devastated and would not be able to handle that he is not going to walk unassisted ever in life.

Doctor—I can see that you care deeply for your sister and want her to be prepared to accept the situation that the amputation is required to save his life. (Empathic and kind manner and allows enough silence)

Patient's brother-in-law (breaks into tears)—She has two small children Doctor, I do not know how she will cope and how she will run the family without my brother-in-law's financial assistance if he loses his job after surgery.

Thus, reflections can convey empathy and allow the family members to steer the conversation and express their concerns.

"Responding to Emotion"

Conversations about major surgeries and their outcome on activities of daily living on patients and their loved ones are very difficult and intensely emotional. As clinicians, not only do we have to contend with anger, sadness, grief, disbelief, hopelessness, and despair that patient's or family members experience, but also with our own feelings around the future.

Being mindful of our own reactions and feelings allows us to actively listen to patients and family members and express empathy. This allows us to focus our energies for eliciting patient/family concerns and addressing their emotional needs.

The expression of emotional needs is usually through nonverbal cues and indirect verbal cues. Identifying and responding to these needs is of paramount importance. Emotional reactions interfere with the ability to understand factual information and significantly affect decision-making ability.

Once an emotional reaction is identified, it must be addressed as soon as possible. One of the described models for this is NURSE (Naming, Understanding, Respecting, Supporting, and Exploring) **(Table 2)**.[8]

The most effective empathic statements are those that link the "I" of the healthcare provider to the "you" of the patient/family. We need to be able to put ourselves in the position of the patient/family and understand them fully. For example, *"I" can understand how difficult this must be for "You"*.

"Assessing the Informational, Coping, Decision-making Style"

Patients and families are not all the same in the way they process information or in the way, they cope with crisis situations. Two typical types of informational coping style "Monitors" and "Blunters" were identified by Miller et al.

Table 2: NURSE model for acknowledging emotions.

Technique	Explanation
Naming	Name the emotion appropriately, e.g., *"Some people in this situation would be upset"* rather than *"I can see that you are angry"*. (People do not like to be told what they are feeling)
Understanding	Understand and appreciate what the patient/family is experiencing, e.g., *"I cannot begin to imagine what it might be like to be in this situation"*. Avoid giving false hope or premature reassurance
Respect	Showing respect can be a nonverbal response but a verbal response can help validate the emotion. Depending on the strength of the expressed emotion, you might want to give an equally strong acknowledgment. Praising the way that the patient/family is coping is a good way of showing respect
Supporting	Support can be expressed in many ways. Willingness to help, being available, expressing your concern, and making statements about working together for resolution are all very useful. E.g., *We have covered a lot of ground today. If you want to ask me anything else, I will be available in my office and of course, we have a scheduled meeting for tomorrow*
Exploring	Exploring what people are feeling with open-ended questions or inviting them to share their story is a good way to help them express their emotions. E.g., *"What has this been like for you?" "I have given you a lot of information? What are you thinking?"*

by using the Miller Behavioural Style Scale.[9] "Monitors" are family decision makers who seek high levels of information and are prone to greater anxiety and depression. They will need identification of their emotions and support in order to prevent depression. On the other hand, "Blunters" avoid information, distance themselves from the situation at hand and tend to be in denial. They will frequently not be able to take decisions. They will require support for going beyond their emotions in order to process information for appropriate decision making.[10] At times, however, decision makers may exhibit a combination of styles. It is important to explore this "Some people prefer having all the information that they can get whereas others get overwhelmed with too much information and are content getting to know about the big picture. What kind of person are you?"

Often we may have to try out one or the other approach and decide which approach is best at that particular time for that particular person.

HOW TO ADDRESS COMMUNICATION FAILURE?

Communication failure is not an uncommon occurrence. It is an important reason for conflict and family dissatisfaction. Occasionally it may lead to violence or litigation.

The reasons for such communication failure include:
- Knowledge gap
- Transference and countertransference
- Surgeons discomfort with bad outcomes
- Lack of training in communication skills.

The ways to address such communication failure include:
- Avoiding false hope
- Controlling communication by identifying a captain of the ship
- Focusing on what the patient would want
- Setting time limited trials for therapy

- Clarifying the available choices
- Being present and expressions of understanding and empathy.[11]

An important way of preventing communication failure in the perioperative period is conducting regular family meetings.

The Family Meeting

It is clear from empiric data that communication is the single most important thing that helps preserve patient autonomy and dignity. Poor communication leads to family dissatisfaction, interferes with shared decision making, and may impose a psychological burden on the family.[12] A recent guideline endorsed by multiple medical societies gives recommendations on shared decision making.[13]

Family meetings should be conducted in the preoperative period and during postoperative care when the patient condition changes, when there is conflict, when the treating team believes that goals of care should be essentially palliative, and whenever the family requests a meeting or if the providers feel it would be helpful.

There are several steps in conducting a structured family meeting:
- *Identify and invite the clinicians/providers involved in the treatment.* This should include the nurses and social worker involved in the management. The primary care clinician or family doctor, if available, should also be invited if desired by the family. Palliative care physicians have a role to play especially if there is conflict. It may make sense to involve them early rather than late.
- *Identify the appropriate surrogates.* If possible, the patient must always be included. In India, surrogates include not only the spouse and immediate family but also the extended family and the community members and religious heads who may be providing financial and social support.

- *Meet prior to meeting the family.* Clarifying doubts about the therapeutic plan within the treating team, eliciting consensus, and setting the agenda are very important. As uncertainty is not uncommon, differences of opinion in prognosis and management should be discussed so that they can be presented in a sensible manner to the family. Clinicians need also to consider and acknowledge their own feeling and beliefs around death and dying so that it does not affect the family meeting. Nurses and social workers can provide important input regarding the family, regarding conflict and regarding their coping styles. It is also important to identify who will expedite the meeting.
- *Decide an appropriate meeting place*
- *Consider and appreciate the family dynamics*
- *Make introductions and explain the goals for the meeting*
- *Ask what the family already knows*
- *Build on what they already know by providing further information.* Provide information in small chunks.
- *Check their understanding.*
- *Summarize the clinical situation including diagnosis prognosis and therapy.* How to discuss prognosis is a matter of debate. Asking families how much information they want would be a useful starting point. Families tend to be more optimistic than clinicians in their prognostic estimates and a greater discordance maybe associated with more conflict. Given the uncertainty surrounding prognosis it is best to keep an open mind and arrive at a shared decision that reflects patient and family interest. A time limited trial of intensive care often helps to clarify uncertainty regarding prognosis.[14] Another way of dealing with uncertainty is to use *"Hope for the Best, Prepare for the Worst"* type of statements.[15] The therapeutic plan should be generated by balancing the clinicians' medical and technical expertise (balance of beneficence and non-maleficence) and the patient and family's values and goals (respect for autonomy). Patient comfort should be regarded as paramount and the tradeoffs of interventions between comfort provided and suffering entailed should be discussed. When the clinician, patient or family goals regarding therapy are not being met, a transition to palliative care must be considered.
- *Consider end-of-life issues.* The important thing is to help surrogate decision makers understand that they should be guided by what the patient would have wanted in a particular situation. Most guidelines suggest making a shared decision based on medical facts and patient values. This helps take away the decision-making burden from the surrogates/family.
- *Manage emotions.* The NURSE mnemonic has already been discussed as an aid for managing emotions.

Another useful mnemonic is VALUE that describes a communication system that enhances harmony between care providers and surrogates/family. Its components include: **V**aluing surrogate/family communication (V), **A**cknowledging their emotions with reflective summary statements (A), **L**istening actively (L), **U**nderstanding the patient as a person with the help of open-ended questions (U), and **E**liciting questions (E).[16]

- *Identify and resolve conflict.* Emotions such as sadness or frustration, stress, denial, guilt, lack trust, and misunderstanding often underlie disagreement between health care providers and surrogates/family. Attending to these emotions sensitively and providing more information often help to resolve conflict. Occasionally a second opinion, ethics consultation or palliative care consultation may be needed.
- *Prepare a summary and further plan.* At the end of the meeting, it is important to summarize the important points that cover the decisions made, the areas of disagreement if any, and the plan for follow-up. Conducting debrief with the team is an important way to teach and learn regarding communication. Ethical issues are also identified and any moral distress felt by the team members is tackled.[17]

AN INTEGRATED FRAMEWORK FOR COMMUNICATION IN THE PERIOPERATIVE PERIOD

Communication in the perioperative period starts from the time of admission and the initial contact with the patient and family by the surgeon, junior doctors, staff nurses, and the housekeeping staff. Throughout the hospital stay multiple specialists, other healthcare professionals, social workers, ancillary staff, administrative personnel, security staff, billing executives, and many others communicate with the patient or more commonly with the surrogates/family. A hospital wide communication policy can help prevent dissatisfaction and conflict. Seaman et al. outlined five goals of clinician-family interaction—establishing trust, providing emotional support, conveying clinical information, understanding the patient as a person, and facilitating careful decision making.[18] They suggest integrating multiple communication platforms such as bedside conversation, telephone discussion, family centered rounds, daily briefing by junior doctors, and well-timed family meetings in order to meet the complex communication needs of patients/families. This helps in maintaining patient satisfaction and avoiding conflicts which may arise due to communication failure. Respectful relationships are created which will help eliminate mistakes and overcome obstacles to communication.

REFERENCES

1. Cvetic E. Communication in the perioperative setting. AORN J. 2011;94:261-70.

2. Definition of communication. [online] Available from https://www.merriam-webster.com/dictionary/communication. [Last accessed March, 2020].

3. Institute of Medicine Committee on Quality of Health Care in America. Crossing the Quality Chasm: A New Health System for the 21st Century. Washington, DC: National Academy Press; 2001.

4. Makoul G. Essential elements of communication in medical encounters: the Kalamazoo consensus statement. Acad Med. 2001;76:390-3.

5. Baile WF, Buckman R, Lenzi R, Glober G, Beale EA Kudelka AP. SPIKES: a six-step protocol for delivering bad news: application to the patient with cancer. Oncologist. 2000;5:302-31.

6. Pease N. Palliative medicine: Communication to promote life near the end of life. In: Kissane D, Bultz B, Butow P, Bylund C, Noble S, Wilkinson S (Eds). Oxford Textbook of Communication in Oncology and Palliative Care, 2nd edition. Oxford: Oxford University Press; 2017.

7. Arnold R, Nelson J, Prendergast T, Emlet L, Weinstein E, Barnato A, et al. Educational Modules for the Critical Care Communication (C3) Course—A Communication Skills Training Program for Intensive Care Fellow. [online] Available from https://www.uclahealth.org/palliative-care/Workfiles/Educational-Modules-Critical-Care-Communication.pdf [Last accessed March, 2020].

8. Smith RC. Patient-Centered Interviewing: An Evidence-Based Method. Philadelphia: Lippincott Williams & Wilkins; 2002.

9. Miller SM. Monitoring versus blunting styles of coping with cancer influence the information patients want and need about their disease. Implications for cancer screening and management. Cancer. 1995;76:167-77.

10. Hickman RL Jr, Daly BJ, Douglas SL, Clochesy JM. Informational coping style and depressive symptoms in family decision makers. Am J Crit Care. 2010;19(5):410-20.

11. Meier DE. Communication failure in the ICU. Virtual Mentor. 2006;8:564-70.

12. Wood GJ , Chaitin E, Arnold RM. Communication in the ICU: Holding a family meeting. [online] Available from https://www.uptodate.com/contents/communication-in-the-icu-holding-a-family-meeting/ [Last accessed March, 2020].

13. Kon AA, Davidson JE, Morrison W, Danis M, White DB; American College of Critical Care Medicine; American Thoracic Society. Shared Decision Making in ICUs: An American College of Critical Care Medicine and American Thoracic Society Policy Statement. Crit Care Med. 2016;44:188-201.

14. Back AL, Arnold RM. Dealing with conflict in caring for the seriously ill: "it was just out of the question". JAMA. 2005;293:1374-81.

15. Back AL, Arnold RM, Quill TE. Hope for the best, and prepare for the worst. Ann Intern Med. 2003;138:439-43.

16. Lautrette A, Darmon M, Megarbane B, Joly LM, Chevret S, Adrie C, et al. A communication strategy and brochure for relatives of patients dying in the ICU. N Engl J Med. 2007;356(5):469-78.

17. Santiago C, Abdool S. Conversations about challenging end-of-life cases: ethics debriefing in the medical surgical intensive care unit. Dynamics. 2011;22:26-30.

18. Seaman JB, Arnold RM, Scheunemann LP, White DB. An integrated framework for effective and efficient communication with families in the adult intensive care unit. Ann Am Thorac Soc. 2017;14:1015-20.

Evaluation and Management of Obstructive Sleep Apnea during Perioperative Period

Sree Kumar EJ, Pon Thelac, Nileena NKM, Nagarajan Ramakrishnan

INTRODUCTION

Sleep-disordered breathing (SDB) is increasingly being recognized and treated in the past few decades. It is an umbrella term to describe disorders characterized by breathing disturbances during sleep. The third edition of International Classification of Sleep Disorders (ICSD-3) classifies SDB into obstructive sleep apnea (OSA) disorders, sleep-related hypoventilation disorders, central sleep apnea syndromes, and sleep-related hypoxemia.[1]

The shared features of sleep and anesthesia make understanding of sleep physiology and SDB in a perioperative scenario crucial. The increased risk of perioperative cardiopulmonary complications has long been recognized in patients with SDB. The prevalence of OSA is more in the surgical population than in the general population.[2] Anesthesiologists are best suited to screen patients for SDB, optimize their perioperative management along with intensivists and other experts, and contribute to their continuum of care and outcomes.[3] There are various practice guidelines given by societies around the world for perioperative management of OSA including American Society of Anesthesiologists, Society of Anesthesia and Sleep Medicine and Indian Initiative of OSA (INOSA) Guidelines.[4-7] The complex challenge of decision making in the midst of increasing number of patients and insufficient evidence on duration of therapy have resulted in a high noncompliance to available guidelines.[2]

OBSTRUCTIVE SLEEP APNEA

Prevalence, Risk Factors, and Associated Comorbidities

Among the various diagnoses of SDB, OSA is the most commonly encountered category. OSA rather than being a disease, is a syndrome characterized by periodic, partial, or complete obstruction in the upper airway during sleep. This, in turn, triggers repetitive arousal from sleep in order to restore airway patency. The resulting interruption in sleep may manifest as excessive daytime somnolence, mood swings, and cognitive disturbances. Such events may also cause episodic sleep-associated oxygen desaturation, hypercarbia, and cardiovascular dysfunction.[7] Patients with OSA have been observed to be at greater perioperative risk due to possible difficult airway management, respiratory, and cardiovascular comorbidities. These factors have been proven to worsen patient outcome even in milder degrees of the disease.[8]

The overall prevalence of OSA has been reported to be around 22% (4–50%) and has been observed to have an increasing trend due to improved diagnostic modalities, changes in the criteria as well as grading of severity of the illness.[9] The prevalence of OSA in pediatric age group alone has been reported to be between 1 and 5%.[10] Risk factors for OSA include male gender, age, obesity, craniofacial and upper-airway abnormalities, smoking, alcohol, and hormonal imbalances.[11] Most commonly observed associations are cardiovascular diseases such as systemic hypertension, coronary artery disease, arrhythmias, ischemic stroke, respiratory diseases such as chronic obstructive pulmonary disease (COPD), bronchial asthma, metabolic disorders such as diabetes mellitus, dyslipidemia, gout, obesity, psychiatric disturbances like depression, anxiety, insomnia, gastroesophageal issues such as reflux disease [gastroesophageal reflux disease (GERD)], chronic liver disease and ophthalmological conditions, e.g., glaucoma, floppy eyelid syndrome, and keratoconus.[12-14] Comprehensive knowledge about OSA (both adult and pediatric categories) and its associations is fundamental for the perioperative management to put together an appropriate strategy for enhanced patient care.

Diagnosis and Evaluation

Diagnosis of OSA is made on the basis of history and investigations **(Table 1)**. The history should encompass:

- Nocturnal symptoms such as snoring, nocturia, witnessed apnea, choking, fragmented sleep.
- Daytime symptoms such as excessive daytime somnolence and other manifestations of sleep fragmentation such as mood swings and cognitive disturbances.
- Associated comorbidities such as hypertension, diabetes, cardiovascular, and cerebrovascular diseases.
- Morbid obesity and COPD which, when present with OSA is referred as overlap syndrome.

Investigation primarily involves polysomnography (PSG), often referred to as sleep study. There are various categories of polysomnography depending on the number and types of parameters measured. Although, PSG performed in a sleep lab attended by a sleep technician is considered to be the gold standard, home sleep testing (HST) or out of center sleep testing (OCST) monitoring fewer parameters might be an acceptable option in appropriately selected candidates. The results of the studies should be scored and subsequently analyzed by the sleep specialist. Using autoscoring and autointerpretation software should be discouraged. The diagnosis and severity stratification **(Table 2)** of OSA requires the apnea hypopnea index (AHI) which is the average number of abnormal respiratory events (apneas and hypopneas per hour of sleep). Apnea refers to air flow cessation for at least 10 seconds and hypopnea represents reduced air flow with associated desaturation of at least 3%.[15]

Obesity Hypoventilation Syndrome

Obstructive sleep apnea is a part of a spectrum ranging from primary snoring to obesity hypoventilation syndrome (OHS) and OHS requires special mention with regards to perioperative management. Criteria for OHS are:

- Body mass index (BMI) of 30 kg/m^2 or greater
- Arterial partial pressure of carbon dioxide (PaCO$_2$) of 45 mm Hg or greater during wakefulness
- Exclusion of other causes of hypercapnia.

Obesity hypoventilation syndrome occurs in 10–20%[16] of patients with known OSA and around 90%[17] of patients with OHS have OSA. OHS is frequently linked to various medical comorbidities and often is undiagnosed or undertreated before elective procedures. In comparison with patients suffering from OSA alone, in the perioperative setting, patients with OHS have an increased risk of respiratory failure, heart failure, prolonged intubation, tracheostomy, and ICU transfer. Active efforts are necessary to diagnose and manage OHS to improve perioperative outcome.[17]

Pathophysiology of Obstructive Sleep Apnea

Individuals with OSA

- Have anatomical small upper airways secondary to a small bony structure, increased soft tissue encompassing the airway.
- Have physiological narrow airways due to increased collapsibility due to lower airway muscular activity or

Table 1: Diagnostic criteria for OSA (adapted from ICSD-3).[1]
Diagnostic criteria for obstructive sleep apnea, adult

A. The presence of at least one of the following:
  i. The patient complains of sleepiness, nonrestorative sleep, fatigue or insomnia symptoms
  ii. The patient wakes up with breath holding, gasping or choking
  iii. The bed partner or observer states snoring, breathing interruptions or both during the patient's sleep
  iv. The patient has been diagnosed with hypertension, mood disorder, cognitive dysfunction, coronary artery disease, stroke, congestive heart failure, atrial fibrillation or type 2 diabetes mellitus
B. Polysomnography (PSG) or (OCST) reveals:
  i. Five or more predominantly obstructive respiratory events [obstructive and mixed apneas, hypopneas or respiratory effort-related arousals (RERAs)] per hour of sleep during a PSG or per hour of monitoring during OCST or
C. PSG or OCST reveals:
  i. Fifteen or more predominantly obstructive respiratory events (apneas, hypopneas or RERAs) per hour of sleep during a PSG or per hour of monitoring (OCST)

Diagnostic criteria for obstructive sleep apnea, pediatric

Criteria A and B must be met
A. The presence of at least one of the following:
  i. Snoring
  ii. Labored, paradoxical or obstructed breathing during sleep
  iii. Sleepiness, hyperactivity, behavioral problems or learning difficulties
B. PSG demonstrates one or more of the following:
  i. One or more obstructive apneas, mixed apneas, or hypopneas, per hour of sleep
  ii. A pattern of obstructive hypoventilation, defined as at least 25% of total sleep time with hypercapnia (PaCO$_2$ >50 mm Hg) along with one or more of the following:
    (a) Snoring
    (b) Flattening of the inspiratory nasal pressure waveform
    (c) Paradoxical thoracoabdominal movement

(ICSD-3: International Classification of Sleep Disorders; OCST: out of center sleep testing; OSA: obstructive sleep apnea)

Table 2: Severity assessment using AHI as per American Academy of Sleep Medicine (AASM) criteria.[46,47]		
OSA severity (AHI)	***Adults***	***Pediatric***
Normal	<5	<1
Mild	5–15	1–5
Moderate	15–30	5–10
Severe	>30	>10

(AHI: apnea hypopnea index; OSA: obstructive sleep apnea)

Flowchart 1: Pathophysiology of perioperative events in OSA.

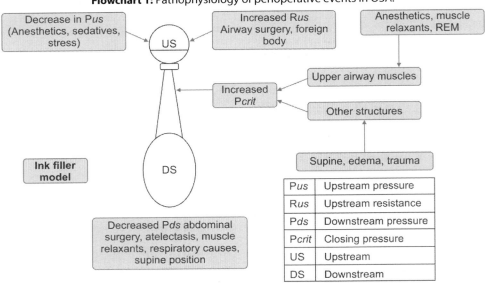

Pus	Upstream pressure
Rus	Upstream resistance
Pds	Downstream pressure
Pcrit	Closing pressure
US	Upstream
DS	Downstream

reduced response to negative upper airway pressure, especially during inspiration.

It requires coordination of approximately 20 pharyngeal muscles to counter the negative pressure created by the diaphragm and intercostal muscles. Some upper airway muscles such as the genioglossus (GG) and palatoglossus show enhanced activity with inspiration (phasic activity). Mechanoreceptors in the upper airway mucosa sense the exaggerated negative pressure, which initiates the traveling of the neural signal to hypoglossal motor neurons through the superior laryngeal or glossopharyngeal nerves and nucleus of the solitary tract. Other muscles such as the tensor veli palatini show tonic activity and are sleep state-dependent [wake >nonrapid eye movement (NREM) > rapid eye movement (REM)]. Physiologically, with sleep onset, there is a diminution in the activity of the upper airway muscles with further worsening during REM sleep.

In people with OSA, it is noticed that there is a greater than normal fall in GG activity with sleep onset. During an event of upper airway obstruction, an increase in GG activity is triggered not only by the hypoxic and hypercapnic drives, but also by the mechanoreceptors below the level of the obstruction. These responses are suppressed during REM sleep and anesthesia. General anesthetics affect the phasic activity more than the tonic activity (**Flowchart 1**). This influence of anesthetics, sedatives, and opioids on ventilatory responsiveness, arousal mechanisms and upper airway muscle tone have been associated with worsening OSA in the postoperative period leading to poor outcome, predominantly in those with unaddressed OSA.

The collapsibility of the upper airway is estimated by the pharyngeal passive closing pressure (Pcrit).

The perioperative factors affecting the upstream and downstream intraluminal pressures are enumerated here.

Obstructive sleep apnea can lead to various cardio-vascular complications which could be either direct consequences of airway collapse and/or obstruction or long-term perpetuation of episodes of hypoxia and hyper-capnia. These could lead to increased sympathetic tone and endothelial dysfunction further progressing to arrhythmias, myocardial ischemia, and even cardiac failure.[8]

OTHER SLEEP DISORDERS

Perioperative immobility, blood loss, iatrogenic sleep loss due to pain, cessation of treatment of preexisting sleep disorder, and use of medications such as metoclopramide can worsen restless leg syndrome. Central disorders of hypersomnolence can result in delayed emergence in patients with the presence of spinal fluid receptors of a positive allosteric modulator of gamma-aminobutyric acid type A (GABA-A).[18]

PREOPERATIVE EVALUATION

Surgery is a substantial physiological stress and is characterized by increased metabolism, oxygen uptake, stress hormone production, and release of inflammatory cytokines.[19] In case of elective surgeries, a comprehensive strategy is to be implemented well in advance of surgery so that all possible comorbidities that may escalate the risk for complications can be identified and intervened. As for emergency cases, rapid screening measures need to be adopted to stratify the risk status of patient and to plan for a safe perioperative period. Studies reveal that about

10–20% of surgical patients are discovered to being at high risk of OSA at preoperative assessment and an alarming 80% of the patients are newly diagnosed.[20] Newly diagnosed patients are at a significantly higher risk of perioperative complications than known cases of OSA.[21] This makes it crucial to have a protocol for effective screening and evaluation for OSA well in advance of the day of surgery to allow preparation of a perioperative management plan. Though recognized as important, OSA is not included in most of the risk predictor scores including American Society of Anaesthesiologists (ASA) physical status classification.

ASSESSMENT OF PATIENTS WITH KNOWN OBSTRUCTIVE SLEEP APNEA

Preoperative assessment of patients already diagnosed with having OSA focuses on the assessment of severity and adequacy of current management. Severity can be assessed by the clinical history and available sleep study reports. Presence of residual symptoms, compliance to mode of treatment (oral appliance or positive airway pressure), and adherence to lifestyle changes such as weight loss, smoking/alcohol cessation will indicate the adequacy of the management. Presence of other aforementioned comorbidities needs to be explored.[22]

ASSESSMENT OF PATIENTS UNKNOWN TO HAVE OBSTRUCTIVE SLEEP APNEA

Whom to Screen?

Though guidelines recommend screening every patient, it might not be feasible and has not shown to improve outcome. However, unrecognized severe OSA was significantly associated with increased risk of 30-day postoperative complications.[23]

The following categories of patients should not be overlooked:
- Obese patients (BMI ≥35 kg/m² especially those scheduled for bariatric surgery)
- Patients with medical conditions in which OSA is prevalent, such as hypertension, type II diabetes, uncontrolled hypothyroidism, congestive heart failure, and stroke.
- Patients with a history of difficult intubation or upper airway characteristics that predict a difficult intubation.

How to Screen?

- *Clinical history*: Interview with patient or family members should focus on nocturnal symptoms such as shortness of breath, snoring, dryness of throat, nocturia and/or diurnal symptoms such as intense sleep inertia (state of impaired cognitive and sensory-motor performance present immediately after awakening), morning headaches, excessive daytime sleepiness, fatigue, mood swings, or cognitive disturbances.
- *Screening tools*: STOP-BANG questionnaire is one of the frequently used questionnaires (**Table 3**), 1 point is added for each positive answer. The questionnaire has demonstrated a high sensitivity, using a cut-off score of at least 3, of 84% in detecting any sleep apnea (AHI >5 events/h), 93% in detecting moderate-to-severe sleep apnea (AHI >15 events/h), and 100% in detecting severe sleep apnea (AHI >30 events/h). The corresponding specificities were 56.4%, 43%, and 37%.[24] Other questionnaires include Epworth sleepiness scale (ESS) and perioperative sleep apnea prediction score (PSAP), Berlin Questionnaire, and ASA risk scoring (**Table 4**). Though no single tool is found to be better than the other, studies have shown that combination of different tools can have a higher sensitivity rate in eliminating moderate-to-severe OSA.[7,25]
- Medical records review and physical examination
  - BMI for obesity.
  - Dyspnea on exertion or at rest, resting hypertension, and tachycardia.
  - Signs of right heart failure such as increased jugular venous pressure, parasternal heave, tricuspid regurgitation murmur, hepatomegaly, and peripheral edema.
  - A full airway assessment evaluating modified Mallampatti scale, nasopharyngeal characteristics, neck circumference, atlanto-occipital mobility, tonsil size, and tongue volume.
- *Investigations*: Investigations are performed to primarily rule out the aforesaid comorbidities and complications of OSA.
  - *Blood tests:* To evaluate for diabetes mellitus, hypothyroidism and acute or chronic kidney disease.
  - *ECG:* Arrhythmias such as atrial fibrillation and right ventricular hypertrophy.
  - *Arterial blood gas (ABG):* A high preoperative value of arterial CO_2 should alert the physician about the possibility of prolonged episodes of desaturation

Table 3: STOP-BANG questionnaire.	
S	Snoring heard through closed doors
T	Tired during daytime
O	Observed apnea (gasp/choke/stop breathing during sleep)
P	High blood pressure with or without treatment
B	BMI >35 kg/m²
A	Age >50
N	Neck circumference >40 cm
G	Male gender

Severity grading: 0–2 (low risk); 3–4 (intermediate risk); 5–8 (high risk).

Table 4: ASA perioperative risk estimation in patients with OSA.[4]

	Variable	Points
A	OSA severity	
	Mild	1
	Moderate	2
	Severe	3
B	Invasiveness of procedure	
	Superficial surgery under LA/PNB without sedation	0
	Superficial surgery with moderate sedation/GA	1
	Peripheral surgery under SAB/EA with no more than moderate sedation	1
	Peripheral surgery under GA	2
	Airway surgery under moderate sedation	2
	Major surgery/airway surgery under GA	3
C	Requirement of postoperative opioids	
	Low-dose oral opioids	1
	High-dose oral opioids/neuraxial or parenteral opioids	3
D	Preoperative CPAP/NIPPV	-1
	Mild or moderate OSA with resting $PaCO_2$ >50 mm Hg	+1
	Total score = A + greater of B and C and consider D	
	Increased risk for score of 4	
	Significantly increased risk >4	

(ASA: American Society of Anaesthesiologists; EA: epidural anesthesia; GA: general anesthesia; LA: local anesthesia; NIPPV: noninvasive positive pressure ventilation; OSA: obstructive sleep apnea; PNB: peripheral nerve block; SAB: subarachnoid block)

postoperatively. The addition of serum HCO_3 (at least 28 mmol/L) to a STOP-BANG score (of at least 3) improves the specificity to predict moderate-to-severe OSA.[26]

- *A baseline oximetry:* Values ≤94% without any other underlying condition may be suggestive of severe OSA.
- *Pulmonary function tests:* When there is a clinical evidence of respiratory disease, poor exercise tolerance or abnormal ABG.

Preoperative Preparation

Use of preoperative empiric positive airway pressure (PAP) therapy is not recommended as there is not much evidence to support the same.[7] However, once diagnosed with OSA, commencement of PAP therapy is recommended, particularly if OSA is moderate or severe with significant oxygen desaturations. The preoperative use of oral appliances, if patient is not able to tolerate PAP therapy, should be deliberated for elective surgeries, which can be delayed. A patient who has undergone corrective airway surgery for OSA should be presumed to remain at risk of OSA-related complications unless a sleep study confirms no evidence of OSA. Known cases of OSA are advised to

Table 5: CPAP duration for optimization.[29,30]

S. No	Complication	Duration of CPAP for improvement	Evidence
1.	Sympathetic over activity	2–4 weeks	Good
2.	Vascular effects	3 months	Insufficient
3.	Endothelial effects	6 weeks–6 months	Insufficient
4.	Coagulation	2 months	Insufficient
5.	Hypertension	6–8 weeks	Good
6.	Pulmonary hypertension	12 weeks–6 months	Insufficient
7.	Cardiac arrhythmias	1 month	Insufficient
8.	Cardiac failure	1–6 months	Moderate
9.	CAD	Not Available	Insufficient
10.	Stroke	Not Available	Insufficient

(CAD: coronary artery disease; CPAP: continuous positive airway pressure)

continue the PAP therapy at the hospital. Preoperative clinic is a potential "awareness moment" for patients with undiagnosed or untreated OSA,[3] who could be convinced of the importance of treatment.

Deciding the Time of the Procedure

The elements which determine timing of the surgery depends on urgency of the procedure, status of OSA management, severity of OSA, comorbidities, invasiveness of the diagnostic or therapeutic procedure, the requirement for postoperative narcotic analgesics, institutional protocol, and infrastructure for evaluation and sleep study. In case of well-controlled OSA and negligible weight gain since sleep study, no further evaluation before the procedure is warranted. Delaying the procedure for further evaluation and management of suspected OSA is justified if there are signs indicating OHS, pulmonary hypertension, heart failure, arrhythmia, or hypoxemia. The decision pertaining to rescheduling the procedure in case of suspected OSA with no complications depends on the risk-benefit of the surgery. But as observed in **Table 5**, the duration of optimization is still controversial.

INTRAOPERATIVE MANAGEMENT OF OBSTRUCTIVE SLEEP APNEA

A patient with OSA on abovementioned grounds ought to be deemed as high risk and various elements have to be specifically kept in mind for risk alleviation.

Premedication

Sedatives and opioids which are routinely used as premedication should be avoided in patients with OSA. If necessary, short-acting preparations are to be administered in minimal doses. Hypnotics

- Suppress central ventilatory drive by binding to benzodiazepine (BZD) receptors, to activate the GABA system in motor neurons, the limbic system, and the dorsal horn of the spinal cord.
- Reduce muscle tone in OSA patients with already functionally morbid upper airway dilator muscles.
- Increase the arousal threshold.
- Decrease the cyclic alternating pattern (CAP) rate in NREM sleep which results in less resilience to adverse respiratory events.[27]

Airway Management

Due to predilection of airway collapse, patients with OSA may have a higher incidence of difficult airway during and after procedure. Difficult intubation, mask ventilation, and both difficult intubation and mask ventilation were 3.4, 3.4 and 4.1-folds higher in OSA patients compared to non-OSA patients, respectively.[28] The patient should be placed in a head-up/ramped position to decrease pharyngeal closing pressure, increase lung volume and for better laryngeal visualization. Preoxygenation with individualized continuous positive airway pressure (CPAP) delays the time for desaturation. Also, the perioperative physician should anticipate GERD due to hypotonia of the lower esophageal sphincter. Lung protective ventilatory strategy may be followed in these patients. Positive end expiratory pressure (PEEP) providing minimum permissible atelectasis and minimum hemodynamic disturbances is advisable in these patients.

CHOICE OF ANESTHETIC AND ANALGESIC TECHNIQUE

Due to tendency of airway collapse and sleep fragmentation, patients with OSA are at enhanced susceptibility to the respiratory depressant and airway effects of sedatives, opioids, and inhaled anesthetics. Regional anesthesia in the form of peripheral nerve blocks and neuraxial blocks are preferred over general anesthesia whenever feasible. Use of opioids in neuraxial blocks can also predispose to delayed respiratory complications (e.g., neuraxial morphine—even after 24 hours). Perioperative hypoxemic events can occur even in patients undergoing regional anesthesia.

Short acting agents such as Desflurane, Remifentanil, and Propofol are preferred as general anesthetics. Propofol might be used as a sedative as it has prompt onset and offset, short context sensitive half-life, and good titratability. Ketamine has sedative, analgesic, and respiratory stimulant properties which also makes it a favored drug. Ketamine anesthesia abolishes the coupling between loss of consciousness and upper dilator muscle dysfunction and thereby protects upper airway patency in OSA patients.[29]

A multimodal approach to analgesia is preferred and analgesics such as nonsteroidal anti-inflammatory drugs (NSAIDs), ketamine, and clonidine are favored over opioids. α-2 agonists such as clonidine, dexmedetomidine can be used as sedatives as they have insignificant respiratory depression. The reduced opioid requirement noticed with clonidine in OSA patients could be due to upregulation of μ-opioid receptors in the brainstem caused by continuous hypoxemia. Use of clonidine in OSA patients has shown less oxygen desaturation in the postoperative period.[30]

Monitoring

Apart from mandatory monitoring of pulse oximetry, ECG, noninvasive blood pressure, capnography and temperature, invasive arterial monitoring, and dynamic indices of hemodynamic monitoring may be considered in severe OSA with cardiovascular complications. Neuromuscular monitoring is also advisable in these patients. Bispectral index (BIS) is also valuable and the scores between 75 and 90 show light sleep and the scores between 20 and 75 indicate a deep sleep wave. This can help in titrated delivery of intravenous and inhalational anesthetics.[31] Use of target control infusion and closed loop anesthesia system may also improve recovery times in these patients.

Intravenous Fluid Management

A restrictive or goal-directed strategy with regards to intraoperative fluids is to be applied in patients with OSA. Preparations with lower salt content are preferred as it may otherwise cause fluid accumulation in the neck and other soft tissues in addition to the same due to the stress response.[32-35]

Extubation

Absence of residual neuromuscular blockade, hypothermia, and achieving optimal ABG should be confirmed and the patient is to be extubated after complete recovery of consciousness. Use of neostigmine should be guided by the neuromuscular recovery values as it can significantly impair GG muscle activity unlike Sugammadex.[36] Extubating directly on to the patients' own CPAP is preferred. However, postoperative airway obstruction may occur in pharyngeal procedures, following edema or nasal packing. In such a scenario, CPAP might not be a practical option. Whenever possible, extubation should be conducted in a nonsupine (semi-upright or lateral) position. This follows the rationale that sleeping in supine position worsens the passive pharyngeal collapsibility and increases rostral fluid shift, and is thereby associated with increased respiratory events.[37]

POSTOPERATIVE MANAGEMENT OF OBSTRUCTIVE SLEEP APNEA

The mode of postoperative management of the OSA patient is decided by various determinants such as the severity of OSA, opioid/sedative requirement during postoperative period, the level of invasiveness of the procedure.[20] Patients with OSA have more than twice the incidence of postoperative oxygen desaturations, respiratory failure, cardiac events, and unplanned intensive care admissions. The main postoperative concern for the OSA patients is opioid-induced ventilatory impairment (OIVI).[38] However, an endotype of OSA where persons having low arousal threshold were found to have less incidence of perioperative complications.[39]

Postanesthesia Care Unit Stay

All known or suspected cases of OSA are to be kept in postanesthesia care unit (PACU) for an extended period (recommended at least 60 minutes) for monitoring for respiratory events. PACU respiratory events include the following:[27]

- Episodes of apnea for 10 seconds
- Bradypnea <8 breaths per minute
- Repeated oxygen desaturation to <90% or
- Pain-sedation mismatch (high pain and sedation scores concurrently).

Oxygenation

Continuous supplemental oxygen is essential for those at increased perioperative risk from OSA until they can preserve baseline oxygen saturation at room air. However, a strategy of titrated low-flow oxygen is to be adopted to prevent hypoventilation, particularly in patients with coexisting OHS and COPD, and prevent subsequent hypercapnia. Supplemental oxygen reduced the AHI significantly in OSA patients with high loop gain (LG), but not in those with low loop gain.[40] Supplemental oxygen effectively reduced the LG in patients with a high LG but had little effect in those with a low LG.[41]

Positive Airway Pressure Therapy

Positive airway pressure (PAP) therapy is preferably initiated in the PACU and continued on the floor through recovery and discharge back home. PAP should be in place or at least within reach of the patient, as postoperative patients may sleep anytime during the day. CPAP treatment can mitigate opioid-induced negative effects on AHI.[42]

If patient has difficulty using CPAP, measures to improve comfort such as better fitting mask, humidifier, pressure ramp may be tried. Patient with history of OSA on PAP therapy may be continued on the same pressures as previously prescribed. However, pressure adjustments may be required in those with perioperative changes such as facial swelling, upper airway edema, and fluid shifts. Sometimes, a fixed CPAP pressure setting may not be sufficient in the perioperative environment and autotitrating positive airway pressure (APAP) may be preferred. Concerns regarding safety of PAP therapy in postoperative interval were alleviated when it was demonstrated in a study that there was no increased risk of anatomic dehiscence in gastrointestinal surgery.[43] As for the patients on oral appliances, they are to continue using those in the PACU, if feasible. As patients with OSA tend to have high pain sensitivity, CPAP might have a role in reducing the same. However, there is not much conclusive evidence supporting this.

It has been noted that only 45% of patients with newly diagnosed OSA were adherent to PAP therapy in the perioperative period.[6] Acceptance of sleep testing, cost, under appreciation of complications of untreated OSA, and the interval between evaluation and actual date of surgery may all be reasons contributing to this.

Discharge to Unmonitored Settings

As already cited, the shifting of patient from PACU is to be delayed and the decision of shifting is based on the confirmation that the patient is able to maintain adequate oxygen saturation, at room air, in an unstimulated setting, especially while sleeping. Patients who have severe OSA, multiple comorbidities, major surgery, substantial opioid/sedative use during perioperative period, experienced respiratory events and with significant pain scores are to be discharged to a monitored setting.

Care in High Dependency/Step-down Units

Postoperative period is associated with various alterations in sleep architecture such as significant decrease in sleep efficiency, REM sleep, and slow-wave sleep in all patients regardless of OSA status and that too predominantly the first night. A study by Chung et al. inferred that there was an increase in AHI during non-REM sleep irrespective of OSA status with the unanticipated increase in N3 and REM sleep during the third night, possibly due to resumption of normal sleep.[44] It is prudent that the patients continue nonsupine positioning if possible, supplemental oxygenation, monitoring of ventilation, tapering of analgesics if feasible, and maintain PAP therapy or oral device.

Complications

Postoperatively, there are alterations in sleep architecture and an increase in the AHI in both patients with and without OSA. Twenty six percent of patients without OSA developed moderate-to-severe SDB in the first 1–3 days after surgery.[3] Another less-recognized cause of sudden death in patients with OSA is arousal failure.[45] It is speculated that an apneic event may not spontaneously terminate because of an ineffective arousal mechanism related to impaired chemosensitivity and/or opioid-induced respiratory depression, leading to profound cerebral hypoxemia, and ultimately death. More than half of the adverse events occurred intraoperatively or in the PACU

and were often related to difficulty with airway management and/or premature extubation. These events were most often associated with a permanent vegetative state or required a permanent tracheostomy. Also majority of the complications reported, occurred in an unmonitored setting, and a substantial minority involved the use of opioids. These cases were most likely to be associated with death as the outcome.[21] Other possible complications anticipated in a postoperative scenario are listed in **Table 6**.[19]

Flowchart 2: Algorithm for decision making in the perioperative period.

Table 6: Complications in postoperative period.

	Complications
Pulmonary	• Hypoxemia • Aspiration pneumonia • Adult respiratory distress syndrome • Prolonged ventilation • Early extubation with failed reintubation
Cardiac	• Dysrhythmias • Abnormal heart rate, myocardial infarction and ischemia • Hypotension • Congestive heart failure
Neurological	• Delirium • Agitation • Confusion • Excessive drowsiness
Others	Unplanned ICU transfer

LEGAL IMPLICATIONS

Perioperative complications directly related to OSA are increasingly recognized in the legal arena as well as with a growing number of medical malpractice suits reaching the courts in the Western countries. It should be noted that the majority of rulings favored the plaintiff and on an average 2 million dollars were claimed.[21] Again, the overlapping responsibilities of the anesthesia service and the otolaryngologist cannot be overemphasized. As the surgeon and the anesthesiologist have a shared responsibility, the plaintiff's claim was charged on the whole operating team. Although litigations related to perioperative complications due to OSA is still being under reported in our country, it is prudent to set up appropriate screening protocols (**Flowchart 2**) and management of the same.

FUTURE

Further research is required in the effect of anesthesia on remodeling of GABA-related neural circuitry and neurotoxicity which may play a role in long-term effects in these patients. There is also a need for monitoring compliance and effect of CPAP in the perioperative period using biomarkers. Further research should also be directed toward the time duration for improvement of symptomatology with treatment in such patients as it will give more information on the risk-benefit in the perioperative period.

REFERENCES

1. Darien I. American Academy of Sleep Medicine. International Classification of Sleep Disorders, 3rd edition. American Academy of Sleep Medicine; 2014.

2. Memtsoudis SG, Besculides MC, Mazumdar M. A rude awakening--the perioperative sleep apnea epidemic. N Engl J Med. 2013;368(25):2352-3.

3. Chung F, Nagappa M, Singh M, Mokhlesi B. CPAP in the perioperative setting. Chest. 2016;149(2):586-97.

4. Nightingale CE, Margarson MP, Shearer E, Redman JW, Lucas DN, Cousins JM, et al. Peri-operative management of the obese surgical patient 2015: Association of Anaesthetists of Great Britain and Ireland Society for Obesity and Bariatric Anaesthesia. Anaesthesia. 2015;70(7):859-76.

5. Memtsoudis SG, Cozowicz C, Nagappa M, Wong J, Joshi GP, Wong DT, et al. Society of Anesthesia and Sleep Medicine Guideline on intraoperative management of adult patients with obstructive sleep apnea. Anesth Analg. 2018;127(4):967-87.

6. Chung F, Memtsoudis SG, Ramachandran SK, Nagappa M, Opperer M, Cozowicz C, et al. Society of Anesthesia and Sleep Medicine Guidelines on preoperative screening and assessment of adult patients with obstructive sleep apnea. Anesth Analg. 2016;123(2):452-73.

7. American Society of Anesthesiologists Task Force on perioperative management of patients with obstructive sleep apnea. Practice guidelines for the perioperative management of patients with obstructive sleep apnea: an updated report by the American Society of Anesthesiologists Task Force on perioperative management of patients with obstructive sleep apnea. Anesthesiology. 2014;120(2):268-86.

8. Corso R, Russotto V, Gregoretti C, Cattano D. Perioperative management of obstructive sleep apnea: a systematic review. Minerva Anestesiol. 2018;84(1):81-93.

9. Franklin KA, Lindberg E. Obstructive sleep apnea is a common disorder in the population—a review on the epidemiology of sleep apnea. J Thorac Dis. 2015;7(8):1311-22.

10. Dehlink E, Tan H-L. Update on paediatric obstructive sleep apnoea. J Thorac Dis. 2016;8(2):224-35.

11. Young T, Skatrud J, Peppard PE. Risk factors for obstructive sleep apnea in adults. JAMA. 2004;291(16):2013-6.

12. Pinto JA, Ribeiro DK, Cavallini AF, Duarte C, Freitas GS. Comorbidities associated with obstructive sleep apnea: a retrospective study. Int Arch Otorhinolaryngol. 2016;20(2): 145-50.

13. Santos M, Hofmann RJ. Ocular manifestations of obstructive sleep apnea. J Clin Sleep Med. 2017;13(11):1345-8.

14. Bonsignore MR, Baiamonte P, Mazzuca E, Castrogiovanni A, Marrone O. Obstructive sleep apnea and comorbidities: a dangerous liaison. Multidiscip Respir Med. 2019;14(1):8.

15. Kapur VK, Auckley DH, Chowdhuri S, Kuhlmann DC, Mehra R, Ramar K, et al. Clinical practice guideline for diagnostic testing for adult obstructive sleep apnea: an American Academy of Sleep Medicine clinical practice guideline. J Clin Sleep Med. 2017;13(3):479-504.

16. Kaw R, Gali B, Collop NA. Perioperative care of patients with obstructive sleep apnea. Curr Treat Options Neurol. 2011;13(5):496-507.

17. Ayas NT, Laratta CR, Coleman JM, Doufas AG, Eikermann M, Gay PC, et al. Knowledge gaps in the perioperative management of adults with obstructive sleep apnea and obesity hypoventilation syndrome. An Official American Thoracic Society Workshop Report. Ann Am Thorac Soc. 2018;15(2):117-26.

18. LaBarbera V, García PS, Bliwise DL, Trotti LM. Central disorders of hypersomnolence, restless legs syndrome, and surgery with general anesthesia: Patient perceptions. Front Hum Neurosci. 2018;12:99.

19. Howard R, Yin YS, McCandless L, Wang S, Englesbe M, Machado-Aranda D. Taking control of your surgery: impact of a prehabilitation program on major abdominal surgery. J Am Coll Surg. 2019;228(1):72-80.

20. Raveendran R, Chung F. Ambulatory anesthesia for patients with sleep apnea. Ambulatory Anesthesia. 2015. [online] Available from https://www.dovepress.com/ambulatory-anesthesia-for-patients-with-sleep-apnea-peer-reviewed-fulltext-article-AA [Last accessed March, 2020].

21. Fernandez-Bustamante A, Bartels K, Clavijo C, Scott BK, Kacmar R, Bullard K, et al. Preoperatively screened obstructive sleep apnea is associated with worse postoperative outcomes than previously diagnosed obstructive sleep apnea. Anesth Analg. 2017;125(2):593-602.

22. Chokroverty S. Sleep disorders medicine: Basic science, technical considerations, and clinical aspects, 4th edition. Boston, New York: Springer; 2017. pp. 647-60.

23. Chan MTV, Wang CY, Seet E, Tam S, Lai HY, Chew EFF, et al. Association of Unrecognized Obstructive Sleep Apnea with Postoperative Cardiovascular Events in Patients Undergoing Major Noncardiac Surgery. JAMA. 2019;321(18):1788-98.

24. Nagappa M, Wong J, Singh M, Wong DT, Chung F. An update on the various practical applications of the STOP-Bang questionnaire in anesthesia, surgery, and perioperative medicine. Curr Opin Anaesthesiol. 2017;30(1):118-25.

25. Saxena M, Gothi D, Sah R, Ojha UC, Gahlot T. Utility of combining Epworth sleepiness scale, STOP-BANG and perioperative sleep apnea prediction score for predicting absence of obstructive sleep apnea. Indian J Sleep Med. 2018;5.

26. Chung F, Chau E, Yang Y, Liao P, Hall R, Mokhlesi B. Serum bicarbonate level improves specificity of STOP-Bang screening for obstructive sleep apnea. Chest. 2013;143(5):1284-93.

27. Wang SH, Chen WS, Tang SE, Lin HC, Peng CK, Chu HT, et al. Benzodiazepines associated with acute respiratory failure in patients with obstructive sleep apnea. Front Pharmacol. 2018;9:1513.

28. Nagappa M, Wong DT, Cozowicz C, Ramachandran SK, Memtsoudis SG, Chung F. Is obstructive sleep apnea associated with difficult airway? Evidence from a systematic review and meta-analysis of prospective and retrospective cohort studies. PLoS One. 2018;13(10):e0204904.

29. Eikermann M, Grosse-Sundrup M, Zaremba S, Henry ME, Bittner EA, Hoffmann U, et al. Ketamine activates breathing and abolishes the coupling between loss of consciousness and upper airway dilator muscle dysfunction. Anesthesiology. 2012;116(1):35-46.

30. Ankichetty S, Wong J, Chung F. A systematic review of the effects of sedatives and anesthetics in patients with obstructive sleep apnea. J Anaesthesiol Clin Pharmacol. 2011;27(4):447-58.

31. Kuyrukluyıldız U, Binici O, Onk D, Ayhan Celik S, Torun MT, Unver E, et al. Comparison of dexmedetomidine and propofol used for drug-induced sleep endoscopy in patients with obstructive sleep apnea syndrome. Int J Clin Exp Med. 2015;8(4):5691-8.

32. Ramachandran SK. Can intravenous fluids explain increased postoperative sleep disordered breathing and airway outcomes? Sleep. 2014;37(10):1587-8.

33. Vena D, Bradley TD, Millar PJ, Floras JS, Rubianto J, Gavrilovic B, et al. Heart rate variability responses of individuals with and without saline-induced obstructive sleep apnea. J Clin Sleep Med. 2018;14(4):503-10.

34. Lam T, Singh M, Yadollahi A, Chung F. Is perioperative fluid and salt balance a contributing factor in postoperative worsening of obstructive sleep apnea? Anesth Analg. 2016;122(5):1335-9.

35. Lam TD, Singh M, Chung F. Salt content in IV fluids given intraoperatively may influence postoperative OSA severity. Sleep. 2015;38(6):989.

36. Hafeez KR, Tuteja A, Singh M, Wong DT, Nagappa M, Chung F, et al. Postoperative complications with neuromuscular blocking drugs and/or reversal agents in obstructive sleep apnea patients: a systematic review. BMC Anesthesiol. 2018;18(1):91.

37. Joosten SA, Landry SA, Sands SA, Terrill PI, Mann D, Andara C, et al. Dynamic loop gain increases upon adopting the supine body position during sleep in patients with obstructive sleep apnoea. Respirol Carlton Vic. 2017;22(8):1662-9.

38. Lam KK, Kunder S, Wong J, Doufas AG, Chung F. Obstructive sleep apnea, pain, and opioids: is the riddle solved? Curr Opin Anaesthesiol. 2016;29(1):134-40.

39. Fouladpour N, Jesudoss R, Bolden N, Shaman Z, Auckley D. Perioperative complications in obstructive sleep apnea patients undergoing surgery: a review of the legal literature. Anesth Analg. 2016;122(1):145-51.

40. Wang D, Marshall NS, Duffin J, Yee BJ, Wong KK, Noori N, et al. Phenotyping interindividual variability in obstructive sleep apnoea response to temazepam using ventilatory chemoreflexes during wakefulness. J Sleep Res. 2011;20(4):526-32.

41. Wellman A, Malhotra A, Jordan AS, Stevenson KE, Gautam S, White DP. Effect of oxygen in obstructive sleep apnea: role of loop gain. Respir Physiol Neurobiol. 2008;162(2):144-51.

42. Gali B, Whalen FX, Schroeder DR, Gay PC, Plevak DJ. Identification of patients at risk for postoperative respiratory complications using a preoperative obstructive sleep apnea screening tool and postanesthesia care assessment. Anesthesiology. 2009;110(4):869-77.

43. Tong S, Gower J, Morgan A, Gadbois K, Wisbach G. Noninvasive positive pressure ventilation in the immediate post-bariatric surgery care of patients with obstructive sleep apnea: a systematic review. Surg Obes Relat Dis. 2017;13(7):1227-33.

44. Chung F, Liao P, Yegneswaran B, Shapiro CM, Kang W. Postoperative changes in sleep-disordered breathing and sleep architecture in patients with obstructive sleep apnea. Anesthesiology. 2014;120(2):287-98.

45. Gami AS, Olson EJ, Shen WK, Wright RS, Ballman KV, Hodge DO, et al. Obstructive sleep apnea and the risk of sudden cardiac death: a longitudinal study of 10,701 adults. J Am Coll Cardiol. 2013;62(7):610-6.

46. Hudgel DW. Sleep apnea severity classification–revisited. Sleep. 2016;39(5):1165-6.

47. Katz ES, Greene MG, Carson KA, Galster P, Loughlin GM, Carroll J, et al. Night-to-night variability of polysomnography in children with suspected obstructive sleep apnea. J Pediatr. 2002;140(5):589-94.

Index

Page numbers followed by *b* refer to box, *f* refer to figure, *fc* refer to flowchart, and *t* refer to table